KU-017-353

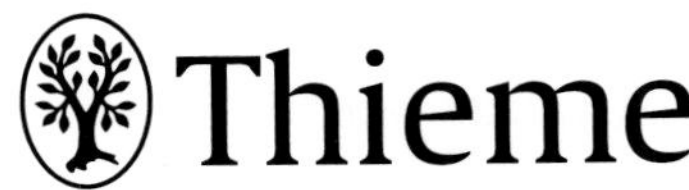
Thieme

# Diagnosis of Breast Diseases

## Integrating the Findings of Clinical Presentation, Mammography, and Ultrasound

Volker Barth

Professor
Breast Imaging Center
Esslingen, Germany

With contributions by

Volker Frohwein, Johannes Herrmann, Brigitte Koellner, Elfi Steinhilber, Oliver Wild, Andrea Barth, Stephan Barth

1560 illustrations

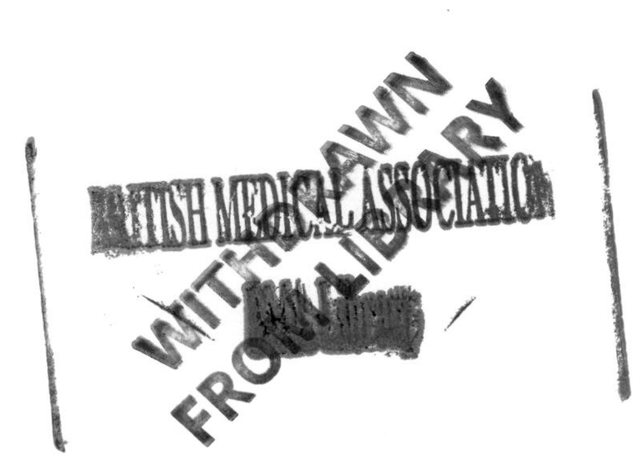

Thieme
Stuttgart · New York

*Library of Congress Cataloging-in-Publication Data*
Barth, Volker.
[Atlas der Mammadiagnostik. English.]
Diagnosis of breast diseases : mammography and ultrasound / Volker Barth ; with contributions by Johannes Herrmann ... [et al.].
p. ; cm.
Includes bibliographical references and index.
Summary: "A practical approach to the early detection and management of breast cancer. This lavishly illustrated atlas provides radiologists with essential information for the differential diagnosis of breast diseases on the basis of clinical presentation, mammography, and ultrasound. The book begins with chapters on tumor biology, prognostic factors, and histology. The authors then provide a thorough evaluation of various methods for early detection and accurate diagnosis, including analog and digital mammography, ultrasound, MR imaging, PET/CT, and interventional procedures. They discuss in detail the strengths and limitations of each imaging modality, aspects of quality control, test intervals, peri- and postoperative management principles, and follow-up care. Highlights: – Presentation of difficult cases that effectively demonstrate the diagnostic hurdles and forensic pitfalls in breast diagnosis – Special sections on breast cancer in men and young women, with discussion of women who are pregnant or lactating – Color-coded practical tips and clinical notes for optimal comprehension of the material – Extensive Q&A sections for self-testing in two major chapters – More than 1,700 high-quality illustrations, including clinical color photographs, ultrasound images, and mammograms" – Provided by publisher.
ISBN 978-3-13-143831-7 (hardback : alk. paper) 1. Breast–Ultrasonic imaging–Atlases. 2. Breast–Diseases–Diagnosis–Atlases. I. Herrmann, Johannes, Dr. med. II. Title.
[DNLM: 1. Breast Diseases–radiography–Atlases. 2. Breast Neoplasms–radiography–Atlases. 3. Diagnosis, Differential–Atlases. 4. Mammography–Atlases. 5. Ultrasonography, Mammary–Atlases. WP 17]
RG493.5.U47B3613 2010
618.1'90754–dc22 2010042870

This book is an authorized, revised, and enlarged translation of the 2nd German edition published and copyrighted 2006 by Georg Thieme Verlag, Stuttgart, Germany. Title of the German edition: Atlas der Mammadiagnostik: Mammographie und Sonographie intensiv trainieren.

Translators: Terry Telger and Julie Foster, Fort Worth, Texas, USA

Illustrators: Angelika Kramer, Stuttgart, Germany, and Andrea Schnitzler, Innsbruck, Austria


Rüdigerstrasse 14, 70469 Stuttgart, Germany
http://www.thieme.de
Thieme New York, 333 Seventh Avenue, New York, NY 10001, USA
http://www.thieme.com

Cover design: Thieme Publishing Group
Typesetting by Ziegler + Müller, Kirchentellinsfurt, Germany
Printed in China by Everbest Printing Co Ltd, Hong Kong

ISBN 978-3-13-143831-7 1 2 3 4 5 6

**Important note:** Medicine is an ever-changing science undergoing continual development. Research and clinical experience are continually expanding our knowledge, in particular our knowledge of proper treatment and drug therapy. Insofar as this book mentions any dosage or application, readers may rest assured that the authors, editors, and publishers have made every effort to ensure that such references are in accordance with **the state of knowledge at the time of production of the book.**

Nevertheless, this does not involve, imply, or express any guarantee or responsibility on the part of the publishers in respect to any dosage instructions and forms of applications stated in the book. **Every user is requested to examine carefully** the manufacturers' leaflets accompanying each drug and to check, if necessary in consultation with a physician or specialist, whether the dosage schedules mentioned therein or the contraindications stated by the manufacturers differ from the statements made in the present book. Such examination is particularly important with drugs that are either rarely used or have been newly released on the market. Every dosage schedule or every form of application used is entirely at the user's own risk and responsibility. The authors and publishers request every user to report to the publishers any discrepancies or inaccuracies noticed. If errors in this work are found after publication, errata will be posted at www.thieme.com on the product description page.

*Dedicated to Klaus-Dieter Schulz (of Marburg), for his decades of commitment to the early detection of breast cancer.*

# Preface

The *European Guidelines for Quality Assurance in Breast Cancer Screening and Diagnosis* of the European Commission (Perry et al. 2004) pertain basically to mammography, and very little to adjunctive methods. But the early detection of breast cancer can be effective only when the three pillars—clinical investigation, mammography, ultrasound—are united within a structured, quality-assured program. The German *S3 guidelines* (Albert et al. 2003, 2008; Kreienberg et al. 2008) come closest to meeting this requirement. The European and American guidelines are very similar to each other but are basically limited to mammography. Professor Klaus-Dieter Schultz and his team were instrumental in introducing the S3 guidelines, which were revised in 2008 to become the quality standard throughout Germany. The German and English editions of this atlas were therefore dedicated to Professor Schultz, whose sudden death left a gaping hole in the German Senology Society. I credit Professor Schultz with many valuable ideas that set my professional horizon during my years of working with him in the Society.

Rigorous efforts at early detection (secondary prevention) as well as adjuvant surgical and medical treatments (tertiary prevention of recurrence and metastasis) have significantly improved the survival rates and mortality rates for breast cancer throughout the world during the past 25 years. These factors do not account for the declining aggressiveness of malignant tumors that has been documented in recent decades.

*Primary* prevention, or the prevention of gradual malignant tumor development in response to tumor-stimulating biological or synthetic agents, is not yet a reality. This atlas is concerned with *secondary* cancer prevention.

The illustrations in this book do not include mammograms that display obvious tumors with associated palpable nodules. There are very good textbooks and atlases of mammography that present images of this kind (for example, Barth and Prechtel 1991; Tabar et al. 2000; Fischer and Baum 2005). A great many of the mammograms in this book show only minimal changes or no abnormalities at all, which makes the ultrasound findings all the more impressive by comparison. This is typical of the cases that are seen outside of screening programs. I have focused mainly on difficult cases illustrating the diagnostic hurdles and forensic pitfalls that are encountered in breast diagnosis. I hope that even experienced colleagues will find this book a valuable teaching aid.

I could not illustrate everything that would be important in routine situations—the scope of modern breast diagnosis is too extensive. But the book is intended to show how important it is to know *all* the diagnostic possibilities in the breast, not only mammography.

Because such high standards are placed on the technical quality of mammograms throughout the world, our radiologic technologist, **Elfi Steinhilber**, contributed a special section dealing with *mammographic positioning and quality assurance*. Using the PGMI system, physicians and their assistants who perform mammography can rate the technical quality of their mammograms as "perfect," "good," "moderate," or "inadequate." This section pertains to both conventional and digital mammography and should be required reading for every breast diagnostician.

My computer expert, **Oliver Wild**, authored the section on *digital full-field mammography*. He explains the advantages of this technology for screening and modern diagnostic testing and for making a detailed comparison of current and previous mammograms—primary digital images as well as images that have been secondarily scanned into the computer.

A section written by my practice partner, **Dr. Johannes Herrmann**, gives readers the opportunity to interpret subtle mammographic changes *(in mammgraphic case presentation and training in interpretation)*. These images simulate a screening situation. Some of the mammograms show only minimal changes or appear normal despite the presence of a breast tumor. This section illustrates the limitations of mammograms and shows that mammography alone is (outside of screening) no longer the gold standard and can yield optimum results only in concert with other modalities. Typical *screening cases* are also illustrated.

Recall the publications of Nakama et al. (1991), Gordon and Goldenberg (1995), Teboul and Halliwell (1995), Kolb et al. (2002), and Leconte et al. 2003 to understand the possibilities of ultrasound, and the 2006 study by Dr. Wendie Berg of Johns Hopkins University (Berg et al. 2008), in which mammography plus breast ultrasound detected almost one-third more cancers than mammography alone. So what are we waiting for?

It should be added that ultrasound may yield false-positives that prompt unnecessary interventions, but this does not alter the fact that ultrasound reduces interval cancers and improves the prospects for a cure. Mammography generates a significantly higher rate of false-positive findings (30%), which cause serious distress for the affected women. The addition of ultrasound eliminates approximately 50% of recalls, fully compensating for the 5% rate of false-positive sonographic findings. *Fine-needle aspiration* (FNA) is particularly useful for identifying false-positive ultrasound findings at low cost and very quickly (Berg et al. 1962; Zajicek 1974; Schöndorf 1977; Lindholm 1999; Orell 1999; Frohwein 2002).

The section on *screening and tumor progression* underscores this theme by showing how tumors that were missed on previous mammograms can be detected retrospectively on the basis of relatively subtle findings. Every breast diagnostician has missed a tumor or delayed its diagnosis at one time or another. This should not be a frequent occurrence, however. We practitioners cannot treat the concept of *interval cancer* as an abstraction; sometimes we must explain in a court of law why we missed a tumor that may have harmed our patient.

Other sections in this book deal with breast cancer in young women and during pregnancy. Diseases of the male breast are also addressed.

We examine the pitfalls of pre- and postoperative diagnosis and the possibilities and limitations of breast diagnosis in the *postoperative care* setting. Performed by nonscreening radiologists and gynecologists, these follow-up examinations require special expertise in the differenzial diagnosis of mammographic, sonographic, and MRI findings.

*Breast implants* are included because of the growing numbers of women who present with these devices after breast-conserving therapy. These cases cannot be adequately evaluated by single-view mammography, and we must obtain a second view or even a third view in selected cases. Familiarity with different types of implant is essential in order to be able to make an accurate differenzial diagnosis.

We take a critical look at imaging modalities that either are used as a matter of course or are withheld from patients due to their high cost. These include *magnetic resonance imaging* (MRI), *positron emission tomography* (PET), and PET/CT. Why should MRI be used only in patients with lobular carcinoma to define tumor extent and evaluate the healthy breast, merely because MRI has been identified as the best *evidence-based* modality for lobular cancer detection? MRI should be available for the preoperative analysis of *all* malignant tumors, especially in younger women, if it will advance treatment planning. Most doctors would not think twice about evaluating the knee joint or a little finger with MRI. Why, then, is there a reluctance to apply this modality to breast cancer, with its many therapeutic challenges and potenzial for recurrence?

We touch on the importance of dedicated, *certified breast centers* as an effective approach to early cancer detection and treatment. These breast centers have been an important factor in the worldwide decline of breast cancer mortality. Centers are springing up everywhere in the world, which is a positive development (Kreienberg et al. 2008).

It is unacceptable for a woman to be referred to a hospital for cancer treatment simply because the referring physician is a friend of the department head. The international care standard for breast cancer treatment is met only at a specialized care center where all diagnostic and therapeutic information is coordinated, archived, and reviewed at multidisciplinary case conferences—a place where all therapeutic options are available and can be practiced in an optimal way. *Digital patient databases* are essential in this setting, although security and confidentially issues have kept them from being established on a broad, interdisciplinary scale.

The *axilla* is a region of profound importance. Untold misery has resulted from aggressive, often unnecessary, axillary lymph node dissections (with or without irradiation) in breast cancer patients. The worldwide introduction of the sentinel node biopsy has spared many women the sufferings of arm edema, axillary foreign-body sensation, and radiating pains. My former colleagues **Dr. Brigitte Koellner** and **Dr. Petra Zimmer** have dealt with this topic for years. They introduced the sentinel node biopsy at Esslingen Hospital 10 years ago and worked with the gynecology chief *Professor Dr. Thorsten Kuehn* and his team to optimize the procedure. I extend special thanks to **Dr. Koellner** for writing the section on the *sentinel lymph node procedure.*

## Acknowledgments

An atlas of this kind is always a team effort. Many have helped me in bringing the book to completion, including those who worked in the background. I am particularly indebted to my secretary, *Cornelia Wahl*, who typed the manuscript and made revisions from her home while caring for her child. I also express sincere thanks to my assistants *Hatice Kara* and *Derya Celik*, *Heide Scherbaum*, *Milka Leovac*, and *Tuğçe Yiğit*. They painstakingly collected the published mammograms and sonograms, scanned them into the computer, and looked up numerous case histories.

I am grateful to my colleagues *Professor Dr. Thorsten Kuehn*, chief of gynecology at Esslingen Hospital, and *Professor Dr. Stefan Kraemer*, who succeeded me as head of the radiology department at Esslingen Hospital, for providing me with valuable suggestions and illustrative materials. I thank *Dr. Hans-Helmut Dahm* and his partner *Dr. Joern Straeter* for providing some of the cytology illustrations and a large portion of the histologic illustrations that were included in this book. I supplemented these illustrations with material from the collections of the leading German breast pathologists of recent decades, *Professor Roland Baessler* (Fulda, Germany) and *Professor Klaus Prechtel* (Starnberg, Germany), with whom I worked for years and still maintain friendly ties. They provided me with illustrations for this atlas, and their contribution is gratefully acknowledged.

I also thank the former director of St. Joseph Hospital in Haan, *Dr. Heinz Uedelhoven*, who left me a large portion of his valuable mammogram and sonogram collection for use in scientific publications. I have put several of these images to excellent use in the atlas.

I express special thanks to the radiologist *Dr. Volker Frohwein* of Landstuhl, Germany, now retired. As a radiologist and cytologist (an extremely rare combination!), he was an enthusiastic, life-long collector of cytologic specimens from the breast. He published his experience with breast cytology in the paper *Frühdiagnostik des Mammakarzinoms* (2002). *Dr. Volker Frohwein* supplied most of the cytologic specimens pictured in this atlas.

One could hardly expect that images collected over a period of decades would consistently satisfy today's quality standards. For this reason, I have replaced earlier images of poorer quality, and the materials from Dr. Frohwein were valuable in this regard. MR images of marginal quality have been replaced wherever possible by similar images acquired with a 1.5-tesla scanner and the latest coil technology. *Dr. Stefan Kraemer* helped me with this task.

I appreciate the help of my two former doctoral candidates *Coscina Weining* and *Oskar Weining-Klemm*, who analyzed my case files from the past 10 years to identify the most economical and effective early detection strategies as part of their doctoral dissertation. I am pleased to note that they found only a 1.5% incidence of interval cancers.

My daughter, **Andrea Barth**, not only edited this book time and again, making stylistic revisions and offering excellent organizational suggestions, but also helped me with the statistical materials. She has thus made a valuable contribution to the concept of the book. My son, **Dr. Stephan Barth** (St. Johann, Austria), did extensive literature research that was necessary to ensure that the contents of the atlas were up to date. He also revised the chapter on breast cancer in males.

I thank the staff at Thieme Publishers, especially *Gabriele Kuhn-Giovannini*, and *Elisabeth Kurz* for their work in producing the English edition. I extend special thanks to the translators of the book, *Terry Telger* and *Julie Foster*, and to the copy editor *Len Cegielka* for his excellent work.

Finally I would like to thank all the retired department heads at Esslingen Hospital for decades of friendly cooperation and wish them all the best.

*Volker Barth, MD*

# List of Contributors

Volker Frohwein, MD
Specialist for Radiology
and Nuclear Medicine
Landstuhl/Pfalz, Germany

Johannes Herrmann, MD
Breast Imaging Center
Esslingen, Germany

Brigitte Koellner, MD
Central Institute for Radiology
Esslingen Hospital
Esslingen, Germany

Elfi Steinhilber
Esslingen, Germany

Oliver Wild
OwiCom
Esslingen, Germany

Andrea Barth
Nutritionist, Editorial Journalist
Breast Imaging Center
Esslingen, Germany

Stephan Barth, MD
Supervising Physician
Department of General Surgery
District Hospital
St. Johann/Tirol, Austria

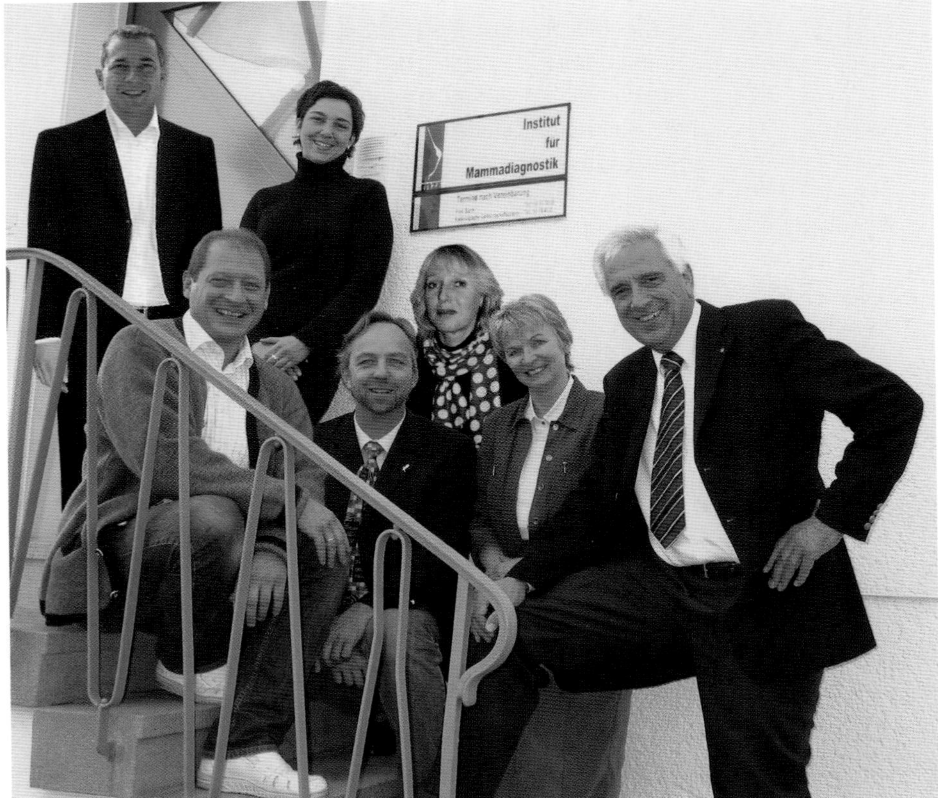


From left to right: Dr. Stephan Barth, Dr. Johannes Herrmann, Andrea Barth, Oliver Wild, Elfi Steinhilber, Dr. Brigitte Koellner, Prof. Volker Barth.

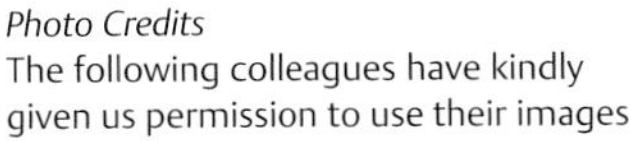

*Photo Credits*
The following colleagues have kindly given us permission to use their images:

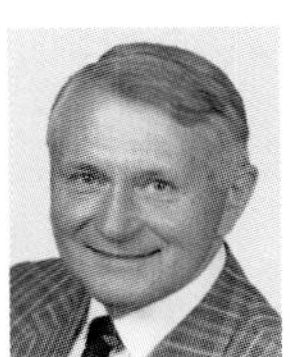

Prof. Roland Baessler, MD
Pathologist
Fulda, Germany

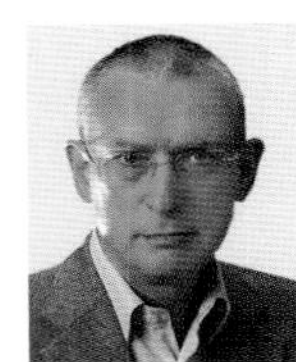

Hans-Helmut Dahm, MD
Assistant Professor
Pathologist
Esslingen, Germany

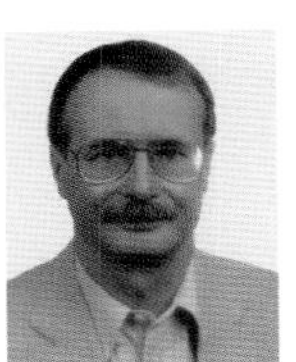

Volker Frohwein, MD
Radiologist/Cytologist
Landstuhl/Pfalz, Germany

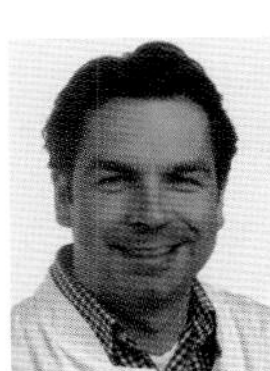

Prof. Stefan Kraemer, MD
Radiologist
Esslingen, Germany

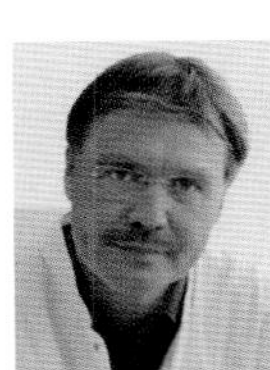

Prof. Thorsten Kuehn, MD
Gynecologist
Esslingen, Germany

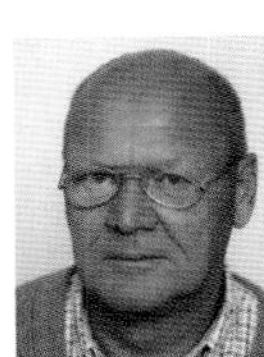

Prof. Klaus Prechtel, MD
Pathologist
Starnberg, Germany

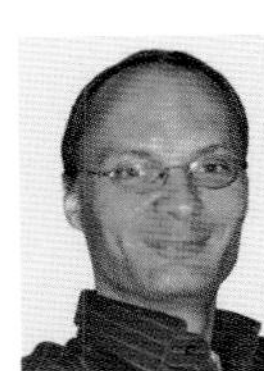

Joern Straeter, MD
Assistant Professor
Pathologist
Esslingen, Germany

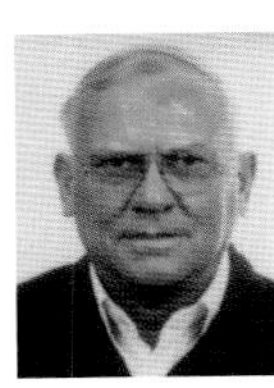

Heinz Uedelhoven, MD
Radiologist
Haan, Germany

# Contents

# Abbreviations

| | |
|---|---|
| ACR | American College of Radiology |
| ACS | American Cancer Society |
| ADH | atypical ductal hyperplasia |
| AFBUS | automated full-field breast ultrasound |
| AGD | average glandular dose |
| ALH | atypical lobular hyperplasia |
| BCT | breast conserving therapy |
| BIRADS | Breast Imaging Reporting and Data System |
| CA | breast cancer |
| CAC | computer-aided classification |
| CAD | computer-aided detection |
| CLIS | carcinoma lobulare in situ |
| CNB | core-needle biopsy |
| CT | computed tomography |
| CUP | carcinoma of unknown primary |
| DCIS | ductal carcinoma in situ |
| DH | ductal hyperplasia |
| DQE | detective quantum efficiency |
| DVB | digital stereotactically guided vacuum biopsy |
| EIC | extensive intraductal component |
| EOD | extent of disease |
| EPCQ | European Protocol for the Quality Control of the Physical and Technical Aspects of Mammography Screening |
| ER | estrogen receptor |
| FASC | full-angle spatial compounding |
| FEA | flat epithelial atypia |
| FNA | fine-needle aspiration |
| FOV | field of view |
| HCG | human chorionic gonadotropin |
| HRT | hormone replacement therapy |
| IGF | insulin-like growth factor |
| IMZE | Interdisciplinary Breast Center of Esslingen |
| IUD | intrauterine device |
| LCIS | lobular carcinoma in situ |
| LIN | lobular intraepithelial neoplasia |
| LN | lymph node; lobular neoplasia |
| LND | lymph node dissection |
| LP/mm | line pairs per millimeter |
| MRI | magnet resonance imaging |
| MRM | magnetic resonance mammography |
| NOS | not otherwise specified |
| NPL | nipple–pectoral line |
| NPV | negative predictive value |
| PACS | Picture Archiving and Communication System |
| PAI | plasminogen activator inhibitor |
| PET | positron emission tomography |
| PGMI | perfect–good–moderate–insufficient quality of mammography |
| PPV | positive predicted value |
| PR | progesterone receptor |
| PSVU | palpation + single-view mammography and ultrasound |
| RR | relative risk |
| RT | radiotherapy |
| SCL | supraclavicular lymph node |
| SLN | sentinel lymph node |
| SLNB | sentinel lymph node biopsy |
| SO-VB | ultrasound-guided vacuum biopsy |
| SPECT | single-photon emission computed tomography |
| ST-CNB | stereotactic core-needle biopsy |
| ST-FNA | stereotactic fine-needle aspiration |
| SV | single-view mammography |
| SVB | sonographically guided biopsy |
| SVB | sonographically guided vacuum biopsy |
| SVU | single-view mammography plus ultrasound |
| TDLU | terminal duct lobular unit |
| TRAM flap | transverse rectus abdominis myocutaneous flap |
| TV | two-view mammography |
| uPA | urokinase plasminogen activator |
| US | ultrasound (sonography) |
| VB | vacuum biopsy |
| VPN | virtual private network |

# 1 Introduction

Breast cancer is the most common form of cancer in women throughout the world. According to statistics from the International Agency for Research on Cancer (IARC), 1.2 million women are diagnosed with breast cancer each year, and 410 000 (35 %) will die from this disease. The American Cancer Society estimates that 200 000 women develop breast cancer annually in the United States, with more than 40 000 deaths (it is estimated that in 2009 192 370 women will be diagnosed with and 40 170 women (37.1 %) will die of breast cancer [Horner et al. 2009]). In Europe, breast cancer is the leading cause of cancer deaths in women (**Fig. 1.1**) (Ferlay et al. 2006). Approximately 350 000 new cases are diagnosed annually in Europe, and 130 000 women will die of this disease. Statistically, every tenth to twelfth woman in Western Europe will develop breast cancer by 80 years of age. Breast cancer is also the leading form of cancer among women in Germany (26% of all cancers), although it ranks far behind cardiovascular disease as a *cause of death*, accounting for just 3.9% of all deaths.

The incidence of breast cancer varies in different countries. Highly developed western countries have a higher incidence and mortality than less-developed regions of the world. More women in the United States die from lung disease (excluding vascular diseases) than from breast cancer (Baines 2000). While the number of new cases is rising in varying degrees throughout the world (showing a slightly downward trend in the United States since 1990), the mortality rates from breast cancer are falling, again in varying degrees.

Besides genetic factors hormonal, environmental and nutritional influences are believed to play an increasingly significant role. This theory is consistent with the rising incidence among women who have emigrated to the United States from Japan. Turkish women who live in Germany have shown a similar trend, with an almost 2-fold increase in breast cancer mortality (Zeeb et al. 2002, Gerber 2003).

Owing to more rigorous efforts at early detection and adjuvant drug therapies, the survival rates for breast cancer patients have improved significantly during the past 25 years. Numerous therapeutic trials have shown not only a decrease in recurrence rates but also a true, long-term reduction in mortality. The early detection of breast cancer is no longer the exclusive domain of mammography. Ultrasound imaging with high-resolution probes can detect a large percentage of tumors that are not visible on mammograms. Similar considerations apply to magnetic resonance imaging in young women who are at risk for developing breast cancer.

The time has come to change our thinking: outside of screening, mammography is currently *the most important adjunct to breast ultrasound, not the other way around.* Current screening practices should be modified to reflect a new concept: **single-view mammography aided by breast ultrasound and physical examination.** There would be no need to obtain a second, craniocaudal mammographic view. This view contributes very little to cancer detection (p. 105). Its loss would be offset by the far more effective ultrasound examination, and the costs of the additional ultrasound scans would be covered.

**Fig. 1.1 Most frequent types of cancer in European women.**

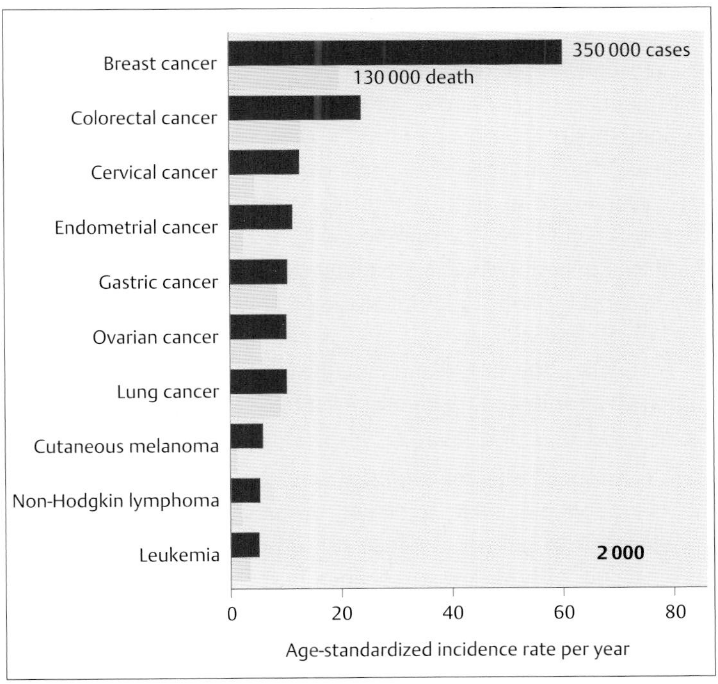


The argument that a new screening model would be too costly and time-consuming is no longer tenable in the age of digital full-field mammography, which has resulted in faster and more efficient workflow.

Today the ultrasound examination can even be automated: new *automated full-field ultrasound scanners* (such as the *AFBUS* system; Yi-Hong Chou et al. 2007, Wenkel et al. 2008) and *full-angle spatial compounding* (*FASC*; Hollenhorst et al. 2008) will enable technologists to perform standard-projection ultrasound screening while the physician reviews mammograms, ultrasound scans, and clinical findings at a workstation. This will result in a more efficient workup at lower cost and less radiation exposure without increasing the length of the examination. Radiodense breasts or suspicious lesions can be examined with ultrasound on site by a trained doctor or technologist and, if necessary, can be biopsied within the next day or two. The double reading of images is a practice that should be maintained.

Palpable abnormalities can also be objectively investigated with the *Sure Touch System*, for example, and represented as a digital image. While these techniques are new and have not yet been clinically proven, those that stand the test of time could also be applicable to regular screening. It is reasonable to predict that this concept will find clinical application in the next 5–10 years.

Understandably, those responsible for breast cancer screening still think in terms of conventional mammography with its relatively complex protocols. This is where our thinking needs to change. The situation is better than we might think. The new fully digital systems have also influenced screening protocols, which traditionally involve the tedious and time-consuming handling of mammographic cassettes, screens, and films and the archiving of film jackets. All of this is eliminated with a fully digital mammography system that includes a scanner for old films and a PACS filing system. Because the images are available in seconds, the first reader can inform the patient of the result on site, if desired, and state the possible need for additional tests. Ultrasound could also be done on site, eliminating costly recalls and sparing women a great deal of emotional distress. The current practice of taking mammograms and having women wait several weeks for a result and suffer the anxiety of a recall visit, not knowing whether it will involve an additional mammogram, ultrasound scan, or breast biopsy, is unsatisfactory for our patients.

These opinions regarding modern screening are of course not yet corroborated in studies, that is, they are not evidence-based. They do however result from 40 years of extensive experience of the author in performing and reading mammography examinations, and in working with additional diagnostic methods in so-called therapeutic breast diagnosis.

For 9 years, the author and his colleagues have had excellent results with a combined regimen consisting of single-view mammography (except for initial mammograms in women over 40 years of age), ultrasound, and visual inspection and palpation of the breasts. Occasionally we add magnetic resonance imaging and interventional procedures for the investigation of suspicious findings. Our rate of interval cancers is 2%. Of course, we cannot equate the operational procedures in a specialized diagnostic breast center with those in a mass screening program. But there are certain aspects of our practice that can be applied to other settings.

> **!**
>
> It is reasonable to ask whether we should maintain the current population-wide screening programs in the future, or change to a system in which risk groups are identified and screened with various modalities based on personal breast cancer risk, regardless of age. One approach would be to use MRI and ultrasound in young women at high risk; single-view mammography and ultrasound in 40- to 60-year-old women at moderate risk; single-view mammograms alone in women over aged 60 with a radiographic breast density of ACR 1 or 2; four-plane mammograms plus ultrasound in women with ACR 3 density, and so on.
>
> Four decades of mammography have led to deeply ingrained attitudes when it comes to breast screening. It is time to muster enough courage and flexibility to look for new approaches and to modify current screening protocols, at least in selected model projects.
>
> These aspects have led the American Cancer Society to rethink screening modalities, not with respect to breast ultrasound (why?) but in its acceptance of magnetic resonance mammography. The Society has recently issued the following recommendations:
>
> - Annual mammograms and MRI for women with a very high personal risk of breast cancer (lifetime risk > 25%)
> - Mammograms once a year and MRI every 2–3 years for women with a markedly increased personal risk (lifetime risk of 15–20%)
> - Annual mammograms without MRI for women at average risk (< 15% lifetime risk) (Saslow et al. 2007)
>
> The rationale for this selective screening approach is open to question, especially when we consider that the ACR recommendations disregard the far more cost-effective modality of ultrasound until 2007 (Mahoney and Mendelson 2007). Nevertheless, it is clear that the rigid attitudes toward screening are beginning to loosen in the right direction. This is an encouraging sign for all those who have begun to feel helpless under pressure from the screening lobby.

The technology for a modern screening design is already available—a fact that should be noted by program planners! The costs are probably not higher than in traditional programs (they are probably lower); radiation exposure of the female population is reduced; the diagnostic yield is increased; and patient acceptance is higher since each breast is compressed only once. But who will have the courage to conduct a model project that parallels regular screening? Almost all screening publications by prominent scientists have reached the same conclusion: mammography is the only evidence-based modality for mass screening. Who could argue with this conclusion?

If mammographic screening alone (with 30% interval cancers) can lower mortality rates by 25%, how much further can mortality be decreased if interval cancers could be reduced from the current 30% rate with conventional mammographic screening to approximately 5% with modified single-view mammographic screening at one-half the usual radiation exposure? Where are the studies that could prove this?

In this book we explore the capabilities of mammography and of complementary diagnostic modalities, especially ultrasound, in the early detection of breast cancer. *Digital full-field mammography* offsets many of the weaknesses of conventional mammography and virtually eliminates the need for magnification mammograms for about 50% of all traditional indications.

Of course, mammography is essential for the detection or exclusion of calcifications in the breast. This requires only *one* well-positioned, high-quality oblique projection, except in selected cases where a second projection is required. Noncalcifying lesions (75% of all malignancies) and especially small invasive tumors are usually demonstrated better by high-resolution (11–15 MHz) ultrasound than by mammography.

Ultrasound does not only optimize early cancer detection. It can also demonstrate physiological changes in the breast parenchyma that affect the radiographic density (ACR value) of the breast. It is known that a radiodense mammogram during menopause is associated with an increased breast cancer risk (Wolfe 1976, Arthur 1990, McCormack et al. 2006). Too little research has been done on why breast density varies from one woman to the next. The *inter*lobular stroma within the breast cannot be the cause, as it does not undergo cyclic changes. But the *intra*lobular stroma distributed around and within the lactiferous ducts and mammary lobules, like the lobules themselves, is subject to hormonal variations.

In this book we seek to explore these relationships in greater detail, recognizing the limits of our knowledge in this area. The *inter*lobular and *intra*lobular stroma are clearly distinguishable from each other sonographically by their different fluid contents. Apparently this is more difficult to do histologically with current staining methods, as most pathology reports do not distinguish between *inter*- and *intra*lobular stroma, classifying all such findings under the heading of *fibrosis*. Thus, pathologists and sonographers should come together in analyzing these basic structures of the breast. They provide important insights into the physiologic changes that occur in response to hormone replacement therapy (HRT), for example, and during the normal menstrual cycle. Mammography and MRI cannot provide this kind of information.

The important links between mammographic breast density and cancer risk can be analyzed only with high-resolution ultrasound scanners (11–18 MHz). Prior sonograms should be displayed on a separate monitor for comparison during the examination (see p. 158). This is possible in the digital age with a **p**icture **a**rchiving and **c**ommunication **s**ystem (PACS), a digital system for storing, retrieving, and displaying diagnostic images. This type of system permits the early and rapid detection of new abnormalities as well as changes in hormonally active glandular tissues (terminal duct lobular units, TDLUs). Standard ultrasound planes must be used (see p. 157) so that the findings at different times are displayed in the same planes of section. Risk groups have actually been eliminated in this way by noting, for example, that detectable stimulation of these anatomic structures occurs in women who are receiving HRT. It is noteworthy that predominantly lobular carcinomas are reported to occur in women on combined estrogen–progestin therapy. These tumors originate from stimulated cells of the TDLUs, which are given special attention in this atlas.

Based on the latest findings from the *Women's Health Initiative (WHI) (2002)* and *Million Women Study (2003)*, estrogens alone do not appear to increase the risk of breast cancer. In many cases estrogen reduces the mammographic density of the breasts, thus helping to lower the cancer risk. The varying radiographic density of the breasts, the proliferation of TDLUs, and the risk of breast cancer should be viewed in a holistic manner, as we have attempted to do in this book.

It is quite possible that the hypotheses advanced here are not entirely valid or correct, especially in cases where they conflict with traditional beliefs about hormonal effects. In years past it has been thought that progestins have a "calming" effect on the glandular breast tissue while estrogens tend to stimulate it. We hope that this book will motivate further research into these pivotal questions, taking note of previous excellent works by other scientists such as Teboul and Halliwell (1995), who performed a detailed sonographic analysis of the TDLUs and made this a basis for breast analysis.

It is only by evaluating the TDLUs, particularly the ducts and lobules, that we can evaluate lobular stimulation and perhaps minimize cancer risks based on the cycle phase of reproductive-age women and the individual hormonal status of menopausal women.

In this atlas we will also explore the typical anatomy of specific tumor entities. *Tumor shape, margins, blood supply,* and *calcification pattern*, along with associated findings such as architectural distortion, skin and nipple retraction, and edema, play a pivotal role in clinical, mammographic, sonographic, and MRI analysis. Anyone who understands the pathology and pathophysiology of the normal and diseased breast will also understand the distinctive contributions of the various diagnostic modalities (Prechtel and Rutzki 1973, Hamperl 1968, Höffken and Lanyi 1973, Tabar and Dean 2000).

Attention is also given to complementary investigations, particularly interventional procedures. Until about 10 years ago, the indications for core-needle biopsy (CNB; also known as fine-needle biopsy, FNB) and vacuum biopsy (VB) were based on the Lanyi analysis of microcalcifications (Lanyi 1986), and too few interventional biopsies were being performed. Today, on the other hand, breast biopsies are too frequent and too invasive. Almost all clustered microcalcifications are biopsied without regard for their form or structure and usually without evaluating prior images. The preferred technique is *vacuum biopsy*, a very costly procedure that imposes a tremendous burden on patients. Along with many harmless lesions, these biopsies naturally yield a large number of ADH and DCIS lesions.

Not all of these preinvasive lesions will develop into invasive cancer, however. With some calcifications, then, it would be appropriate to take a less aggressive approach or at least proceed as noninvasively as possible. It is difficult to understand why so many scientists (and so few pathologists) recommend vacuum biopsy for the investigation of microcalcifications, when a simple and far less costly *core-needle biopsy (CNB)* would be sufficient to make a benign–malignant differentiation. For decades, we have performed fine-needle aspiration biopsies (FNA) at our center without missing cancers at all, and this experience is reflected in the present atlas. Ultimately it is important that the biopsy cores contain calcifications, not whether the histologic examination reveals ADH or DCIS. Surgery will be done in any case, and the histologic result will be modified accordingly with no further therapeutic implications (except perhaps in sentinel node biopsies). Given the current situation of dwindling finances and high funding needs in this and other health-care sectors, we must ask ourselves whether we can still afford these cost-intensive frills.

Some readers of this book will wonder why so many cytologic specimens are shown, given the fact that percutaneous biopsies are more reliable. This is because FNA performed by an experienced examiner is such a fast, simple, and cost-effective tool that it should not be withheld. FNA can quickly clarify indeterminate clinical and/or sonographic findings with minimum cost and effort. It would be a great shame if this procedure were forgotten, as current trends in Germany seem to indicate (Decker and Böcker 2008).

Cytology is so valuable that it should continue to be developed along with fine-needle core and vacuum biopsies. It is easy, for example, to prepare an *imprint specimen* for cytologic analysis during a core or vacuum biopsy (p. 230). Cytology can supply an immediate diagnosis with 95% accuracy and can provide the patient with an on-site benign–malignant differentiation. The cytologic result is then confirmed by core tissue histology, providing significant emotional relief for anxious patients. This is the only way that cytology can continue to evolve. If pathologists and cytologists follow the current trend of investigating everything by vacuum biopsy and are no longer given cellular material for analysis, this would eventually mean the end of sound, substantive cytodiagnosis. It is unfortunate that cytologists as a professional group have not made a scientific effort to rescue breast cytology.

Interventional procedures for screening purposes are used with different frequencies in the United States and in the United Kingdom. Smith-Bindman et al. (2003) compared the results of mammographic screening in the United States and in the United Kingdom. While the cancer detection rates were the same, the recall and negative open-biopsy rates were twice as high in the United States as in the United Kingdom. This suggests that there is a great need in the United States for interventional procedures as an alternative to open biopsies.

This book is concerned less with the epidemiology of breast cancer than with its early detection and optimum treatment and the diagnostic problems that may arise in the postoperative breast. Nevertheless, a section has been devoted to the questions that women commonly *ask their doctors about breast cancer and tumorbiologic aspects.* We seek to give authoritative answers to questions that breast diagnosticians must address with respect to hormone replacement therapy, genetic concerns (What is my daughter's risk if I have breast cancer? When should she start having mammograms? etc.) (see p. 7).

Screening examinations reduce breast cancer mortality and allow for breast-conserving therapies, but only if the screening tests (mammography, ultrasound, MRI, interventional procedures) conform to proper guidelines and yield quality results, if the physicians and assistants performing and interpreting the tests are properly trained, and if surgeons respect the limits of breast-conserving operability. But these are areas in which quality training has been lacking—for, aside from some university facilities, teaching hospitals in Europe have performed fewer and fewer mammographic examinations during the past 20 years that would provide learning opportunities for young doctors. Mammography has been practiced more and more at ambulatory centers, and the Europe-wide mammographic screening programs have contributed to the fact that fewer doctors are being trained in mammography and there are fewer and fewer mammographic specialists.

Radiologic technologists are already being trained and employed as double-readers of screening mammograms (Duijm et al. 2007). This is a disturbing development.

This atlas is intended to close the gap in physician education. Our goal is not to teach the fundamentals based on impressive mammograms showing typical benign and malignant lesions but to explore the full spectrum of breast examinations including the many pitfalls that are encountered in various methods. There are many breast diseases outside screening programs for which patients visit their doctors seeking a competent evaluation and, if possible, a cure. Screening programs are legally mandated tests that employ a single method (mammography) and are geared toward *asymptomatic* women in a specific age group (Koubenec 2000, Peer et al 1994, Poplack et al 2000, Sickles et al. 2002, Butz 2003). But women under 50 and over 70 years of age may also have breast cancer, which may be asymptomatic or may produce clinical complaints. Approximately 35% of all breast cancer patients seen by the author and his colleagues are under age of 50 years, and this percentage has shown a rising trend.

It is important to know not just the mammographic but also the clinical, sonographic, MRI, and cytologic features of affected breasts in order to avoid missing a malignancy or overdiagnosing a benign condition.

To make the teaching process as concise as possible, the case presentations are followed by *multiple-choice questions.* The answers contain additional illustrations on the current status and further course of the illustrative cases. The edges of the pages in the Questions section are marked with alphanumeric coordinates (1–28 and A–t) so that specific points in the images can be located without using arrows that might give away the answer. The Answers section of the book does use arrows.

This book, then, is an interactive guide that trains the reader in differential diagnosis and is intended more for experienced breast diagnosticians than for students learning the basics of mammography and other modalities. All in all, this atlas is not an "easy read" but a very challenging work. Note, however, that each *case history* includes a typical criterion that points the way to the correct diagnosis.

The only exception to this question-and-answer format is breast ultrasound (p. 153). With this modality, an effort is made to teach the fundamentals of the TDLU wherever possible. Greater emphasis is placed on physiologic changes in the breast parenchyma relating to the normal menstrual cycle and HRT, because in the past too little attention has been given to the sonographic aspects of these changes. Each sonogram is accompanied by a correlative drawing that identifies key anatomic structures. This section naturally includes a great deal of author speculation based on 35 years of comparative observations regarding hormonal status, cycle phase, pregnancy, and so on, as they are reflected in mammograms and sonograms. This part of the book is intended mainly as a stimulus for further research in this area. It seeks to draw a correlation between the mammographic density of the breast (an indicator of breast cancer risk) and the proliferation of hormonally active breast parenchyma that can be seen on sonograms. Ultrasound is still an evolving tool and still has many aspects that need to be explored more fully.

Owing to European and American quality guidelines, an outstanding quality level has been achieved in screening facilities and in the new breast centers that are springing up everywhere. It remains to be seen whether enough personnel can be trained for these facilities to maintain these high quality standards on a population-wide scale.

At any rate, it is becoming increasingly difficult for these centers to recruit physicians who have a comprehensive understanding of breast diagnosis, are proficient in mammography, ultrasound, interventional procedures, and magnetic resonance mammography (MRM), and know the capabilities and limitations of these procedures. These skills are essential when it comes to detecting and interpreting *postoperative changes.* Consequently, considerable space is devoted to examining the postoperative breast and recognizing typical changes (p. 313). Essential pretherapeutic procedures such *as preoperative localization* and *specimen radiography* are also addressed in this context. *Sentinel node biopsy* (p. 307) is included because it is a diagnostic procedure that can definitely be done preoperatively in outpatient nuclear medicine facilities. It is generally scheduled the day before the operation in coordination with the surgeon.

Apart from digitization, there have been no major technical advances in mammography during recent years. As a result of *digital* technology and especially *fully digital* systems, mammography is now undergoing a renaissance. This results partly from costly innovations such as *digital tomosynthesis* but relates mainly to new capabilities for image interpretation, improved image quality, and new workflow procedures within breast departments. The mammograms presented in this atlas either are fully digital images (*Giotto Image*, IMS, Bologna, Italy) or were digitally scanned into a computer with the *Lumisys scanner.* Using this scanner and the workstation supplied by Image Diagnost International (Munich, Germany), we can also document the clinical appearance of the breast, scan the pictures into a computer, and place them in the patients' files. A large number of these photographs are included in this atlas. Of course, we routinely practice the double reading of mammograms.

It is time to rethink the diagnostic methods that are used. It bears repeating—though many scientists do not like to hear it—that mammography is *no longer the gold standard of breast imaging* as it was in the 1970s and 1980s. Ultrasound (and even MRI) has

**Fig. 1.2 Fruits of the breast cancer awareness movement.** The activities of medical and lay societies throughout the world have substantially reduced the treatment-related morbidity and emotional distress suffered by women with breast cancer. In cases where mastectomy is necessary, scars are placed in such a way that they are concealed by clothing, troublesome skin folds and fat folds are eliminated, and patients do not experience a foreign-body sensation from fat deposits or other causes. The SLN procedure has limited axillary surgery to the removal of sentinel lymph node metastases, thereby reducing the incidence of lymphedema. Computer-assisted radiotherapy allows for precise dose calculation and distribution within the residual breast, avoiding radiation injuries. Even bilateral breast-conserving surgery can yield a satisfying cosmetic result that helps to maintain the patient's feeling of self-worth.

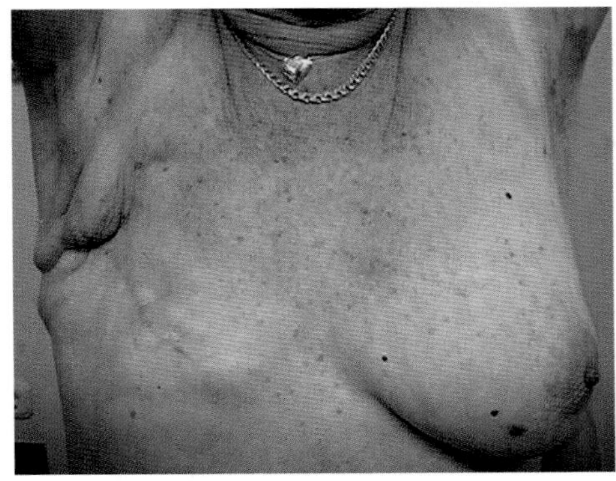

**a** This 76-year-old woman underwent mastectomy in 1997. Two fat deposits in the scarred area restrict arm mobility and create a constant foreign-body sensation below the axilla.

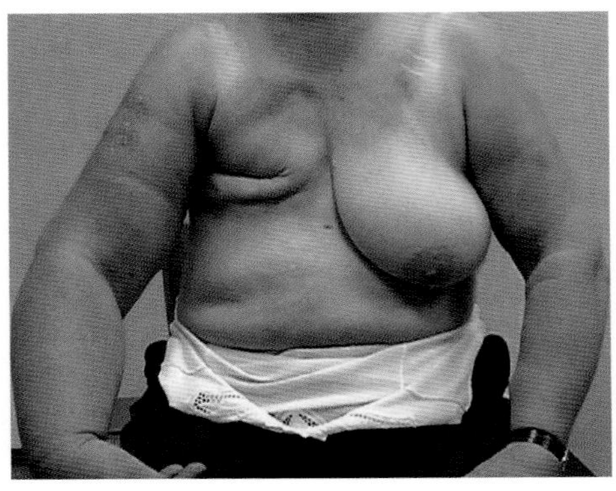

**b** A 72-year-old woman underwent right mastectomy and radical axillary dissection. Two years later she has massive edema of the right arm.

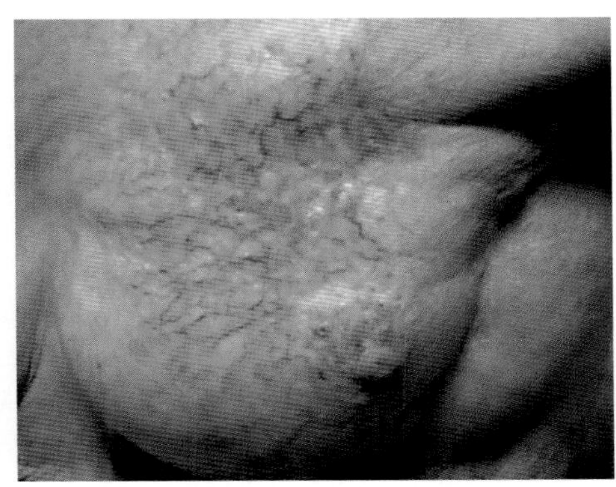

**c** A 76-year-old woman underwent breast-conserving surgery 15 years earlier and sustained tissue damage due to radiation overdose. There is plaquelike scarring of the supra-areolar breast with extensive telangiectasis.

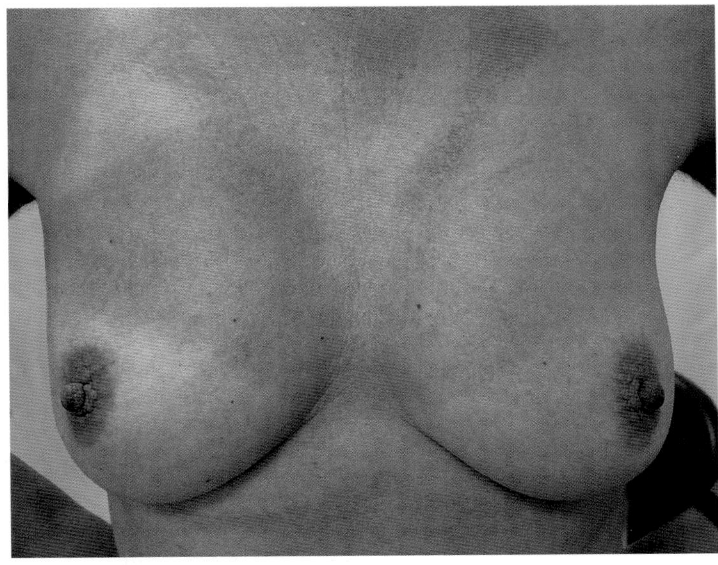

**d** This 40-year-old woman underwent bilateral breast-conserving treatment. She has an excellent cosmetic result that preserves her sense of self-worth. (A local recurrence developed on the right side 10 years after primary treatment.)

The goal of modern breast cancer treatment is to preserve the breast while respecting oncologic principles, avoiding the destruction of axillary structures, and achieving a good cosmetic result. There is no guarantee of permanent success, as disease may recur even years or decades after treatment. But the time gained can contribute greatly to the enhancement of self-worth, especially in younger women.

made tremendous strides, and today it should be used routinely in the early detection of breast cancer. At our center we have already detected more cancers with routine breast ultrasound than we have with mammograms. All guidelines repeat the stereotypical claim that mammography is the only evidence-based method for the early detection of breast cancer. This is true, of course, because ultrasound has not had a chance to prove its evidential value. There is no screening program or model project—except that of Wendie Berg and her colleagues (Berg et al. 2008)—in which single-view mammograms are being supplemented by ultrasound. Dr. Berg had also used biplane mammography for screening of women with an elevated risk of breast cancer. Adding a single screening ultrasound to mammography yielded for mammography 7.2 cancers per 1000 high-risk women, which increased to 11.8 cancers with mammography and ultrasound combined, with a substantially increased number of false positives (4.4%). However, the mammographic and sonographic investigations were performed by different physicians who did not know each others' results. Therefore, there were more false positives for the ultrasound studies (without reduction of false positives in mammography), in the presence of a relatively long examination time (19 mins) for the ultrasound. In our clinic, we perform combined mammography and ultrasound routinely within 20 minutes, including a physical examination and the "small talk." It is the physician who reads the mammograms, and performs the ultrasound and physical examination. What country will have the courage to initiate a model project of this kind in parallel with regular screening?

The 50% dose reduction with single-view mammograms means that even women under age 50 years could be included in screening. This is significant, because 35% of all breast cancer cases affect women between 30 and 50 years of age. Nevertheless, women in this age group are still excluded from diagnosis and treatment in many countries with established screening programs. There is no screening program for these women in Germany, for example, and only women with a high familial risk (approximately 10% of all women) may present for mammographic screening. All that remain for the other 90% of women aged 30–50 are the unsatisfactory options of self-examination and manual examination by their doctor. There are better alternatives. In Scandinavia, for example, screening begins at 45 years of age and continues through age 75.

*Lest I create the wrong impression*—I have been a friend of mammography for 40 years; but, as in most old friendships, I have come to see not just its positive qualities but also its flaws. I no longer look at mammography through rose-colored glasses, though I can see its substantial merits as well as its weaknesses. We need mammography *and* ultrasound if cure rates are to be improved.

I am also a friend of vacuum biopsy and core-needle biopsy, but I know the inestimable value of fine-needle aspiration (cytology) in routine diagnosis and as a screening method. While I am a friend of old and new techniques, I am also mindful of the costs and of the distress that women experience from a particular examination method and from needlessly long waits for their test results.

With integrated care at *certified breast centers*, we can ensure that cancers detected at an early stage will be referred for optimum treatment. Better cure rates are attributable to the optimized treatment that is provided at certified breast centers, which have become more numerous over the past decade and are being established throughout the world.

The images in this book are intended to illustrate the modern chain of care from early detection to optimum treatment, to review the diagnostic equipment necessary for this level of care, and to show how services can be interlinked to create diagnostic and therapeutic networks. Today these concepts are not taught at many teaching facilities, yet they are becoming increasingly important.

Modern antibody therapies have brought changes in postoperative morbidity. For example, peripheral tumors show very good response to *trastuzumab* (Herceptin) even in seemingly hopeless cases, but a certain percentage of breast cancer patients treated with this drug develop cerebral metastases (see **Fig. 5.188**) (Siekiera 2006). Formerly, patients did not live long enough to develop these metastases because they died from peripheral disease. These relationships must be explored more fully and integrated into the differential diagnosis (see p. 410).

It is hoped that this newly revised atlas will bolster the concept of quality-assured care and expand our differential diagnostic horizon beyond the limits of mammography. Breast cancer is not as aggressive as it was 30 years ago. Its incidence is already trending downward in the United States, for example, and mortality rates are showing an even sharper decline. The earlier a breast tumor is detected (by whatever method) and treated at a specialized, certified care facility, the better the chance for a cure. Our task is to further optimize what has already been accomplished and improve the odds for the women of today, especially those who entrust their health to population-wide screening. The success of the worldwide breast cancer awareness movement has become clear to everyone (**Fig. 1.2**).

One goal of this atlas is to stimulate a change in thinking that is appropriate for the new technologies. Naturally this will require some effort. There is still much groundwork to be done in developing a *standard protocol* for breast ultrasound examinations (p. 158). Digitization makes this possible.

In the interest of the female population in all countries, the least we can ask is that population-wide screening detect as many disease cases as possible with the lowest possible radiation exposure. *There is much work to be done, so let's get started!*

May all of our readers enjoy a fascinating learning experience!

# 2 Aspects of Tumor Biology

**"Doctor, I have one last question ..."**

Does this sound familiar? The examination is over and the patient has gotten dressed. Before leaving the office, she says casually, "Doctor, I have one last question...," such as:

- *What causes breast cancer?*
- *Can breast cancer be prevented?*
- *Do contraceptives cause breast cancer?*
- *If you take hormones during menopause, is that really as dangerous as people say?*

It is extremely common for women to present their family doctor, gynecologist, or radiologist with questions of this kind. It is important, therefore, to be aware of the latest scientific discoveries in these areas so that you can provide your patients with accurate information. Thus, we open this book on the early detection and differential diagnosis of breast cancer with a look at the most important aspects of tumor biology. Admittedly, the contents of this chapter have been influenced by the author's 35 years of experience in the diagnosis of breast diseases.

## Causes, Growth Factors, Endocrine and Exocrine Influences

The pathogenesis of breast cancer is based on a variety of nongenetic, ethnic, geographic, and biogenetic factors. The current annual death toll from breast cancer is 229 000 in the United States and 59 000 in Germany. Breast cancer mortality is still rising slightly in Germany, while it has been declining in the United States since 1990.

Of all cancers in women, 32% are breast cancers. The risk of breast cancer is highest (12.5%) among white North American women, followed by African-American women. The breast cancer risk is lowest among women living in Asia. Interestingly, the risk among Asian women who live in the United States rises to the general risk level for the North American population within a few generations.

According to Hesch et al. (1997), the female body is not "designed" to withstand an intense barrage of cyclical hormonal changes every month. They argue that the menstrual cycle is an evolutionary mistake, and that numerous ovulatory cycles and their effects on the breast tissue can be damaging to a woman's health. The longer the ovaries continue to function during a woman's lifetime, the more damaging the effects on the breast. The menstrual cycle has but *one* function—to prepare for pregnancy. In centuries past, the "natural" reproductive life of women included decades of anovulatory cycles because multiple consecutive pregnancies were separated by long intervals of breastfeeding.

Today this phenomenon is still encountered in Inuit women who become pregnant, nurse for a year, become pregnant again, nurse for another year, and so on. While the *long-term* risk of breast cancer is significantly reduced in these women following multiple childbirths and prolonged nursing, their *short-term* risk is actually slightly increased during the first 10–15 years in comparison to Canadian women (Harris et al. 2004).

As well as the frequency of menstrual cycles and the density of the breast, the biology of the menstrual cycle also plays a key role in the pathogenesis of breast cancer. The proliferative cell changes that take place during the menstrual cycle create a window for mutagenic attacks on the cells by harmful exogenous agents. Throughout the cycle the breast parenchyma is constantly stimulated to undergo mitosis, and this increases the likelihood that parenchymal cells may undergo somatic mutations. While women under "natural" conditions (frequent pregnancies, prolonged breastfeeding) formerly had no more than 50 menstrual cycles in their lifetime, women in modern society experience up to 500 cycles—each one opening a new window of opportunity for cellular mutations to occur. The incidence of breast cancer correlates with the number of menstrual cycles. It correlates with continuous hyperstimulation by estrogen and progesterone as well, which can also lead to genetic mutations. The breast tissue is most vulnerable to mutations in young women during the years between menarche and their first pregnancy (see p. 9).

According to Hesch et al. (1997), ovulation inhibitors have a range of beneficial health effects for women, reducing the risk of various diseases by the following percentages:

- Benign breast disorders: 14%
- Fibrous nodules: 17%
- Ovarian and endometrial cancer: 40%
- Pelvic inflammatory disease, menorrhagia, and iron deficiency: 50%
- Dysmenorrhea: 40%

Large scientific studies to date have not shown an increased breast cancer risk in women who take oral contraceptives. Mammograms do not show an increase in breast density, because ovulation inhibitors suppress lobular proliferation during the second half of the cycle. If Hesch's theory is correct, the risk of breast cancer should be reduced in women who take the pill. Other factors also influence breast cancer risk, however.

This is evidenced by the fact that women with *BRCA1* gene mutations are at greater risk for breast cancer than women with the *BRCA2* gene, especially if they take oral contraceptives.

Many women suffer episodes of severe mastodynia, which are permanently improved by the use of ovulation inhibitors. By the end of the menstrual cycle, the breast has undergone an approximately 20% increase in volume. In our experience, this increase is most pronounced in women who have ovulated during the cycle. Ovulations become less frequent in later reproductive life, and mastodynia is less severe in anovulatory cycles.

Ovulation inhibitors reduce the impact of endogenous hormones on the breast parenchyma. In theory, then, oral contraceptives may help to prevent breast cancer. In our small case–control study about sport and breast-cancer (see p. 17) this was obviously not the case. Women who took the "pill" developed breast-cancer about 5 years earlier than women without any anticonceptives (see **Fig. 2.6**).

Ovulation inhibitors do not interfere with breast imaging. It should be added, however, that the breast is inherently difficult to evaluate mammographically in women of reproductive age. The examination should be limited to **single-view mammograms** for the detection or exclusion of calcifying tumors. Breast ultrasound should also be performed as an adjunct to radiography.

> **!** **The optimum time for all breast examinations (palpation, mammography, ultrasound, MRI) is at the end of the first half of the menstrual cycle, corresponding to days 7–12 of the cycle (first day of menstrual bleeding = first day of the cycle). This is true regardless of whether the patient is on the pill.**

It is likely that an abundance of fatty tissue in the female body, especially in the breast, contributes to the development of breast cancer. This is because mammary fat, which is not involved in lactation, is hormone-sensitive and is itself a source of estrogen synthesis. We know that estrogen levels in breast cancers and the surrounding parenchyma (including fat-tissue) are relatively high compared with serum estrogen levels. Breast fat also tends to accumulate environmental toxins.

Women with large breasts have a significantly greater risk of developing breast cancer, as do obese women in general. The risk is particularly high in breast tissue that is very radiodense owing to hormonal stimulation (Harvey and Bovbjerg 2004). Hunt and Sickles (2000) studied the effect of obesity on tumor growth, aggressiveness, recurrence rates, and recall rates in 88 364 consecutive mammographic screening examinations. Greater obesity was found to correlate with higher recall rates, biopsy rates, and the number of screening-detected cancers. The tumors detected in obese women tended to be larger and more advanced than tumors detected in normal-weight and underweight women. Interval cancers were also slightly more prevalent in obese women, which is consistent with data published elsewhere (Harris et al. 2004). Because mammograms are less specific in obese women, obesity leads to a 20% increase in false-positive screening mammograms (Elmore, Carney, Abraham et al. 2004). The authors attribute the increased breast cancer risk in obese women to higher estrogen levels. Androstenedione is converted to estrogen in the fatty tissue of menopausal women. Obesity is also associated with a decline in the production of sex hormone-binding globulins, resulting in higher levels of biologically active free estradiol.

Body weight in itself appears to be a less dominant factor than the type of diet leading to obesity. According to the German Institute of Nutritional Research in Potsdam-Rebrücke, women who consume large amounts of fat, butter, margarine, and processed meats and sausages while consuming only small amounts of bread or fruit juices are twice as likely to develop breast cancer within a 6-year period as women with the opposite nutritional pattern. Body weight and menopausal status are far less important factors. There are still a number of unanswered questions concerning the role of obesity. Carcinogenesis is obviously a multifactorial process in which individual factors such as obesity have a limited influence. Gerber (2003) correctly states that even well-designed epidemiologic studies have a number of biases that can affect the study outcome. For example, *nonobese* women with a "normal" body weight tend to eat healthier foods, are more likely to be physically active, avoid alcohol and nicotine, and generally take better care of their health than women who are overweight. The *insulin metabolism* in these women may play a major role, and this is currently the subject of intensive research. The beneficial effect of a healthy lifestyle on an abnormal insulin metabolism is comparable to the effect of adjuvant endocrine and/or cytostatic therapy in women with hormone-receptor-negative breast cancer (Kleeberg 2008). New discoveries on insulin-like growth factors (IGFs) in oncogenesis are also important in the setting of breast cancer follow-up.

According to Wolfe (1976), Gram et al. (1997), Harvey and Bovbjerg (2004), the risk of breast cancer increases with the radiographic density of the breast. A radiographically dense breast results either from an abundance of connective tissue in the breast or from the stimulation and proliferation of breast lobules (inside terminal ductal lobular units, TDLUs) in response to endogenous or exogenous hormones and noxious agents (including alcohol, nicotine, saturated fatty acids, and high doses of vitamin C and E). Harvey and Bovbjerg (2004) found that high doses of vitamin A tended to reduce breast density.

In a study by Lee et al. (1997), experienced mammographers estimated the average fat content of the breast to be 42%, while MR imaging experts calculated a fat content of 66%. In evaluating radiodense areas seen on mammograms, neither mammography nor MRI allow reliable differentiation between connective tissue and breast parenchyma. It is correct, then, to classify breast density into ACR grades I through IV based on the proportions of glandular and fatty tissue:

- I The breast is almost entirely fat (< 25% glandular);
- II There are scattered fibroglandular densities (approx. 26–50% glandular);
- III The breast tissue is heterogeneously dense, which can hinder the detection of small masses (approx. 51–75% glandular);
- IV The breast is extremely dense. This may reduce the sensitivity of mammography (> 75% glandular) (ACR BIRADS®). This is because what appears to be the *glandular* component on mammograms is actually a combination of connective tissue and hormonally active glandular tissue (TDLU). This combination varies from one patient to the next. It would be more accurate to define the four ACR grades as less than 25% breast *parenchyma*, i.e., fibrous tissue and TDLU, and so on (see p. 98 and **Table 5.7**).

The proportion of fat in the breast increases with aging, doing so at a rate of approximately 6% per decade. The Wolfe and Tabar classification pertains only to mammographically visible structural patterns (see p. 98); it does not tell us the actual percentage of fat in the breast or the amount of hormonally active glandular tissue (TDLU), from which breast cancer may arise. In any case, it is only by combining mammography and ultrasound and correlating their findings that we can confirm or exclude the presence of proliferating breast parenchyma that is capable of undergoing malignant change; this cannot be accomplished with mammograms alone. As our own ultrasound studies have shown, a radiographically dense breast may consist not only of fibrofatty tissue and normal or harmlessly enlarged mammary ducts and cysts, but also of proliferation within the terminal duct lobular unit (TDLU). These lobules may create a nidus for carcinogenesis due to fat-induced cell proliferation.

Ultrasound is the only imaging modality that can consistently differentiate among connective tissue, fat, and glandular tissue (see p. 156).

The breast is exposed to a wide range of endocrine, paracrine, and exocrine influences. Besides the hormones that control the cell cycle, we find that growth factors, proto-oncogenes (oncogene precursors), oncogenes, tumor suppressors, cyclins, and other regulatory agents also play a role. Taken together, they constitute a signaling system that regulates the division and differentiation of cells.

**Prolactin** has a key role in initiating the formation of estrogen receptors. This hormone promotes physiologic lobular proliferation in premenopausal women, and it does not have carcinogenic activity. After menopause, however, elevated prolactin levels in the blood are associated with increased breast density due to greater lobular proliferation—a circumstance that triples the risk of developing breast cancer (Hankinson et al. 1999).

During the period of sexual maturation from 10 to 19 years of age, the breast tissue is particularly sensitive to the effects of endogenous and exogenous agents. **Endogenous agents** include elevated serum estradiol levels. Not only the so-called coma-drinking but even moderate alcohol consumption can double or triple the active estradiol level in the blood, thereby increasing the cyclic stimulation of the breast. On the other hand, an endogenous estrogen metabolite, 2-methoxyestradiol, inhibits angiogenesis and thus has an inhibitory effect on tumor growth. Xenoestrogens are potentially hazardous compounds that are abundant in our modern environment. They possess carcinogenic activity, they bind to estrogen receptors, and they can induce changes in cell biology. Many other carcinogens are present in the environment, including:

- Nicotine
- Atrazine and other pesticides
- Insecticides such as endosulfan, methoxychlor, DDT, and chlordane
- Liquid coolants such as polychlorinate and biphenyl
- The softening agent nonylphenol
- Bisphenol a (a breakdown product of polycarbonate)
- Aromatic hydrocarbons from petroleum products

The high content of *isoflavones and lignans in soy* may be one reason why the incidence of breast cancer is significantly lower in Southeast Asia (especially Japan) than in western countries (Vachon et al. 2000). It is noteworthy that the daughters of Japanese families who emigrate to the United States have the same incidence of breast cancer after two generations as American women. The incidence of breast cancer in Japan has also risen, presumably due to changes in dietary habits. Researchers have also studied the effect of soy products on lobular stimulation of the breast parenchyma and thus on the radiographic density of the breast. The consumption of soy products and soy isoflavones by Chinese women in Hong Kong was found to cause a regression of radiographic density on mammograms. This suggests that soy products may protect against breast cancer in addition to their possible benefit in relieving menopausal complaints (Jakes et al. 2002). A particularly significant decrease in mammographic breast density has been found in 56- to 65-year-old women, with an apparent reduction in breast cancer risk. Soy products may also be beneficial in girls and young women, especially those from high-risk families, as the period between puberty and first pregnancy is the most vulnerable period for the breast parenchyma (Key et al. 1999).

### Tip

**The consumption of soy-containing foods protects the estradiol receptors, because the phytoestrogens in these foods bind to the receptors and keep them from being occupied by xenoestrogens. Thus, women under 30 years of age are encouraged to consume 30 g of soy each day in the form of tofu or soybeans, for example, to reduce their risk of developing breast cancer. Dietary soy intake no longer has a protective effect after age 40.**

*Women who had their ovaries removed* at a young age have a 50% lower risk of developing breast cancer in later life. Because a woman's age at the birth of her first child is an important risk factor, the extension of the reproductive period by 10 years or more may be one reason for the rising incidence of breast cancer of younger women in our society. As noted earlier, the number of menstrual cycles during a woman's lifetime correlates with breast cancer risk. For this reason, early menarche (before 11 years of age) and late menopause (after 50 years of age) constitute additional risk factors. Women who experience natural menopause after age 55 develop breast cancer at twice the rate of women who enter menopause at age 45.

*Intrauterine exposure of the fetus to estrogen* may also play a role in the etiology of breast cancer. The daughters of women with preeclampsia (characterized by a very low maternal estrogen level) were found to have a 50% lower risk of developing breast cancer.

While a great many risk factors for breast cancer have been identified, only one **protective factor** has definitely been established: pregnancy at a young age (Hesch et al. 1997). The glandular epithelium of the breast is most vulnerable when the lobules are still in the formative budding stage and have not yet fully matured (**Fig. 2.1**). The first pregnancy forces this maturation to occur. Only *developing* lobules are vulnerable to endogenous and exogenous toxins; fully *mature* lobules are immune to their effects. Thus, an early pregnancy (at 15–23 years of age) will presumably protect against breast cancer.

Analysis of the authors' own case material has not confirmed this protective effect of early pregnancy, but in a relatively small number of patients.

**Progestins** are also known to confer a certain protective effect, at least during the premenstrual period.

**Human chorionic gonadotropin** (HCG) promotes budding, arborization, and differentiation of the mammary lobules (TDLUs) along with well-ordered cellular proliferation and timely cell death by apoptosis. If a carcinogen acts on the cell at a stage when the alveolar bud is fully mature, the cell will not become malignant. If the TDLUs were previously exposed to a carcinogen at an earlier stage, they may still undergo malignant change. Thus, the longer the duration of the maturation process, the greater the chance that mutations may occur. But hormones and antihormones do not cause cancer cells to form, nor do they kill them. The regulatory mechanism is based on cell inhibitors. The first step, according to Hesch et al. (1997), is intraductal proliferation, followed by the development of carcinoma in situ (DCIS, LCIS), which eventually progresses to invasive cancer (see p. 397). HCG can halt the exacerbation of intraductal proliferation to intraductal carcinoma and arrest its progression to invasive cancer, presumably by stimulating lobular maturation. This suggests that HCG could be administered to **high-risk patients** (see p. 13) in their younger years in order to accelerate budding

**Fig. 2.1** **Microanatomy of TDLU in adolescent and mature breasts.**

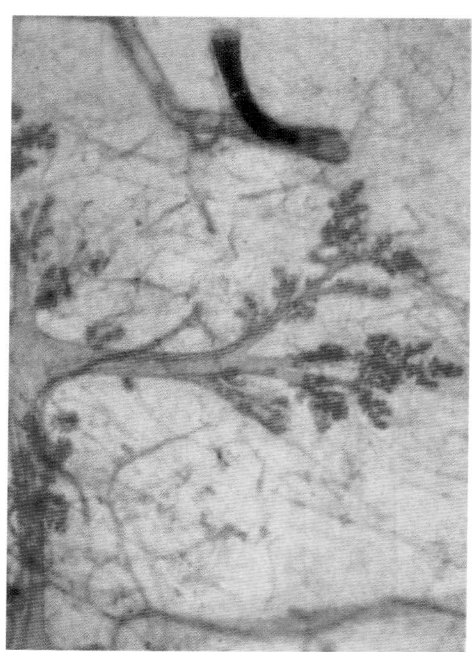

**a** Microanatomy of the terminal duct in an *immature adolescent breast.* Maturing lobules are surrounded by a fine network of capillaries and precapillaries that supply the **t**erminal **d**uct **l**obular **u**nit (TDLU).

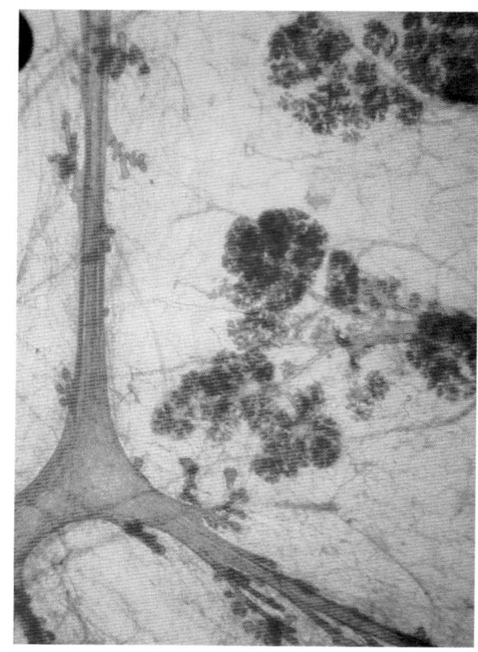

**b** Microanatomy of the TDLU in a *mature breast.* The lobules and acini are fully developed. Exposure to harmful endogenous and exogenous agents at this stage can no longer damage the epithelium or induce mutations. Mutations may occur during the development and breakdown of cells in the normal cycle, however, in circumstances where the cells are exposed to potentially harmful agents. The duct supplying the TDLU is visible in the left and lower part of the section (courtesy of Bässler, 2002) (see **Fig. 4.40**, p. 68).

and maturation of the breast lobules and protect them from harmful endogenous and exogenous agents. Oral contraceptives may inhibit the budding and maturation process in young women and, when combined with exogenous agents such as alcohol or nicotine, may actually promote mutagenesis. These properties tend to lessen the protective role of oral contraceptives in suppressing cyclic proliferative changes. The particular hormonal combination that is used, along with the patient's specific genotype and phenotype, will determine what effect predominates in any given case.

## Oral Contraceptives in Women at Risk

It is still unclear whether oral contraceptives lead to breast cancer in women at risk. A team of physicians led by Steven Narod at the University of Toronto compared the data for 2600 women from 11 different countries (Narod et al. 2002). Half of the women carried mutations in the *BRCA1* or *BRCA2* gene. Women who had a mutation on the *BRCA2* gene and took the "pill" did not have an increased risk of breast cancer. However, 33% more women who had the *BRCA1* gene mutation developed breast cancer if they had used oral contraceptives when they were young, compared with women who had the same mutation but had never taken the pill. It is possible that early contraceptive use in *BRCA1* gene carriers inhibits maturation of the breast lobules, making these women more vulnerable to the effects of potentially harmful endogenous and exogenous agents. This suggests that women under 30 years of age who know that they are *BRCA1* carriers should not use oral contraceptives. The researchers found no risk correlation in women who began taking the pill after 30 years of age.

Regional differences have been documented as well. For example, women in Europe have a slightly lower risk than women from Israel or North America. Asian women have the lowest risk. Oral contraceptives vary from country to country in their formulations, and this could account for some of the differences. Other studies on ovarian cancer yielded an opposite result: The pill actually reduced the risk of developing this type of cancer in women who carried the *BRCA1* mutation.

## Does Smoking Prevent or Promote Breast Cancer?

As a general rule, addictive substances are harmful to the body and mind—not only because of their possible physical effects but also because they induce dependency. The effect of smoking on breast cancer risk is a controversial issue. Does it increase risk, especially in younger women during the vulnerable phase of lobular maturation (see p. 9), or does it have an antiestrogenic effect that actually reduces risk? Biological mechanisms in the development of the female breast play a fundamental role (see pp. 9, 11) and have prompted a retrospective case–control study by Band et al. (2002). Questionnaires from 318 premenopausal and 700 postmenopausal women with breast cancer were compared with a control group of 340 premenopausal and 658 postmenopausal women. The questionnaire covered factors such as ethnicity, family situation, education, alcohol use, age at menarche and menopause, and the use of contraceptives or hormone replacement therapy. A comparison of "ever smokers" and "never smokers" showed that there was an **increased breast cancer risk** in perimenopausal women with at least one full-term pregnancy who began smoking within 5 years after menarche and also for nulliparae who smoked more than 20 cigarettes a day. Postmenopausal women, on the other hand, were not found to have an increased risk. In fact, women who had carried at least one pregnancy to term were actually found to have a reduced risk. These findings suggest that lobular breast tissue is most vulnerable to tobacco and other environmental toxins between menarche and the first pregnancy.

Surprisingly, women who smoked and who had continually gained weight after 18 years of age showed a 50% reduction in risk, regardless of their menopause status. This paradoxical risk reduction points to another effect of smoking: a *nicotine-induced reduction of endogenous estrogen activity.* This effect is particularly striking in obese women because estrogen is synthesized in fatty tissue (and subsequently converted to estriol). This "dual effect" of smoking may account for the controversial study results on breast cancer risk in obese female smokers.

A 7-fold risk increase faced by young nulliparous smokers was recently reported in a study by Kobaa (2003, quoted by Mueck and Wallwiener 2004). This emphasizes the importance of educating young women about the dangers of smoking, particularly with regard to subsequent breast cancer risk. Not all studies reported a reduction of estriol levels because the effects of smoking vary in different age groups. Smoking was found to inhibit the aromatization of androgens, induce androgen stimulation, and cause changes in renal clearance.

**It is important to educate young women—not only BRCA carriers—about the complex risks of smoking.**

Thus, issues relating to maturation of the breast parenchyma, harmful endogenous agents, and breast cancer risk are of major concern in cancer prevention and are likely to prompt many new and interesting discoveries in the future.

## Hormone Replacement Therapy in Menopause

Glandular tissue may undergo local or diffuse proliferation in response to hormonal stimulation. This means that the breast lobules (TDLU) enlarge and proliferate much as they do during pregnancy. The breast becomes more radiographically dense, and proliferating structures scanned with a high-resolution ultrasound probe appear as small, confluent zones of low echogenicity. Some of these areas show focal enhancement on postgadolinium MRI. The phenomenon of increasing mammographic density during hormone therapy and diminishing density after hormone withdrawal can be explained by the waxing and waning of breast lobules and by interstitial edema in the *intra*lobular stroma (TDLU) (see **Fig. 2.1**).

### Advantages

The risks and hazards of hormone replacement therapy (HRT) have become a "hot topic" in the media and in many doctor-patient consultations. Some women even say that they no longer talk about using HRT with their friends because many women would condemn them and as being reckless with their own health and irresponsible toward their families. Given this level of controversy, doctors should be careful to discuss not only the risks of HRT with their patients but also its benefits.

A range of benefits have been identified:

- HRT is still the most effective treatment available for relieving **menopausal complaints** and improving quality-of-life issues relating to estrogen deficiency. Several other options are available for minor complaints, such as herbal products (phytoestrogens). Hot flashes respond well to serotonin reuptake inhibitors (Fluxetin and Trevilor), which also provide an antidepressant side-benefit. The antihypertensive agent Catapresan has similar properties (Rauthe et al. 2003). HRT should always have a definite medical indication. The risks and benefits should be individually assessed, and comprehensive patient education should be provided.
- Long-term HRT is justified in patients with an increased **osteoporosis risk** and for the prevention of osteoporosis. Other treatment options are calcium, vitamin D, and oral bisphosphonate in cases where HRT is contraindicated (e.g., due to high thrombosis risk, migraines, and so on). Estrogens can relieve osteoporosis symptoms, although acute local pain (e.g., spinal pain) responds well to adjuvant radiation therapy (orthovolt therapy), especially when combined with bisphosphonates. The results of the **Women's Health Initiative** (Reeves et al. 2006) and **Million Women Study** (Beral 2003) should not be applied to women who experience *early* menopause (40–50 years of age) or *premature* menopause (before age 40), nor are they applicable to symptomatic perimenopausal or early postmenopausal women who experience menopause at a normal age.
- HRT improves **urogenital complaints** and can also improve sexual relations by relieving dyspareunia. If systemic therapy is contraindicated, estrogens should be administered by topical vaginal application.
- The effect of estrogen therapy on **libido** is controversial. Tibolone and androgens are better for this indication.
- Nonspecific joint and limb pain improve in response to hormone therapy. Skin, mucous membranes, and connective tissues respond favorably to estrogens. HRT can slow but not prevent skin aging. It cannot reverse skin damage due to sun exposure. Hair loss can be arrested or slowed by the topical application of estrogens to the scalp when alopecia is caused by an estradiol deficiency (treatable with alfatradiol) or in cases with an androgenic cause (treatable with minoxidil). Some hair tonics contain a combination of both agents.
- **Cerebral (cognitive) memory functions** improve in response to estrogens. Unlike endogenous depression, postmenopausal depression responds well to estrogens. Additionally, estrogens can enhance the effect of certain antidepressants.
- Based on data from the WHI and other studies, HRT is not indicated solely for the prevention of cardiovascular disease. However, well-designed observational studies have shown that women with an increased **risk of cardiovascular disease** who are treated with estrogens for menopausal complaints tend to have lower long-term rates of cardiovascular disease. HRT should not be used solely for cardiovascular disease prevention, however, until this potential indication has been confirmed by new data.
- Cyclical or continuous progestin therapy is appropriate for endometrial protection in women with an intact uterus who are receiving HRT with estrogen. Estrogen therapy alone, as in patients who have undergone hysterectomy, appears to reduce the risk of breast cancer. Intrauterine progestin application is a possible alternative to systemic dosing. Progestin therapy is unnecessary in women who are already receiving local vaginal estrogen therapy (Birkhäuser et al. 2006).

## Risks

In the past, experience and studies indicated that progestins tend to protect against breast cancer more than promote its growth. The results of the WHI (2002) and the MWS (2003) seem all the more remarkable when viewed in this light. According to these questionnaire-based observational studies, women who received *combined estrogen–progestin HRT* for longer than 5 years had a 30–45% higher incidence of breast cancer than women who did not take hormones. *Estrogen-only therapy* was found to have a protective effect, but it was surprising to find that women who took *tibolone* (Liviella) had a higher risk of developing the disease (WHI 2006). There is no difference, then, between estrogen–progestin combinations and tibolone in terms of breast cancer risk. Tibolone and combination products can both have a stimulatory effect on TDLUs during menopause (see **Fig. 5.81**, p. 187).

When we look at the numbers, we find that 80 out of every 10 000 women in the MWS (as of 2003) who were not on HRT developed breast cancer, while 85 of every 10 000 women who did receive HRT developed the disease. These numbers as well as the short duration of the study (2 years) are cause for critical concern. The breast cancer risk returned to normal only 6 months after the discontinuation of hormone therapy. These periods are really too short to be able to detect all cancer occurrences (detected tumors plus interval cancers) in screening examinations, even in the nonhormone group (the MWS parallels the British national screening program). The first 2-year interval between the start of the study and breast cancer diagnosis is simply too short when we consider that it takes years or decades for breast cancer to develop following tumor inception (von Fournier et al. 1980). It is reasonable to assume, therefore, that the diagnosed tumors were already present when the study began but were still mammographically occult. It should be added that two dozen other studies conducted in the United States on breast cancer and HRT found little or no increase in risk (Harris et al. 2004).

In the British national screening program, women are screened for breast cancer every 3 years. Thirty-one percent of the incident cancers diagnosed in the first year, 52% in the second year, and 82% in the third year are interval cancers, i.e., tumors that are not detected mammographically but are discovered clinically between screening rounds (Woodman et al. 1995). This represents a significant number of malignancies that were missed at screening or first became detectable after completion of the 2-year MWS study (the estrogen–progestin arm and, recently, the estrogen-only arm as well). It may be that participants in the control groups had tumors that were missed on mammograms, and that the results will need to be revised in 2–3 years. Even now, the data from the WHI data suggest that an estrogen-only treatment regimen (e.g., after hysterectomy) reduces the risk of breast cancer, heart attack, colorectal cancer, osteoporosis, and even mortality rates by 30–40%. The effects of progestins is still uncertain. Apparently they increase the risk of thromboembolism, and they appear to increase the breast cancer risk after 5 years of use (Mueck 2005). The biggest surprise from the interim results of the WHI is that there were obviously more instances of breast cancer among women treated with tibolone (Liviella) than among women taking estrogen only (Singer 2005).

A major shortcoming of the MWS is that it excluded women with serious menopausal complaints. As a result, the efficacy of HRT in relieving menopausal symptoms—the prime motivation for women to undergo treatment—could not be investigated. For this reason alone, any overall assessment of the risks and benefits of HRT is already on shaky ground. It is based solely on the results of breast cancer incidence, which in turn were drawn from questionnaires and were not acquired in a randomized study. Another troubling aspect of the MWS is the fact that significantly more women (40%) were informed about the risks and benefits of the hormone product they were taking than the women who received placebos (7%). This in itself probably introduced a systematic error in which the more rigorous evaluation of the hormone group very likely affected the number of cancers that were diagnosed. Moreover, these cancers were diagnosed in the setting of a mammogram-only screening regimen, the efficacy of which remains unclear.

We already know that receptor-positive malignancies grow in response to hormone therapy. We do not know whether this therapy cause the tumors to spread and metastasize at an earlier stage. If the only effect is to stimulate tumor growth, it should be possible to detect the tumors earlier in regular screening examinations.

When we look at the mortality rates in both studies, we find that the studies excluded not only women with menopausal complaints but also women with a prior history of breast cancer. If all cases had been included in the analysis of breast cancer mortality, this would have resulted in a much lower mortality rate for women on HRT than for women who had never taken HRT. Based on the published data, women who did not take HRT would have had up to a 50% higher mortality rate (Schering AG 2003). Thus, the duration of the study is much too short to draw reliable conclusions on the incidence of new cancer cases and the resulting deaths. This could be one reason why the authors of the MWS relied more heavily on data published in the literature than on their own very low incidence when estimating the cancer cases caused by HRT—a practice that could lead to questionable conclusions. The Schering Corporation was correct in pointing out that, if the authors' calculations were correct, the incidence of breast cancer in the UK should have risen as the number of HRT users increased. In reality, however, breast cancer incidence has remained stable during the past 10 years. The further course of this study is certain to bring some significant modifications in the results. For example, as of 2005, fewer breast cancers had been recorded in the discontinued estrogen arm of the study than in the control group. At present the "culprit" appears to be progestins. It will be interesting to see what the future course of the study will bring.

The author's own study on sports and breast cancer in 1260 women has shown that HRT tends to protect against breast cancer rather than promote it. Women on HRT developed the disease 7 years later on average than in the control group without HRT (see **Fig. 2.7**, p. 18).

HRT causes the breast parenchyma to become more radiographically dense in many women, even during menopause. Apparently this effect limits diagnostic accuracy only in screening programs (Elmore, Carney, Abraham et al. 2004) that rely entirely on mammograms. It is not a problem in multimodal evaluations that include breast inspection, palpation, mammography, and ultrasound. It is more important to determine whether the increased density is caused by stimulation of the breast parenchyma, as this would imply an increased risk of breast cancer. Ultrasound is effective in differentiating interlobular stroma from proliferating glandular tissue and (indirectly) from proliferating intralobular stroma. Whenever increased mammographic density is noted in a patient on HRT, hormonal lobular stimulation should be excluded. If the breast parenchyma becomes stimulated in response to a particular HRT, that hormone should be discontinued or a different combination should be instituted (e.g., an estrogen-only product). In some cases this will cause a decline in lobular stimulation. The same applies to MRI: if the breast parenchyma shows intense gadolinium enhancement in response to HRT, the therapy should be reconsidered.

To avoid any misunderstanding, it should be stressed that the indiscriminate use of hormones during menopause should definitely be avoided. Women who do not need hormones should not take them, and age-related problems such as osteoporosis and cardiovascular disease should be managed whenever possible by regular exercise and a healthful, calcium-rich diet. But women who suffer from depression, sleeplessness, and hot flashes that are responsive to HRT should take hormones without concern—preferably an estrogen-only product (e.g., after hysterectomy) and preferably in transdermal form to reduce the risk of thrombosis. If the uterus is present, a progestin is indicated and should be given by the topical intravaginal route or by intrauterine administration (hormone-releasing IUD). We cannot assure these women that they will be protected from breast cancer simply by foregoing what is, for them, a necessary therapy.

However the data are interpreted, large studies show that the declining use of HRT has been accompanied by a decrease in the incidence of breast cancer. The greatest decrease (12%) has been documented for receptor-positive tumors in the 50- to 69-year age group (Emons 2008). This means that a certain percentage of women in perimenopause and early menopause have occult breast cancers or their precursors whose progression to clinically apparent cancer is arrested by physiologic menopause. HRT may preempt this protective effect. It is unclear at present whether this is a permanent effect or simply reflects a shift in the time at which occult cancers become clinically overt. The blockage of estrogen or progesterone effects may lead to the permanent death (apoptosis) of occult cancer cells, similar to the effects observed with tamoxifen.

The incidence of breast cancer has been declining in the United States. It rose by 40% from 1980 to 1998 and has fallen since 1999, most notably between 2002 and 2003. This coincides with a cutback in the prescribing of HRT and has been marked by a particularly sharp decline of estrogen-receptor-positive cancers in women 50 years of age or older (Ravdin et al. 2007, Clarke et al. 2006). Prescriptions for the two leading hormone-replacement products in the United States, Premarin (conjugated estrogen) and Prempro (conjugated estrogen plus medroxyprogesterone acetate), showed a particularly sharp drop in 2002 and 2004 (falling from 60 million to 20 million prescriptions; Stang 2008).

Also, the cancer registries of the German states of *Saarland* and *Schleswig-Holstein* report that the incidence of breast cancer declined from 2003 to 2005, falling each year by an average rate of 5.7% in Saarland (1 million population) and 6.5% in Schleswig-Holstein (2.8 million population). The reasons for this are unknown. If it cannot be related to the decreased use of HRT described in 2002 publications, it must be linked to the stimulation of hormone-receptor-positive, clinically occult cancers and precancerous lesions. It cannot be based on a true increase in new malignancies, which take 5 to 15 years to grow from the first atypical cell to a diagnosable tumor (von Fournier 1980).

A current population-based case–control study in the United States supports the hypothesis that the combined use of estrogen and progestins may promote the growth of lobular breast cancers, while estrogen-only therapy appears to reduce the risk of invasive ductal breast cancers by 30%. Ductal tumors account for approximately 70% of breast cancers, and lobular tumors account for approximately one-third.

Lobular cancers are often more difficult to diagnose than ductal tumors (see **Fig. 4.31**, p. 60; **Fig. 5.10**, pp. 87 and 352 ff; **Fig. 5.34**; p. 120 f; **Fig. 5.128**, p. 260; **Fig. 5.188**, p. 342 ff) and are more frequently bilateral. They have a better prognosis if they are receptor-positive. Usually they are difficult to see on mammograms but are more easily detected by ultrasound (and MRI). An answer to this problem will be found in the future. Today it is still unclear why progestins, but not estrogen, should incite rapid tumor growth. In any case, the two large studies have fostered useful discussions on the optimization of HRT, which are becoming more rational and objective after an initial period of emotionally charged debate.

After all, the average life expectancy for women has increased from 40 years (early 20th century) to 80 years (early 21st century) despite world wars, famine, poverty, air pollution, the hole in the ozone layer, pesticides in food, and hormone replacement. Obviously the human body is more robust than is commonly believed.

## Predisposing Genetic Factors

It is likely that genetic factors play a more important role in the development of breast cancer than does HRT. Genetic factors are believed to be responsible for approximately 5–10% of all breast cancers and are based on a variety of exogenous mutations. It is believed that environmental factors (carcinogens like nicotine), cultural factors (such as age at first pregnancy), and socioeconomic factors (such as dietary habits) all play a role.

Apparently, the genes that predispose to the development of breast cancer, ovarian cancer, and endometrial cancer include five genes of varying dominance: *BRCA1, BRCA2, p-53, HRAS1*, and the *PTEN* gene (Cowden syndrome) (Beckmann et al. 1997).

With regard to the incidence of breast cancer, it is still unclear what percentage of cancer patients actually have a genetic predisposition. Fifteen percent of all cancer carriers and approximately 20–40% of all women diagnosed with breast cancer before 35 years of age develop the disease because of a genetic predisposition. This etiology should definitely be considered in patients under 50 years of age (35% in our own case material), as it is likely that the tumor began to form 5–15 years prior to diagnosis, or between 30 and 45 years of age.

Thus, it does not appear to be true that only breast cancer in first- and second-degree relatives under age 50 can have a genetic cause. This cause may also apply to cancers in women over age 50, albeit to a lesser degree. The younger the patient at the time of the disease, the greater the likelihood of a genetic predisposition.

> **!** We know that certain genes launch cancer cells on their aggressive path. Scientists have broken the genetic code of cancer cells and have discovered how genes suddenly become active when "quiescent" cancer cells become aggressive. The research group led by Todd Golub of the Dana Farber Cancer Institute at Harvard University compared genes in "sleeping" tumors with genes in aggressive, metastasizing tumors. Aided by DNA chip technology, they analyzed thousands of genes from 279 cancer specimens and systematically arranged the DNA fragments on a glass slide. Then they wetted this biochip with a solution containing genetic products from the patient's own cancer cells. The amount of genetic material that binds to the standard DNA of the chip depends on which genes in the cancer cell are active. This binding is then quantified. Using this technique, Shridhar Ramaswamy and Todd Golub were able to identify a characteristic molecular signature that predicted whether a tumor would metastasize in a particular patient (Ramaswamy et al. 2003).

Our case–control study on the link between sports and breast cancer, conducted in a total of 1269 women, supports the notion that genetic risk is probably more important than formerly believed (Beyer 2003) (see p. 17). The case group in our study consisted of 869 women who had been treated for breast cancer, and the control group consisted of 360 athletically active women without breast cancer. The goal of the study was to investigate the possible role of sports activities, especially those involving direct trauma to the breast, in the pathogenesis of breast cancer. The participants were also questioned about a possible family history of breast cancer in grandmothers, mothers, sisters, aunts, or cousins. Thirty-eight percent of the women in the case group had a positive family history of breast cancer, compared with 24% in the control group. This is consistent with epidemiological studies in which 10–30% of breast cancer patients reported a positive family history with at least one affected first-degree relative (Kiechle et al. 2003). Because of this link, all women with a family history of breast cancer *at our institution* are screened at 12-month intervals, whereas women with a negative family history are screened every 18 months. The screening examinations consist of single-view mammograms supplemented by breast ultrasound (see pp. 105 ff, 193).

The genes mainly responsible for familial breast cancer are designated as tumor suppressor genes *BRCA1* (43% of breast or ovarian cancers) and *BRCA2* (10%). These are defective genes that can no longer regulate cell growth because of their mutated form. Located on chromosomes 13 and 17, they are transmitted as a dominant trait, and the sex of the carrier is irrelevant to transmission. It does not matter whether the family history of breast cancer is on the maternal or paternal side. Both lines transmit the same risk to their offspring.

A very complicated analysis is necessary to determine whether or not a mutation is present. When a defective gene is present, it allows unrestricted cellular proliferation to occur as long as the intact gene from the other parent does not prevent it. If that gene is also inactive or damaged (mutated) due to an exogenous insult, loss of heterozygosity will result and the cells will acquire a malignant phenotype.

Based on current statistical data, **carriers of a BRCA1 gene defect** have a > 80% risk of developing predominantly *hormone-receptor-negative breast cancer* by 80 years of age (versus 10% in the normal population). More than 60% of these women are diagnosed before 50 years of age. They also have a 44% risk of developing ovarian cancer by age 70. Additionally, a remarkably high incidence of pancreatic and colon cancers has been documented in the families of these women (Langenbeck 1995).

**Carriers of a BRCA2 mutation** have an increased familial incidence of cancers of the prostate (RR: 4.69), pancreas (RR: 3.51), bile ducts (RR: 4.97), stomach (RR: 2.59), and uterus (RR: 2.38) (Runnebaum et al. 2001). Reportedly, up to 19% of all patients with a *BRCA2* gene mutation have a positive family history of pancreatic cancer (Hahn et al. 2003).

Besides carriers of the above gene mutations, women with the following characteristics are also considered to be **at high cancer risk** and should undergo regular screening examinations starting at 30 (or preferably 25) years of age:

- At least two first-degree relatives with breast cancer or ovarian cancer, one diagnosed before age 50 years
- One first-degree relative with bilateral breast cancer or unilateral breast cancer and ovarian cancer before age 40 years
- One family member who developed unilateral breast cancer by age 30 years
- One family member who developed ovarian cancer by age 40 years
- One family member who developed breast and ovarian cancer at any age
- One family member who developed male breast cancer

Family members may also be referred for genetic counseling (Schmutzler et al. 2002; Wagner 2005).

Based on current estimates, a positive family history is associated with the following risks:

- If two instances of breast cancer and two instances of ovarian cancer have been documented in family members, the risk of developing breast cancer is 91%.
- With two instances of breast cancer in relatives under 50 years of age, the risk of developing breast cancer is 25%.
- With one instance of breast cancer and one of ovarian cancer in relatives under 50 years of age, the risk of developing breast cancer is 10%.

For example, if a 35-year-old healthy woman has a mother who had breast cancer at the same age (35 years), she runs an 11% risk of developing the disease sometime in the next 35 years. If her sister also had breast cancer at that age, her risk increases to 33%. The risk does not increase if a first-degree relative develops breast cancer after age 50 or even if two first-degree relatives develop the disease after age 70 (Langenbeck 1995).

Many breast cancer patients ask whether their children should have genetic testing. In the author's experience, genetic testing is not advisable in most cases. Most women will not consent to a prophylactic bilateral subcutaneous mastectomy or oophorectomy even when a *BRCA1* or *BRCA2* defect has been identified. Many women are also reluctant to begin "prophylactic" antiestrogen therapy while in their reproductive years because of the associated side-

**Table 2.1 Screening program for the early detection of breast and ovarian cancer in women at high risk (modified from Kiechle et al. 2003)**

| | |
|---|---|
| **Breast cancer** | |
| Initial screen | At age 25 years, or 5 years before cancer was detected in a family member, but not before 18 years of age. |
| Palpation | Monthly self-examination as instructed; clinical examination every 6 months. |
| Breast ultrasound | Every 6 months, using a 7.5 MHz or higher-frequency probe. May reduce to once yearly after age 50 years. |
| Mammography | Start at age 30 years (single views are sufficient!); repeat every year if readability is good. |
| Magnetic resonance imaging | Yearly starting at age 25 years. |
| **Ovarian cancer** | |
| • Gynecologic examination and transvaginal ultrasound every 6 months. | |
| • CA-125 serum assay every 6 months. | |

effects (menopausal complaints). Tamoxifen, while considered relatively effective in women under 50 years of age, is not recommended in *BRCA1* carriers. However, every woman should decide for herself, in consultation with her gynecologist, whether antiestrogen therapy is appropriate for her, especially since it can be discontinued at any time and its effects are reversible.

> **!** **Psychological testing should precede genetic testing. The awareness of a genetic predisposition for breast cancer may cause severe anxiety in many women (though it should pass within a few weeks; Kiechle et al. 2003). Not all women can cope with a positive test result.**

More and more, women are asking their doctors about the option of genetic testing. This type of consultation is never neutral, because our personal opinion will always color the advice that we give our patients. Given the complexity of a risk–benefit analysis for an individual woman at risk, we feel that the patient should have more than her doctor's opinion; she should also be referred to a reputable counseling service, which is available at any cancer center. All university hospitals and larger breast centers have counseling offices staffed by personnel from various disciplines who are familiar with the criteria for genetic testing. In all genetic tests, it should be considered that a positive result may lead to employment discrimination or may be used as a basis for raising life- and health-insurance premiums or denying coverage. Additionally, some uncertainties still remain in the interpretation and specific implications of genetic test results.

Special screening programs have been developed for women considered to be at high cancer risk, as illustrated in **Table 2.1**.

As well as family history and the presence of mutated genes, there are several additional parameters that may affect the individual risk of breast cancer:

- Early menarche (before 12 years of age)
- Late menopause (after age 50)
- Nulliparity or late first pregnancy (after age 30)
- Detection of atypical breast cells at biopsy
- Personal prior history of breast- or other cancer
- Age > 60 years

**Fig. 2.2 Age distribution of the whole study population and of breast cancer patients based on data from the authors' own files.**

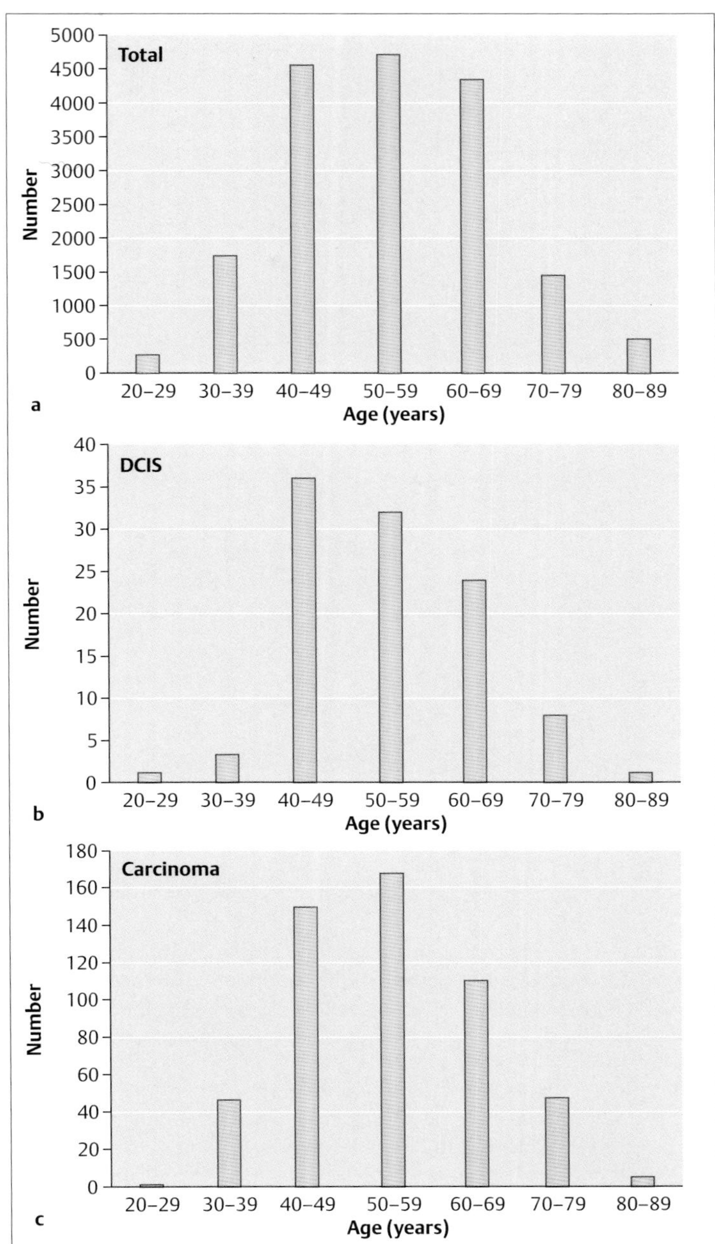


**a** Age distribution of 18 222 patients from the Center for Breast Diagnosis in Esslingen, Germany, during 10 years (1996–2005). The great majority of patients examined were between 40 and 69 years of age.
**b** Age distribution of 105 DCIS patients during these 10 years. 35 % of all DCIS cases occur in women 30–49 years of age.
**c** Age distribution of 525 patients with invasive breast cancer. 38 % of our own patients are less than 50 years of age. Breast cancer is rare from age 20 to 29, but in our statistic, women in the 30–39 age group have the same incidence of breast cancer as women 70–79 years of age (in the USA about 14 % of the patients are younger than 50 years [see p. 43]). **This raises the question**: Why wait until age 50 to begin routine screening when so many cancers and precancerous lesions are already present before 50 years of age? The answer lies in the *costs* and the radiation risk of *two-view mammograms* for younger women.

**Fig. 2.3** **Methods of breast cancer detection and age distribution.**

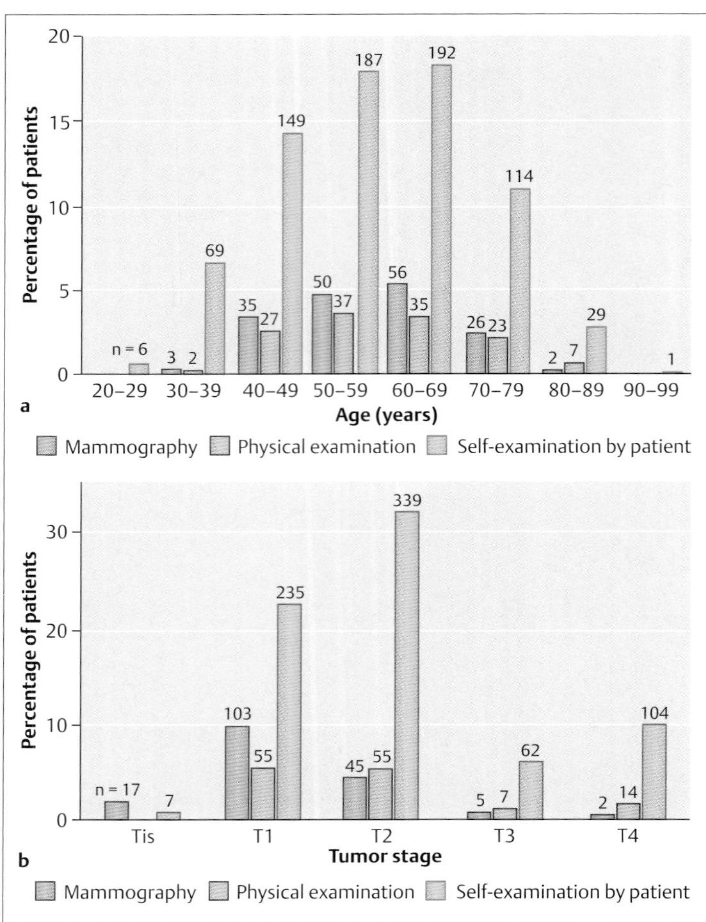


**a** By what tests is breast cancer detected in different age groups, and with what frequency? Comparison of mammography, physical examination by the physician, and self-examination by the patient. We see that tumors are first detected outside of screening by physical examination in all age groups.
**b** What tumor stages are detected by mammography, office examination, and self-examination? In situ carcinomas are the only stages that are detected more frequently by mammography than by self-examination. All other tumor stages are detected by palpation outside of screening (from Schleicher 1995).

To evaluate breast cancer risk in an individual patient, Kaufmann (Frankfurt) and Eiermann (Munich) devised a relatively simple breast cancer risk test and posted it on their website (www.brustkrebsvorbeugen.de). According to their criteria, however, all women over 60 years of age have a high cancer risk. While this is technically correct, it is too superficial for an individual risk assessment.

Although the cancer registry of the German state of Saarland shows that breast cancer is most prevalent between 60 and 85 years of age and least prevalent between 25 and 39 years, the author's own statistics are quite different. In a series of 630 diagnosed cases of breast cancer, 35% were diagnosed under 50 years of age. When precancerous lesions are included, this figure rises to 65% (**Fig. 2.2**).

In cases where a high cancer risk has been confirmed, regular screening examinations should begin at 25 years of age. The young woman should learn **self-examination** in order to develop **breast awareness**. She should keep a careful record of all cyclical changes in her breasts so that she will be able to detect a suspicious mass at the earliest possible stage.

**Fig. 2.4** **Relative risk for *radiation-induced breast cancer at 1 Sv*** ($ERR_{1Sv}$) as a function of age at radiation exposure. The data are from the latest analysis of the Japanese study and are summarized at 5-year intervals (red bar graph) and 10-year (green bar graph) intervals. The function **e**xcess **r**elative **r**isk = $ERR_{1Sv} = 3.6 \exp(-0.0374 \times E)$, where $E$ = age at radiation exposure) was used to curve-fit the date (from Jung 2001). Blue curve shows relationship between age and radiation exposure at 1 Sv.

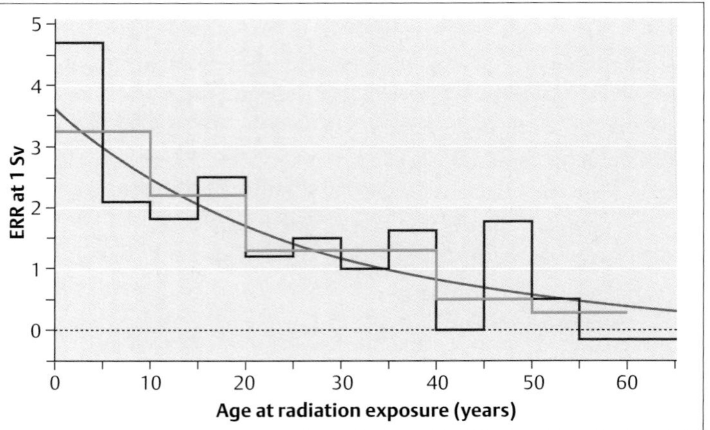


At most, however, only about 10% of women conduct thorough, systematic self-examinations on a regular basis; the rest leave this task to their gynecologists. Unfortunately, the fact that 80% of all cancers, including those in younger women, are first detected by self-examination or office palpation does not mean that women are particularly diligent with self-examination or that self-examination is particularly effective. Nor does it mean that women present for regular screening examinations, although some 60% of state-insured women in Germany do this. The fact that 80% of breast cancers are detected by palpation is due solely to the fact that malignant tumors eventually grow so large that they must become palpable (**Fig. 2.3**) (Schleicher 1995).

Women are being diagnosed with breast cancer at an increasingly young age. They are developing their cancer between 30 and 50 years of age. Breast cancer is still rare in women between 20 and 30 years of age, although early cancers (DCIS) are becoming more common in that age group (**Fig. 2.2 c**). The youngest of the author's patients to be diagnosed with breast cancer was only 18 years old—an extreme rarity (see **Fig. 5.65**). This young woman had no precancerous disease, just a locally advanced tumor. She did not have a family history of breast cancer.

***Tip***

**Single-view mammography (a good oblique view!) is sufficient for excluding microcalcifications in young women. Noncalcifying tumors in young women can be detected earlier with high-resolution ultrasound and/or MRI than by mammography.**

**Single-view mammograms** should be obtained in women *at high risk*. The examination should be scheduled every 2 years initially (beginning at age 25), then once a year after age 30, in each case supplementing the mammograms with breast ultrasound (every 6 months). MRI should also be done once a year or every other year, depending on payor policies and restrictions, and should be scheduled between the other screenings (see **Table 2.1**, p. 15).

MRI is especially rewarding in younger women because of their radiodense parenchyma (Kuhl et al. 2000) and should be done at the end of the first half of the menstrual cycle (7th to 12th day of the cycle) every 1–2 years, depending on the individual risk (see p. 14).

Single-view mammography reduces the potential radiation risk (30–50% lower dose, distributed over a lifetime), which is a more serious threat to younger women than to older women (**Fig. 2.4**) (Jung 2001). Breast compression causes significant discomfort for many women, and single-view mammograms are easier to tolerate since each breast is compressed only once.

Frankenberg et al. (1996) published figures indicating that women with a mutation in one of the breast cancer genes, *BRCA1* or *BRCA2*, have a 10 million times higher radiation risk than other women. Leading radiation biologists (for example Jung 1997) dispute the accuracy of this claim. The possibility of a higher radiation risk based on current data (which are still incomplete) does not justify withholding a rigorous screening program, including mammograms, from women with a known *BRCA gene mutation*. Studies by Dörk et al. (2002) are of interest in this regard. According to these authors, previously known genetic predispositions to breast cancer show an interesting correlation between the repair of radiation-induced chromosome breaks and an increased breast cancer risk. Epidemiological studies suggest that many cases of breast cancer are not based on a single gene but have a polygenic cause. If 40% of all breast cancer patients have increased cellular radiosensitivity, it is likely that additional mutations, possibly associated with a moderate cancer risk, may be found in other genes concerned with DNA repair. Heredity and environment do not operate independently of each another. While carriers of a genetic predisposition may not manifest increased toxicity during radiation therapy, it is possible that this therapy may induce clinically silent chromosome changes in particularly sensitive individuals—changes that could initiate a malignancy following a latent period of many years. On the other hand, it is hoped that the tumor cells of affected carriers are exceptionally sensitive to local radiation therapy. There is already initial evidence of a reduced recurrence rate after radiation therapy in breast cancer patients with an ATM (Ataxia Telangiectasia Mutation) gene mutation.

While it is possible that a common genetic disposition may exist for breast cancer and radiosensitivity, a 10 million times higher radiation risk seems, to put it mildly, a slight exaggeration. In any event, it is wise to keep radiation exposure to a minimum in young patients and especially in gene carriers (single-view mammography, ultrasound, MRI).

## Case–Control Study on Sports and Breast Cancer

There is no question that large studies are necessary to assess the risks posed by contraceptive and hormone-replacement therapies. Nonetheless, studies in smaller case numbers often yield results that contradict larger studies but are not necessarily false.

For completeness, we shall review the most important anamnestic data from a study on sports and breast cancer that was conducted by the author and his colleagues (Beyer 2004).

The goal of our case–control study was to investigate the general role of accidental or sports-related trauma in the pathogenesis of breast cancer. The study also addresses the question whether "compression trauma" from mammography has causal significance in breast cancer, as many patients believe. A total of 1269 women participated in the study, and the results are summarized below (see also **Figs. 2.5, 2.6**):

- Regular athletic activity protects against breast cancer.
- Women who engage in regular athletic activity at least one hour per week develop breast cancer an average of 4 years later than women who have never been active in sports.
- Women who engage in sports only sporadically (once a month or seasonally) have only a 1-year advantage over women who do not.
- There is no evidence of an increased breast cancer risk in women who engage in sports involving repetitive trauma to the breast (e.g., handball, tennis, judo, boxing, wrestling).
- Women who are not athletically active have a 1.35 times higher risk of developing breast cancer than female athletes who have sustained violent trauma to the breast.

**Fig. 2.5 Likelihood of developing breast cancer after participation in sports** involving trauma to the breast (blue) compared with other sports activities (red).

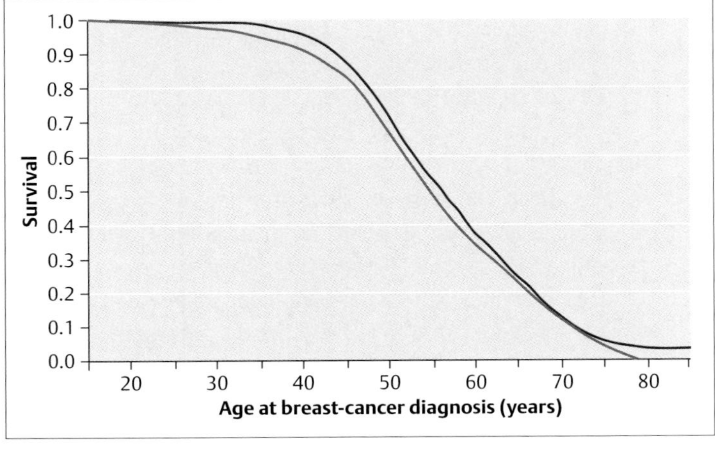


**Fig. 2.6 Likelihood of developing breast cancer in regular sports activities,** including sports involving trauma to the breast (blue), compared with sporadic sports activity or no activity (red).

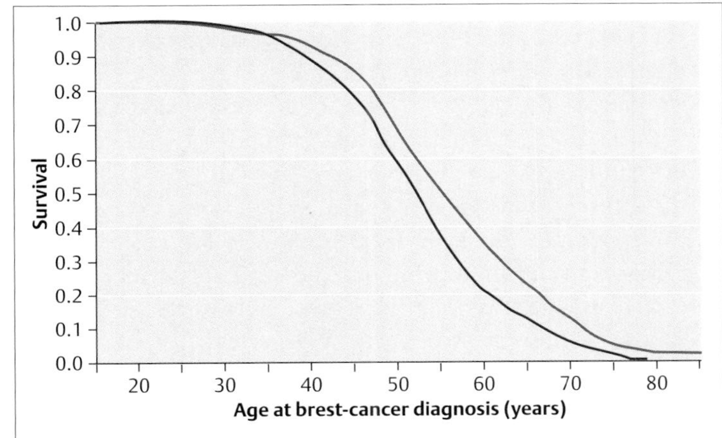

- Based on our results, there should be no risk associated with a uniform force of 4–14 kilopond (kp) applied to the breast in compression mammography. Extreme compression with prolonged pain should definitely be avoided, however. **Even mammograms with a light to medium exposure level are still readable!**
- There appears to be a certain risk associated with a single episode of severe sports-related or non-sports-related trauma to the breast. If the trauma is severe enough to cause protracted pain, we cannot rule out a certain increase in risk.

Regular athletic activity, regardless of whether it involves contact with the breast, is definitely effective in the prevention of breast cancer. On the other hand, the possibility of significant accidental trauma to the breast exists in every sport, as it does in ordinary life. For the participants in this study, these accidents were isolated and at times very painful incidents that consisted mainly of horseback riding accidents (falls or bite injuries), skiing accidents involving blows from ski poles or chest contusions, bicycle accidents (handlebar injuries to the chest), falls during rock concerts, thoracic injuries caused by falls during mountain hikes, automobile seatbelt injuries, backpack strap injuries, and sledding injuries. Physical-education instructors reported impact trauma while spotting athletes, and some developed hematomas caused by a high-energy ball impact. Our results indicate that a single, severe traumatic event was associated with a statistically significant ($p = 0.0224$) increase in breast cancer risk: A single severe trauma may, along with many other factors, constitute an additional risk factor. It should be noted that biopsy also represents a severe trauma to the breast, although it does not lead to future breast cancer. Like other "traumatic events," breast biopsy should be kept to a minimum.

Thus, severe trauma to the female breast during competitive sports or even during sexual activity should be avoided. Women who have experienced an isolated incident of severe and painful breast trauma should immediately be referred for regular screening examinations (yearly single-view mammograms plus ultrasound for at least 5 years).

**Fig. 2.7 Sports and Breast Cancer Study:** hormone replacement therapy (HRT) and oral contraceptives in breast cancer patients.

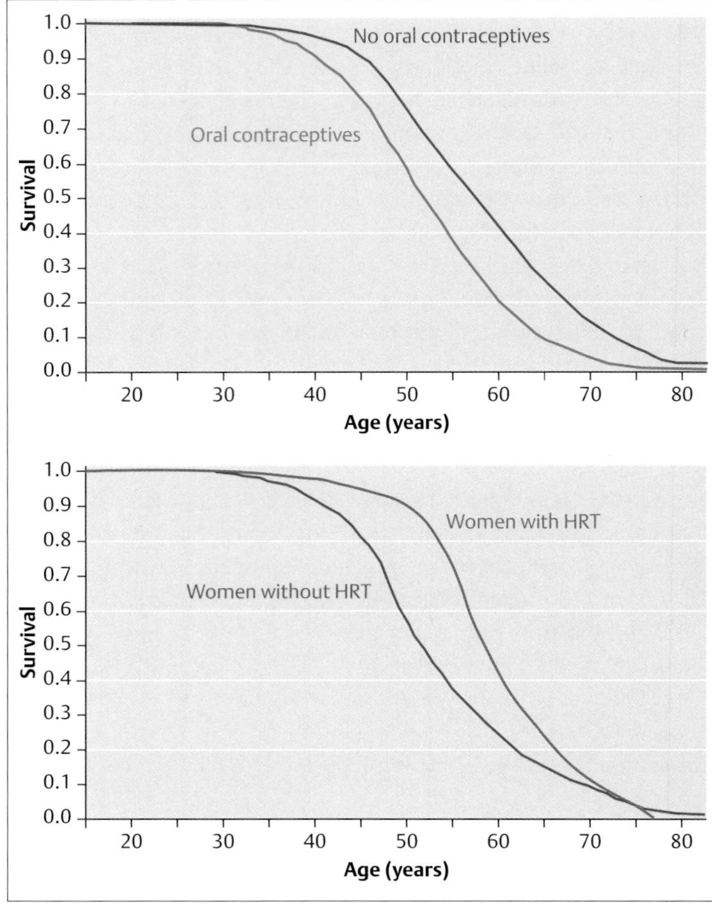


Women on hormonal contraception develop breast cancer approximately 5 years earlier than women who do not take the pill. Women who receive HRT during menopause develop breast cancer approximately 7 years later than women not on HRT.

Further results of the study can be summarized as follows:

- Contrary to reports in the literature, **smoking** was found to be a significant risk factor. Smokers developed breast cancer an average of 5 years earlier than nonsmokers. **Alcohol consumption**, on the other hand, did not appear to be a significant risk factor based on our results. In interpreting our results, however, it should be considered that some breast cancer patients may well have curtailed or eliminated their alcohol intake after they had been diagnosed with the disease.
- Women in the breast cancer group took **oral contraceptives** less often than women in the control group (53% vs. 69%;). They began taking "the pill" at 27 years of age on average, compared with about 22 years in the control group. The average duration of contraceptive use was the same in both groups. Based on these results, the study concluded that women who used oral contraceptives developed breast cancer an average of 5 years earlier than women who did not. This suggests that oral contraceptive use is a significant risk factor for breast cancer. This is in contrast to the opinion of Hesch (1997), see pp. 7 ff, 10.
- With regard to **HRT**, our study yielded different results from the 2004 studies discussed earlier (see p. 11). Twenty-three percent of the cancer patients were on HRT for an average of 7.3 years, while 31% of women in the control group received the therapy for 8.2 years. Women who took hormones during menopause developed breast cancer an average of 7 years later than those who did not (**Fig. 2.7**). Moreover, the participants with breast cancer nursed their children significantly less often and for shorter periods than women in the control group.
- Almost half (48%) of the participants in our cancer group offered a **subjective explanation for their disease**. They mostly described emotional strain and stressful situations in their family lives, especially relating to marital problems, unreconciled separations, death or serious illness of family members, and depression. Other explanations included stress and overwork on the job, loss of employment, and physical and emotional exhaustion relating to the dual burden of a family and a career. These stress factors play an important role in the psychosocial management of patients undergoing rehabilitation and aftercare. It is still unclear whether these types of stressful situations have any etiologic relevance to breast cancer. The many studies published on this topic often lack adequate controls. In our study as well, only women with breast cancer were asked to state other possible reasons for their disease. As a result, we do not know how many women from the control group were exposed to similar stressful situations.

Incidentally, remarkably little information has been published on the link between sports and breast cancer in women.

## Summary

In conclusion, we can offer the following answers, with modifications, to our patients' questions.

- Women who experience many menstrual cycles during their reproductive years (approximately 400) have a higher risk of breast cancer than those who have only about 50 cycles.
- Pregnancy at a young age may reduce the risk of breast cancer because the breast lobules mature earlier and become invulnerable to mutagenic insults. So far, surveys of our own patients (perhaps since today a too small number) have not confirmed the protective effect of early pregnancy.
- Multiple pregnancies and prolonged nursing (6–9 months) are thought to reduce the number of menstrual cycles and shorten the proliferative periods in the second half of the menstrual cycle in which cells are vulnerable to damage from estrogens and/or gestins as well as harmful endogenous and exogenous agents.
- On the basis of our research, hormone replacement therapy protects against breast cancer in postmenopausal or oophorectomized women (Beyer 2004). This contradicts larger studies (WHI/MWS) that were discontinued after 1.5 to 3 years—too early, as current evidence appears to indicate that it may be that HRT in perimenopausal women stimulates the growth of hormone-receptor-positive cancers and preempts the physiologic apoptosis of tumors that would otherwise occur during menopause.
- Reanalysis of the WHI and MWS studies suggests that HRT with estrogen-alone therapy reduces the risk of breast cancer developing to about 30% against women without any HRT. Estrogen sometimes reduces the density of breast tissue in postmenopausal women. The lower the density, the more reduced is the proliferation of TDLU, and the more reduced is the breast cancer risk.
- Postmenopausal women with combined estrogen/gestin therapy for longer than 5 years had a 30–45% higher incidence of breast cancer. Estrogen-only therapy seems to have a protective effect (WHI 2006).
- Postmenopausal gestins especially seem to enhance the density of breast tissue, and simultaneously the risk of lobular breast cancer, which is may be overlooked at mammography and is better detected by ultrasound and MRI.
- Premenopausal gestins seems to have a protective function for the breast tissue and reduce the number of complaints (mastodynia, premenstrual syndrome, etc.).
- Genetic factors contribute greatly to the risk of breast cancer and are probably more important than formerly believed.
- Sports involving repetitive trauma to the breast are more protective than harmful. On the other hand, isolated severe traumatic events causing prolonged pain may constitute an additional risk factor. This suggests that open and percutaneous breast biopsies should be kept to a minimum.
- Women who are considered at risk or at high risk for breast cancer should begin regular screening examinations at age 25 years whenever possible. For high-risk groups, we recommend *single-view mammograms* supplemented by *high-resolution breast ultrasound* (11–13 MHz) and *magnetic resonance imaging.* Additionally, women who have experienced a single episode of severe breast trauma should also be referred for regular screening for about 5 years.
- Our own data indicate that surgical procedures on the breast—ultimately the most severe trauma to the breast parenchyma—do not increase the long-term risk of breast cancer.
- There is no risk of induction of breast cancer, even in younger women, by gentle, graded compression during mammography—especially when mammographic exposures are limited to single views.
- The pressure normally used in compression mammography does not cause breast cancer. Extreme force causing prolonged pain should be avoided.

# 3 Prognostic Factors

## Growth Rate, Tumor Size, Lymph Node Involvement, and Prognosis

In recent decades, the treatment options for breast cancer have been more vigorously debated and more rigorously analyzed than for any other type of tumor. Despite remarkable successes, however, a serious hurdle remains: Once distant hematogenous metastasis has occurred, a definitive cure is no longer possible unless adjuvant therapies (hormone therapy, chemotherapy, etc.) can destroy the disseminated cancer cells or inactivate them so that they cannot metastasize further.

> **!** **A significant improvement in cure rates can be achieved only by detecting the disease at an earlier stage.**

By the time clinical symptoms appear, 60% of patients have already developed axillary lymph node metastases. This percentage increases over time:

- 70% after 12 months
- 73% after 24 months
- 74% after 36 months (Park and Lees 1951).

Generally (though exceptions are possible), the metastasis proceeds relative slowly.

Tumors that measure approximately 1 cm have already metastasized to the axillary lymph nodes in approximately 30% of cases. When the tumor measures 5 cm, axillary metastases are present in 80% of cases. When clinical symptoms begin to appear, the average tumor diameter is 3 cm. The tumor gradually enlarges over time, measuring

- 3.4 cm after an additional 12 months
- 3.8 cm after 24 months
- 4.2 cm after 36 months

While Park and Lees (1951) state that tumors grow at a rate of only about 0.4 cm per year of nontreatment, Richards (1948) estimates that tumors with a moderate growth rate enlarge by approximately 1 cm every 6 months. How quickly a nodule enlarges depends on its individual growth rate, called the tumor doubling time. Von Fournier et al. (1980) made a detailed analysis of tumor growth rates based on mammographic progression.

The growth rate of a tumor is affected by its cellularity, local aggressiveness (G1 to G3), rate of mitosis, hormonal dependency, and host defense mechanisms. In their final stages, some tumors fairly "explode" and grow very swiftly through unrestricted mitosis. This phenomenon is particularly common in very cellular tumors. These final growth spurts are more conspicuous on palpation than in diagnostic images. The annual growth rate from 3–4 cm reported by Park and Lees (1951) is true of hypocellular, well-differentiated G1 tumors but not for hypercellular, undifferentiated malignancies that have a volume doubling time of 40–100 days. The rate of 1 cm every 6 months described by Richards (1948) applies mainly to G2 and G3 tumors.

The **grading** system used by pathologists (see p. 74) describes a tumor at the time of its detection. But it says nothing about the time preceding its detection—whether, for example, the tumor was always a G3 lesion or whether it progressed from a G1 to a G2 and then a G3. All formulas for predicting tumor growth rate are hypothetical. It is surprising how long tumors can grow in the breast before they metastasize to the axilla or other sites in the body (see **Fig. 5.128**, p. 260).

### Tumor Doubling Time

The tumor doubling time (volume doubling) ranges from 1869 days (approximately 5 years) for less aggressive, very slow-growing tumors (G1) to 44 days for fast-growing aggressive lesions (G3) (**Table 3.1**). The average doubling time is 212 days. At that rate, a tumor takes an average of about 4 years to enlarge from 2 mm to 10 mm and approximately 20 years to develop from a single cell to a 2 cm mass. In light of this information, the results of the most recent breast cancer studies (Million Women Study, MWS; Women's Health Initiative, WHI) are surprising. These studies were discontinued after 1–3 years because it appeared that too many malignancies were developing in response to hormone replacement therapy.

A malignant tumor 1 cm in diameter contains approximately 17 million cells (**Fig. 3.1**). Apparently it takes an average of 8–10 years for that many cells to be produced. Rapidly growing tumors double their volume within one year. But a cancerous nodule 2 mm in diameter cannot be reliably demonstrated or detected with an

**Table 3.1 Volume doubling times for G1 to G3 tumors** (modified from von Fournier et al. 1980)

| Tumor growth | Tumor doubling time (days) | Percentage of all tumors | Time needed for the tumor to reach 1 cm (years) |
|---|---|---|---|
| Rapid (G3) | < 150 | 28 | 10 |
| Moderately rapid (G2) | 150–300 | 39 | 15 |
| Slow (G1) | > 300 | 33 | 20 |

**Fig. 3.1 Relationship between growth, metastasis, and detectability of breast cancer** (from Krokowski 1964).

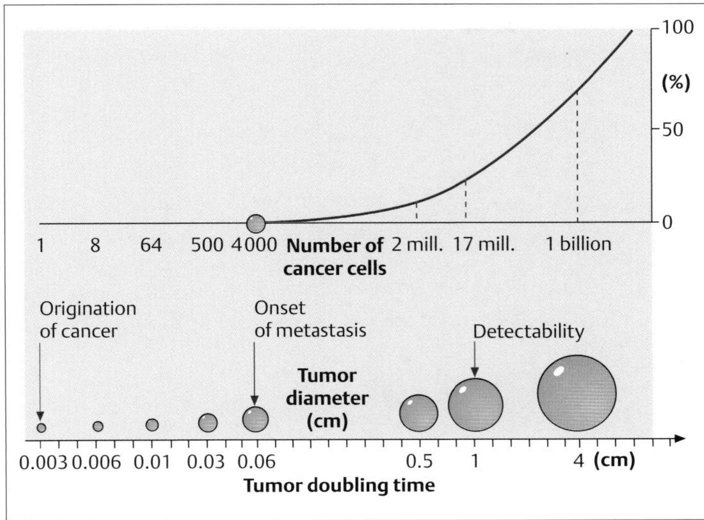


imaging procedure; the minimum detectable lesion size is 4 mm. A radiologically occult nodule 2 mm in diameter grows to approximately 4 mm in one year, presumably after undergoing two doubling phases. A tumor at this stage can be detected with high-resolution ultrasound, regardless of the thickness of the breast parenchyma or the age of the patient. A lesion as small as 3–4 mm can be detected mammographically if it is associated with visible microcalcifications or is located in a fatty area of the affected breast.

Reports of fast-growing tumors that appear "out of nowhere" and reach a size of 2–3 cm within a few weeks or months after medical examination are not realistic. Generally these lesions are cancer nodules that were simply missed in previous examinations. It is reasonable to estimate that a 2 cm cancer nodule growing at an average rate is approximately 15–20 years old (von Fournier et al. 1980).

With an average tumor doubling time of 212 days, most breast cancers are likely to reach an invasive stage when the patient is between 30 and 40 years of age. They will usually be detected as 1–2 cm breast nodules in the 50- to 60-year-old patient by mammography, ultrasound, and/or physical examination.

> **!** **Once a tumor reaches a diameter of approximately 0.6 mm, it is already able to metastasize (Krokowski 1964) (Fig. 3.1).**

In the near future, we may be able to determine through genetic testing which tumors have significant metastatic potential and which do not (see p. 14).

## Lymph Node Involvement, Tumor Size, and Survival Time

> ***Tip***
>
> Lymph node status is currently the most important indicator for the staging of breast cancer and the selection of treatment modalities.

It should be noted, however, that 30% of all N0 cancers metastasize and that cancer cells are often overlooked in the lymph nodes or enter the bloodstream directly without traversing the lymph nodes. As a result, lymph node status is a relatively uncertain prognostic indicator.

Alan Ashworth of Duke University Medical Center in North Carolina developed a technique for investigating the activity of 50–100 key genes. These genes have a different activity profile in normal cells from that do in cancer cells. In addition, different types of breast cancer have different gene activity profiles. This makes it possible to predict how a tumor will behave, i.e., whether it will grow slowly without metastasizing or whether it will be an aggressive, fast-growing cancer with very strong metastatic potential. The researchers tested their methods in women who had no signs of lymph node metastasis. By analyzing the **gene activity profiles**, they could predict with 90% accuracy whether a cancer would recur within 3 years. The researchers believe their results to be an important step toward **personalized medicine**, in which treatment is tailored to the individual course of a patient's illness. Every woman should be able to assess her own personal risk based on her unique genetic profile. Guided by this approach, treatment could be made more selective and specific than in previous years, significantly improving the prospects for a cure. Aggressive therapies could be avoided in patients who would still be selected today for an aggressive adjuvant therapy based on conventional profiling criteria.

> **!** **Even when breast cancer is detected at a very early stage by screening, there is no guarantee that the patient can be cured.**

Although lymph node status is a relatively uncertain prognostic factor, it is still the only factor that can determine how far a tumor has advanced with a reasonable degree of confidence. Lymph node status has become an important tool in deciding how aggressively the disease should be treated. Thus, it was extremely common in past years to remove the axillary lymph nodes routinely in breast cancer operations. An increasingly conservative approach has been taken to axillary lymphadenectomy, however, as this procedure is associated with high morbidity (10%) and many women still suffer from its after-effects, which range from arm edema to neurogenic disorders (see **Fig. 5.159**).

The relationship between 5-year survival rate, tumor size, and extent of axillary involvement is summarized in **Table 3.2**.

The incidence of axillary lymph node metastasis rises by 5–10% per year following the onset of clinical manifestations in the breast. Assuming a constant growth rate, the lymph nodes are still mostly clear 6–12 years before a *clinical* diagnosis is made.

Normally, then, it takes several years for a tumor to produce clinical manifestations, and a relatively long time is needed for the tumor to undergo axillary or retrosternal metastasis.

> **!** **While breast cancers detected by their *clinical* manifestations have an average diameter of 2 cm, tumors detected by screening average 1 cm and have only a 30% rate of axillary involvement versus 60% with clinically detected tumors and interval cancers. The extent of axillary metastasis is far more important than tumor size in assessing the chance for a cure.**

**Sentinel lymph node identification**, in which the lymph node draining the tumor (the "sentinel node") is analyzed, selectively removed and histologically examined (see p. 307), is likely to significantly reduce morbidity and make the analysis of lymph node status more precise. This is because tumors located in the inner breast quadrants do not always metastasize to the axilla; they may spread to retrosternal and infraclavicular nodes (see **Fig. 5.186**). This may partially account for the 30% incidence of distant metastasis that occurs despite a negative lymph node status.

Bone marrow biopsies are increasingly being used for disease staging because tumor cells are detectable in bone marrow at an early stage. Lymph node analysis, "genetic fingerprinting" (of the tumor), and the sentinel lymph node procedure are likely to make the treatment of breast cancer more individualized, sparing some women the ordeal of undergoing aggressive postoperative treatments with their added morbidity (see **Fig. 1.2**). It should also be noted that tumor protease determination can predict whether adjuvant chemotherapy would be beneficial in any given case (Harbeck 2002).

The **10-year cure rate** is approximately 80% in patients who have clear axillary lymph nodes. It is approximately 70% in patients with three affected lymph nodes and falls to approximately 15% in patients with more than four positive axillary nodes (Carter et al. 1989) (**Table 3.2**). Both lymph node status and tumor grade (see p. 76) have a crucial bearing on 5- and 10-year survival rates. The lower the tumor grade (G1–G3), the better the prognosis in terms of cure rates and survival (**Table 3.3**).

The average length of survival in women with untreated breast cancer was in earlier time 3–4 years after onset of symptoms. In a study by Daland (1927) in 100 patients with untreated breast cancer, 40% of the women were still alive at 3 years and 22% were still alive at 5 years. The average survival time from symptom onset to death was 40 months. It should be added, however, that in the past two decades breast cancer has become a less aggressive disease worldwide, and so these numbers do not accurately reflect present-day reality.

Today we have achieved an 85% 10-year cure rate for small tumors that are detected at screening, have not undergone nodal metastasis, and are managed with up-to-date treatment modalities and adjunctive systemic therapies. Approximately 80% of these women undergo breast-conserving surgery. In cases that require mastectomy (due to tumor spread or multicentric disease), various **esthetic breast reconstruction** options are available that can yield excellent results (**Figs. 1.2** and **5.82**, p. 188 ff). We may credit this in part to the worldwide success of the breast cancer movement.

When distant metastases occur, curative treatment is no longer a realistic goal, although palliative measures can still be provided to prolong the patient's survival and improve her quality of life.

**Table 3.2 Five-year survival rates as a function of tumor size and lymph node status in 24 740 women with breast cancer** (from Carter et al. 1989)

| Lymph node status | n | Relative survival rate (%) |
|---|---|---|
| **Tumor size < 2.0 cm** | | |
| Total | 8319 | 91.3 |
| Negative lymph nodes | 5728 | 96.3 |
| 1–3 positive lymph nodes | 1767 | 87.4 |
| 4 or more positive lymph nodes | 824 | 66.0 |
| **Tumor size 2–5 cm** | | |
| Total | 13 723 | 79.8 |
| Negative lymph nodes | 6927 | 89.4 |
| 1–3 positive lymph nodes | 3622 | 79.9 |
| 4 or more positive lymph nodes | 3174 | 58.7 |
| **Tumor size > 5 cm** | | |
| Total | 2698 | 62.7 |
| Negative lymph nodes | 809 | 82.2 |
| 1–3 positive lymph nodes | 630 | 73.0 |
| 4 or more positive lymph nodes | 1259 | 45.5 |

**Table 3.3 Relative 5- and 10-year breast cancer survival rates (in %) according to UICC stage and tumor grade (G1/G2 or G3)**, based on data from the Münster Cancer Registry for the period 2002–2004 (invasive tumors only) (with courtesy of Epidemiologisches Krebsregister NRW GMbH, Germany, Klaus Kraywinkel)

| UICC stage | Relative 5-year survival rate | | Relative 10-year survival rate | |
|---|---|---|---|---|
| | G1/G2 | G3 | G1/G2 | G3 |
| I | 98.0 | 93.2 | 97.0 | 88.5 |
| IIA | 95.3 | 88.4 | 83.8 | 68.8 |
| IIB | 85.6 | 74.6 | 64.0 | 48.3 |
| III | 76.1 | 57.8 | 44.8 | 45.2 |
| IV | 29.9 | 10.4 | 15.4 | 2.4 |
| Unknown | 88.0 | 72.8 | 84.4 | 66.4 |
| Overall | 89.9 | 71.9 | 79.3 | 57.7 |

# 4 Macroanatomy, Histology, Radiography, and Ultrasound

## Anatomy of the Breast: Lobes, Lobules, and the Terminal Duct Lobular Unit (TDLU)

The breast parenchyma is divided into 12–15 lobes that are arranged radially within the breast. Their lactiferous ducts open on the nipple. The longest and broadest lobes are located in the upper outer quadrant of the breast. The longest lobe is directed toward the axillary recess; it may extend into the axilla and terminate in heterotopic glandular tissue (**Fig. 4.1 a**).

The lobe is the physiologic unit of the breast parenchyma. The multiple lobes present in the breast cannot be differentiated from one another during adolescence or during the reproductive years (**Fig. 4.1 b**). Only the main ducts can be identified, especially in the periareolar region. The mammary lobes are subdivided into lobules, which are most abundant in the peripheral portion of the lobe during each phase of life (see **Figs. 5.63 c, 5.66 d**). As a result, the majority of lobular neoplasms develop in that region. Tumors detected in that area by screening are called "no man's land" cancers, although the origin of this term is uncertain (see **Fig. 4.12**).

After menopause, the mammary lobules atrophy back from the periphery of the breast toward the nipple (opposite to their sequence of development in young breasts). The main ducts remain intact for life, marking the original extent of the mammary lobes even after the lobes have atrophied.

## Terminal Duct Lobular Unit: Microradiography, Mammography, and Sonography

The lobules contain the intralobular terminal ducts and the terminal ductules, also called acini (**Figs. 4.2, 4.3**). The space between the terminal duct and acini is occupied by loose ***intra*lobular stroma**, which proliferates in response to hormones, may swell with mucoid material, and regresses with aging. While this intralobular stroma is located *inside* and immediately around the lobules, tough ***inter*lobular stroma** is located *between* the lobules and is not responsive to hormonal stimulation. The lobules, the intra- and perilobular stroma, and the interlobular stroma together comprise a functional unit called "mastion" (Rahn 1972), meaning the **terminal duct lobular unit (TDLU)**. The importance of the TDLU is summarized below.

- Ozzello (1970) showed by electron microscopy that the boundary zone between the epithelium and stroma is occupied by a functional unit consisting of epithelial and myoepithelial cell membranes, the intercellular spaces, the lamina lucida, the basement membrane, fibrillated connective tissue, and a surrounding fibroblastic layer. Active metabolic exchange takes place between the blood vessels and epithelium in this area. It appears that any disturbance of this transport function leads to fibrosis and calcifications due to a change in mucopolysaccharide content (see **Fig. 5.149 i, j**, p. 395).
- The lobules of the breast are rarely visible on x-ray films. Instead, the complete TDLU and the surrounding interlobular stroma usually appear mammographically as opacities of varying size. The TDLU is easier to identify in breasts that contain smaller amounts of supportive tissue. The TDLU cannot be differentiated in cases where the *inter*lobular stroma is confluent between adjacent TDLUs (**Fig. 4.4 a, e**).
- The TDLU appears at **ultrasound** as a small, hypoechoic zone with smooth margins (**Fig. 4.3 c**). The *intra*lobular stroma has the same echogenicity as the lobular acini and cannot be differentiated from them. If heavy stromal proliferation has occurred along the main ducts, it may resemble glandular tissue proliferation (e.g., adenosis) at ultrasound. This phenomenon can be distinguished from lobular proliferation, however, by noting that the ducts within the intralobular stroma appear as fine *echogenic* lines (**Fig. 4.5**). This is opposite to the pattern normally seen, in which the ducts have a hypoechoic (dark) appearance (see **Fig. 4.13c**) due to the presence of watery fluid inside the ducts.
- The TDLU appears sonographically as a hypoechoic zone that contrasts sharply with the hyperechoic interlobular stroma of the breast. The TDLU derives its **blood supply** from branches of the internal mammary artery and intercostal arteries (3–7). The outer quadrants of the breast are supplied by the lateral thoracic artery. These large vessels are interconnected by numerous anastomoses. Each TDLU is supplied by its own blood vessel and has its own nerve supply (**Fig. 4.6**). Metabolic exchange is carried out through these blood vessels. They also create a pathway by which endogenous and exogenous toxins can reach the TDLU, damaging the immature acini and possibly inducing cellular mutations (see p. 9).

Each TDLU contains a main duct, to which the lobules are connected almost at right angles (see **Fig. 2.1, Figs. 4.7–4.10, Fig. 4.13**). As a result, high-resolution ultrasound (12–18 MHz) can define the TDLU and its main duct only when the transducer is directed radially to the nipple. In practice, the probe must be slightly rotated in the vertical and radial axis to delineate the ducts. It should be added that the ducts do not always follow a direct centripetal path from the periphery of the breast to the nipple. Duct tortuosity is common, especially at the retroareolar level.

The anatomical relationships of the lobes, ducts, and lobules and their involvement by ductal and lobular carcinoma are vividly depicted in the drawings by Dabelow and Bässler (**Figs. 4.11, 4.12**).

**Figures 4.10** and **5.69 b, f** show microradiographs of TDLUs.

**Fig. 4.1 Diagram of the terminal duct lobular unit (TDLU).** The mammary lobes are 12 to 15 in number and are the basic anatomical unit of the breast. Viewed from the front, they display a radial arrangement in which the ducts converge toward the nipple (modified from Teboul and Halliwell 1995).

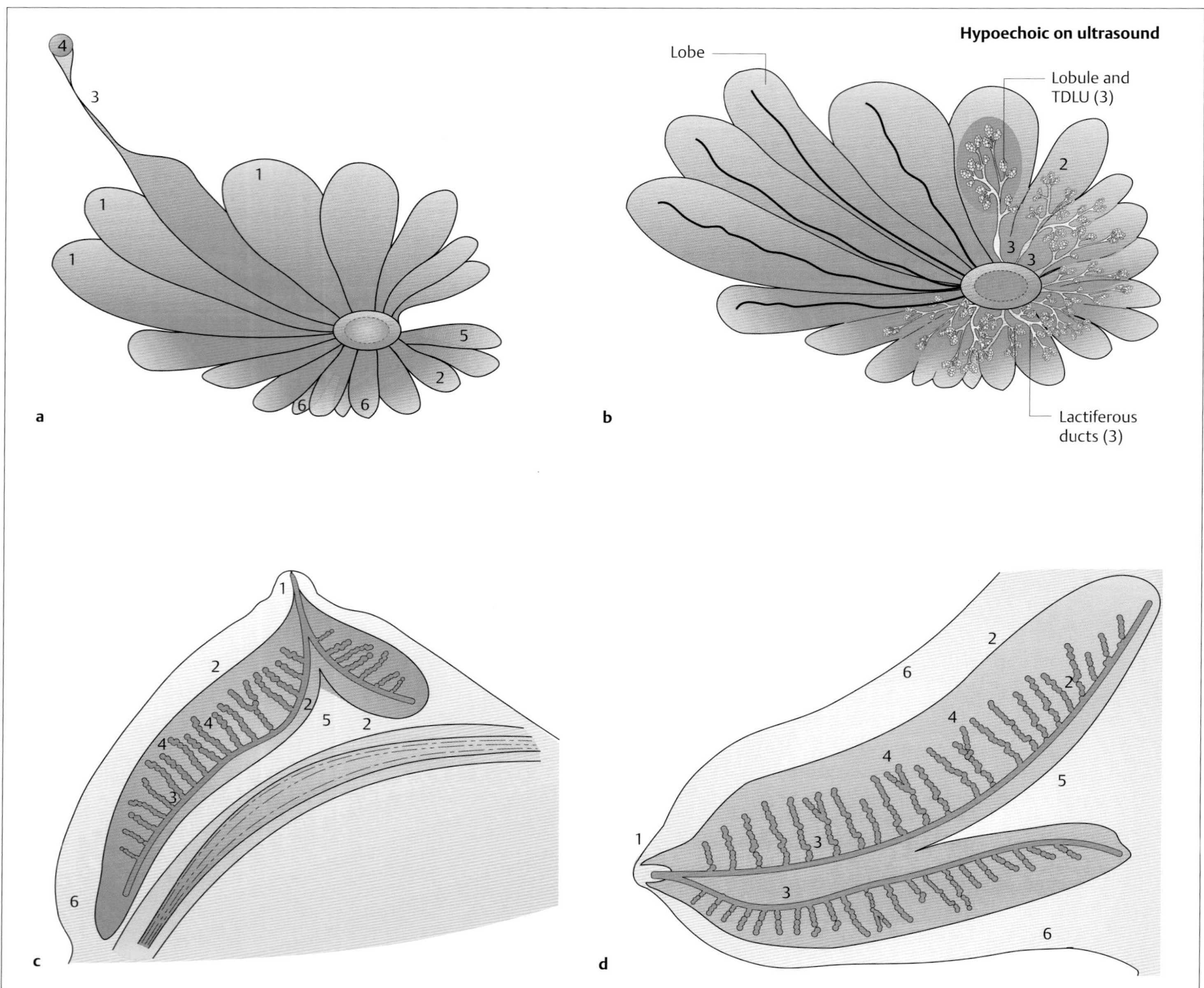


**a** The ducts in the upper outer quadrant of the breast (1) are larger than in the inner quadrant. A long duct may extend to the axilla (3) and communicate with heterotopic glandular tissue (4). Thus, it is important in some cases to trace the ducts back to the periphery when the breast is examined with ultrasound. The lobes in the upper inner quadrant (5) are easily missed and appear to be the first lobes to atrophy with aging. Some lobes overlap one another, especially in the lower quadrants (2, 6).
**b** The lobes form an overlapping arrangement that is particularly dense in the lateral quadrants, where they cannot be distinguished from one another, especially in the young breast. They undergo a progressive involution from the periphery of the breast toward the nipple. The ducts maintain their original arrangement for life.

**c, d** The lobes (4) are the physiologic unit of the breast parenchyma. Viewed in three dimensions, they form a cone that is centered on the lactiferous duct (3) and around which the lobules and TDLUs (2) are arranged at right angles. The duct is backed by fatty tissue (5). The individual lobes (4) converge toward the areola and open into the nipple (1). The superficial portions of the lobes are separated from the skin by fat (6). The lobes are traversed by the main lactiferous ducts (3), which run almost through the center of each lobe from the nipple (1) toward the periphery. Normally the lobules show a "brush border" arrangement that is directed toward the skin. The microanatomy of the breast parenchyma is explored more fully in **Fig. 5.69 c**, p. 170.

**Fig. 4.2 Terminal duct lobular unit (TDLU).**

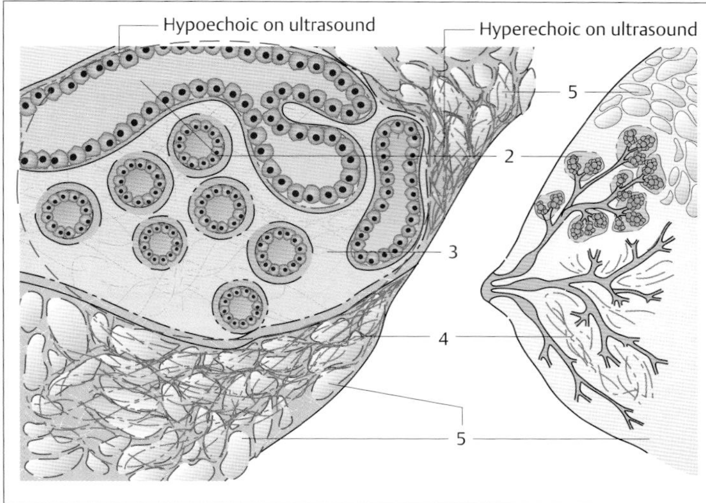


**a** Diagrammatic representation of the terminal duct lobular unit (TDLU). The lobules contain the terminal ducts and their associated acini (2), which are hypoechoic on ultrasound. The acini are embedded in a loose intralobular stroma (3) which also appears *hypo*echoic on ultrasound and may proliferate in response to hormones and regresses with aging. While *intra*lobular stroma is located within the lobules and is hypoechoic, the space between the lobules is occupied by tough *inter*lobular stroma (4), which appears *hyper*echoic at ultrasound, and fatty tissue, neither of which is responsive to hormones. The acini and *intra*lobular stroma have the same acoustic characteristics and are indistinguishable from each other by ultrasound.

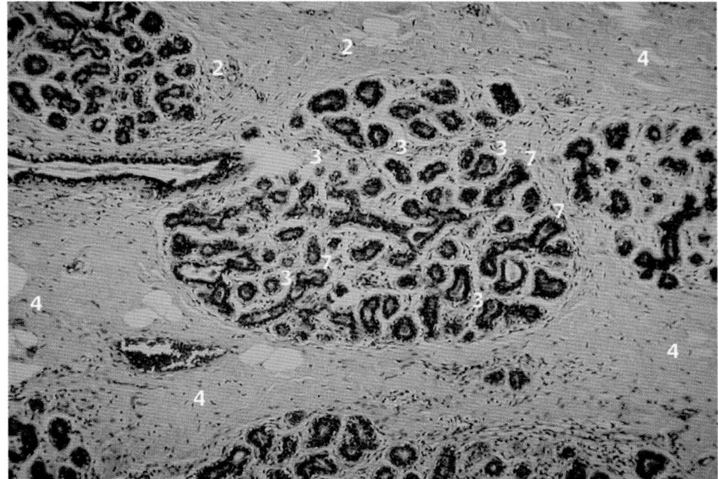

**b** Histology of a terminal duct lobular unit. Lobules and terminal duct (2), acini (7), and intralobular stroma (3). Tough *inter*lobular stroma (4) is present between the TDLUs (4).

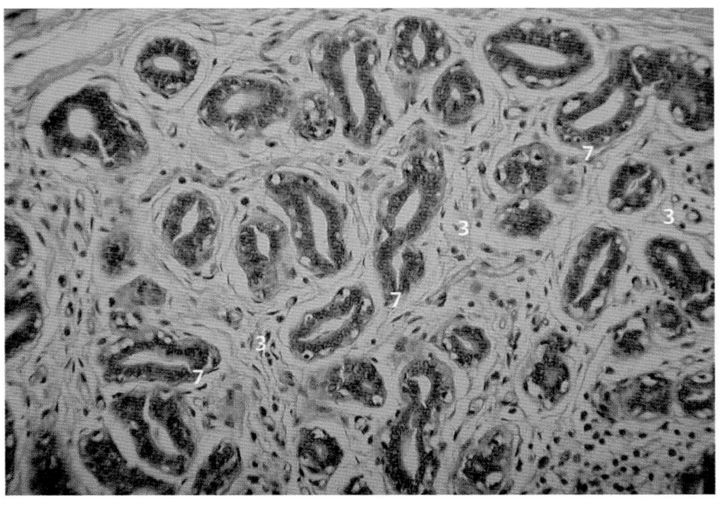

**Fig. 4.3 Three-dimensional representation of the peripheral and terminal ducts (TDLU) and their ultrasound characteristics.**

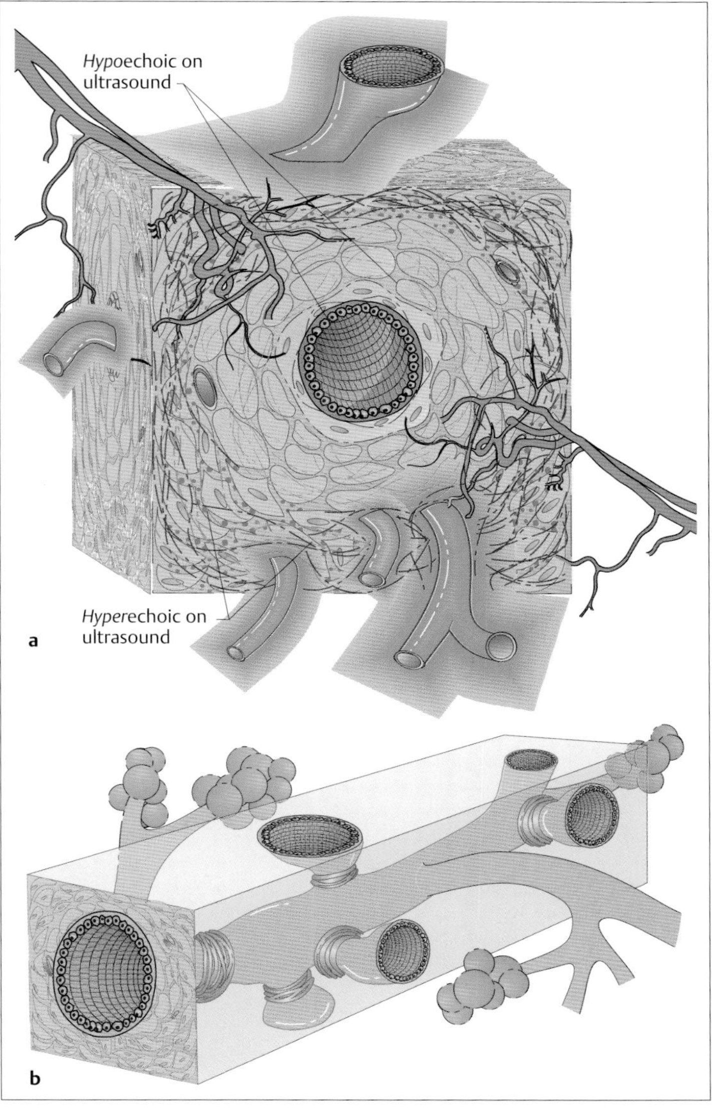


**a** Acinus (columnar epithelium) surrounded by basket cells and intralobular stroma. At the center of the tissue block (and protruding from the top) are blood vessels and nerves. Interlobular stroma is visible at the edge of the tissue block.
**b** Glandular duct with multiple peripheral TDLU. A cross section of the opened duct is visible on the left side of the tissue block (after Lamarque et al. 1976). The orange-colored structures are *hypo*echoic at ultrasound, and the blue structures are *hyper*echoic.

▶ **Fig. 4.3 c**

**c** Histology of a lobule. The functional unit (TDLU) consists of acini (7) with loose *intra*lobular stroma (3).

**Fig. 4.3 Ultrasound of TDLU.** *(continued)*

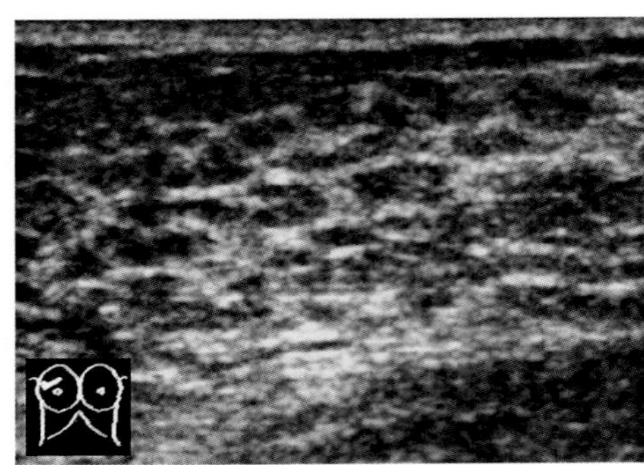

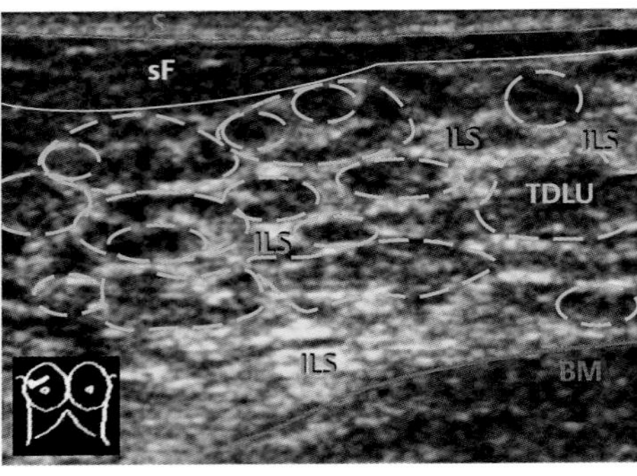


S = skin
sF = subcutaneous fat
TDLU = terminal duct lobular unit
ILS = interlobular stroma
BM = breast muscle

**c** Prominent TDLU in the second half of the cycle in B-mode sonography. Transverse sonogram through the upper outer quadrant of the right breast in a 24-year-old woman who was not on hormone therapy. The scan demonstrates connective tissue with central, thickened TDLUs. As higher-frequency ultrasound transducers are developed (preferably over 18 MHz), these structures of the TDLUs can be analyzed with greater precision. Ultrasound is still far from reaching its diagnostic potential.

**Fig. 4.4 Radiographic and sonographic features of the terminal duct lobular unit (TDLU) in breasts with different amounts of interlobular stroma.**

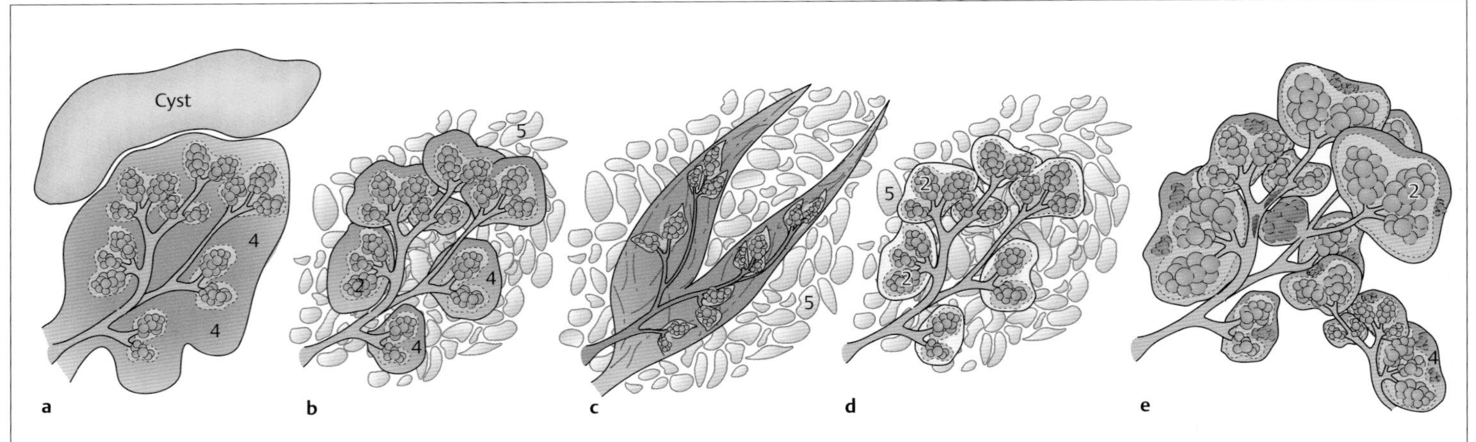


**a Terminal duct lobular unit (TDLU) with copious interlobular stroma (4)** and an adjacent cyst (fibrocystic change). *Radiography* shows homogenous opacity (ACR 3–4) in which the TDLU cannot be identified as it can with ultrasound (**Fig. 5.67 a**, p. 166).

**b Scant interlobular stroma in the breast** (normal breast in a woman of reproductive age, ACR 2–3). The TDLU and the surrounding interlobular stroma (4) appear *radiographically* and *sonographically* as focal opacities (see **Fig. 5.81**, p. 187).

**c** Interlobular stroma in the form of stromal septa with TDLUs (e.g., involuted breast-ACR1). The radiograph shows linear and bandlike opacities. Only larger lactiferous ducts are visible with ultrasound. The TDLUs are difficult to distinguish from surrounding fat (5) (see **Fig. 5.78**, p. 181).

**d Absence of interlobular stroma** (e.g., congenital or ACR 1). The TDLUs are surrounded by fat (5). The radiograph shows fine nodular opacities 1–2 mm in size. Ultrasound gives poor differentiation between fat and TDLUs (see **Fig. 4.31 b, c**, p. 60). Adenosis and lobular neoplasia are poorly visualized by ultrasound.

**e Irregularly enlarged TDLUs with scant interlobular stroma** (e.g., due to pregnancy, adenosis, or lobular carcinoma ACR 3 + 4). Radiography shows either a homogeneous density or an irregular, partly confluent focal opacities up to 10 mm in size in the periphery of the breast parenchyma. Proliferating TDLUs are clearly demonstrated by ultrasound (see **Figs. 5.66**, p. 165; **5.68b, c, d**, p. 168 f; **5.74 a, b**, p. 175; **5.145c**, p. 285; **5.146 d, e**, p. 287).

**Fig. 4.5 Periductal proliferation of intralobular stroma.** Ultrasound shows proliferating stromal tissue with linear ducts of high echo contrast. This is opposite to the pattern seen in a normal sonogram (see **Figs. 4.7 b, 4.10 c**, and **5.149 i, j**).

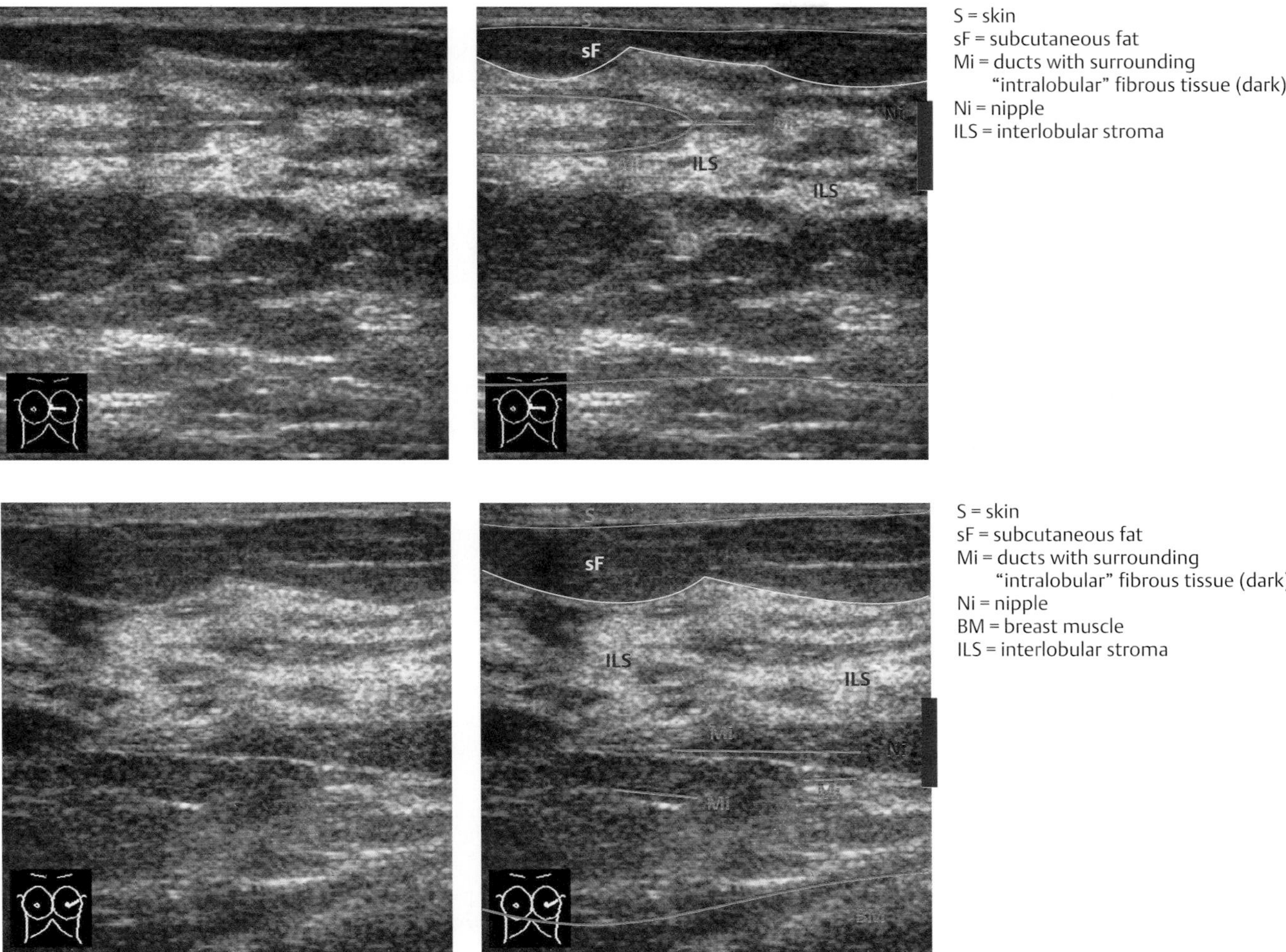


**Fig. 4.6 Histologic section stained with India ink** (Courtesy of Bässler, Fulda) to demonstrate the neurovascular supply of the terminal duct lobular unit (TDLU) (2). A heavily branched capillary network in the interlobular stroma (4) supplies blood to the lobules. The intramammary nerves have little importance in the transmission of pain sensation (except in the retro- and periareolar regions), and percutaneous needle insertion in the breast generally is not painful except skin, nipple, and retroareolar region.

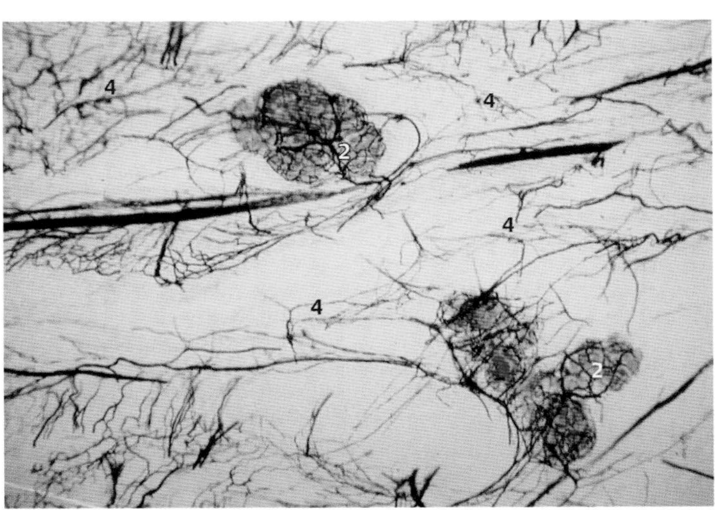


**Fig. 4.7 Ductography and sonography of the TDLUs.**

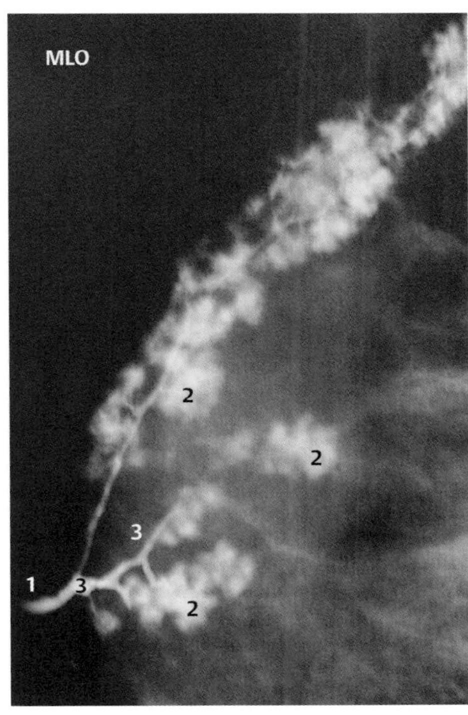


**a** Ductogram of a healthy breast demonstrates the main duct (1, 3), branching ducts, and opacified terminal duct lobular units (TDLUs, 2).

▶ Fig. 4.7 b

**Fig. 4.7 Ductography and sonography of the TDLUs.** *(continued)*

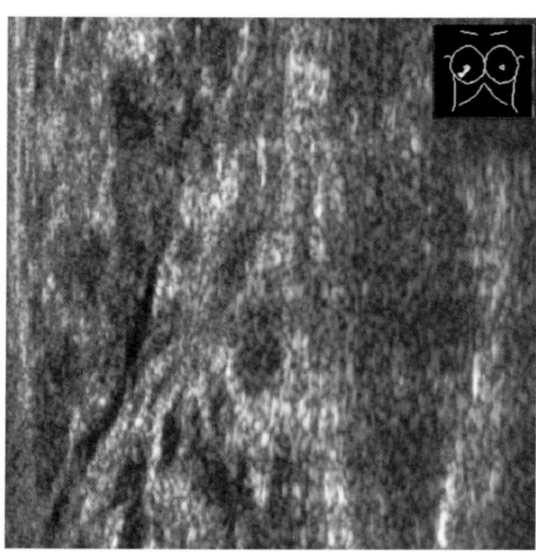

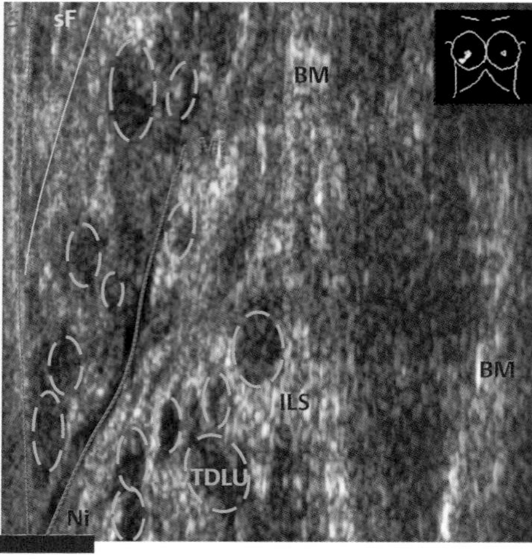


S = skin
sF = subcutaneous fat
Mi = lactiferous duct(s)
Ni = nipple
TDLU = terminal duct lobular unit
BM = breast muscle
ILS = interlobular stroma

**b** Sonogram of a lactiferous duct (hypoechoic, dark) with enlarged terminal duct lobular units. The TDLUs appear as rounded, hypoechoic areas that contrast with the hyperechoic (lighter) interlobular stroma (compare with diagram to the right).

**Fig. 4.8 Lactiferous ducts: normal ducts and appearance in ductectasia.** Normally the fluid-filled ducts are not visible on *mammography*, even when mildly enlarged, due to insufficient contrast between the radiographic density of fluid (1.0) and that of the breast (0.95). If the ducts are enlarged (ductectasia) and filled with fatty debris (density of 0.7), they will appear darker (more lucent) than the rest of the breast parenchyma, especially if the breast is very rich in connective tissue (density of 0.95). Air is as lucent as fatty debris (**b**). *Sonographically*, the ducts are hypoechoic (dark) when viewed in longitudinal and transverse section. If debris has collected in the ducts, it will appear as a round or oval zone of increased echogenicity, similar to the pattern of the breast parenchyma (**d**).

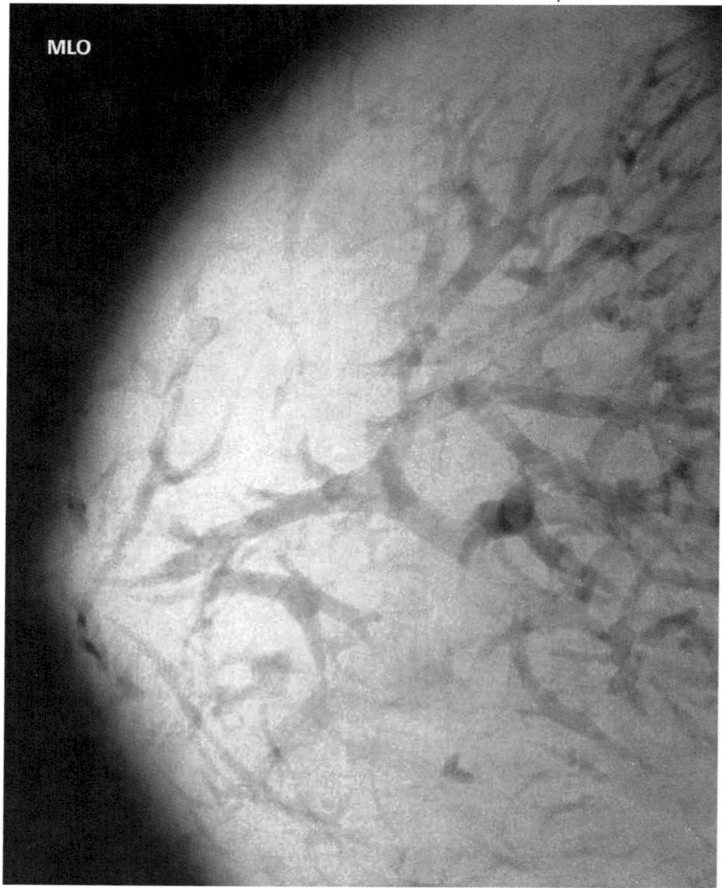


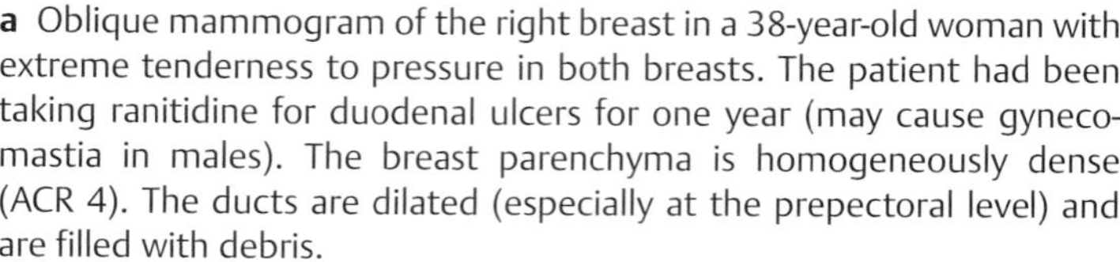

**a** Oblique mammogram of the right breast in a 38-year-old woman with extreme tenderness to pressure in both breasts. The patient had been taking ranitidine for duodenal ulcers for one year (may cause gynecomastia in males). The breast parenchyma is homogeneously dense (ACR 4). The ducts are dilated (especially at the prepectoral level) and are filled with debris.

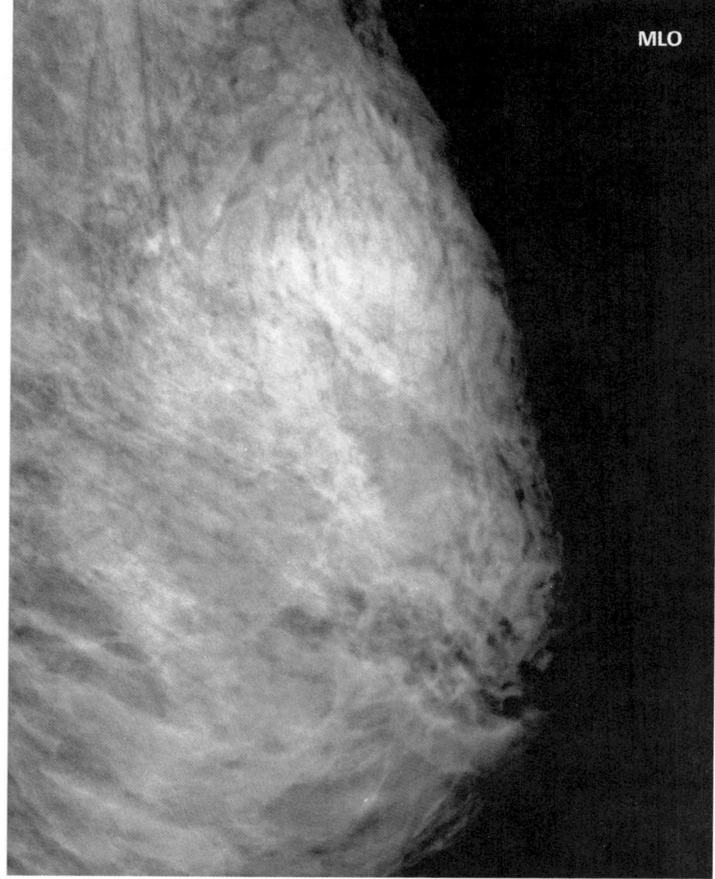


**b** Oblique mammogram of the left breast in a 38-year-old woman demonstrates an enlarged duct system filled with air, the cause of which is unknown (erotic practices?).

**Fig. 4.8 Duct system in galactogram: Ductectasia with detritis in sonogram.** *(continued)*

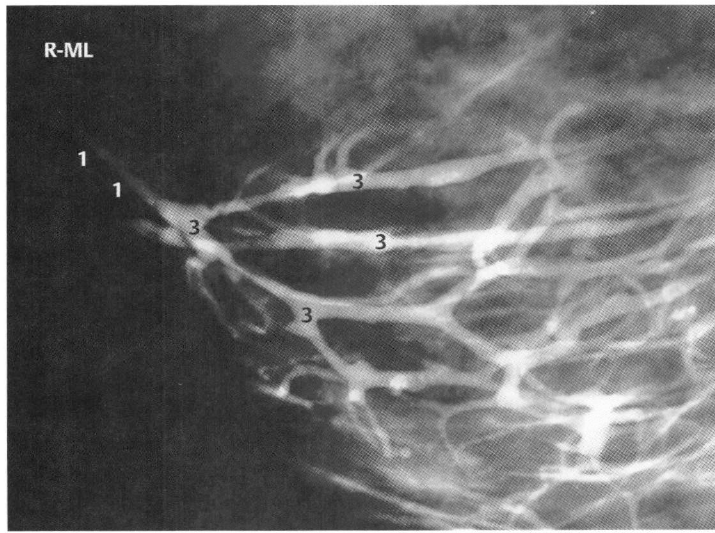


**c** Ductogram of the right breast in a 64-year-old woman shows a retroareolar sinus (1) and main ducts (3) with smooth contours and homogeneous density.

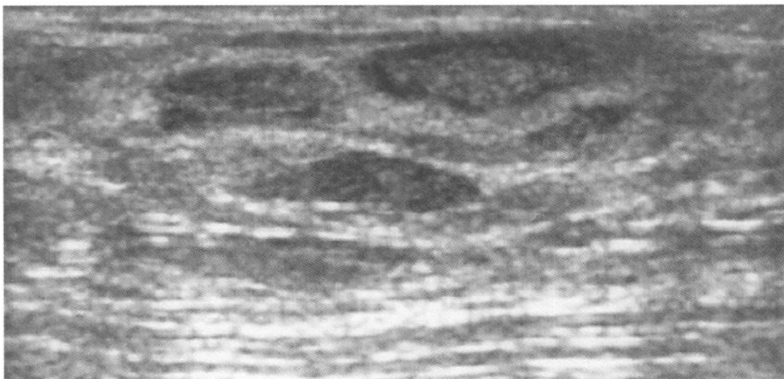

**d** Transverse sonogram shows enlarged retroareolar ducts with hyperechoic intraductal debris. The debris is slightly inhomogeneous and is not adherent to the duct wall. Papilloma may have a similar ultrasound appearance (debris was cytologically confirmed in the present case).

**Fig. 4.9 Macerate preparation specimen to demonstrate the duct system and TDLUs.**

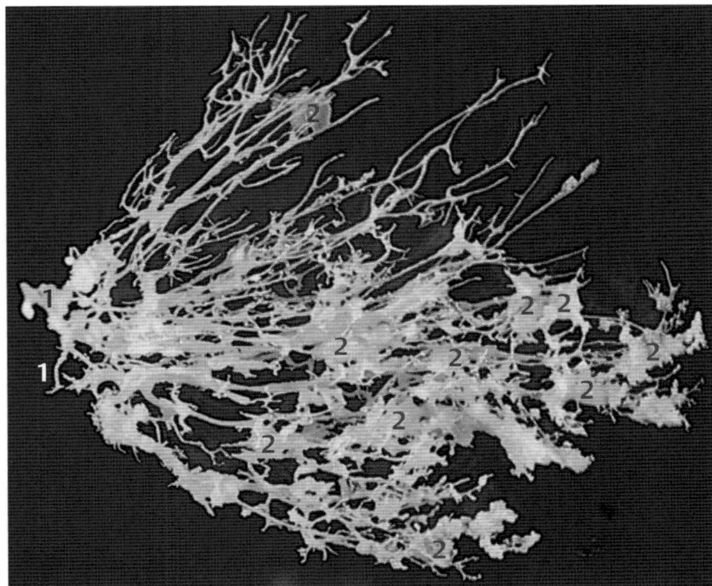


**a** Maceration of the duct system and lobules in a woman of reproductive age (Courtesy of Prechtel, Starnberg). The nipple-areola (1) is on the left. The duct system of the mammary lobes is splayed out in the periphery. Few TDLUs (2) are visible, especially in the periphery (lower part of photograph).

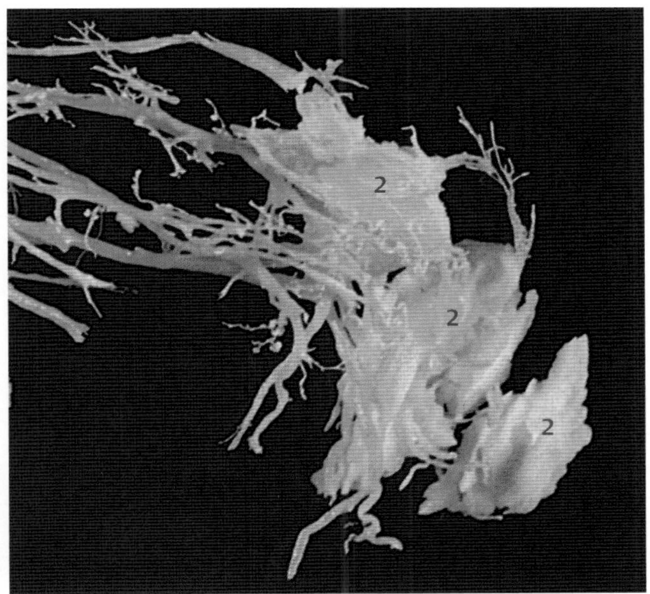


**b** Maceration specimen of a terminal duct lobular unit (Courtesy of Prechtel, Starnberg). After maceration of the breast tissue, the plastic-filled lactiferous ducts and lobules (TDLUs) in the periphery have much the same appearance as they would have in an ultrasound image.

**Fig. 4.10** Microradiograph and histologic section of the TDLU.

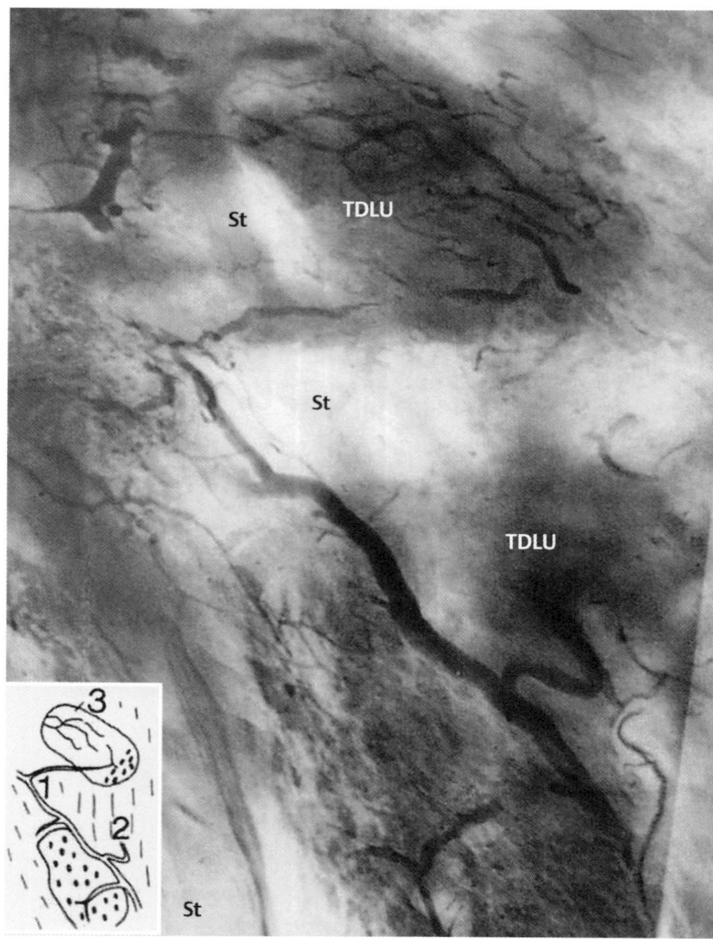


**a** Microradiograph of the terminal duct lobular unit (TDLU). Radiograph of a tissue slice 50 µm thick shows the main duct with branching ducts (1, dark because it contains air). The lobules appear dark (3) because of the acini, terminal ducts, and intralobular stroma. Interlobular stroma (St) appears light. The ultrasound image is similar in appearance to the microradiograph.

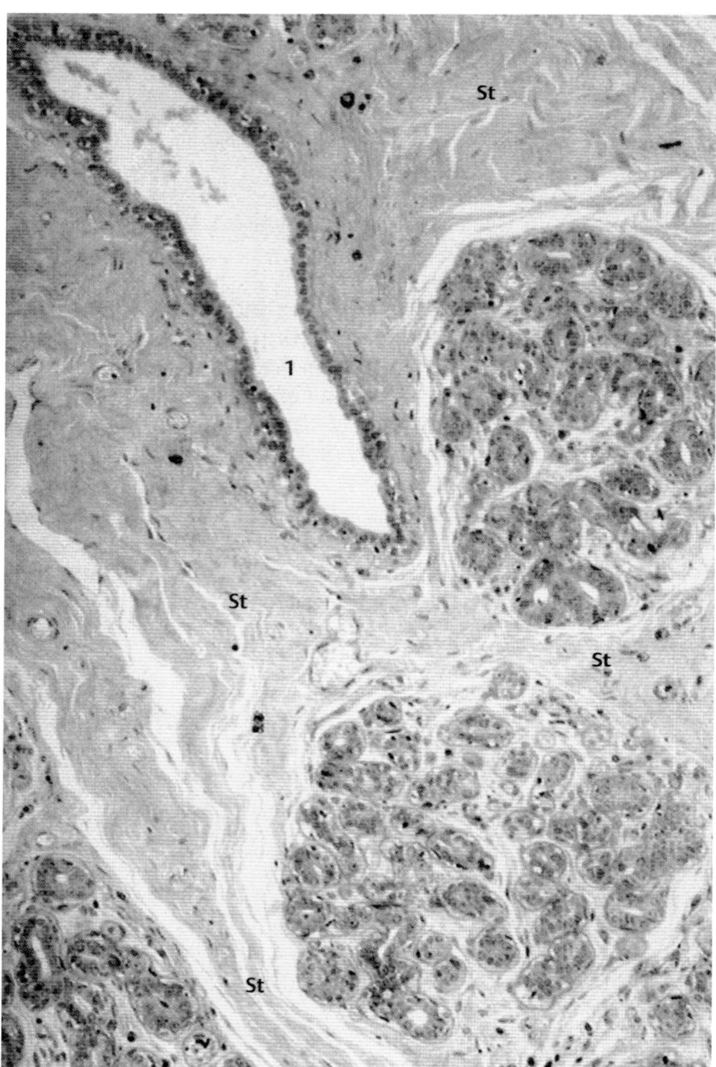


**b** Histologic section of a TDLU with ductules (acini) and intralobular stroma. Terminal duct (1) surrounded by interlobular fibrous tissue (St).

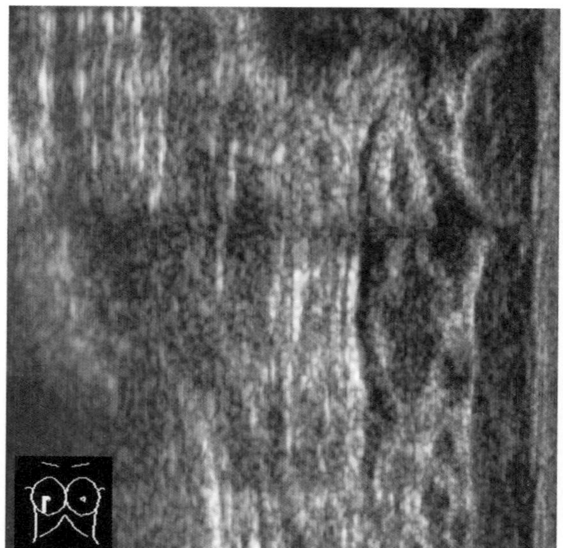

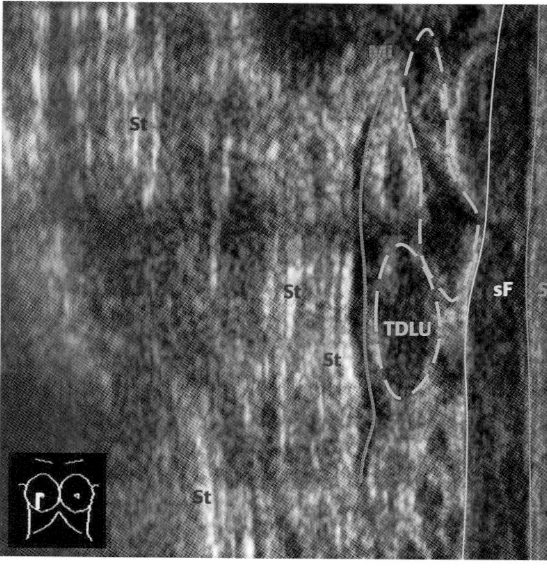


S = skin
sF = subcutaneous fat
Mi = lactiferous duct
TDLU = terminal duct lobular unit
St = interlobular stroma

**c** Ultrasound. The sonographic appearance of the TDLU resembles its appearance on the microradiograph. The lobules with intra- and perilobular stroma appear hypoechoic, while the interlobular stroma between the TDLUs appears hyperechoic and light.

**Fig. 4.11 Ductal carcinoma originating from a large central duct and spreading toward the periphery** (light blue) with secondary (retrograde) lobular malignant transformation (Courtesy of Dabelow and Bässler, Fulda).

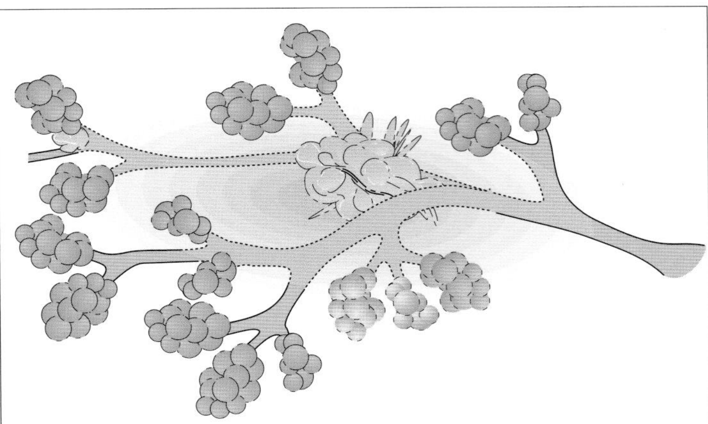

**Fig. 4.12 Lobular carcinoma originating in the peripheral lobules** with secondary cancerization of the ducts (light blue) and lobules (Courtesy of Dabelow and Bässler, Fulda).

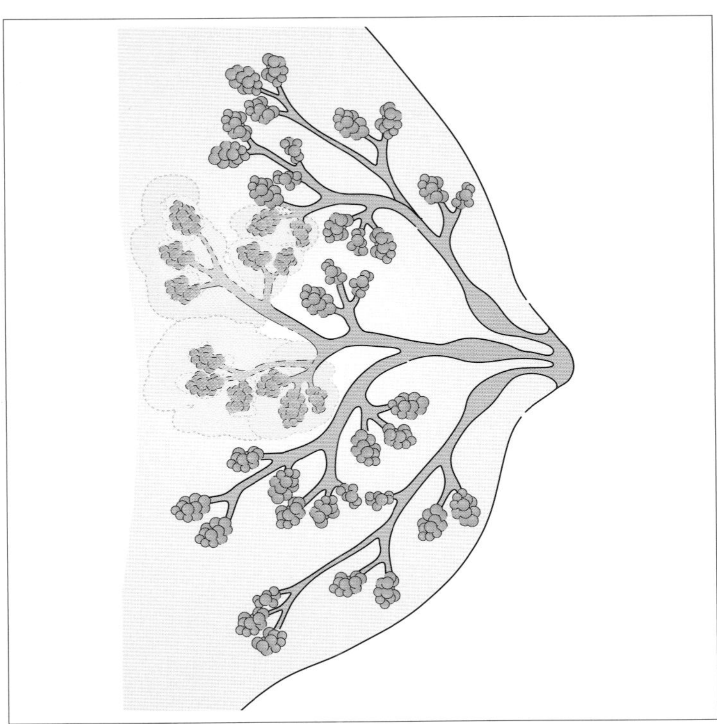

## Hormone-Induced Proliferation

The breast in women of reproductive age undergoes cyclic changes during the course of the menstrual cycle. Estrogen increases cellular proliferation and progesterone promotes this effect, apparently with greater potency than estrogen (Harvey and Bovbjerg 2004). Cellular proliferation is stimulated during the follicular phase of the cycle and is sustained during the luteal phase. As the TDLUs enlarge, water accumulates in the intralobular stroma, leading to overall breast enlargement. This effect occurs during the luteal phase but is most pronounced during the premenstrual phase (see **Figs. 4.3 c, 4.13 c**). The acute fall in plasma estrogen and progesterone levels causes a regression of proliferative cellular tissue (apoptosis), which is maximal just before menstruation. These cyclic changes in the TDLUs have the result of increasing the mammographic density of the breast, especially during the premenstrual phase. Ultrasound imaging at this time may define the TDLUs as small hypoechoic foci in the peripheral portions of the mammary lobes (see **Fig. 4.13**).

This is the least favorable time for mammography as well as for MRI. The breast tissue is relatively radiodense, and mammography is even more painful and unpleasant than at midcycle, for example (7th–12th days of cycle). Because blood flow to the breast is also increased during the second half of the cycle, MRI is unfavorable as it tends to produce more false-positive findings (see p. 203).

The menstrual cycles shorten as menopause approaches. The follicular phase becomes less intense, while the luteal phase shows no significant change. During the perimenopausal years, the preovulatory serum estradiol levels are higher than in younger women, while the progesterone levels remain the same before declining at menopause. It is very common for breast cysts to develop during this period. They may be caused by the shortened follicular phase accompanied by a premenstrual rise in estrogen levels. Cysts and ductasia may also occur in response to progestin administration, however.

In theory, the relative fall of progesterone during perimenopause could not only promote the atrophy of hormonally active breast parenchyma but could also lead to the regression (apoptosis) of very small intramammary tumors. Again in theory, progesterone administration during HRT could preempt this natural tumor regression and could even stimulate the growth of receptor-positive cancers. This in turn could explain the results of the Million Women Study and Women's Health Initiative studies and would also explain why the incidence of breast cancer has fallen with the worldwide decline of HRT (see p. 11). All of this is purely hypothetical, however.

At menopause, only about 34% of women 75–79 years of age have fully involuted (atrophied) breasts, compared with 11% of women in the 25–29 age group. Thirty percent of women in the 75–79-year age group still have breasts that are as dense as those of younger women.

Ultrasound scanning at 5–7 MHz cannot adequately document the cyclical changes in the TDLUs in pre- and postmenopausal women. Specifically, scanning at these frequencies cannot distinguish between connective tissue and glandular breast tissue. This can be accomplished to some degree with high-resolution probes (11–13 MHz), however, and ultrasound is better than mammography for defining the TDLUs within their stroma-rich surroundings. Higher-frequency ultrasound scanners may be able to shed more light on the dramatic cyclical changes that occur in the TDLUs and throughout the breast (see also "Basic Structures of the Breast and their Variants on Ultrasound" in Chapter 5, p. 156).

Pathologic changes are most likely to develop in areas where TDLUs are most abundant, i.e., the periphery of the lobes (see **Fig. 5.66 d**, p. 165) (Harvey et al. 2004). The main types of pathology are adenosis, fibroadenoma, and especially lobular carcinoma. Areas that require special attention at mammographic screening are called "no man's land" in the craniocaudal projection and the "milky way" in the oblique projection.

**Fig. 4.13** Ultrasound in different phases of the menstrual cycle.

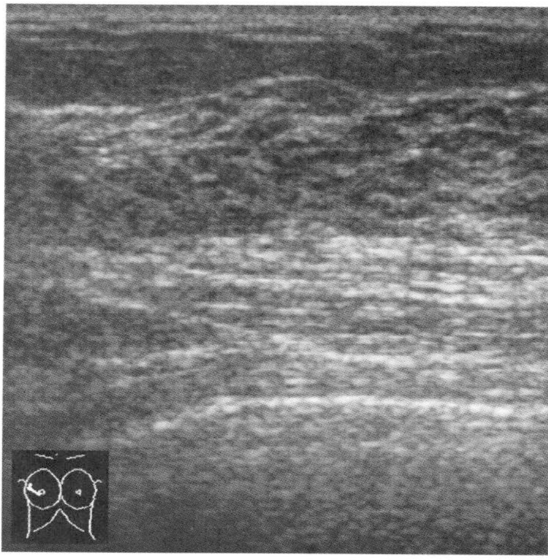

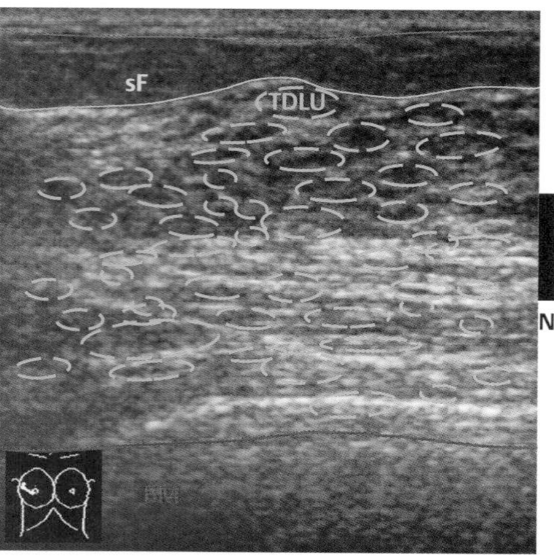


S = skin
sF = subcutaneous fat
TDLU = terminal duct lobular unit
Ni = nipple
BM = breast muscle

**a** TDLUs are well delineated relative to the interlobular stroma in the early second half of the cycle.

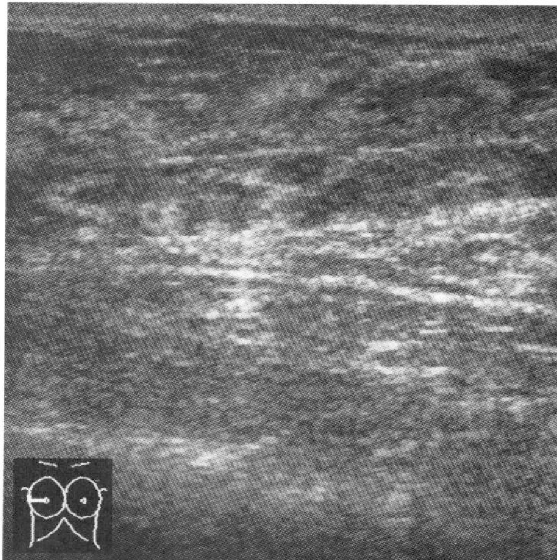

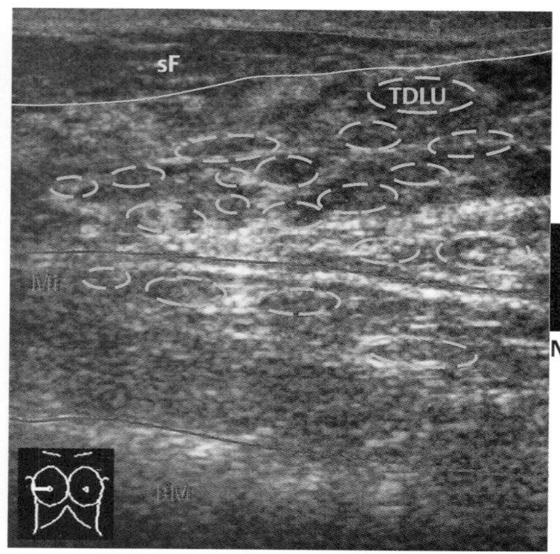


S = skin
sF = subcutaneous fat
TDLU = terminal duct lobular unit
Mi = lactiferous duct
Ni = nipple
BM = breast muscle

**b** Ultrasound in a more lateral plane. The TDLUs show a much less compact arrangement at the same point in the cycle.

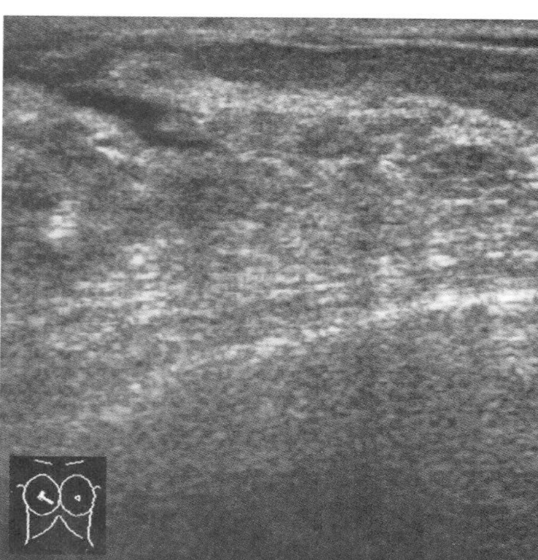

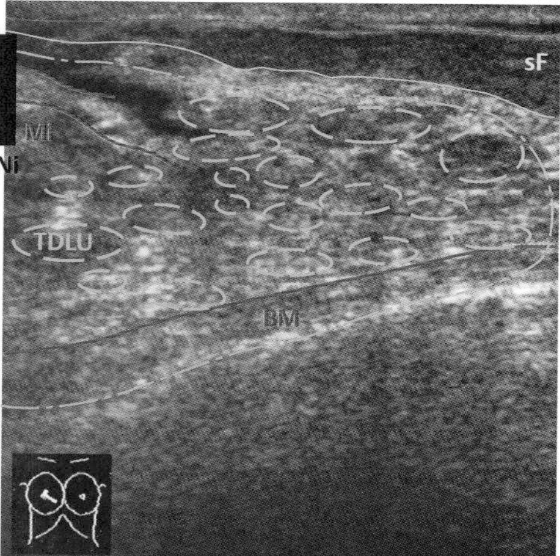


S = skin
sF = subcutaneous fat
TDLU = terminal duct lobular unit
Mi = lactiferous duct
Ni = nipple
BM = breast muscle

**c** Ultrasound near the nipple shows greater lobular proliferation (enlarged TDLUs) around the slightly expanded duct during the premenstrual phase of the cycle.

## Mammographic Density and Cancer Risk

Wolfe (1976) was the first author to note a correlation between mammographic density and an increased risk of breast cancer. An increase in mammographic density and especially short-term changes in density result from proliferation of the TDLUs—basically the lobules and *intra*lobular stroma but not the *inter*lobular stroma (see pp. 98, 156).

> **Tip**
>
> **An increase in mammographic breast density correlates very well with the size and contents of the TDLUs, which can be demonstrated by high-resolution ultrasound (11–18 MHz).**

Proliferation of the acini within the TDLUs (see p. 156), accompanied by an increase in mammographic density, apparently results from hormonal stimulation of the breast, with an associated increase in cancer risk. Harvey et al. (2004) correlated mammographic breast density with the relative risk of breast cancer and enumerated the causes of increased breast density. According to these authors, induced ductal hyperplasia (DH) and adenosis with the development of premalignant lesions such as atypical ductal hyperplasia (ADH) offer a plausible explanation for the relationship between breast density and increased cancer risk. They attribute these conditions to the effects of stimulating growth factors, increased intramammary production of estrogen, and activated aromatases. In many studies the breast cancer risk is 4–6 times higher in radiographically dense breasts than in radiolucent breasts. While Harvey et al. (2004) do not believe that breast density can be quantified with ultrasound, they state that digital mammography may offer a means of objective quantification. Studies, especially follow-up studies, using full-field digital mammographic systems (Giotto, I.M.S., Italy) could yield further information that may enable us to define standard hypo- and hyperdensity values as potential risk factors.

> **!** **Women whose breasts show fading radiographic density during menopause have significantly less risk of developing breast cancer than women whose breasts remain dense.**

The four ACR grades of breast density (see p. 98 and **Tab. 5.7**) are based on the concept that hormonally active glandular tissue is scant in the radiolucent breast (ACR 1) but abundant in the very radiodense breast (ACR 4). This is correct only to a degree, however. An ACR 4 breast may consist largely of unresponsive interlobular stroma, which does not increase breast cancer risk, or it may consist mainly of proliferating TDLUs (similar to the pregnant breast with extensive adenosis and other fibrocystic changes), which do increase cancer risk. Only ultrasound can differentiate between abundant stromal tissue and abundant glandular tissue, thus permitting an accurate risk assessment.

Despite the skepticism of Harvey et al. (2004), it is definitely possible to analyze and in some cases quantify the density of the breast by using 12 MHz or 13 MHz ultrasound probes. A breast that is dense due to the proliferation of interlobular stroma is distinguishable from a breast that is dense due to proliferation of the TDLUs (see **Figs. 5.70–5.80**). Breast cancer does not develop from interlobular stroma.

Thus, a "glandular" breast that is dense due to TDLU proliferation can be distinguished sonographically from a stroma-rich breast, a fact that has significant implications for hormone replacement therapy, for example. *Postmenopausal* women with radiographically dense breasts have a greater risk of breast cancer than reproductive-age women with dense breasts. Lobular proliferation in *premenopausal* women is a physiologic process. Neither hyperestrogenemia nor hyperprogesteronemia affects their risk of breast cancer. On the other hand, increased breast density in postmenopausal women is most likely due to endogenous hyperprogesteronemia and the resulting stimulation of the TDLUs, which increases the risk of breast cancer (Key et al. 1999 a). Hyperprogesteronemia causes not only TDLU-stimulation but also cysts and ductectasia which further increase the breast density. Opinions differ, however, with regard to radiodensity and breast cancer risk and whether the increased density is due to stimulation of the TDLUs. The research team headed by Watson (quoted by Warren and Lakhani 2003) studied the stromal proteins **lumican** and **decorin** in normal breast tissue and in breast cancer. The concentrations of the compounds were found to be markedly higher in malignant tumors. According to Watson and colleagues, stimulation of connective tissue by these two proteins can lead to increased breast density in the absence of lobular or ductal proliferation. Perhaps the elevated stromal protein levels originate from the intralobular stroma and exert their carcinogenic effect on the breast lobules. All in all, these interrelationships should provide fertile ground for future research. Ultrasound studies may help to shed additional light on mammographic density.

Breastfeeding activity provides an indirect measure of the number of TDLUs in the breast. Women who are or were capable of effective nursing probably have a greater density of TDLUs than women who were unable to nurse at all, or for just a few days, due to a deficiency of milk production. It is unknown whether this could serve as a potential indicator of breast cancer risk.

A relationship also exists between body weight, radiographic density, and breast cancer risk. Obesity is a well-known risk factor for breast cancer.

> **Obese women with radiographically dense breasts have a higher risk of breast cancer, especially during and after menopause, than obese women with radiolucent breasts.**

**Alcohol** also appears to play a role in breast density, as higher alcohol consumption is generally associated with greater breast density. White wine in particular increases breast density in postmenopausal women, whereas the consumption of red wine is believed to be associated with a decrease in breast density (Vachon et al. 2000).

**Athletic activity** appears to have a nonspecific effect on breast density (see p. 17).

**Hormone replacement therapy** plays a major role as well. HRT delays involution of the breast and increases mammographic breast density in up to 73% of women 67–72 years of age. In most cases the increased density is diffuse, but sometimes it is focal or multifocal.

Treatment with an estrogen–progestin combination results in higher breast density than estrogen-only therapy. This density increase occurs in both continuous and cyclical hormone regimens. The greatest density increase occurs during the first year after the initiation of HRT. Breast tissue is relatively quick to respond to hormones. A visible decrease in breast density is noted just 2 weeks after the discontinuation of HRT and is most evident after a period of months or years (see **Figs. 5.72** and **5.75**). These density changes are probably unrelated to the interlobular stroma and are most likely due to changes in the size of the TDLUs.

If mammographic breast density and the TDLU pattern at ultrasound do not change during HRT, it is reasonable to assume that the breast parenchyma is not responding to hormonal stimulation. A decrease in breast density would suggest a calming effect after a period of hormonal stimulation with an associated reduction in cancer risk. Digital radiography is better than ultrasound for the objective documentation of increasing or decreasing radiodensity. Radiation to one breast, incidentally, will cause a regression of TDLUs relative to the unirriadiated side, and usually this is easily detectable with ultrasound. Mammography, on the other hand, will tend to show increased density on the irradiated side due to radiation-induced fibrosis. This density increase does not imply an increased risk of breast cancer.

Histologic studies of benign breast changes in women on estrogen–progestin HRT show a greater degree of lobular proliferation than in women on estrogen-only therapy or women not receiving HRT. The proliferative changes predominantly affect the TDLUs. Women from the Canadian breast cancer screening program who had extremely dense breasts were 12 times more likely to have epithelial hyperplasia, albeit without atypia, than women with normally dense breasts. When breast discharge was present, cellular atypias were significantly more common in the discharge from women who had radiographically dense breasts.

**Antiestrogens** have a positive effect on radiographic breast density. Forty-four percent of women taking tamoxifen were found to have decreased mammographic density compared with only 15% of women taking a placebo. Raloxifene, used mainly in the treatment of osteoporosis, also leads to a significant reduction in breast density, comparable to that produced by tamoxifen. Tamoxifen reduces breast cancer risk by 32% in high-risk women, raloxifene by 50%, and Arimidex (anastrozole) by 58% (Eiermann et al. 2004). But only women with high serum estradiol levels respond well to tamoxifen and raloxifene, while women with low estradiol levels already have a lower risk of breast cancer. Radiographic density in these women is not further decreased by antiestrogen therapy, providing indirect evidence that the interlobular stroma is not affected by hormones.

**Gonadotropin agonists** inhibit ovarian function, thereby reducing breast density and lowering the risk of breast cancer.

**Tibolone** (Liviella) blocks estrogen synthesis and has androgenic activity. In 6% of women, however, tibolone metabolites produce a breast density similar to that associated with estrogen–progestin therapy (see **Fig. 5.81**).

The effects of **oral contraceptives** and androgens on breast density have not yet been investigated.

**Elevated prolactin levels** in postmenopausal women may lead to a radiodense breast with a heightened risk of breast cancer.

Thus, increased breast density due to stimulation of the TDLUs is likely to provide an important key in the evaluation of risk factors and may prove to be more important than previously thought. The TDLUs and related mammographic breast density may also become an important consideration in the search for an optimum HRT that does not induce breast cancer. If breast density increases or if ultrasound shows lobular (TDLU) proliferation in response to HRT, then that therapy should either be discontinued or replaced with an estrogen-only regimen whenever possible (**caution:** uterine mucosa, see p. 11). The potential increase in breast cancer risk associated with HRT does not occur until a few months or years after treatment is initiated. This leaves ample time to explore HRT modifications and other options that do not increase breast density (lifestyle modification, chemoprevention, antiestrogens, hormone-releasing IUDs, etc.). The radiographic density of the breast is the most frequently overlooked risk factor in research on the causes of breast cancer (Harvey et al. 2004).

Digital mammography could provide an objective tool for measuring changes in breast density in response to various influences (Schreer et al. 2004).

## Precancerous Lesions: Atypical Ductal Hyperplasia and Noninvasive Carcinoma (Carcinoma In Situ)

*Atypical ductal hyperplasia (ADH) or lobular hyperplasia* and *noninvasive or preinvasive carcinoma (DCIS, LCIS)* are confined to the ductolobular structures of the breast. They are characterized by the intracanalicular spread of epithelial cell masses that have undergone malignant transformation. These types of lesions will be fully explored in this section because the goal of screening programs—especially mammography and ultrasound—is to detect cancers and their precursors at the earliest possible stage. In the author's own case material, precursor lesions (ADH, DCIS, LCIS) account for at least 30% of all breast malignancies and are most commonly detected in women under 50 years of age (60%). By contrast, most of the invasive cancers in his cases were found in women over 50 years of age (62%). Nevertheless, 38% of all breast cancers that he diagnosed during one decade were found in women under 50 years of age (see **Fig. 2.2**, p. 15). In this analysis of data from the authors' own files, he did not include ADH or atypical proliferative forms of fibrocystic change (formerly classified as Prechtel grade III disease). These conditions were evaluated and treated as precursors of carcinoma in situ.

Other researchers with larger study populations ($n = 1179$) have published their results on age distribution. Evans et al. (1997) compared the incidence of clinically occult DCIS and invasive carcinomas in women under and over 50 years of age (**Tables 4.1, 4.2**).

Twenty-five percent of all women with preinvasive and invasive breast cancer concern the age group under 50 years. DCIS was found in 46% of the women under age 50, while 36% were found in the older group. Invasive carcinomas (including invasive lobular carcinomas), on the other hand, were diagnosed in 63% of the women over age 50 and in 53% of the women under age 50. Invasive lobular carcinoma was found in 3% of the women under age 50 and in 8% over age 50. On the basis of these numbers (1179 carcinomas in 3734 patients), Evans et al. (1997) recommend that systematic screening should begin at 40 years of age. The author agrees with this recommendation and would actually suggest because of his own results (see pp. 15, 105, 107) the beginning of screening with single-view mammography (plus ultrasound) at age 35, even in the absence of known familial risk factors. This is because many tumors that are detected between 50 and 69 years of age may already be detectable as precursor lesions by 35 years of age, and unfortunately breast cancer is no longer a rarity among 30- to 40-year-olds. *Single-view mammograms*, which reduce the radiation dose by half,

**Table 4.1 Malignant breast tumors in women under 50 years of age** (Evans et al. 1997)

| Malignancy | n | % |
|---|---|---|
| Invasive ductal carcinoma | 144 | 49.0 |
| DCIS | 137 | 46.6 |
| Invasive lobular carcinoma | 9 | 3.1 |
| Metastases | 0 | 0.0 |
| Lymphoma | 0 | 0.0 |
| Colloid (mucinous) carcinoma | 4 | 1.3 |
| Tubular carcinoma | 0 | 0.0 |
| Medullary carcinoma | 0 | 0.0 |
| Total | 294 | 100.0 |

**Table 4.2 Malignant breast tumors in women 50 years of age or older** (Evans et al. 1997)

| Malignancy | n | % |
|---|---|---|
| Invasive ductal carcinoma | 475 | 53.7 |
| DCIS | 325 | 36.7 |
| Invasive lobular carcinoma | 49 | 5.6 |
| Metastases | 1 | 0.1 |
| Lymphoma | 1 | 0.1 |
| Colloid (mucinous) carcinoma | 15 | 1.7 |
| Tubular carcinoma | 17 | 1.9 |
| Medullary carcinoma | 1 | 0.1 |
| Paget carcinoma | 1 | 0.1 |
| Total | 885 | 100.0 |

are appropriate for the higher radiosensitivity of the breast parenchyma in women under age 50. Moreover, the breast lobules are fully mature by age 35 and are no longer vulnerable to potentially harmful endogenous and exogenous agents (see p. 9).

At this point it must be mentioned, that the main reason of screening at age 50–69 comes predominantly from financial criteria combined with radiation-dose-aspects of a double-view mammography.

## Flat Epithelial Atypia (FEA) and Other Cylindrical Cell Lesions of the Breast

Besides the various forms of ductal and lobular carcinoma in situ (DCIS, LCIS), interest has also focused on cylindrical cell lesions of the breast. There are cytologic, architectural, molecular biological, and prognostic differences that distinguish these lesions from carcinoma in situ. The intraluminal cells in FEA exhibit low-grade cytologic atypias that develop in previously normal small mammary ducts and TDLUs. Hence the process involves the transformation of normal ductal structures rather than the formation of new structures. FEA is an incidental pathology finding in numerous biopsy samples but has no significance for the diagnostic radiologist. Management depends on other diagnostic factors (nodularity, microcalcifications, etc.; Fritzsche et al. 2006). There is no need to discuss FEA further in this context, but it does appear useful to divide the ductal intraepithelial neoplasias into two groups:

- Low-risk lesions (FEA, ADH, low-grade DCIS)
- High-risk lesions (intermediate- and high-grade DCIS)

This would allow for greater consistency in the diagnosis of breast cancer and could simplify further diagnostic and therapeutic decision making (Bonk et al. 2005).

## Atypical Ductal Hyperplasia

**ADH is associated with a 4-fold increase in cancer risk, and that heightened risk is doubled in women who have a positive family history. ADH is therefore definitely a precancerous lesion.**

ADH and DCIS are mammographically indistinguishable from each another on the basis of their calcification patterns, and noncalcifying forms are not detectable. ADH has no sonographic characteristics and shows nonspecific gadolinium enhancement on MRI. The growth characteristics of ADH are similar to those of DCIS. According to molecular genetic studies, ADH is a neoplastic epithelial process with the histological features of a low-grade DCIS. ADH is characterized histologically by the proliferation of atypical cells with solid or cribriform growth patterns and the partial or complete involvement of ducts, lobules, or even entire lobes (Böcker et al. 1997) (see **Fig. 4.22**). For the radiologist, then, there is no difference whatsoever between ADH and DCIS as far as routine diagnosis and treatment are concerned.

Differentiation from simple benign **ductal hyperplasia** (DH) is based histologically on *qualitative* features (cellular morphology), while differentiation from DCIS it is based on *quantitative* criteria (number of cells, tumor extent). According to Page et al. (1995), the incidence of ADH in the screened population is 2% of all breast biopsies, rising to 4% in perimenopausal women and 6% in postmenopausal women. Today the term ADH is used in preference to the older concept of Prechtel grade III atypical fibrocystic change (Prechtel 1971, 1976).

Immunohistochemical analyses and molecular genetic studies in recent decades have increasingly deepened our knowledge of ADH. An important step was the histologic definition of ADH by Page and Rogers in 1992. The most important differentiating criteria between ADH and simple DH are based on qualitative differences in cell proliferation. *ADH* is distinguished by atypical monomorphic cells and cribriform growth, while *DH* is characterized by a more mixed, variegated cell pattern and fenestrating growth.

The differentiation of ADH from low-grade and intermediate-grade DCIS is based on quantitative criteria. This means that a radiologist cannot differentiate between DH, ADH, and DCIS on the basis of mammographic microcalcifications or atypical proliferation of TDLUs at ultrasound. In all cases it is important to differentiate ADH from DH and treat it the same as DCIS, i.e., by complete excision and histologic evaluation. Small, low-risk ADH lesions are an exception to this rule if they have been removed with clear margins by vacuum biopsy and show no atypia on histologic examination in the surrounding tissue.

**Fig. 4.14** **A 49-year-old woman presented with a 1-year history of progressive enlargement of the right breast** and a palpable supra-areolar nodule at the 12-o'clock position (**b**). For the previous 8 days there has been redness of the right areolar region between the 3 and 7-o'clock positions (**c**). Fine-needle aspiration (FNA) of the supra-areolar nodule yielded Pap IV atypical cells (**g**). A core-needle biopsy revealed atypical ductal hyperplasia (ADH). A previous core-needle biopsy from the inflamed area indicated an acute exacerbation of chronic mastitis.

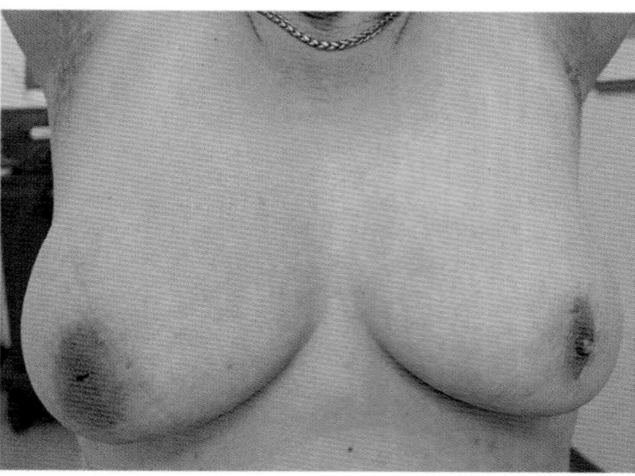

**a** Clinical appearance of both breasts in 2002. Diffuse enlargement of the right breast (two years before, the right breast had been exactly the same size as the left breast).

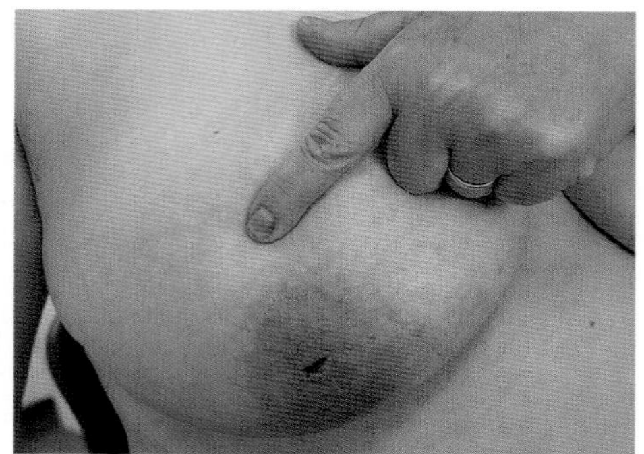

**b** Palpable supra-areolar mass at the 12-o'clock position in the right breast with no associated skin changes.

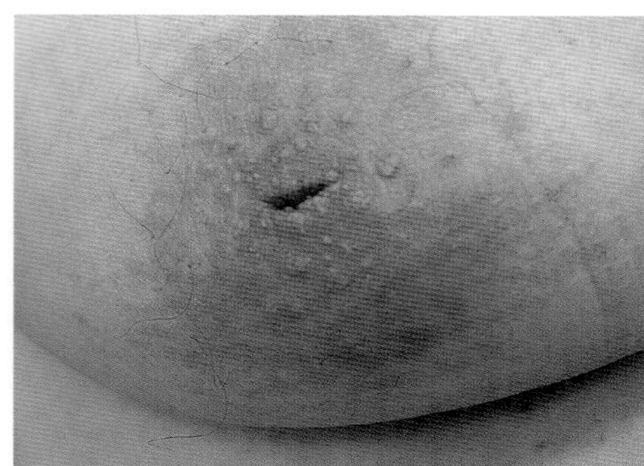

**c** View of the areola. Nipple retraction had been present for several years. Areolar skin redness and warmth are noted in the lower inner quadrant.

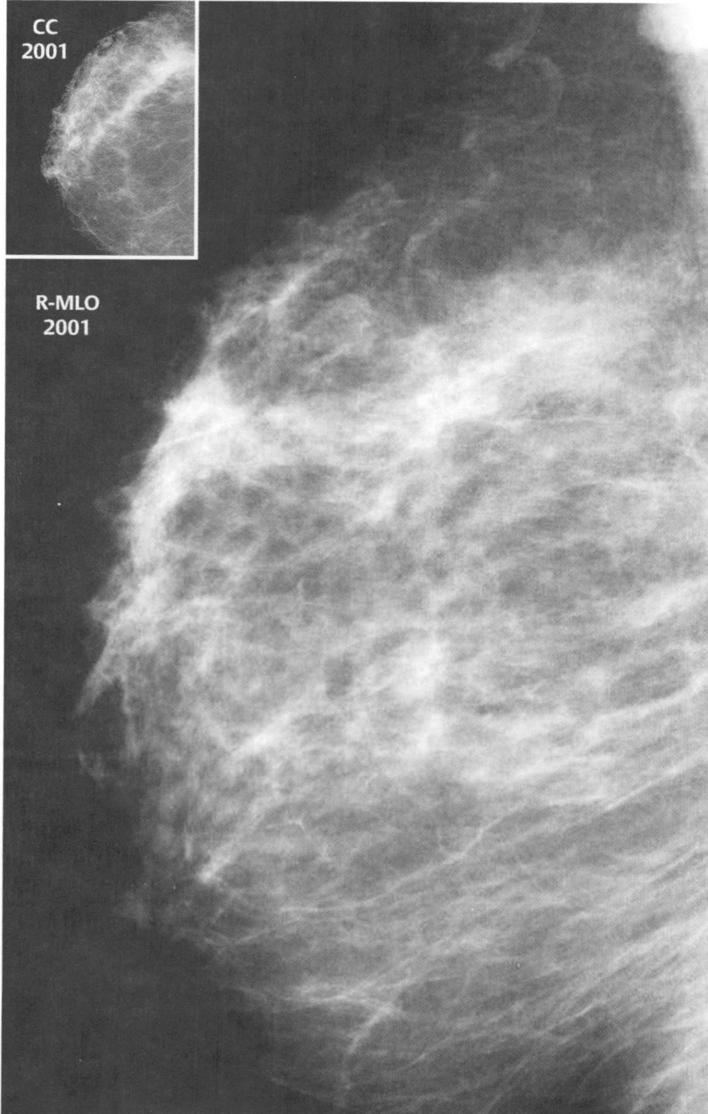


**d** Oblique mammogram of the right breast in 2001. Compared with the left side (**e**), the right breast is inhomogeneously dense with a 1 cm round opacity in the axilla (**0/19**) (ACR2, BIRADS 3, PGMI). The inset at upper left shows the corresponding craniocaudal view.

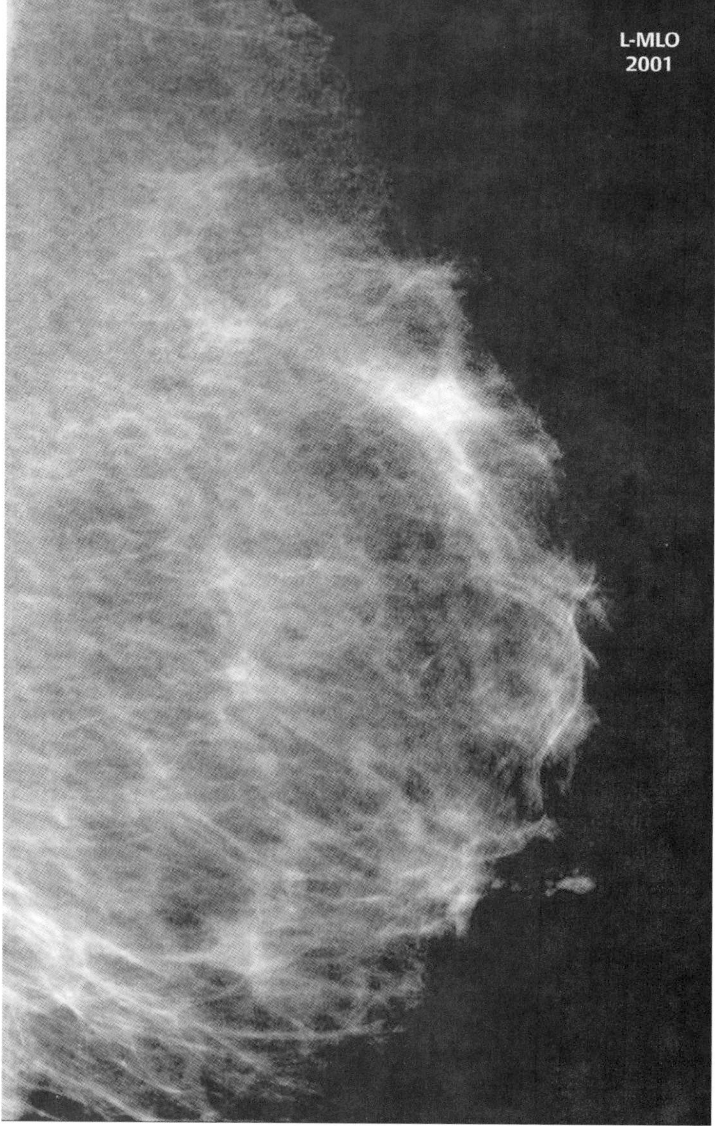


**e** Left oblique mammogram in 2001. The breast parenchyma shows no abnormalities (ACR 2, BIRADS 1, PGMI).

**Fig. 4.14** **A 49-year-old woman presented with a 1-year history of progressive enlargement of the right breast.** *(continued)*

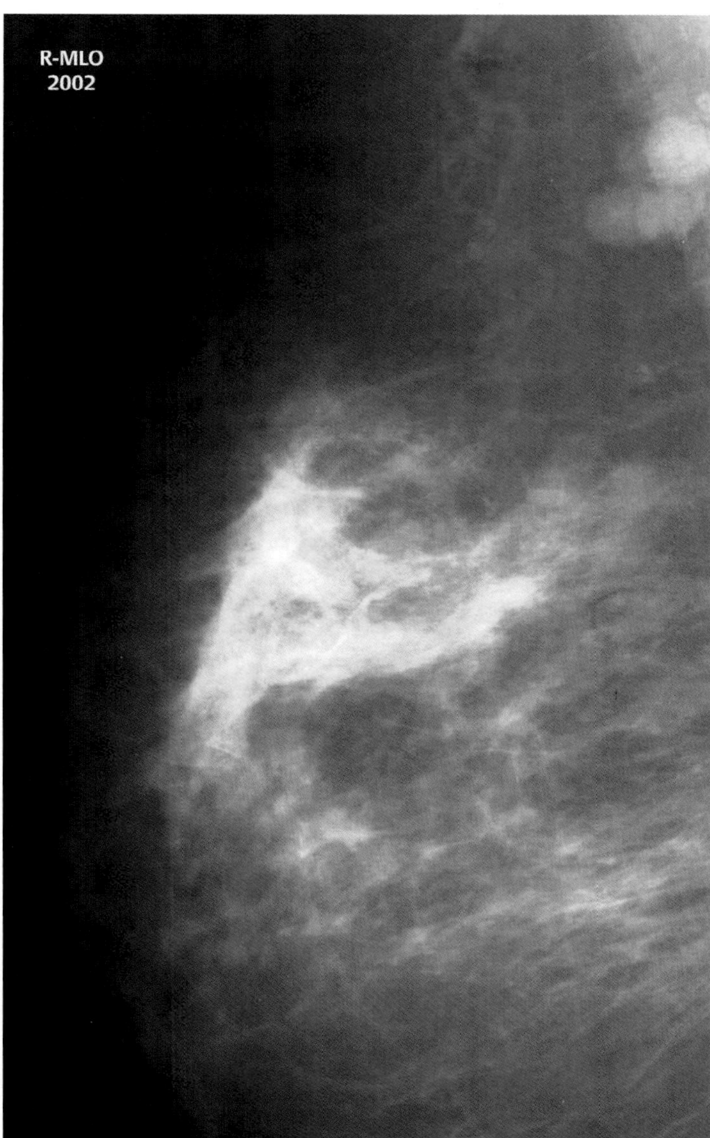


**f** Oblique mammogram of the right breast in 2002. The glandular tissue appears more dense than in the 2001 film (**d**). A right axillary lymph node is enlarged and shows no fatty degeneration (ACR 2, BIRADS?, PGMI). The left breast was unchanged relative to the 2001 mammogram.

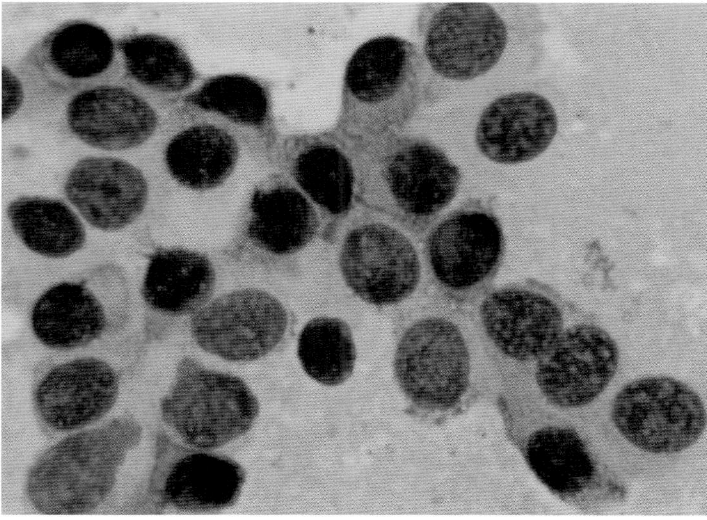

**g** Cytologic smear shows a stellate cluster of ductal epithelial cells with large pleomorphic nuclei in a loose chromatin framework of varying density. The nuclear–cytoplasmic ratio was omitted to preserve the nuclei.

**Question on Fig. 4.14**

*Given the patient's case history, what would you recommend?*

(**a**) Follow-up in 6 months.

(**b**) Open biopsy including investigation of the increased parenchymal density.

(**c**) Anti-inflammatory therapy with follow-up at 4 weeks.

→ **Answer on p. 345**

As a general rule, however, diagnostic *vacuum biopsy* (VB, see p. 230) as described in the German S3 guidelines should not be considered a therapeutic procedure for ADH (or DCIS). Cases where ADH (or DCIS) has been confirmed by core-needle or vacuum biopsy should be managed by surgical excision and complete removal with a margin of healthy tissue (Schulz et al. 2003, Albert et al. 2008).

If ADH is found on the margin of a surgical specimen (DCIS, invasive carcinoma), reexcision should be performed for the definitive exclusion of adjacent DCIS (Decker et al. 1997). If the ADH lesion in the specimen is small and is surrounded by at least a 5 mm margin of healthy tissue, reexcision may be omitted but the patient should be followed with biannual mammograms for 2 years, followed by annual mammograms, especially if the lesion was detected based on the presence of calcifications (Faverly et al. 1994; Ohtake et al. 1995; Decker et al. 1997) (**Fig. 4.14**). Mammography should in every case be combined with ultrasound.

## Ductal Carcinoma In Situ

Three-fifths of all in situ carcinomas are ductal (DCIS) and one-fifth are lobular (LCIS). DCIS and LCIS coexist as adjacent lesions in 20% of cases.

Special variants of DCIS are *Paget carcinoma* with centripetal spread and involvement of the nipple epidermis (differential diagnosis: eczema, see **Figs. 5.1, 5.52c**, p. 364) and *intracystic papillary carcinoma* (see **Fig. 5.138**, pp. 274, 389f), which has a longer in situ phase (differential diagnosis: papillary cyst). Only about one-fourth of noninfiltrating carcinomas are grossly detectable as circumscribed densities. The majority are detected as single or multiple microscopic foci occurring in small areas (usually with diffuse intracanalicular growth), and more than half of cases are detected on the basis of microcalcifications (**Figs. 4.15–4.19**).

*(continued on p. 40)*

**Fig. 4.15** **Noninvasive ductal carcinoma (DCIS).**

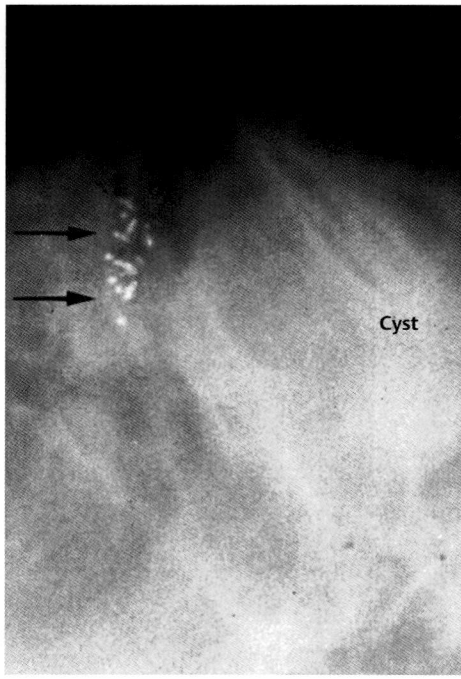


**a** Mammogram shows an oblong cluster of pleomorphic calcifications (arrows) to the left of a well-circumscribed cyst of homogeneous density.

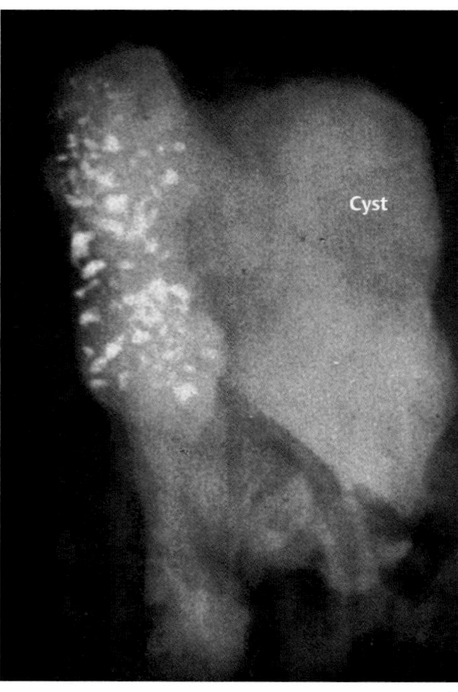


**b** Specimen radiograph of a duct (5 × magnification) shows an isolated duct with coarse, pleomorphic calcifications beside the cyst.

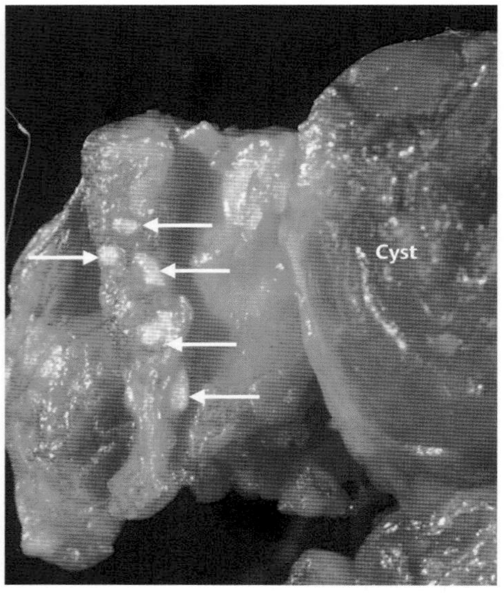


**c** Gross specimen of an isolated broad, thickened duct. Yellowish-white flocculent calcifications (arrows) are visible next to the isolated cyst.

**Fig. 4.16** **Small focus microcalcification of noninvasive ductal carcinoma beside adenosis.**

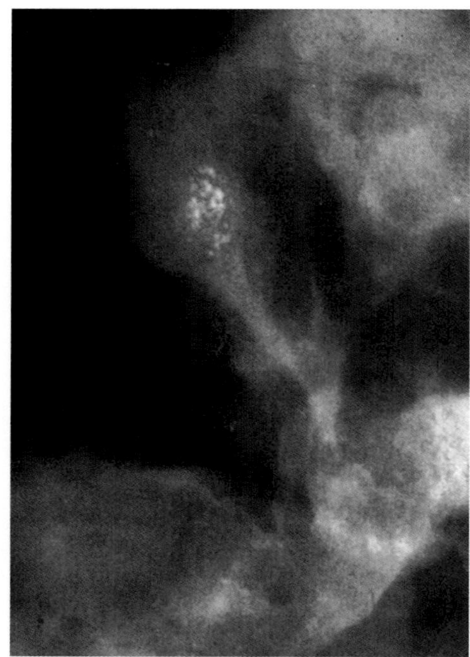

**a** Specimen radiograph (3 × magnification) shows a cluster of mixed flocculent and dust-like microcalcifications in an area of 3 × 4 mm. The particles are definitely pleomorphic and form a lentil-sized cluster (similar to **Figs. 4.15** and **4.17**).

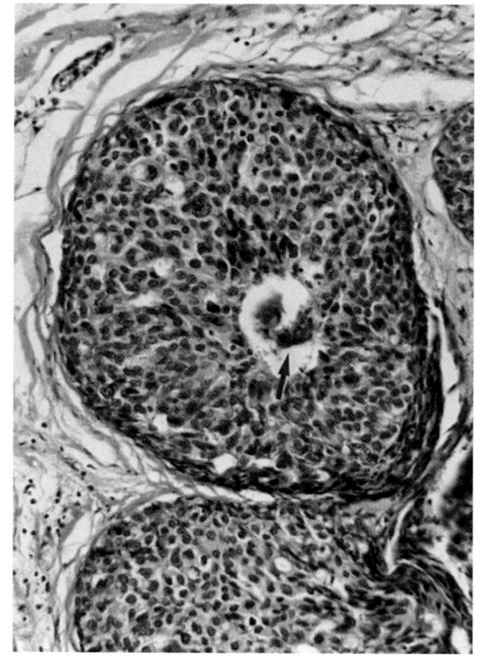

**b** Histologic section (approximately 160 × magnification) of intraductal carcinoma (monomorphic DCIS) shows central calcification of scant debris.

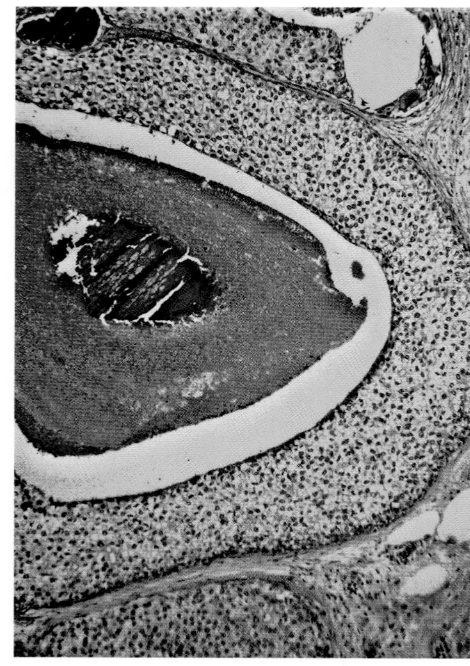

**c** Histologic section (approximately 250 × magnification) of a ductal carcinoma in situ (DCIS) shows atypical intraductal epithelial proliferation with calcifying dystrophic comedo necrosis.

**Fig. 4.17 Multifocal noninvasive lobular carcinoma next to infiltrating lobular carcinoma.**

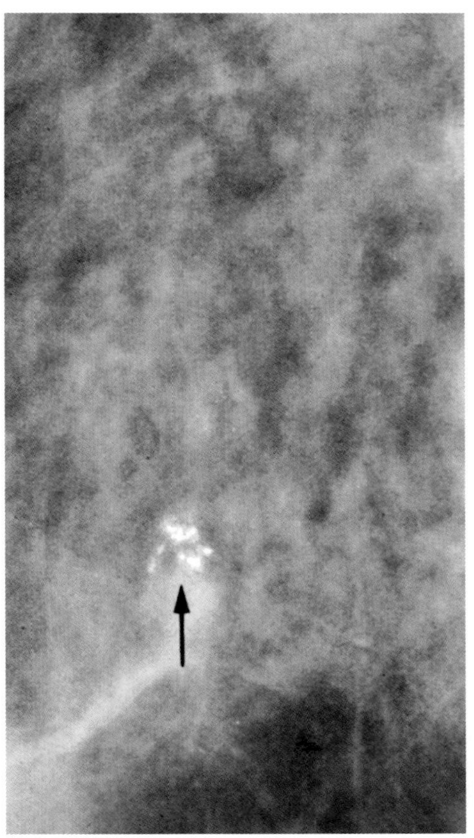

**a** Mammogram (magnified view) shows a small area of clustered microcalcifications, 3 mm in diameter in an otherwise normal-appearing breast.

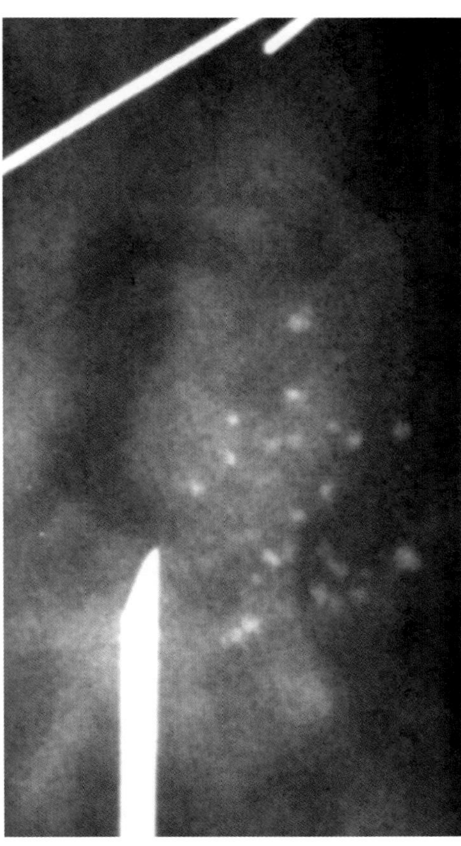

**b** Specimen radiograph (10 × magnification) shows clustered, moderately pleomorphic microcalcifications in a circumscribed area marked with a metal wire and hypodermic needle.

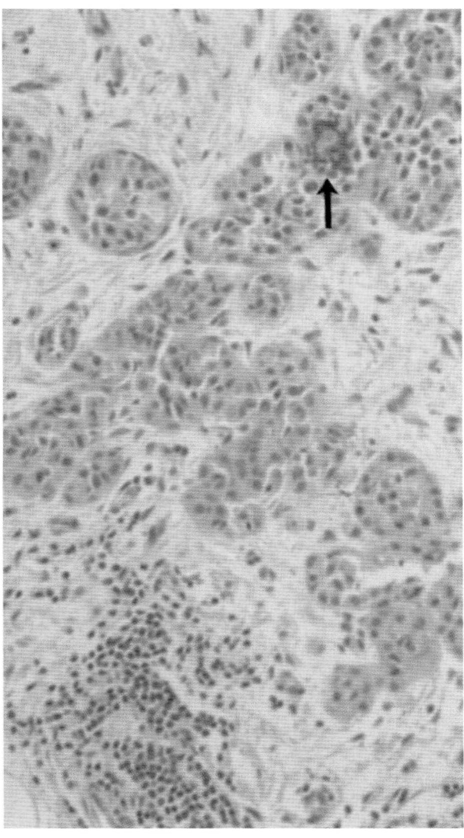

**c** Histologic specimen (approximately 160 × magnification) shows *atypical lobular hyperplasia* (LIN3 bordering on LCIS) with microcalcifications in an acinus (arrow) (courtesy of Dahm, Esslingen). **Note:** LIN-lesions sometimes show microcalcification like DCIS.

**Fig. 4.18 Noninvasive ductal carcinoma (DCIS).**

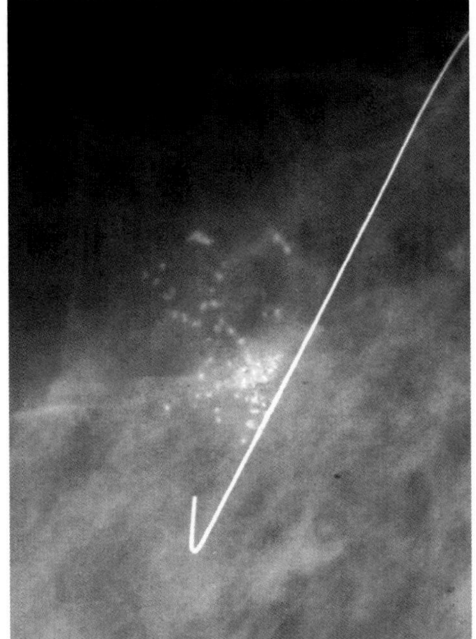

**a** Mammogram (magnified view) shows clustered pleomorphic microcalcifications following preoperative wire localization.

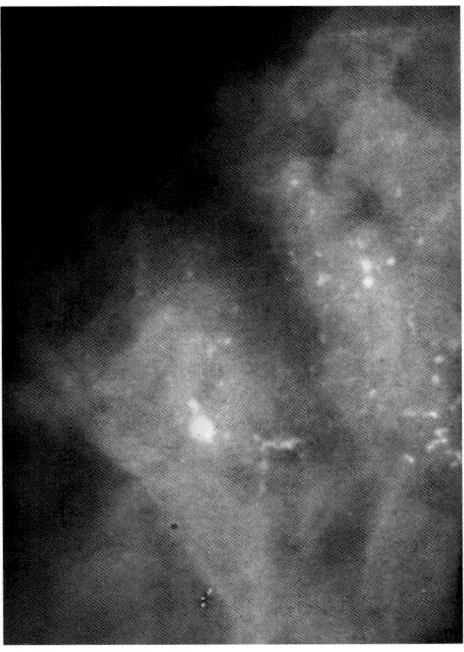

**b** Specimen radiograph (detail, 3 × magnification). Very pleomorphic calcifications show a combination of stippled, rounded, and crescent shapes.

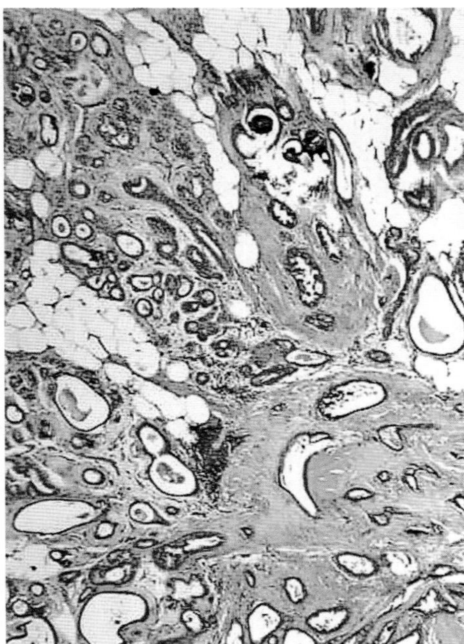

**c** Histologic section (approximately 120 × magnification) shows *blunt adenosis* in proximity to the carcinoma. Intrastromal calcium is visible at epithelial and luminal sites. **Note:** This case illustrates that clustered calcifications may occur next to carcinoma. Not all calcification seen in atypical mammograms must be malignant.

*(continued from p. 37)*

Noncalcifying in situ carcinomas cannot be detected mammographically in radiodense areas of the breast. DCIS may appear sonographically as ill-defined hypoechoic areas 5–15 mm in diameter. Because ultrasound cannot detect calcifying DCIS and LCIS, it will never replace mammography as a screening test. Ultrasound is an effective adjunct to mammography, however, significantly increasing the sensitivity not only of screening mammograms but of all screening tests such as MR mammography and interventional procedures (Hille et al. 2004 b, Yang and Tse 2004).

In a properly exposed mammogram of DCIS, only the "tip of the calcium iceberg" is visible when the lesion has reached a size of 100 µm or more. DCIS is displayed better and more accurately by **magnification mammography** (2–3 × magnification), biplane mammography, or digital mammography. **C**omputer-**a**ided **d**etection **(CAD)** in digital mammography enables the viewer to zoom in on all breast areas and reduces the false-negative rate of mammography from 31 % to 19 % (Destounis et al. 2004, Helvie et al. 2004). During preoperative localization, at least 1 cm should be added to the mammography-visible lesion margins in all planes to ensure that the DCIS is surgically encompassed with adequate margins (see **Fig. 4.22**). Magnetic resonance imaging occasionally defines the extent of DCIS better than mammography, although gadolinium enhancement does not always accurately reflect anatomical relationships, and time–density curves are not helpful in narrowing the differential diagnosis (DCIS, ADH, and DH all show similar gadolinium enhancement kinetics; see **Fig. 5.139** (p. 275).

DCIS has an impressive variety of histologic patterns that affect radiographic findings. Some lesions have a pleomorphic cell pattern with a propensity for cellular dissociation and necrosis with subsequent calcification (**Fig. 4.18b**), while others have a more monotonic, uniform cell pattern with very little calcification and debris formation (**Fig. 4.16b**). **Pleomorphic, usually large-cell DCIS** tends to show such intense calcification of debris that it is clearly visible on radiographs (see **Figs. 4.21–4.25, 4.28**). These relatively coarse flecks of calcification are typical of a solid carcinoma with calcifications. The calcifications of **papillary DCIS** have a coarse but less pleomorphic pattern and are difficult to detect on mammograms. **Cribriform DCIS**, by contrast, contains punctate calcifications. These calcifications are of a **monomorphic type** with more coherent, medium-sized cells that are slightly pleomorphic or monomorphic. The rather subtle calcifications of these cribriform tumors (**Fig. 4.19 b**) form within the pores of the tumor, as in a sponge. This form of DCIS is extremely difficult to detect on mammograms, the digital technique being better than the conventional.

Thus, the mammographically visible calcifications correlate with the histologic subtypes of DCIS. Extensive calcifications usually correlate with high-grade DCIS (G3). The calcium particles are pleomorphic; they may be linear and branched, may form coarse clumps, or may show a ductal or segmental arrangement according to Lanyi's criteria (Lanyi 1986) (see **Figs. 4.19 a, 4.20**). By contrast, the calcifications in low-grade DCIS (G1) are more often punctate and show a uniform ductal or lobular arrangement similar to secretory calcifications, for which they are often mistaken. In some cases these calcifications are associated with other, noncalcifying DCIS lesions that are detectable by ultrasound. A continuum of forms exist between the two extremes.

We occasionally see reports, especially from "progressive" epidemiologists, that DCIS is an inactive, dormant breast lesion that may never become malignant—similar to the "docile" form of prostatic cancer described by Hackethal (1977). They support their theory by noting that autopsy findings often include cancer precursors (ADH, DCIS, LCIS) that show no signs of invasiveness. This theory conflicts with numerous observations indicating that a missed or misinterpreted DCIS will often develop into invasive cancer with a latent period ranging from several months to 25 years. As a general rule of thumb, the more differentiated the DCIS is, the longer it takes to become invasive (Page et al. 1995). If the patient should happen to die for other reasons before an invasive tumor develops, then naturally the pathologist will find a DCIS in the breast at autopsy. This does not imply that every breast contains a DCIS that will never become invasive. The "snapshot" taken at autopsy cannot tell us how long the DCIS has lain dormant in the breast, whether and when it developed from an ADH, and when it will become invasive. Age is the greatest risk factor for any type of cancer. The malignant potential of DCIS is often speculated about in the popular media and in professional circles, and many women are needlessly alarmed.

**Fig. 4.19 Diagrammatic representation of microcalcifications in ducts infiltrated by the main types of ductal carcinoma** (from Lanyi 1986).

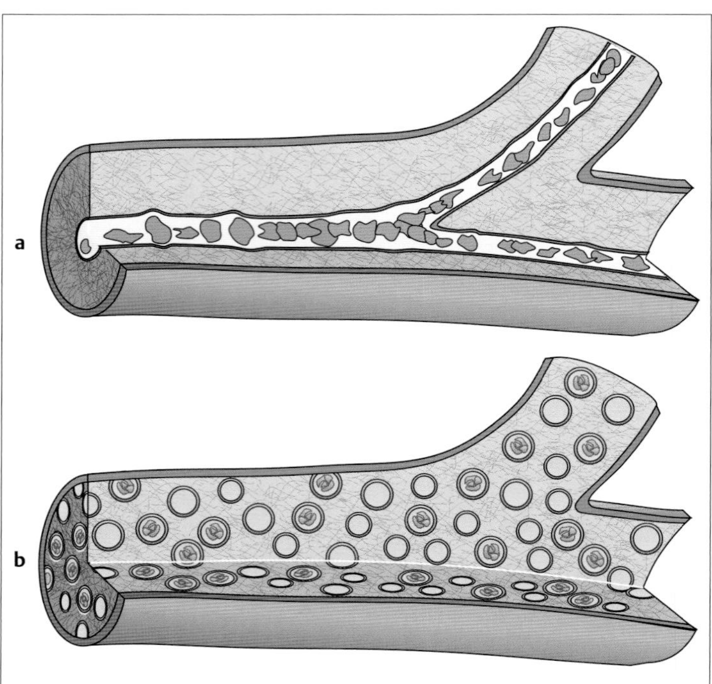


**a** Comedo carcinoma with central coarse calcifications including Y-shaped forms at the center of the intraductal tumor masses (see **Figs. 4.15, 4.16, 4.21**).
**b** Cribriform carcinoma with psammomatous calcifications in the small cavities of the spongy, cribriform tumor (see **Fig. 4.22 c**). This type of malignant calcifications is hard to see visible on conventional mammograms.
Most of ductal tumors have a mixed pathology in which areas of comedo carcinoma coexist with cribriform and papillary elements.

> **!** **Every DCIS should be surgically removed with at least a 10 mm margin of healthy tissue. The removal of this precursor lesion means that a carcinoma will never be able to develop at that site.**

What woman (and what doctor) would accept the risk of a confirmed but untreated ADH or DCIS and wait for invasive cancer to develop?

The fact that the peak incidence of DCIS is between 40 and 50 years of age while that of invasive carcinoma is between 50 and 60 years of age (see **Fig. 2.2 b, c**, p. 15) supports the contention that DCIS is a precursor to invasive disease. It is widely known that benign calcifications may spontaneously regress. It is less well known that calcifications in DCIS may disappear as the lesion progresses to invasive cancer. The reason for this is not yet fully understood. The angiogenesis factor may play a role, with vascular invasion causing the calcifications to disintegrate. The authors' own observations are confirmed in a case described by Schwarz et al. (1999): In a 64-year-old woman who declined to have her DCIS removed, the regression of calcifications did not indicate resolution of the DCIS but signaled its progression to invasive cancer over an 8-year period (**Fig. 4.21**).

**Fig. 4.20 Progression of microcalcifications in a 46-year-old woman with no palpable breast abnormalities.** The patient presented for a regular screening examination and had no family history of breast cancer.

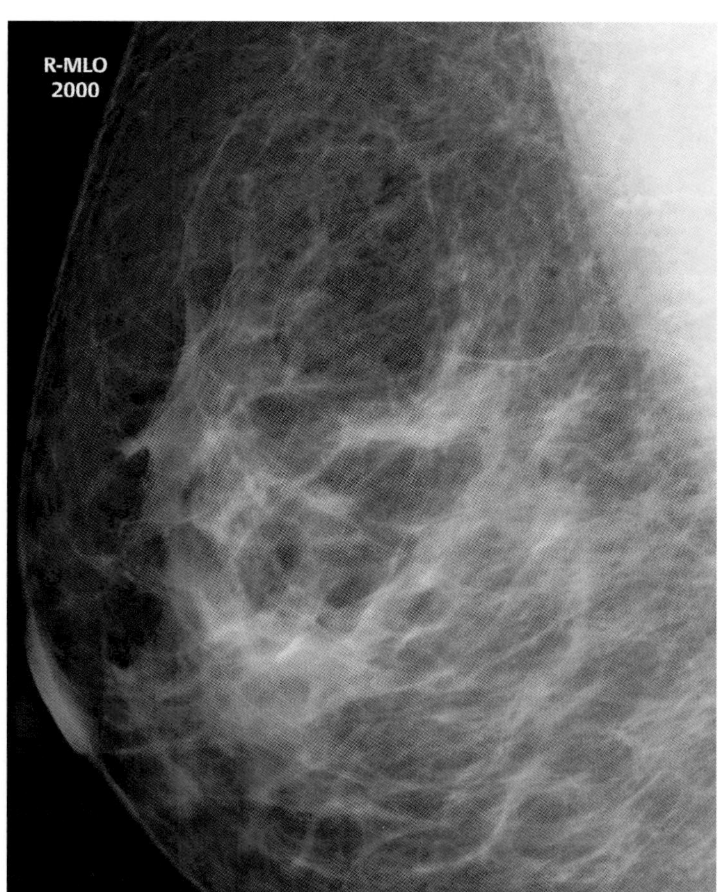


**a** Oblique mammogram of the right breast in June, 2000, shows normal-appearing glandular parenchyma (ACR 2, BIRADS 1, P**G**MI).

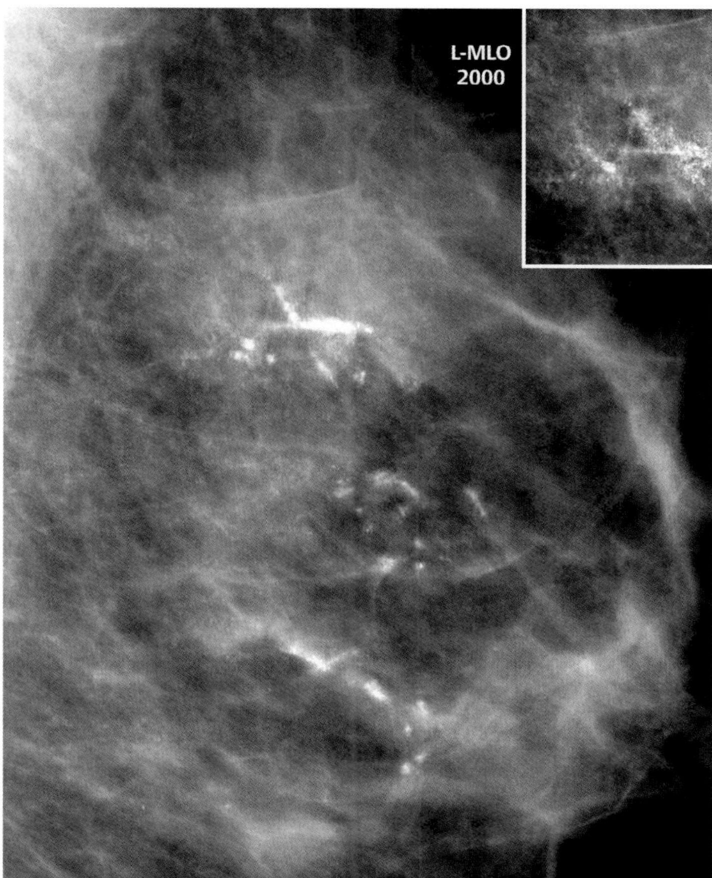


**b** Oblique mammogram of the left breast in June, 2000. Microcalcifications are scattered throughout the radiodense breast and are most numerous in the outer quadrants (ACR 3). *Inset:* Digital magnification mammogram taken in June, 2000 gives better delineation of the particles.

**Question on Fig. 4.20**

*How would you interpret the calcifications?*

(**a**) Benign
(**b**) Malignant
(**c**) uncertain

→ **Answer on p. 345**

**Fig. 4.21 Progression of malignant calcifications** in a 53-year-old woman who presented for a regular screening examination with no palpable abnormalities. During mammography, clustered microcalcifications were noted at the boundary between the upper inner and lower inner quadrants of the right breast. Surgery was recommended, but the patient refused consent. Seven and a half years later she came to follow-up with a palpable, locally advanced tumor at the same location with associated nipple retraction. The microcalcifications detected in 1989 had completely disappeared within the tumor, and some comedo calcifications were visible at the periphery of the mass (Schwarz, Austria, 1999).

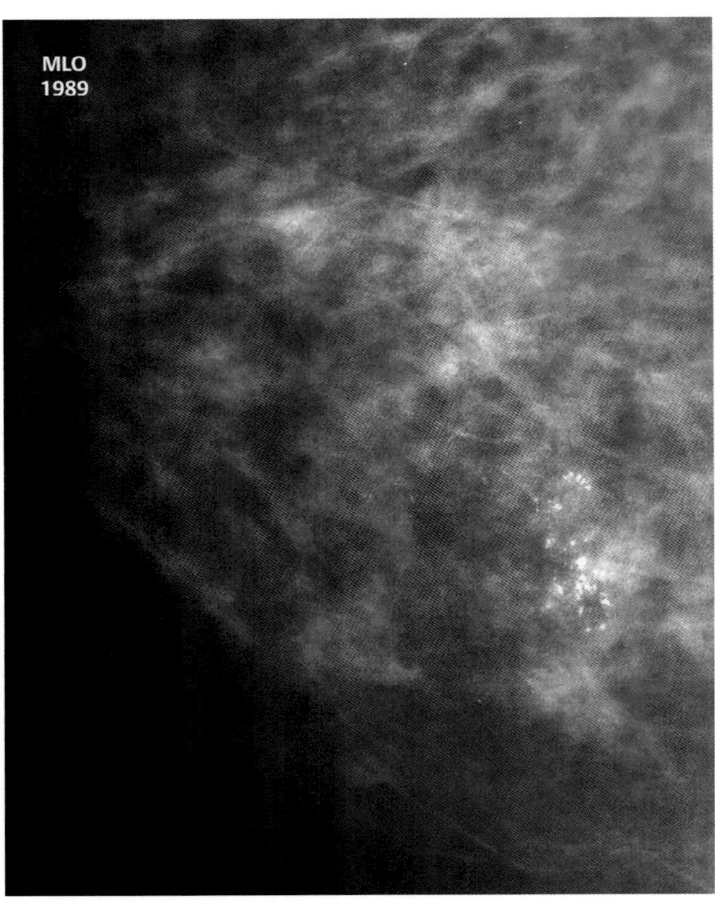


**a** Oblique mammogram of the right breast in December, 1989. The breast parenchyma is relatively dense and shows nonspecific opacities and clustered microcalcifications occupying an area 1 cm × 1.5 cm × 2 cm in size. The calcifications are pleomorphic and suspicious (ACR 3, BIRADS 4b).

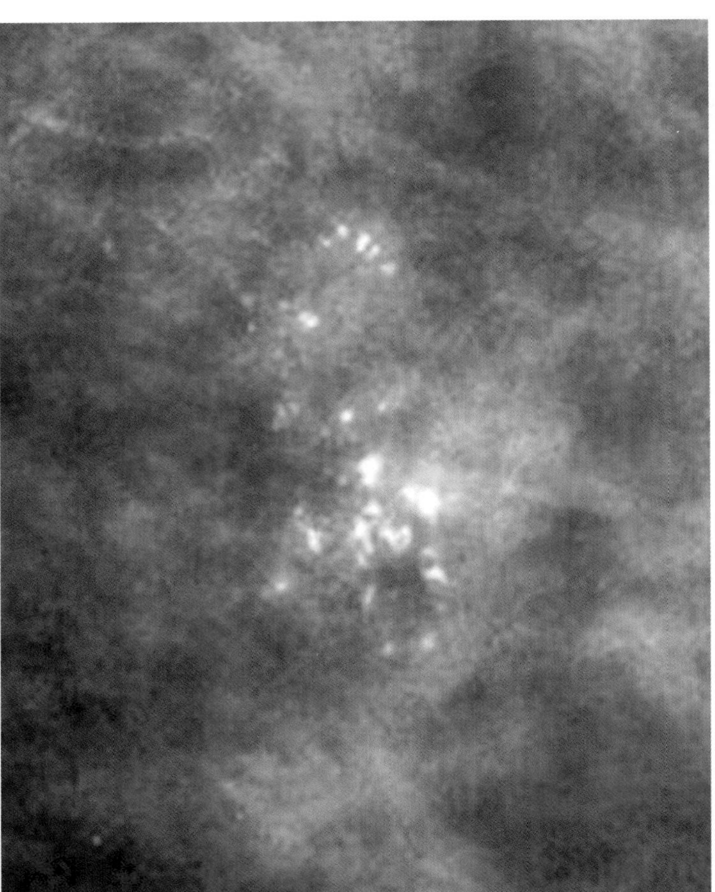

**b** Magnified view of the calcifications (5 ×).

**Fig. 4.21 Progression of malignant calcifications.** *(continued)*

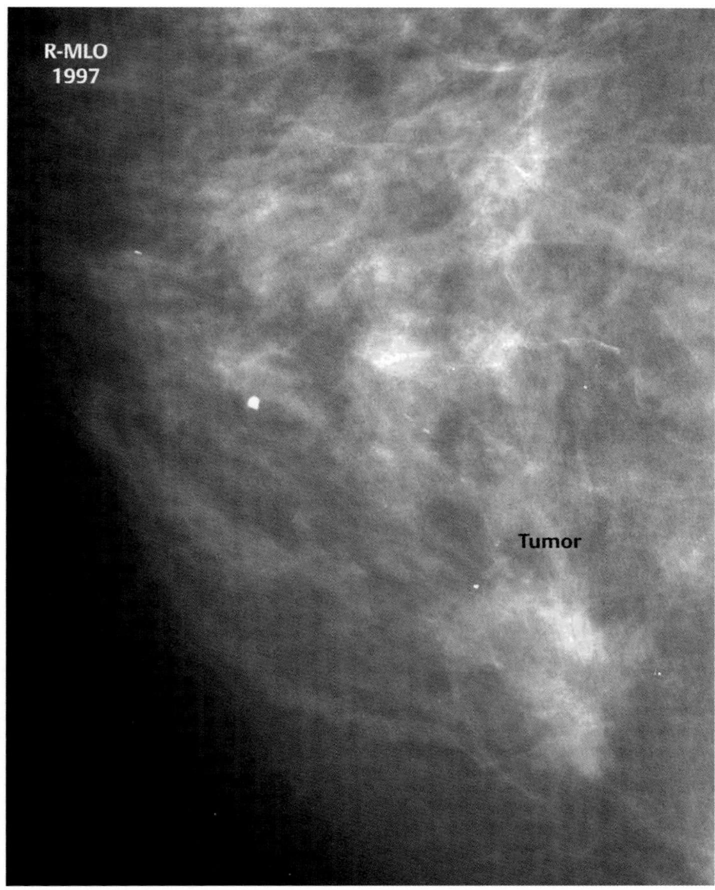


**c** Oblique mammogram of the right breast in June, 1997. The area that formerly contained calcifications is now occupied by an inhomogeneous, spiculated tumor measuring 2.5 cm × 2.5 cm × 5 cm. Calcifications are no longer present in that area. Isolated comedo calcifications are visible toward the nipple (ACR 3, BIRADS 5).
**Note:** Microcalcifications of DCIS can disappear when this precancerous stage changes in invasive cancer!

This observation cannot be an isolated incident. Otherwise, given the great many DCIS lesions that are diagnosed purely on the basis of calcifications, we would expect to find considerably more calcium in invasive neoplasms than is actually the case—assuming the invasive tumor originated from DCIS. This explains why calcifying ADH and in situ carcinomas are the domain of *mammography*, while invasive, early noncalcifying carcinomas and their precursors are the domain of *ultrasound*, and MRI should be combined in screening programs and should begin by age 40 whenever possible (see **Fig. 2.2 c**).

DCIS accounts for 25% of all breast neoplasms identified by pathologists (American Cancer Society, 1997). Approximately 20 years ago this rate was only about 6%. The increase has been documented not only in the United States but also in Europe (Svane 2004) and in those European countries without screening-programs like Switzerland (Levi et al. 1997). The increase in the United States in recent decades can be explained by the implementation of screening programs. In Germany it is explained by the "Gray Breast Screening" program in which approximately 5 million mammograms are taken annually. This has been paralleled by an increased rate of open breast biopsies in women with harmless calcifications—a significant cost obstacle to early detection (to say nothing of the psychological distress to patients). Women should no longer have to undergo primary excisional biopsy for the histologic investigation of breast microcalcifications. This can easily be accomplished by ambulatory interventions (digital stereotactic core-needle or vacuum-biopsy, see p. 230).

It has been estimated that only about 30% of all DCIS lesions contain calcifications. The majority are noncalcifying precursors that remain silent and undetected in the breast. From time to time they are discovered as a result of increased duct density, nipple retraction, a bloody or serous nipple discharge, or—in involuted breasts—by small, ill-defined focal opacities on mammograms or ill-defined hypoechoic areas at ultrasound (see **Figs. 4.26, 4.27**) or at MRI with local gadolinium spots (see **Figs. 5.36 e, 5.79, 5.124 b**).

The increased rate of detection of DCIS is one reason for the decline in breast cancer mortality. In the United States, for example, the *total cancer mortality* curve is trending downward for the first time. After decades of steady increase, the age-standardized cancer mortality rate fell by 3.1% between 1990 and 1995, to a total of 24% in 2003 (Koch 1996, Jatoi et al. 2007).

From 2002 to 2006 the average age of patients presenting with breast cancer in the United States was 68 years (1% between *age 20 and 34*, 6% between *age 35 and 44*, 15% between *age 45 and 54*, 20% between *age 55 and 64*, 20% between *age 65 and 74*, 23% between *age 75 and 84*, and 15% above *age 85*). About 14% of the affected women were under 50 years of age.

On January 1, 2006 in the Unites States there were approximately 2 533 193 women alive with a history of breast cancer (SEER statistics, Horner et al. 2009).

Experts claim that the decline in breast cancer mortality is due largely to effective screening programs and optimized treatment protocols resulting in higher cure rates. The declining use of HRT based on the WHI study results is probably related to the falling incidence of breast cancer. The decrease had already begun in 1999, but after 2002 the incidence rose by 11%, paralleling a sharp decline in HRT based on the WHI study (Emons 2008).

Breast cancer mortality in Germany declined from 28.7% (per 100 000 deaths) to 25.9% during the period from 1995 to 1999. The trend should continue with an increasing frequency of DCIS removals, but while breast cancer and its precursors are being diagnosed with greater frequency, the mortality rate from this disease remains the same. Mortality rates should improve as screening mammography is instituted on a broader scale. The increased utilization of magnetic resonance imaging in younger women with a family history of breast cancer should help as well, although the implementation of screening MRI is still constrained by high costs (Kuhl et al. 2007). Approximately 50% of all DCIS lesions show preoperative gadolinium enhancement. Recurrent lesions have similar enhancement characteristics to the original tumors. The larger the DCIS and the closer it is to a high-grade lesion (G3), the more it enhances. Gilles et al. (1995) noted early postgadolinium enhancement in 34 of 36 ductal carcinomas in situ, although two of these high-grade lesions conspicuously did not enhance. The fact that certain low-grade DCIS (G1; Van-Nuys Index 1–3, see p. 58) are not visible on MR mammograms does not weaken the rationale for performing breast MRI (especially for cost reasons). The value of MR mammography in an individual case can be determined only after the examination has been completed. Disadvantages of postoperative MR mammography are the potential for surgically induced gadolinium enhancement and the frequent lack of preoperative images for comparison.

**Fig. 4.22 Fibroadenoma or ADH?** A 51-year-old woman with no family history of breast cancer presented for a screening examination. She had no palpable abnormalities but did have a previously known fibroadenoma at the 2-o'clock position in the outer upper quadrant of the left breast.

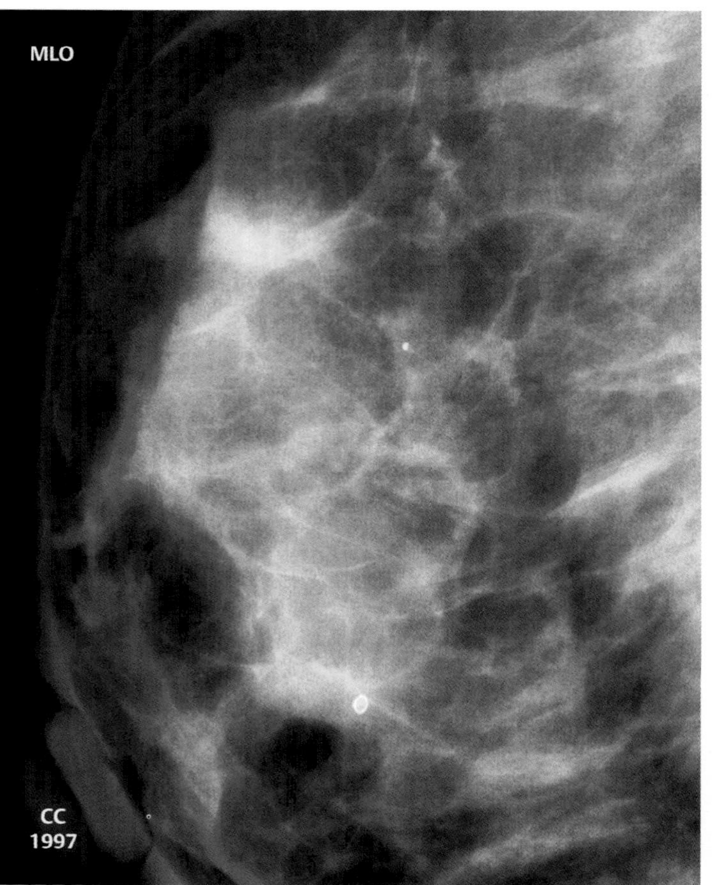


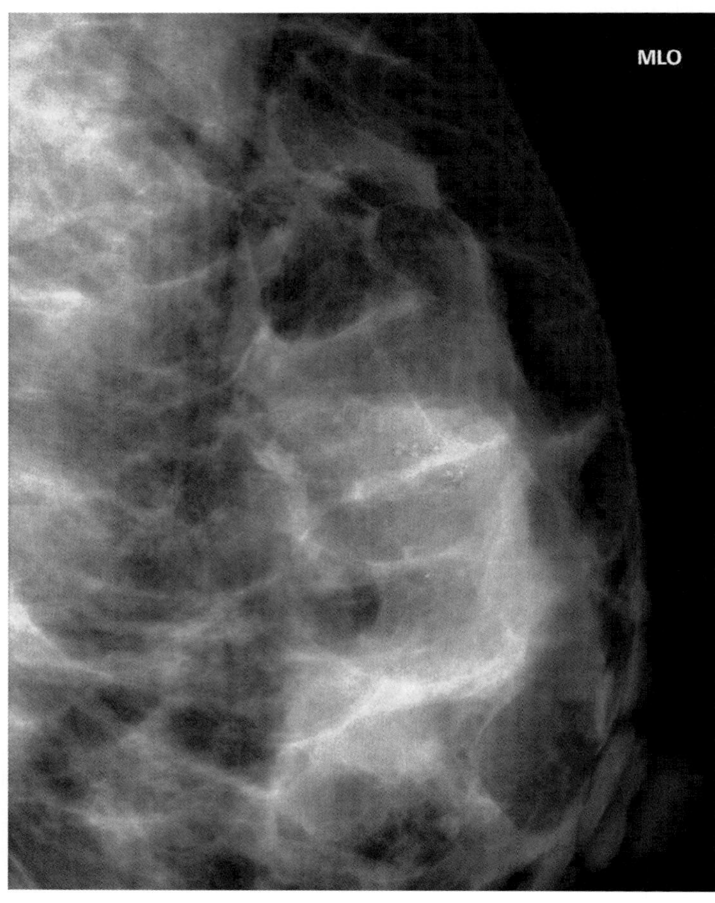


**a, b** Bilateral oblique mammograms. New clustered microcalcifications are visible in the upper portion of the left breast at the 11-o'clock position (**I/21**). They are relatively pleomorphic and occupy an area approximately 1 cm in diameter (ACR3, BIRADS?, **P**GMI).

The enhancement characteristics and margins of gadolinium-enhancing foci are extremely important in MR mammography, as ill-defined margins are suspicious for malignancy. Like conventional mammography and ultrasound, MR mammography cannot distinguish among ductal hyperplasia (DH), DCIS, and microinvasive or invasive carcinoma.

DCIS displays many variants that can be appreciated in mammography, ultrasound, MRI, and cytology. All physicians who deal with breast imaging should understand the pathology of these lesions so that they can properly interpret mammograms, sonograms, and MR images singly or in combination.

### Tip

**If the nature of clustered microcalcifications remains uncertain, it is better to recommend a core-needle or vacuum biopsy under digital stereotactic guidance than the usual short-term follow-ups. The biopsy can be done quickly on an outpatient basis, is well tolerated, and can provide a definitive diagnosis. It also relieves patient anxiety by eliminating the waiting time for future follow-ups. Moreover, follow-ups are often unrewarding because benign adenosis and particularly low-grade (G1) in situ carcinomas calcify very slowly over a period of years or even decades, and the calcifications may regress or disappear completely on progression to an invasive neoplasm. Short-term follow-ups tend to increase more than allay the patient's (and doctor's) level of uncertainty.**

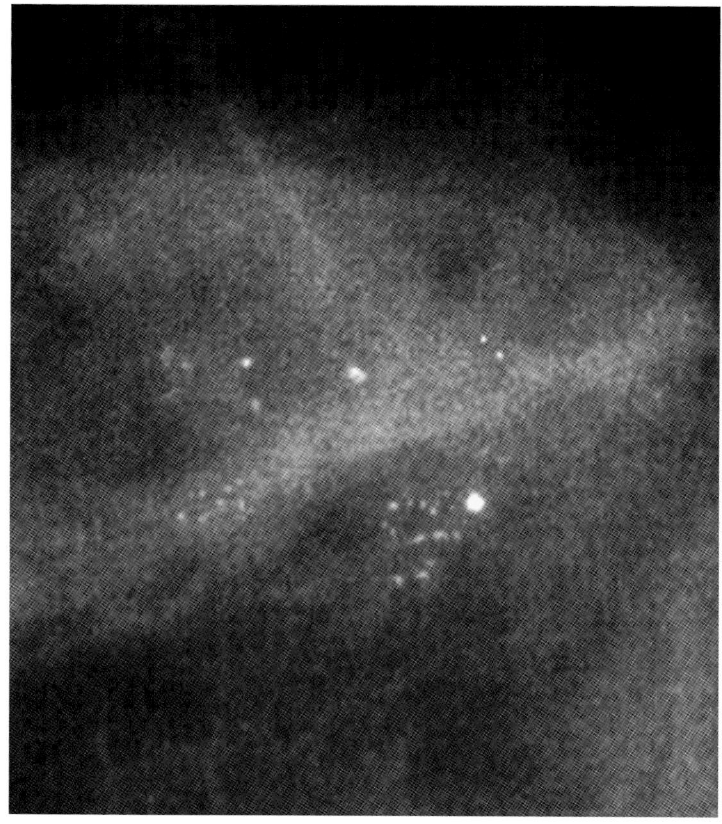

**c** Magnified view of the calcifications in mediolateral oblique view.

**Fig. 4.22 Fibroadenoma or ADH?** *(continued)*

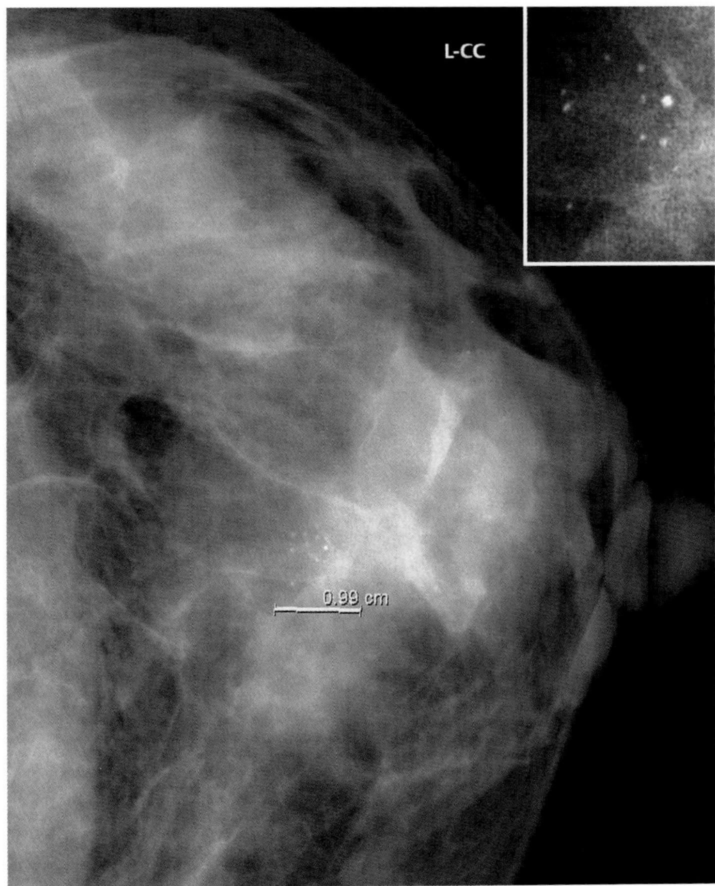


**d** Craniocaudal mammogram of the left breast shows clustered microcalcifications located at approximately the 11-o'clock position (**M/20**) (ACR3, BIRADS?, **P**GMI). The inset at upper right is a magnified view of the calcifications.

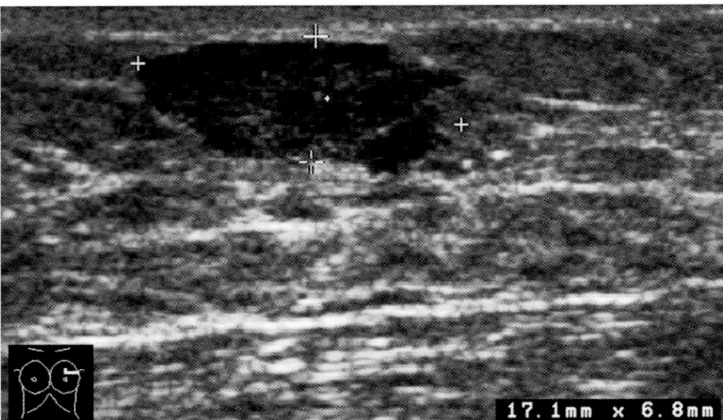


**e** Ultrasound scan of the left breast shows a 1.7 × 0.4 × 0.4 cm fibroadenoma at the 2-o'clock position with smooth margins and internal echoes. The benign tumor shows no change in size or shape relative to the previous examination.

**Question on Fig. 4.22**

*How would you interpret the calcifications?*

(**a**) Fibroadenoma
(**b**) ADH/DCIS
(**c**) Blunt duct adenosis

→ **Answer on p. 346**

### Therapeutic Implications

Despite the absence of invasiveness on pathologic examination, a 1–6% incidence of axillary lymph node metastasis has been reported in the literature (Holland et al. 1990). These figures include metastases from DCIS lesions larger than 2 cm.

> **!** **The detection of lymph node metastasis always signifies an invasive tumor (see Fig. 5.87, p. 199).**

According to Holland et al. (1990), the metastasis rate is very low for DCIS lesions smaller than 2 cm. It rises sharply with lesions more than 2.5 cm in diameter, however. The risk of nipple involvement increases as well. Every DCIS lesion, regardless of its size, should receive postoperative radiation to the breast of 50 Gy without a boost. This has been shown to reduce the invasive and noninvasive recurrence rate from 4.8% to 1.9% (Julien et al. 2000). Postoperative radiotherapy has very little effect on recurrence rate when applied to low-grade malignancies. Thus, postoperative radiation may be omitted for tumors smaller than 2 cm (low-grade G1) that have been encompassed with a 10 mm margin of healthy tissue (according to AGO, German Cancer Society).

Böcker et al. (1997) state that, as a general rule, DCIS is already large at the time of its detection (see **Figs. 4.22, 4.23**). While it is true that invasive cancers are being detected at a significantly smaller size than previously because of the increased use of mammography, this is not the case with DCIS. Improved diagnosis has led to an absolute and relative increase in the diagnosis of DCIS, but there has been no trend toward the detection of smaller lesions. Most DCIS lesions involve an area approximately 5 cm in diameter; smaller lesions are much less common. All DCIS lesions may be multicentric. DCIS is described as **multifocal** when there is a distance of at least 4 cm between individual foci. It is **multicentric** only when lesions are distributed over multiple breast quadrants.

> ***Tip***
>
> **If histopathologic analysis (after core-needle or vacuum biopsy) shows evidence of multicentric DCIS, the possibility of bilateral lesions should also be considered (MRI is recommended).**

Ninety percent of poorly differentiated (G3) DCIS lesions undergo **contiguous** intraductal spread (see **Fig. 4.28**), while 70% of well-differentiated (G1) DCIS arise as **multifocal** lesions. A possible reason for this phenomenon is that as the acini and alveoli mature in both breasts, they are vulnerable to the effects of potentially harmful endogenous and exogenous agents (see p. 9).

The distances between the individual foci, called “gaps” by pathologists, are usually very small. Approximately 82% of the gaps are smaller than 4 mm, 10% are from 5 to 9 mm, and 8% are 10 mm or larger. This means that the radiologist should mark or otherwise indicate for the surgeon all calcifications or sonographic/MRI abnormalities in the area surrounding the main calcification cluster. Additional lesions can be detected with digital full-field (microspot) mammography or conventional biplane magnification mammography for inclusion in the biopsy specimen. Thus, ultrasound and magnetic resonance imaging should definitely be used in patients who are found to have relatively large areas of calcification.

For the surgeon, this means that ADH and DCIS should be encompassed as widely as possible, giving attention to areas that may lie outside the mammographically visible focus (**Figs. 4.22, 4.23**). Breast-conserving surgery should always take precedence over subcutaneous or total mastectomy (which is necessary at multicentricity)—for if ADH or DCIS has been detected by the presence of microcalcifications, any local recurrence is also likely to develop calcifications after a certain latent period, enabling it to be detected and reexcised at an early stage. Local recurrences are sometimes difficult to distinguish from postsurgical fat necrosis, but this is facilitated by noting that recurrences take longer to develop than fat necrosis. Every operation that removes breast calcifications requires follow-up. This may be done immediately after the operation (especially if there is doubt that the calcifications were completely removed) or by 3 months at the latest in order to detect any residual calcifications and subsequently distinguish recurrences from fat necrosis. Follow-up mammograms should consist of biplane views since postoperative calcifications are sometimes obscured by organized bloody effusions and scars and may be invisible in just one plane. Additional follow-ups should then be scheduled at 6 months or 12 months (depending on the recommendation of the country’s own guidelines) using the view that best displayed the operative area. Magnification mammography or digital full-field mammography with CAD (see p. 100) is recommended to allow for maximum magnification. Surgeons and radiologists are generally held responsible for local recurrences because they were unsuccessful in removing all neoplasia from the breast. The pathologist is considered blameless.

In a study by Liberman et al. (1997), local recurrences of DCIS were detected an average of 26 months after surgery (range from 6 to 198 months). Eighty-five percent were detected by mammography alone, 10% by palpation and mammography, and 5% by physical examination alone. Ninety percent of local recurrences developed the same microcalcifications as the primary tumor.

*(continued on p. 48)*

**Fig. 4.23 Asymmetry, inhomogeneities, and calcifications** in the breast of a 68-year-old woman. The patient presented for routine screening. Mammography 3 years ago was normal.

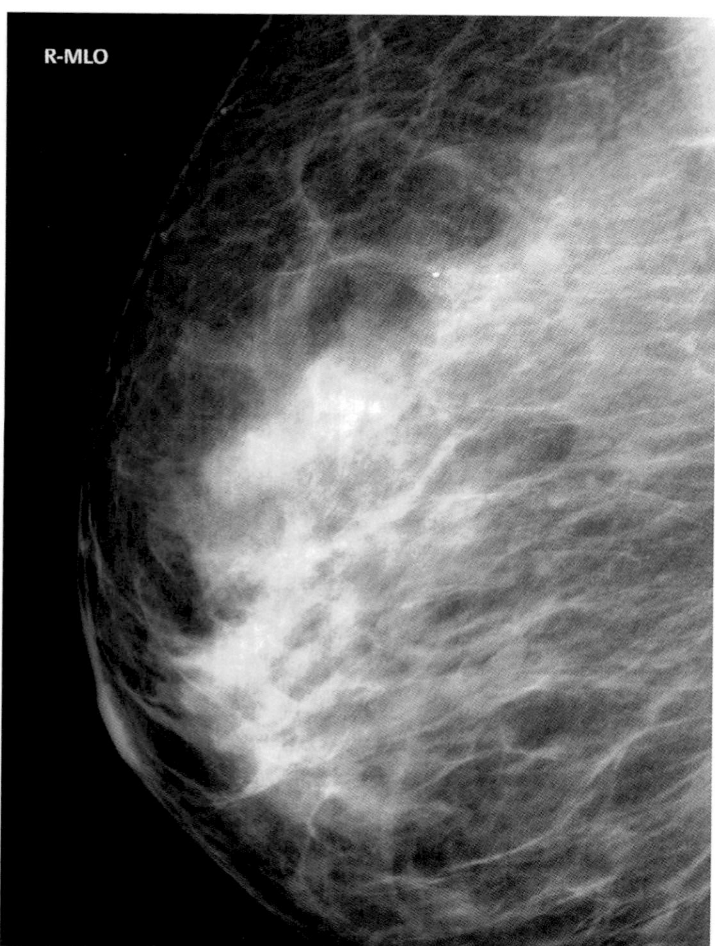


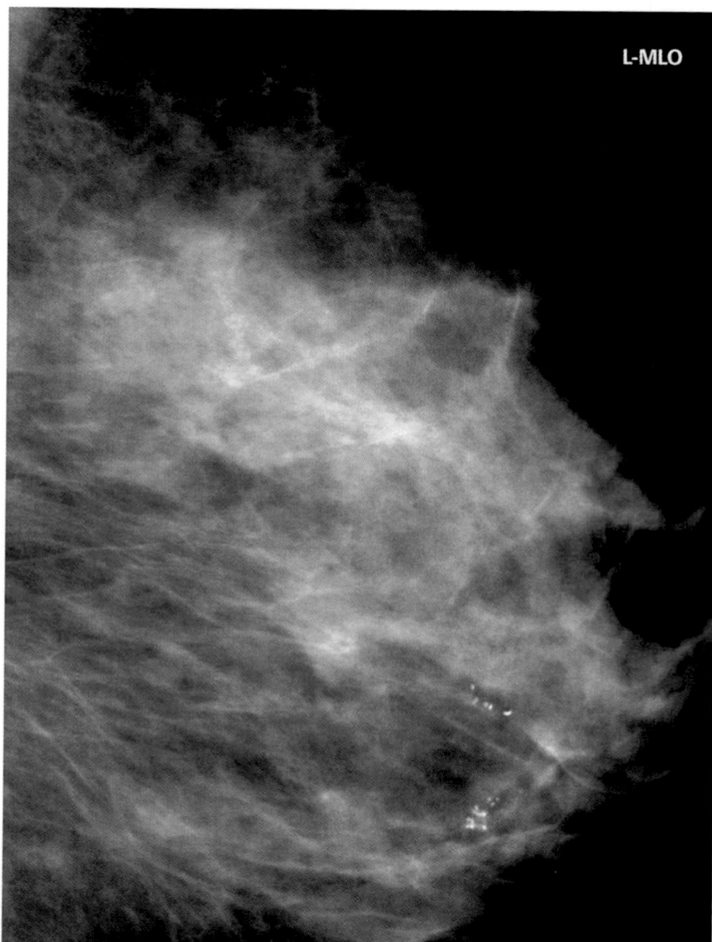


**a, b** Bilateral oblique mammograms show dense breasts with nonvisualization of the pectoral muscle (ACR 2, BIRADS?, PGMI).

**Fig. 4.23 Asymmetry, inhomogeneities, and calcifications.** *(continued)*

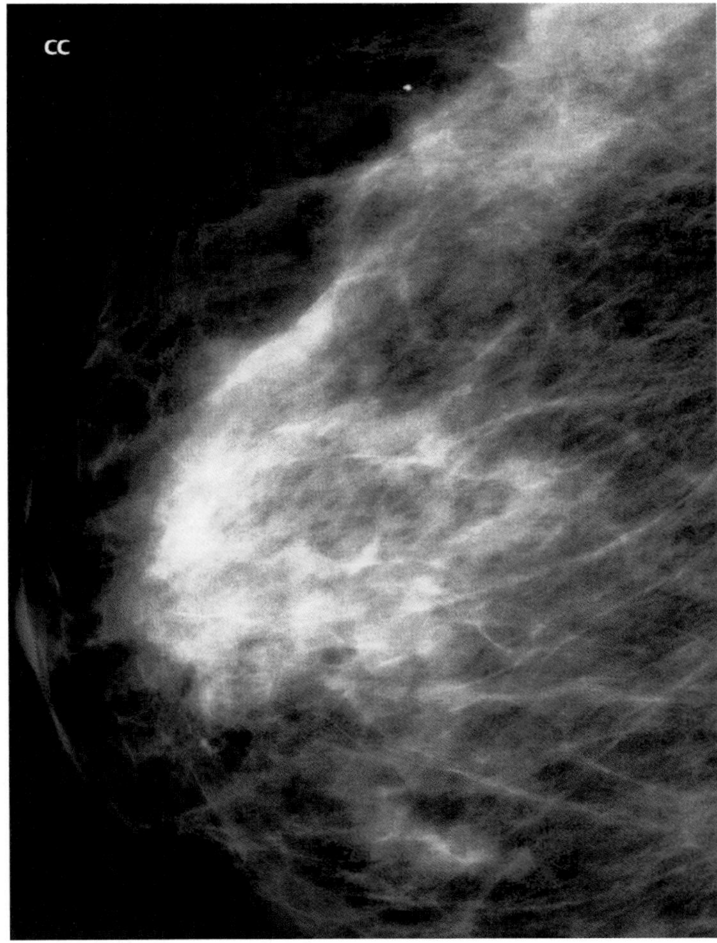


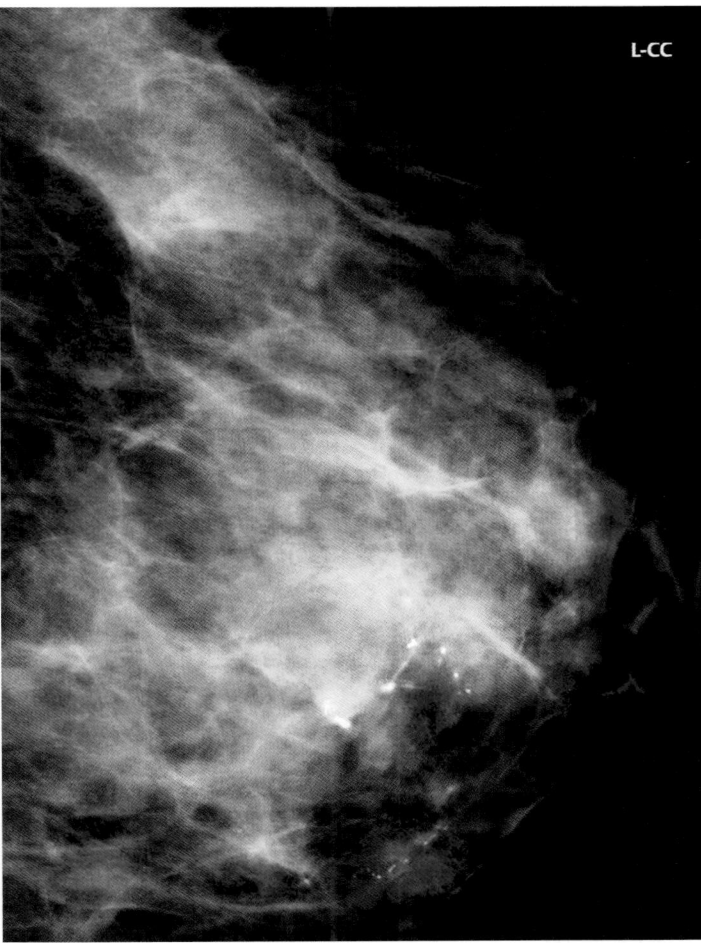


**c, d** Bilateral craniocaudal mammograms. The breast parenchyma appears less dense than in the oblique projection. The pectoral muscle is not visualized. Calcifications at **r/18–19** (ACR 2, BIRADS?, PGMI).

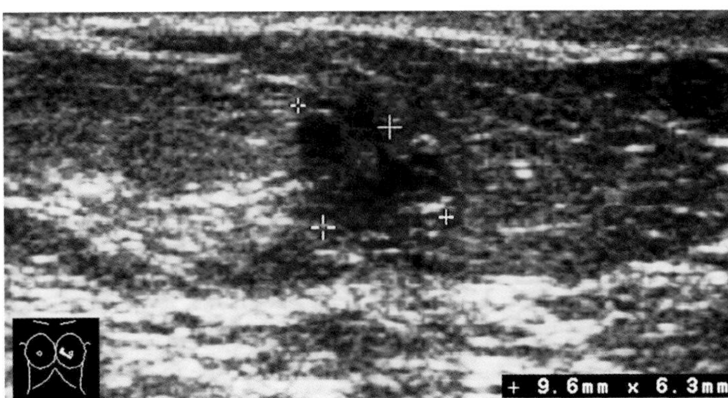


**e** Ultrasound demonstrates small, hypoechoic foci in the inner quadrant of the left breast (**l–m/10–11**) (see marker inside the image).

**Question 1 on Fig. 4.23**

*Is there a pathologic process in either breast at mammography? (Give coordinates.)*

(**a**) No

(**b**) Yes

**Question 2 on Fig. 4.23**

*How would you interpret the calcifications in the left breast according to the ultrasound examination (**e**)?*

(**a**) Benign microcystic calcification

(**b**) Malignant calcification

**Question 3 on Fig. 4.23**

*How would you describe the structural pattern of both breasts based on a careful comparison of both sides?*

(**a**) Both breasts are homogeneous.

(**b**) One side is a little bit more inhomogeneous (left or right?).

→ **Answers on p. 346**

*(continued from p. 46)*

In situ carcinomas that accompany invasive carcinoma are a major consideration in selecting patients for breast-conserving therapy. This is reflected in the term **"extensive intraductal component"** (EIC). EIC was formerly viewed as a contraindication to breast-conserving therapy because of the risk of local recurrence. Today this is no longer the case, although EIC may be an indication for postoperative radiotherapy, even in patients with very small, low-grade invasive carcinomas (**Fig. 4.24**).

*(continued on p. 51)*

**Fig. 4.24 Mammograms in a 47-year-old woman with breast-conserving therapy (BCT) in February, 1998.** The patient detected a nodule herself at the 2-o'clock position in the upper outer quadrant of the left breast. The mammogram shows a small spiculated density with microcalcifications (**a–d**). After several reexcisions for new calcifications, three uneventful years passed until a follow-up in June, 2004 (**e–k**), when new microcalcifications were found in a small nodule that was also visible sonographically in the upper outer quadrant (**h**). Nonspecific firmness was noted in the sternal recess on the right side.

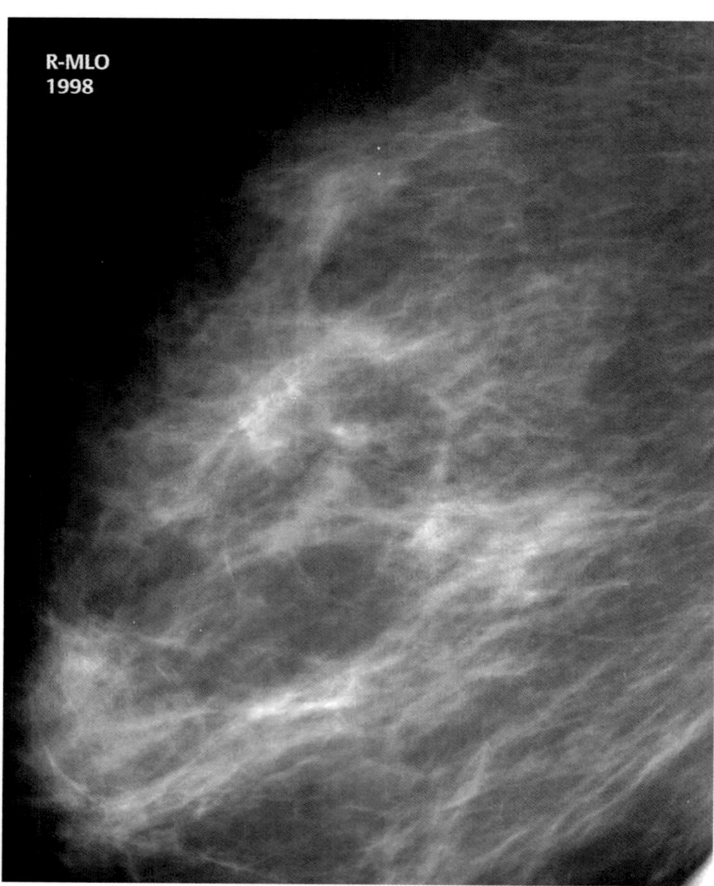


**a** Oblique mammogram of the right breast in February, 1998 shows normal radiolucent breast parenchyma.

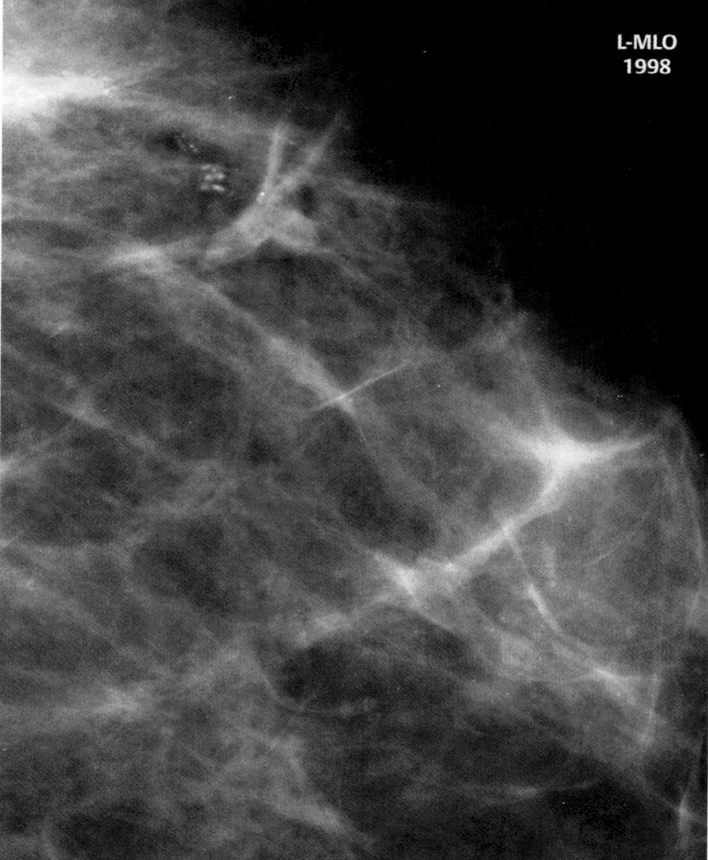


**b** Oblique mammogram of the left breast (magnified view of the upper portion) shows a spiculated density with clustered atypical microcalcifications (**g–h/18–20**) (ACR 2, BIRADS 4, PG**M**I).

**Fig. 4.24 BCT without radiation in the presence of EIC.** *(continued)*

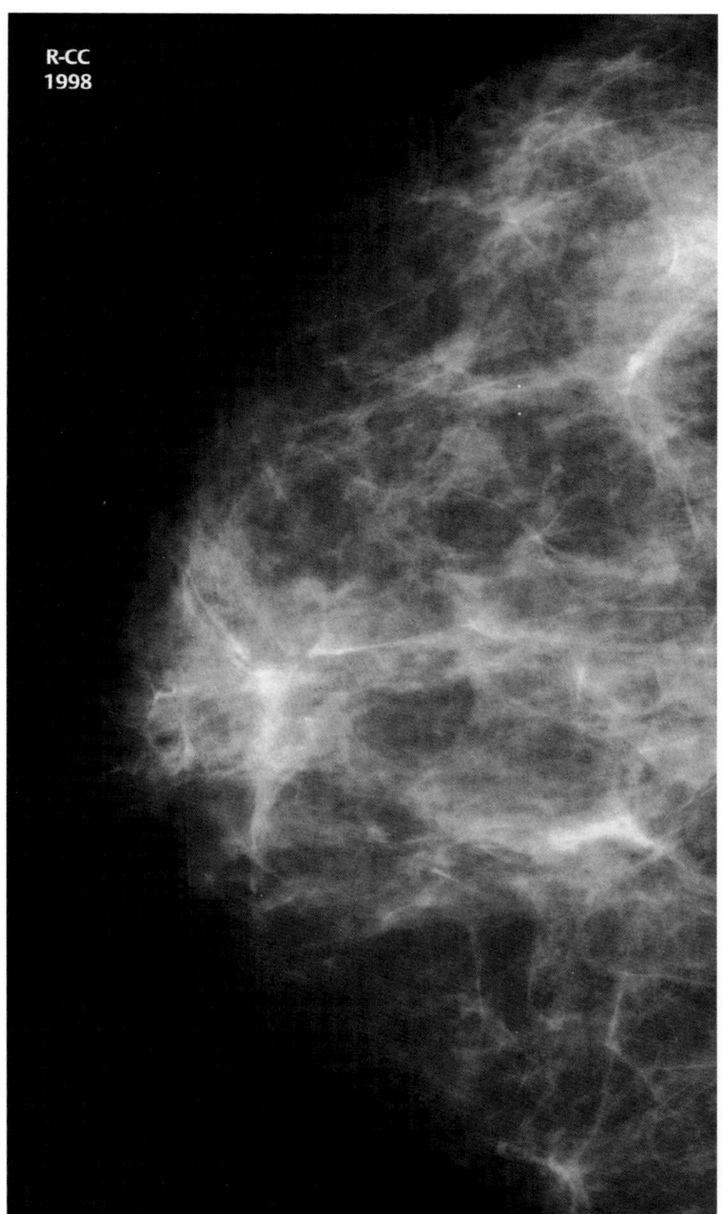


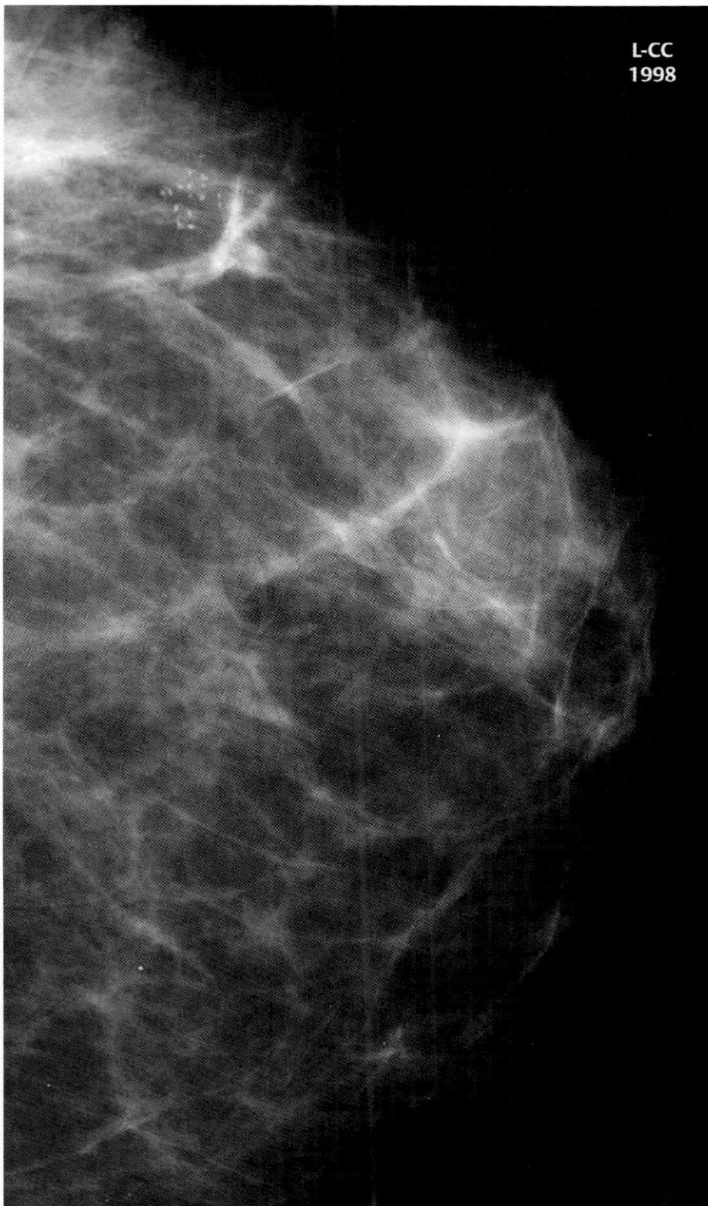


**c, d** Bilateral craniocaudal mammograms in February, 1998 show moderate radiodensity with markedly increased parenchymal density at the site of the palpable left breast nodule (**Q, 24–25**). Some microcalcifications are visible. **Histology** revealed *poorly differentiated invasive ductal carcinoma with a pronounced extensive intraductal components* (EIC, see pp. 48, 75) and focal microcalcifications. The tumor was easily demonstrated by ultrasound and MRI. No additional foci were detected on either side in 1998. The patient (a surgeon) refused radiation and other additional therapies!

▶ Fig. 4.24 e–h

**Fig. 4.24 Follow-up after BCT without radiation in the presence of EIC.** *(continued)*

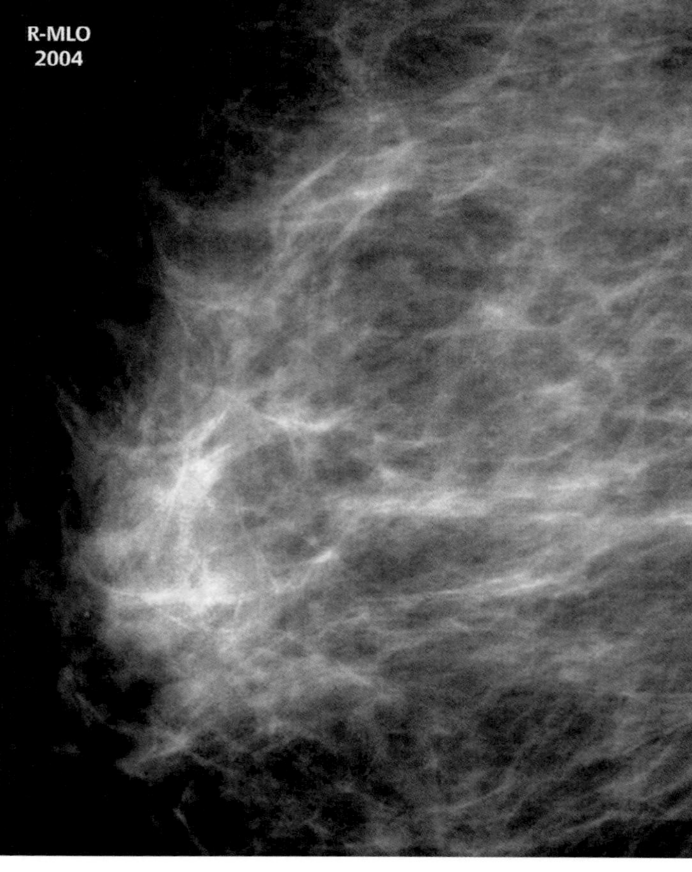


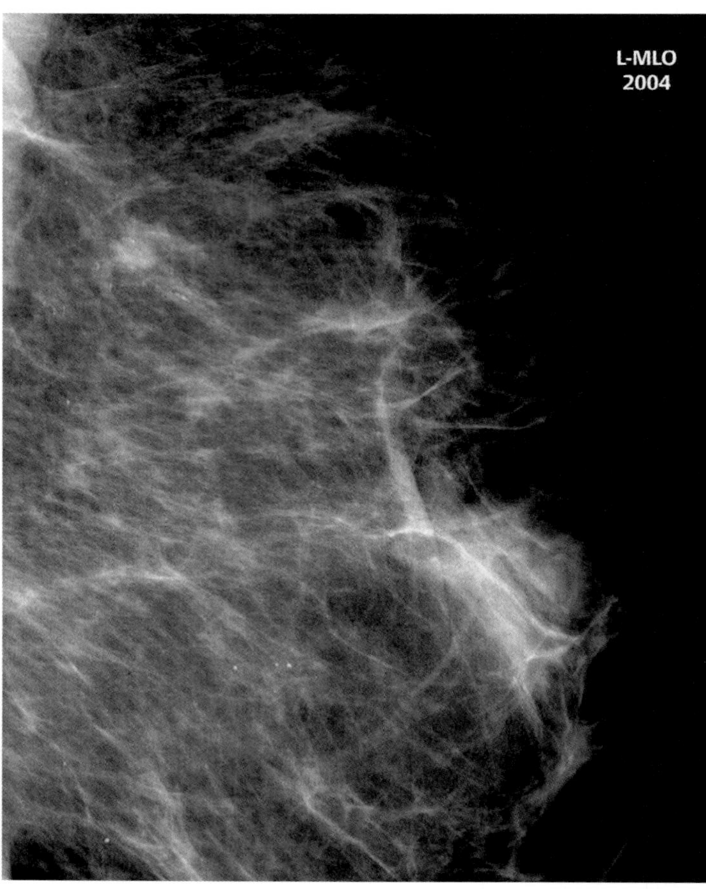


**e, f** Bilateral oblique mammograms in June, 2004 show small focal opacities in the left breast with extensive atypical microcalcifications (**G/24–25**).

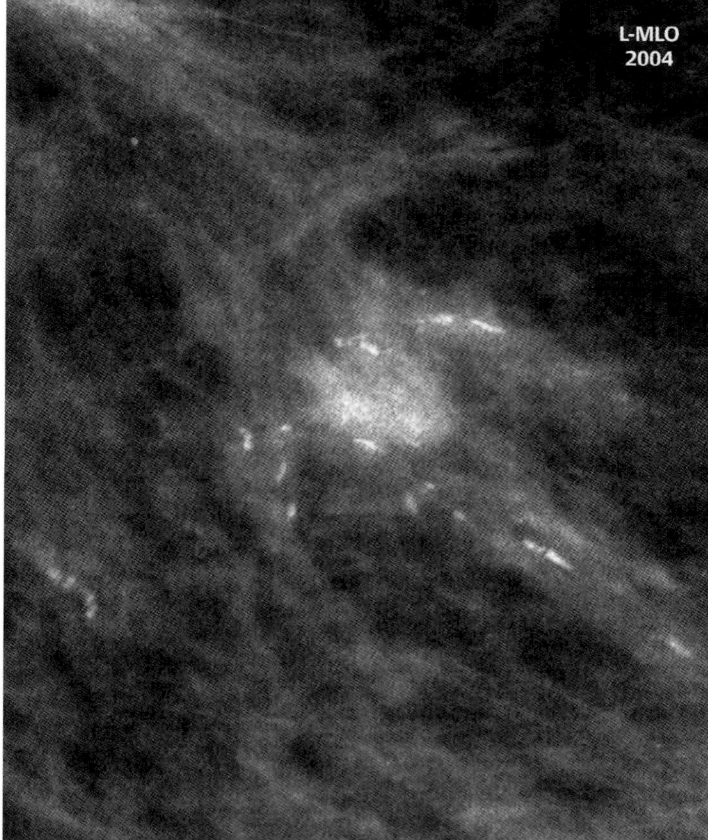


**g** Digital magnification mammogram shows a small unsharp nodule with surrounding microcalcifications (**b–e/5–10**). **Histology** revealed invasive ductal carcinoma with an EIC.

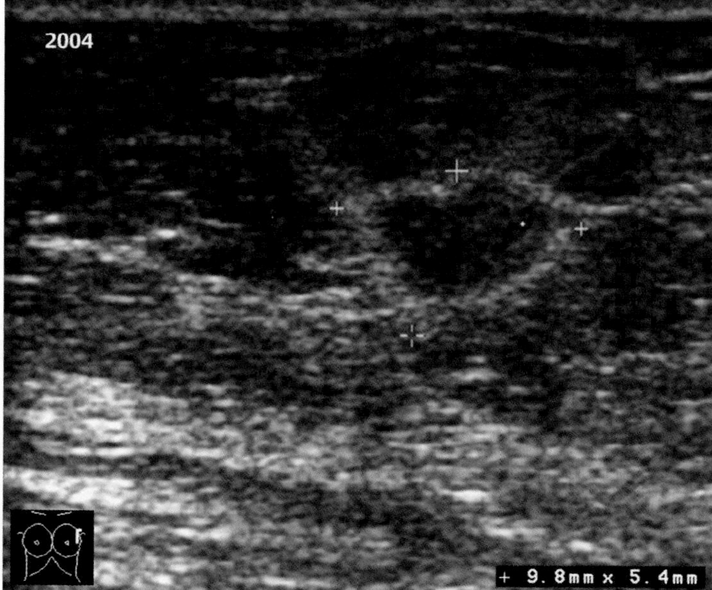


**h** Sonogram of the left outer quadrant (see marker) shows an 8 mm hypoechoic area with irregular margins (**h–j/11–12**). The area was investigated by ultrasound-guided core-needle biopsy and again reveals an *invasive ductal carcinoma with EIC and comedo-calcifications*.

**Question on Fig. 4.24**

*Do the mammograms from 2004 show any other abnormality in the left or right breast?*

(**a**) No

(**b**) Yes (coordinates?)

→ **Answer on p. 346**

*(continued from p. 48)*
Böcker et al. (1997) conclude that noninvasive ductal neoplasms represent a morphologically and biologically diverse spectrum of diseases ranging from focal ADH to advanced DCIS. A large percentage of the lesions are **focal processes** that can be managed with breast-conserving therapy. The pathologist may find it difficult to distinguish these lesions from hyperplasia, identify the exact subtype of ductal neoplasia, and confirm negative margins. This extra preoperative work (for the radiologist and the surgeon) and the increased difficulty of differential diagnosis place high demands on modern breast pathologists. It is with good reason that European guidelines prescribe a second opinion on histologic specimens during the first two years of screening, with a requirement that the corresponding paraffin blocks be submitted in the case of nonmalignant lesions. In lesions with microcalcifications, a radiograph of the paraffin block prepared by the pathologist should always be taken in addition to the specimen radiograph so that it can be compared with the calcifications found at histology. **Paraffin-block radiography** should be done prospectively, i.e., concurrently with each work-up. This will provide good orientation for pathologists, enabling them to determine whether they are evaluating the center or periphery of the calcifications. A "post-section" radiograph of the paraffin block is difficult to interpret unless a "pre-section" radiograph is also available. This requires considerable extra logistical work and staffing, however, and this is rarely possible or cost-effective in most hospital settings.

During a 5-year screening period in Sweden (Uppsala), 474 DCIS and invasive neoplasms were diagnosed in a series of 75 000 women. Eighty-five of those cases involved nonpalpable lesions and atypical microcalcifications. Only one in five screening-detected neoplasms was detected due to the presence of atypical microcalcifications. *Paraffin-block radiography* was a valuable adjunct in these cases to ensure that the areas bearing calcifications were actually examined. Interestingly, six women in this study with an initial benign diagnosis were later given a malignant diagnosis based solely on paraffin-block radiography and further processing.

The selective removal of a lesion with clear margins and the specific identification of DH, FEA, ADH, DCIS, or invasive carcinoma by the pathologist have significant therapeutic implications for the patient. Pathologists may differ significantly in their interpretations of cancer precursor lesions, however, as **Fig. 4.25** illustrates (see also **Figs. 4.26–4.29**).

**Fig. 4.25 The difficulty of diagnosis in the borderline area between DH, ADH, and carcinoma** is illustrated by the case of a 51-year-old woman with microcalcifications in the right breast. Three pathologists gave three different histologic diagnoses.

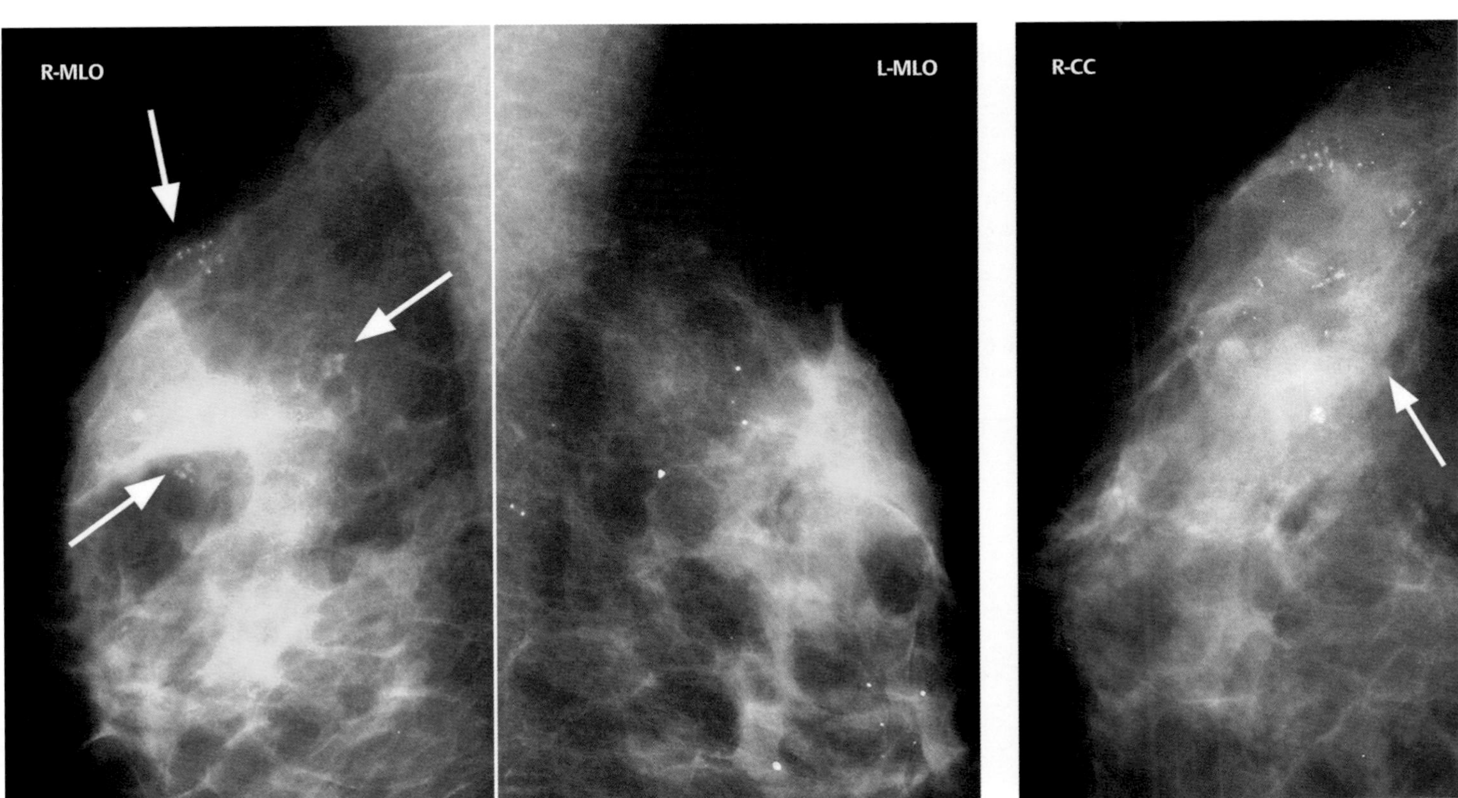


**a** Bilateral oblique mammograms in April, 2002 show disseminated microcalcifications in the upper portion of the right breast (arrows) (ACR 2, BIRADS 4, PGMI). The calcifications were not present in prior mammograms from February, 1998. The image of the left breast shows small cysts with coarse calcifications.

**b** Craniocaudal mammogram shows microcalcifications in the lateral portion of the right breast (arrow) (ACR 2, BIRADS 4, PGMI).

▶ **Fig. 4.25 c, d**

**Fig. 4.25 Borderline area between DH, ADH, and carcinoma.** *(continued)*

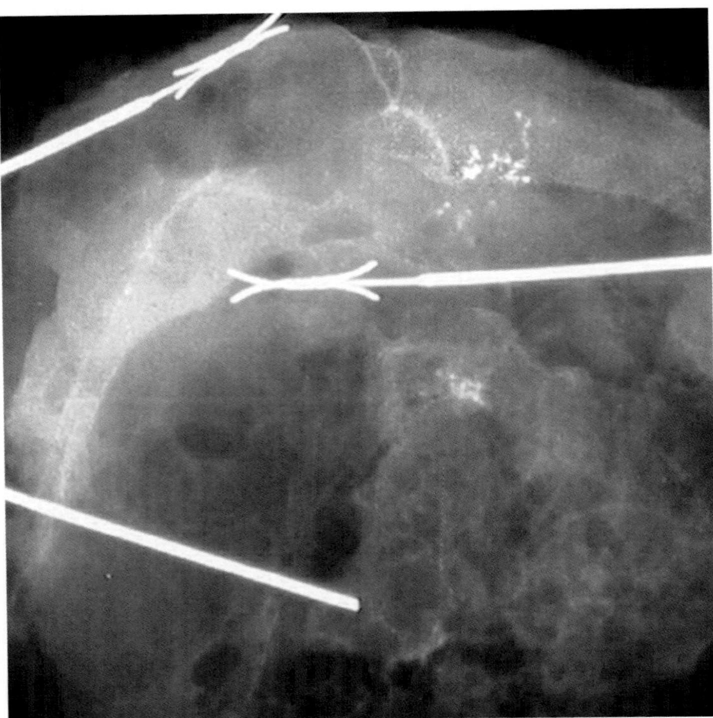

**c** Specimen radiograph with three localizing wires and the main calcification cluster.

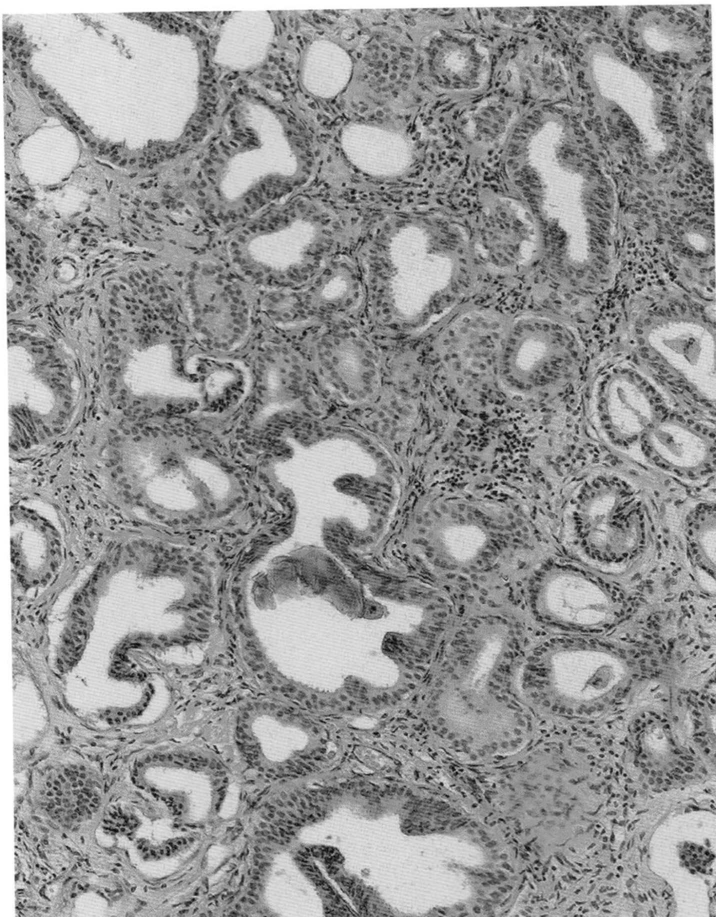

**d** Histologic section of the calcifications. The sections were evaluated by three pathologists.

**Question on Fig. 4.25**

*Which statement is correct?*

(**a**) Benign calcifications were removed with clear margins.
(**b**) Malignant calcifications were removed with clear margins.
(**c**) Benign calcifications were not removed with clear margins.
(**d**) Malignant calcifications were not removed with clear margins.

→ **Answer on p. 347**

**Fig. 4.26 A 62-year-old woman with an 18-month history of recurrent galactorrhea** from a single duct in one breast. She had no other clinical abnormalities and no family history of breast cancer (similar to the case in **Fig. 5.114 a**, p. 245).

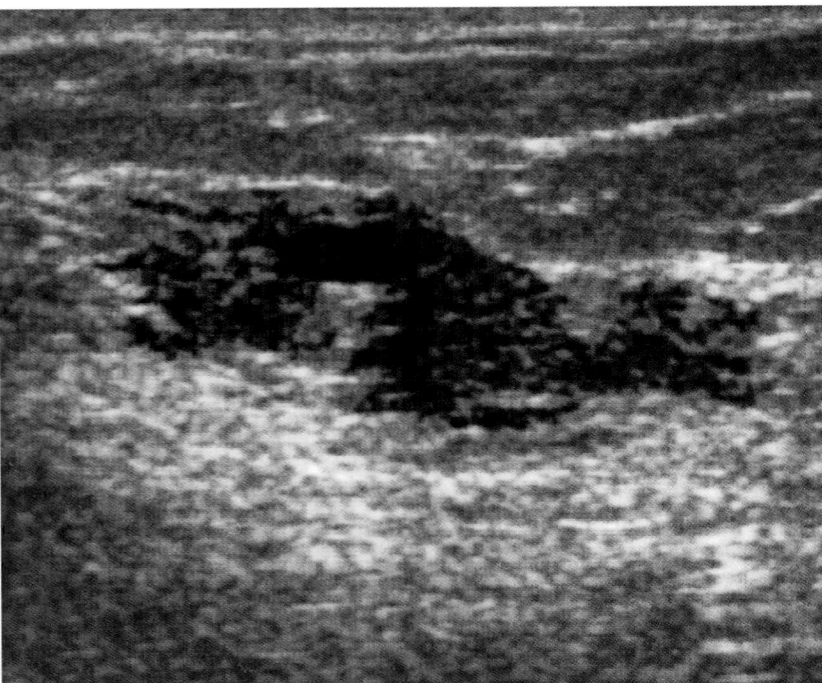

**a** Ultrasound scan of shows a 1.2 × 0.8 × 0.8 cm nodule with smooth margins and a well-circumscribed central hypoechoic cyst. The surrounding tissue is rich in stroma and appears normal.

**Fig. 4.26 Recurrent galactorrhea.** *(continued)*

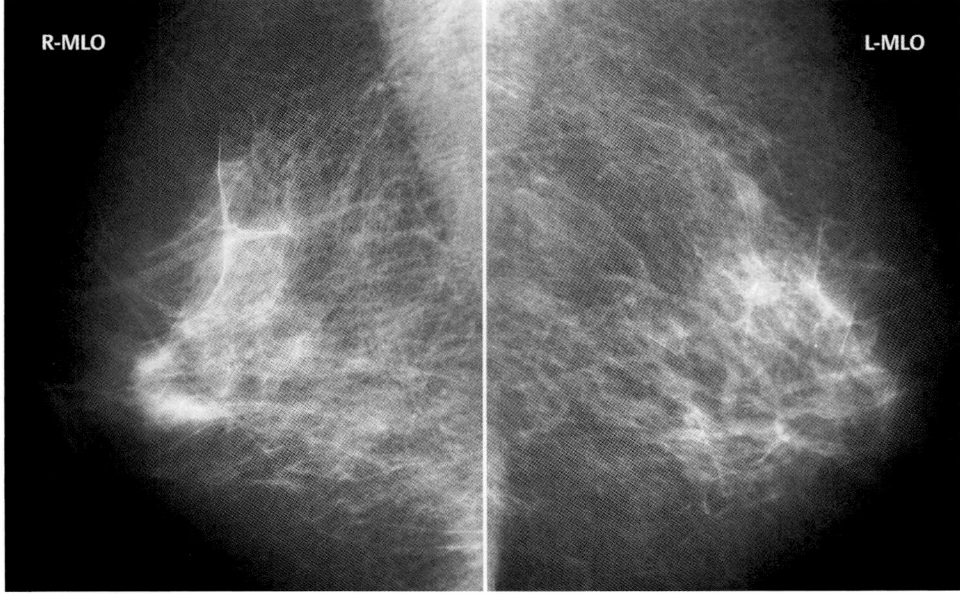


**b** Bilateral oblique mammograms (magnified views). (ACR 2, BIRADS?, P**G**MI).

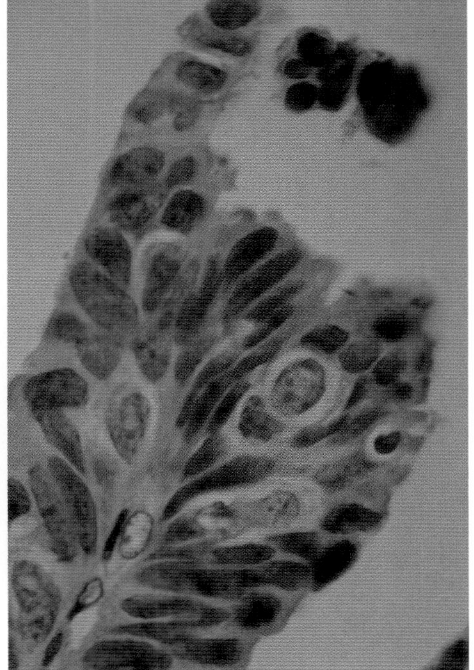

**d** Cytology: fine-needle aspiration (FNA) yields elongated cells with a narrow cytoplasmic rim that are arranged in a "school of fish" pattern.

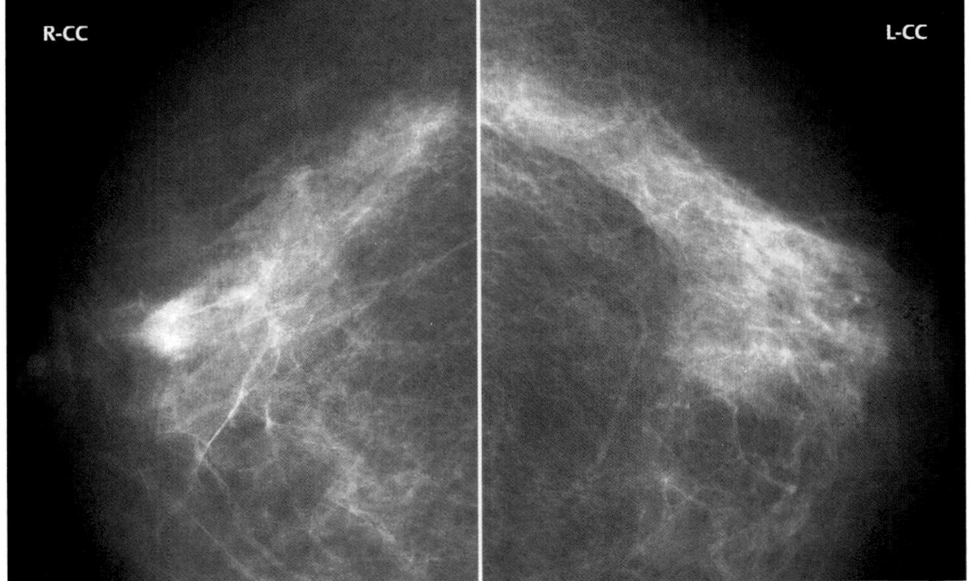


**c** Bilateral craniocaudal mammograms (PG**M**I).

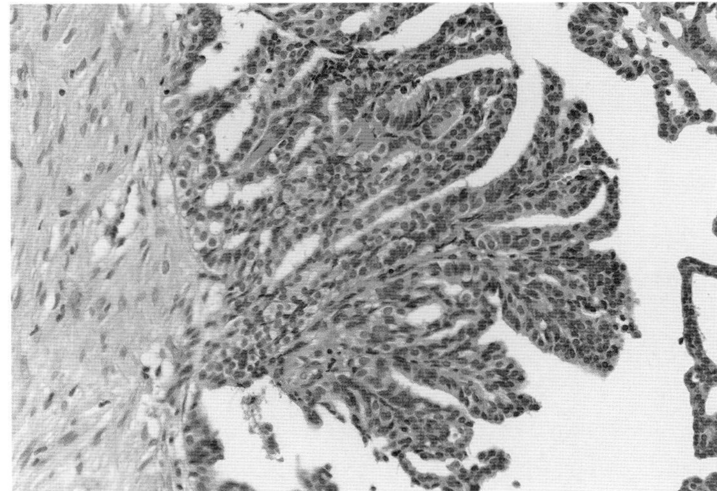

**e** Histologic section shows intraductal proliferation with cells similar to those in **d**.

**Question 1 on Fig. 4.26**

*Where is the tumor located in the mammogram?* (Give coordinates.)

**Question 2 on Fig. 4.26**

*How would you interpret the lesion based on clinical, cytological, sonographic, and mammographic findings?*

(**a**) Fibroadenoma
(**b**) Medullary carcinoma
(**c**) Intacystic or intraductal papilloma

→ **Answers on p. 347**

28 27 26 25 24 23 22 21 20 19 18 17 16 15 14 13 12 11 10 9 8 7 6 5 4 3 2 1

K k L l M m N n O o P p Q q R r S s T t

**Fig. 4.27 A 46-year-old woman with recurrent bilateral galactorrhea**, greater on the right side than on the left. She had no palpable abnormalities, no nipple retraction, and no regional lymph node enlargement.

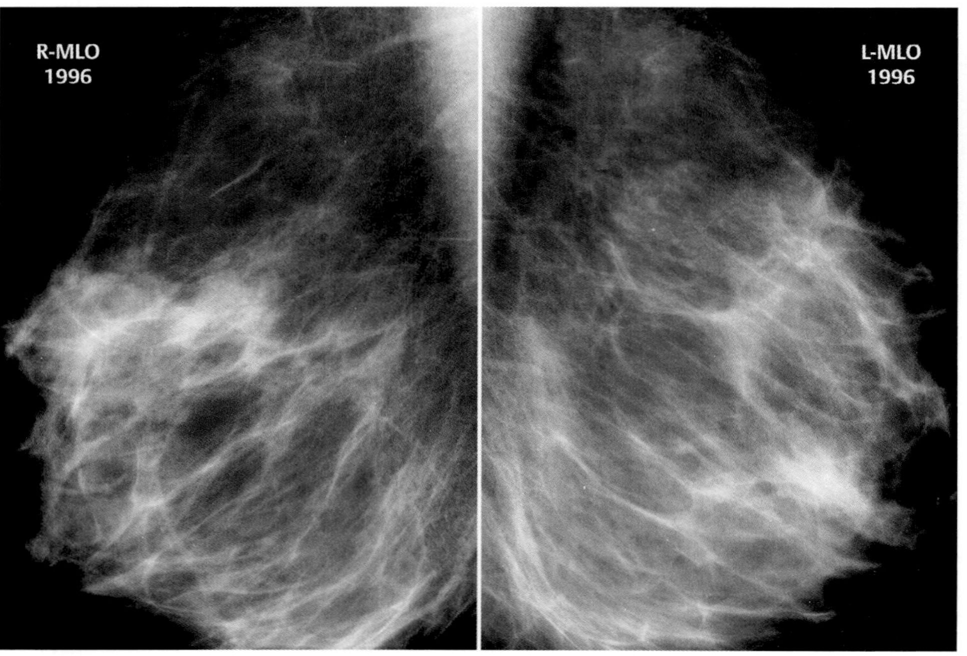


**a, b** Bilateral mediolateral oblique mammograms in November, 1996 show nonspecific opacities and no microcalcifications (ACR 2, BIRADS?, PGMI).

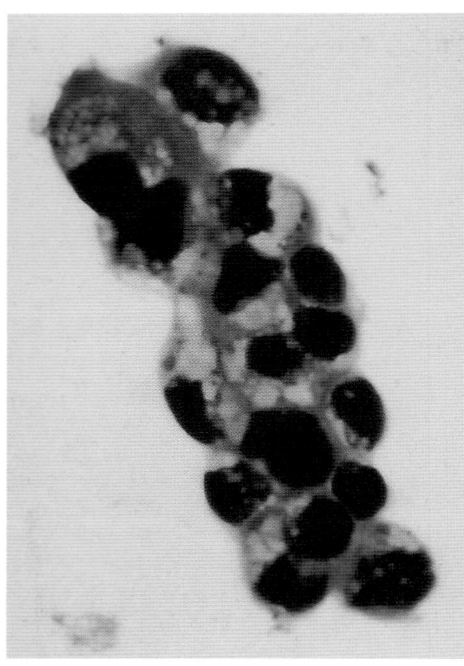

**e** Cytologic smear of discharge from the right breast shows proliferative cells sloughed from the ductal epithelium with pleomorphic, hyperchromatic nuclei.

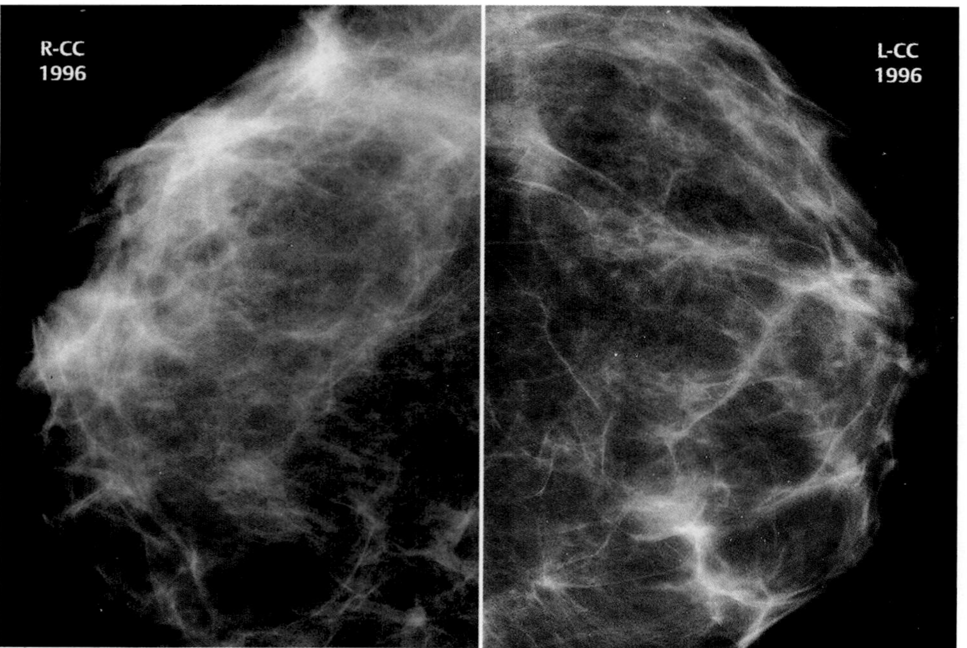


**c, d** Bilateral craniocaudal mammograms in November, 1996 (ACR 2, BIRADS?, PGMI).

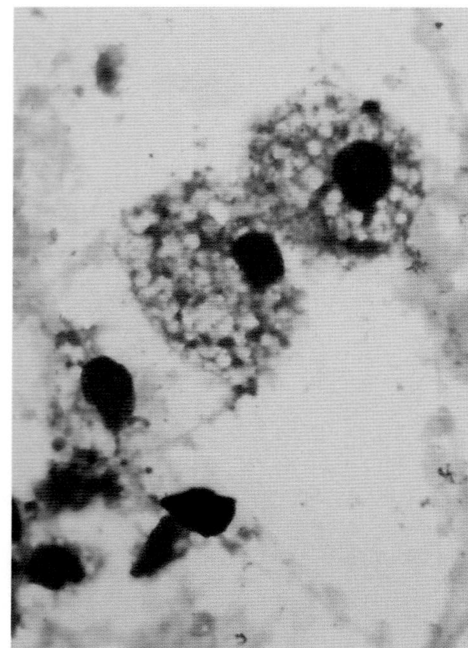

**f** Cytologic smear of discharge from the left breast demonstrates "foam cells."

**Question 1 on Fig. 4.27**

*Where do you see an abnormality (coordinates)?*

*What would you recommend?*

(**a**) Follow-up in 12 months
(**b**) Ductography (left? right?)
(**c**) Magnetic resonance imaging
(**d**) Ductography (left? right?) and magnetic resonance imaging

→ **Answer on p. 347**

**Question 2 on Fig. 4.27**

*What is your presumptive diagnosis?*

(**a**) Incipient involution of the left breast
(**b**) Diffuse ductal neoplasm in the right breast
(**c**) Bilateral ductectasia with mastitis on the right side

→ **Answer on p. 347**

**Fig. 4.28 A 41-year-old woman with no palpable breast mass and no nipple changes or discharge.** Mammography revealed clustered calcifications in the upper outer quadrant.

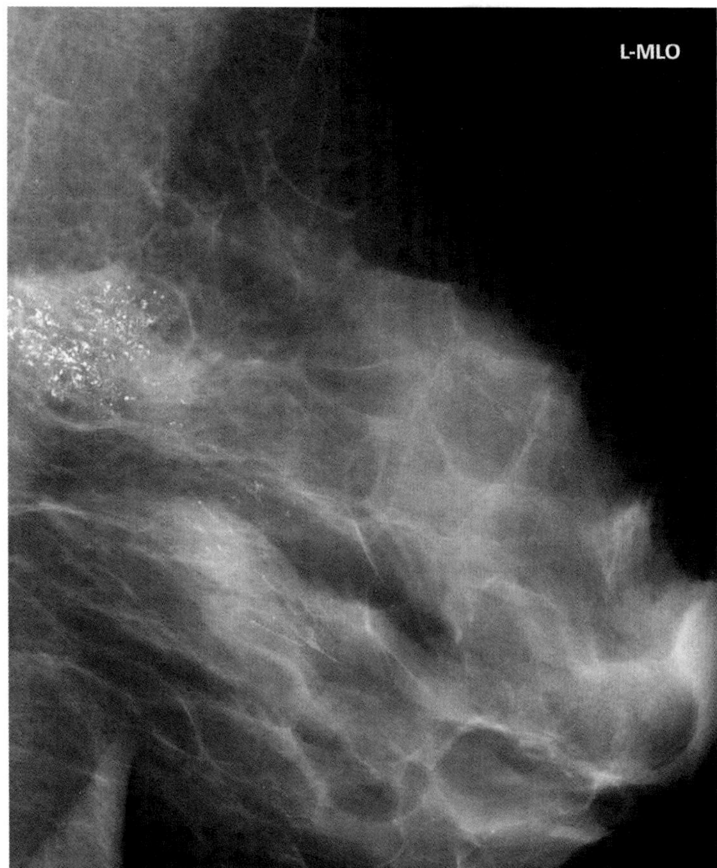


**a** Oblique mammogram of the left breast shows clustered calcifications occupying an area of 2 $cm^2$. The calcifications are atypical and pleomorphic (ACR 3, BIRADS 5, P**G**MI).

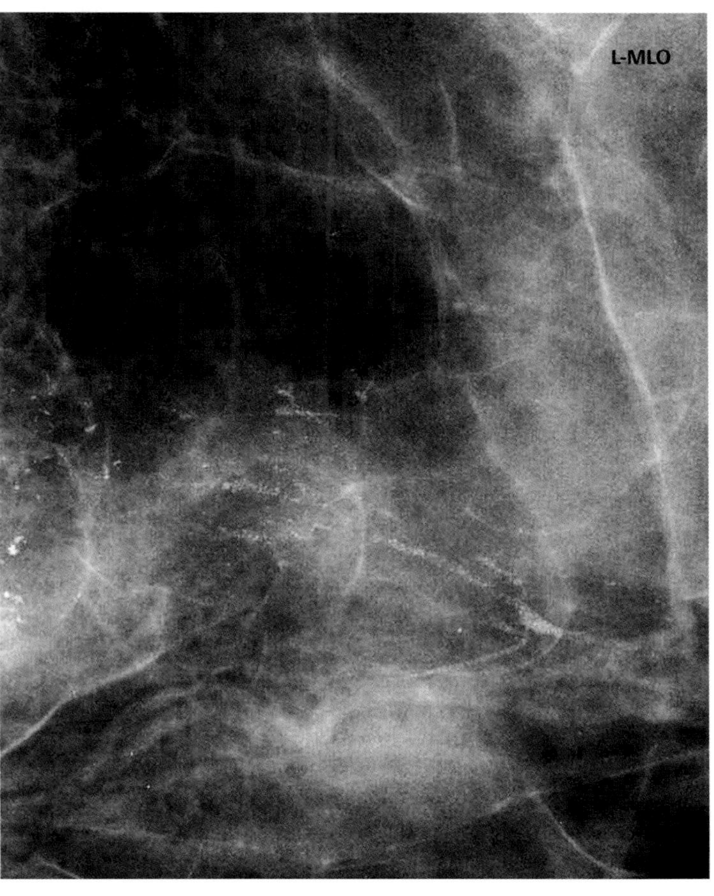


**c** Digital magnification mammogram of the retroareolar region (nipple on right at **t/17**) (coordinates **l–n/16–20** relative to **a**).

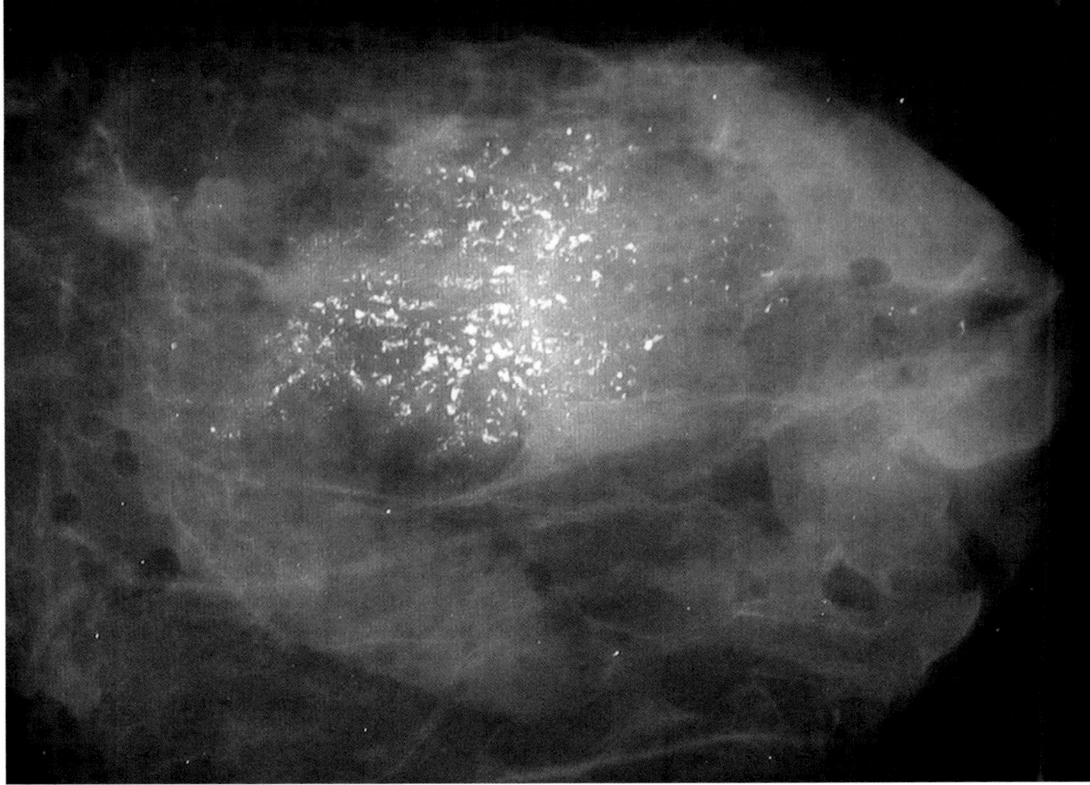

**b** Specimen radiograph shows pleomorphic malignant-type calcifications. The histologic diagnosis is DCIS with a small invasive component (T1a, see p. 73).

**Question on Fig. 4.28**

*Was the DCIS removed with adequate margins?*

(**a**) Yes
(**b**) No
(**c**) Cannot be evaluated

→ **Answer on p. 349**

**Fig. 4.29 Findings in the right breast of a 75-year-old woman in 1997.** Bloody crusts were found on the right nipple at physical examination. Digital stereotactic fine-needle aspiration of a 1 cm opacity in the right breast showed the cytologic features of papilloma, but excisional histology identified the lesion as DCIS. Bleeding from the duct subsided over time. The patient had no further complaints and presented for routine follow-up 1 year later in 1999, when microcalcifications were detected at the operative site. A small second nodule in the lateral portion of the breast had not been removed in the first operation, despite wire localization, and was found to be unchanged.

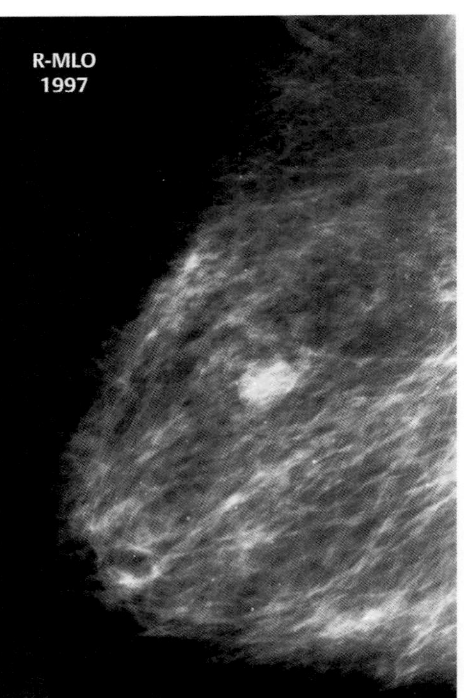


**a** Oblique mammogram of the right breast in 1997, shows an approximately 1 cm opacity with predominantly smooth margins at the 1-o'clock position (**C/20–21**) (ACR 2, BIRADS 3, PGMI).

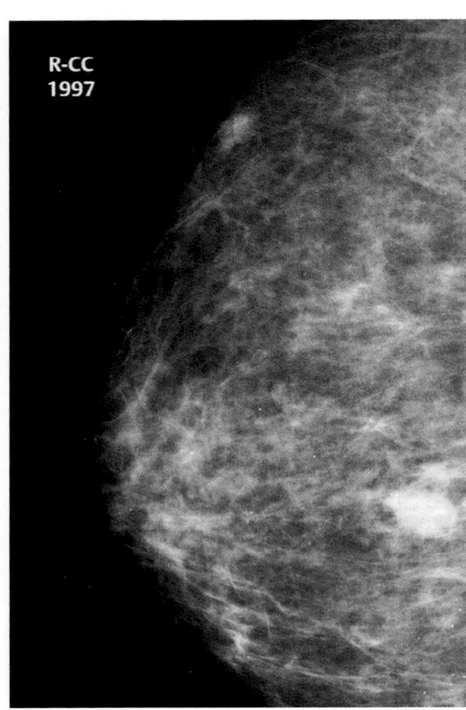


**b** Craniocaudal mammogram of the right breast in 1997, shows an ill-defined lesion at **G/19** (ACR 1, BIRADS 4, PGMI) and a second 4-mm focus at **e–f/24**.

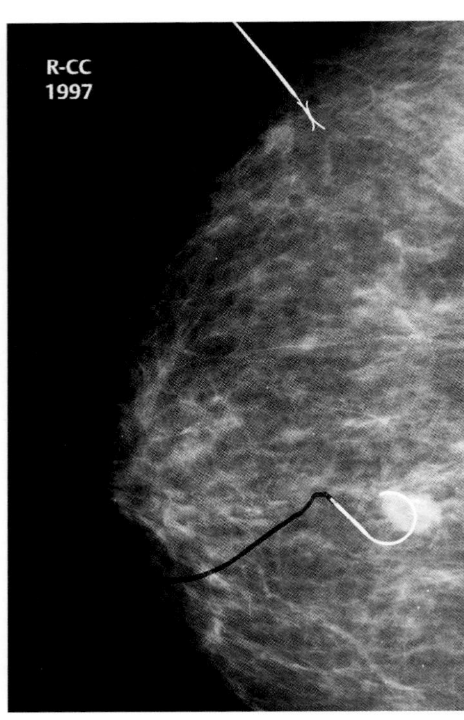


**c** Localization film of the right breast taken in 1997. Cytology identified the nodule (**n/19**) marked with a wire hook as a papilloma. The localization is correct. The second lateral nodule is improperly localized with a hookwire. The wire is behind the nodule toward the edge of the breast, making it difficult to access through a periareolar incision (see p. 299).

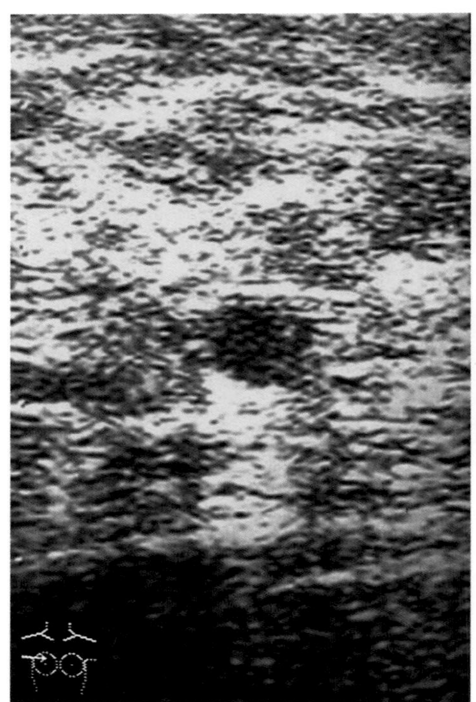

**d** Sonogram of the right breast in 1997 shows a 0.8 cm nodule at the 1-o'clock position with irregular margins, internal echoes, and posterior acoustic enhancement.

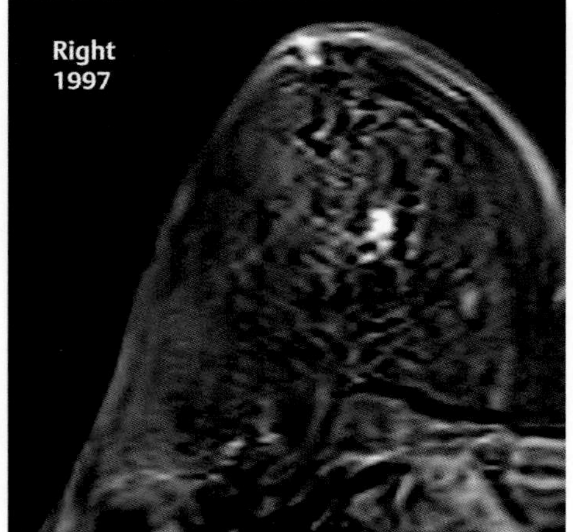


**e** MRI in December, 1997. The nodule is suspicious for papilloma or DCIS and shows intense gadolinium enhancement with surrounding small enhancing foci. Nonspecific retroareolar linear enhancement is also seen.

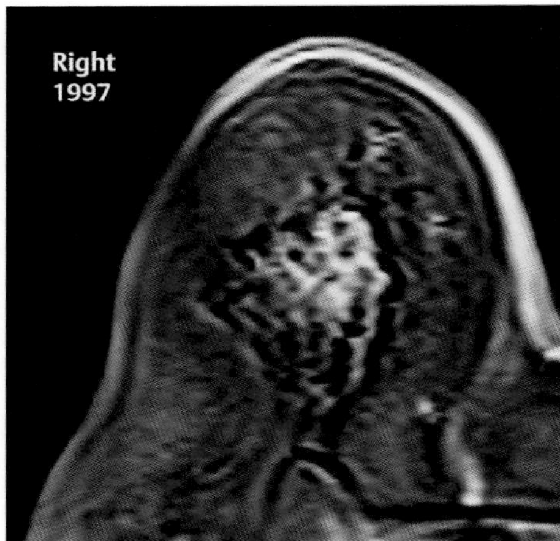


**f** MRI in a plane *4 mm lower than in* **e** shows irregular linear gadolinium enhancement in the vicinity of adjacent ducts (EIC?). The left breast appeared normal.

**Fig. 4.29** **75 year-old woman with DCIS and questionable EIC.** *(continued)*

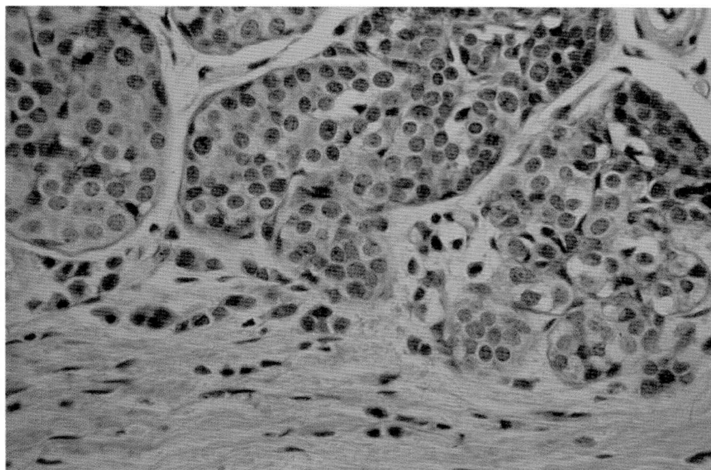

**g** Histologic section of the larger nodule in July, 1997 shows a *well-differentiated, intracystic 0.5 cm carcinoma in situ* (G1) with papillary and cribriform features. There is concomitant fibrocystic change with focal ductal hyperplasia and signs of recurrent intraductal bleeding. There is no evidence of invasive cancer (Dahm, Esslingen).

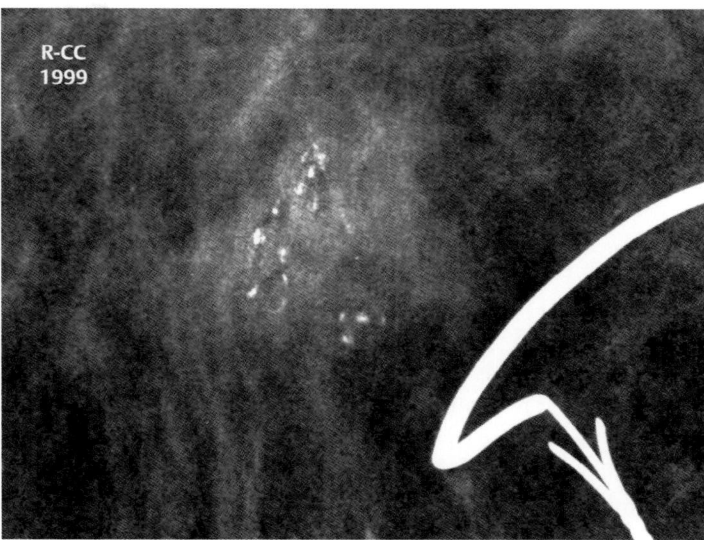


**h** Right craniocaudal mammogram (spot film after localization in 1999) shows a nonspecific, 1 cm area of increased tissue density with microcalcifications a little bit lower than the DCIS from 1997.

**The following images (h–k) are from an examination done 14 months later in February, 1999.**

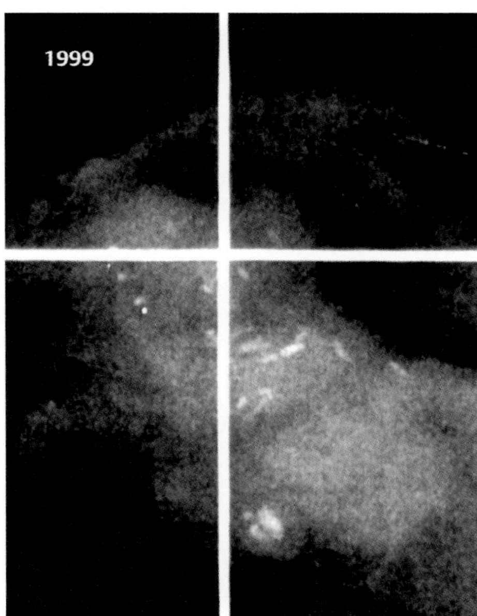


**i** Specimen radiograph of the calcifications, 1999, shows nonspecific increased density with coarse opacities.

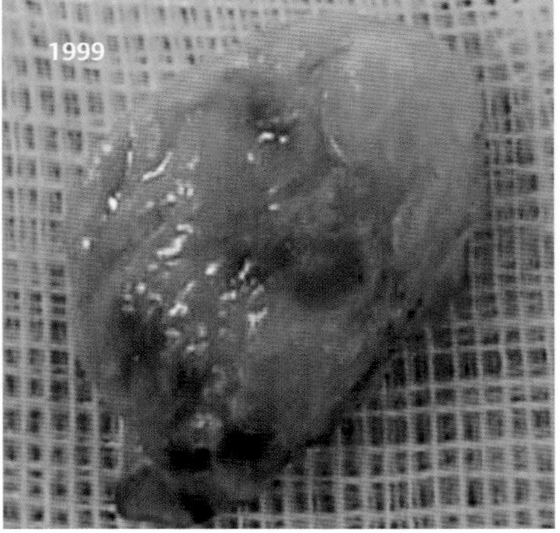


**j** Surgical specimen of the new change shows a glassy nodule with greenish pigmented tumor structures. and no visible signs of a surgical scar.

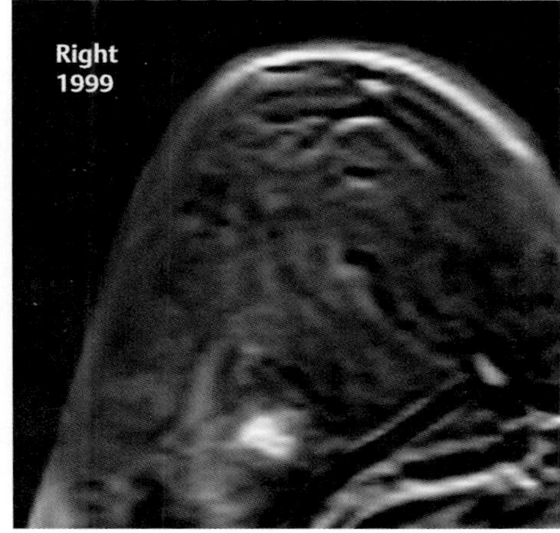


**k** MRI, 1999, shows a faint stellate pattern of prepectoral gadolinium enhancement behind the lesion of 1997 (see **Figs. 4.29 e, f**) (neoplasm? fat necrosis?).

**Question on Fig. 4.29**

*Based on the clinical symptoms, primary histology and MRI, especially before 1997, how would you interpret the microcalcifications that appeared one year later?*

(**a**) Fat necrosis
(**b**) DCIS or invasive carcinoma
(**c**) Ductal papilloma

→ **Answer on p. 350**

### Prognosis

The prognosis of DCIS depends on whether clinical manifestations are present. The size of the lesion, the degree of multicentricity, bilaterality, and other factors (see Van-Nuys Grading System, below) are less important as prognostic indicators. The axillary lymph nodes are, of course, unaffected by DCIS. In the case of extensive DCIS, however, removal of at least the sentinel lymph nodes is recommended to exclude a locally invasive metastatic process (see **Fig. 4.22**).

### Van Nuys Grading System

The **Van Nuys index** is a classification and grading system for DCIS that is useful in therapeutic planning. Applying the criteria of **tumor size, margin width** and **pathologic classification**, points are scored that predict the risk of tumor recurrence. The Van Nuys index ranges from a minimum of 3 points to a maximum of 9 points and is divided into three grades:

- **G1**: 3–4 points; the recurrence rate is 4%
- **G2**: 5–7 points; the recurrence rate is 11%
- **G3**: 8–9 points; the recurrence rate is 26%

The parameters used to determine the Van Nuys index and their interpretation are summarized below:

- **DCIS tumor size.** A strong correlation exists between tumor size, the risk of tumor recurrence, and the likelihood that the tumor has already penetrated the duct and invaded healthy breast tissue (microinvasion). Because most DCIS lesions are not palpable, the exact tumor size usually cannot be determined until the affected tissue area has been completely removed from the breast and thoroughly evaluated by a pathologist. A DCIS smaller than 15 mm scores *1 point*, a lesion from 15 to 40 mm scores *2 points*, and a lesion larger than 40 mm scores *3 points*.
- **Margin width (margin clearance).** The criteria used to evaluate surgical margin width are not standardized. The minimum clear margin, or the margin of healthy tissue resected with the tumor, should be greater than 10 mm whenever possible. A margin width less than 10 mm adds one point to the index because it is associated with a higher risk of local recurrence.
- **Pathologic classification (nuclear grade).** This criterion is interpreted as high grade (very aggressive) or non-high grade (less aggressive) based on evaluation of the tumor cell nuclei and the presence of cell necrosis with or without calcification. Non-high grade without necrosis scores *1 point*, non-high grade with necrosis scores *2 points*, and high grade with or without necrosis scores *3 points*.

Additional fine points in the differentiation of DCIS are described in the "S3 Guidelines for Breast Cancer Screening in Germany" (Schulz and Albert 2003, pp. 169–199).

The higher the point value of the Van Nuys index, the more aggressively the disease should be treated. Treatment options range from simple tumor removal without postoperative radiotherapy (G1) and tumor removal with radiotherapy (G2) to subcutaneous or total mastectomy (G3). Recently, age has been included as a criterion in the Van Nuys index. Age over 60 years scores 1 point, 40–60 scores 2 points, and under 40 scores 3 points.

**The Van Nuys index is valid only for cancer precursors like DCIS. It is not valid for invasive breast cancer.**

## Lobular Neoplasias: Atypic Lobular Hyperplasia/ Lobular Carcinoma In Situ (LIN 1–3)

Lobular hyperplasia (LH) is characterized by an atypical, monotonic, small-cell epithelial proliferation that begins in the acini or terminal ductules.

Lobular neoplasia (LN), which includes lobular carcinoma in situ (LCIS) and atypical lobular neoplasia (ALH), is generally considered a high-risk lesion rather than an obligate precursor to the development of invasive cancer. The term "LN" is synonymous with lobular intraepithelial neoplasia (LIN). A morphologic grading system (LIN 1 to LIN 3) has been proposed as an aid to individual risk assessment. When LN has been confirmed by core biopsy, subsequent open biopsy reveals a coexisting higher-grade lesion in approximately 17% of cases, justifying the indication for surgical investigation. LIN 3 (pleomorphic LN, extensive LN, signet-ring-cell LN) is considered to have a higher risk of progression than LIN 1 or LIN 2 (Sinn et al. 2006). The LIN 1–3 categories are of no importance for the diagnostic radiologist but are important for the treating physician.

Most of these LIN lesions (atypical lobular hyperplasia (ALH), lobular carcinoma in situ/carcinoma lobulare in situ (LCIS/CLIS) remain intraluminal for some time, then spread centripetally to the smaller milk ducts, and finally penetrate the basement membrane and progresses to invasive lobular carcinoma, although this apparently takes years or even decades to occur. Simultaneous and successive multifocal and multicentric occurrence in one (65%) or both breasts (30%) is far more common with LN than with DCIS. Endogenous and exogenous insults to the maturing alveoli in various regions of the developing breast apparently contribute to pathogenesis of LCIS (see p. 9).

LIN lesions are usually detected fortuitously. They may be discovered near small benign microcystic microcalcifications, during the removal of fibrocystic nodules and fibroadenomas, or in association with invasive carcinoma. Otherwise as DCIS, LIN rarely produces micro-calcifications (**Fig. 4.30**).

**Fig. 4.30** **Findings in the left breast of a 52-year-old woman.** The patient presented for screening with a negative prior examination in 1998. New microcalcifications were detected in 2002.

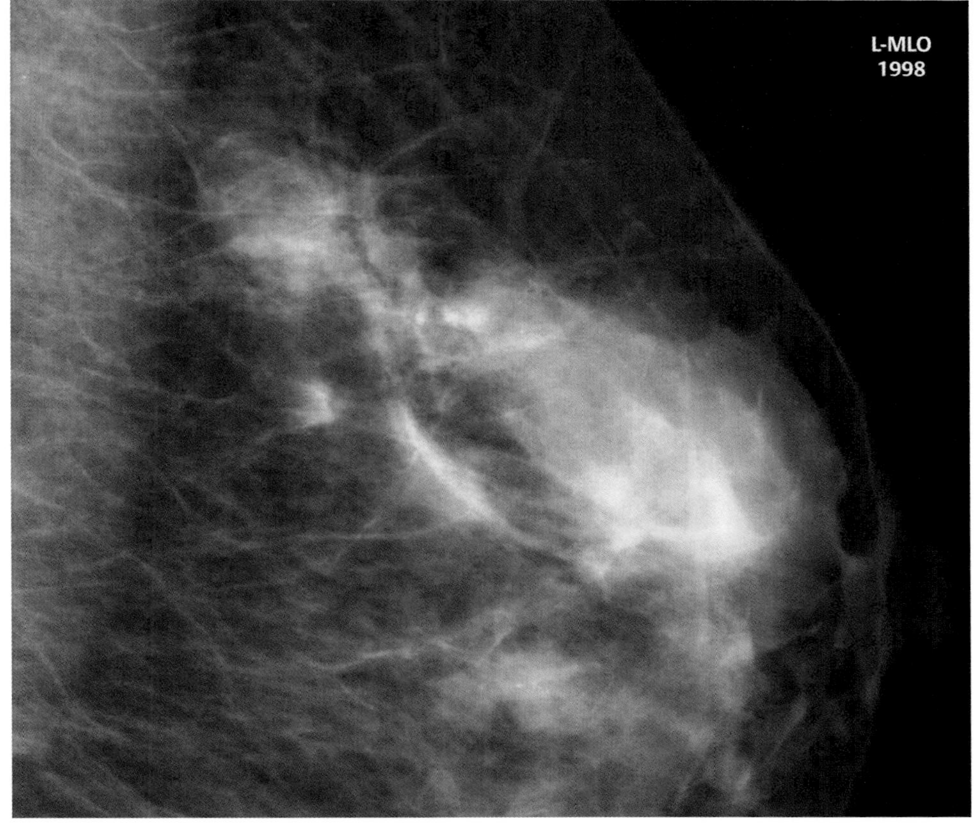


**a** Oblique mammogram of the left breast in 1998 shows stroma-rich breast parenchyma with no visible abnormalities (ACR 2, BIRADS 1, PGMI).

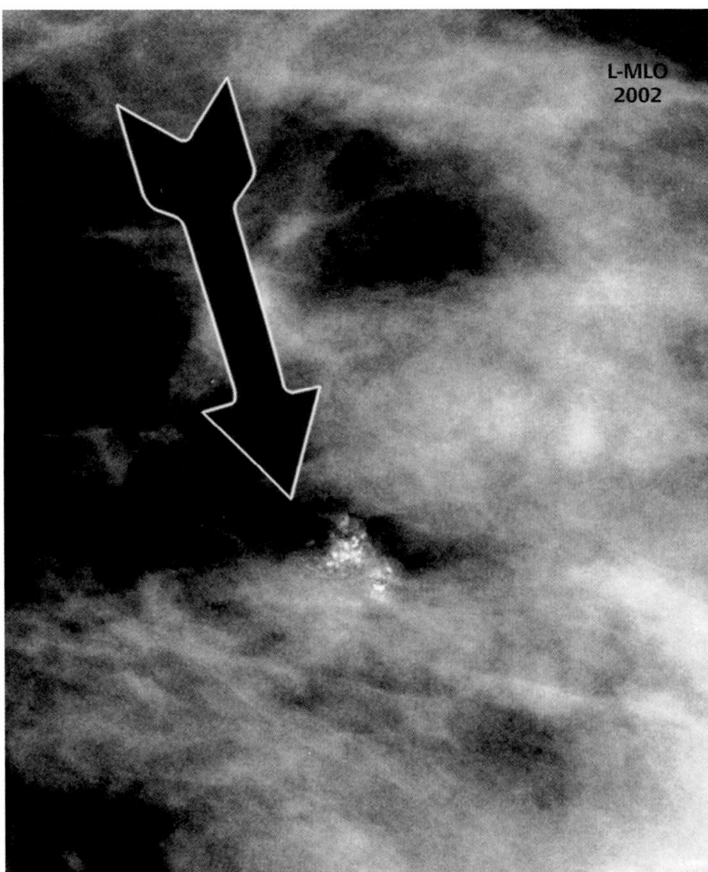


**b** Oblique mammogram of the left breast in 2002 (magnified view) shows new, atypical clustered microcalcifications in the upper outer quadrant requiring histologic evaluation (BIRADS 4). The parenchymal tissue is generally more dense than in 1998 (ACR 3).

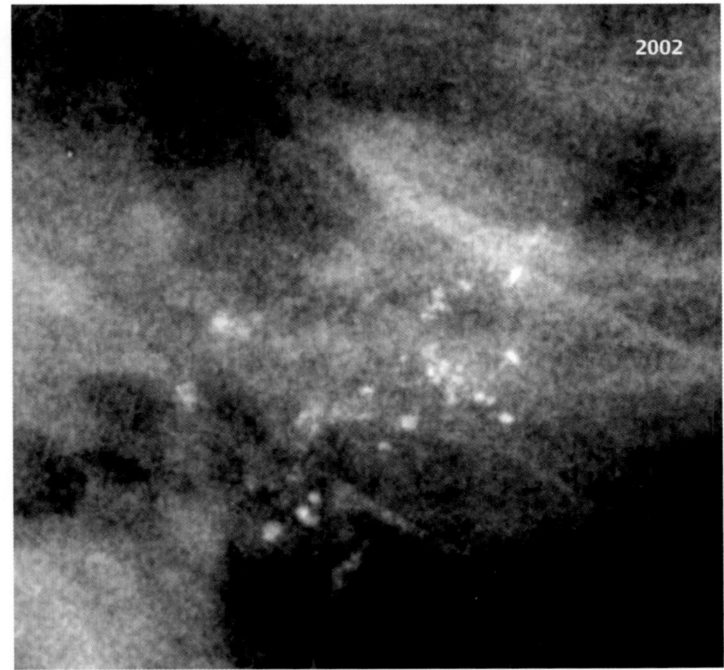


**c** Oblique magnification mammogram in 2002 shows atypical microcalcifications, mostly rounded.

**Question on Fig. 4.30**

*Which of these conditions could **not** account for the new calcifications?*

(**a**) Lobular carcinoma in situ (LCIS)

(**b**) Ductal Carcinoma in situ (DCIS)

(**c**) Medullary carcinoma

→ **Answer on p. 350**

LIN lesions do not have typical radiographic features (except for rare atypical calcifications), as the calcifications are often located next to the tumor and are usually benign. Lobular enlargement occasionally occurs but is so nonspecific that it often goes undetected in dense breasts, and even when detected it has no therapeutic implications (**Figs. 4.31, 4.32**). High-resolution ultrasound would be best for identifying areas of focal glandular proliferation (**Fig. 4.33**), but this is such an extremely common finding that LCIS would not be suspected on that basis alone. Pope et al. (1988) described the mammographic appearance of 26 LCIS lesions from 820 biopsies in 8628 women who underwent mammography. Carcinoma was detected in 3.8% of the biopsies. LCIS was not found as a concomitant or satellite lesion of the malignancies, although mirror-image biopsy of the clinically healthy breast in women with breast cancer revealed LCIS next to benign lesions and in one fibroadenoma. Not infrequently, palpable lesions were excised and incidental LCIS was discovered in or around the lesions. Three women with metastatic adenocarcinoma and an unknown primary tumor underwent breast biopsies for a palpable mass or mammographic asymmetry with microcalcifications. In these cases as well, LCIS was found to be located in healthy tissue or in a fibroadenoma. It is likely that LCIS will be diagnosed less often in the future because the excision of benign breast changes is becoming obsolete as excisional biopsies are replaced by less invasive interventional procedures (see p. 230). Even fibroadenomas and papillomas 2 cm in diameter can be selectively removed by a tissue-conserving vacuum biopsy performed under sonographic or digital stereotactic guidance.

LCIS is a remarkably common finding in stroma-rich breasts with prominent ducts and focal opacities (P2 or DY pattern described by Wolfe [1976]; see p. 98). High-resolution ultrasound can define proliferative lobules in these radiodense areas—a probable nidus for LCIS and eventual invasive lobular carcinoma (see **Fig. 4.33**) and distinguish them from intramammary connective tissue. Ultrasound-guided core-needle biopsy (CNB) is recommended in cases where the lobules are unusually large (differential diagnosis: adenosis).

**Fig. 4.31** **Lobular carcinoma in situ (radiographic features).**

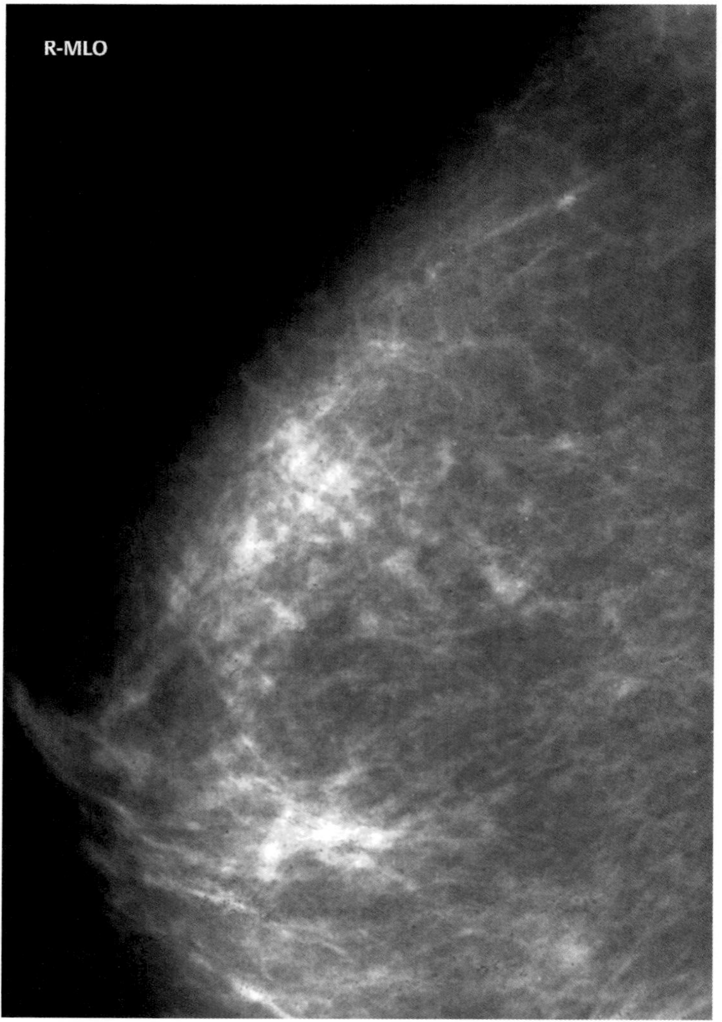


**a** Oblique mammogram of the right breast (magnified view) shows numerous enlarged TDLUs in the upper portion of the breast (see **Fig. 4.4 d**, p. 26).

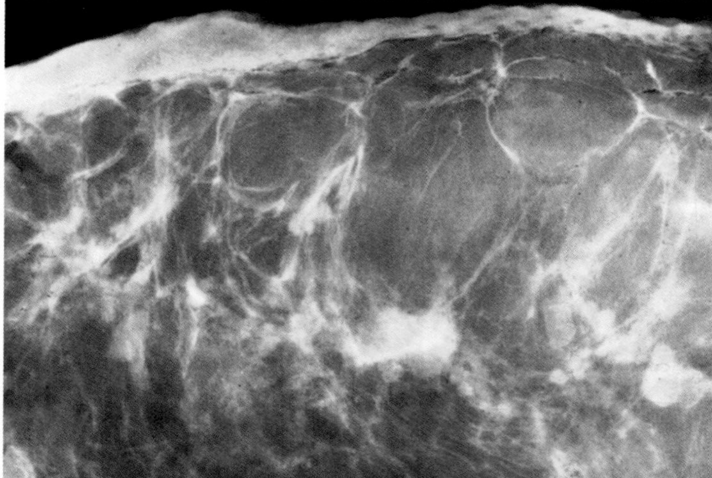

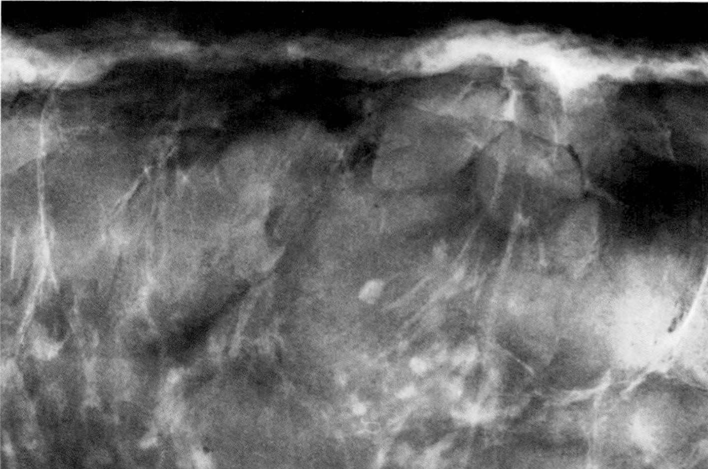

**b, c** Specimen radiograph of lobular carcinoma in situ (LCIS) shows additional enlarged TDLUs in two different specimens. Image **c** shows a duct with (TDLUs). All areas were identified histologically as lobular carcinoma in situ.

**Fig. 4.32 Lobular carcinoma in situ (LCIS).**

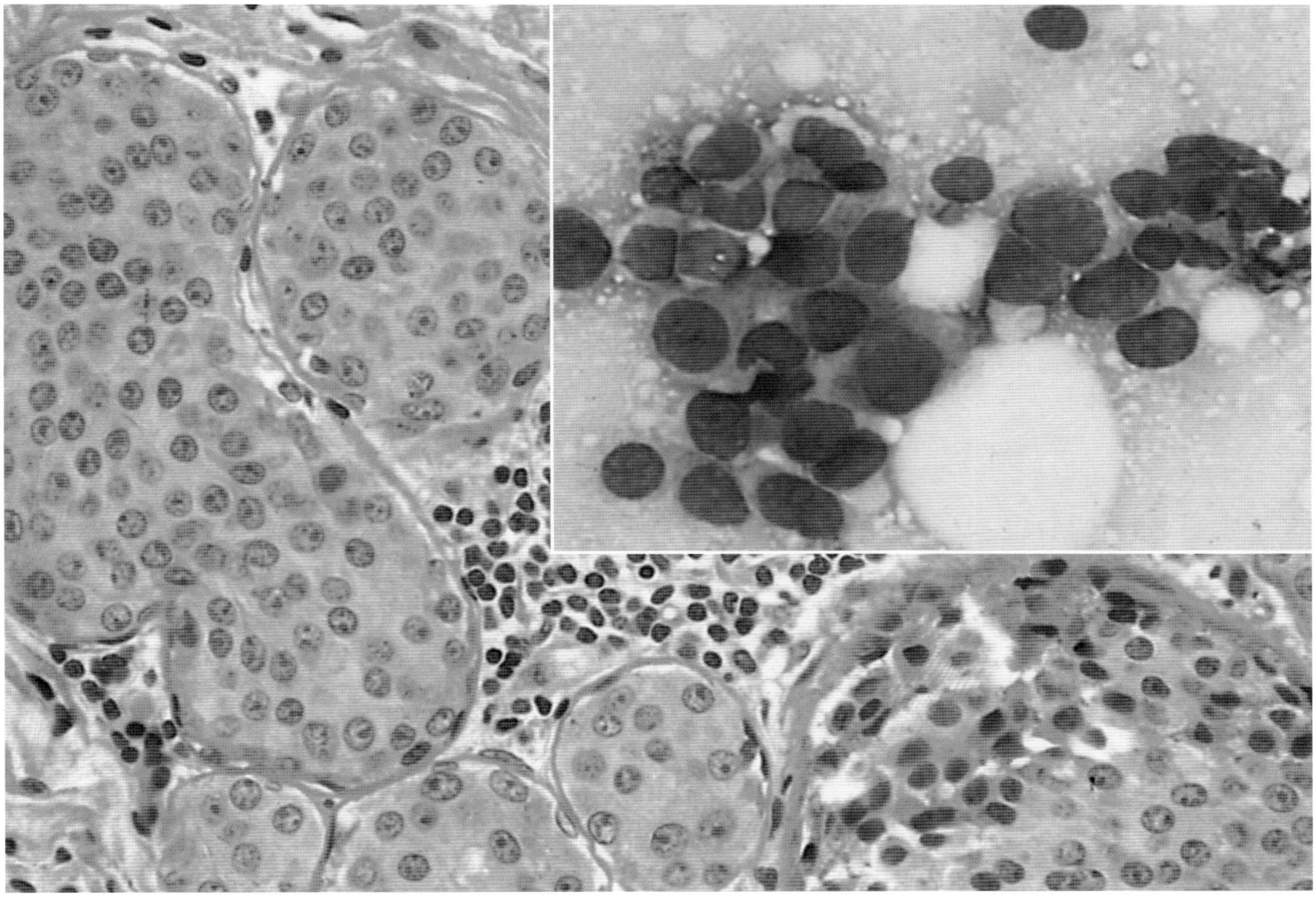

**a** Histologic section (250 × magnification) shows broadened acini in a lobular segment obstructed by small, slightly pleomorphic epithelial round cells with a nest of lymph cells embedded in the intralobular stroma. Corresponding aspiration cytology (inset) shows small pleomorphic cells with a dense, fine reticular chromatin pattern.

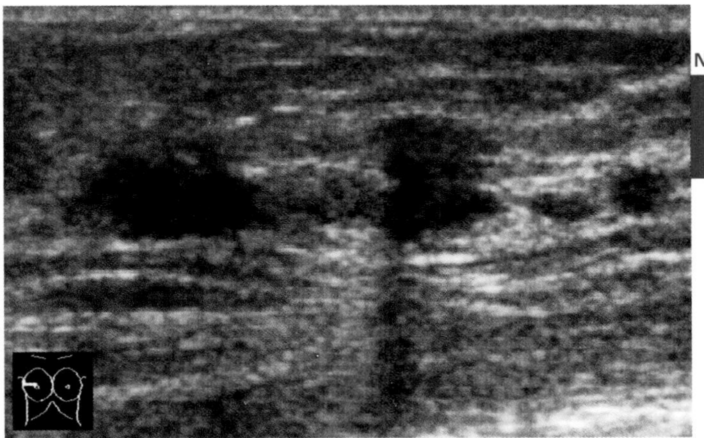


**b** Ultrasound shows two foci of lobular carcinoma at the distal edge of the breast parenchyma. Additional enlarged TDLUs (arrows) are visible toward the nipple (right side of the picture).

**Fig. 4.33 Adenosis and lobular neoplasms.**

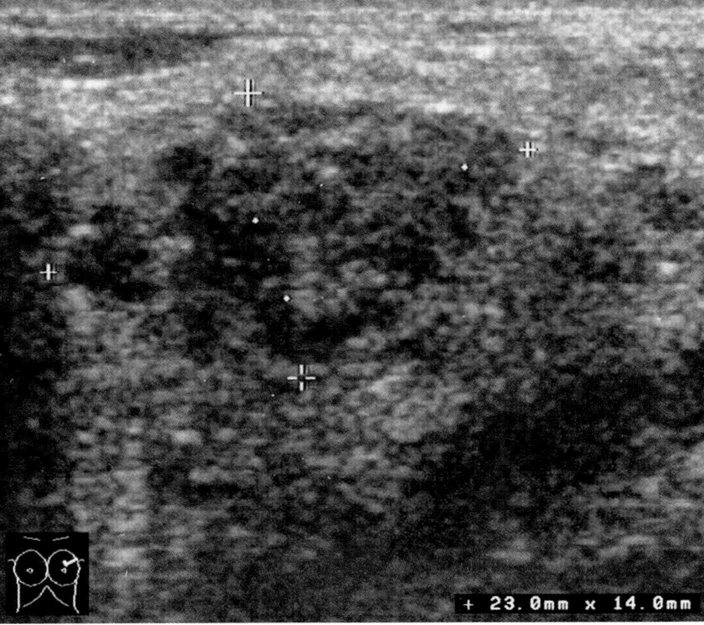


Sonogram of fibrocystic change with circumscribed adenosis (thickened, confluent TDLUs in a circumscribed area of the breast parenchyma) with scalloped margins (DD: LIN, lobular carcinoma).

#### Therapeutic Implications

The treatment of LINs is more conservative than that of DCIS. Ipsilateral mastectomy with axillary dissection and mirror-image biopsy of the healthy breast is increasingly uncommon. Long-term studies indicate a 6.8–25% risk of invasive carcinoma developing in the ipsilateral breast and a 9.2–25% risk in the contralateral breast. There is no therapeutic urgency, as these lesions tend to develop slowly over a period of years.

> **Tip**
>
> **The average risk increases by approximately 1% each year, so the patient's age should also be considered in therapeutic decision making (McDivitt et al. 1968; Rosen et al. 1978, 1981).**

Given its low propensity for malignant transformation, LCIS is basically considered a high-risk indicator that should be followed clinically, mammographically, and sonographically at yearly intervals (Lattes et al. 1980, Powers et al. 1980). It should be noted at mammography, however, that these women often have very dense breasts in which calcifications may be the only appreciable finding. Single-view mammography, supplemented by ultrasound and occasionally by MRI, provides an alternative to mammography alone and local excision. This is because invasive lobular carcinoma is easier to detect by sonography and MRI than by mammography. If LCIS has been diagnosed by CNB or vacuum biopsy, reexcision should be performed. Seventeen percent of LCIS cases progress to invasive lobular carcinoma. As this is the same rate at which ADH upgrades to DCIS (where excision is also indicated), LCIS should be managed by reexcision (Foster et al. 2004). It may be difficult in these cases for the surgeon and radiologist to relocate the precise site of origin of the initially diagnosed LCIS. It is frequently difficult to distinguish residual LCIS or a recurrence from postoperative fat necrosis.

#### Local Recurrence of DCIS and LCIS and Follow-Ups

Ninety percent of all recurrences of calcifying DCIS and LCIS are detected on the basis of atypical microcalcifications that develop at the lesion margins and require differentiation from postoperative fat necrosis (see **Fig. 4.29**). Conventional mammography of microcalcifications should generally be performed with molybdenum anodes and filters (MO-MO) at 25 kV. This combination is excellent for displaying microcalcifications. This also applies to magnification mammography but not to digital mammography.

Recurrences of LCIS are more common than DCIS recurrences, while subsequent invasive carcinoma is less common, despite the fact that LCIS is more frequently multifocal and bilateral than DCIS. The incidence of occult microinvasions in DCIS increases with tumor extent, and so an important issue in treatment planning is how extensive surgery should be for DCIS and how sparing it should be for LCIS. High-resolution ultrasound and magnetic resonance imaging should be consistently utilized in screening examinations for recurrences. Ultrasound imaging should be done concurrently with mammography, and magnetic resonance imaging should be performed every 1–2 years, depending on breast radiodensity, and should be scheduled 6 months apart from mammographic examinations.

Thus, mammography has a major role in the perioperative period and also in the follow-up of ADH, LCIS, DCIS, and calcifying invasive carcinoma. The follow-up intervals after removal of LCIS/DCIS are the same as after the breast-conserving treatment of carcinoma (see p. 328). The first follow-up examination to exclude residual calcifications should be scheduled for 3 months after the operation, especially if the calcifications were extensive and may not have been fully covered in the specimen radiograph. Immediate postoperative mammography is necessary in special cases where calcifications are incomplete in the specimen radiograph and absent in the reexcision specimen. This eliminates the common (and for patients, very distressful) discussion about whether calcifications detected later were missed initially or did not form until after the surgery. Subsequent to this immediate postoperative or 3-month follow-up, further examinations should be scheduled every 6 months for the next 2 years and then once yearly. At some centers, close-interval follow-ups are performed for 3 years rather than for 2 years. The exact schedule should be tailored to the individual risk of recurrence.

Postoperative follow-ups are even more important with LCIS/DCIS than with invasive cancers. This is because local recurrence is extremely unlikely to develop during the first 2 years after removal of invasive carcinoma—postoperative radiotherapy and adjuvant treatments will generally prevent it. By contrast, local or systemic adjuvant therapies are usually not given to control the growth of LCIS/DCIS (although postoperative radiation is recommended for DCIS), and rapid flare-ups may occur. The appropriate treatment for a recurrence—mastectomy or breast-conserving therapy—will depend on the extent of the recurrence, its grade, and the attitude and willingness of the patient (and doctor) to assume risk. Because in situ carcinoma does not metastasize, breast conservation may be tried in cases where the breast is closely followed and has not yet received postoperative radiation.

Postoperative radiotherapy is generally unnecessary for LCIS.

> **!**
>
> **In specimen radiography, it is important to accurately mark the anterior, superior, and lateral portions of the specimen (see p. 305) to direct the surgeon to the proposed reexcision site in case the calcifications or tumor foci are at the edge of the specimen or have been incompletely removed.**

### Invasive Carcinoma

As with in situ carcinomas, a basic knowledge of pathoanatomy is necessary to understand the imaging appearances of different tumors: which features are typical and which are not. This will increase diagnostic accuracy and prevent many errors of interpretation. Round or lobulated tumors typically contain abundant stroma, while spiculated lesions are hypocellular. We can recognize typical patterns of tumor spread based on clinical, mammographic, sonographic, and MRI findings and draw appropriate conclusions.

It is occasionally difficult to relate structures detected on mammograms to a particular morphologic substrate, especially in the case of malignant tumors. Generally the histologic type of an underlying tumor cannot be accurately determined on mammograms. Accordingly, radiographic tumor criteria should be based on structures that the pathologist can see and evaluate histologically.

### Gross Morphology

The pathologist should provide the diagnosing and treating physician with a TNM classification of the carcinoma as well as detailed information on its growth characteristics and immunohistochemistry (see p. 74).

First it is determined whether the tumors are discrete solitary or multifocal masses as opposed to multicentric or diffuse lesions. The definitive tumor margins are confirmed or adjusted on the basis of histologic assessment of the surgical margins. Most breast cancers are not spherical but are **stellate and spiculated** with associated areas of retraction. Others are **lobular and scalloped** and grow by expansion. Breast cancers are commonly associated with a fibrous stromal reaction of varying intensity and may show central regressive fibrosclerotic changes.

Infiltrating margins explain why malignant tumors do not have a peripheral halo like that seen with cysts or some fibroadenomas, and so the absence of a halo is an important differentiating sign. Central fibrosclerosis and the proliferation of tumor epithelium at the edges of malignancies help to explain why certain tumors show peripheral rim enhancement on MRI.

It is important that **spiculated margins** be recognized clinically. Their differential diagnosis includes sclerosing adenosis and radial scars in a fibrocystic breast. The differential diagnosis of tumors with **scalloped margins** includes fibroadenomas, papillomas, phylloides tumors, inflammatory pseudotumors, and lymphomas.

Peritumoral linear calcifications (see **Fig. 4.24 g**) or a slight diffuse gadolinium enhancement (see **Fig. 4.29 f**) are a sign of associated intraductal cancer spread (EIC, see p. 48) outside the actual tumor region. It is important to recognize EIC because breast-conserving therapy may be inappropriate for these tumors.

Carcinomas that appear to have **rounded, pushing margins or sharply defined contours** are rare and are most likely to be medullary or mucinous carcinomas. Their gross differential diagnosis includes fibroadenomas, adenomas, hamartomas, and papillomas. Macrocystic carcinomas are occasionally encountered and are difficult to distinguish radiographically from benign cysts with intraluminal benign epitheliosis (papillary cystadenoma) (see **Fig. 5.138**, p. 274). Cysts with inspissated, protein-rich contents are equally difficult to evaluate. They also have smooth margins but meet all the sonographic criteria of a solid nodule (e.g., apocrine carcinoma, see **Fig. 5.49**, p. 140).

**Diffuse involvement** by lobular, small-cell ductal or inflammatory carcinoma with severe carcinomatous lymphangitis can be difficult to interpret on mammograms, especially in dense breasts with abundant fibroglandular tissue. Size and growth are closely linked to the classic prognostic indicator of axillary lymph node status (see **Fig. 4.43** and p. 73). The occurrence of axillary lymph node metastases depends on the size and location of the tumor and its mode of spread. This determines the success of sentinel lymph node biopsy (see p. 307). Tumors located in the inner quadrants are often drained more by the retrosternal or infraclavicular lymph nodes than by axillary nodes.

Comparing different nodular lesions with a uni- or multilobular configuration (in multifocal lesions, the largest discrete focus determines the pT stage), we find that multifocal carcinomas are associated with a greater frequency of metastasis (Barth and Prechtel 1991).

The **TNM classification** of breast lesions is reviewed on p. 75.

As far as mammographic findings are concerned, pathologists and radiologists have identified **five radiographic types** of malignancy based on microradiographic-histologic analyses (Barth 1979a), electron microscopic analysis of calcifications (Barth et al. 1977), and comparative anatomic and radiographic studies (Bässler 1978, Bjurstam 1978, Ingleby and Gershon-Cohen 1960, among numerous others). These varying patterns are based on different underlying tumor histologies (**Fig. 4.34**):

- Predominantly ductal carcinomas (with or without calcifications) (p. 64 ff)
- Predominantly round to lobular malignancies (p. 69)
- Predominantly stellate malignancies (p. 71)
- Mixed (lobular and stellate) malignancies (p. 72)
- Diffuse malignancies (p. 72)

The **radiographic** tumor types are defined on the basis of their growth and resulting configuration and occupy a continuum. While these patterns do correlate with specific **histologic** tumor entities, radiologists cannot determine histologic type based on mammograms alone—they can only form an impression. For example, the radiologist can differentiate among tumors that show a predominant **ductal distribution**; lesions that present as a **circumscribed tumor mass** at mammography, sonography, or MRI; and tumors that **grow diffusely** in the breast. Ductal tumors may be calcifying or noncalcifying on mammograms, but calcifications cannot be consistently identified with ultrasound. The diagnostic work-up should definitely include mammography, especially in patients with DCIS. In a series of 60 confirmed carcinomas in situ, Yang and Tse (2004) detected 42% of the lesions mammographically but only 22% by ultrasound. The sonographic detection of calcifications is most likely to be successful if the examiner knows their location based on previous mammograms. Circumscribed tumor shadows usually originate from invasive ductal carcinomas NOS ("not otherwise specified") such as solid and scirrhous carcinoma (older nomenclature). Lesions such as medullary and anaplastic tumors are classified as special forms rather than NOS tumors. The **radiographic and sonographic features** of NOS tumors and special forms vary according to the relative proportions of cells and stroma in the tumor:

- **Cellular tumors with scant stroma** are lobulated and are delineated from the surrounding parenchyma by smooth or scalloped margins. Spontaneous hemorrhage occasionally occurs. These tumors appear to have pushing margins and grow at a relatively rapid rate.
- **Hypocellular, stroma-rich (scirrhous) tumors** have stellate or spiculated margins, distort surrounding structures, and cause skin and nipple retraction. Calcifications are common, especially at the tumor periphery (EIC) (**Fig. 4.24 g**, p. 50). Spontaneous hematomas do not occur. These lesions have a slower growth rate than cellular tumors.

Approximately 0.7% of all carcinomas have smooth margins, 15% have mixed margins (smooth and spiculated), and 84% are spiculated (Barth et al. 1979b; Castano-Almendral et al. 1971; Gallager and Martin 1969; Hamperl 1968).

**Diffuse malignancies** (usually special forms) often do not produce a nodular tumor mass on mammograms. They infiltrate the breast parenchyma without definite boundaries, usually appearing on sonograms as ill-defined areas of low echogenicity. They appear on MRI as focal areas of intense gadolinium enhancement. These tumors include invasive lobular neoplasms, small-cell carcinomas, anaplastic carcinomas, and especially the clinical type of inflamma-

**Fig. 4.34** Types of breast malignancy.

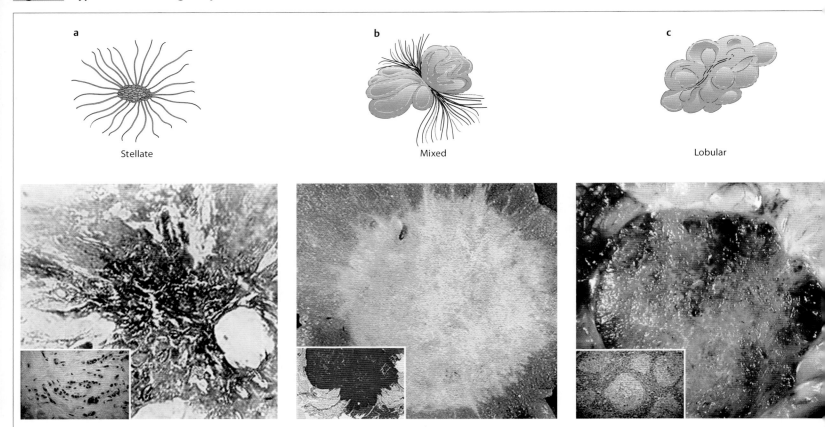


**a** *Stellate.* Fibrous (scirrhous) tumour with low cell content in the fibrotic center of the lump. Tumor cells are present in the long spicula (see inset below). MRI therefore very often shows broad *ringlike gadolinium enhancement* (see p. 71; **Fig. 5.90 g**, p. 372).
**b** *Mixed lobular/stellate.* Partly lobulated, partly stellate tumor growth. The tumor center has more tumor cells and a lower fibrous tissue content than in stellate tumours. The spicula are smaller than in stellate tumours (see inset). Mammography and MRI show partly smooth, partly stellate irregular margins. MRI shows a sp ical tumor with inhomogeneous gadolinium enhancement in the center and tional small, ringlike peripheral contrast enhancement (see p. 72).
**c** *Lobulated* tumor-cell-rich with small fibrous septa in the center of the knot lilac network in inset). On ultrasound and MRI we see smooth contours as wi fibroadenoma (see p. 69; **Fig. 5.36 e**, p. 357). Very quick homogeneous gad um enhancement on MRI.

tory carcinoma. Diffuse malignancies are usually detected at a late stage on mammograms, especially when calcifications are absent, and have become a major source of malpractice litigation (**Fig. 5.143d**, p. 282).

### Predominantly Ductal Growth

Two morphologic patterns are distinguished with regard to their mammographic, sonographic, and MRI appearance:

- Tumors without calcifications
- Tumors with calcifications

#### *Ductal Spread Without Calcifications* (see **Fig. 4.34 e**)

Ductal spread occurs when tumor cells proliferate within the lactiferous ducts, spreading at first only within the ductal system (noninvasive in-situ form, see p. 37) and later infiltrating its surroundings (invasive form, **Figs. 4.35, 4.36**). The lesion then assumes the features of an undifferentiated NOS carcinoma (e.g., solid carcinoma). The infiltrated ducts appear mammographically as a circumscribed mass in no more than 25% of all ductal tumors. They also form linear, reticular, or comet-tail opacities resulting from their transverse and oblique orientation in the breast parenchyma with or without nipple retraction (depending on the distance to the nipple) (**Fig. 4.37**).

Individual ducts may be enlarged and therefore detectable. The greater the amount of fatty tissue surrounding the infiltrated ducts, the more clearly the changes can be seen on radiographs.

> **Tip**
>
> **A noncalcifying ductal lesion surrounded by connective tissue is mammographically detectable only when it is located at the edge of the breast parenchyma and has caused parenchymal asymmetry or nipple retraction. Often this type of lesion is already palpable, however. It cannot be detected when located at the center of the breast. Like diffuse malignancies, noncalcifying ductal carcinomas are frequently missed by radiologists who do not supplement mammograms with ultrasound. This is one reason why mammography should be combined with ultrasound and if necessary with MRI, especially in dense breasts.**

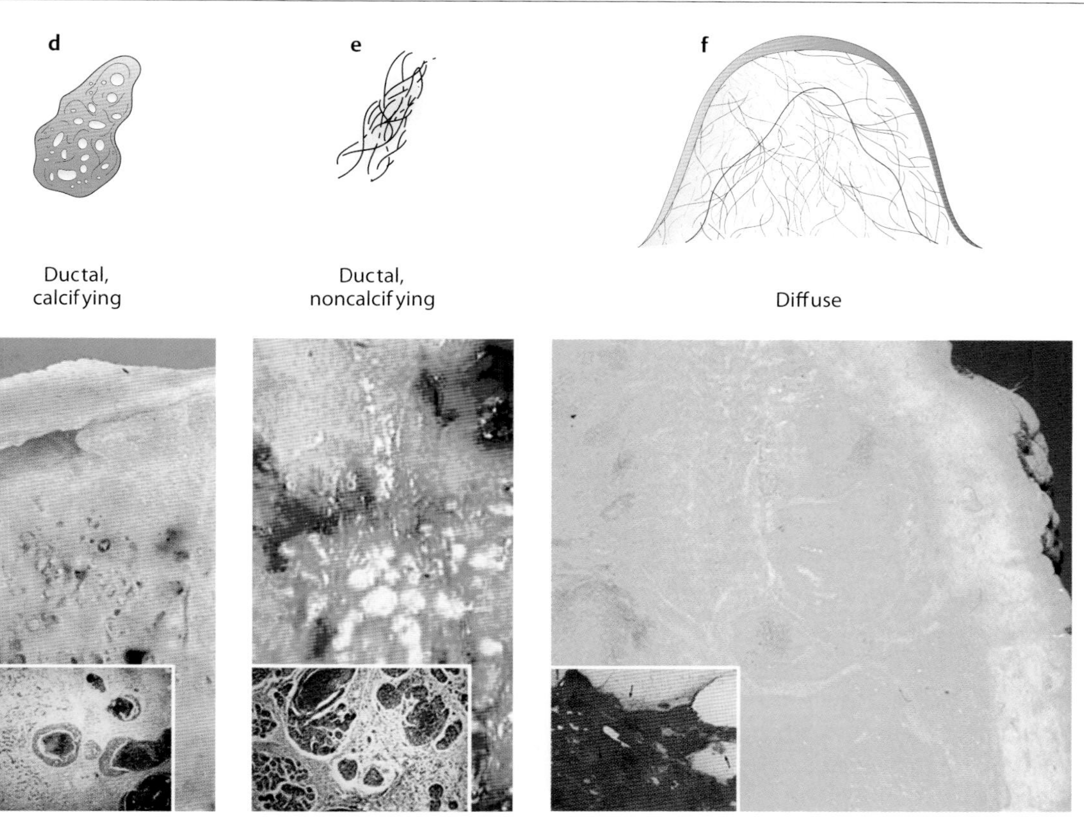


**d** *Ductal carcinoma with microcalcifications.* Tumor masses can be seen in the dilated ducts (see inset) widening the duct lumen and shortening it (nipple retraction!). Early detection is possible with mammography because of the calcifications (see **Figs. 4.15 a, b**, p. 38, and p. 67); this is not the case with ultrasound and even MRI (see p. 201).
**e** *Ductal noncalcifying.* Diffuse infiltration of milk ducts with widening of the lumen and shortening of the ducts (see inset and **Fig. 4.35 b**). On palpation there is uncharacteristic resistance of skin near growth (**Fig. 5.90 d**, p. 372). The first clinical sign is deviation and/or retraction of the nipple (**Figs. 4.37 b, c**, p. 66; **Figs. 5.11 a, b**, p. 88; **Fig. 5.57 e**, p. 367). Mammographically late identification, irregular margins. Better visualized on ultrasound, ideally on MRI with inhomogeneous gadolinium enhancement (**Figs. 5.11 d, e**, p. 354; **Fig. 5.124 b**, p. 255).
**f** *Diffuse.* Tumor spread is diffuse along the ducts and lymphatic vessels (lymphangiosis carcinomatosa) (see p. 75). There may be shrinking or enlargement of the breast (depending on tumor-induced fibrosis). MRI shows a more diffuse, not very strong gadolinium enhancement (see **Fig. 5.173**, p. 320; **Fig. 5.178 f**, p. 326) except lobular invasive cancer (**Fig. 5.188**, p. 342 f).

**Fig. 4.35 Ductal carcinoma, noncalcifying.**

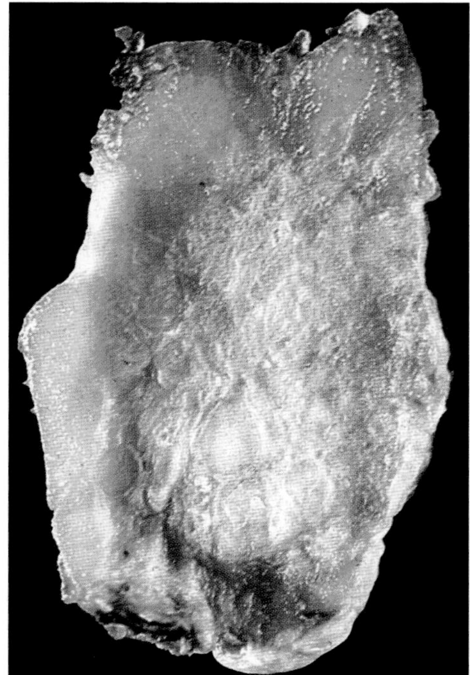

**a** Gross tissue specimen contains a grayish-white area with partially scalloped and partially ill-defined margins. End-on sections of dilated, tumor-filled ducts are visible in the specimen.

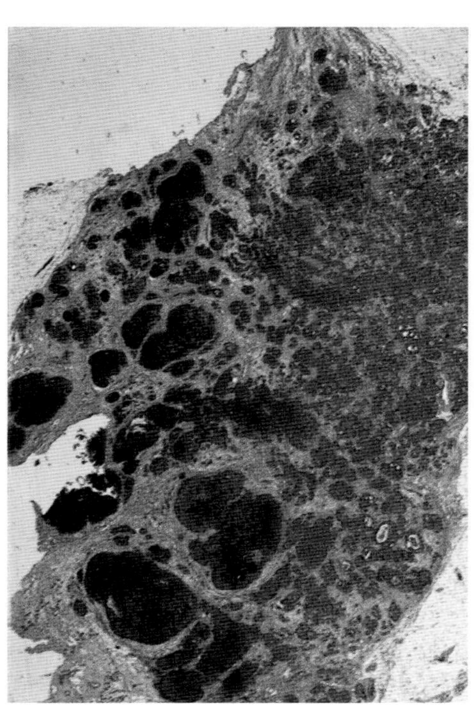

**b** Histologic section (40 × magnification) with Van Gieson stain. Connective tissue appears brownish-red. The ducts and TDLUs are distended by dark tumor masses (lower half of section) and have fibrotic walls.

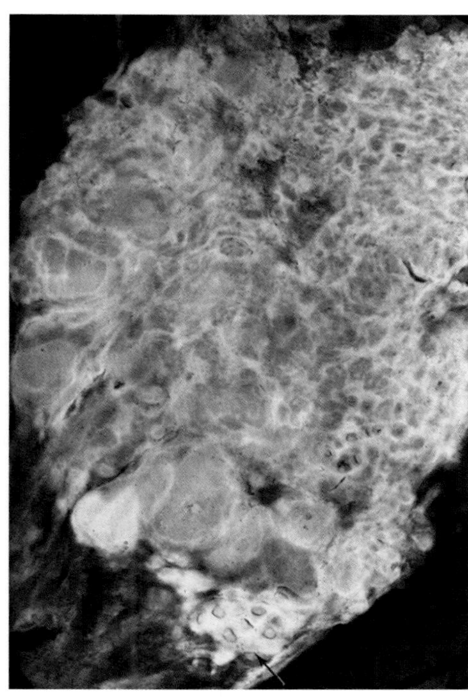

**c** Microradiograph (30 × magnification). Radiograph of a 50 µm thick tissue. Tumor masses in dilated ducts are radiographically less dense than the fibrotic duct wall. The specimen has a similar sonographic and microradiographic appearance (see **Fig. 4.36**).

**Fig. 4.36 Ultrasound displays noncalcifying ductal carcinoma** as a scalloped, hypoechoic nodule measuring 1.8 × 1.2 cm. Faint acoustic shadows are visible at the edges of the lesion. Adjacent glandular tissue is rich in connective tissue (interlobular stroma).

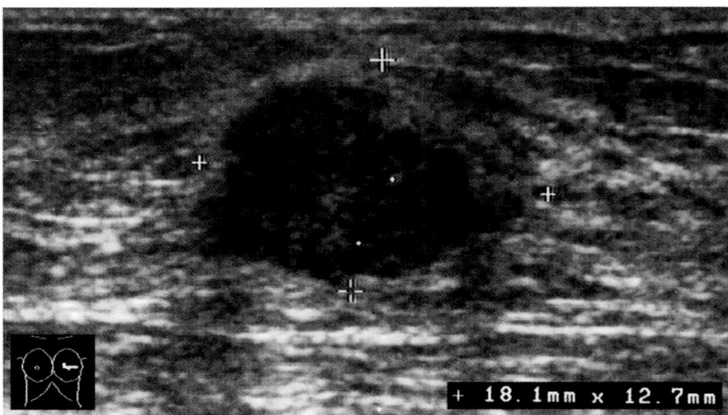


Noncalcifying ductal carcinoma is not detectable at ultrasound, even with a high-resolution probe (11–13 MHz), until it reaches at least 5 mm in diameter. This is still significantly earlier than it can be detected on mammograms. Vignal et al. (2002) conducted a histopathologic study to determine why ultrasound is superior to mammography in detecting some carcinomas. They found that with certain early carcinomas, hyaluronic acid is stored within the tumor tissue and its surroundings. While this process is visible sonographically, appearing as a hypoechoic focal mass, it is mammographically occult. Only when fibrotic structures containing actin (desmoid reactions) or microcalcifications form do they become visible on mammograms. However, these structures were present in only 13 of the 22 carcinomas that were investigated in the study.

When the tumor is in close contract with a TDLU or main duct (see p. 23), ultrasound displays an ill-defined area that may or may not have a hyperechoic rim. The lesion increases in size until it crosses into neighboring septa and undergoes asymmetric spread (see **Fig. 5.64 d**, p. 162). This opacity may be round or elliptical, or it may have a triangular shape with the apex pointing toward the nipple (segmental tumor involvement).

Noncalcifying ductal carcinoma appears on gadolinium-enhanced T1-weighted MR subtraction images as an ill-defined area of contrast uptake (detectable when 1 cm or larger). The degree of enhancement depends on the degree of tumor differentiation. Poorly differentiated (G3) tumors show intense enhancement, intermediate-grade (G2) tumors show moderate enhancement, and well-differentiated (G1) tumors show little or no enhancement. This method is not entirely reliable, therefore (see **Figs. 4.27 k**, p. 349 and **Figs. 4.29 e, k**, p. 56 f) and correlates with tumor vascularity.

The first **clinical manifestation** of ductal carcinoma is nipple retraction (see **Fig. 4.37 b, c**). Ten percent of cases present with a bloody or brownish watery discharge, which means that the tumor can be visualized by **ductography** (see **Fig. 4.27 l, m**, p. 349).

The morphologic, clinical, radiographic, sonographic, and MR imaging features of early **noncalcifying ductal carcinoma** are listed below:

- **Morphologic features:** tumor proliferation within the ducts.
- **Radiographic features:** increased duct density, reticular opacities, asymmetries, frequent absence of radiographic signs.

**Fig. 4.37 A 59-year-old woman who presented with a nonspecific mass at the 12-o'clock position in the upper quadrant of the left breast.** There was no skin or nipple retraction and no discharge. The lesion was identified histologically as *noncalcifying invasive ductal carcinoma*.

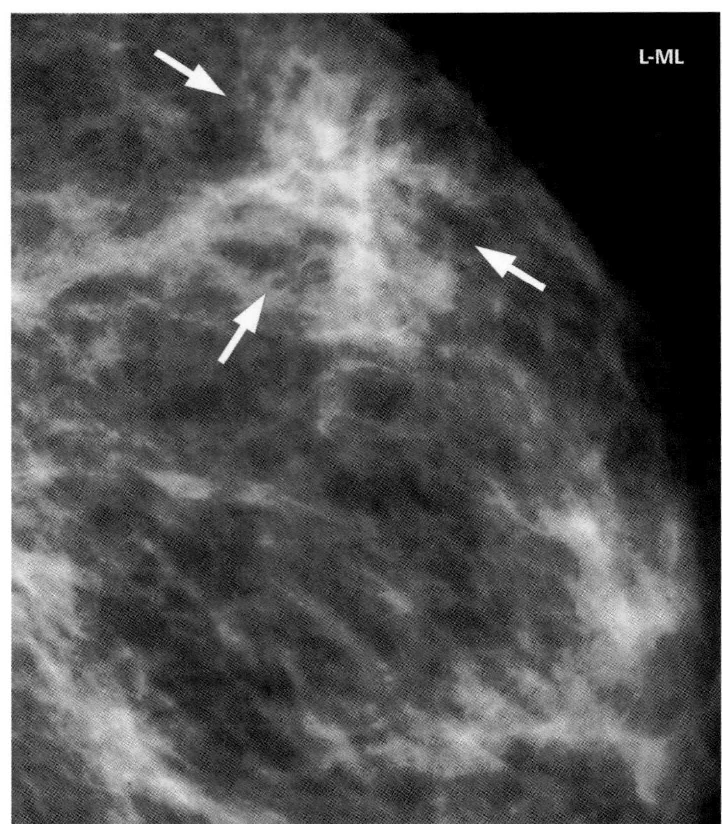


**a** Mammography showing left oblique view: inhomogeneous linear opacities a great distance from the nipple (thus no nipple retraction).

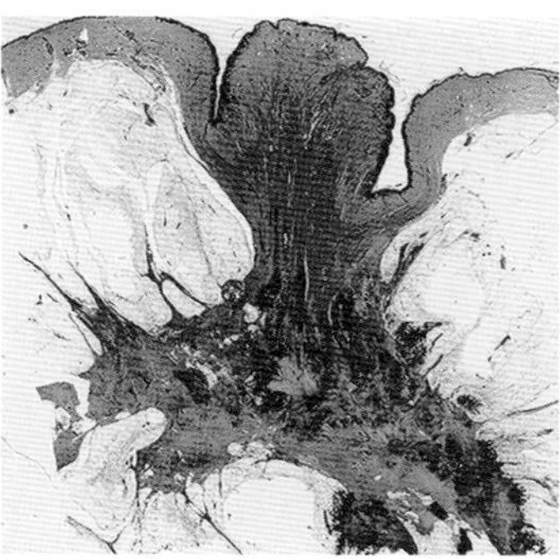

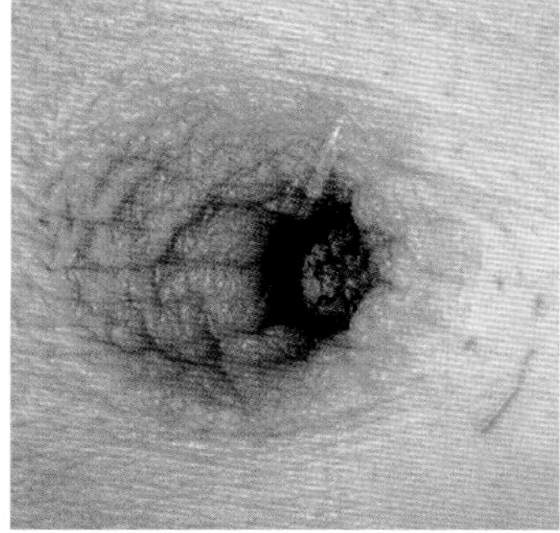

**b** Histologic section of the areola (a different patient) shows a retroareolar noncalcifying tumor infiltrating the milk ducts, with nipple retraction as a first clinical sign of malignancy. **c** Clinical aspect of tumor-induced nipple retraction.

- **Clinical features:** no palpable mass, nonspecific doughy firmness of the glandular tissue, nipple retraction, discharge (bloody or watery).
- **Sonographic features:** ductectasia with intraductal proliferation.
- **MRI features:** predominantly ductal gadolinium enhancement.

It is not unusual to find intraductal carcinomas in proximity to a cyst, or a cyst may develop next to the intraductal tumor when the tumor mass obstructs the draining duct (**Fig. 4.15**). In extremely rare cases carcinomas develop in the wall of duct cysts, creating the appearance of a cystic carcinoma (see **Fig. 5.138**, p. 274).

**Fig. 4.38** **Comedocarcinoma.**

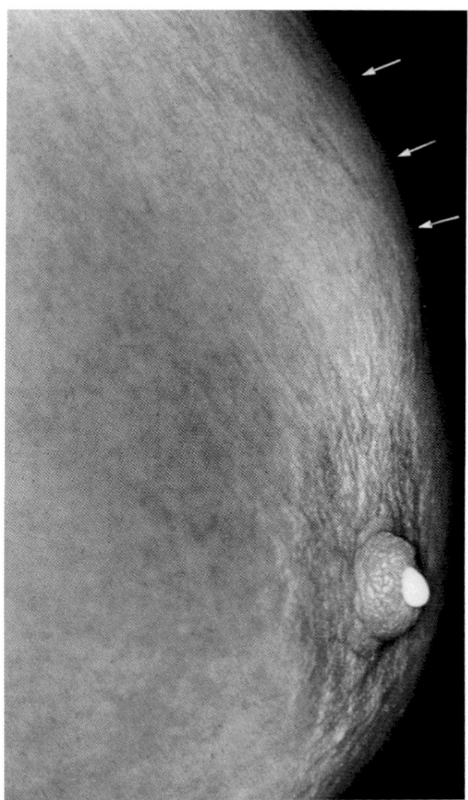

**a** Clinical appearance of the breast shows a tumor bulging beneath the skin (arrows) and a milky white nipple discharge (milk of calcium).

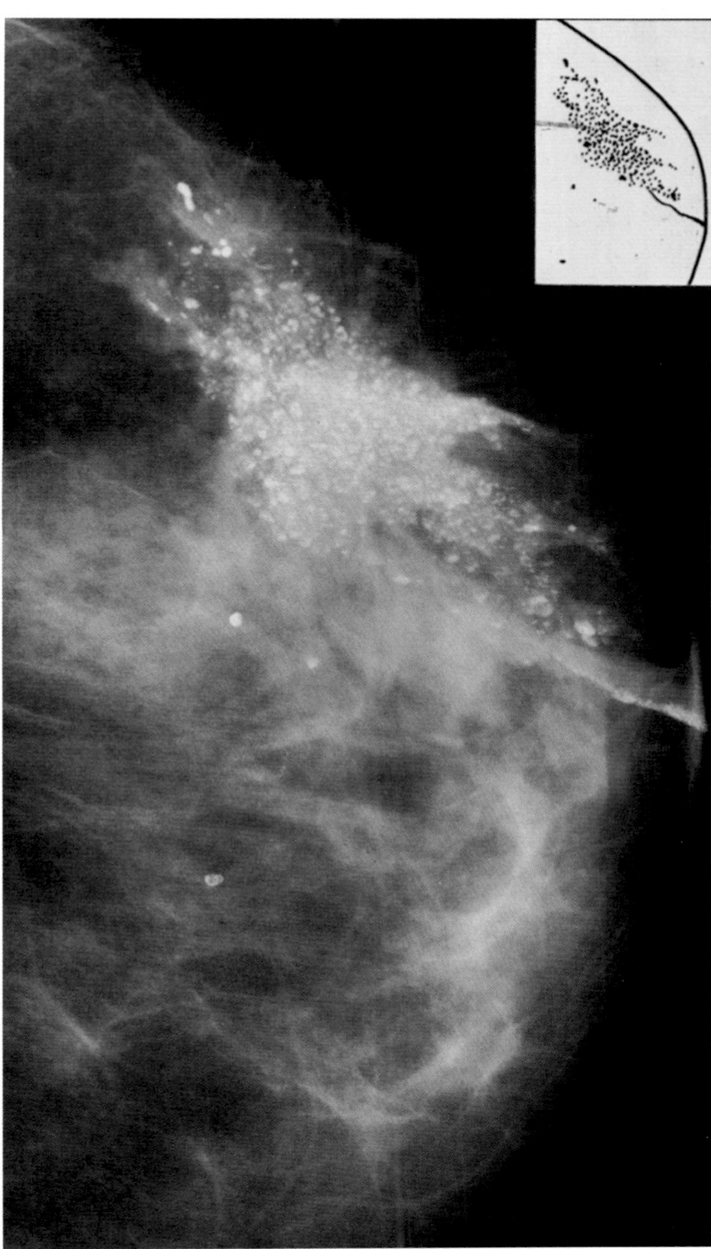

**b** Mediolateral mammogram shows massive coarse calcifications with pleomorphic particles. The Cooper ligaments of the nipple also show calcifications (tumor involves the entire lobe and has spread into surrounding tissues).

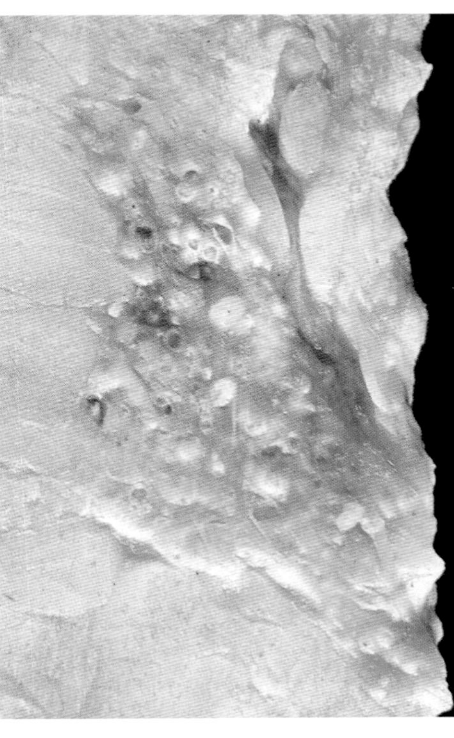

**c** Cut surface of the tumor shows ectatic grayish-white ducts, some ruptured, with yellow comedone plugs that can be popped like acne blackheads and squeezed from the cut surface (hence the name "comedone").

### *Ductal Spread with Calcifications*

See **Fig. 4.34 d**, p. 65.

The pathologist finds calcifications or hydroxyapatite in approximately two-thirds of all ductal carcinomas (Barth et al. 1977), while the radiologists finds them in only one-third of cases. This relates to the resolution limits of radiographs and to particle size. The particles are smaller and more numerous in calcifying ductal carcinoma than in other infiltrating malignancies (Hassler 1969). They are pleomorphic in the **comedo type**, flocculent in the **papillary type**, and punctate in the **cribriform type.** They present a variety of cluster shapes within the lobes and lobules including triangular (**Fig. 4.38**) and dovetail configurations. Lanyi refers to these configurations again and again in his numerous publications (Lanyi 1986, 2003; Lanyi et al. 1994). The calcifications occur not only in the lumina of the ducts and lobules but also—with benign lesions—in the interlobular stroma (Barth 1979 a). The particles vary in size and present bizarre

**Fig. 4.39 Microcalcification.** Scanning electron micrograph of a 0.1 mm calcium particle (comedo plug, 50 × magnification) taken from the center of a duct. Several small calcium flecks are visible on the surface of the particle and enlarge the plug through accretion.

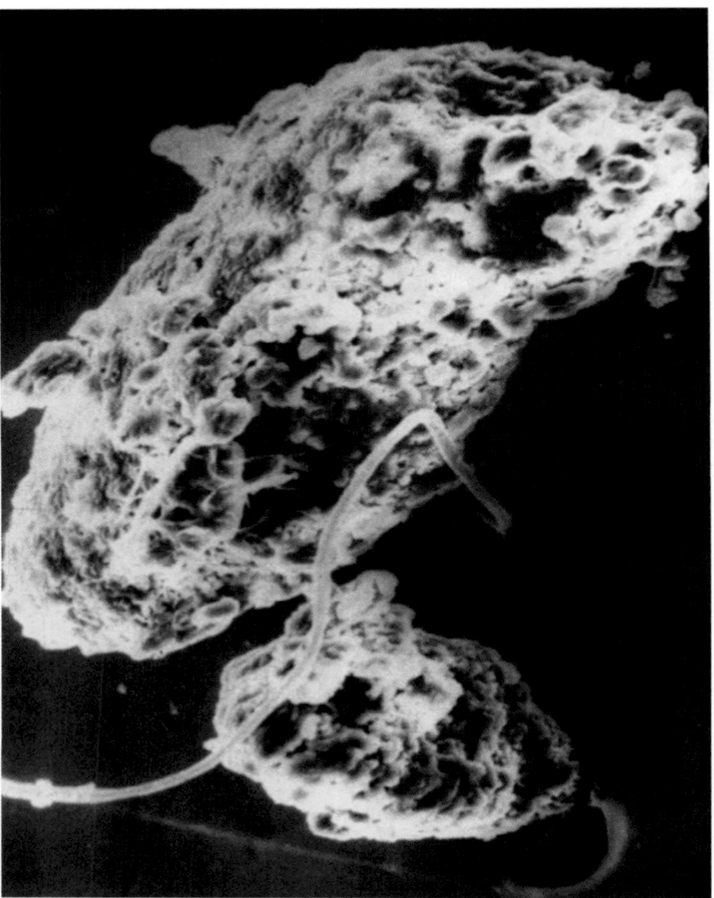

**Fig. 4.40 Scanning electron micrograph** of the surface of a 0.4 mm calcium particle (1000× magnification). The filigreed "branches and twigs" most likely originate from small side-branches of the duct system (see TDLU, p. 23 and the small ducts of TDLU, **Fig. 2.1 b**, p. 10).

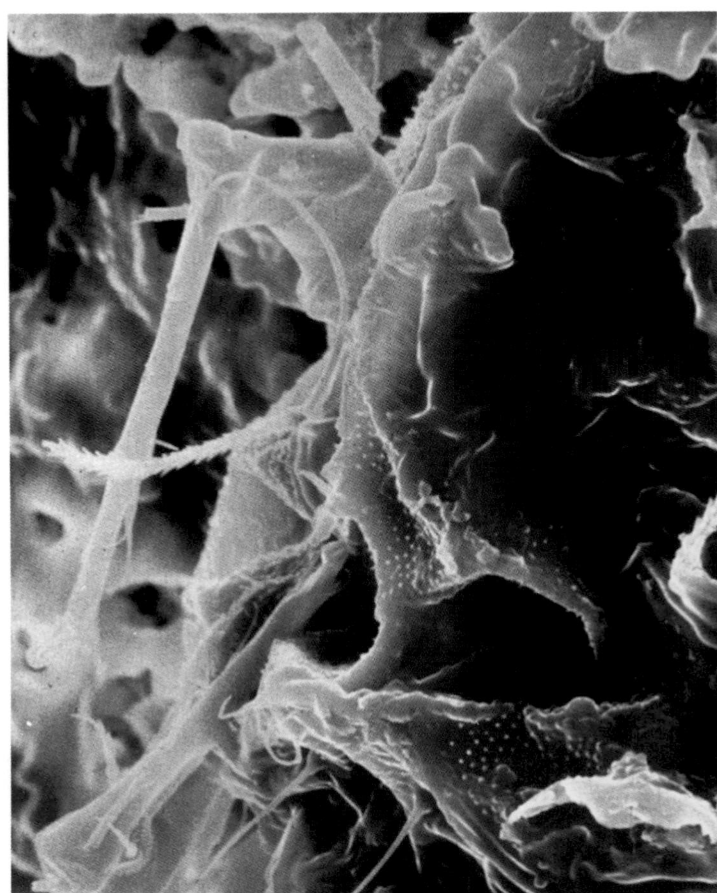

shapes. They enlarge through appositional growth (calcium accretion), becoming detectable on conventional mammograms when they reach a diameter of approximately 0.1 mm and even earlier on digital mammograms (**Figs. 4.39, 4.40**).

The calcifications occasionally extend as far as the nipple or the Cooper ligaments (see **Fig. 4.38 b**).

Not all mammographically suspicious calcifications originate from epithelial necrosis. Microradiographic studies show that calcium occasionally precipitates in an apatite-rich milieu ("milk of calcium"). These precipitates enlarge by appositional growth, becoming mammographically visible calcifications. The cause of this process is unknown, however. It is conceivable that disturbances in the electrical membrane potential consisting of abnormal or locally absent electric currents in the breast may cause this precipitation to occur.

One-fourth of all mammographically detected atypical calcifications in the breast are malignant. The most common histologic findings are listed below:

- Carcinoma (23%)
- Adenosis (60%)
- Apocrine epithelial proliferation (5%) (microcystic calcifications)
- Ductal papilloma (2%)
- Fibroadenoma (7%)
- Fat necrosis (2%)
- Scars and connective-tissue calcifications (1%)

> **!** **Calcifying neoplasms, unlike noncalcifying ductal carcinomas, are radiographically detectable at a relatively early stage—long before they are manifested clinically by nipple or skin retraction, a palpable mass, or discharge and long before they exhibit tumor criteria at ultrasound or MRI. These relatively slow-growing lesions are definitely in the domain of mammography, and this modality is still essential for the early detection of breast cancer.**

Underlying tumor morphology cannot always be determined solely from the number and arrangement of the calcifications and the apparent shape of the lesion, although Lanyi (1986) established a practical system that is very useful for radiologists. Even with apparently benign calcifications, however, there is always the possibility of an unpleasant surprise.

Ultrasound is of little help in the differential diagnosis of calcium deposits. When an invasive neoplasm is already present, hypoechoic areas with ill-defined margins may be seen within the calcified region. Occasionally this allows us to distinguish DCIS from an invasive tumor, but the hypoechoic areas may also stem from the calcifications themselves.

One of the most difficult decisions for the radiologist is to determine which calcifications require further investigation. Short-term follow-ups are of no value, and only follow-ups from 6 to 12 months could supply useful information on calcium progression. From the standpoint of the patient's emotional health, however, it is desirable to obtain immediate clarification. Questionable calcification clusters can be quickly and almost painlessly biopsied on an ambulatory basis by digital stereotactic core-needle biopsy (CNB) or vacuum biopsy to establish a histologic diagnosis. Fine-needle aspiration (FNA) should not be used for the analysis of calcifications because of the frequent aspiration of cellular debris, which is difficult to evaluate. If CNB reveals DCIS or an invasive malignancy, the core biopsy sample can also be used for the immunohistochemical analysis of prognostic factors.

**Tip**

**Ductal neoplasia should be suspected whenever a new microcalcification cluster appears within a short period of time (months).**

Digital mammography with calcification detection software (computer-aided detection, CAD) can be helpful in finding very small calcification clusters that show little contrast with surrounding tissues. CAD is particularly helpful in screening, where many images must be analyzed within a limited time (see p. 126). The human eye and the attentiveness of the examiner can quickly tire in situations where up to 800 images from 200 women must be analyzed every hour (Heinlein et al. 2001).

If microcalcifications have been classified as benign by stereotactic CNB but continue to increase, they should be completely removed by vacuum biopsy. According to German quality guidelines, the diagnosis in 80% of all operations should be confirmed by preoperative interventional procedures, which raises the question why this should not be done in 100% of operations. Because the differential diagnosis of breast calcifications is a difficult task, many women undergo unnecessary surgery. Unfortunately, too few radiologists and gynecologists opt for interventional procedures (except in screening, where there is a tendency to overuse percutaneous biopsy), despite the fact that interventional procedures could eliminate the need for 25% of all operations

The morphologic, radiographic, sonographic, MRI and clinical features of early **calcifying ductal carcinoma** are listed below:

- **Morphologic features:** predominantly intraductal tumor growth.
- **Radiographic features:** clustered (pleo- or isomorphic) microcalcifications (needle-shaped, flocculent), arranged along a duct, next to a cyst, segmental within a lobule (e.g., triangular), or in the nipple; no circumscribed tumor mass.
- **Clinical features:** no palpable mass and no skin or nipple retraction. Discharge is rare.
- **Sonographic features:** no change in the early stage. Coarse flocculent calcifications seldom appear as hypoechoic areas.
- **MRI features:** no change initially. Larger areas cause a focal, predominantly ductal pattern of gadolinium enhancement.

### Predominantly Round to Lobulated Growth

See **Fig. 4.34 c**, p. 64.

**Ductal** and **lobular** carcinomas may both be lobulated, but this morphology is more common with advanced ductal tumors. Advanced lobular neoplasms usually undergo spiculated or diffuse spread.

Common examples of lobulated tumors are very cellular neoplasms with a high fluid content such as **medullary carcinoma** (see **Fig. 4.34 c**), **mucinous carcinoma** (see **Figs. 4.41; 5.169 b**, p. 314), **intracystic carcinoma** (see **Fig. 5.138**, p. 274), **papillomatous carcinoma** (see **Fig. 4.26**, p. 53) and **apocrine carcinoma** (see **Fig. 5.49**, p. 140). Radiographically, the tumor has relatively smooth margins that may be scalloped, rounded, or partially ill-defined. Unlike cysts, it does not have a halo.

It has homogeneous density and usually does not contain microcalcifications. Only papillary carcinomas may contain fine or coarse calcifications. Peritumoral retraction is absent, although a fast-growing peripheral tumor may expand sufficiently to cause a lump in the skin.

Very cellular neoplasms may "explode" in the preclinical phase through exuberant cell growth and rapid volume doubling. The question has not yet been researched whether rapid growth is associated with earlier metastasis. This does not appear to be the case, however, as medullary neoplasms have a relatively favorable prognosis. In the debate regarding the link between hormone replacement therapy and the growth stimulation of receptor-positive tumors, it is reasonable to suggest that rapid tumor growth not accompanied by distal or nodal metastasis could actually be helpful for early detection—provided the patient presents for regular screening examinations at 12- to 18-month intervals, depending on the familial predisposition to breast cancer.

**The slower a tumor grows, the greater its metastatic potential.**

The ability to detect lobulated tumors on mammograms depends on the density of the surrounding parenchyma. Nodules are clearly visible in breasts that consist predominantly of fatty tissue (ACR 1, see Fig. **4.31**). On the other hand, nodules are frequently missed in stroma-rich breasts (ACR 2–4), even when they are clinically palpable (6% of all breast carcinomas), due to a lack of contrast with surrounding connective tissue (see **Fig. 5.140**). This does not mean, however, that all malignancies that are missed in the breast are of the lobulated cellular type and have a correspondingly good prognosis. The interval cancers that were missed in radiodense breasts (121 of 239) during screening by Roubidoux et al. (2004) tended to be very aggressive (G3) estrogen-receptor-negative tumors with relatively large diameters and a relatively high incidence of axillary lymph node metastasis. Thus, **radiographically dense breasts** with a density of ACR 2 or higher should additionally be investigated by **ultrasound** (tumors up to 0.5 cm may be missed mammographically in ACR 2 breasts) to minimize the number of tumors that are missed by mammography.

As a general rule, every **palpable breast mass** should be morphologically confirmed, regardless of whether or not it is mammography visible—unless it has been positively identified as a cyst or lipoma by ultrasound. Mainly for psychological reasons (and not because something malignant might develop from a cyst), the cyst should be percutaneously aspirated and completely drained so that the palpable nodule is gone. A pneumocystogram is unnecessary when ultrasound findings are innocent. Lobulated tumors can be detected at ultrasound when they measure at least 5 mm in diameter. They appear as hypoechoic lesions with relatively smooth or indistinct margins. The smaller they are, the more closely they may

**Fig. 4.41** Anatomic–radiographic comparison of spiculated and lobulated tumors.

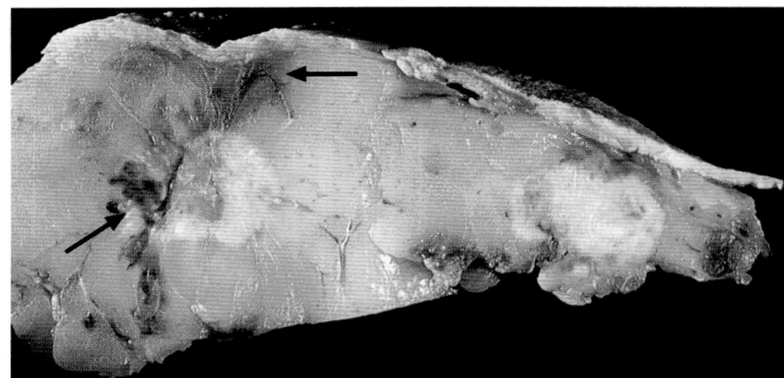

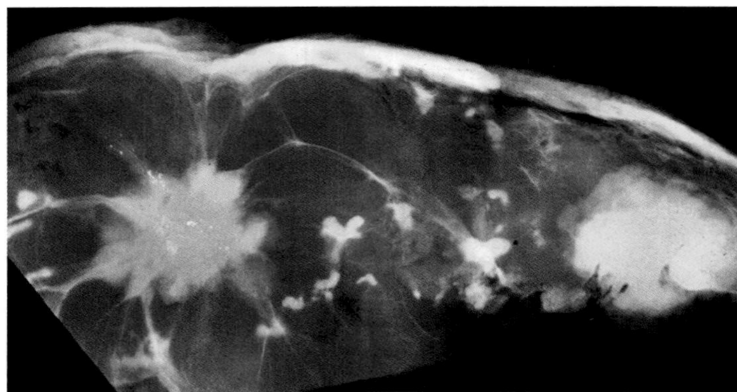

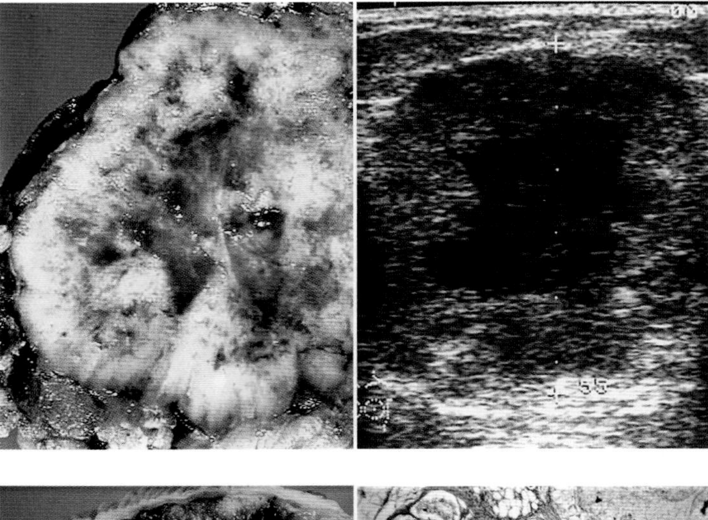

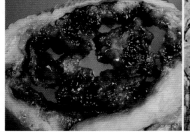

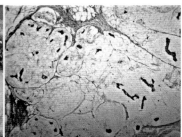

**a** The *cut surface of a gross specimen* reveals two grayish-white tumors, one spiculated (left) and the other scalloped (right), embedded in yellow fat. Hemorrhagic areas are visible on the left side (arrows) following fine-needle aspiration. The spiculated tumor is probably an older, slower-growing lesion while the lobulated tumor is younger and faster growing. *Specimen radiograph* (below) shows the typical characteristics of stellate (see p. 72) and lobular (see p. 71) tumors.

**b** *Anatomical/ultrasound correlation* of *lobular tumors. Image upper left:* Macroview of a lobular tumor with central necrosis. Ultrasound shows the necrosis very clearly with the smooth outer contours of the tumor *(image upper right)*. *Image below left:* Macroview of a *mucinous carcinoma* with shrunken tumor masses in the center and smooth contours. *Histology (below right)* shows expanding mucus, inside tender fibrous septa.

resemble a fibroadenoma or cyst (see **Fig. 5.49**, p. 140). Ninety percent of neoplasms measuring at least 1 cm in diameter do not present completely smooth or scalloped margins but are surrounded by a echogenic rim of variable thickness (1–5 mm). This rim is caused by tumor infiltration of surrounding tissues and should be included in measurements of tumor size. Measuring only the central mass would underestimate the actual tumor size. Even the pathologist can determine actual tumor size only by working with unfixed material. Tumors shrink when they are fixed in formalin, becoming approximately 10% smaller than in the unfixed state. The echogenic rim is often visible in the cut surface of the surgical specimen as a pale yellow zone located at the interface with fatty tissue.

Incidentally, ductal growth does not occur with **medullary carcinoma**, which is why atypical microcalcifications are not often found in this type of tumor.

Lobulated tumors have smooth margins like fibroadenomas on MR images and usually show intense gadolinium enhancement, also like fibroadenomas. Perifocal satellite tumors usually do not accompany medullary carcinoma, but their presence in association with very cellular ductal tumors may signify DCIS. Lobulated tumors cannot be positively distinguished from fibroadenoma in **time–density curves** (see **Fig. 5.91**, p. 205), and it may be dangerous to rely only on enhancement kinetics. Generally, a nodule must be diagnosed morphologically rather than by magnetic resonance imaging, mammography, or ultrasound.

Magnetic resonance imaging may be useful in a neoplasm that has already been histologically confirmed in order to detect or exclude multi- and plurifocality in the affected breast and to exclude a second carcinoma in the healthy breast. This is important, as concomitant carcinomas in the opposite breast are found in up to 12% of cases.

A lobulated tumor can be distinguished from fibroadenoma cytologically from cysts with debris inside the lumen with 98% confidence by FNA. Approximately 2% of fibroadenomas have a cellular pattern closely resembling that of a polymorphocellular malignancy.

Suspicious FNA findings (Pap III–V cytology) can be definitively confirmed by CNB. Malignancies are excised while fibroadenoma (or papilloma) should be removed by vacuum biopsy whenever possible (see p. 230). Removal is not necessary for every fibroadenoma. If CNB or FNA shows no evidence of atypias, the risk of malignant transformation is no higher than in healthy breast parenchyma.

Cellular tumors grow rapidly and are prone to **spontaneous hemorrhage**. This bleeding does not always present as a typical "blue spot," however; sometimes it appears as skin redness, similar to mastitis in ductectasia, for example. Thus, hemorrhagic and inflammatory skin redness cannot be distinguished clinically, particularly since the patient does not always know whether trauma to the breast has occurred. Moreover, the patient does not always see a doctor right away but often waits until the cutaneous symptoms have subsided. With a purely traumatic hematoma, a nodule may form at the center of the hemorrhage due to fat necrosis and clot formation. Without CNB or FNA, it may be difficult to distinguish this type of nodule from a spontaneously bleeding malignant tumor. A useful clinical criterion is that the palpable and radiographic tumor sizes are approximately equal.

The morphologic, radiographic, sonographic, clinical, and MRI features of *lobulated malignancies* are summarized below:

- **Morphologic features:** high cellularity and fluid content, scant stroma, tendency to form nodules.
- **Radiographic features:** smooth margins with possible short extensions, homogeneous radiodensity, no microcalcifications; contrasts poorly with breast parenchyma.
- **Clinical features:** lobulated, frequently mobile mass with no skin or nipple retraction, equal palpable and radiographic tumor sizes, proneness to spontaneous hemorrhage, rapid growth. Markedly less compliant than normal or surrounding glandular tissue.
- **Sonographic features:** hypoechoic nodule with smooth, scalloped, indistinct margins; little posterior acoustic enhancement; usually has a hyperechoic rim.
- **MRI features:** intensely enhancing nodule with smooth or ill-defined margins.

Cellular metastases from carcinomas in other organs (kidney, thyroid gland, lung, stomach) or from melanoma are very rare in the breast. The metastases also have smooth margins and homogeneous density, making them indistinguishable from medullary and mucinous carcinoma. They are usually bilateral and multifocal, however. They are invariably round.

Some cellular types of **sarcoma** are also lobulated. They can mimic the radiographic appearance of a fibroadenoma, cyst, mucinous tumor, or papilloma but are distinguished from these by their very rapid rate of growth. Their margins show a mixed smooth and scalloped pattern on ultrasound with only minimal unsharpness. There are no mammographic or sonographic findings that are pathognomonic for sarcoma. Microcalcifications are absent. Radiation-induced Kaposi sarcoma—an angiosarcoma that spreads mainly in the skin—is rare (see **Fig. 5.180**).

### Predominantly Stellate or Spiculated Growth

See **Fig. 4.34 a**, p. 64.

The group of predominantly stellate tumors most notably includes **stroma-rich (scirrhous) ductal carcinoma**, formerly called hypocellular solid carcinoma. Some **lobular carcinomas** (30%) are also stellate while the rest are more diffuse. Well-differentiated (G1) **tubular carcinomas** may also have stellate and radial features, although lobulated forms also occur. They must be differentiated from radial scars (see below). Tubular carcinomas metastasize very rarely.

These stellate tumors are characterized by a heavy stromal reaction. They grow more slowly than very cellular tumors, are more prone to calcification, and are associated with skin and nipple retraction (see **Fig. 4.41 a**).

Their slow growth presumably makes them—except for tubular tumors (see **Fig. 5.97**, p. 216)—more dangerous than lobulated tumors because undetected lesions as small as 0.6 mm are able to metastasize to other body sites at a relatively early stage (see **Fig. 3.1**, p. 21). The prognosis is less favorable than with ductal calcifying and lobulated tumors. In advanced cases the breast may become significantly smaller due to stromal proliferation and eventually may undergo complete involution. Mixed stellate and diffuse lobular carcinomas are especially likely to cause a decrease in breast size, which is clearly appreciated in oblique mammograms by comparison with previous films (Harvey et al. 2000). In some cases the affected breast may become stony hard. Not only is it firmer on palpation, but mammograms demonstrate small, somewhat nonspecific focal densities that may be well-delineated or may be indistinguishable from the breast parenchyma. Clustered microcalcifications mark the site where the tumor originated.

Tumors with a greater stromal content tend to develop longer spicules. Not all stellate densities on mammograms are malignant tumors. Differentiation is mainly required from **radial scars, sclerosing adenosis**, and scar-forming processes such as **hematomas, mastitis,** and **fibrosis**.

> **Tip**
>
> **Palpation is important in assessing the benignancy or malignancy of a spiculated mammographic density. If a palpable mass is not found in a patient whose mammograms show a subcutaneous stellate density or a large focal density with ill-defined margins, it is unlikely that a malignant tumor is present—although this cannot be stated with absolute certainty.**

A discrepancy between clinical and radiographic size is typical of scirrhous tumors. The tumor often seems larger clinically than radiographically due to increased peritumoral cellularity and its infiltration of ducts and lymphatic channels. Lanyi et al. (1994) stress the importance of a complete resection, as they found that 91% of these tumors were associated with foci of DCIS. These authors felt that spicules at the tumor margins were of greater diagnostic importance than microcalcifications (**Fig. 4.42**).

Most scirrhous cancers appear sonographically as hypoechoic lesions with irregular margins and a dense posterior acoustic shadow. In the author's experience, the more sonodense features described in some textbooks are seen only in diffusely infiltrating lobular malignancies, not in scirrhous stellate nodules. An echogenic rim like that of very cellular tumors is somewhat rare with stellate carcinomas and is usually narrower.

Magnetic resonance imaging shows a variable degree of gadolinium enhancement, depending on the tumor grade (G1–G3, see **Fig. 5.105 i**, p. 228) and receptor status. Marklund et al. (2008) observed very intense peripheral contrast enhancement in receptor-positive carcinomas but did not find this enhancement in receptor-negative tumors. So far this observation has not been explained.

The lesion extent shown by MR mammography more accurately depicts the pathoanatomy of the tumor than mammography or ultrasound, especially in radiographically dense breasts, because the surrounding EIC usually enhances along with the rest of the tumor (see **Fig. 4.29 e, f**, p. 56). Magnetic resonance imaging, with its unlimited capacity for magnification, is ideal for distinguishing affected from healthy tissue, especially in breasts with extensive tumor involvement (see **Fig. 5.188 e**, p. 343). Spiculated tumor margins are a typical MRI finding. Thus, margins are a more important criterion for malignancies than gadolinium enhancement kinetics, and they are most clearly demonstrated in sagittal images. The morphologic, radiographic, sonographic, clinical and MRI features of *stellate malignancies* are summarized below:

**Fig. 4.42 Palpable mass in the upper outer quadrant of the right breast in a 63-year-old woman.** Mediolateral mammogram of the upper portion of the breast (magnified view) shows numerous oblong, pleomorphic comedo calcifications with a 1 cm central nodule consistent with infiltrative growth. The tumor has broken out of the duct system at this site and has formed a solid cancer nodule with broad linear opacities.

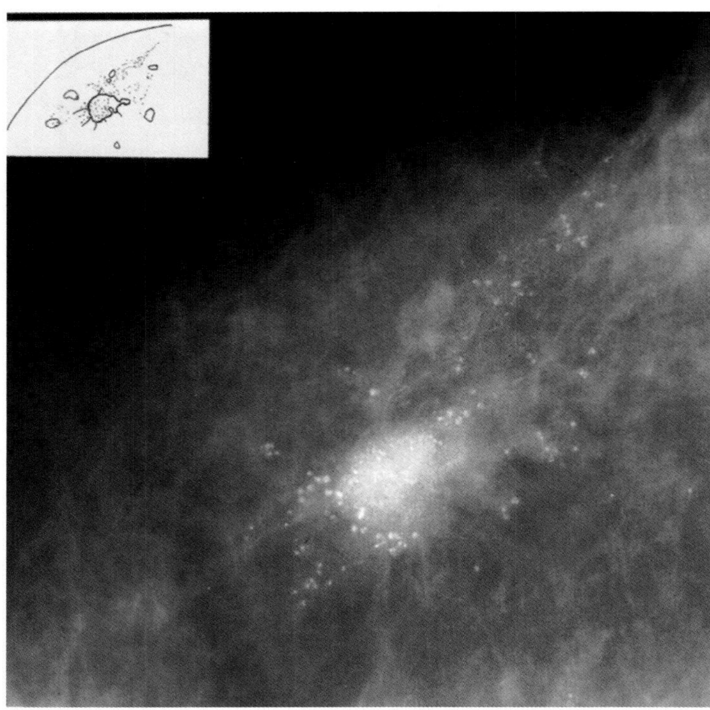

- **Morphologic features:** abundant stroma; extensive local tissue infiltration with associated retraction and elastosis; infiltration of the ducts, lymphatics, and fatty tissue.
- Radiographic features: stellate densities, spiculations of varying length, microcalcifications, and linear opacities.
- **Clinical features:** skin and nipple retraction, discrepancy between palpable and radiographic tumor size, slow growth. Significantly less compliant than normal glandular tissue.
- **Sonographic features:** hypoechoic focal densities with irregular, spiculated margins and a posterior acoustic shadow. Architectural distortion toward the tumor.
- **MRI features:** usually intense gadolinium enhancement, even in the tumor periphery. Possible satellite lesions or atypias in the clinically healthy breast.

Occasionally, stellate and lobulated tumors may both be elements of the same tumor mass or may occur separately as adjacent nodules in the same breast (see **Fig. 4.41**). The stellate tumor in these cases is most likely to be the primary tumor (slower growth), while the lobulated tumor presumably developed later and grew more rapidly.

### Mixed (Lobulated-Stellate-Ductal) Tumors

See **Fig. 4.34 b**, p. 64.

Approximately 15% of all tumors are not purely stellate, lobulated, or ductal but involve a combination of these forms. This is explained by the fact that 80% of invasive cancers originate from intraductal carcinoma. The greater the stromal content of the tumor, the greater its spiculation and the slower its rate of growth.

During its invasive stage, ductal carcinoma gives rise to circumscribed tumor nodules in which the thickened and expanded ducts can be identified on histologic examination (**Fig. 4.42**).

While calcifications are absent or rare in lobulated tumors, they frequently accompany all other forms (except diffuse lobular and inflammatory neoplasms). Calcifications may occur in the peripheral portions of stellate or mixed nodules or in proximity to DCIS satellite lesions. EIC frequently accompanies these tumors (see p. 75), in contrast to lobulated medullary tumors.

**Tumors with greater spiculation should be excised with a broader healthy tissue margin.**

### Diffuse Spread

See **Fig. 4.34 f**, p. 65.

Approximately 10% of all breast carcinomas are in this category. Typical examples are listed below:

- Invasive lobular carcinoma
- Diffuse small-cell carcinoma
- Inflammatory carcinoma
- Diffuse anaplastic tumor

No visible breast changes are present in the early stages. As the disease progresses, the tissue becomes smaller and begins to harden. Breast enlargement is rare and occurs most often with inflammatory carcinoma and occasionally with invasive lobular carcinoma. While **inflammatory carcinoma** of the breast is manifested by rapid changes such as redness, swelling, increased warmth, and enlarged skin pores, especially about the nipple see **Figs. 5.147, 5.148**), the breast changes associated with other diffuse neoplasms are insidious and may go undetected for some time. The changes develop slowly and diffusely, without forming a palpable nodule, in one quadrant of the breast. From there they spread throughout the breast over a period of months or years. The process is so insidious that huge tumors may develop literally under the nose of various doctors and go undetected in multiple examinations. Often it is the patient herself who finally insists on having a breast biopsy to investigate a palpable mass. Even the typical "orange-peel skin" like that seen in inflammatory carcinoma does not accompany the other entities, especially diffuse lobular carcinomas. Similarly, skin or nipple retraction is rare and occurs only at very advanced stages. The parenchyma is palpably firm and lobulated. The axillary lymph nodes are generally enlarged due to reactive lymphadenectomy or metastatic involvement. **Diffuse tumor growth is usually missed on mammograms and is therefore a major factor in malpractice suits.**

Diffuse tumors appear sonographically as ill-defined hypoechoic areas that may have scalloped or irregular wavy margins. Comparison with the opposite breast (if unaffected) will show evidence of a diffusely invasive neoplasm, usually with a lobular origin, prompting a recommendation for ultrasound-guided CNB. Nine percent of all diffuse or focal lobular carcinomas in our practice were detected sonographically in a breast with normal mammograms.

The diffuse lesions show intense gadolinium uptake on contrast-enhanced MRI and appear to have relatively smooth margins. This examination can accurately define the extent of breast infiltration (see **Fig. 5.148 f**, p. 290).

**Fig. 4.43** Mediolateral mammogram of the right and left breast.

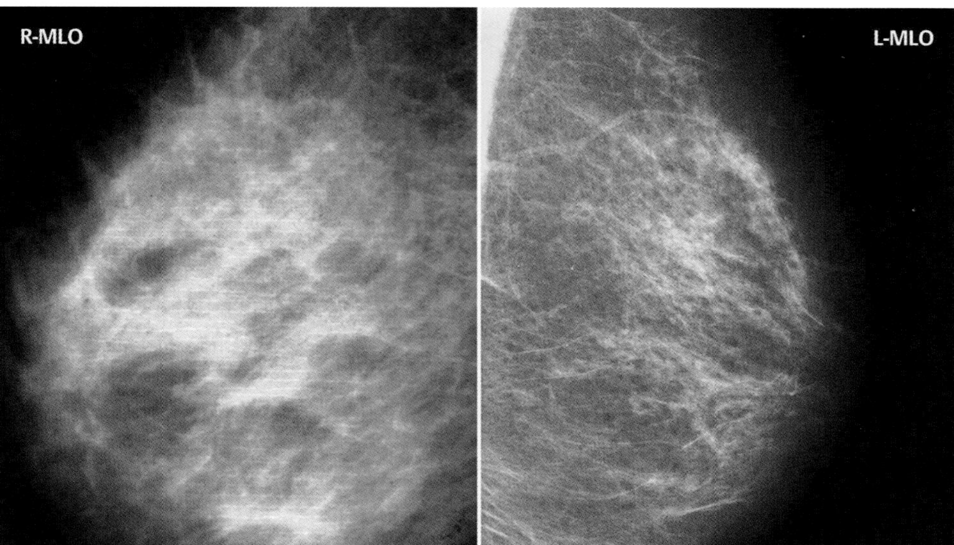


**a** *Left (right breast):* Inflammatory carcinoma has caused substantial breast enlargement with increased inhomogeneous reticular density in the breast parenchyma and typical increased markings in the subcutaneous fat in the lower half of the breast (enlarged lymphatics). *Right (left breast):* Mammography of the left breast for comparison.

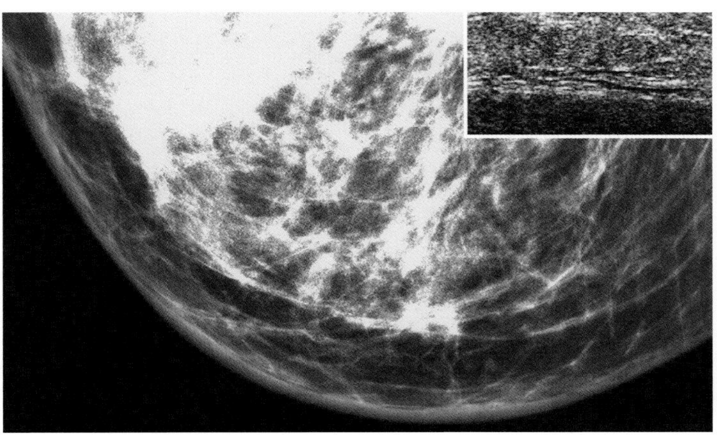

**b** *Mammography:* Lower part of right breast (magnified view). Enlarged subcutaneous lymphatics with thickening of the skin. *Insert:* Enlarged lymphatics (skin at bottom of image).

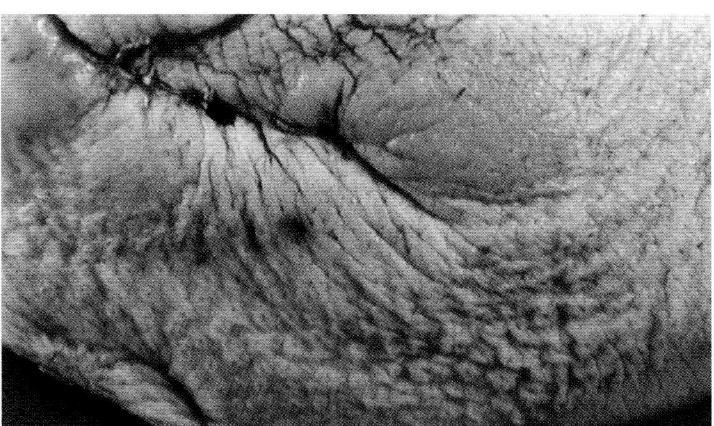

**c** Massive orange-peel dimpling of the skin associated with an advanced neoplasm.

The diagnosis is histologically best established by the ultrasound-guided core-needle or vacuum biopsy of sites localized by ultrasound findings or nonspecific firmness.

**Inflammatory carcinoma** is associated with redness and swelling of the skin, especially in the periareolar region. **Orange-peel skin** with dimpled pores is another common finding (see **Fig. 4.43 c** and **5.148 a, b**, p. 289). The swollen skin tends to protrude around the nipple, causing the nipple to appear retracted even though it is not. This condition is difficult to distinguish clinically and mammographically from obstructed axillary lymphatic drainage, which may also cause skin redness but does not enlarge the pores. Mammography is not useful for differentiation, since even nonneoplastic lymphatic obstruction (due to scarring, lymphoma, vascular aneurysm, or seroma) may present with retriculostriate densities in the tissue (see **Fig. 4.43 a, b**). Ultrasound in these conditions shows enlarged lymphatics in the axillary recess—the most reliable indicator of axillary lymphatic obstruction. Inflammatory carcinoma, on the other hand, tends to cause diffuse, peripheral infiltration of lymphatics in the breast and may enlarge them in the direction of the nipple but not toward the axilla (see **Fig. 5.179 d**). Neoplastic obstruction of intramammary lymphatics, like axillary obstruction, does cause mammographically visible skin thickening about the nipple but does not produce the reticular markings in the subcutaneous fat that are typical of inflammatory carcinoma (see **Fig. 4.43 b**).

Otherwise, ultrasound supplies little information on inflammatory carcinoma, although it may show typical enlargement of the axillary lymph nodes with or without extended intracutaneous lymphatics (see p. 194). Magnetic resonance imaging of inflammatory carcinoma can occasionally define the primary tumor, but the most common finding is diffuse gadolinium enhancement distributed throughout the breast (see **Fig. 5.147 e**, p. 288). If breast biopsy is indicated, a vacuum biopsy is preferred over CNB and is definitely superior to FNA. Vacuum biopsy yields a larger tissue sample for evaluation. A punch biopsy of the skin is sometimes useful in cases where the tumor has actually infiltrated the skin. If skin swelling is due solely to lymphedema, however, it can be dangerous to try to exclude inflammatory carcinoma by performing a skin biopsy (see **Fig. 5.179**, p. 327).

Preoperative staging by positron emission tomography (PET) is recommended for locally advanced invasive lobular carcinoma as well as anaplastic carcinoma and clinically pronounced inflammatory carcinoma that has been confirmed by biopsy. This imaging modality can detect tumor deposits outside the breast that will influence treatment planning.

The morphologic, radiographic, sonographic, clinical, and MRI features of *inflammatory carcinoma* are listed below. (Note that there may be other small, circumscribed neoplasms associated with histologically confirmed lymphatic invasion. These lesions are characteristic of inflammatory carcinoma in a strict pathoanatomic sense but do not always produce the same clinical features as inflammatory carcinoma—redness, swelling, orange-peel skin dimpling—due to more limited involvement of the lymphatic system.)

- **Morphologic features**: diffuse lymphatic invasion in the breast parenchyma, enlarged lymphatics, rapid lymph node involvement.
- **Radiographic features:** prominent reticular markings in the breast, especially subcutaneously, caused by the enlarged lymphatics (see **Fig. 5.5a**). There are no microcalcifications and no circumscribed tumor mass.
- **Clinical features:** rapid increase in breast size, orange-peel skin, apparent nipple retraction, enlarged axillary lymph nodes.
- **Sonographic features:** nonspecific changes. Many cases have no sonographic abnormalities.
- **MRI features:** diffuse, slightly reticular pattern of gadolinium enhancement, somewhat nonspecific, with increased subcutaneous markings in the T1-weighted image.

The morphologic, radiographic, clinical, sonographic, and MRI features of *diffuse lobular carcinoma* are summarized below:

- **Morphologic features:** diffuse focal and sometimes small-cell infiltration of the breast parenchyma and fat; eventual lymph node involvement.
- **Radiographic features:** usually no visible changes and no circumscribed tumor mass. Microcalcifications may form in rare cases. Tumor is frequently obscured by radiodense parenchyma.
- **Clinical features:** gradual induration with a progressive decrease in breast size. Nodular and enlarging areas are sometimes present. Slow growth, no nipple retraction, rare skin retraction, no axillary lymph node enlargement.
- **Sonographic features:** atypical hypoechoic areas with smooth or ill-defined margins, possible posterior acoustic shadow, possible acoustic enhancement. Other show extended intra- and/or subcutaneous lymphatics.
- **MRI features:** usually intense gadolinium enhancement in areas of variable size with smooth or ill-defined margins.

Thus, the external form of the carcinoma generally results from the relative proportions of cells and stroma in the tumor and its mode of spread in the breast.

The degree of tubular differentiation, cellular pleomorphism and hyperchromasia, and rate of mitosis are important considerations in planning the mode and aggressiveness of treatment, which are determined by the histologic grade and stage of the tumor and by its immunohistochemical features.

### Histologic Classification, Staging, and Grading

An invasive cancer has penetrated the basement membrane of the duct and lobules and has infiltrated the surrounding healthy tissue. The most widely used classification differentiates between **ductal and lobular tumor types**. According to Sainsbury et al. (2000), this classification is based on the concept that ductal carcinomas arise from the epithelium of the ducts while lobular carcinomas arise from the epithelium of the acini (lobules) (see **Figs. 4.11, 4.12**). Both types originate in the terminal duct lobular unit (TDLU), however, suggesting that conventional terminologies are not entirely correct from a pathologic and anatomic standpoint. Some tumors show distinctive growth patterns and changes by which they can be identified. Tumors with specific features are called "invasive carcinomas of a specific type" while others are classified as "NOS," meaning that they have no specific type. This classification is less important for the diagnostic radiologist. It is important for clinical and adjuvant therapies, however, because specific tumor types usually have a better prognosis than NOS tumors.

The **classification of invasive carcinomas** is outlined below:

- Specific types
  - Tubular
  - Cribriform
  - Medullary
  - Mucinous
  - Papillary
  - Classic lobular
- NOS types

Prognostic information can be obtained by tumor grading. The **Bloom–Richardson grading system** (Bloom and Richardson 1957) is the most familiar and is based on the grade of tubular differentiation, nuclear grade, mitosis rate, and similar factors.

The German S3 guidelines recommend the **Elston-Ellis grading system** (Elston and Ellis1991), which is a modification of the Bloom–Richardson system. The Elston–Ellis system is outlined in **Table 4.3.** A more detailed classification, the Nottingham Prognostic Index (Galea et al. 1992), additionally takes into account lymph node status. The index scores range from good (G 1) to poor (G 3), with corresponding 15-year survival rates of 80% to 13% **(Table 4.4).**

Grading provides parameters that are important in predicting disease-free survival (no recurrences or metastases) and overall survival. Approximately 10% of breast cancers fall within the G1 risk category, 70% in G 2, and 20% in G 3 (Harbeck 2002).

Immunohistochemical analysis of the tumor is closely related to grading and is part of the standard histopathologic work-up. The immunohistochemistry result is essential in the selection of treatment modalities. It provides information on hormone receptors, HER-2 determination, and the analysis of protease activity (if all these parameters are negative, the tumor is described as *triple negative* and warrants special therapeutic measures).

The levels of **urokinase plasminogen activator** (uPA) and **plasminogen activator inhibitor** (PAI) are useful in assessing the need for chemotherapy in the G 2 risk group (G 1 does not require chemotherapy and G 3 almost always requires it). The protease level, for example, identifies patients in the G 2 group who will need chemotherapy. Fifty-five percent of G 2 patients will require this therapy and 45% will not (Harbeck 2002).

**Table 4.3 Grading criteria for breast cancer** (Elston and Ellis 1991)

| Features | Criteria | Points |
|---|---|---|
| Tubule formation | > 75% | 1 |
| | 10–75% | 2 |
| | < 10% | 3 |
| Nuclear pleomorphism | Slight | 1 |
| | Moderate | 2 |
| | Pronounced | 3 |
| Mitosis rate | 0–5/10 HPF | 1 |
| | 6–11/10 HPF | 2 |
| | ≥ 12/10 HPR | 3 |
| Total score | | 3–9 |

**Groupings based on total score**

| Total score | Degree of malignancy | Group | Definition |
|---|---|---|---|
| 3–5 | Low | G1 | Well differentiated |
| 6–7 | Medium | G2 | Moderately differentiated |
| 8–9 | High | G3 | Poorly differentiated |

HPF = high-power field: the criteria stated here are for a visual field diameter of 0.45 mm, corresponding to a field setting of 18 on a standard light microscope without a wide-field tube.

**Table 4.4 Nottingham Prognostic Index** (Galea et al. 1992)

| Feature | Criterion | Points |
|---|---|---|
| Elston–Ellis tumor grade (1991) | G1 | 1 |
| | G2 | 2 |
| | G3 | 3 |
| Lymph node status | pN0 | 1 |
| | 1–3 positive lymph nodes | 2 |
| | 4 or more positive lymph nodes | 3 |

**Groupings based on index score**

| Index score | Prognosis | 15 year survival rate (%) |
|---|---|---|
| ≤ 3.4 | Good | 80 |
| 3.41–5.40 | Intermediate | 42 |
| < 5.40 | Poor | 13 |

**Tip**

**Every breast diagnostician should know these parameters, because close attention should be given to the breast parenchyma and surrounding lymph nodes during the follow-up of prognostically unfavorable tumors. Even subtle clinical, mammographic, sonographic and MRI changes should be investigated by biopsy whenever possible.**

Other histologic factors are also extremely important in making a prognosis and determining the aggressiveness of treatment:

- The histologic detection of tumor invasion of blood vessels and lymphatics is crucial. Even small, clinically occult tumors may present the histologic features of *inflammatory carcinoma.*
- The *extensive intraductal component* (EIC) occasionally precludes breast-conserving surgery or may necessitate postoperative radiotherapy with a local boost to the former tumor site.

The presence of EIC correlates with an increased risk of local recurrence. Postoperative follow-ups should be scheduled at shorter intervals and for a longer time (every 6 months for 3 years) than in patients with clear margins.

### *Staging: TNM and pTNM classification, UICC Staging*

The most widely used system for the classification of invasive carcinomas is the TNM classification (T = tumor, N = lymph nodes, M = metastasis). This system is based on clinical parameters and has therefore been modified according to pathoanatomic criteria (p).

The **T classification** is outlined below:

- **TX**: Primary tumor cannot be assessed
- **TO**: No evidence of primary tumor
- **Tis**: Carcinoma in situ
- **Tis (DCIS)**: Ductal carcinoma in situ
- **Tis (LCIS)**: Lobular carcinoma in situ
- **Tis (Paget):** Paget disease of the nipple with no detectable tumor (Paget disease combined with a detectable tumor is classified according to tumor size)
- **T1**: Tumor 2 cm or less in its greatest dimension
- **T1a**: Tumor more than 0.1 cm but not more than 0.5 cm in its greatest dimension
- **T1b**: Tumor more than 0.5 cm but not more than 1 cm in its greatest dimension
- **T1c**: Tumor more than 1 cm but not more than 2 cm in its greatest dimension
- **T2**: Tumor more than 2 cm but not more than 5 cm in its greatest dimension
- **T3**: Tumor more than 5 cm in its greatest dimension
- **T4**: Tumor of any size with direct extension to the chest wall or skin
- **T4a**: Extension to the chest wall (ribs, intercostal muscles and serratus anterior, but *not* the pectoral muscle)
- **T4b**: Edema (including orange-peel skin) or ulceration of the skin of the breast or satellite skin nodules confined to the same breast
- **T4c**: Both of the above (T4a and T4b)
- **T4 d**: Inflammatory carcinoma

The **pT classification** includes the **"pT1 mic"** category. "Microinvasion" is defined as the extension of cancer cells beyond the basement membrane into adjacent tissues with no focus more than 0.1 cm in greatest dimension. When there are multiple foci of microinvasion, the size of only the largest focus is used to classify the microinvasion. A sum of the size of all the microinvasion foci may not be used. The presence of *multiple* microinvasion foci and of multiple larger carcinomas should be recorded and classified according to the size categories of the T classification.

**Table 4.5 N classification of regional lymph node involvement**

| | Axillary lymph node involvement | | |
|---|---|---|---|
| **Internal mammary lymph nodes** | **Clear** | **Involved, mobile** | **Involved, fixed** |
| Clear | N0 | N1 | N2a |
| Involved | N2b | N3b | N3b |

N3a: clinical involvement of ipsilateral infraclavicular lymph nodes.
N3c: clinical involvement of ipsilateral supraclavicular lymph nodes.

**Table 4.6 pN classification of lymph node metastases larger than 2 mm**

| | Axillary lymph node involvement | | | |
|---|---|---|---|---|
| **Internal mammary lymph nodes** | **Clear** | **1–3 nodes involved** | **4–9 nodes involved** | **10 or more nodes involved** |
| Clear or not evaluated | pN0 | pN1a | pN2a | pN3a |
| Only histologic involvement | pN1b | pN1c | pN3b | pN3b |
| Clinical or microscopic involvement | pN2b | pN3b | pN3b | pN3b |

pN3a: involvement of infraclavicular lymph nodes.
pN3c: involvement of supraclavicular lymph nodes.

In the **N classification, "NX"** means that the **regional lymph nodes were not assessed**. Only clinical involvement is taken into account based on clinical examination or imaging procedures except for lymphatic scintigraphy. Sentinel lymph node biopsy findings are always classified as **"pN"** or **"SN"** and are disregarded in the clinical N classification.

**Assessment of regional lymph node status** is reviewed in **Table 4.5.**

Regional lymph nodes include the ipsilateral axillary lymph nodes (including intramammary and interpectoral "Rotter" nodes), infraclavicular and supraclavicular lymph nodes, as well as the internal mammary nodes. Any other nodal involvement is classified as distant metastasis.

Lymph nodes that appear suspicious at ultrasound should be morphologically evaluated by preoperative FNA cytology or CNB histology.

The **pN classification** is shown in **Table 4.6**. The pN classification requires resection and histologic evaluation of at least the lower axillary lymph nodes (level 1). At least 10 lymph nodes should be histologically evaluated. The number of lymph nodes evaluated should also be recorded. Evaluation of one or more sentinel lymph nodes may be used for pathologic classification and is described, for example, as pN1 (sn). The **"pN1 mi"** stage means involvement only by micrometastases no larger than 2 mm. Axillary dissection is unnecessary for metastases smaller than 0.2 mm.

The **M classification** is used for staging distant metastases:

- **MX:** Presence of distant metastases cannot be assessed
- **M0:** No distant metastases
- **M1:** Distant metastases present (includes metastasis to ipsilateral supraclavicular lymph nodes)

The **UICC staging system** is outlined below (Sobin and Wittekind 2002):

- **Stage 0:** Tis N0 M0
- **Stage I:** T1 mic/T1 N0 M0
- **Stage II**
  **a** T0/T1 mic/T1 N1 M0 and T2 N0 M0
  **b** T2 N1 M0 and T3 N0 M0
- **Stage III**
  **a** T0/T1 mic/T1/T2 N2 M0 and T3 N0/N1 M0
  **b** T4 N0/N1/N2 M0
  **c** all T N3 M0
- **Stage IV:** all T, all N, M1

**Table 3.2** underscores the importance of the early detection of breast cancer. For example, a tumor smaller than 2 cm without axillary lymph node involvement has a 5-year cure rate of 96%. With a locally advanced IIIc tumor that has spread to the lymph nodes, the 5-year cure rate falls to 45%.

The risk of **local recurrence** increases with the following factors:

- **The tumor was not excised with clear margins:** 3- to 4-fold increase in relative risk.
- **EIC:** 3-fold increase in relative risk.
- **Patient age < 35 years versus > 50 years:** 3-fold increase in relative risk for women under age 35.
- **Vascular or lymphatic invasion:** 2-fold increase in relative risk.

It is important for radiologists to be aware of these factors, as they are known by many patients and should be discussed with them in some circumstances.

More information on TNM classification and staging can be found on our homepage at **www.brustkrebs.de.**

## Conclusions

The radiographic classification of breast cancer as *ductal* (with or without calcifications), *lobulated, stellate*, or *diffuse* is based on the cellularity of the tumor, its susceptibility to necrosis, the affinity of the tumor for certain parenchymal structures (ducts, interstitium, lymphatics, etc.), and in large part on the connective-tissue response of the host.

The more cellular the tumor, the more lobulated its appearance and the more rapid its growth, resulting in a better prognosis compared with scirrhous tumors. Calcifying tumors are most easily detected by mammography, especially preinvasive lesions such as ADH and DCIS. Diagnosis is most difficult for noncalcifying ductal and diffuse lobular neoplasms and inflammatory carcinoma, which are usually diagnosed clinically by inspection and palpation. Diffuse invasive noncalcifying ductal and lobular carcinomas are very difficult to detect mammographically. Generally they go undetected unless mammograms are supplemented by ultrasound and/or MRI.

The current gold standard of modern breast imaging is high-resolution ultrasound (11–13 MHz). This modality can detect all lobulated and stellate neoplasms 5 mm or more in diameter, even in radiographically dense breasts and without intratumoral calcifications. While mammography cannot match ultrasound in terms of early diagnostic precision, it is still an indispensable tool because microcalcifications are visible only on mammograms.

Without supplementary mammograms, approximately 25% of tumors and their precursors would be missed. This may sound blasphemous to the proponents of a "mammogram-only" approach, especially since mammography is still the only evidence-based modality for detecting breast cancer at a curable stage. But once the capabilities of ultrasound have been established on an evidential basis, attitudes toward ultrasound should quickly change.

Breast ultrasound has a 5% rate of false-positive diagnoses, and this circumstance should be considered in cost–benefit analyses (Buchberger 2005).

The contributions of MRI relate less to the appearance and growth of tumors than to their blood supply (neoangiogenesis) and histologic grade. Aggressive, poorly differentiated malignancies (G3) show intense gadolinium enhancement, whereas well-differentiated tumors (G1) show little or no enhancement. MRI is not useful for screening women 40–70 years of age, but it is important in the early evaluation of young women considered to be at high risk for breast cancer (Kuhl et al. 2000, 2007). It should be performed in this group *independently* of mammography and ultrasound, though even when mammography and ultrasound show no suspect changes.

Noncalcifying ductal carcinoma still presents a diagnostic challenge. It cannot be detected clinically or mammographically. A tumor at least 5 mm in diameter can be detected by ultrasound or MRI, provided the breast is scanned between days 7 and 12 of the menstrual cycle. In the second part of the menstrual cycle about 20% false-positive results are possible (Kuhl 1995).

Intervention is justified whenever a malignant process (preinvasive as well as invasive) is suspected. The possibilities and limitations of various interventional techniques are explored in Chapter 5 (see p. 230). A finding that is suspicious for malignancy should never be followed; it should be morphologically investigated without delay. Controls after 3, 6, or 12 months are obsolete.

# 5 Early Detection and Appropriate Treatment

## Diagnostic Options

Eighty percent of all breast cancers are detected by inspection and palpation, usually by the women themselves. This does not mean that these methods are particularly effective, only that most women do not present for regular breast screening examinations. Mass screening programs open to entire populations are a step in the right direction (Elmore et al. 2005; Becker 2008; Becker and Junkermann 2008). These programs target everyone who has not previously been screened. Early carcinomas can be detected by palpation and inspection only when they are subcutaneous or are located just deep to the nipple-areola. When they develop at the center of the breast, diagnostic imaging is the only way of detecting them at an early stage.

Although mammography was once considered the "gold standard" for early detection, this is no longer true. Only die-hard advocates still believe in the infallibility of mammography as a standalone screening test.

Mammography is definitely necessary for the detection of preinvasive tumors (DCIS) and their calcifications, but in recent years it has been joined by other modalities that have gained an established role in early breast cancer detection. The most important of these is ultrasound, followed by magnetic resonance imaging (MRI) and interventional procedures (find-needle aspiration [FNA]; core-needle biopsy [CNB]; vacuum biopsy [VB]; and sonographically or digital stereotactically guided vacuum biopsy [SVB, DVB]). It is assumed that the reader has a basic knowledge of these procedures, which will be described more fully in later sections of the book. Particular emphasis will be placed on points that are important in screening as well as routine diagnostic investigations.

Other procedures such as thermography, transillumination, and electrical potential measurements are of no importance in breast cancer screening, although tests such as **computer regulation thermography**, for example, are occasionally successful, as the author of this book was surprised to discover in one patient.

### Physical Examination: Visual Inspection

> **!** Every patient and every examining physician should be proficient in breast inspection and palpation.

Although **breast self-examination** is advocated by the media, doctors and women's organizations, only about 10% of women between 25 and 70 years of age perform regular self-examinations. For that reason alone, this method is ineffective. The fact that women show very little interest in self-examination has been personally and painfully experienced by the author. He produced a video on the subject titled "The Breast: Between Fear and Eroticism" and advertised it nationally in women's magazines, on television, over the internet, etc., only to see it flop with only 160 copies sold. Indeed, almost all women admit to their doctors that they do not palpate their breasts regularly because they are more frightened than reassured by the frequent presence of firmness and nodularity even in objectively soft breasts. They would rather leave this chore to their gynecologists. Self-examination, then, will not be explored further in this book. It is fully described and illustrated in numerous publications (Ohlinger et al. 2003). Women can be trained in the specific skills needed for breast self-examination in "MammaCare" courses. This program was developed in Gainesville, Florida, by Dr. Mary Mehn, Dr. Mark Goldstein, and Prof. Henry Pennypacker, who were awarded the US Cancer Prevention Prize in 1990 for their work. **MammaCare** is a method for training and heightening the sense of touch in order to optimize clinical breast examinations and breast self-examinations. Just as the blind can learn to read Braille with their fingertips, women and health professionals can hone their manual sense of touch. Additional information can be found on the internet at *www.mammacare.com*.

Inspection and palpation by radiologists are also somewhat precarious, and unfortunately these examinations are not always done properly even by gynecologists. It is alarming how many women are sent for screening with no apparent palpable abnormalities, when even a glance at the breast, nipple, and supraclavicular fossa would suggest the correct diagnosis (see **Fig. 5.184**, p. 335).

> **Tip**
> **Inspection and palpation are always essential in breast diagnosis, for sometimes very slight skin or nipple retraction or nonspecific firmness can raise suspicion of a pathologic process and prompt additional testing (see Fig. 5.11, p. 88).**

Visual inspection of the breasts occasionally reveals changes that are difficult to classify and require differentiation from breast cancer and systemic malignancies. These changes must be recognized and correctly classified. **Figures 5.1–5.12**, p. 79ff illustrate some common and some rarer types of skin and nipple changes.

*(continued on p. 90)*

**Fig. 5.1 Right breast of a 66-year-old woman.** Nonspecific, wartlike eruptions cover an area of approximately 2 × 3 cm in the areola. The lesions are not itchy or painful. Both breasts appear normal, and slight crusting is noted on the nipple.

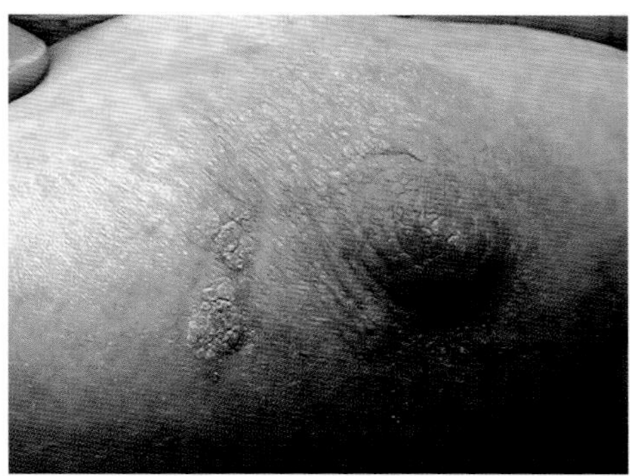

**a** *Visual inspection* reveals small, wartlike lesions with eruptions at the border of the areola (**L/24**). Crusts are visible on the nipple.

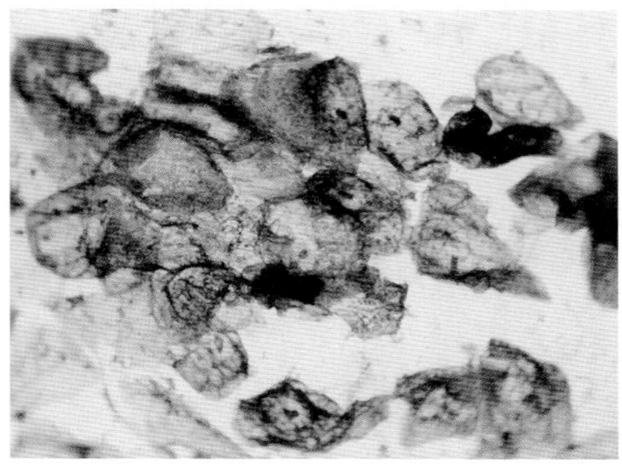

**b** *Cytologic scrapings* from the hyperkeratotic lesions contain numerous keratin scales.

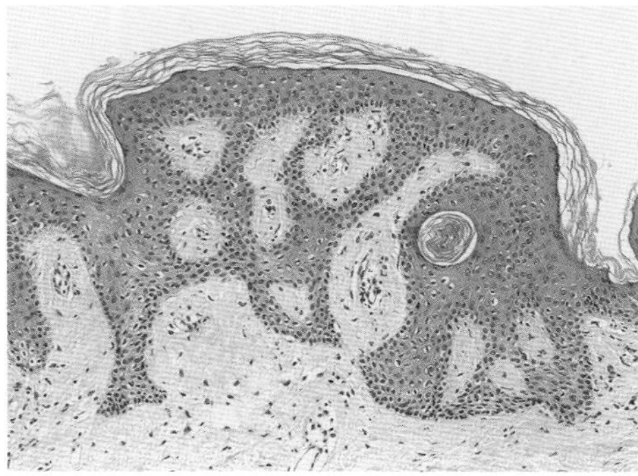

**c** *Histologic examination* shows a thickened epidermis with a greatly thickened horny covering and keratin pearls within the epidermis.

**Question on Fig. 5.1**

*How would you interpret the changes in the right areola?*

(**a**) Paget disease

(**b**) Seborrheic keratosis and seborrheic wart

(**c**) Shingles

→ **Answer on p. 350**

**Fig. 5.2 A 26-year-old woman with a congenital hemangioma on the left side of her body** (**a**). The patient underwent multiple laser treatments, the most recent a few weeks previously. A retroareolar nodule was later detected on the left side. The skin around the nipple-areola is sclerotic (**b**). Extensive liponecrotic calcifications are present in the left breast and increased significantly from 2001 (**c**) to 2002 (**d**). Fine-needle aspiration of the nodule yields great numbers of cells with pale cytoplasm and small nuclei (**e**). Ultrasound scan at the site of the palpable nodule shows nonspecific echogenic densities with posterior acoustic shadows (**f**).

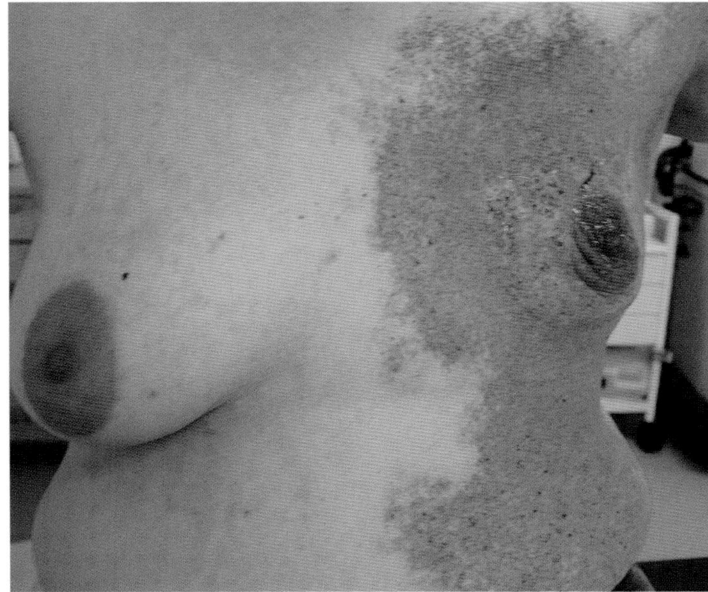

**a** *Physical aspect:* Congenital hemangioma on the left side with brownish-purple skin discoloration and angiomatous changes covering the upper inner quadrant of the left breast. The left breast is markedly smaller than the right breast. The hemangioma also extends over the upper abdomen and left upper arm.

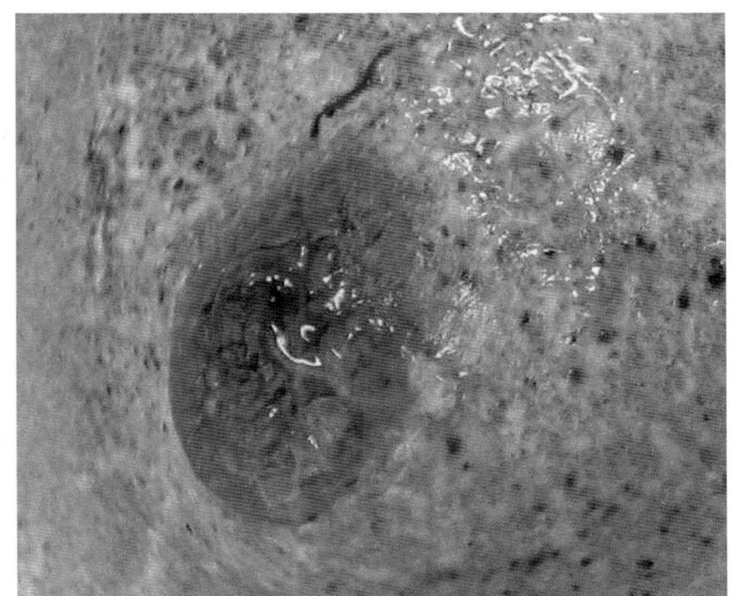

**b** *Close-up view* of the left periareolar region. The skin is shiny, the nipple is scarred, and multiple angiomatous skin lesions are visible.

▶ **Fig. 5.2 c–g**

**Fig. 5.2** **A 26-year-old woman with a congenital hemangioma on the left side of her body.** *(continued)*

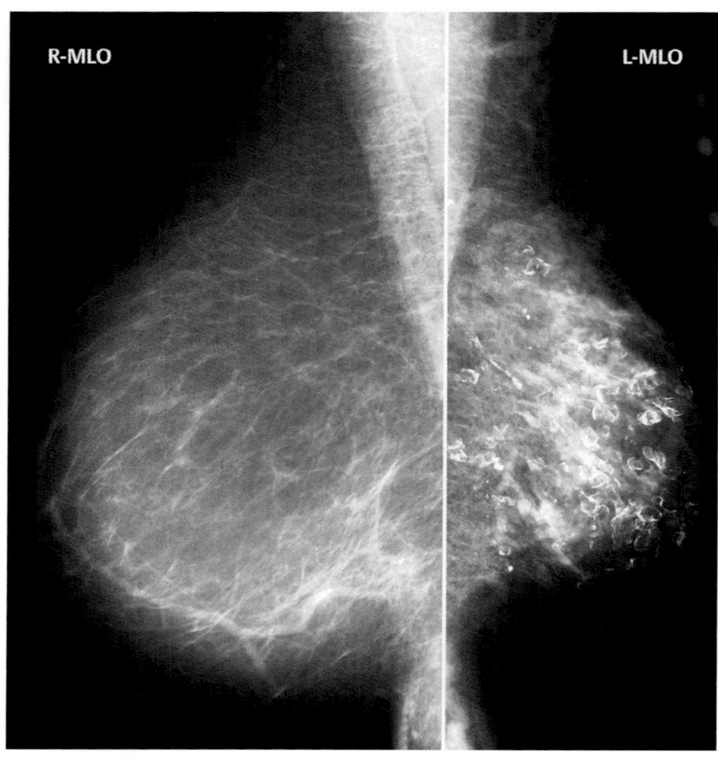


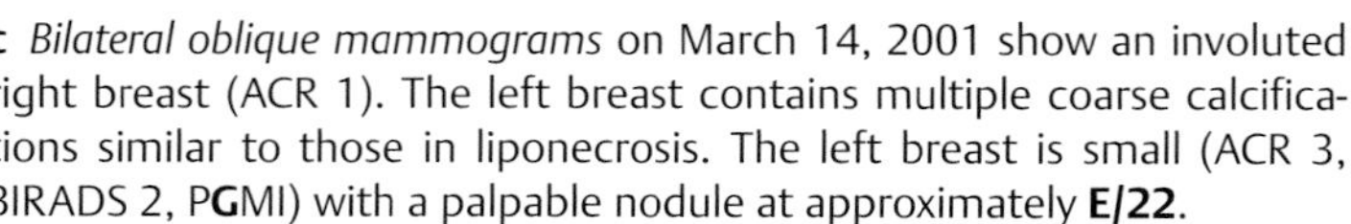

**c** *Bilateral oblique mammograms* on March 14, 2001 show an involuted right breast (ACR 1). The left breast contains multiple coarse calcifications similar to those in liponecrosis. The left breast is small (ACR 3, BIRADS 2, P**G**MI) with a palpable nodule at approximately **E/22**.

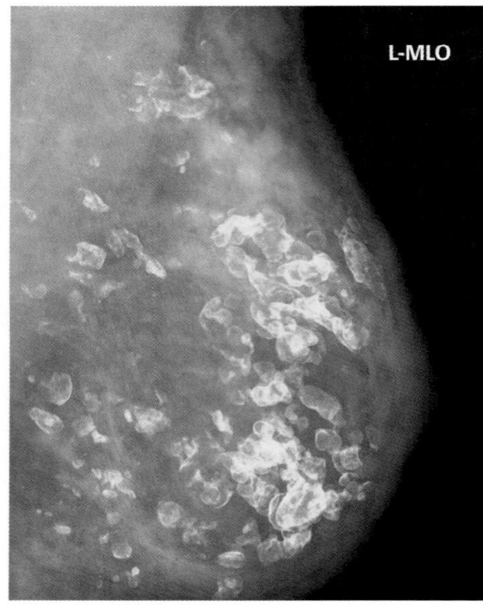


**d** *Oblique mammogram* of the left breast on December 30, 2002 shows a marked increase in calcifications. No other changes are apparent.

**Question on Fig. 5.2**

*The retroareolar nodule is most likely:*

(**a**) A hemangiosarcoma

(**b**) Fat necrosis

(**c**) Paget disease with invasive retroareolar ductal carcinoma

→ **Answer on p. 350**

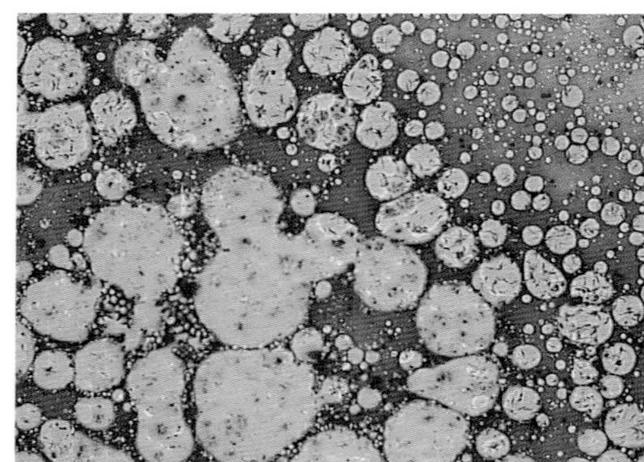

**e** *Cytology.* Rapid stain of fine-needle aspirate shows multiple cells with broad, foamy cytoplasm and some with multiple small nuclei.

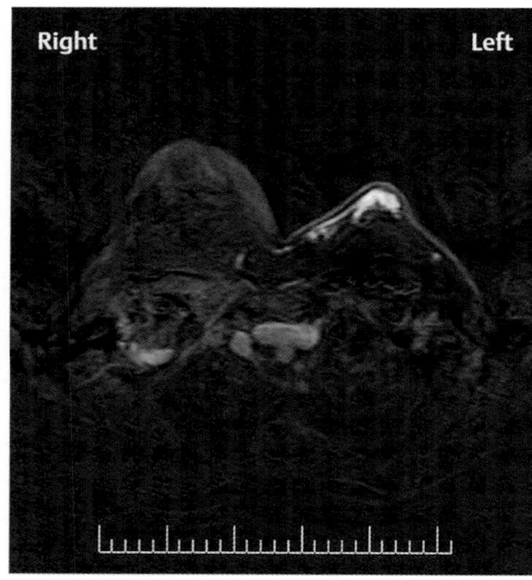


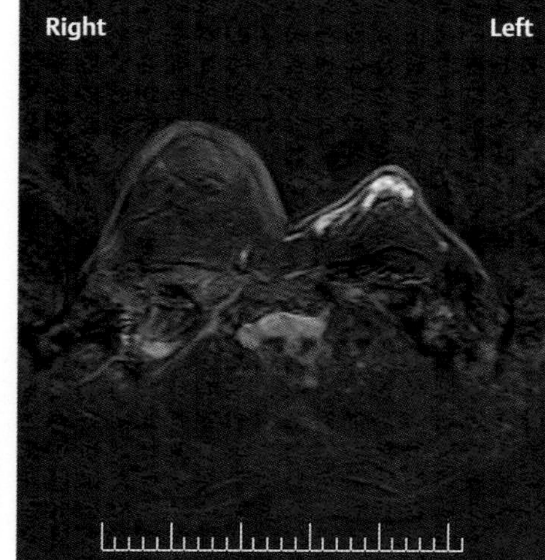


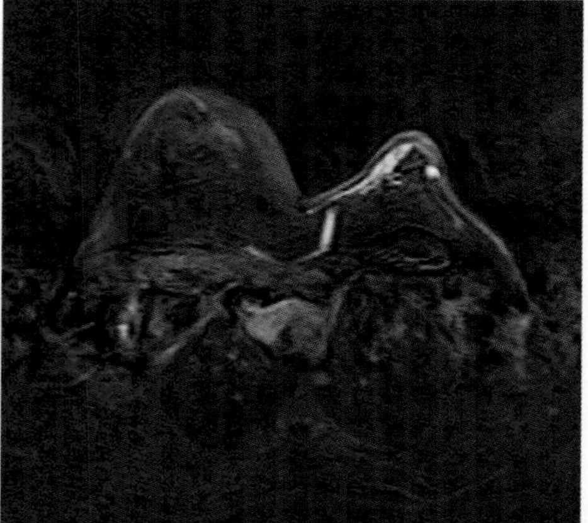

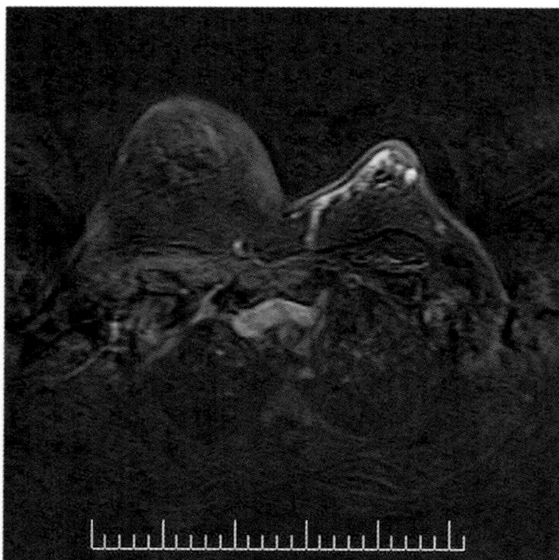

**f** *Periareolar sonogram* of the left breast shows multiple posterior acoustic shadows in the area of the nodule.

**g** *MR images* show subcutaneous linear gadolinium enhancement on the left side with no other abnormalities on either side.

**Fig. 5.3 A 35-year-old woman with severe neurodermatitis,** which is especially pronounced in the axillae (**a**). She has enlarged axillary lymph nodes and recurrent abscesses in the sweat glands. Neurodermatitis is present on the right breast (**b**). One year previously a periareolar abscess developed in the right breast. It was incised and drained but continued to yield a purulent discharge. Fistulography reveals a fine network of smaller ducts that do not communicate with the main ducts (**c**). Galactorrhea is also present.

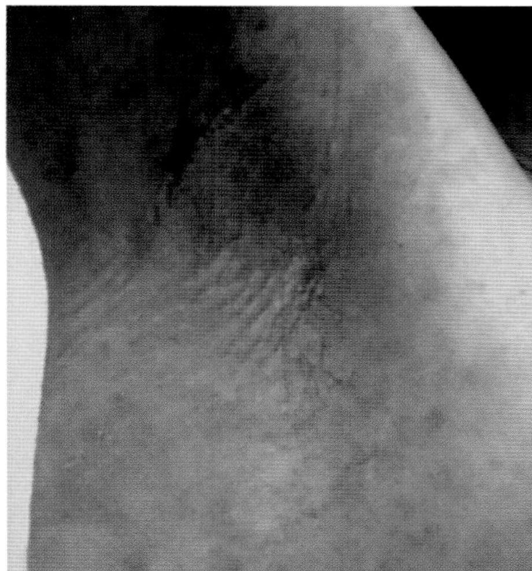

**a** *Inspection* of the right axilla shows neurodermatitis with reddened skin and small focal eruptions.

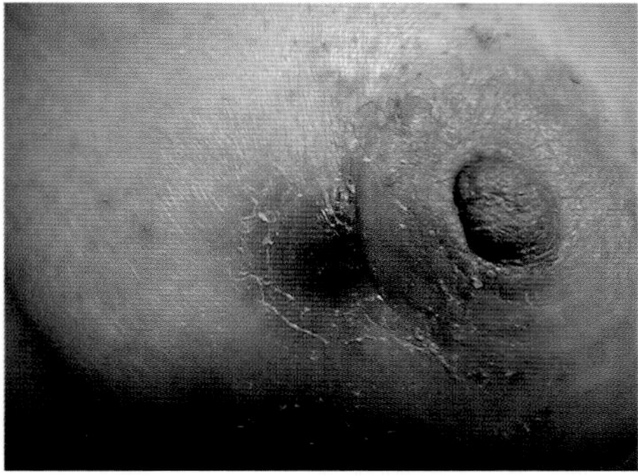

**b** *Inspection* of the right breast shows neurodermatitis with small focal skin eruptions in the upper outer quadrant. Next to the nipple is a circumscribed red nodule with a fistulous opening.

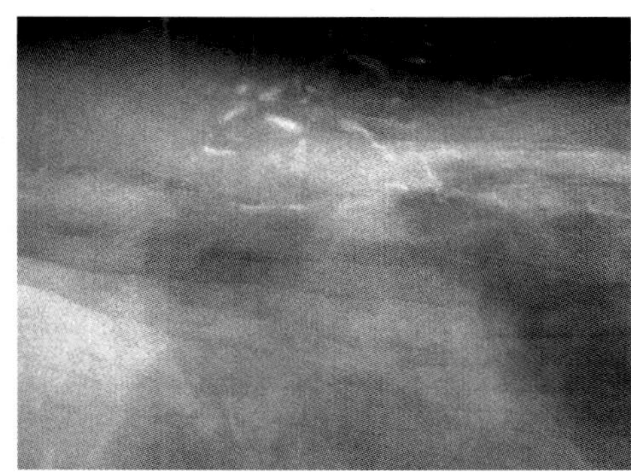

**c** *Fistulography* reveals shell-like pockets of opacity that do not communicate with the main ducts.

**Question on Fig. 5.3**

*How would you interpret the periareolar changes?*

(**a**) Paget disease
(**b**) Folliculitis
(**c**) Ductectasia with plasma cell mastitis and a periductal abscess

→ **Answer on p. 350**

**Fig. 5.4 A 46-year-old woman presents with deep red skin eruptions with a scaly surface and occasional itching.** She has no breast nodularity, no discharge, and no known history of neoplasia.

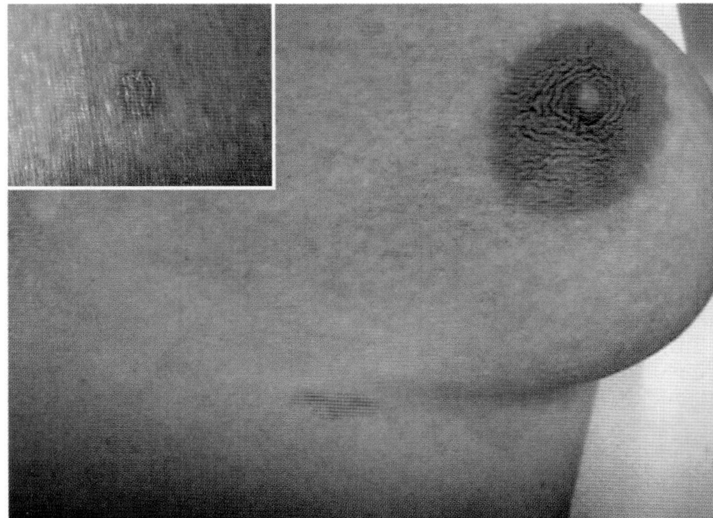

**a** *Inspection* of the left breast reveals skin eruptions in the inframammary fold (**M/7**). A skin lesion 5 mm in diameter is visible above the nipple (see close-up at upper left).

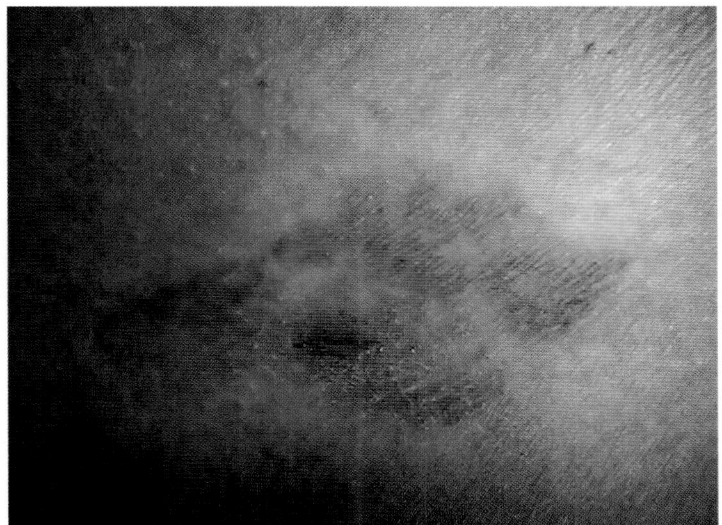

**b** *Close-up view* of the skin lesion.

**Question on Fig. 5.4**

*How would you interpret the skin lesion?*

(**a**) Psoriasis
(**b**) Neurodermatitis
(**c**) Shingles

→ **Answer on p. 350**

**Fig. 5.5 Several months previously a 39-year-old woman noticed a nonspecific firmness over the upper inner quadrant of her left breast associated with slight skin discoloration.** Mammograms and ultrasound show no abnormalities. The firmness has a mostly intra- to subcutaneous location. The patient has no skin changes elsewhere on the body and no known history of neoplasia.

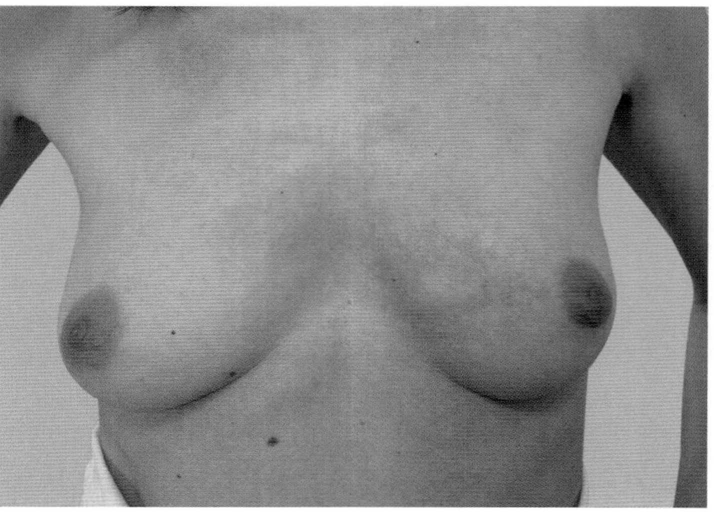

**a** *Visual inspection* reveals a circumscribed pale area with livid borders over the upper inner quadrant of the left breast (**D–d/22–23**). The area is not itchy or painful.

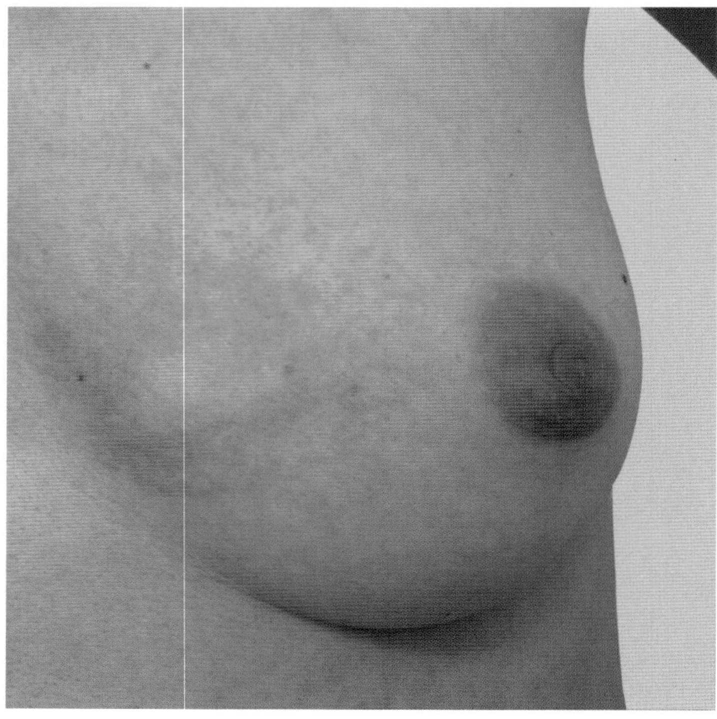

**b** *Close-up view* of the skin lesion.

**Question on Fig. 5.5**

*How would you interpret the skin lesion?*

(**a**) Neurodermatitis
(**b**) Carcinomatous lymphangitis
(**c**) Circumscribed scleroderma

→ **Answer on p. 350**

**Fig. 5.6 Diagnostic nightmare: a 63-year-old woman noticed a slowly progressive change in her left breast.** She describes the chronology of her illness and tests as follows:

- **October, 2003.** The gynecologist orders ultrasound of the left breast to investigate a strange pallor (whitish discoloration) of the nipple and surrounding area. The gynecologist attributes the pallor to poor circulation.
- **February 17, 2004.** Gynecologist orders ultrasound of the left breast for redness and swelling. Sonograms are negative. A topical ointment is prescribed, and mammography is scheduled for March 4, 2004.
- **March 4, 2004.** Mammograms show a suspicious finding in the left breast. The patient is scheduled for a core needle biopsy at a local hospital on March 9, 2004.
- **March 9, 2004.** Hospital: ultrasound scanning and percutaneous biopsy of the left breast are performed under local anesthesia. Although vacuum biopsy was scheduled, it is canceled due to a heavy case load in the outpatient unit.
- **March 11, 2004.** Outpatient unit: A vacuum biopsy is performed on the left breast because the result of the core biopsy on March 9, 2004 was benign.
- **March 17, 2004.** Outpatient unit: vacuum biopsy also yields a benign result. The patient's case is presented at a multidisciplinary case conference. To the patient's surprise, the treating physician notes that the redness is gone although the left breast still shows considerable blue, green, and yellowish discoloration due to hemorrhagic effusions.
- **March 29, 2004.** Hospital staff physician telephones with the result of the case conference: The patient does not have breast cancer, and follow-up is recommended. Breast ultrasound is scheduled for April 7, 2004, and additional mammograms and MRI are scheduled in 6 weeks.
- **April 4, 2004.** The hospital physician calls again (at about 20:00 on Sunday) to say that he is preparing reports for the patient's family doctor and gynecologist and wants to discuss the matter again with the patient. The patient asks whether the previously scheduled appointments still stand and the physician confirms them but states that he forgot to note the dates. The patient mentions that she still has redness of the left breast.
- **April 7, 2004.** The patient cancels her appointment because of severe diarrhea (chronic colitis). The attending physician emphasizes the importance of further testing and suggests April 13, 2004, for the next appointment.
- **April 13, 2004.** Outpatient unit: The attending physician sees the redness and orders another ultrasound scan. On the basis of the ultrasound findings, the physician recommends surgery under general anesthesia to remove a large amount of tissue. The patient points out that the previous tissue samples were normal. The physician responds that the pathologist probably did not have enough tissue and that the findings definitely warrant surgery, regardless of whether the condition is benign or malignant.
- **April 14, 2004.** The patient returns to her family doctor and explains what has happened thus far. Her doctor advises her to pick up her images from the hospital and seek a second opinion.
- **April 15, 2004.** The patient is unable to pick up her mammograms at the hospital. She is surprised to learn that the hospital physician had them sent back to the imaging center on **April 1, 2004**, despite the alleged need for an operation. The patient picks up her mammograms at the imaging center on April 16, 2004. During an unplanned interview with the hospital physician on the same day, he is frankly baffled by the delays in the case. He states that there is no need for MRI or a second opinion, as neither would supply any new information. He reemphasizes the urgent need for a breast operation.

**Fig. 5.6 Diagnostic nightmare** *(continued).* The patient's skepticism toward surgery stems from an incident that occurred several years before. The patient was scheduled for gallbladder surgery, and tissue samples were to be taken from her ovary because elevated tumor markers had been found. When her case was under discussion, a gynecologist at the same hospital insisted that her uterus should also be removed (without medical indication), arguing that she no longer needed the organ and that its removal would eliminate all risk of cervical cancer. The patient had some difficulty in preventing the hysterectomy. So much for the history from the patient's perspective. A total of 7 months elapsed between the initial clinical visit and a definitive diagnosis. This lengthy process jeopardizes the chance for a cure.

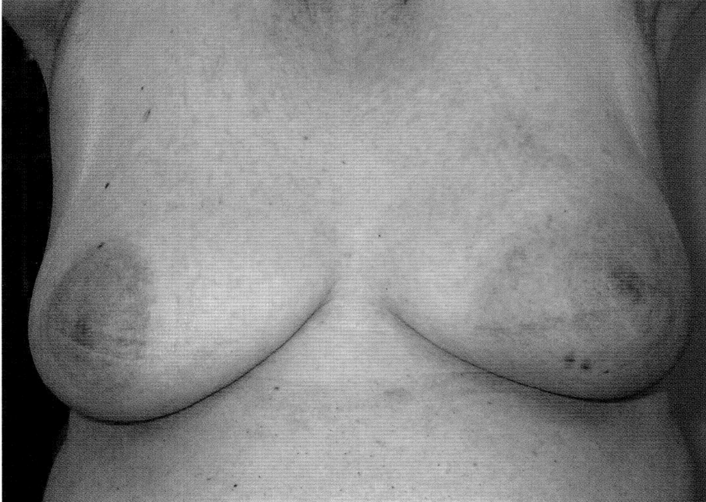

**a** *Clinical appearance* on April 20, 2004. A purplish discolored area on the periareolar left breast is relatively sharply demarcated from the surrounding skin (**N–o/21–23**). There is no orange-peel dimpling of the skin. The right breast appears normal.

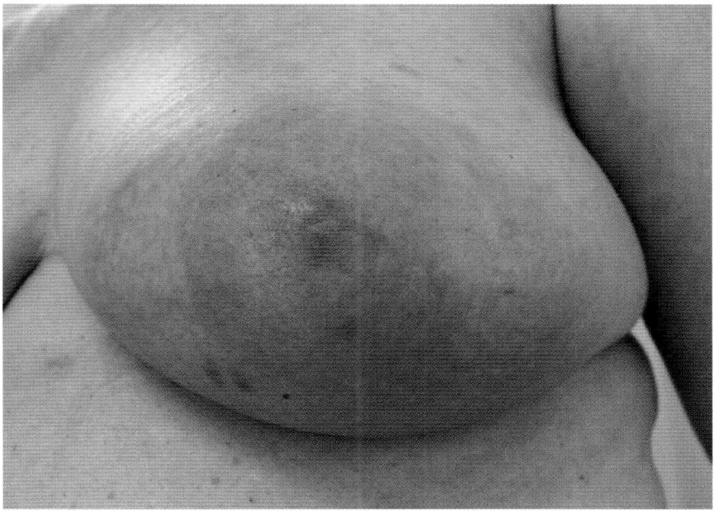

**b** *The left areolar* region is enlarged.

R-MLO L-MLO

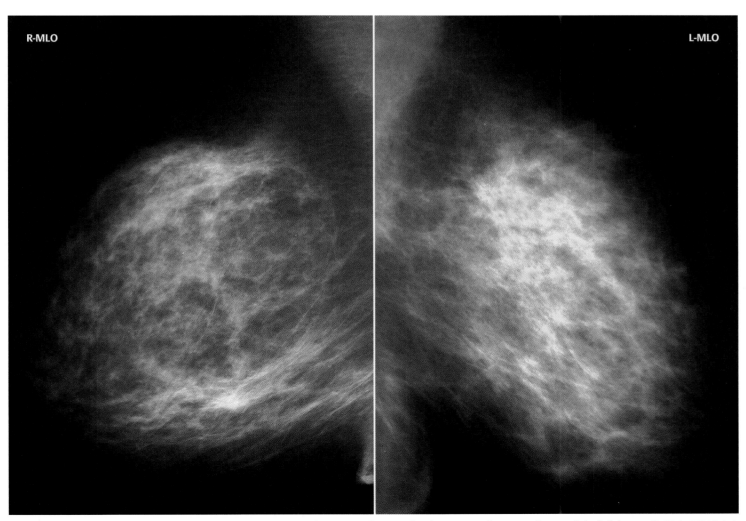

**c** *Bilateral oblique mammograms* show a stroma-rich breast with nonspecific reticular densities in the parenchyma of the left breast (ACR 3, BIRADS 4, PGMI). Circumscribed densities are also visible in the upper and lower portions of the right breast (**m–N/5–6; 11–12**).

▶ **Fig. 5.6 d–f**

**Fig. 5.6 Diagnostic nightmare.** *(continued)*

R-CC L-CC

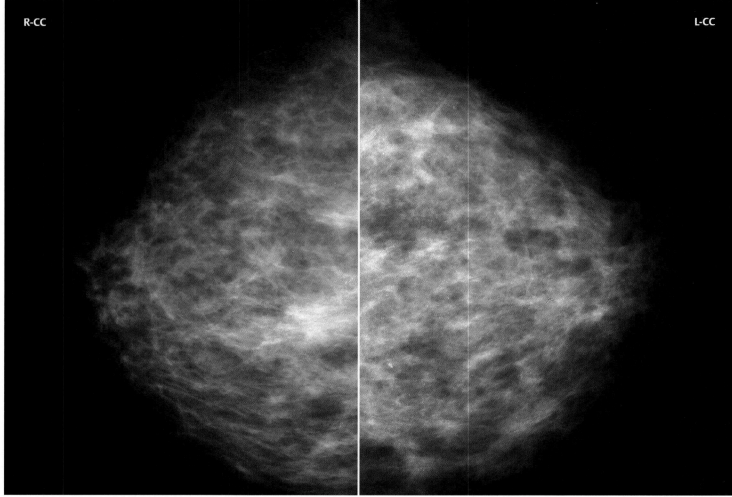

**d** *Bilateral craniocaudal mammograms* show a stroma-rich breast with a nonspecific diffuse parenchymal density on the left side and a less pronounced density on the right side occupying a 2 cm × 4 cm × 4 cm area (**d–e/18–19**) (ACR 4, BIRADS?, PG**M**I).

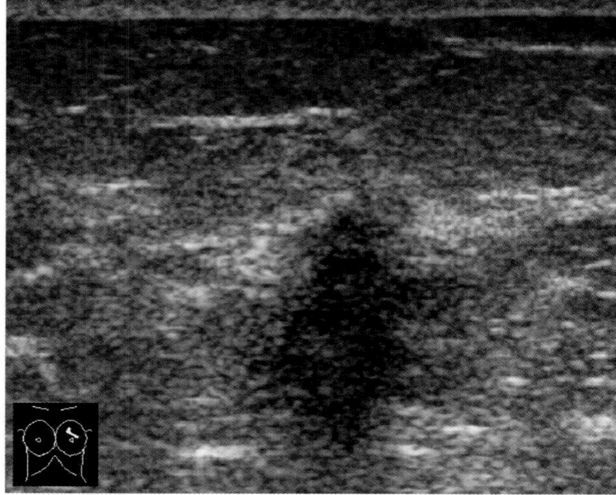

**e** *Bilateral ultrasound* reveals several small, hypoechoic foci in the upper portion of the left breast.

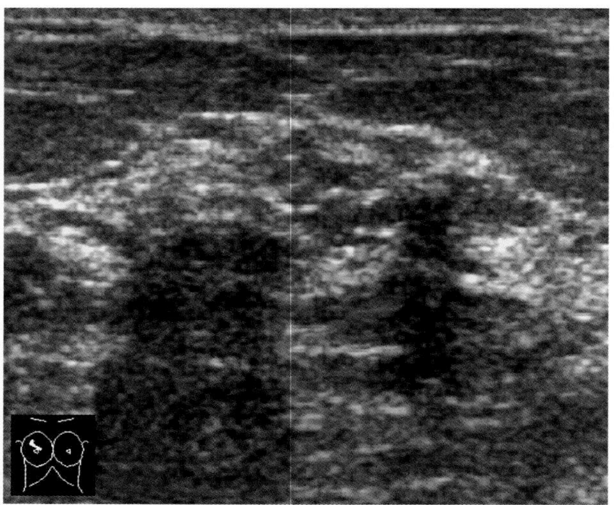

**f** *Sonogram* of the right breast at the 12-o'clock position.

**Question on Fig. 5.6**

*What is the most likely diagnosis?*

(**a**) Inflammatory tumor in the left breast

(**b**) Obstruction of lymphatic drainage in the left axilla

(**c**) Thrombosis of the left subclavian vein

→ **Answer on p. 350**

**Fig. 5.7** **A 77-year-old woman 3 years after breast-conserving therapy (1995).** Physical examination shows induration of the right breast with depigmentation of the nipple and nonspecific skin redness over the upper and lower outer quadrants (**a**). The patient describes severe back pain radiating to the right breast and also to the upper abdomen. The left breast appears normal. Small, focal, nonpruritic skin eruptions are visible on the patient's back (**c**). Mammographic and ultrasound findings are normal in both breasts.

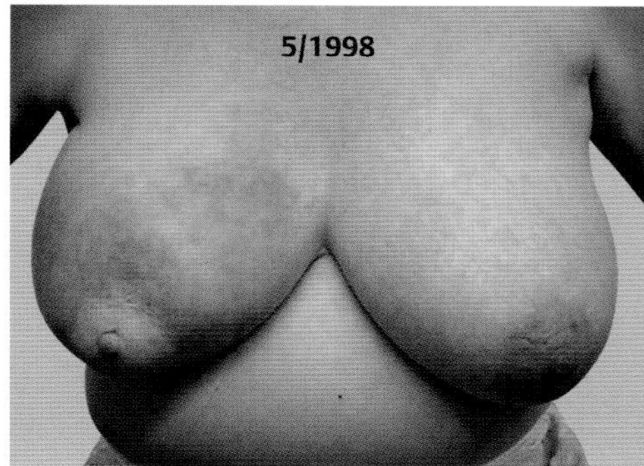


**a** *Clinical inspection* in May, 1998 shows a small right breast with skin redness and depigmentation of the nipple 3 years after radiotherapy. The left breast appears normal.

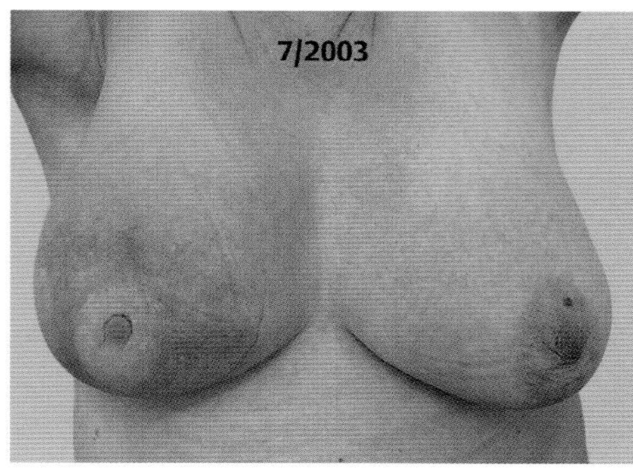


**b** *Clinical appearance* in July, 2003. Skin redness on the right breast has regressed somewhat, but otherwise there are no significant changes relative to 1998.

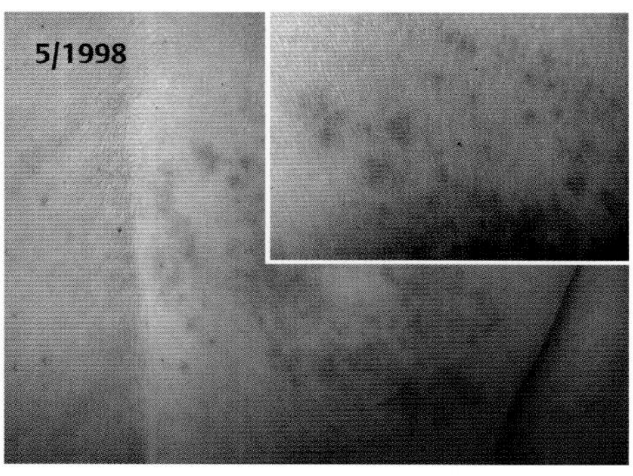


**c** *Inspection* of the back reveals small focal skin eruptions showing a bandlike and segmental arrangement. Inset at upper right: close-up view of the skin lesions.

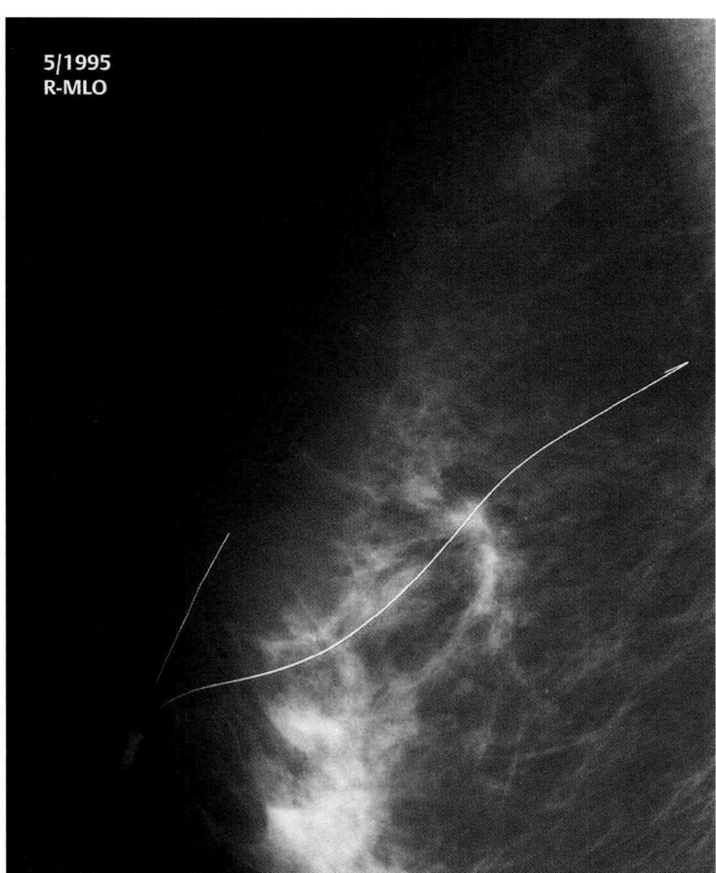


**d** *Mammogram* taken in August, 1995, shows a 1 cm × 3 cm spiculated density that has been marked with a localizing wire (**N/12**).

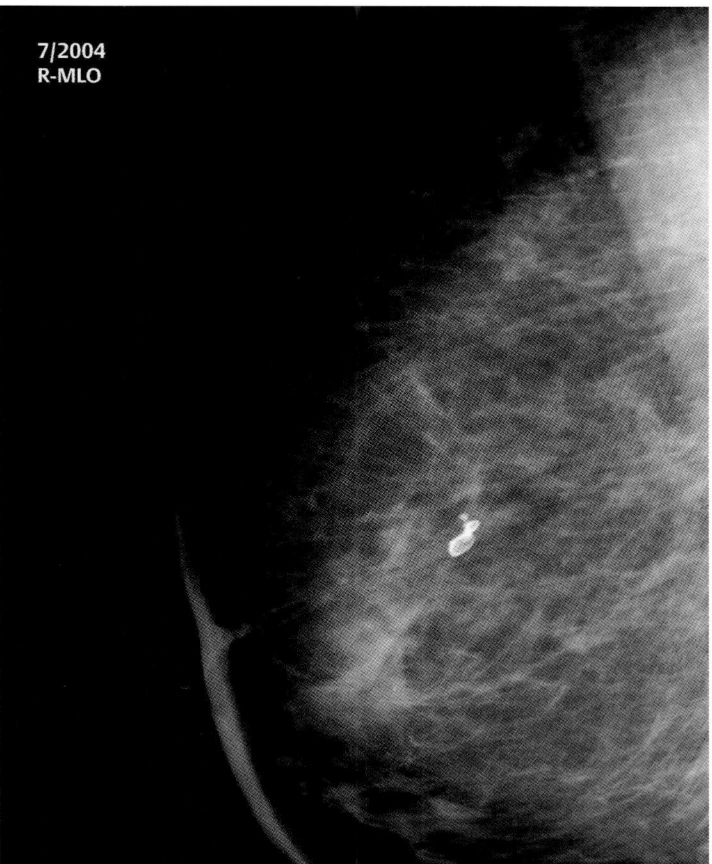


**e** *Mammogram* taken in July, 2004, shows radiation-induced fibrosis with calcified liponecrosis (**S/12**) and cutaneous sclerosis.

**Question on Fig. 5.7**

*How would you interpret the lesions on the patient's back 1998?*

(**a**) Cutaneous metastases

(**b**) Shingles

(**c**) Postirradiation changes

→ **Answer on p. 351**

**Fig. 5.8 A 67-year-old woman with a slightly mobile 2 cm nodule in the upper outer quadrant of her left breast.** There is no skin or nipple retraction and no regional lymph node enlargement. Ultrasound reveals cysts in both breasts. Mammography shows a nonspecific density in the upper outer quadrant of the left breast in which homogeneous opacity is combined with ground-glass opacity. Ultrasound also shows a hypoechoic area measuring 7 mm × 10 mm at the location of the palpable nodule. Ultrasound-guided fine-needle aspiration of the nodule yields a bloody and purulent material. Bacteriologic tests of the aspirate are negative. Cytology yields cells showing inflammatory changes. After the fine-needle aspiration, a standard pressure dressing was applied (see **Fig. 5.107**) and the patient was told to leave the dressing on for 4 hours and apply a cooling pack to the biopsy site. A follow-up examination was scheduled for 4 weeks after FNA. The patient returned before the scheduled follow-up date because of suspicious skin changes (**a, b**).

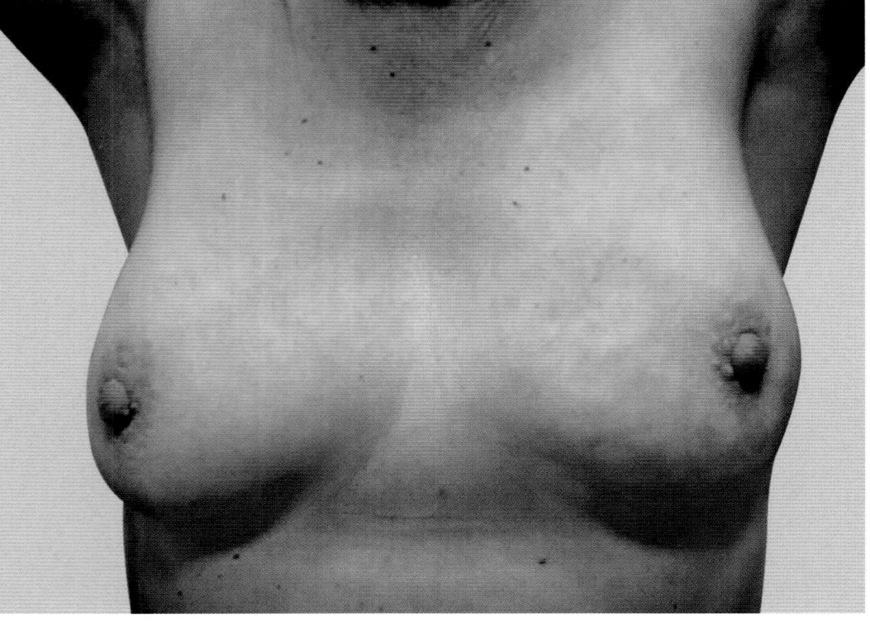

**a** *Bilateral inspection* reveals patchy redness of the left breast following FNA at the 2-o'clock position in the upper outer quadrant.

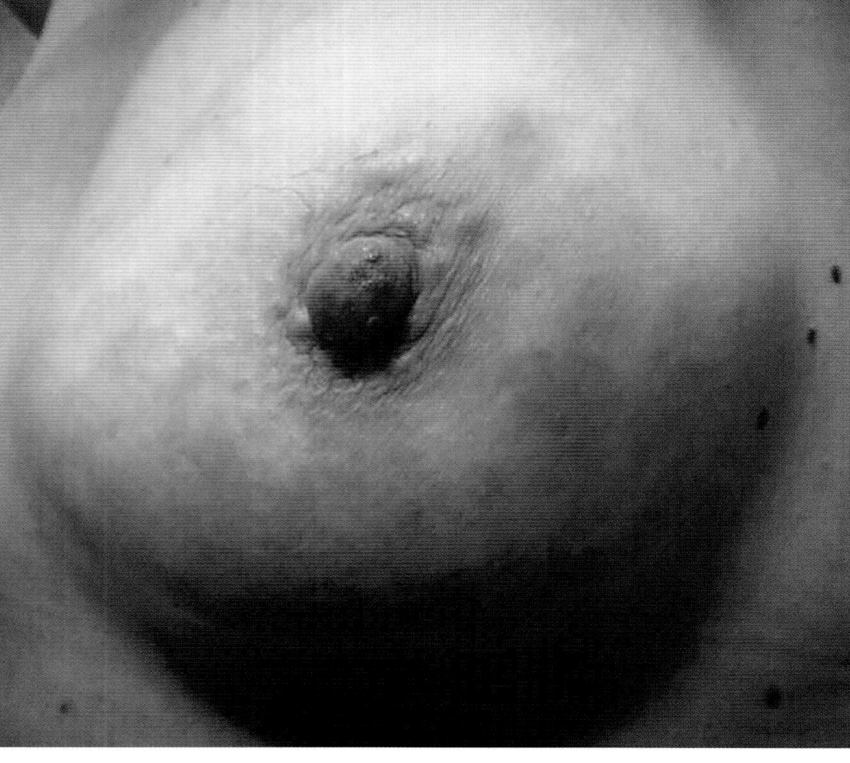

**b** *Close-up view* of the left breast shows uniform redness of the skin approximately 1–2 cm from the areola (**a–F/7–14; 17–21**).

**Question on Fig. 5.8**

*How would you interpret the skin changes?*

(**a**) Carcinomatous lymphangitis

(**b**) Inflammatory infiltrates following puncture of an abscess (intramammary spread?)

(**c**) First-degree frostbite

→ **Answer on p. 351**

**Fig. 5.9** **A 60-year-old woman has nonspecific palpable masses in both breasts** and bilateral breast redness that has been gradually increasing for weeks. The patient has normal mammograms and sonograms and no regional lymph node enlargement. She is clinically healthy.

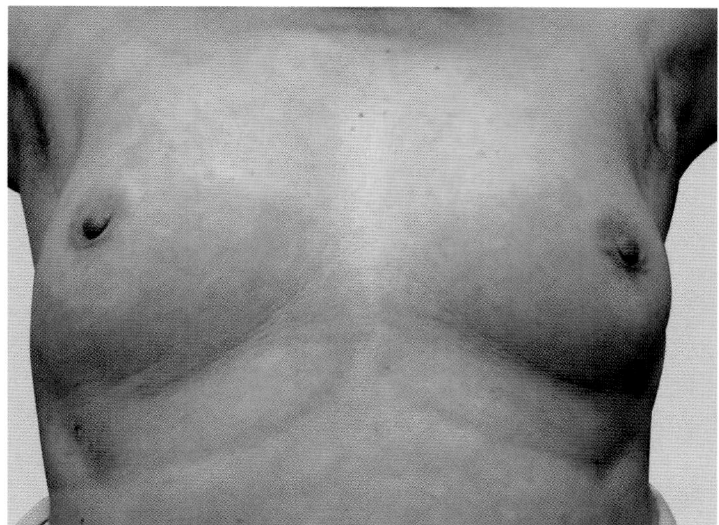

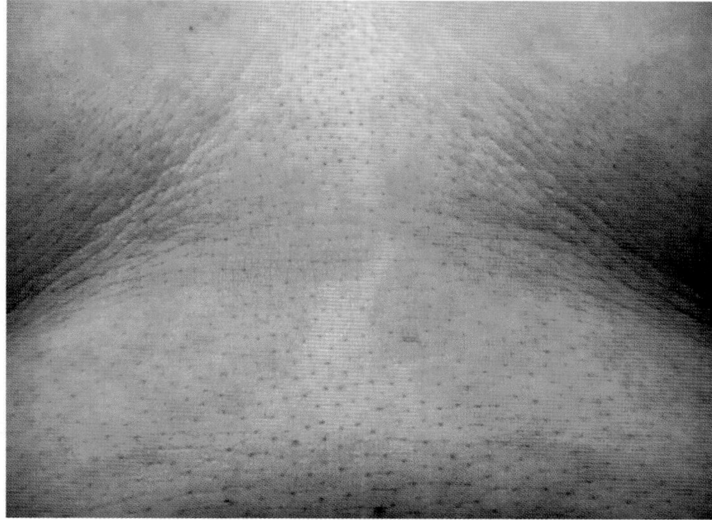

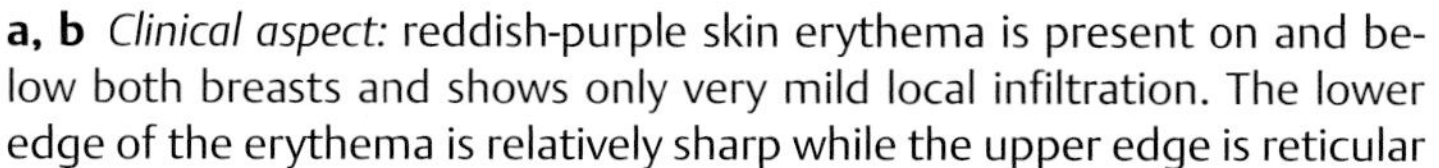

**a, b** *Clinical aspect:* reddish-purple skin erythema is present on and below both breasts and shows only very mild local infiltration. The lower edge of the erythema is relatively sharp while the upper edge is reticular and indistinct. **Histology** reveals mucus between connective-tissue fibers, T-lymphocytes, and small numbers of B-lymphocytes.

**Question on Fig. 5.9**

*What is the most likely cause of the changes?*

(**a**) Lupus erythematosus
(**b**) REM syndrome (reticular erythematous mucinosis)
(**c**) Bilateral shingles

→ **Answer on p. 352**

**Fig. 5.10** **A 49-year-old woman 6 years after bilateral reduction mammoplasty (in 1995).** The surgical specimens weighed 1.9 kg on the right side and 1.6 kg on the left side. The breast tissue contained innumerable cysts up to 3.5 cm in diameter, most filled with a brownish material, and several rubbery nodules up to 2 cm in diameter. **Histology** revealed *cystic ductectasia with apocrine metaplasia accompanied by epitheliosis, adenosis, and sclerosis. Diagnosis:* Prechtel grade II fibrocystic change with *heavy proliferative foci but no evidence of malignancy.* Mammography shows very radiodense breasts. Regular mammographic and ultrasound follow-ups have shown no abnormalities. Cranial CT and a thyroid scintiscan were ordered due to ocular changes, and both tests were normal.

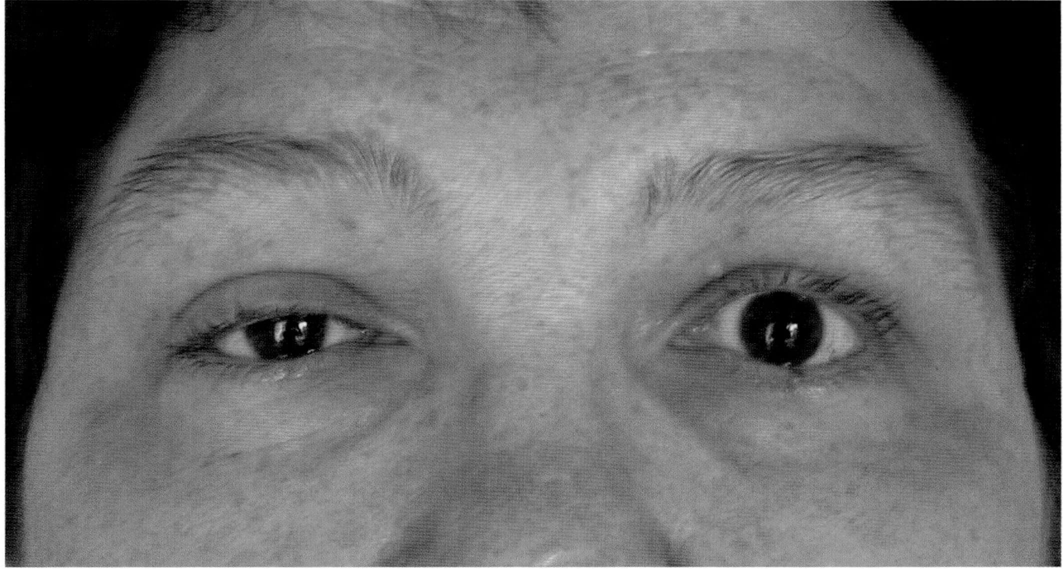

**a** *Clinical appearance* of the eyes (2002).

**Question on Fig. 5.10**

*The findings are consistent with what syndrome?*

(**a**) Horner syndrome
(**b**) Cervical sympathetic paralysis syndrome
(**c**) Hutchinson syndrome

→ **Answer on p. 352**

**Fig. 5.11 A 56-year-old woman with equivocal ultrasound findings.** The patient has no palpable breast abnormalities and no regional lymph node enlargement. Subjectively, the patient reports having no breast problems since her prior examinations in 1998 and 1999, with no indication of nodules, firmness, or discharge. There is an apparent shallow scar retraction on the medial side of the right nipple-areola, and the patient claims that it has been there for years without change. An incisional biopsy was done on both breasts in 1983, with benign results. There is a positive family history of breast cancer, as the patient's mother was diagnosed with the disease 2 years before.

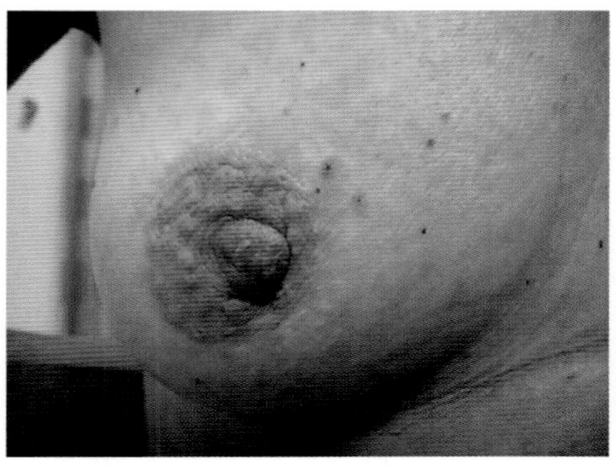

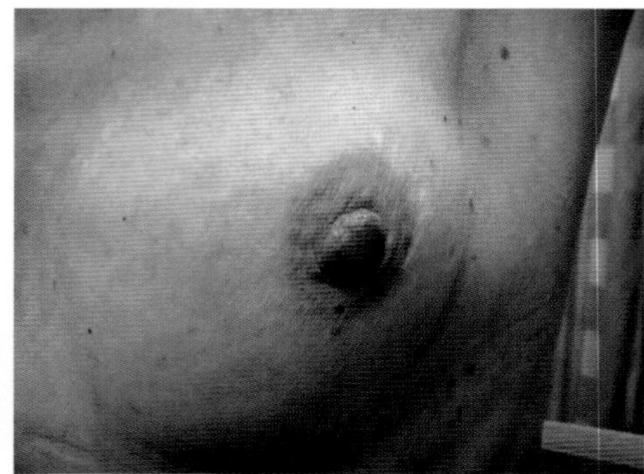

**a** *Clinical appearance* of both breasts several years after incisional biopsy of the left breast. A nonpruritic periareolar scar is present at the 3-o'clock position.

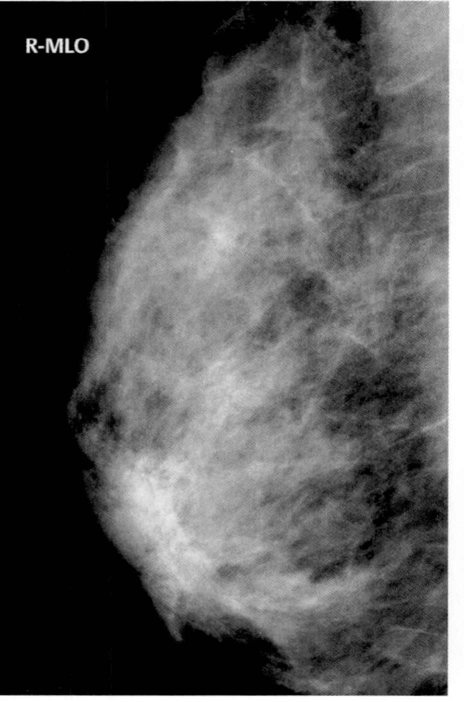


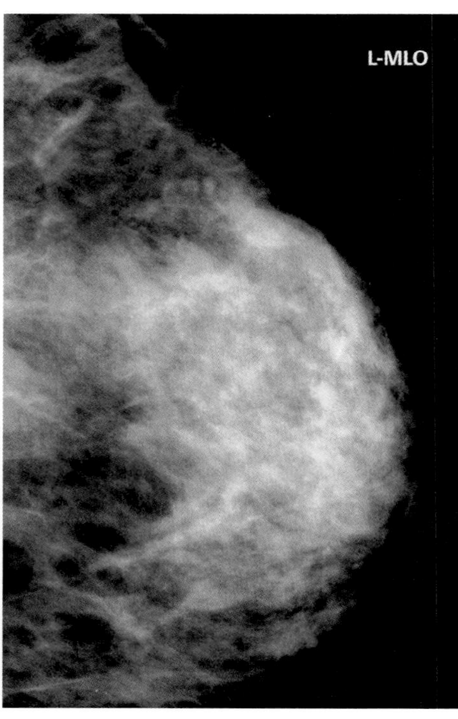


**b** *Bilateral oblique mammograms* show nonspecific focal densities in both breasts.

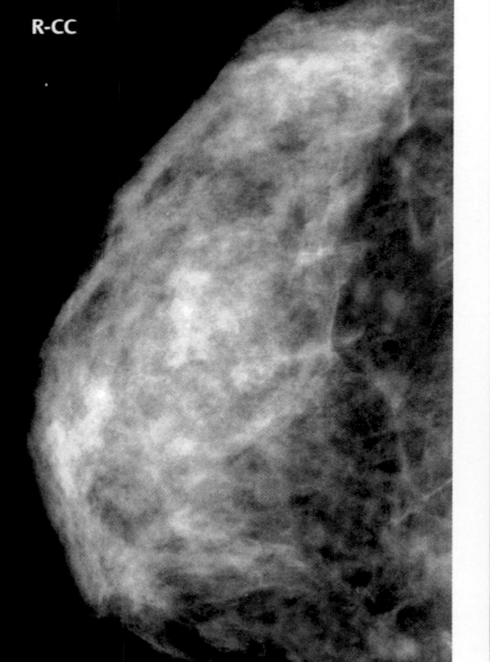


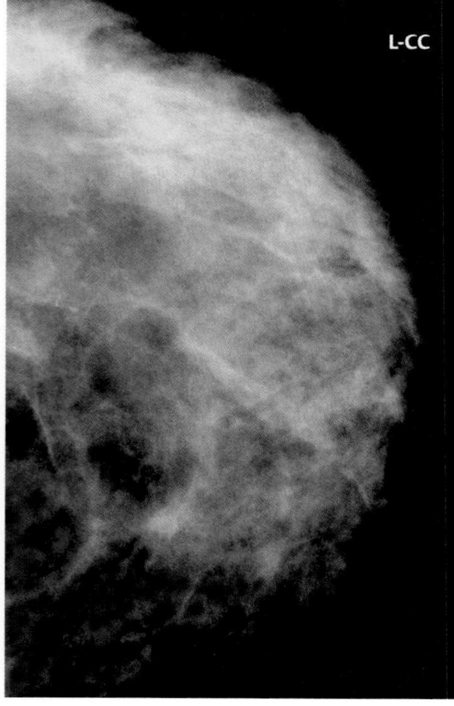


**c** *Bilateral craniocaudal mammograms* (ACR 2, BIRADS 3) (courtesy of Walter Seyferth, Ansbach).

**Question on Fig. 5.11**

*What course of action would you recommended?*

(**a**) Routine follow-up in 12 months

(**b**) Further investigation of the left breast

(**c**) Further investigation of the right breast

→ **Answer on p. 354**

**Fig. 5.12 A 68-year-old woman with a palpable retroareolar nodule in the right breast** and a smooth, plaquelike area on the areola at the 6-o'clock position (**a**).

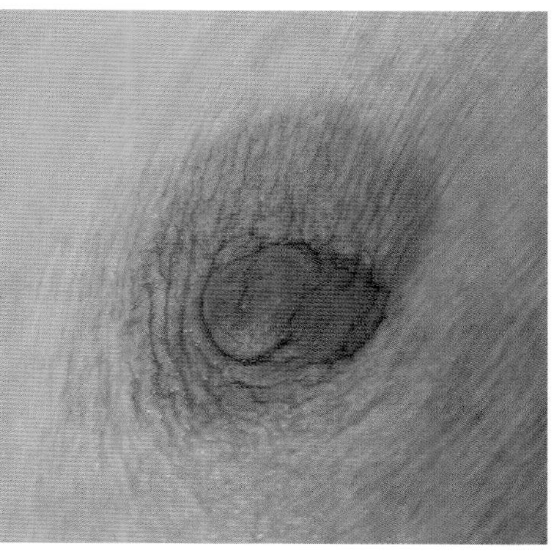

**a** *Inspection of the nipple-areola* reveals a very small, raised smooth area at the 6-o'clock position (**s/23–24**).

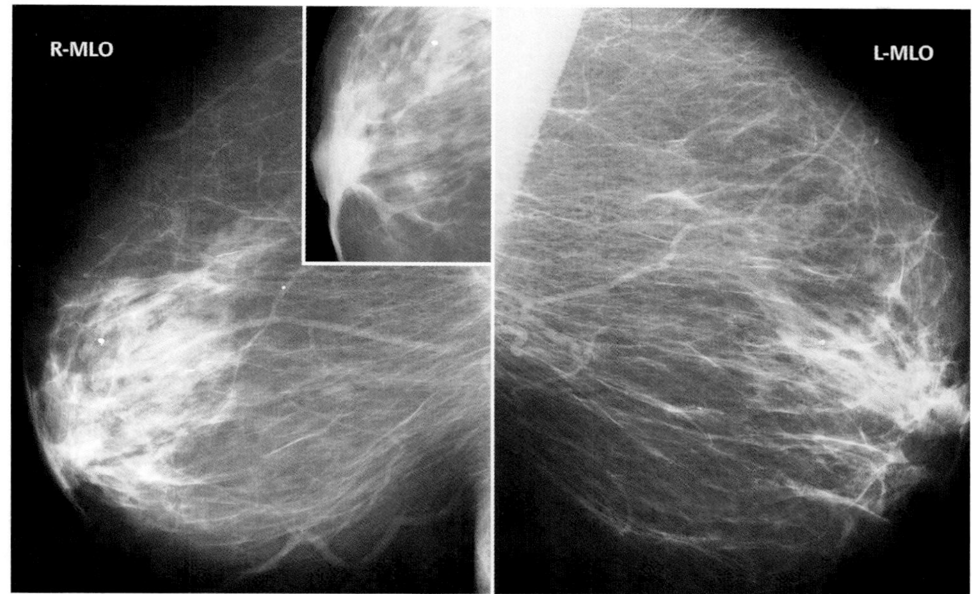


**b** *Bilateral oblique mammograms* show a cloudy opacity with no microcalcifications in the retroareolar region of the right breast. The nipple is thickened and there is increased retroareolar density (inset: magnified view) (ACR 2, BIRADS 4b, **P**GMI).

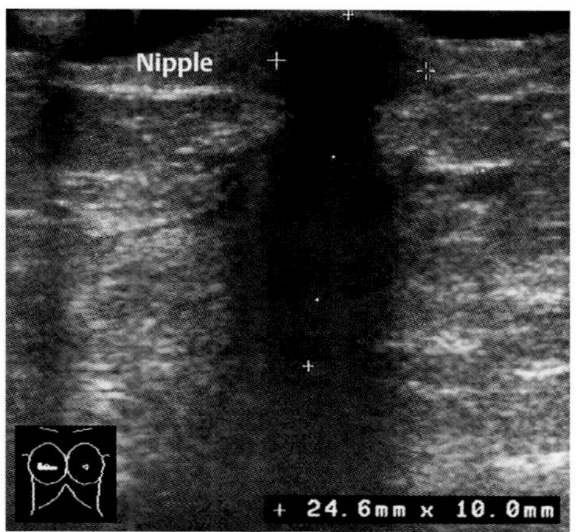


**d** *Sonogram* of the right breast shows a 1 cm hypoechoic area with ill-defined margins below the nipple associated with a dense retroareolar posterior acoustic shadow.

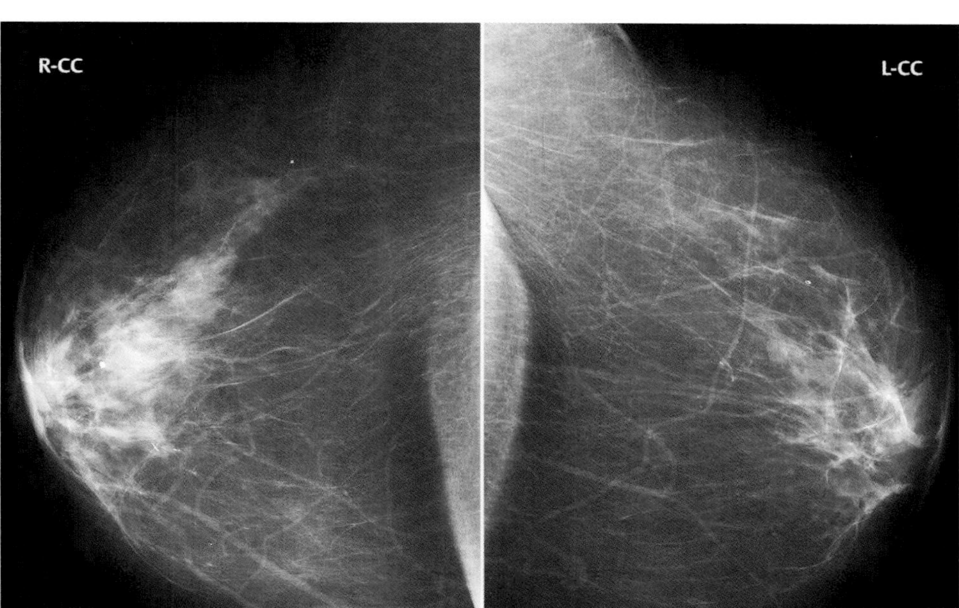


**c** *Craniocaudal mammograms* shows the same findings as in **b** (ACR 2, BIRADS 4b, **P**GMI).

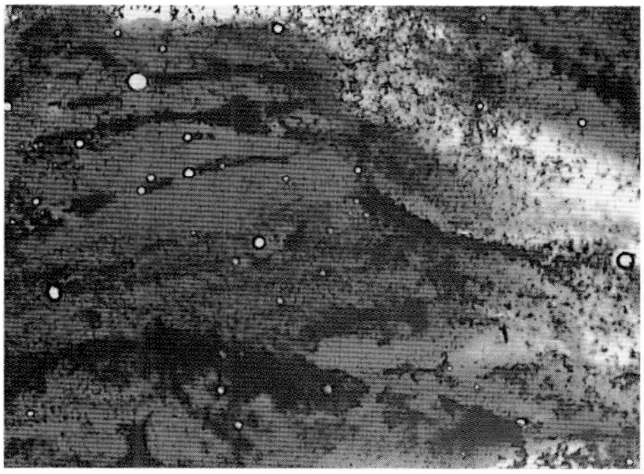

**e** *Cytology.* Needle aspiration of the retroareolar area elicits retained mucus, which also drains from the nipple. The material does not contain tumor cells.

**Question on Fig. 5.12**

*What is the cause of the changes?*

(**a**) Paget disease
(**b**) Invasion of the nipple by a malignant tumor with mucocele
(**c**) An inflammatory process in ductectasia with retained secretions

→ **Answer on p. 355**

*(continued from p. 78)*

Palpation should be carried out with the patient's arm extended above the head or with the hands clasped behind the neck. These positions place tension on the pectoral muscles and make it easier to detect any areas of firmness by palpating the breasts with circular movements of the hands. This is much better than placing the hands on the hips or letting the arms hang freely at the sides. All quadrants of the breast should be systematically palpated on the pectoral muscle. Particular attention should be given to the retroareolar area, all recesses—axillary, clavicular, sternal, abdominal (see **Fig. 5.61 a**)—and to the inframammary fold (see **Figs. 5.59 c, 5.91 i**).

### *Tip*

**Palpation should include the careful application of pressure to the retroareolar region, including the lactiferous sinuses in that area, to check for abnormal discharge (see Ductography, p. 241). For anatomic reasons, the patient herself is better able to apply concentric pressure to the retroareolar region than is a doctor seated in front of her. Thus, if questionable discharge is noted, the patient should compress the breast herself. If she has noticed the discharge at home, she has usually trained herself over a period of weeks to know exactly where she must push to elicit the discharge.**

Retroareolar nodules in the breast are easily missed at mammography (see **Fig. 5.11 b, c**, p. 88). If bilateral discharge is present, the patient should be asked whether she has been taking **tranquilizers** or other medications that may cause nipple discharge. The overuse of **"nutritional supplements"** such as growth hormones and DHEA should be excluded, or the products should be temporarily withdrawn for 3 months to see whether the discharge stops. Patients are generally unaware of the side-effects that these products may cause.

Clinical inspection and palpation are skills that should be the object of rigorous training, especially in screening situations. The gynecologist should never assume that the radiologist performed a physical examination when the mammograms were taken, even if the radiologist is capable of doing so or if such an examination was expected. Because radiologists rarely have personal contact with patients during routine screening, radiologic technologists should be well trained in physical examination and palpation. Radiologists usually concentrate far more on diagnostic imaging than on physical findings. The tendency of physicians to rely blindly on the judgment of other physicians is a common source of malpractice litigation. Most patients can credibly claim that a nodule or mass had been palpable in their breast for some time.

Palpable and visible findings should be noted on every conventional mammogram (by applying an adhesive label, see **Fig. 5.59 f–i**, p. 370) or in the radiology report. Even nonspecific descriptions (a scar on the upper outer quadrant of the left breast, eczema, moles, goiter scar, and so on) should be recorded. In the event of a malpractice suit, this type of information can prove that the radiologist did examine and palpate the breast.

It is wise, especially for legal reasons, to document any special physical findings with a digital camera (a large percentage of the pictures in this book were taken in that way). Digital photographs can be scanned into medical records using the Workstation software developed for example by Image Diagnost International (Munich, Germany) and will then be available for comparison during all subsequent examinations (see p. 78). For other issues relating to legal liability and the problem of "missed" breast cancers, including the four common ways that doctors may become involved, see the excellent work of Harder and Ratzel (1999). This topic was also covered extensively in an earlier edition of this book, and it would go beyond our present scope to reexplore it here.

Factors that play a major role in almost every lawsuit are poor technical quality, inadequate physical examination, and failure to take the patient's complaints seriously.

During inspection of the woman's upper body, it is also important to check for pigmented tumors, thyroid changes, and possible cervical lymphadenopathy. More than a few malignant melanomas have been detected in this way, and a great many cold and hot thyroid nodules have been identified. Goiters that are hidden in the retrosternal region are especially likely to be discovered in a thorough breast examination that includes a "swallow test."

It is important to palpate the **supraclavicular fossa** and especially the **infraclavicular fossa**. These areas are particularly important in follow-up care, since radical axillary lymphadenectomy is becoming less and less common. When there is an axillary lymph node metastasis or if only the sentinel lymph node has been removed (see p. 307), undetected metastases may still (seldom) develop in level II or level III nodes (see **Fig. 5.184 j**, p. 408). These metastases first become palpable in the infraclavicular fossa, appearing as slight protrusions of the pectoral muscle rather than mobile subcutaneous nodules as in the case of lipoma (see **Fig. 5.184 e**, p. 407). The neck, throat, clavicular fossae, and skin receive relatively little attention during breast examinations.

Many women 40–60 years of age complain of noncyclical pains, often projecting into the axillae, during breast examinations, but these pains rarely originate in the breast itself. It is important to thoroughly investigate painful areas using imaging procedures in order to exclude a breast tumor. This is the only way to allay a patient's fears. Often these pains provide a rationale for obtaining initial mammograms. Most breast pains are vertebrogenic (originating from the thoracic spine and typically involving the axilla), and pain on the left side may have a cardiac cause. For this reason, women over 40 years of age who have unexplained left-sided chest pain should be referred to a cardiologist, regardless of whether their mammograms show vascular calcifications. If mammograms do show vascular calcifications, cardiac examination is recommended for all women 40–60 years of age, even those who do not complain of chest pain. Approximately 20% of these women will be found to have coronary heart disease and/or a disorder of lipid metabolism.

**Remember that heart attacks are responsible for 50% of deaths in women 25–50 years of age, whereas breast cancer kills "only" 1 of every 200 women in this age group.**

Many complaints in women 40–50 years of age stem from an altered hormone balance and may be associated with signs of impending menopause (minor symptoms may include sleeplessness and irritability). Breast pain in younger women is often referable to menstrual disorders. Premenstrual syndrome (which occasionally begins just after ovulation) is detectable sonographically by the proliferation of TDLUs, which is the leading cause of these complaints.

Many women misinterpret breast pain (mastodynia) as a sign of breast cancer. Physicians are obliged to take this pain seriously, however. The explanation of mastodynia by Peters (1992) is recommended reading for radiologists. In cases where the cause of mastodynia is unexplained, the physician should *tactfully* inquire into possible sexual abuse during the patient's childhood (Glück 2005).

Occasionally a woman concentrates so much on the pain in one breast that she disregards the opposite breast. This unilateral fixation is dangerous because even the physician may thoroughly examine only the painful breast. Contralateral breast examination is equally important, however, as it is not uncommon for the opposite breast to harbor painless and undetected tumors (see **Fig. 5.136**).

When gynecologists detect a palpable nodule during physical examination, they will generally order mammograms and then proceed with immediate breast ultrasound while the patient is still in their office. Ultrasound imaging allows the physician to make an immediate tentative diagnosis, which can then be confirmed by a morphologic (interventional) test procedure. The tendency to order mammograms for a palpable nodule is remarkable and stems from a time when ultrasound was in its infancy and largely unknown. Today, however, the first step in the diagnostic algorithm should be breast ultrasound, followed by mammography and then, if malignancy is suspected, by magnetic resonance imaging. Ohlinger et al. (2003) conducted a study in 184 women—97 with palpable breast nodules and 87 without. Mammograms taken by experienced mammographers showed a sensitivity of only 53.3%, whereas ultrasound scanning by experienced sonographers achieved a sensitivity of 86%. Ultrasound increased the sensitivity of mammography by 35%, while mammography increased the sensitivity of ultrasound by only 1.6%. In a study comparing the ability of magnetic resonance imaging, ultrasound, and mammography to define the extent of breast cancers in 183 women, the detection rates were 93.7% with MRI, 97.3% with ultrasound, and 84.6% with mammography (Hata et al. 2004).

A palpable breast nodule should at least be morphologically investigated by FNA (see p. 230), even when imaging results are negative. All of these diagnostic procedures should be done by one person, and biopsy should be performed at an accredited breast center (see p. 290). Physical examination is particularly important in breast screening, and the breasts should at least be palpated by the mammographic technologist. The screening physician rarely comes in direct contact with patients (except in certain investigations) and only reads mammograms. Ultrasound is not performed until the patient has been "recalled" for the investigation of a suspicious mammogram. It is likely that some *interval cancers* (see p. 126) could have been detected by inspection and palpation, since up to 10% of all palpable neoplasms are not mammographically detectable for various reasons (radiodense breast), even by highly trained screening physicians. In a study of 60 palpable DCIS lesions by Yang et al. (2004), 10% of the lesions were sonographically occult and 20% were not visible on mammograms.

> **!** **Physical examination is an integral and essential part of breast diagnosis, especially in the age of screening. It should be learned and practiced by technologists.**

The optimum timing for all breast examinations in women of childbearing age is at the midpoint of the cycle (days 7–12). At that time the breasts are least painful and easiest to palpate, and yield the most reliable results in complementary investigations (mammography, ultrasound, MRI). Compression mammography is least painful during this phase of the cycle. Magnetic resonance imaging often yields a false-positive result when performed during the second half of the cycle (see p. 201).

## Mammography

Of all breast imaging procedures, high-resolution mammography (including magnification mammography) is the modality of choice for detecting nonpalpable breast cancers with calcifications, despite its relatively low specificity.

First a word about the *sensitivity* and *specificity* of mammography: In a meta-analysis, Muschlin (quoted by Hille et al. 2004a) found that mammography had a sensitivity in the range of 83–95% and a specificity of 93.5–99.1% (which seems rather optimistic!). Because the sensitivity of mammography depends strongly on the radiographic density of the breast, these values should be broken down into specific groups (age, ACR breast density). In a series of 11 130 women studied by Kolb, the overall sensitivity of mammography was 77.6% and its overall specificity was 98.8% (Kolb et al. 2002). The sensitivity actually varied between 47.8% and 98%, however, in relation to breast density. Age was also important: Sensitivity was 58% in women under 50 years of age but 82.7% in women over age 50. These figures show that mammography is most effective as a screening tool in women with a radiographic breast density of ACR 1 or 2. This subgroup of patients consists mainly of postmenopausal women with involuted breasts. Between 15% and 40% of all carcinomas (depending on the age and breast density of the women studied) are mammographically occult and are detectable only by ultrasound (Hille et al. 2004b). Generally speaking, screening mammography has a reported sensitivity of 72.4%, a specificity of 97.3%, and a positive predictive value of 10.6%. Diagnostic mammography has a sensitivity of 78.1%, a specificity of 89.3%, and a positive predictive value of 17.1%. In every 1000 women who are screened, 3.3 carcinomas are detected while 1.2 are missed and later classified as interval cancers. Eighty percent of screening-detected neoplasms are not associated with axillary lymph node metastases. The rate at which screening requires additional testing is 8.3%. When screening includes ultrasound scans, that rate falls to 3.5%. "Curative" mammography requires the use of additional tests in 17.5% of cases (Poplack et al. 2000).

The sensitivity and specificity of mammography are always high in the diagnosis of calcifying breast lesions. Noncalcifying tumors are the domain of ultrasound (see p. 193) and MRI (see p. 201) rather than mammography.

The standard mammographic protocol consists of two views:

- An oblique (45°) view that covers the axillary recess and preferably the entire breast to the level of the pectoral muscle
- A craniocaudal view that covers the entire breast from its medial to lateral border

**Fig. 5.13 Compression pads for mammography.**

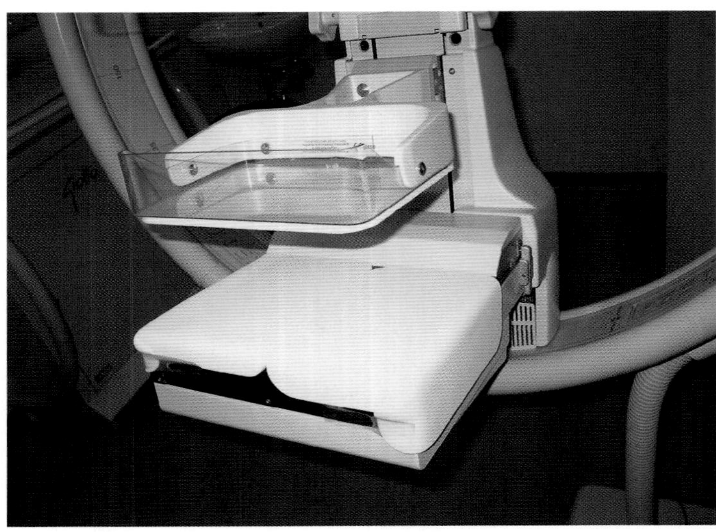

**a** *MammoPads* manufactured by Hologic/Biolucent Inc., Aliso Vieja, California, USA.

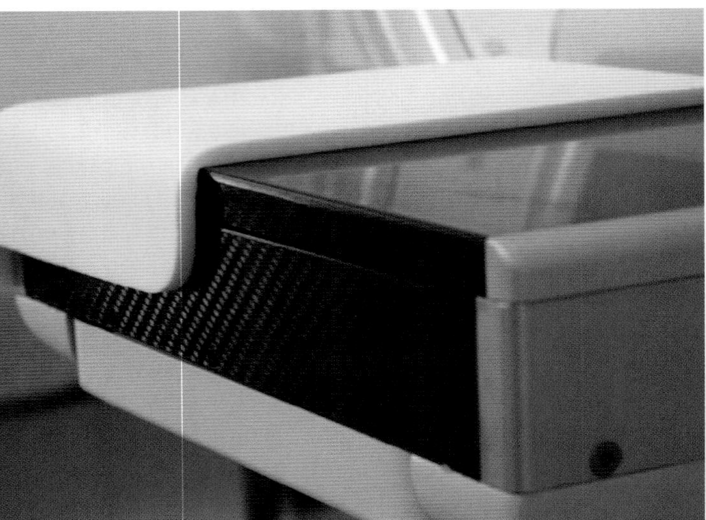

**b** *Edges and corners* are padded with soft, washable, self-adhesive foam pads. This makes mammography less painful while increasing the radiation dose by only 2–3%.

> **!** **The third view (straight mediolateral projection) taken by some radiologists is not recommended, as it adds no information and unnecessarily increases radiation exposure.**

The standard mammographic film size is 18 cm × 24 cm. Larger breasts should be exposed on 24 cm × 30 cm film. If this film size is not available, a standard oblique view should be taken that displays all of the pectoral muscle. This view "cuts off" the nipple-areola, but that region can still be captured in the craniocaudal view.

There is hardly any standard work on mammography or set of guidelines that does not underscore the importance of mammography as the internationally recognized standard for breast diagnosis. But at the same time, modern ultrasound scanners and high-resolution transducers (at least 7.5 MHz, preferably 11–13 MHz) permit such a detailed analysis of the breast parenchyma that mammography cannot keep pace with this technology (except in the diagnosis of calcifying lesions). For the past 8 years, it has been the practice of the author and his colleagues to obtain biplane mammograms only in the initial examination. Follow-up mammograms are limited to the one view that best demonstrated the breast parenchyma. In 95% of cases this is the oblique view (see p. 105). Mammograms in women under 40 years of age are generally limited to one view per breast, thus reducing the patient's radiation exposure by half.

Women have shown a very high acceptance of single-view mammograms. They are more likely to keep their appointments for scheduled follow-ups, because missing an appointment by more than 2 months generally means that their next examination will have to include two mammographic views.

Single-view mammography reduces radiation exposure and limits painful breast compressions to one compression per breast. When combined with high-resolution ultrasound, single-view mammography has a greater impact on early breast cancer detection than two-view mammograms alone.

Instead of 2-year intervals between examinations, we feel that women with *no* family history of breast cancer should be screened every 1.5 years while women with a positive family history should be screened once a year. The usual 2- to 3-year intervals between screening examinations are too long for the early detection of breast cancer. Shortening the screening interval from 24 months to 12 months increases the sensitivity of mammography from 70% to 85% (Kolb et al. 2002). In addition, women have a greater tendency to miss appointments that are scheduled at longer intervals, often missing them by months or even years. Eighty percent of women miss their appointments by at least 6 months. The incentive offered in our practice, where women are notified that they will be "rewarded" with just one compression per breast if they keep their appointments, has been very effective. This campaign has shortened the average appointment delay to only 2 months.

Many women avoid having mammograms because they are painful. The discomfort of breast compression can be reduced by padding the film tray and compression paddle with adhesive foam pads that soften the hard edges of the compression device (**Fig. 5.13**). The manufacturers of mammographic equipment should design units with rounded edges and corners to eliminate one source of discomfort. Unfortunately, a "painful experience" is not the only reason women opt out of mammographic screening. For many women, the fear that the compression itself increases the risk of breast cancer is a major concern. A dissertation by one of the author's colleagues has demonstrated that such fears are unfounded (see p. 17; Beyer 2004).

As a matter of policy, every technologist and medical assistant should be instructed to stop compression when the patient tells them to. Even a lightly compressed mammogram can be evaluated. On the other hand, the degree of compression must be sufficient to enable x-ray beam emission. Most units are set to a minimum force of 4 kilopond (kp). The most common range of compression is 4–15 kp, and the amount of pressure is individually controlled with a foot pedal. Breast compression is necessary to reduce the radiation dose and optimize the quality of the image.

Since "bare-breasted" examinations are uncomfortable for many women, disposable gowns can be provided. This is ultimately, but not entirely, a matter of cost. Patients find it reassuring when the technologist cleans the film tray and compression paddle with alcohol in the patient's presence before use.

**Tip**

**Women with long hair (both patients and technologists) should tie their hair back if possible to keep stray hairs out of the radiation field. Hairspray can mimic microcalcifications and has caused confusion in the past. Powder should not be used in the axillae or inframammary fold, as it may resemble microcalcifications (see Fig. 5.42). Too much deodorant can produce a similar effect.**

A special problem in breast imaging (as well as radiology in general) concerns organizational details. For over 12 years, it has been our policy to let our privately insured patients take their mammograms home with them. This saves filing space in the office and gives women the flexibility to take their mammograms to their gynecologist, family doctor, or treatment facility at any time. This system also eliminates postal fees. At-home filing of mammograms generally works very well. Only about 5% of women forget to bring previous mammograms (or cannot find them because of a recent move, etc.) to their follow-up visits. If a change is found in new mammograms, the patient is told to mail all of her previous images to the medical office. Since the women must pay the postage themselves, they usually remember to bring their pictures with them to the next appointment. Of course, digital mammography solves these problems by eliminating the need for x-ray filing jackets. Relevant conventional mammograms can be scanned into the patient's data file (see p. 100).

When the costs associated with x-ray image filing by hospital and office staff are taken into account, we must ask whether it would be advantageous to have all patients keep their diagnostic images (including mammograms) at home. Certain policy guidelines would have to be changed, but the savings would be well worth the effort and expense.

It has also proven very advantageous to mail a copy of the physician's letter to every woman after her appointment. This gets patients involved in the examination process and reminds them what their physician has found and recommended. It also frees the doctor from liability when, say, a woman is found to have a tumor but is long overdue for her next scheduled mammogram or did not present for recommended additional tests (MRI, interventional procedures, etc.).

## Technical Aspects of an Optimum Mammogram

*E. Steinhilber*

### *Quality Control*

Since 2003; the technical quality of mammograms in Germany has been checked by a random sampling process that is mandated by law. The quality criteria are basically the same as in Britain's national screening program. The four-part quality rating system used in the British program is called the PGMI system, which indicates:

- **P**erfect
- **G**ood
- **M**oderate
- **I**nsufficient

In our practice, every mammogram taken during the past 8 years has been rated according to the PGMI system and recorded in a log. This gives our technologists feedback on how the physicians rated each mammogram, helping them to correct any flaws in their technique. At the end of a specified period, the log entries are evaluated and an average performance rating is determined for the department (at our center: 60% P, 30% G, 10% M, 0% I). Approximately 6500 mammograms are taken each year at our institute, and the data show that physician assistants and radiologic technologists have produced images of equal quality.

The Breast Imaging Committee of the German Radiology Society has developed a mammographic quality standard based on the experience of the British national screening program. Their standard is based on the four levels described above and is not valid for breasts that have undergone excisional surgery, implantation, or reduction mammoplasty. The quality standards are as follows:

- 75% of the images must receive a G or P rating.
- 97% of the images must be rated P, G, or M.
- Less than 3% of the images may be rated I.

Overall, 75% of the images must be good or perfect, 22% may be moderate, and only 3% may be insufficient.

### *Quality Criteria for Craniocaudal Mammograms*

**Perfect:**

- Breast is correctly imaged:
  - Pectoral muscle is shown near the chest wall
  - Nipple is shown in profile
  - Axillary tail is shown without losing the medial portions of the breast
- Correct annotations
- Correct exposure
- Appropriate compression (parenchymal structures are sharply displayed and there is adequate spreading of the breast tissue)
- No motion unsharpness
- Correct processing
- No artifacts
- No skin folds
- Symmetrical images (see **Fig. 5.15**)

**Good:** A *good* mammogram shows deficiencies in some of the criteria of a *perfect* mammogram.

- Breast is adequately imaged:
  - Pectoral muscles are not shown near the chest wall
  - The nipple–pectoral line (NPL) should be such that b > a – 15 mm (**Fig. 5.14**). Lateral portions of the axillary tail are shown without losing the medial portions. Often the pectoral muscle is not visible in the craniocaudal view but is usually visible in the oblique view, so: a – b ≤ 15 mm.
- Minor processing and handling artifacts
- Skin folds
- Slightly asymmetrical images

**Fig. 5.14 Diagrammatic representation of the nipple–pectoral line (NPL).** *a–b* should be < 15 mm.

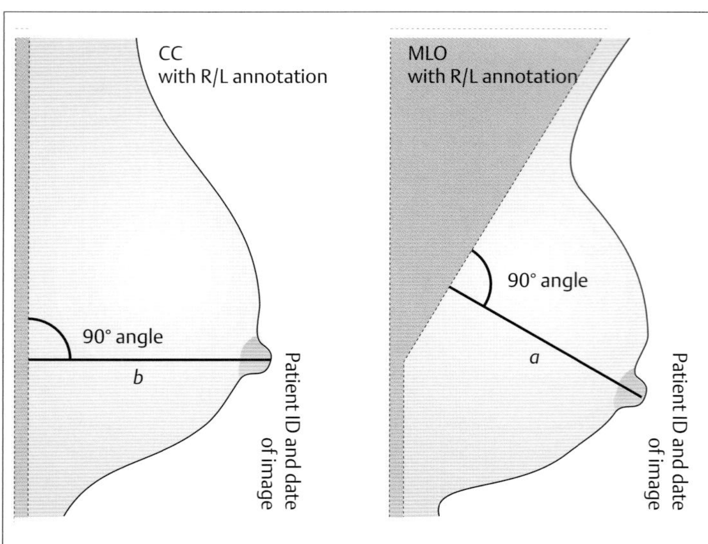


**Moderate:** Image meet criteria 2–6 but show deficiencies in 7 and do not fully meet 1 and 8.

- Breast is not completely imaged:
  - Pectoral muscle is not shown (NPL: b see **Fig. 5.14**) is unmeasurable
  - Large portions of the axillary tail are not shown
- Skin folds are present but do not obscure breast tissue

**Inadequate:** Inadequate mammograms meet one of the following criteria:

- Part of the breast is not imaged
- Inadequate compression
- Incorrect exposure
- Incorrect processing
- Artifacts (e.g., skin folds) are present and obscure the breast tissue
- Inadequate identification

Inadequate mammograms must be repeated.

Quality criteria for the craniocaudal view are shown diagrammatically in **Fig. 5.15**.

**Errors in the craniocaudal view and possible causes:**

- Tissue near the chest wall is not completely imaged
  - Film tray height is incorrect
  - Breast is not pulled far enough forward
- Skin folds:
  - Fat pad on the upper outer quadrant
  - Too much medial shoulder rotation; inferior breast tissue is not pulled far enough forward
  - Nipple is not shown in profile
  - Film tray height is incorrect (if the film tray is too high, the nipple points downward; if the film tray is too low, the nipple points upward)
  - Inferior breast tissue is not pulled far enough forward
  - Congenital anomaly

**Fig. 5.15 Quality criteria for craniocaudal mammograms.**

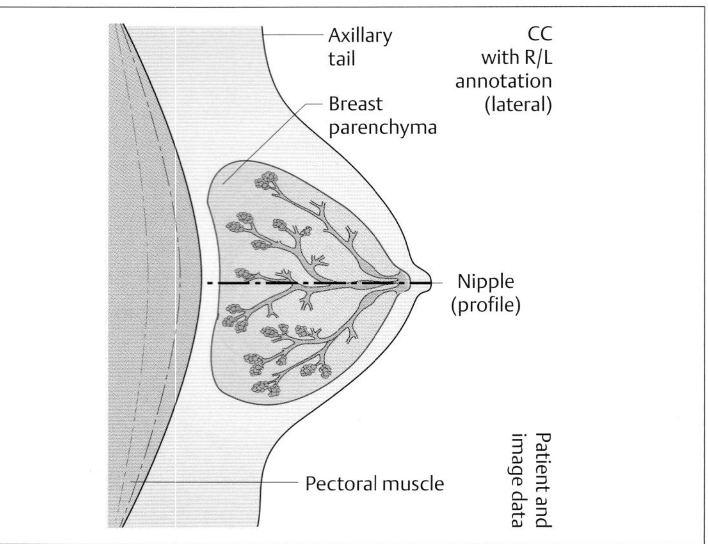


**a** Diagrammatic representation of quality criteria for craniocaudal mammograms.

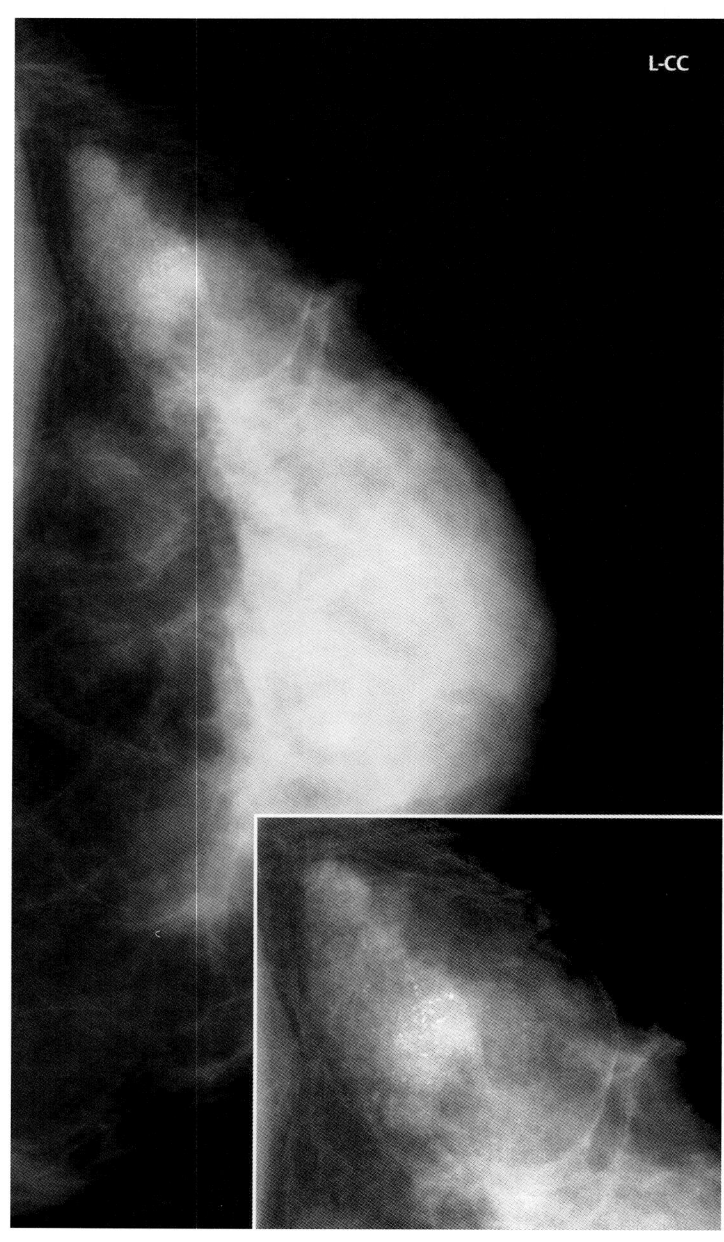


**b** Perfectly positioned *craniocaudal mammogram of the left breast* clearly demonstrates the axillary recess with ductal comedocarcinoma (compare with **Fig. 5.16 b**).

*Quality Criteria for Mediolateral Oblique Mammograms*

The advantage of the 45° oblique projection is that it provides good visualization of the upper outer quadrant, the axillary tail, and the inframammary fold. It is the second standard view in breast cancer screening mammography.

**Perfect:**

- Whole breast is imaged:
  - Pectoral muscle is shown at least to nipple level
  - Pectoral muscle is slightly convex and at an approximately 20° angle
  - Nipple in shown in profile
  - Clear view of inframammary fold
- Views are correctly annotated:
  - Patient identification
  - Examiner identification
  - Date
  - Side and projection
- Appropriate exposure
- Appropriate compression
- No motion unsharpness
- Correct processing
- Absence of artifacts
- No skin folds
- Symmetrical images

**Good:** A good mammogram meets the first 6 criteria for a perfect mammogram:

- Breast is correctly imaged
- Correct annotation
- Appropriate exposure
- Appropriate compression
- No motion unsharpness
- Correct processing
- Minor artifacts
- Minimal skin folds
- Slightly asymmetrical images

**Moderate:** Image meets criteria 2–6 but shows deficiencies in 7 and does not fully meet 1 and 8

- Breast is not correctly imaged:
  - Pectoral muscle is not shown to nipple level, or
  - Pectoral muscle is not at the correct angle, or
  - Nipple is not shown in profile, or
  - Inframammary fold is not shown
- Correct annotation
- Appropriate exposure
- Appropriate compression
- No motion unsharpness
- Minor processing and handling artifacts
- Skin folds are present but do not obscure breast tissue

**Inadequate:** At least one of the following criteria is present:

- Parts of the breast are not imaged
- Inadequate annotation
- Incorrect exposure
- Inadequate compression
- Motion unsharpness
- Incorrect processing
- Artifacts
- Skin folds obscuring the breast tissue

Quality criteria for the mediolateral oblique view are shown diagrammatically in Fig. **5.16**.

**Fig. 5.16 Quality criteria for mediolateral (oblique) mammograms.**

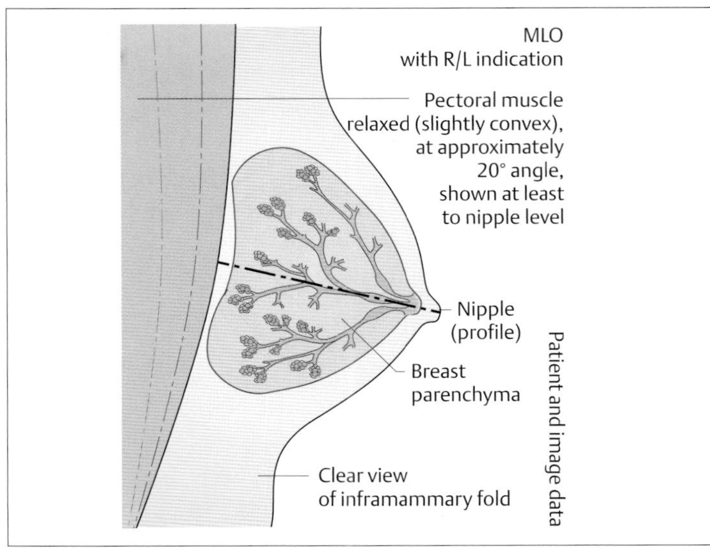


**a** Diagrammatic representation of quality criteria for mediolateral (oblique) mammograms.

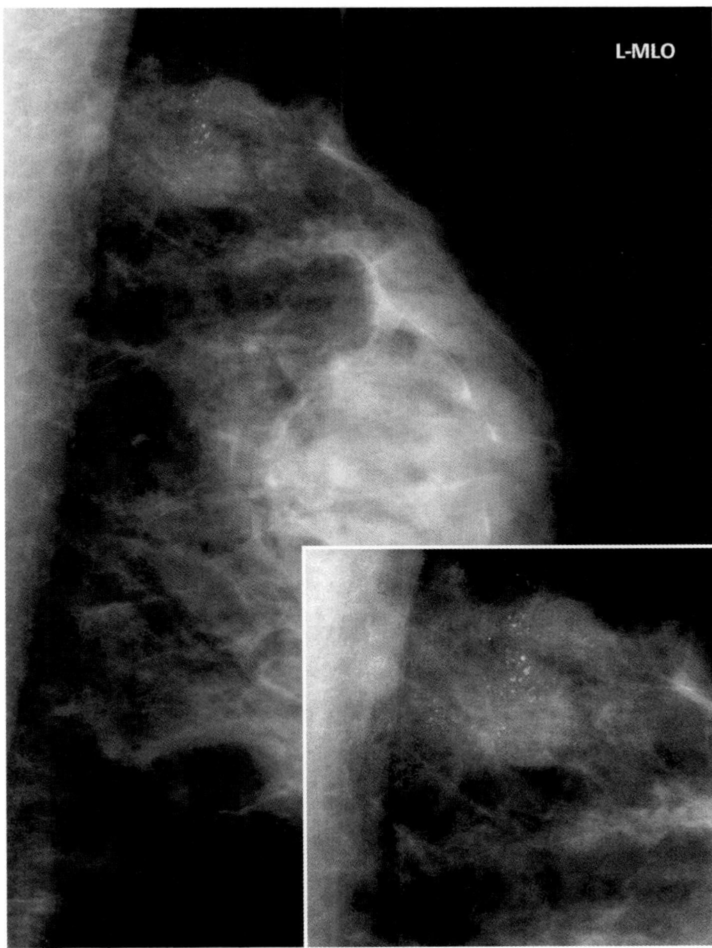


**b** *Oblique mammogram of the left breast.* This is a perfectly positioned view in which the tumor is clearly visible in the upper outer quadrant at the junction with the axillary recess (insets at lower right).

**Errors in the mediolateral oblique view and possible causes:**

- Pectoral muscle is not completely imaged:
  - Film tray is too anterior
  - Upper corner of the film tray should be in front of the posterior axillary fold
  - Shoulder is not relaxed
- Whole breast is not imaged:
  - Axillary tail is not pulled far enough outward
  - Inadequate rotation into the film plane
  - Film tray is too high and too much of the compression plate is on the pectoral muscle
- Inframammary fold is not shown:
  - Hip and feet are turned away from the unit
  - Hip is behind the film tray (the whole body should be turned toward the unit), whole lateral side is against the film tray
- Inframammary fold is not opened up:
  - Breast is not pulled away from the chest wall
  - Breast is too low
  - Nipple is not shown in profile
  - Lower breast tissue is not pulled far enough forward
  - The patient is not turned sufficiently toward the unit

Separate criteria have not yet been established for the true lateral (**ml**) view, but most of the criteria for the oblique view also apply to the lateral projection.

The author has produced a video that covers other aspects of a quality mammogram such as physical facilities, physician examination, and additional tests (www.brustkrebs.de, website in German).

*Test Intervals and Limits Based on the European Protocol for the Quality Control of the Physical and Technical Aspects of Mammographic Screening (EPQC)*

The following abbreviations are used:

- OD = optical density
- Lp/mm = line-pair/mm
- cd = candela
- N = newton

Guidelines for periodic testing of x-ray equipment are given in **Table 5.1. Daily tests** are listed in **Table 5.2; weekly** tests are listed in **Table 5.3**.

**Monthly tests** (summary evaluation): Test results are the maximum deviations of daily sensitometry of individual measurements for fog, sensitivity, and contrast (or mean gradient) as well as deviations of maximum blackening from the mean expressed as optical densities (without a unit) (**Table 5.4**).

**Annual tests** are listed in **Table 5.5**.

The EPQC recommends additional tests at startup and whenever changes are suspected (**Table 5.6**).

On reviewing national and international standards for the testing of mammographic systems, Ewen and Blendl (2004) described an "equivalence between the European guidelines (EPQC) and national quality assurance (QA) guidelines. When it comes to quality assurance in curative or screening mammography, there is no need to draw a distinction between the EPQC and national guidelines regarding the level of quality control. An institution that performs quality assurance under national guidelines is acting in full accordance with the EPQC." These statements are based on experience with the New Hampshire Screening Project in 35 803 women.

**Table 5.1 Guidelines for the periodic testing of x-ray equipment**

| Number | Description | Test intervals |
|---|---|---|
| 6.1 | Visual and function testing | Monthly |
| 6.2 | Optical density | Daily |
| 6.2.1 | Density adjustment (maintenance of required density with the aid of a correction key) | Daily |
| 6.2.2 | Stable equipment operation (maintenance of required density with correct key at zero position) | Monthly |
| 6.3 | Artifacts | Daily |
| 6.4 | Spatial resolution | |
| | • With most commonly used focal spot | • Weekly/yearly |
| | • With other focal spots | • Yearly |
| 6.5 | Contrast resolution (evaluation of low contrast resolution) | |
| | • With most commonly used filter/target | • Weekly |
| | • With other filters/anode targets | • Yearly |
| 6.6 | Image contrast (evaluation of coarse contrast) | Monthly |
| 6.7 | Object and tube voltage compensation (conformance to density requirements in different operating modes) | Monthly |
| 6.8 | Correction key for automatic exposure control | Yearly |
| 6.9 | Dose | |
| | • Automatic exposure control | • Monthly |
| | • With manual setting | • Yearly |
| 6.10 | Useful field | Monthly |
| 6.11 (DIN 6832-2) | Cassettes: beam attenuation and amplification factor | Yearly |
| 6.12 (DIN 6832-2) | Cassettes: film-screen contact pressure | Yearly |
| DIN 6868-2 | • Periodic testing of film processing | • Daily |
| | • Testing of dark room | • Yearly |
| DIN 6856-2 | Film view box (luminous density and uniformity) | Yearly |
| DIN 6868-152 | Compression device | Not stipulated |

**Table 5.2 Daily tests**

| Test | Acceptable limits |
|---|---|
| **Film processing** | |
| OD fog | < 20 |
| Sensitivity | ± 0.10 of reference value |
| Contrast | ± 0.10 of reference value |
| Mean gradient | 3.0–4.0 |
| **Automatic exposure control** | |
| Long-term reproducibility of dose over mean OD | ± 0.15 |
| Reproducibility of mean OD | ± 0.15 |
| Artifacts | No artifacts |

OD = optical density.

**Table 5.3 Weekly tests**

| Test | Acceptable limits |
|---|---|
| **Automatic exposure control** | |
| Object thickness compensation with various phantom thicknesses and varying voltage series | ± 0.15 |
| **Image quality** | |
| Image contrast through aluminum step wedge | Less than ± 0.10 % deviation from reference values |
| High contrast (spatial resolution) | > 12 Lp/mm |
| Low contrast | 10 Lp/mm, vertically and horizontally; visible image of low-contrast wedge must be at least 5 cm long |
| Exposure time | < 2 seconds |
| Deviation near the chest wall (5 spheres) | The number of spheres should match the acceptance test (complete visualization of 3 of the 5 spheres) |

**Table 5.4 Monthly tests**

| Test | Acceptable limits |
|---|---|
| **Variation of processing conditions** | |
| Variation of fog density | < 0.03 |
| Variation of sensitivity | < 0.05 |
| Variation of mean gradient | < 0.20 |
| Variation of maximum blackening | < 0.30 |

**Table 5.5 Annual tests**

| Test | Acceptable limits |
|---|---|
| **Mammographic unit** | |
| Dose limit | < 10 mGy |
| Discrepancy between x-ray field and light field | < 5 mm lateral discrepancy to end of film |
| Half-value layer Mo/Mo | < 0.3 mm Al |
| Compression force | 130–200 N* (ca. 13–20 kp) |
| Uniformity of compression | With nonuniform load: < 15 mm with uniform load: < 5 mm |
| Exposure time | < 2 seconds (< 1.5 seconds) |
| **View box** | |
| Luminous density | 2000–6000 cd/m² |
| Homogeneity | ± 30 % |
| Variation between different view boxes | ± 15 % |
| **Cassettes** | |
| Comparison of different cassettes | < 0.10 discrepancy, < 5 % |
| Film-screen contact | No sites of inadequate contact |
| Ambient light | < 50 lux |

* 1 Newton (force) = 102 gram (weight)

**Table 5.6 Additional tests (initially and for suspected changes)**

| Test | Acceptable limits |
|---|---|
| **Film processing** | |
| Processing time and temperature | 90 seconds at 34–36 °C |
| **Radiation source** | |
| Leakage radiation from the x-ray tube | 1 mGy/hour |
| Focal spot size (pinhole camera method) | 0.3 (0.4) mm |
| Focal spot-film distance | At least 600 mm |
| **Dark room** | |
| Dark room lighting, light tightness | < 0.10 OD |
| Film storage containers | < 0.02 OD |
| Cassettes | No additional fog |
| **Grid** | |
| Attenuation factor | < 3.0 |
| Visible grid lines | None |
| **View box** | |
| Homogeneity/luminous density | ± 30 %/2000–6000 cd/m² |
| **Compression** | |
| With nonuniform load<br>With uniform load | < 15 mm<br>< 5 mm |

### BIRADS Classification and Grading of Breast Density

#### *Breast Density and Cancer Risk*

Leborgne (1953) and Wolfe (1967) described an increased risk of breast cancer in radiographically dense breasts (see pp. 91, 156, 192). Based on an analysis of 7214 examinations, Wolfe developed a classification made up of four basic patterns:

- **N1** (38%): The breast consists mainly of fat (N = normal), corresponding to ACR 1 (lowest risk for breast cancer).
- **P1** (24%): This pattern includes fat as well as linear densities (enlarged ducts) occupying no more than 25% of the breast, corresponding to ACR 2 (low risk for breast cancer).
- **P2** (27%): The linear densities (from enlarged ducts) occupy more than 25% of the breast. They are predominantly in the upper outer quadrant but may be distributed throughout the breast (P = prominent ducts), corresponding to ACR 3 (high risk for breast cancer.
- **Dy** (10%): Dense, radiopaque breasts (Dy = dysplasia) corresponding to ACR 4 (highest risk for breast cancer).

Wolfe added a fifth category to these four:

- **Qdy** (quasi-dysplasia): This group consists of young women whose dense breasts have a somewhat spongy texture due to fatty infiltration.

Wolfe found 76 breast cancers in 7214 examinations. The key results of his study are summarized below:

- Although the **Dy** group (**ACR 4**) made up only 10% of all cases, it accounted for 41% of all cancers.
- The **P2** group (**ACR 3**), which made up 27% of all cases, accounted for a full 45% of the cancers.
- Only 11 cancers were found in the other two groups (**N1** and **P1**) (**ACR 1 + 2**), which together comprised 63% of the patients examined.

Wolfe concluded that the P2 and Dy groups are at high risk for breast cancer, while the N1 and P1 groups have a low risk.

No practical applications were drawn from Wolfe's findings for many years, especially when some authors expressed serious doubts about his conclusions (Arthur et al. 1990, Sickles 2007). The density issue has experienced a resurgence in recent years, because obviously there is something to it (Harvey et al. 2004). The problem of the dense breast goes deeper, therefore.

If we grant that breast density is indeed associated with an increased cancer risk, then the proliferation of glandular parenchyma leading to a more radiodense breast may be the solution to the puzzle. For if copious amounts of proliferating lobular parenchyma are present during menopause, this could be the result of an hormonal stimulus suggesting that the development of lobular carcinoma is a real possibility. Sixteen percent of all malignancies are lobular carcinomas—the type most frequently missed on mammograms. Approximately 60% of all breast cancers develop in P2 and Dy breasts (ACR 3 + 4). These breasts also show varying degrees of lobular proliferation (i.e., enlarged TDLUs) when examined by ultrasound. If P2, Dy, and Qdy breasts could be selected for ultrasound evaluation to determine whether their density results from lobular proliferation—meaning that they are responding to some kind of hormonal stimulus—this would identify not only a risk group but also a group that would require more careful selection for *hormone replacement therapy* (HRT). Additionally, a hormone regimen could be prescribed with the intent to reduce lobular proliferation (tamoxifen, for example, or estrogen-only therapy with a progesterone IUD instead of systemic estrogen and progesterone), and ultrasound could be used to monitor response.

The discoveries of Leborgne and Wolfe on the risk of radiographically dense breasts have taken on new meaning in the era of high-resolution ultrasound. These authors conducted a detailed analysis without knowing exactly what they were seeing. They drew the right conclusions, but for the wrong patients (see p. 192).

The classification system used by leading American breast experts, which appeared in the ACR-BIRADS Report (2003; 2006), is distinguished by its relative clarity and simplicity. It distinguishes four main types of breast composition:

- Fatty (involuted) breast (ACR 1)
- Scattered fibroglandular tissue (ACR 2)
- Heterogeneously dense breast (ACR 3)
- Extremely dense breast (ACR 4)

This system was not correlated with cancer risk (Lanyi 2003).

All the illustrations in this book indicate the ACR classification of the imaged breast and the PGMI rating of the image.

#### *ACR Density Grades*

The American College of Radiology (**ACR**) established the four grades of breast density that are described above (ACR 1–4). About 60% of our own mammograms belong to ACR 3 and 4 (see p. 373). When the breast parenchyma is strongly involuted (ACR 1), malignant processes can be detected mammographically at a very early stage when they are only 2–3 mm in size. In some cases, however, they are detected only by the presence of microcalcifications. The involuted breast **ACR 1** is easy to evaluate mammographically, quite unlike the very radiodense breast **ACR 4.** In extreme cases the breast may be so dense that nodules and tumors are not detectable even when they *exceed 2 cm in diameter.* The high radiographic density of these breasts results from the presence of intra- and interlobular stroma. Intramammary fat contrasts poorly with these tissues but is still present. Between these two extremes are two other grades: **ACR 2** applies to breasts with radiodense areas in which *tumors 5 mm in diameter* may be missed unless they are associated with microcalcifications. Radiodense breasts classified as **ACR 3** consist of two-thirds parenchyma and one-third fat. *Tumors as large as 2 cm* may be missed in ACR 3 breasts (density and visibility of TDLUs, see **Fig. 4.4**, p. 26). The ACR density grades are summarized in **Table 5.7**.

**Table 5.7 ACR (American College of Radiology) density grades**

| Category | Density of breast tissue | Assessability |
|---|---|---|
| ACR 1 | Mostly fat (radiolucent) | Very good |
| ACR 2 | Scattered fibroglandular tissue (moderately radiolucent) | Good |
| ACR 3 | Heterogeneously dense (reduces the sensitivity of mammography) | Limited |
| ACR 4 | Extremely or very dense (malignancies and other lesions are not always detectable) | Limited |

The classification of mammograms into various density grades should be noted in every radiology report so that the referring physician can know how reliably the mammogram reflects the patient's diagnosis.

**Tip**

**A breast with a radiographic density of ACR 3–4 should always be evaluated by ultrasound in addition to mammography. This ensures detection of any malignancy at least 5 mm in size.**

*BIRADS Classification*

BIRADS, an acronym for *Breast Imaging Reporting and Data System*, classifies mammographic findings into six categories based on risk of malignancy:

- **BIRADS 0:** incomplete: definitive diagnosis not possible; further investigations (extra mammography view, ultrasound, or MRI) are necessary.
- **BIRADS 1:** negative: normal breast tissue with no evidence of benign or malignant lesions.
- **BIRADS 2:** normal mammogram wiht benign findings such as cysts, focal fibrosis, benign calcifications, but without signs of malignancy.
- **BIRADS 3:** probably normal but with a 2% risk of malignancy. Repeat mammogram recommended at 6 months. The biopsy rate for BIRADS 3 cases should be no more than 1%. In retrospect, there should be no more than a 3% incidence of malignant findings in follow-ups. This category include cysts, fibroadenomas, ductectasia, clustered calcifications suspicious for a benign process, etc. The ACR discourages the assignment of BIRADS 3 to a screening mammogram. Any findings that require follow-up are BIRADS 2, and all presumably benign findings that still require biopsy are classified as BIRADS 4a.
- **BIRADS 4:** suspicious abnormality with 23% to 34% chance of malignancy. Biopsy necessary for diagnosis. Histologic evaluation would result in a 25% incidence of breast cancer detection. This category includes suspicious clustered calcifications, architectural distortion, nonspecific atypical parenchymal densities, suspicious opacities, etc. It is further differentiated into BIRADS **4a** (identical to BIRADS 3) and BIRADS 4b and c. 4a indicates a mammographically benign lesion (e.g., increasing fibroadenoma), which should be removed surgically or by vacuum biopsy. **4b** indicates a suspicious abnormality, and **4c** is highly suspicious for malignancy.
- **BIRADS 5:** highly suggestive of malignancy (> 95% risk of malignancy). Biopsy is mandatory. 98% of cases should yield a histologic diagnosis of malignancy. Typical changes in this category are stellate densities with microcalcifications, very suspicious densities with radiating spicules, solid nodules with or without calcifications with scalloped margins and focal unsharpness, and atypical patchy calcifications.
- **BIRADS 6:** known biopsy-proven malignancy (histologically confirmed). Treatment plan to be discussed.

Part of the BIRADS classification includes terminology used for mammographic interpretation. Intended to permit a clear and accurate description of findings, the terms describe the **size and shape** of focal lesions (e.g., **round, oval, lobular, irregular**), their **margins** (e.g., **circumscribed, microlobulated, ill-defined margins, spiculated**), and their **relative radiographic density** (e.g., **hyperdense, isodense, hypodense**). These characteristics are generally recognized to describe and differentiate benign and malignant focal lesions. The various types of **calcification** are classified by their appearance as typically benign calcifications (e.g., **cutaneous calcifications, vascular calcifications**), moderately suspicious calcifications (e.g., **amorphous calcifications**), and highly suspicious calcifications (e.g., **pleomorphic or heterogeneous calcifications**). Calcifications that are strongly suspicious for malignancy require a description of their distribution pattern (e.g., **clustered, linear, segmental, regional, diffuse**). These findings can all be assigned to one of the seven BIRADS categories.

The BIRADS classification pertains exclusively to mammography. Problems arise when a suspicious focus is detected sonographically in a patient with negative mammograms. It would be incorrect to classify this case as BIRADS 5, since the BIRADS system was developed to interpret mammograms, which in this case missed the tumor. One solution is to add prefix letters indicating the modality that detected the change:

- M-BIRADS: mammography
- S-BIRADS: sonography
- MRI-BIRADS: magnetic resonance imaging
- PH-BIRADS: physical examination (inspection, palpation)

There are no clear guidelines on this practice, and even the S-3 guidelines do not address it.

The method by which a tumor is detected is irrelevant to referring physicians, who care more about lesion classification and the treatment recommendations that are derived from it (**Table 5.8**).

**Table 5.8 BIRADS categories, actions, and probability of cancer (from Weining 2004)**

| Category | BIRADS description | Action | Probability of cancer (%) |
|---|---|---|---|
| 0 | Incomplete; requires additional imaging evaluation | Order additional imaging studies | N/A |
| 1 | Negative | No follow-up | < 1 |
| 2 | Benign | No follow-up | < 1 |
| 3 | Probably benign | Follow-up in 6 months | 1–3 |
| 4 (a–c) | Suspicious, probably malignant | Percutaneous or excisional biopsy | 20–30 |
| 5 | Highly suggestive of malignancy | Biopsy and appropriate multimodal treatment | > 90 |
| 6 | Histologically confirmed malignancy | Treatment | 100 |

### Digital Mammography

Over the years, conventional mammography has developed a high international standard for positioning technique, magnification imaging, and technical protocols. Highly sensitive film–screen combinations (class 25) have come into use. The focal spot size is very small (0.3/0.1 mm). It has become standard practice to use bimetallic rhodium/molybdenum filters. A very high standard has been developed across Europe and the US as well for the various technical aspects of film processing and image generation.

Digital mammography, on the other hand, still employs a variety of *cassette-based (off-line) and integrated (online) systems.* The cassette-based systems in turn may use "high-resolution" or "transparent" storage plates. Integrated systems may employ TFT flat-panel detectors, CCD detectors, or photon counting detectors. Flat-panel detectors with a cesium iodide-based system and a selenium-based system are currently on the market, while CCD detectors are used in two scanner systems (Fischer and Spectra). This variety in systems and the current lack of quality standards, plus safety concerns, still pose an obstacle to the routine clinical use of digital mammography (Müller-Schimpfle et al. 2003).

The era of film–screen mammography is coming to an end, and digital mammography is on the rise. In the past, the advantages of conventional mammography have still outweighed those of digital systems, especially with regard to resolution (line pairs) and contrast. But microcalcifications are easier to detect with digital mammography than with conventional film–screen mammography. Various search factors (**CAD** systems) and setting parameters for density and contrast have placed digital mammography on an equal footing with conventional mammography in terms of image interpretation and diagnostic accuracy (Shalom et al. 2004). This also applies to screening, where digital mammography offers significant logistical advantages (Skaane et al. 2003). Destounis et al. (2004), for example, were able to detect 81% of missed tumors by using their **CAD** system to evaluate initial mammograms.

Digital technology can greatly facilitate handling and workflow in mammographic departments. This does require some change on the part of the physician, for example, because there is no longer a hard-copy x-ray image to read, only a soft-copy image displayed on a high-resolution monitor. Physicians can no longer send films home with their patients, they do not store them in office files, and earlier mammograms are retrieved from the PACS (Picture Archiving and Communication System) system and not from a file folder. Physicians have much less contact with technologists and medical assistants because images are sent to them in the form of electronic data. More importantly, soft-copy image interpretation on a high-resolution monitor always entails a learning curve, although this process is relatively painless with today's modern workstations (like the one from Image-Diagnost-International, Munich, Germany).

For patients, digital mammography does not seem very different from conventional mammography, although the "Aha!" effect from seeing images manipulated on a monitor (enlargement, inversion, annotation, etc.) is often striking. The positioning technique is usually identical, depending on the particular system being used. It is still essential to use optimum positioning and imaging technique (see p. 93). Breast compression is still necessary in digital mammography, although less pressure needs to be applied. The radiation dose to the patient may be up to 10% lower, depending on individual breast composition and image quality. The examination itself proceeds more swiftly because there is no need to develop cassettes (at least with pure digital technology, not with a storage plate system). Presumably this will shorten the waiting time between mammography and examination by a physician. Digital technology has already been approved for screening use in Germany and has been effective in streamlining examinations.

For radiology technologists and medical assistants, working in pure digital mode means a greater work load. They examine more patients per unit time than before, and their work routine is not interrupted by pausing to develop cassettes—which some view as a positive development and others as negative. They can concentrate more on positioning technique but may tire more quickly than with conventional technology, which has inherent waiting periods that provide breaks in the routine. Technologists see a constant flow of patients, but they no longer see doctors to discuss images with them. They also have less contact with office staff, since most data are accessed through PACS and worklists. These potential drawbacks are balanced by many positive changes: Much less work is devoted to the handling of mammograms (developing, filing, and transport), and workflow is improved. The general atmosphere in the department is less hectic, and digital technology eliminates costs for film, file jackets, developing chemicals and their disposal, leading to a substantial reduction in operating costs. Admittedly, this reduction does not offset the purchase price of the system, at least in the short term. For digital mammography to become widely utilized, it must become even less expensive or health insurers must be willing to cover the examination costs.

Three main types of digital equipment configuration are available:

- Storage plate system
- Digital full-field mammography
- Digital stereotactic units

#### *Storage Plate System*

Cassettes are still used in the storage plate system. Storage plates convert the x-rays to electrical impulses that are evaluated by a digital reading device. Very often the end product is a hard-copy x-ray film, as in conventional mammography. This technology is currently represented in the HR System developed and marketed by Fuji. In general, the storage plate system is well established and can provide a resolution of approximately 8.5 LP/mm, corresponding to the lower standard for conventional mammograms. This does not mean that digital mammograms are difficult to read. On the contrary, the author's experience with the full-field system from Giotto (Internazionale Medico Scientifica [IMS], Italy) has been very positive. Most of the images in this book were obtained with this system—not a storage plate system, but still with 8 LP/mm resolution.

Because the storage plate system is an "off-line" system, it is less elegant than online systems in terms of workflow and is similar to conventional mammography, at least until the film is input into the digital reader.

There are no real advantages to the storage plate system compared with conventional mammography. The images are digitally produced (which has its own pros and cons), but the output still consists often of hard-copy images or CDs, although the images are stored in the PACS archive. It is unclear why this practice is followed. Aside from complicated handling, the other parameters (CAD, PACS archiving, 3-D imaging, etc.) are all identical to full-field online digital mammography. For this reason, the storage plate system will not be described more fully in this section, as it is certain to be replaced by online systems in the near future.

### *Full-Field Online Mammography*

Full-field digital mammography is revolutionizing the practice of mammography owing to its dose advantages and improved contrast. Digital technology allows for automated computer assistance in radiographic image analysis (Helvie et al. 2004) as well as teleradiography and more. New flat-panel x-ray detectors offer extremely high quantum utilization and high-resolution capability. This results in a lower radiation dose with better and more permanent image quality. Both direct and indirect conversion detectors are available. The various techniques will not be explored here, as they have been described extremely well by Smith (2003) and other authors.

The advantage of digital mammography over film-screen imaging is the **linear relationship** that exists between the receiver-level dose and signal intensity over a very **large dose range**. According to Schultz-Wendtland (2003), *conventional film-screen systems* have linear contrast characteristics over a very narrow dose range, making them less sensitive in the detection of subtle microcalcifications in radiodense breasts. Like exposure errors and film processing errors, this leads to a reduction in sensitivity—problems that do not exist in *digital mammography.* While providing the same detail definition and diagnostic accuracy as film-screen systems, some (but not all!) digital mammographic systems can reduce the radiation dose to the patient by up to 20%. The argument that conventional mammography can provide higher spatial resolution (> 15 LP/mm) than digital technology, resulting in better diagnostic accuracy, is no longer valid since digital systems can now achieve spatial resolutions as high as 12.5 LP/mm. The number of line pairs is no longer a key parameter in digital technology, especially regarding the ability to detect microcalcifications. In comparing the resolution of conventional versus digital mammography, it is important to consider the **modulation transfer function** of each system. The slope of the modulation transfer function of both conventional and digital imaging systems, and hence their image quality, is determined by a factor called **detective quantum efficiency** (DQE). Modern digital mammographic systems have a much higher DQE (45–65) and thus a better signal-to-noise ratio than conventional mammographic systems, and this greatly affects their ability to detect preinvasive cancers by the presence of microcalcifications.

Other capabilities of digital mammography without special views include postprocessing options such as *image enlargement, screen shots* (captured regions of interest), *CAD, teleradiography, digital subtraction* after intravenous contrast administration, and *tomosynthesis.*

Two types of digital detector are used in mammography: indirect conversion detectors, which are generally **silicon-based**, and direct conversion detectors, which are **selenium-based**.

**Indirect conversion** is similar to a film–screen system. A scintillator absorbs x-rays and converts them to visible light, which is picked up by photodetectors. This conversion process degrades resolution, resulting in poor quantum utilization by the thin scintillators. **Direct conversion digital detectors** convert x-rays to electrical signals in one step. This system employs amorphous selenium, an ideal material for mammographic detectors since it transforms 100% of incident x-ray energy into electrical signals and thus ensures very high spatial resolution, low noise, and low radiation dose in a relatively trouble-free process. Pixel size and various other factors also play a role but will not be addressed here.

The most widely used indirect conversion system based on *amorphous silicon* detectors is the General Electric Senograph 2000 D, which has a resolution of 6 LP/mm, a 100 µm pixel size, and a field size of 19 cm × 23 cm. One advantage of this system is that it is used all over the world, even in screening programs. At our center we use the selenium-based digital mammographic system from Giotto (IMS, Italy) combined with workstations from Image Diagnost International (Munich, Germany) as well as Mini-PACS from General Electric (GE) (USA). The Mini-PACS was recently replaced by a Tele-PACS system, in which images from various digital users are stored centrally and can be accessed as needed. The IMS Giotto detector has a 24 cm × 30 cm image format.

**Regardless of which company and which mammographic system is used, all manufacturers should round off the edges and corners of the imaging table (detector) to make the examination more comfortable for the women. The edges on the patient's side of the table tend to press into the axilla when the patient is correctly positioned and are the greatest source of pain.**

With its generally lower radiation dose and somewhat higher rates of breast cancer detection, digital full-field mammography represents a major advance in breast care. It will become more widely utilized in the coming years, although its practical implementation is hampered at present by high costs. Insurers as of the time of writing (2009) ought to reimburse digital mammography in nearly the same way as traditional film–screen mammography.

### Model of a Fully Digital Breast Diagnostic Service

*O. Wild*

Digital technology is opening up new ways to improve efficiency in mammographic imaging, especially in cases where all image data, including previous mammograms, are available in digital form. Thus, a fully digital system goes beyond digital mammography itself to include the secondary digitization of previous mammograms and the maximum availability of relevant image data in digital form (clinical photos, sonograms, MR images, digital stereotaxy, cytohistologic findings). The image data are stored internally or externally in a PACS and are organized in patient folders so that they can be accessed and reviewed at any time.

The basic components of a fully digital breast imaging service are shown in **Fig. 5.17**.

This is illustrated by the fully digital mammographic service of the *Breast Imaging Department of the Interdisciplinary Breast Center in Esslingen* (Germany). The heart of the facility, which opened in March, 2004, is the Giotto Image MD digital full-field mammography system manufactured by IMS (**Fig. 5.18**). This system employs an amorphous selenium-based detector that directly converts x-rays to digital image signals. The system conforms to all new German industry standards. The images are sent via data links to review consoles (supplied by Image Diagnost International, Munich). If necessary, hard-copy mammograms can be created with a Kodak digital printer, which requires no chemicals.

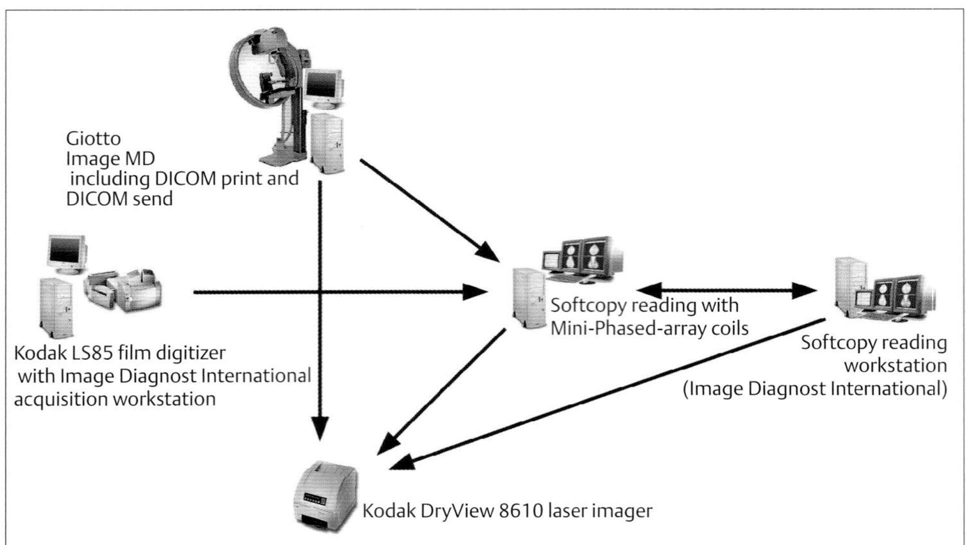


**Fig. 5.17 Basic components of a fully digital breast imaging service** with a full-field digital mammographic unit (upper left), digitizing station (center left), two review workstations (right), an archiving system (center), and a laser imager (below).

Existing imaging modalities (MRI, ultrasound, digital stereotactic core-needle biopsy, etc.) have been integrated into the system so that all relevant images can be accessed at physician workstations for review (**Fig. 5.19**).

Digital technology is changing the way mammographic units work. Previous conventional mammograms are digitized when the patient arrives and are returned to her, if she has brought them along, or they can be returned to office files. As soon as the mammographic examination is completed, the images are instantly available at workstations for immediate physician review. The mammographic unit is again ready for use in approximately 20 seconds, during which time the patient can be repositioned for the next view.

High-resolution monitors and software support for diagnostic workflow make it easier to conduct a complete diagnostic assessment (**Fig. 5.20**). The breast images can be digitally manipulated by adjusting the contrast and brightness (window leveling) to highlight different structures. The images can be enlarged, reduced, or even inverted, and if necessary stored as individual "screen shots." These techniques, not available with conventional mammography, are a valuable aid to visual image interpretation and follow-up. The mammograms are automatically organized and displayed in the proper order, and selected sequences can be accessed and run at the touch of a button. As a result, any abnormalities in the breast can be quickly located and displayed, leaving more time for interviewing the patient and conducting a physical and ultrasound examination. In addition, more than one physician can access the images at the same time, making it easy to consult with colleagues by phone and request second readings.

Digitization can have a major impact on diagnostic workflow, especially in the long term. All relevant image data can be accessed within seconds. Digital technology eliminates the need to hunt for earlier mammograms. This frees office assistants from having to make tedious searches and carry x-ray images back and forth, enabling them to spend more time tending to patients' needs.

Another theoretical advantage of digital mammography is a reduction in radiation dose, especially when selenium detectors are used. Past a certain point, however, the dose reduction may cause degradation of image quality due to increased image noise. This can be a significant problem in cases where the radiologist must locate and identify very fine calcifications to detect or exclude preinvasive disease. *The Esslingen Breast Imaging Center* in Germany has followed a different practice for some years now: apart from the initial mammograms, in which two views are taken of each breast, all follow-up examinations consist of single-view mammograms for each breast whenever possible. This reduces the radiation dose by 50%.

**Fig. 5.18 Giotto Image MD digital mammography system** (Internazionale Medico Scientifica [IMS], Bologna, Italy). Italian design with a circular gantry that contains the rotating x-ray tube. The gantry can be tilted to conform to individual patient anatomy. It can also be turned horizontally, converting to a digital stereotactic biopsy unit that is used with a special height-adjustable biopsy table (see **Figs. 5.22**, p. 104; **5.107**, p. 233).

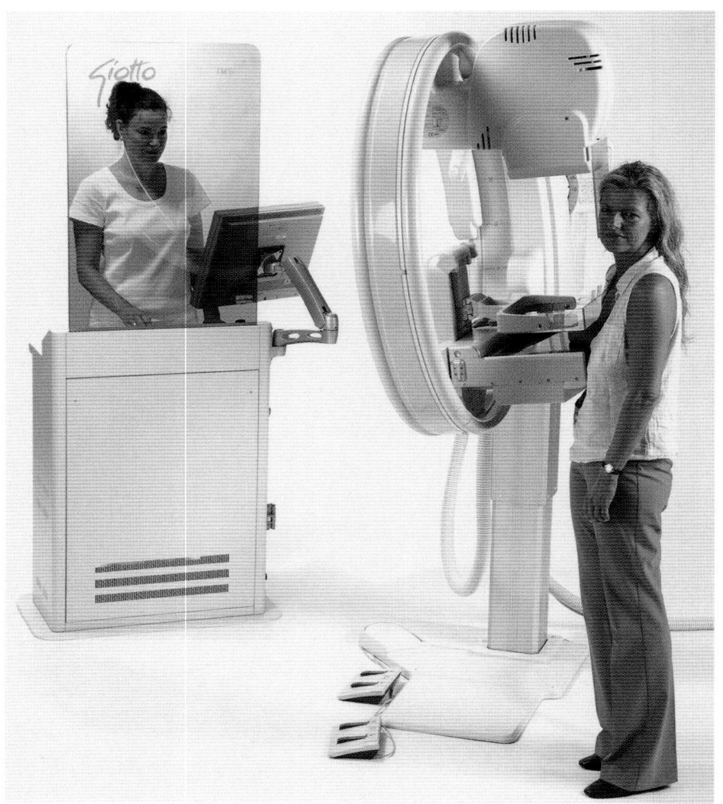

**Fig. 5.19 Integration of mammography, ultrasound, digital stereotactic fine-needle or vacuum biopsy, magnetic resonance imaging, and cytology.**

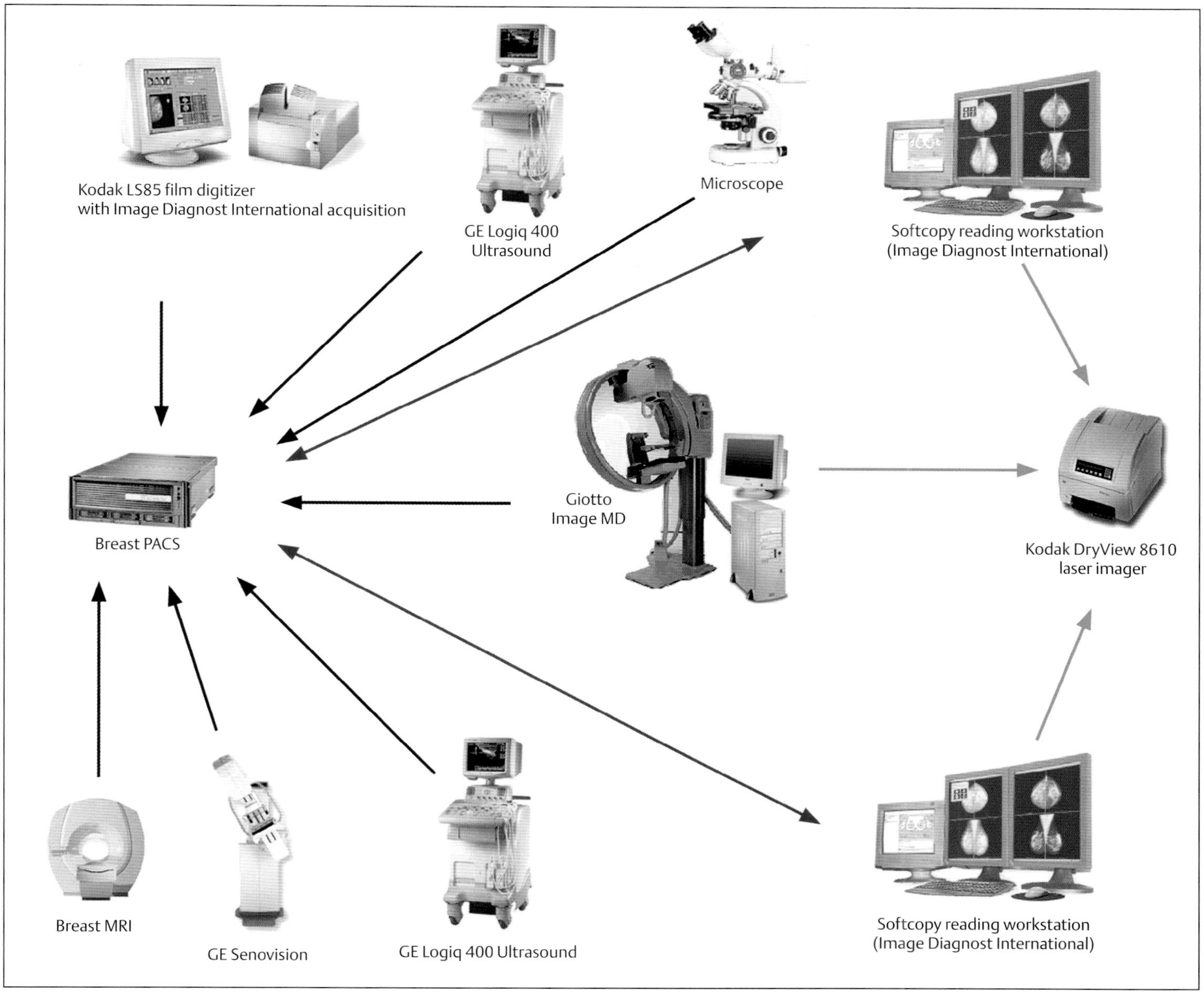

Kodak LS85 film digitizer
with Image Diagnost International acquisition
GE Logiq 400
Ultrasound
Microscope
Softcopy reading workstation
(Image Diagnost International)
Breast PACS
Giotto
Image MD
Kodak DryView 8610
laser imager
Breast MRI
GE Senovision
GE Logiq 400 Ultrasound
Softcopy reading workstation
(Image Diagnost International)

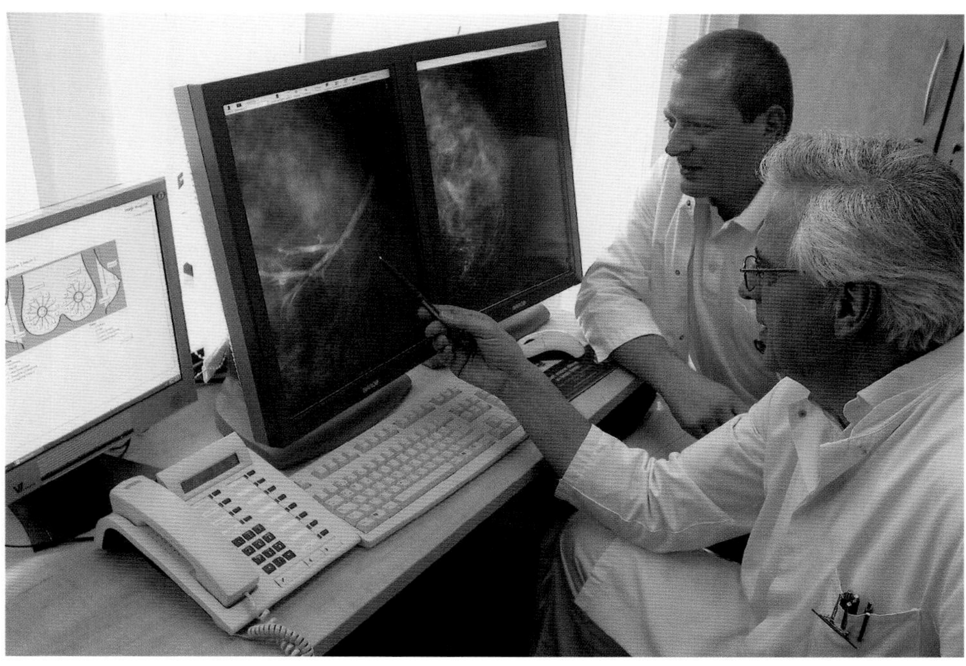

**Fig. 5.20 High-resolution monitors** with optical aids, magnification options, and computer-assisted workflow improve diagnostic capabilities and facilitate double reading. At the Image Diagnost International workstation, even digital clinical photographs (e.g., skin and nipple changes) can easily be placed in the patient's digital record.

Another advantage of digital technology is that the image data can be shared with other computers via networks. Different physicians can join to form specialty-based networks that facilitate information sharing. There are still technical and legal hurdles to overcome, as different digital systems may have trouble "reading" one another, and standard data security measures can make it extremely difficult for different doctors and hospitals to communicate with one another.

> **!** **Digital technology cannot replace personal care by doctors and their assistants. The goal of digital technology is to help optimize treatment protocols, facilitate diagnosis, and streamline hectic work schedules. Rapid data flow in a fully digital mammographic facility can support this process.**

**Fig. 5.21** **Senovision.**

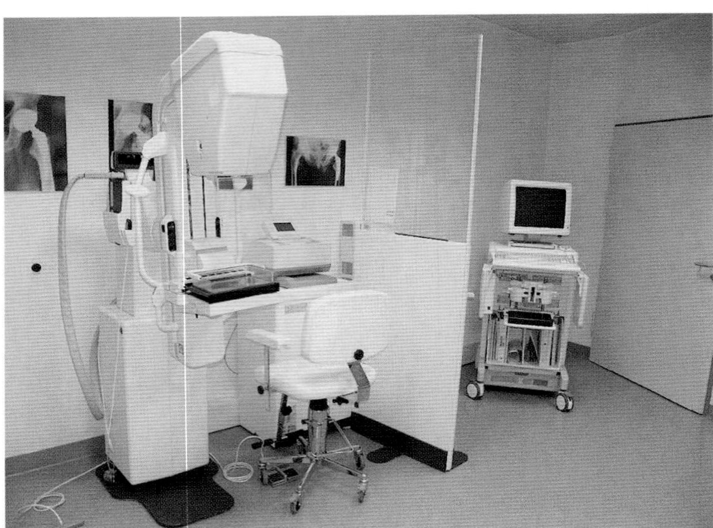

*Digital Stereotactic Biopsy Systems*

Digital stereotactic biopsy technology has already become a routine tool in many hospital and office settings around the world. It has largely replaced nondigital stereotaxy.

Digital biopsy systems permit the rapid performance of FNA, CNB, and VB (see p. 230) with relatively good visualization of fine details. Preoperative wire localization can also be carried out accurately and efficiently with digital stereotaxy.

Below we shall describe the operation of a partially digital system as illustrated by the GE Senovision. This system adds a component to the conventional mammographic unit, enabling the examiner to perform localizations and biopsies within a limited field of 6 × 8 cm (**Fig. 5.21**). Because the mammographic unit can also be used for routine imaging, the utilization level and costs are more favorable than with a dedicated stereotactic unit like the Fischer table. The unit can serve equally well for FNA, CNB, and VB with a mammotome. A similar but more elegant concept is embodied in the IMS Giotto system. The gantry is tilted 90°, and a table is wheeled over the tube and stereotactic unit to create a prone stereotactic system providing a degree of precision comparable to that of a traditional biopsy table (see **Fig. 5.22**; **Fig. 5.107 g**, p. 233). We perform most digital interventions not in the patient-prone but the supine position, as shown in **Fig. 5.22 d**. This position is more comfortable for the patient, poses no problem with the Giotto equipment, and

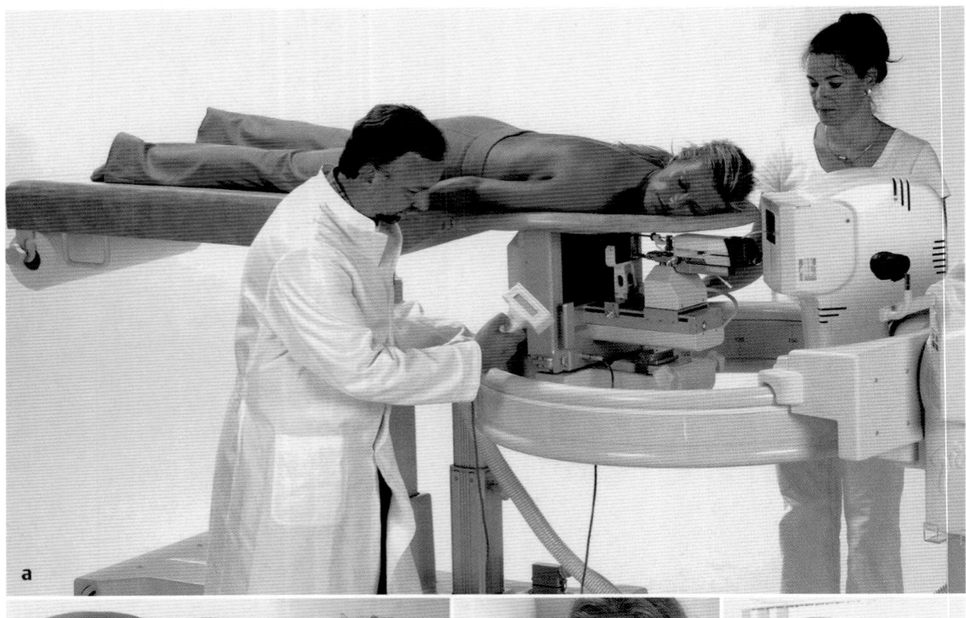

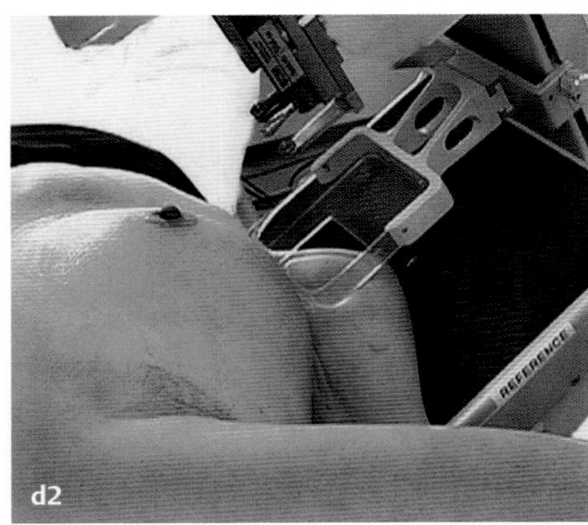

**Fig. 5.22** **Digital mammograpgy Giotto (IMS Italy).**
**a** *Full-field digital mammography unit with patient table.*
**b** *Mammotome biopsy in the prone position.* The biopsy apparatus is mounted below the table.
**c** *Mammotome biopsy in the sitting position*, oblique projection.
**d 1, 2** *Core-needle biopsy (CNB)* in the supine position with angled x-ray tube. This position is very comfortable for the patient, and even lesions deep to the nipple or near the chest wall can be investigated by CNB or VB.

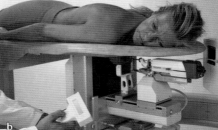

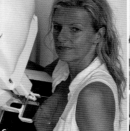

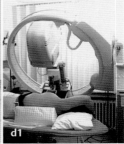

has advantages with lesions near the chest wall and behind the nipple.

The advantage of stereotaxy is that the target lesion can be localized in three planes. The author and his colleagues have documented an approximately 90% rate of agreement between the results of 270 digital stereotactic CNBs and histologic findings (Weining-Klemm 2004; see p. 251).

Stereotaxy with the Senovision system or the Giotto system can be applied to all mammographic findings, especially clustered and suspicious microcalcifications. It can be performed in the sitting or prone position using a standard adjustable-height table (**Fig. 5.22**). We use CNB and occasionally FNA for diagnostic interventions in the breast, and we prefer VB for the removal of benign lesions (fibroadenoma, papilloma) and occasional small foci of FEA and ADH (see p. 35). Digital stereotactic FNA is reserved for unfavorable cases in which the lesion is subcutaneous or otherwise located outside the coordinates that are accessible to CNB.

The digital biopsy systems from Giotto and other manufacturers can be linked to a picture archiving and communication system (PACS). With Senovision, however, the images cannot be retrieved from the PACS and returned to the workstation for subsequent review. It is likely that future technical refinements in the system will address this problem.

With the Senovision digital spot system, the patient is placed in a sitting position for VB. This is accomplished with a simple add-on device (**Fig. 5.23**).

The author and his colleagues investigate all lesions by CNB. Malignant lesions are excised, benign lesions are left alone, and semimalignant lesions (e.g., small foci of ADH) are removed from the breast by VB. Fibroadenomas and papillomas are also removed by VB, but papilloma removals are preceded by ductographic imaging with patent blue dye injection (see **Figs. 5.119 a, e**, p. 252).

The digital biopsy systems eliminate the need for many operations and contribute significantly to cost containment. This has been demonstrated in a model project sponsored by the AOK health insurance group of the German state of Baden-Württemberg and the Association of Statutory Health Insurance Physicians (KV) of that state. Interventional procedures eliminated the need for 25% of the operations recommended by radiologists and gynecologists and led to a 27% cost reduction for in-hospital treatments. The implantation of a metal coil or clip at the biopsy site following *every* CNB or VB has also been omitted to save costs. Most biopsy sites are easy to locate mammographically, and the costs for localization coils are disproportionately high. But note that a clip or coil is a “must” for *very small* (T1a) and any local advanced breast cancer with neoadjuvant (primary) chemotherapy because after tumor-reduction the surgeon may not be able to determine the primary tumor's location.

Additionally, mammography is not performed after CNB or VB as recommended in the European Guidelines unless a discrepancy is found between mammograms and histologic findings. The biopsied calcifications should, however, be visualized in a specimen radiograph of the tissue core and assessed by the pathologist. Otherwise the biopsy is repeated (see p. 230). If the biopsied calcifications are benign, the remaining calcifications are left alone; if they are malignant, the lesion should be excised. To date, two tumors have been missed in approximately 1500 biopsies, but they were subsequently detected at 6-month follow-up.

**Fig. 5.23 Senovision. Vacuum biopsy in the sitting position.**

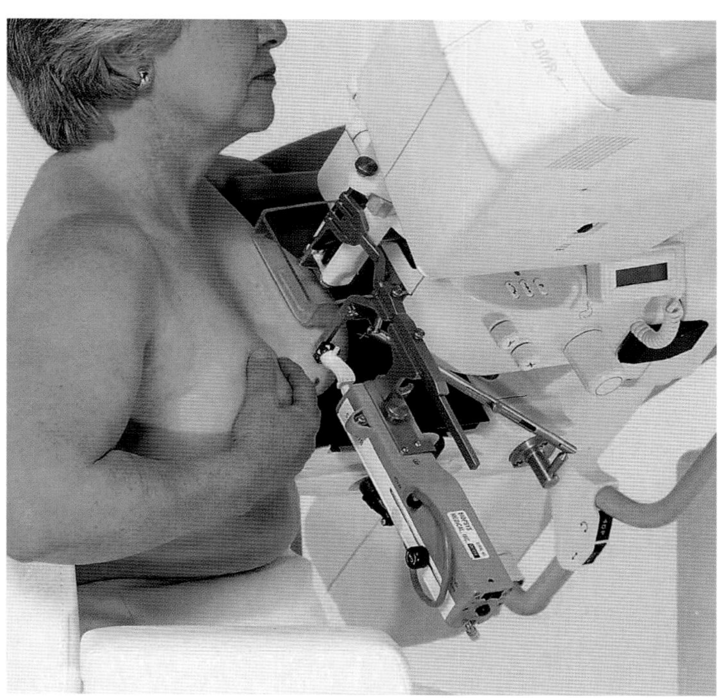

### Future Trends

#### *Single-View Mammography plus Ultrasound versus Two-View Mammography*

The dissertation of Weining (2004) analyzed the results of single-view and two-view mammography, with and without supplementary ultrasound (ACR 2–4). The study was based on a retrospective analysis of the results in 3743 women examined by two-view mammography plus ultrasound at the Esslingen Breast Center between 1993 and 2003. All patients were examined by the same physician (the author of this book).

A total of 334 women had a histologically confirmed malignancy: 267 with ductal carcinoma, 34 with lobular carcinoma, 3 with tubular carcinoma, 5 with ductolobular carcinoma, 2 with inflammatory carcinoma, 1 with adenocarcinoma, 1 with apocrine carcinoma, 1 with cystosarcoma phylloides, 1 with squamous cell carcinoma, 15 with DCIS, and 5 with LCIS. Nine of the 334 women underwent surgery for presumed benign disease (5 had fibrocystic change, 3 had fibroadenoma, 1 had ductal hyperplasia).

The women were classified into five age groups (25–39, 40–49, 50–59, 60–69, and 70 years or older). The positive predictive value (PPV) and negative predictive value (NPV) were determined along with sensitivity, specificity, false-negative rates, and false-positive rates for the following examinations: single-view mammography (SV), two-view mammography (TV), ultrasound (US), single-view mammography plus ultrasound (SVU), and a combination of palpation (P), single-view mammography and ultrasound (PSVU).

The analysis of single-view mammography was based on oblique views taken from available two-view mammograms. Also, some patients were evaluated by additional modalities such as MRI, CT, and PET, including biopsies, in order to document a possible improvement in diagnostic accuracy.

The results were as follows. The oblique view was generally superior to the craniocaudal view. A malignant process was detected in 83% of cases on oblique mammograms compared with 81% on craniocaudal mammograms. There were 8 cases in which a definitive diagnosis could be made from the oblique view, versus 3 cases using the craniocaudal view. Both planes were diagnostically equivalent in all other respects. On average, this applied equally to all five age groups. This means that 331 women received a craniocaudal mammogram, with the attendant increase in radiation exposure, with no appreciable diagnostic gain.

> **!** **No significant difference was found between single-view mammography and two-view mammography with regard to sensitivity and specificity.**

**Ultrasound** was found to be very effective in the detection of breast cancer. It had a sensitivity of 91%, surpassing that of two-view mammography by 8% Expressed in numbers of patients, ultrasound detected 304 malignancies in 334 patients (91%) while two-view mammography without ultrasound detected 227 malignancies (83%). Thus, 27 more malignancies were detected by ultrasound alone than by two-view mammography. The false-negative rate, or the percentage of malignancies missed by each modality, was 16% with two-view mammography and 9% with ultrasound.

A major strength of ultrasound was its ability to detect noncalcifying ductal carcinomas and especially lobular carcinomas. This was a particular advantage in radiographically dense breasts. Ultrasound had an 8% sensitivity advantage in the detection of ductal breast carcinoma and a 9% advantage in the detection of lobular carcinoma.

Ultrasound is not superior to mammography in all situations. Two-view mammography was more sensitive than ultrasound in the detection of DCIS, LCIS, and tubular carcinoma. With a sensitivity of 93% for DCIS and 100% for LCIS, all mammographic projections were found to be particularly useful in the detection of high-risk lesions with *microcalcifications*. Ultrasound ranked far behind mammography with a 57% sensitivity for DCIS and 60% for LCIS (**Table 5.9**).

The **combination of ultrasound and single-view mammography** yielded a high sensitivity of 97% for all age groups, especially women 25–39 years of age. This is 13% higher than the sensitivity of two-view mammography (84%) without ultrasound. Expressed in numbers of patients, this means that ultrasound missed the tumor in only 10 of 334 breast cancer patients, while two-view mammography missed it in 53.

**Physical examination** consisting of inspection and palpation was the weak link in the diagnostic chain, with a sensitivity of only 67% and a specificity of 22%. Sensitivity rose to 98% when physical examination was combined with **single-view mammography** and **ultrasound**. In five women (1.5%), even the combination of all three modalities (PSVU) failed to detect a tumor. In reality there were only four false-negatives because one patient's tumor was detected by craniocaudal mammography. Thus, the other four patients (1.2%) had interval cancers that became palpable several months after negative physical examination + mammography + ultrasound. Tumors may still be missed even in a very thorough examination using several modalities. The lowest rate of 1.5% was achieved with *one* examiner using single-view mammograms plus ultrasound and physical examination at 1- to 1.5-year intervals. The highest rate of missed tumors was 30–40% in mammographic-only screening with a number of experienced examiners interpreting two-view mammograms obtained at 2-year intervals without ultrasound. This high figure occurred only in women 50–69 years of age.

MRI was performed a total of 177 times in the 334 breast cancer patients. With a sensitivity of 89%, MRI was better than two-view mammography (84%) but did not match the sensitivity of breast ultrasound (91%). MRI had a specificity of 40% in patients with normal findings or benign lesions. While better than physical examination (22%), MRI was inferior to the other imaging modalities in its specificity. MRI rarely detected a carcinoma that was clinically, mammographically or sonographically occult, although it did add considerable information on multifocality or the presence of a second tumor in the opposite breast (see p. 201 and **Figs. 5.79g**, p. 184; **5.124b**, p. 255; **5.36e**, p. 357).

**Table 5.9 Comparison of mammography and ultrasound for evaluating various breast morphologies and tumor types** (from Weining 2004)

| General composition of the breast parenchyma | Mammography | Ultrasound |
|---|---|---|
| Fatty breast | + | Hypoechoic tumors: –<br>Hyperechoic tumors: + |
| Copious glandular and connective tissue | – | Hypoechoic tumors (most): +<br>Hypoechoic tumors (some early carcinomas): – |
| Presence of microcalcifications | + | – |
| **Specific tumor types** | | |
| LCIS | Usually nonspecific | Usually not detectable |
| DCIS | Clearly detectable in most cases (approximately 80% have microcalcifications) | Frequently nonspecific or undetectable |
| Ductal breast carcinoma | Clearly detectable in most cases. Diffuse forms without microcalcifications are difficult to detect. | Particularly useful adjunct in breasts difficult to evaluate by mammography |
| Lobular breast carcinoma | Often detected late due to diffuse growth and absence of microcalcifications | Excellent detectability, especially with an indeterminate palpable mass that is mammographically occult |

+ = good analysis, – = poor analysis

**Fig. 5.24 Sensitivity of various diagnostic modalities.** SVMG = single-view mammography, P = palpation, USMG = ultrasound plus mammography, TVMG = two-view mammography.

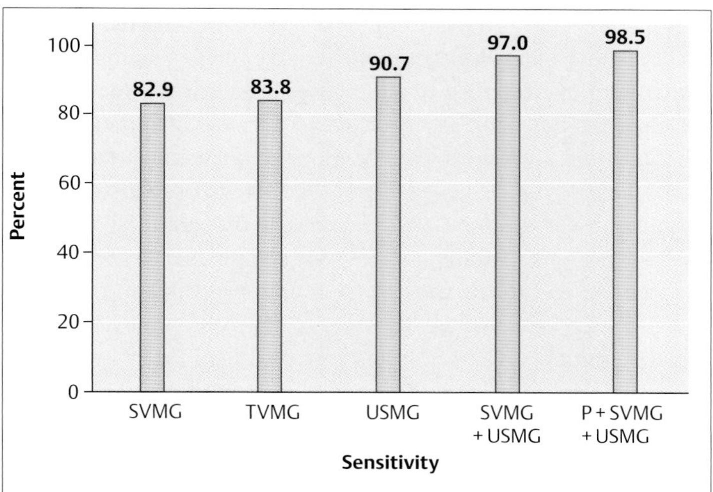


**Fig. 5.25 Comparison of the false-negative rates of various diagnostic modalities.** SVMG = single-view mammography, P = palpation, USMG = ultrasound plus mammography, TVMG = two-view mammography.

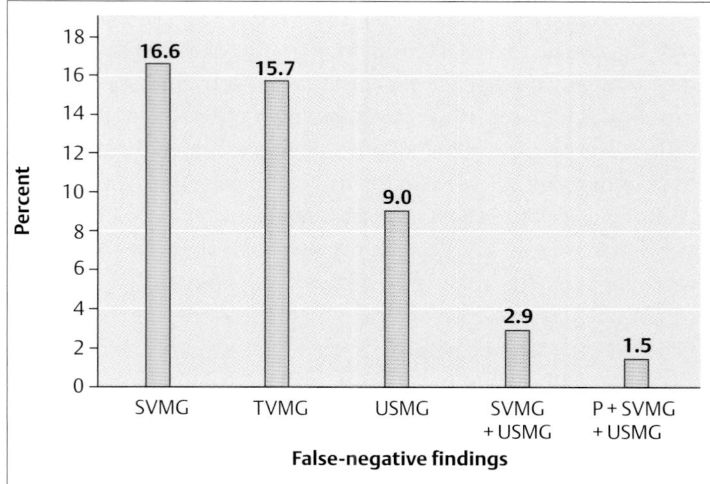


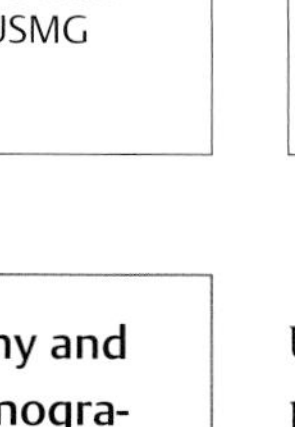

**Overall, the combination of single-view mammography and ultrasound was definitely superior to two-view mammography alone. This applied to all age groups and all malignant diagnoses (two-view mammograms plus ultrasound would have yielded only marginally better results!).**

The results are summarized in **Figs. 5.24** and **5.25**.

In some cases the combined use of single-view mammography and ultrasound provided up to 100% sensitivity for various diagnoses. An example is **lobular carcinoma**, which is generally considered a difficult diagnosis. Physical examination was particularly helpful for detecting tumors in women over 50 years of age. A palpable breast mass in this age group combined with a normal single-view mammogram and normal sonograms indicated absence of disease or a benign diagnosis with a reasonably high degree of confidence. This combination of modalities has significant benefits for patients, which include an almost 50% reduction in radiation dose and a single breast compression. Lower examination costs are a benefit for payors. There is a negative impact on the examining physician's budget, as the addition of breast ultrasound approximately doubles the total examination time compared with two-view mammography alone. Thus, reimbursement rates will have to be modified to ensure that women gain maximum benefit from this combination of modalities.

Two-view mammograms may well become obsolete in the next few years, due largely to economic constraints. For the sake of the insured, it is incumbent upon health insurers to define reasonable physician reimbursement rates that are commensurate with the time requirements and technical costs of multimodal examinations.

Single-view mammography and ultrasound could be supplemented by physical examination in screening situations without having to alter the current reimbursement system. The basic problem is time, since breast ultrasound is more time-consuming than mammography, and the examination of several million women would push physicians' capacities to their limits. But why not train radiology technologists and physician assistants for these extra tasks (inspection, palpation, ultrasound)? The usual practice in the United States is for physicians to read the images that have been produced by technologists according to a standard protocol (Delorme 2004). While this is not an optimum solution, it is one approach. Tonita et al. (1999) described the integration of radiologic technologists into breast cancer screening. Even with second readings and third opinions, the technologist review was still responsible for detecting a significant number of cancers (9) missed by the initial radiologist. This same approach could be used to integrate physical examination and breast ultrasound into a screening program at minimal cost. An experienced on-side radiologist would be needed only for the interpretation of an indeterminate or suspicious sonogram or to render a second or third opinion. We physicians had to learn these examinations as well, and the technologist approach would definitely be worth a try.

### *History of Mammography and Future Outlook*

The development of mammography was *the* diagnostic breakthrough of the twentieth century, for it enabled breast cancer to be detected at an early, curable stage. The evolution of mammography was accompanied by an improvement in survival rates not attainable by any other diagnostic or therapeutic method. Mammographic screening programs in Scandinavia, Holland, the United Kingdom, and the United States have improved 10-year survival rates by 15–40%, aided in part by the development of improved treatment protocols.

In 1913, the Berlin surgeon Salomon became the first physician to examine complete mastectomy specimens by x-ray. He also examined 3000 histologic specimens to analyze the growth and spread of breast cancer and study its behavior in relation to normal breast tissue. He concluded from his studies that as much skin as possible should be removed along with the cancerous breast (Salomon 1913). Salomon's specimen studies enabled him to identify the radiographic hallmarks of breast cancer that are still used in mammographic interpretation (microcalcifications, spiculated densities, architectural distortion, etc.). By better understanding tumor spread, he hoped to find optimum surgical incisions for mastectomy that would include as much skin as possible in radical excisions.

Kleinschmidt in Germany was the first to perform mammography in a patient in 1927. He published his report in a textbook by Zweifelt and Payr (1927), *Clinical Aspects of Malignant Tumors* (in German).

The pathologist Ingleby and the radiologist Gershon-Cohen wrote the classic textbook on mammography that has remained a model for many textbooks over the years (Ingleby and Gershon-Cohen 1960). Starting in 1951, the Frenchman Charles Gros established the scientific principles for introducing a molybdenum anode into mammography. Gros was the driving force behind the European Senology Society, which united all specialties involved in the diagnosis and treatment of breast diseases, and he even coined the term "senology" from the French *le sein*, meaning breast. The first German-language textbook of mammography, by Buttenberg and Werner in 1962, was heavily influenced by Gershon-Cohen.

Doctors Höffken and Lanyi of Cologne helped mammography to become a routine clinical examination and screening method in Germany. Collaborating with the gynecologist Kaufmann and the pathologist Hamperl in 1959, they described the possibility of diagnosing breast cancer while it was still in the clinically occult stage of preinvasive carcinoma in situ. With their *Röntgen Examination of the Breast, Höffken and Lanyi* (1973) created a standard textbook of mammography that has been updated by Lanyi in two subsequent monographs (Lanyi 1986, 2003). The Houston radiologist Egan (1969) popularized the technique of mammography in the United States.

Seifert (1975) was a prodigious German researcher who wrote another classic textbook during the "formative years" of mammography titled *The Mammogram and its Interpretation*.

Höffken (Cologne) and Frischbier (Hamburg) worked with Fournier (Heidelberg), Barth (Esslingen), and private practitioners in Braunschweig and Aurich from 1989 to 1993 to conduct the **first German study of mammography** (Robra et al. 1993), where our institute was also involved. This study did not prompt the immediate implementation of mammography as a general screening test, for it revealed significant qualitative problems, especially relating to mammographic equipment, that were addressed and resolved over the next 10 years. Even so, screening was not introduced in Germany in the late 1990s. There was too much resistance from physicians to a model like that in Sweden and Holland, and this fostered an unwillingness among payors to reimburse screening mammograms. On the other hand, "opportunistic" screening mammography without quality control standards has been practiced for decades and has been quietly tolerated.

Breast cancer is the fifth leading cause of death among women, ranking just below cardiovascular diseases. This is one reason why mammography has become the single most common radiographic service. In 1990, for example, a total of 40% of all radiographic services provided by radiologists in private practice were mammograms. Since then, this percentage has grown smaller for a variety of reasons. Because opportunistic screening mammography is no longer accepted by payors, the numbers of mammograms performed by office radiologists have fallen sharply since the year 2000. Mammography in hospital settings has also declined over the past 20 years due to the sharp division between the outpatient and in-patient sectors and the renewed authority of department heads, with a resulting surge of poorly trained young colleagues going into office practice. They are unfamiliar with optimum mammographic techniques and the fine points of image interpretation.

There is no question that mammography has revolutionized early cancer detection and, combined with improved treatment regimens, has been a tremendous blessing for women whose breast cancers were diagnosed at a curable stage. **But where do we go from here?** Again and again, we hear reports of tumors appearing suddenly just a few weeks or months after a negative screening examination. More than a few malpractice suits have resulted from the delayed detection of breast cancer despite regular mammograms. At the same time, suspicious mammograms prompt many unnecessary breast biopsies that yield negative results and may cause pain or disfigurement. The dean of German senology, Walter Höffken, one remarked that "most women, on hearing the news that their biopsy was benign, will throw their arms around the surgeon out of joy and gratitude. Very few will fly into a rage because they had unnecessary surgery."

The incidence of missed cancers and true interval cancers is alarmingly high (20–50%) in national and regional screening programs throughout the world. These undetected cancers undercut the rationale for having regular screening examinations: the reduction of cancer mortality in clinically healthy women. Some experts even question the inherent value of screening, arguing that it does not statistically benefit the women who are screened (Baines 2000; Sjönell and Stähle 1999). The intense international promotional efforts that have been made in recent decades to encourage women to have regular screening mammograms should now be followed by a more sober phase in which the limits of mammography are seriously discussed.

Between 2000 and 2005, the number of mammographic examinations in the United States declined by 4% in women over 40 years of age and by 7% in women 50–64 years of age (Wolf et al. 2009).

The author of this book has worked intensively in the diagnosis of breast diseases since 1970 and is currently one of the most senior active "mammographers" of his generation. From the outset he has pursued the scientific aspects of mammography, conducted rigorous pathoanatomic studies, and published numerous papers and monographs on this procedure. Because of his experience with and great love for mammography, he continues to favor it as the method of choice for cancer screening and for investigating all palpable and visible changes in the breast. As a result, the author is deeply impressed in cases where ultrasound clearly demonstrates a malignant lesion that was completely invisible on radiographs despite optimum mammographic technique. It has been known for years that even visible and palpable breast malignancies are missed by mammography at a rate of approximately 6–10%. Ultrasound and/or magnetic resonance imaging of clinically healthy breasts or breasts with known carcinoma will often demonstrate focal lesions that are mammographically occult despite very close scrutiny of the image (see **Fig. 5.143**). It is also fascinating to see how ultrasound can provide highly detailed anatomic images of radiographically dense breasts. Many a case of "diffuse fibrosis" is identified as the proliferation of terminal duct lobular units (TDLUs, see **Fig. 5.70**) or the presence of numerous ectatic ducts with clinically occult intraductal papillomas, even though an optimum mammogram shows no discrete abnormalities and the location of the lesion is known (see **Fig. 5.74**).

**Tip**

**Often it is only by applying all diagnostic modalities—especially mammography and ultrasound—that a correct diagnosis can be made.**

For approximately 8 years the author of this book, for the reasons stated above, has adopted a policy of obtaining two mammographic views (craniocaudal and oblique) only during the initial examination of patients over age 40 years, and then limiting follow-up examinations to a single view. The specific view depends on the plane in which the breast parenchyma is most clearly and completely depicted. This is the oblique view in most cases. A second projection is obtained only if the oblique view shows a significant change (e.g., microcalcifications or suspicious densities). If breast density is ACR 2 or higher, high-resolution ultrasound is always added to the examination (formerly 7.5 MHz, currently 11–13 MHz). We see to it that the same physician inspects and palpates the breast, analyzes the mammogram, and performs the ultrasound scan. When this protocol is followed, the rate of interval cancers is extremely low (1.5%) compared with the rate generally reported for screening examinations (20–50%) (see single-view mammography on pp. 14, 106).

We use primary two-view mammography (also known as "curative" mammography) in patients with a palpable breast abnormality or to investigate atypical skin or nipple retraction or abnormal discharge. But regardless of whether single-view or two-view mammograms are obtained, ultrasound is always added in patients whose breast density is ACR 2 or higher.

The **future development of mammography** will no longer focus on positioning techniques and issues of differential diagnosis, which were of primary concern during the twentieth century. Results and facts are extremely well documented in numerous publications (e.g., Duda and Schultz-Wendtland 2004; Heywang-Köbrunner 2003; Lanyi 2003; and many more). Future developments will center on digital technology and optimized screening for calcifications aided by CAD systems, for example (see p. 100). Transfer and archiving problems are currently being resolved in large-scale screening programs, and teleradiographic image transfers to specialty offices and PACS units will become practical in the near future, making it possible to obtain double readings and second opinions at least in patients with BIRADS 3–5 lesions. Optimization and documentation in the setting of *disease management programs, screening*, and interactions with *certificated breast centers* will also play an important role. Not least the optimization of the technique of *tomosynthesis* is important today and will play a great role in the future. This technique means *more* mammography instead less and requires *greater* x-ray-dose instead of smaller (the same dose as one two-view-mammography (Andersson et al 2008)). On the other hand, tomosynthesis is perhaps valuable when the single-view-mammogram shows atypical changes and the technical assistant can carry out tomosynthesis immediately in the screening situation. With this technique and ultrasound (and/or MRI in younger women), the screening results should be excellent. We will see!

#### Conclusions

- **Two-view mammography** is recommended in patients with clinical, sonographic and MRI **abnormalities**. Single-view mammography for all routine controls.
- **Two-view mammography** should be the initial examination for breast cancer **screening** in women 40 years of age or older. Follow-ups should consist of single-view mammograms every 1.5 years
- **Single-view mammography should** be started at age 30 or earlier for **at-risk patients** (5 years before the youngest relation became ill). Single-view mammographic follow-ups should generally be started at age 35 and scheduled at 1.5-year intervals. They should be done yearly in high-risk patients.
- In patients whose breast density is ACR 3 or higher, mammography must be **supplemented by high-resolution ultrasound scans** (preferably an 11–13 MHz transducer).
- **In risk and high-risk adolescent patients, MRI** should be initiated by 25 years of age and repeated every 1–2 years between mammographic examinations.

Screening mammography without a physical examination and without ultrasound, as currently practiced in most screening programs, will probably be modified within 5–10 years because it is too costly, too ineffectual, and too stressful for patients. The current introduction of screening in Europe (EU) and developed countries is definitely a step in the right direction, but the road ahead is rocky and implementation is proceeding at a snail's pace. The Federal Collective Agreement that has been negotiated for example by German doctors and health insurers is a comprehensive but very precise instrument that defines screening modalities. The Agreement is very well conceived and interprets screening not as a fixed protocol but as a process that is subject to further development.

### Double Reading

Double reading of mammograms is effective. Double reading requires a complex logistical setup whose fee structures and technical details have yet to be elaborated and which is not currently supported by many gynecologists and radiologists who perform mammography. Some independent-minded physicians would rather not "show their hand to another player".

Some radiologists in private practice had a similar reaction to the **Model Project on Quality Assurance in Breast Diagnosis and Treatment** conducted by the AOK Regional Federation and Physicians' Association of the German state of Baden-Württemberg. This project ran from 2000 to 2004 and was subsequently extended by one year. Only 10 of 42 physicians in the Stuttgart/Esslingen region participated, although this was due partly to the bureaucratic red tape associated with the project. It was also found, however, that referring radiologists benefited most from a second opinion in the interpretation of BIRADS 3 and 4 lesions and would avail themselves of double readings in those cases. An analysis by Buchbinder et al. (2004) shows how deceptive BIRADS 3 lesions (1.4–14% of all findings) can be. Using a computer-aided classification (CAC) program, these authors analyzed 106 BIRADS 3 cases and detected 42 neoplasms. Double readings identified 6 carcinomas in a series of 146 (38%) BIRADS 3 cases that were evaluated in the model project. There appears to be less rationale for the double reading of BIRADS 5 lesions, even for referring gynecologists, who generally will hospitalize patients at once due to the very high index of suspicion for malignancy. Once a malignant diagnosis has been established, the woman should have several days to come to terms with her situation mentally and emotionally (and perhaps contact a support group) before presenting for surgery. We know from experience that this preparatory phase will help her in coping with her illness.

Thus, double reading should cover all BIRADS mammograms and should include an opportunity to advance the diagnosis by an interventional procedure or special images without having to secure approval from the insurance provider for "noncovered" services (MRI, interventional procedures, PET)—a time-consuming process that can be burdensome for patients and hospital staff. This means referral to a diagnostic breast center (see p. 299), which ideally will have its own budget for a specified number of patients who are members of a certain health plan. This budget will pay for tests that are considered necessary and appropriate.

The second reader should place special emphasis on the clinically healthy breast in the double reading of BIRADS 4 and 5 cases. The "furor" created by the original tumor tends to draw attention away from the apparently healthy breast, and it is easy to miss small contralateral tumors. In the model project described above, second readers detected three malignant tumors in the clinically healthy breast of 298 patients. All three of the tumors had been missed by the initial reader.

### Mammographic Case Presentations and Training in Interpretation

*J. Herrmann*

Both the quality of mammograms and the proficiency of readers have been legally mandated in Germany since 2003. All breast diagnosticians who are involved in patient care must pass an accreditation test in which they are presented with 50 mammograms and 30 pathologic findings. The test is repeated every two years. As this test is a rewarding exercise in itself and is an accurate measure of proficiency in mammogram interpretation, we have selected a number of representative images, which are presented below for training purposes (see **Figs. 5.26 – 5.39**).

Invasive ductal breast carcinoma in an involuted breast, the new occurrence of 1–2 cm spiculated densities in an involuted breast, and large clusters of pleomorphic microcalcifications are relatively easy for the breast diagnostician to classify as malignant. Misinterpretations and missed cancers are more likely to result from tissue asymmetries caused by invasive lobular carcinoma and from the lack of visible details in a radiographically dense breast (ACR 3–4). Of course, the examiner in a screening facility also has access to inspection, palpation, ultrasound, MRI, and interventional procedures to further investigate the breast and make a definitive diagnosis. These tools are not available in test-taking, where the only visual cues are mammographic changes that may include minute lesions, asymmetries, and structural irregularities.

Excessive recall rates lead to exorbitant screening costs, while too few recalls result in greater numbers of interval cancers. It is important, therefore, that subtle changes be correctly interpreted, and this can be accomplished only through experience and constant training.

The domain of mammography is calcifying in-situ carcinoma (DCIS, LCIS), which is often manifested only by a small number of new isomorphic or pleomorphic microcalcifications or, with larger lesions, by a typical distribution pattern within the breast (triangular, linear, diamond-shaped, or conical). Lanyi (1986) described and documented these typical calcification patterns extensively in his publications.

Calcifications are not detectable by ultrasound or MRI, which is why these modalities are not suitable as stand-alone screening tests. Calcifications are mammographically detectable in 30% of all small and medium-sized invasive carcinomas and provide a hallmark for recognizing these tumors—a unique domain of mammography. But what about noncalcifying preinvasive and invasive tumors, lobular malignancies, and noncalcifying tumors in breasts with a radiographic density of ACR 2–4? Sometimes these lesions produce only subtle structural changes that are visible to the trained eye but may be missed by an untrained eye. This chapter is a challenge for both trained and untrained readers.

Occult carcinoma less than 3 mm in diameter is not detectable by any method, and even very fast-growing neoplasms (doubling time < 40 days) will fall through the screening grid. To ensure that no detectable cancers are missed, double reading is recommended for both curative and screening mammography. Even with double reading, however, retrospective studies show that small cancers are still undetected or misinterpreted. Thus, training based on illustrative case material continues to be an important element in the training of breast diagnosticians and screening physicians. We refer the reader to the outstanding book by Uwe Fischer and Friedemann Baum *Mammography Case Book—100 Studies in Breast Imaging* (Thieme 2006).

The following case collection is designed to help train the eye for screening tasks and also to illustrate the capabilities and limitations of mammography as a stand-alone screening test. The collection includes normal mammograms and bilateral neoplasms. As you work through the material, you may increasingly realize that mammograms alone may be insufficient for the confident detection or exclusion of breast cancer. It is noteworthy that all the screening mammograms shown here are an indication for recall. Cases in which the patient was not recalled or ultrasound was not added resulted in a serious misdiagnosis—i.e., an existing tumor was missed. Remember that interval cancers are tumors that were missed at mammography! They were already present in the breast during mammography but were not detectable by that method.

In the cases that follow, we also indicate the ACR density of the mammograms (see p. 98), their PGMI quality rating (see p. 93), and the BIRADS classification of the mammographic findings (see p. 99).

It should be noted that all of the images shown in this chapter are full-field digital mammograms taken with the Giotto Image system (IMS, Italy) (see p. 102 and **Fig. 5.18**).

*(continued on p. 127)*

**Fig. 5.26 Case presentation for training mammographic interpretation. Case 1:** A 69-year-old woman presents for mammographic screening.

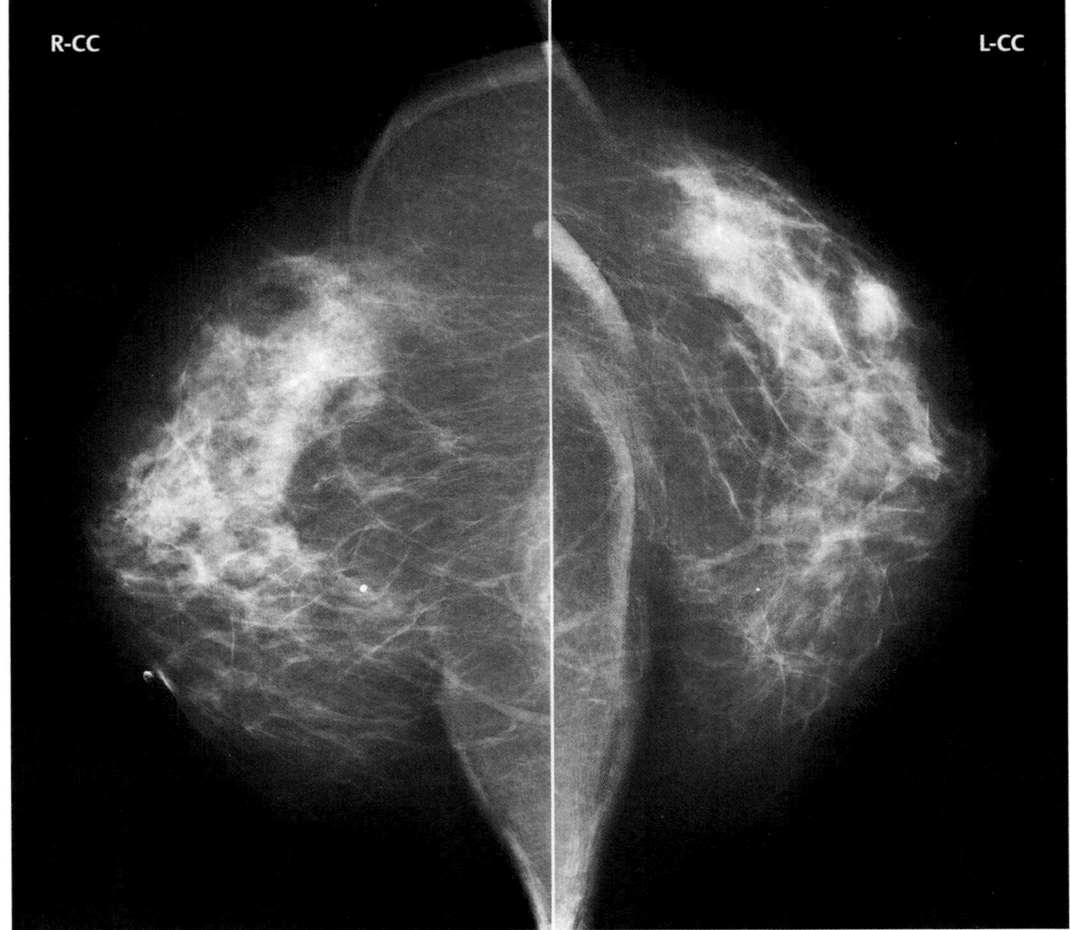


**a** *Bilateral craniocaudal mammograms.*

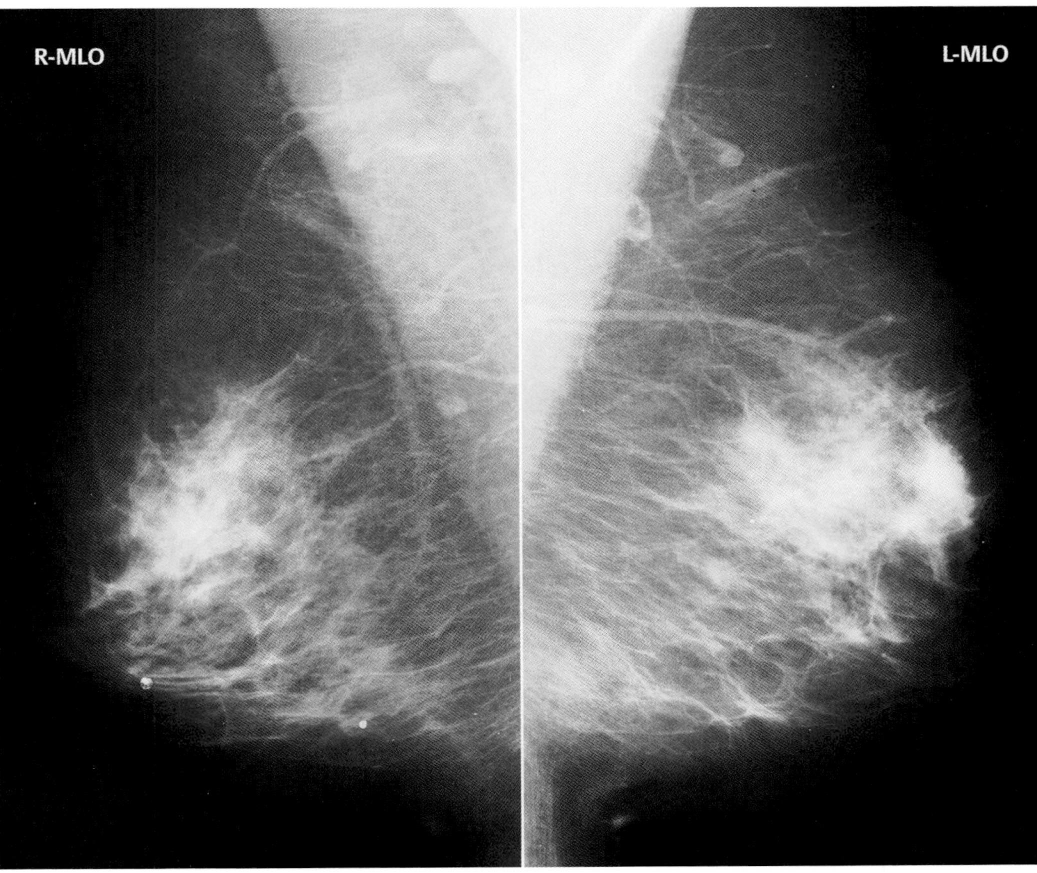


**b** *Bilateral oblique mediolateral mammograms.*

**Question on Fig. 5.26**

(**a**) PGMI?
(**b**) ACR?
(**c**) BIRADS?*
(**d**) Recall?

→ **Answer on p. 355**

* BIRADS 1 & 2 = normal
BIRADS 4 a = follow-up at 6 months
BIRADS 4 b = histologic or cytologic confirmation
BIRADS 5 = histologic confirmation

**Fig. 5.27 Case presentation for training mammographic interpretation. Case 2:** A 55-year-old woman presents for mammographic screening.

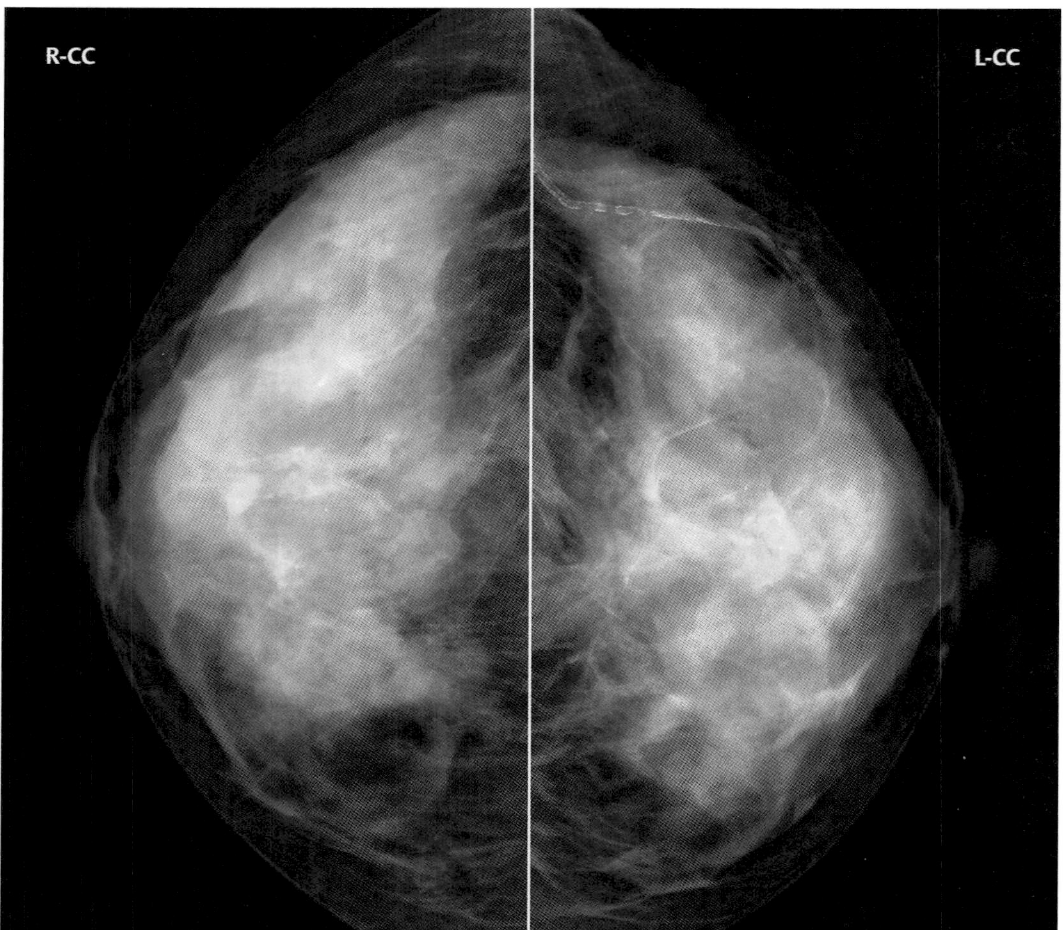


**a** *Bilateral craniocaudal mammograms.*

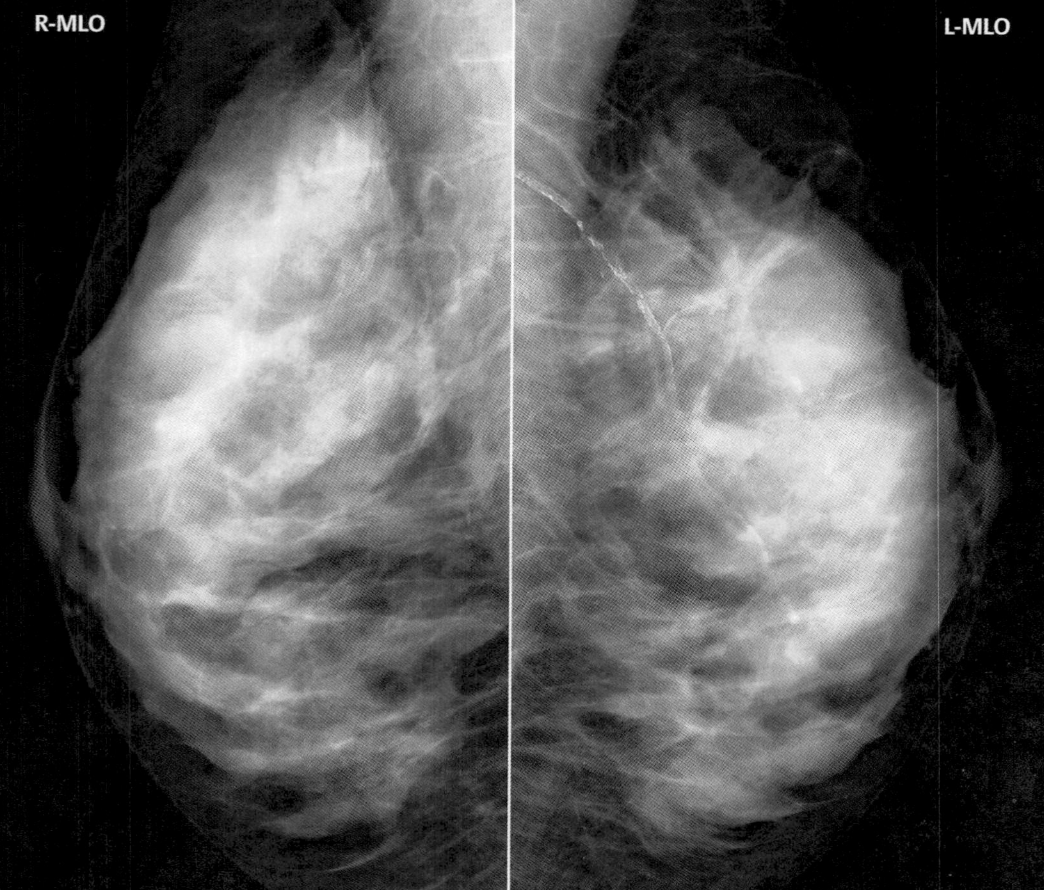


**b** *Bilateral oblique mediolateral mammograms.*

**Question on Fig. 5.27**

(**a**) PGMI?
(**b**) ACR?
(**c**) BIRADS?
(**d**) Recall?

→ **Answer on p. 355**

**Fig. 5.28 Case presentation for training mammographic interpretation. Case 3:** A 59-year-old woman presents for mammographic screening.

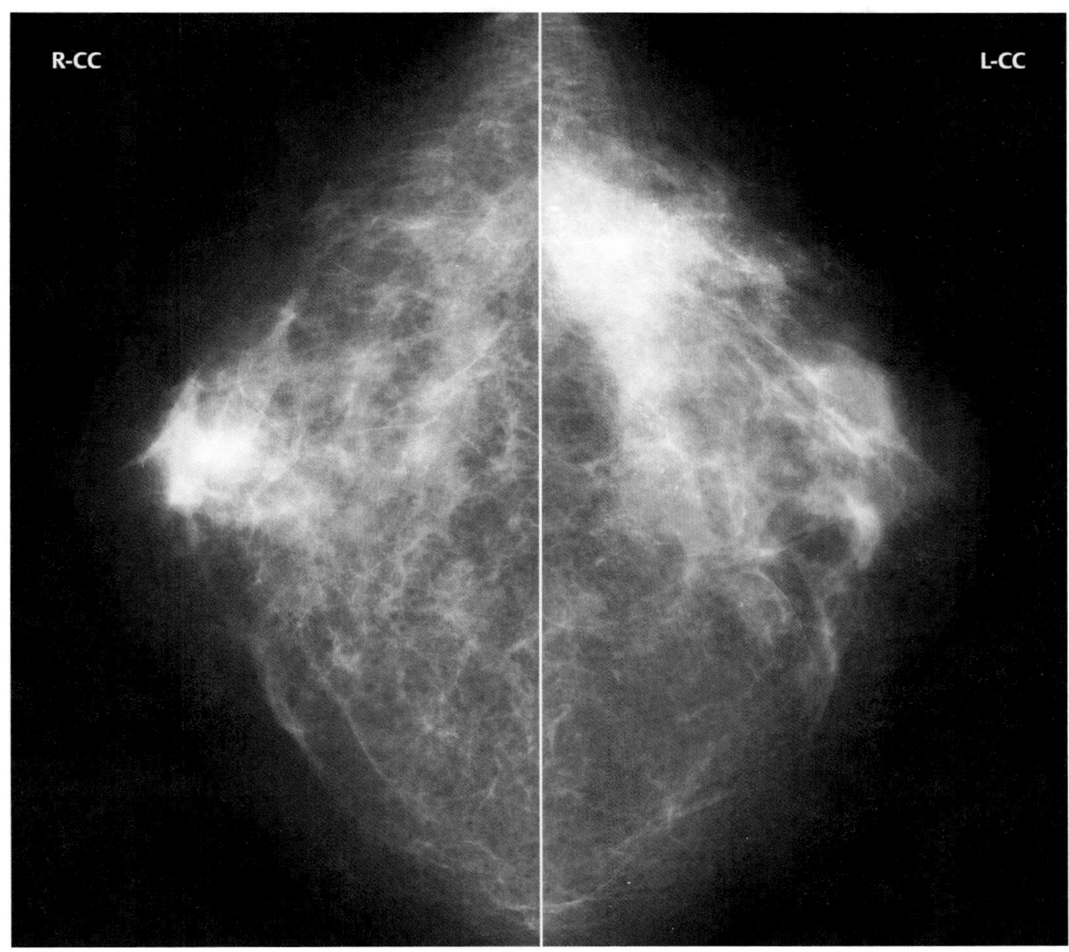


**a** *Bilateral craniocaudal mammograms.*

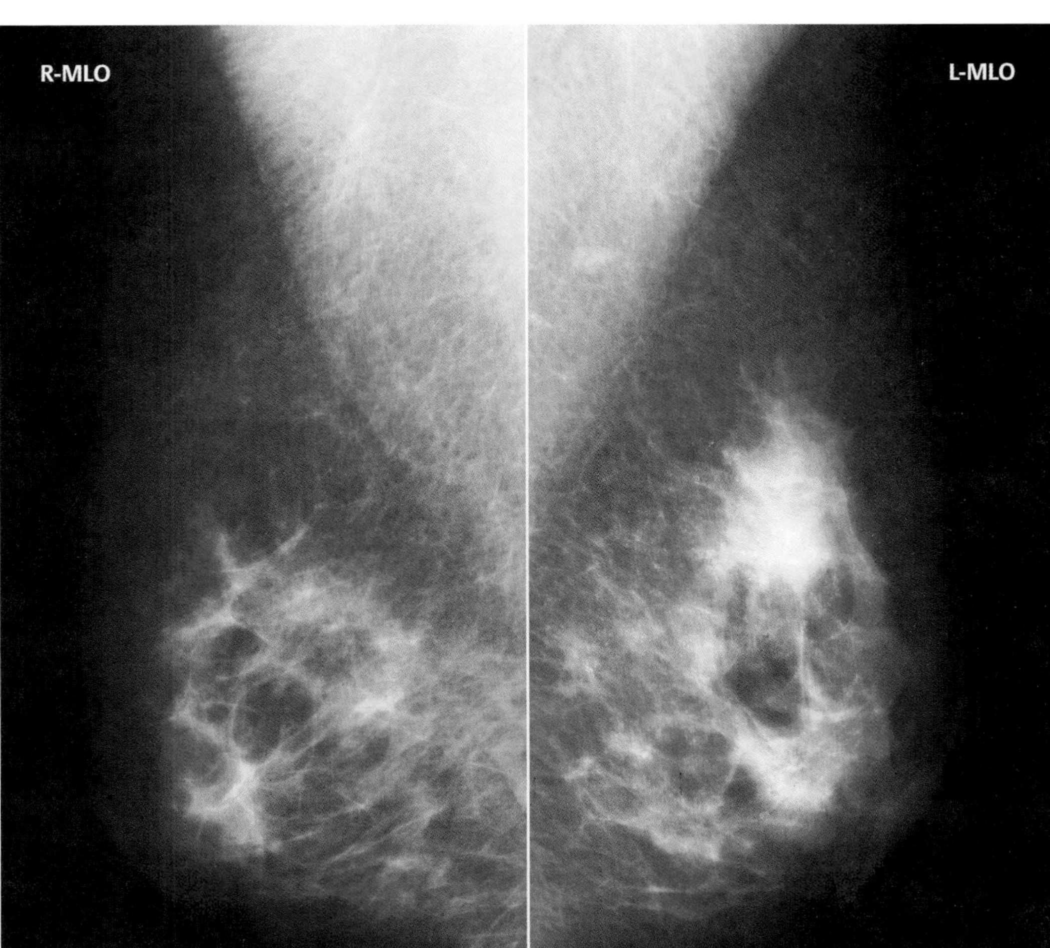


**b** *Bilateral oblique mammograms.*

**Question on Fig. 5.28**

(**a**) PGMI?
(**b**) ACR?
(**c**) BIRADS?
(**d**) Recall?

→ **Answer on p. 355**

**Fig. 5.29 Case presentation for training mammographic interpretation. Case 4:** A 43-year-old woman presents for mammographic screening.

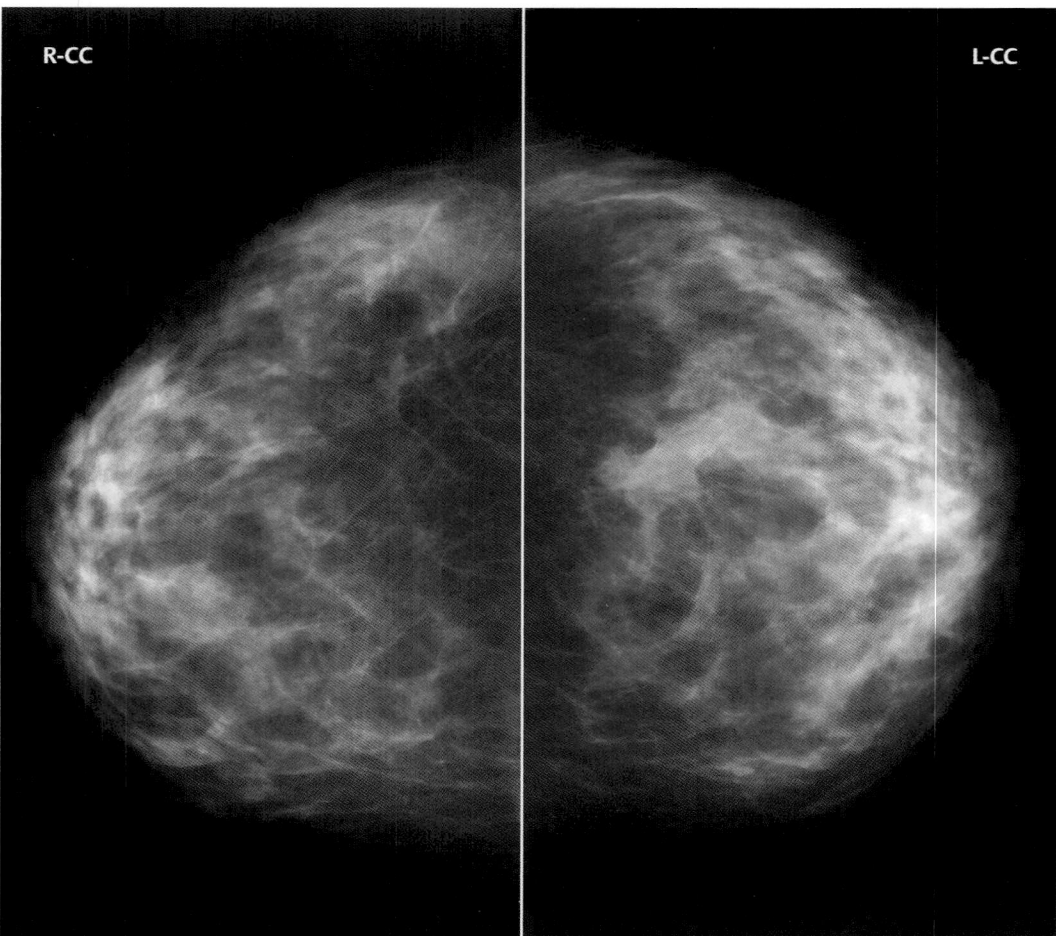


**a** *Bilateral craniocaudal mammograms.*

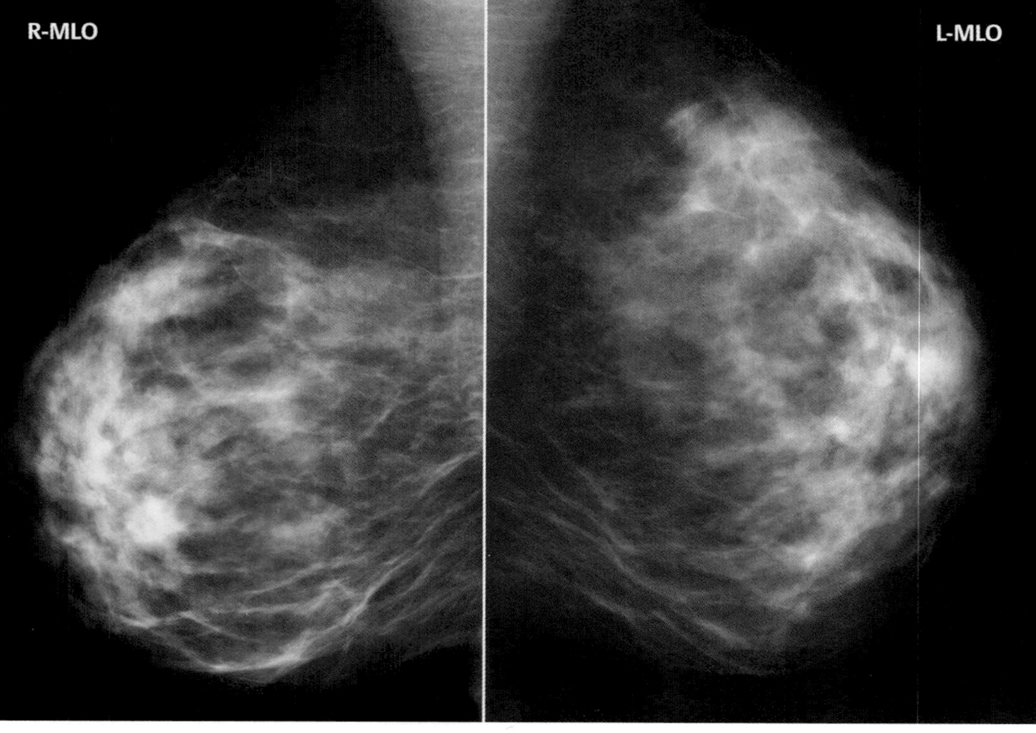


**b** *Bilateral oblique mammograms.*

**Question on Fig. 5.29**

(**a**) PGMI?
(**b**) ACR?
(**c**) BIRADS?
(**d**) Recall?

→ **Answer on p. 355**

**Fig. 5.30 Case presentation for training mammographic interpretation. Case 5:** A 46-year-old woman presents for mammographic screening.

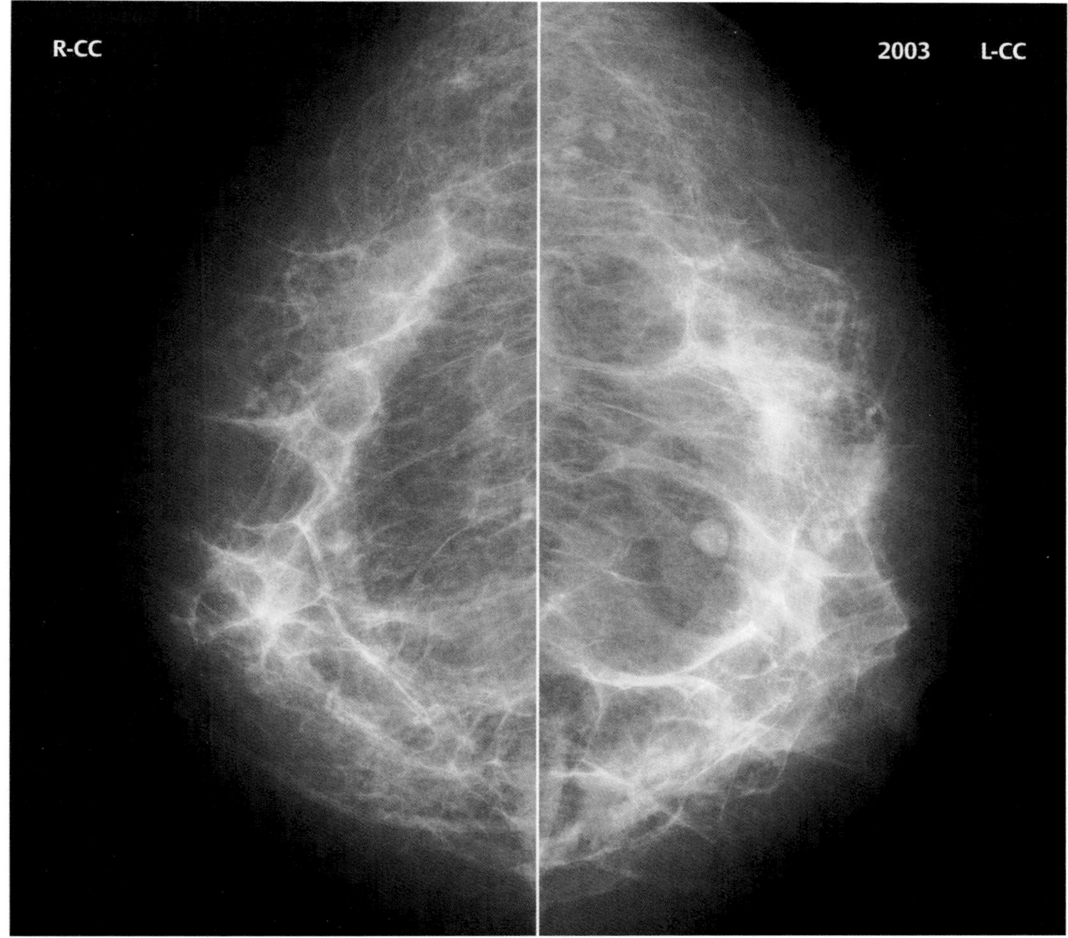


**a** *Bilateral craniocaudal mammograms* in 2003.

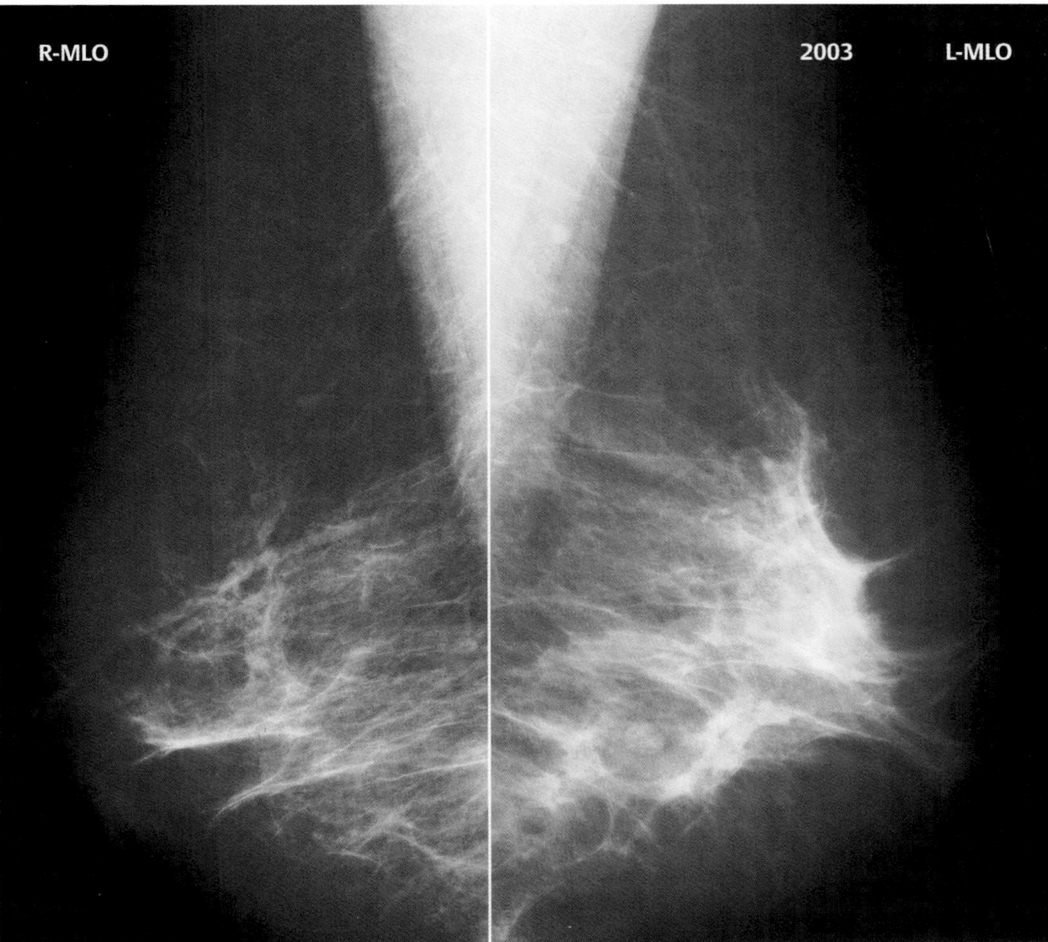


**b** *Bilateral oblique mammograms* in 2003.

**Question on Fig. 5.30**

(**a**) PGMI?

(**b**) ACR?

(**c**) BIRADS?

(**d**) Recall?

→ **Answer on p. 355**

▶ **Fig. 5.30 c**

**Fig. 5.30 Case presentation for training mammographic interpretation. Case 5.** *(continued)*

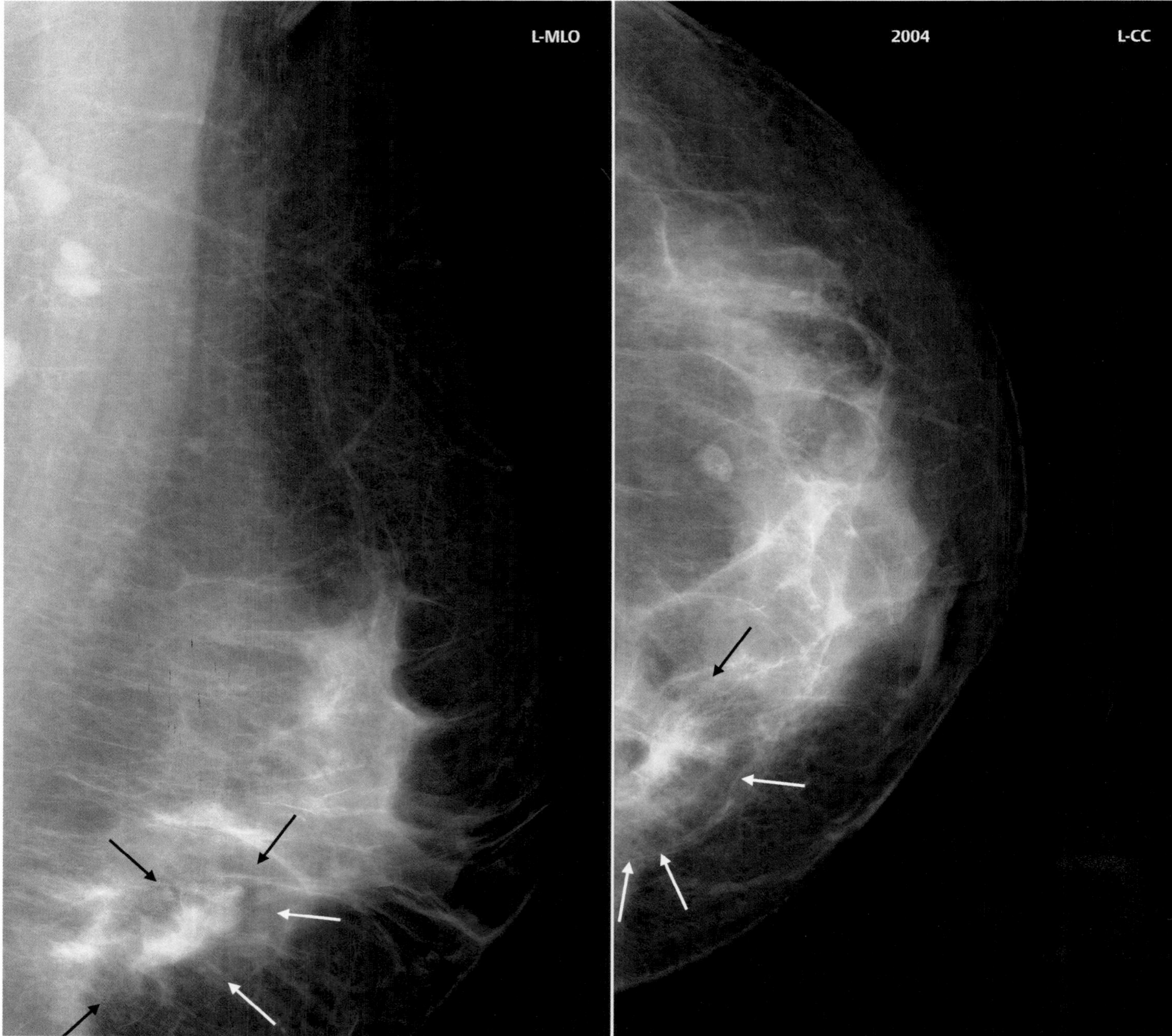


**c** *Oblique mammogram* of the left breast in 2004. *Right:* craniocaudal mammogram of the left breast in 2004. A malignancy is present in the lower inner quadrant (BIRADS 5) (**a–c/11–12** oblique; **f–g/14–15** craniocaudal). MLO: **P**GMI. CC: PG**M**I; **n**ipple–**p**ectoral **l**ine (NPL) is less than 15 mm (see **Fig. 5.14**, p. 94). The 2004 images are of better quality and are easier to compare, identifying the lesion as a scirrhous malignancy with obvious perifocal retraction (typical pseudohalo or pseudolipomatosis around the tumor) (arrows).

**Fig. 5.31 Case presentation for training mammographic interpretation. Case 6:** A 45-year-old woman presents with palpable nodules in both breasts.

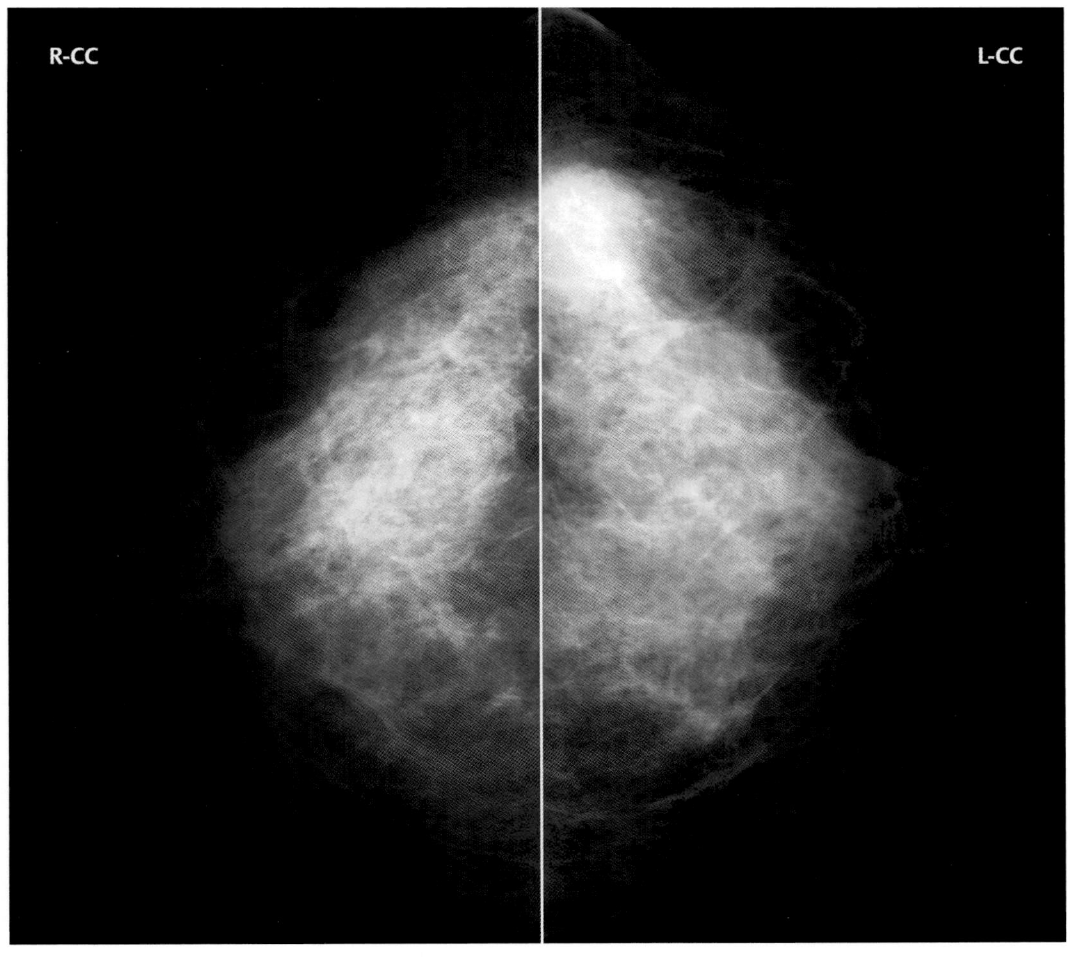


**a** *Bilateral craniocaudal mammograms.*

R-MLO
L-MLO

**b** *Bilateral oblique mammograms.*

**Question on Fig. 5.31**

(**a**) PGMI?
(**b**) ACR?
(**c**) BIRADS?
(**d**) Recall?

→ **Answer on p. 355**

**Fig. 5.32 Case presentation for training mammographic interpretation. Case 7:** A 60-year-old woman presents with a history of breast-conserving treatment for right-sided breast cancer 5 years before. New changes appeared in 2003 and were followed in 2004.

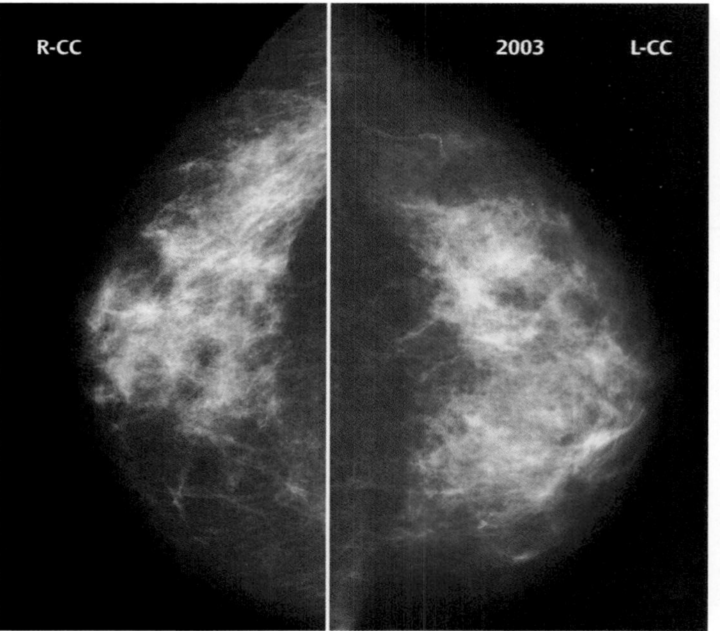


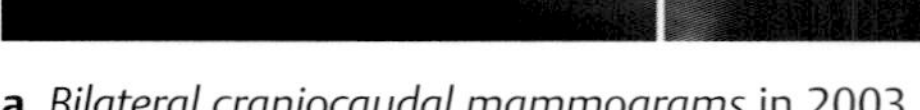

**a** *Bilateral craniocaudal mammograms* in 2003.

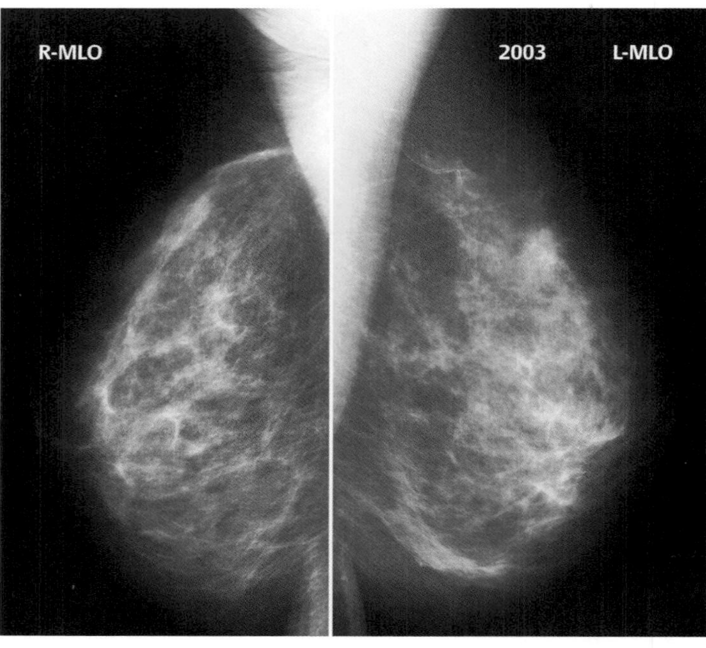


**b** *Bilateral oblique mammograms* in 2003.

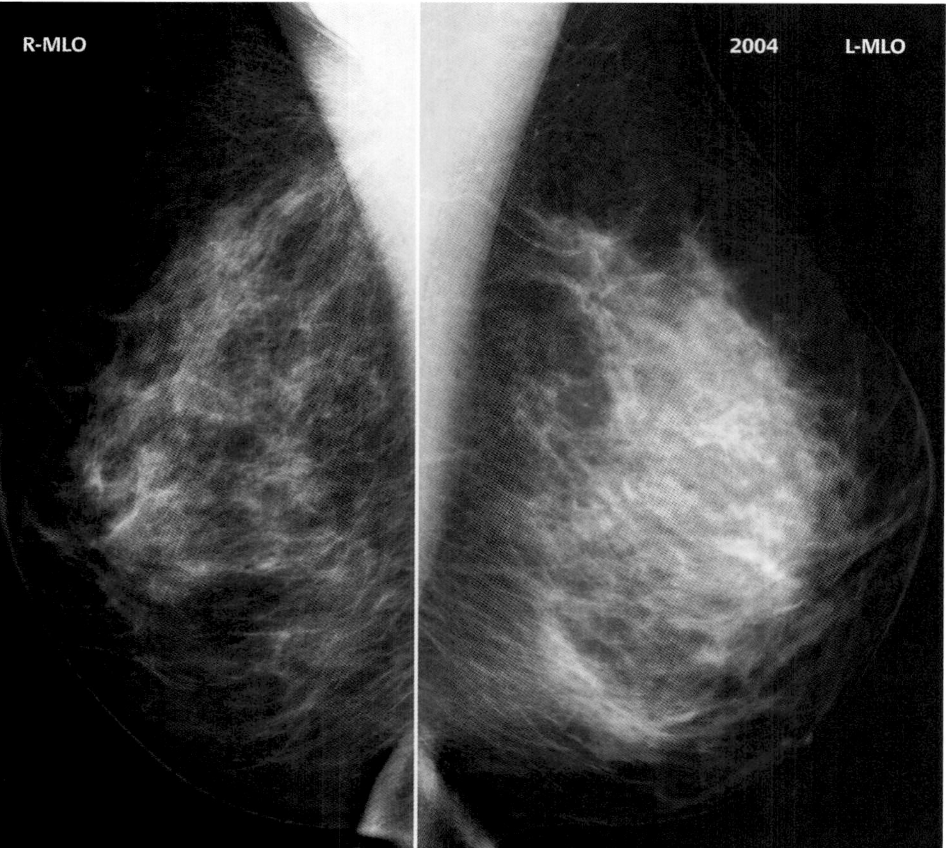


**c** *Bilateral oblique mammograms* in 2004.

**Question on Fig. 5.32**

(**a**) PGMI?
(**b**) ACR?
(**c**) BIRADS?
(**d**) Recall?

→ **Answer on p. 355**

**Fig. 5.33 Case presentation for training mammographic interpretation. Case 8:** A 52-year-old woman presents for mammographic screening.

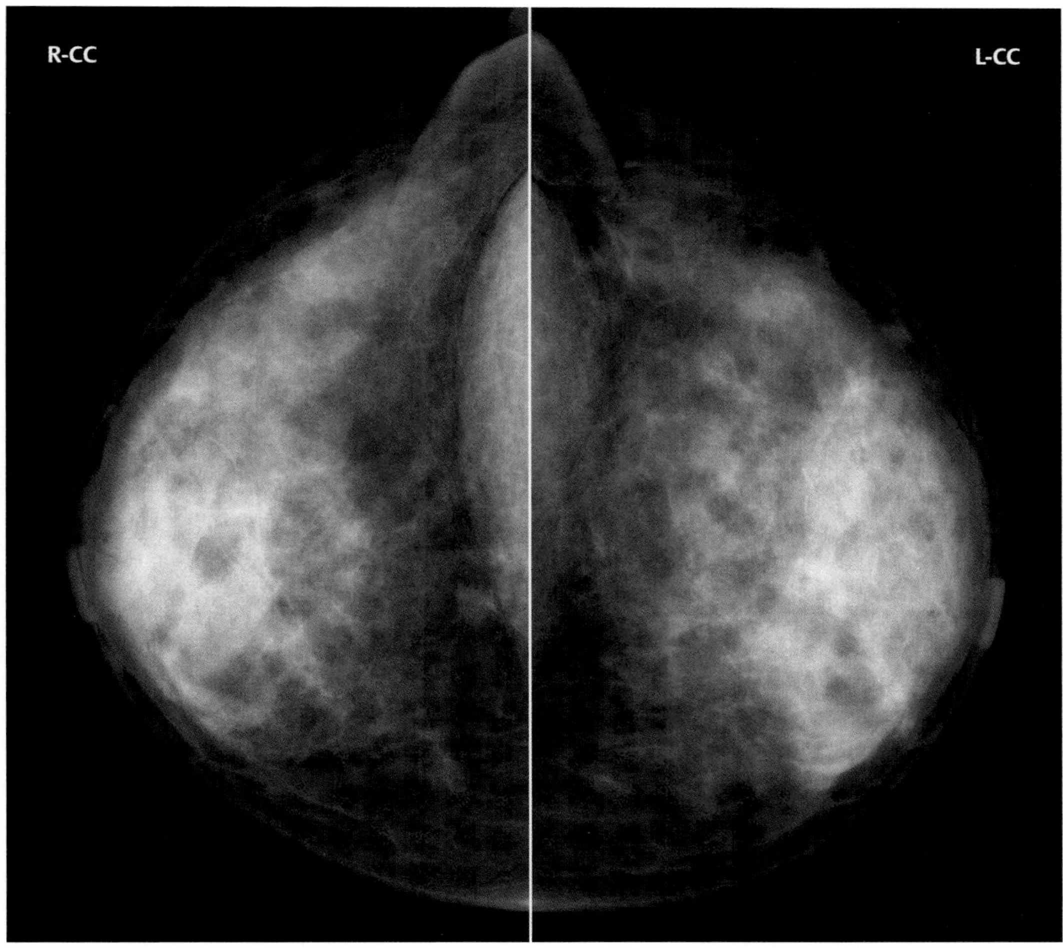


**a** *Bilateral craniocaudal mammograms.*

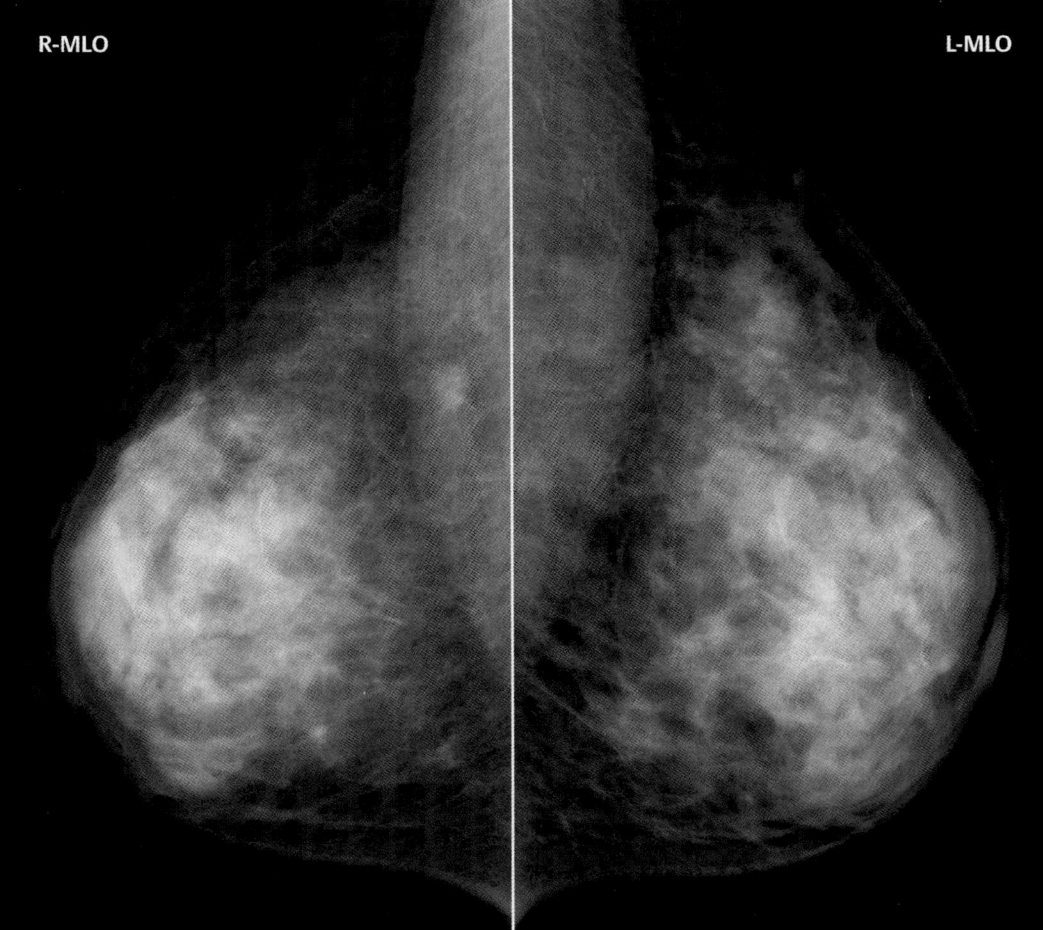


**b** *Bilateral oblique mammograms.*

**Question on Fig. 5.33**

(**a**) PGMI?
(**b**) ACR?
(**c**) BIRADS?
(**d**) Recall?

→ **Answer on p. 355**

**Fig. 5.34 Case presentation for training mammographic interpretation. Case 9:** A 68-year-old woman with fibrocystic breast changes and no palpable abnormalities presents for routine follow-up.

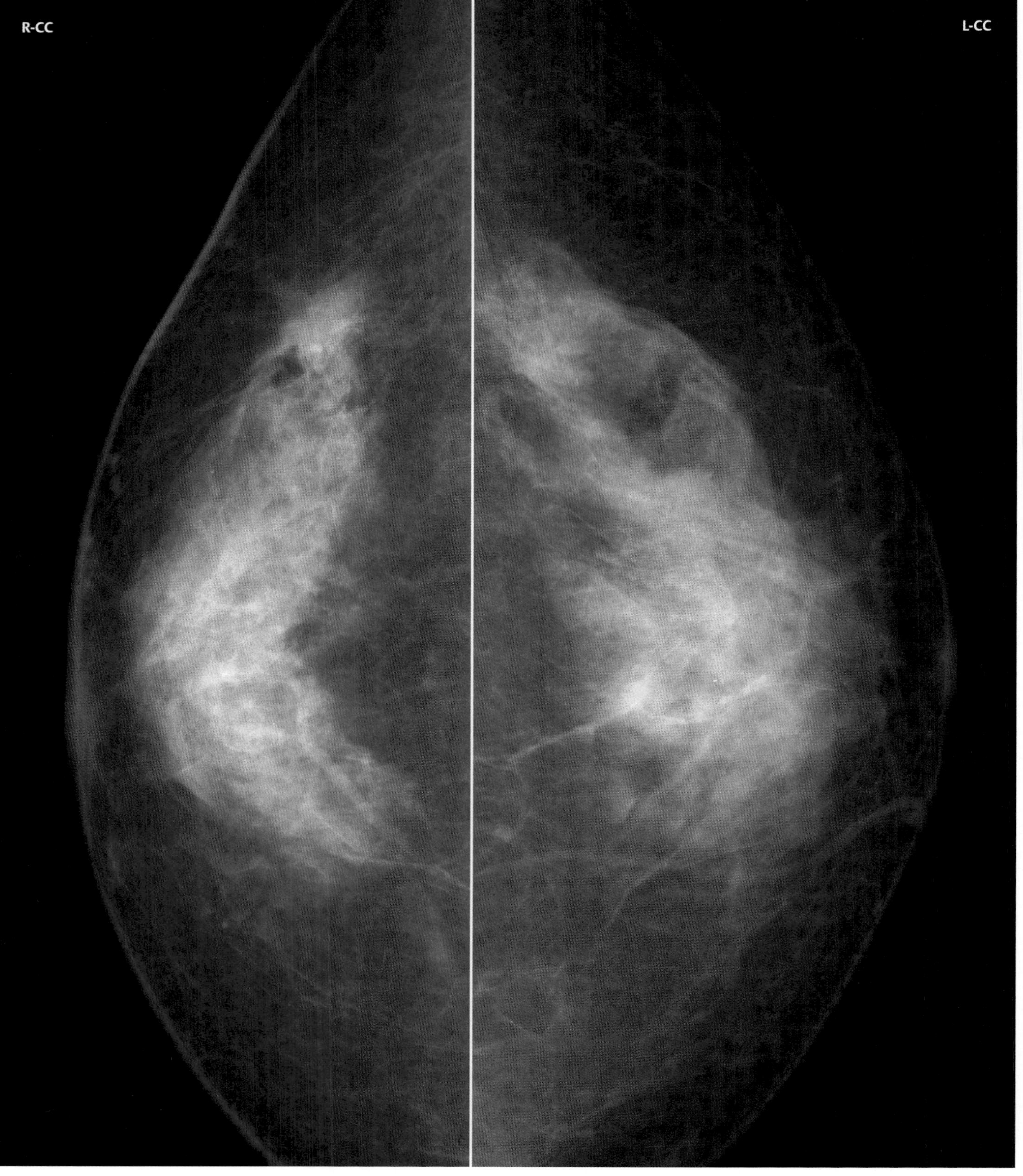


**a** *Bilateral craniocaudal mammograms.*

**Question on Fig. 5.34**

(**a**) PGMI?

(**b**) ACR?

(**c**) BIRADS?

(**d**) Recall?

→ **Answer on p. 355**

**Fig. 5.34** **Case presentation for training mammographic interpretation. Case 9.** *(continued)*

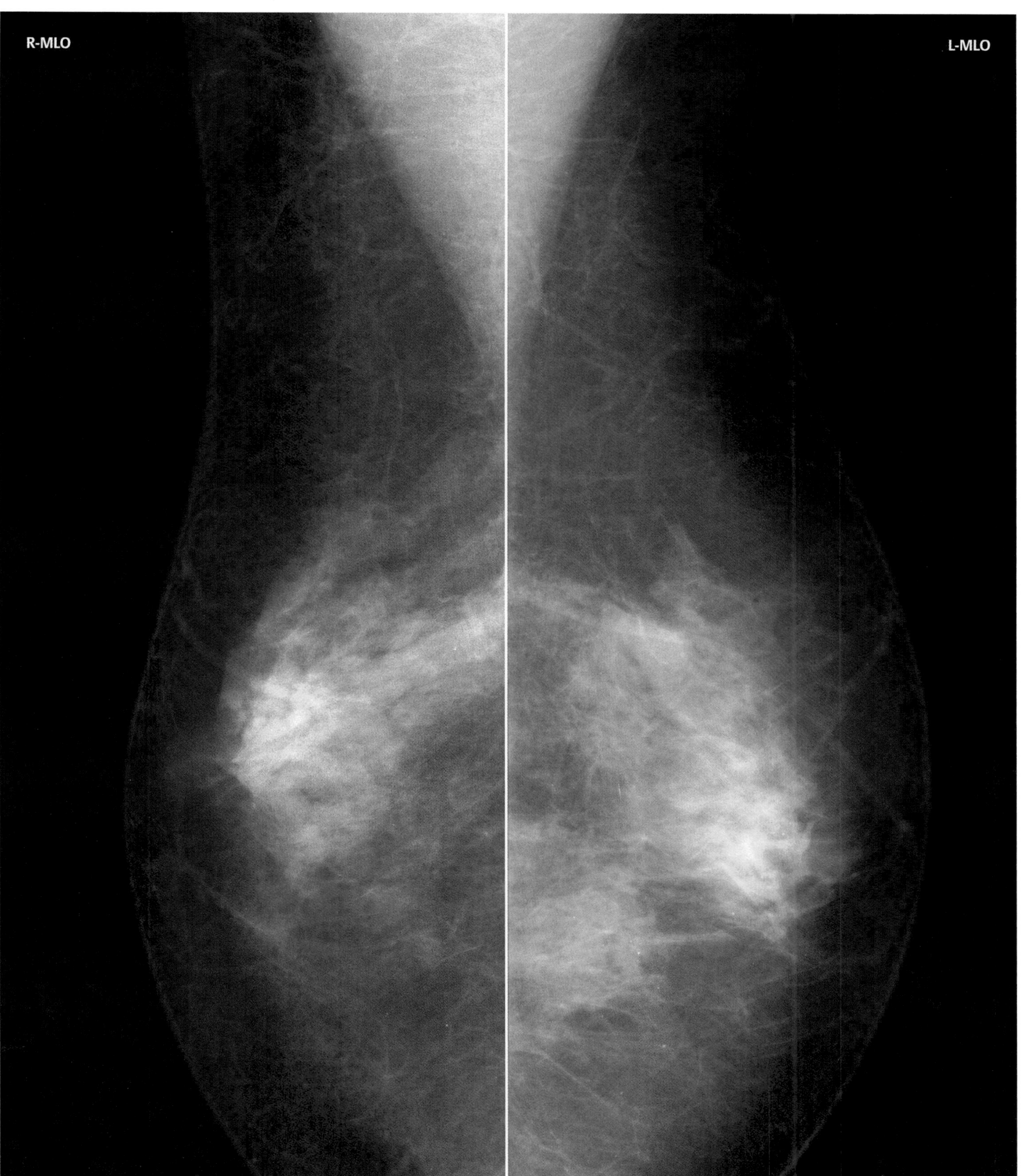


**b** *Bilateral oblique mammograms.*

**Fig. 5.35 Mammographic case presentation for training in interpretation. Case 10:** Screening and follow-up in a 44-year-old woman.

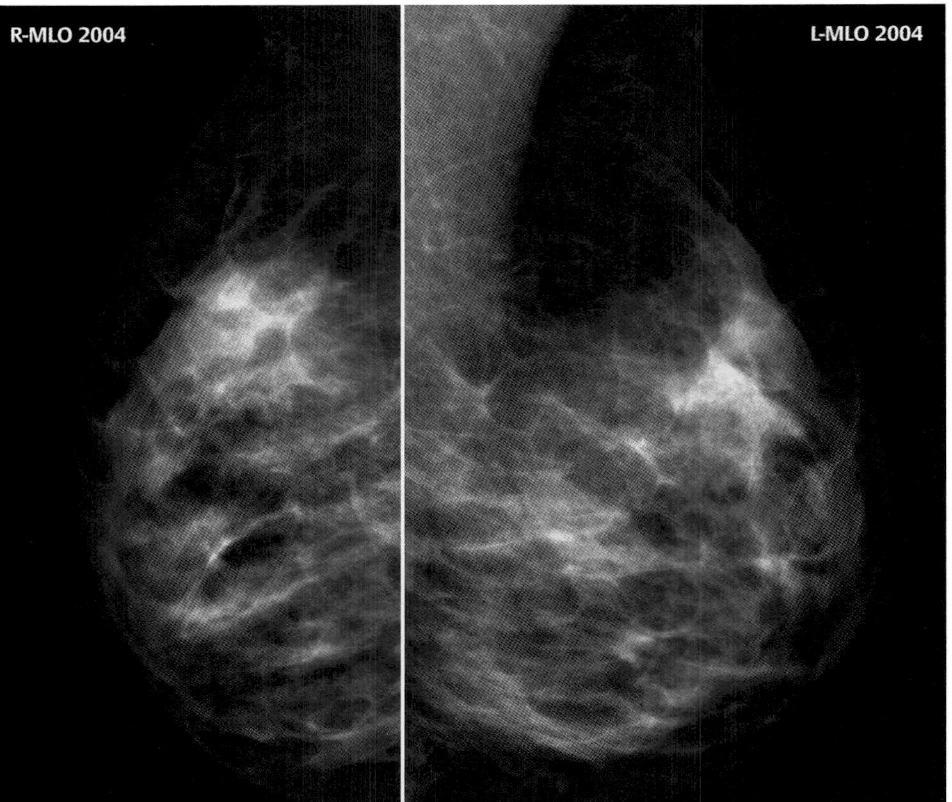


**a** *Bilateral oblique mammograms* in 2004.

**Question on Fig. 5.35**

(**a**) PGMI?
(**b**) ACR?
(**c**) BIRADS?
(**d**) Recall in 2006?

→ **Answer on p. 356**

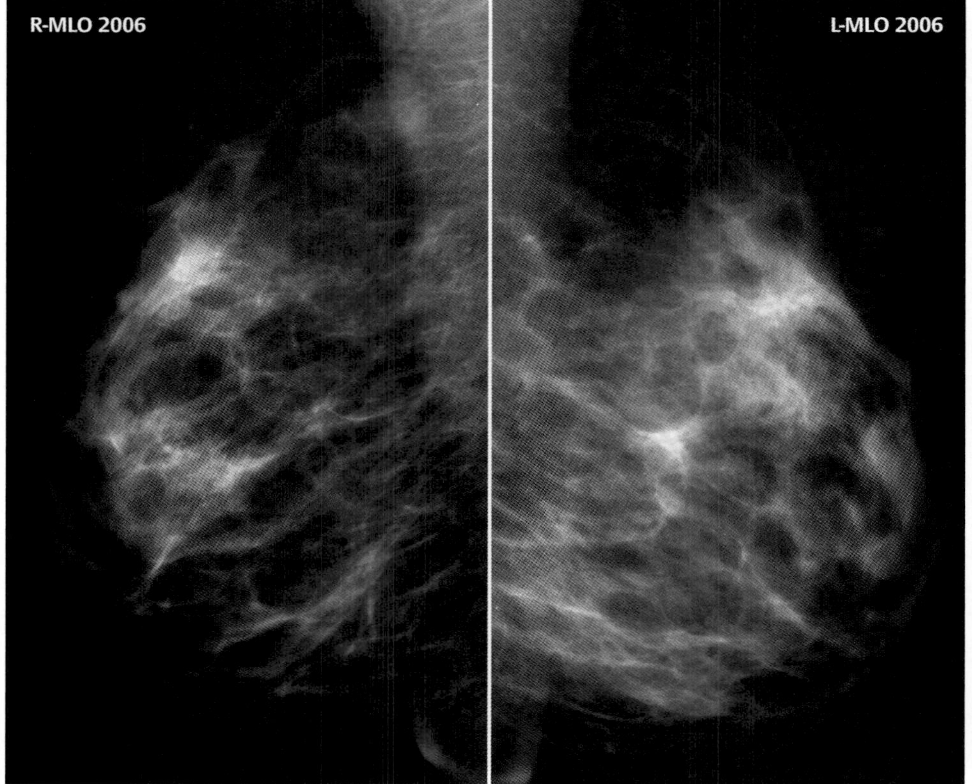


**b** *Bilateral oblique mammograms* in 2006.

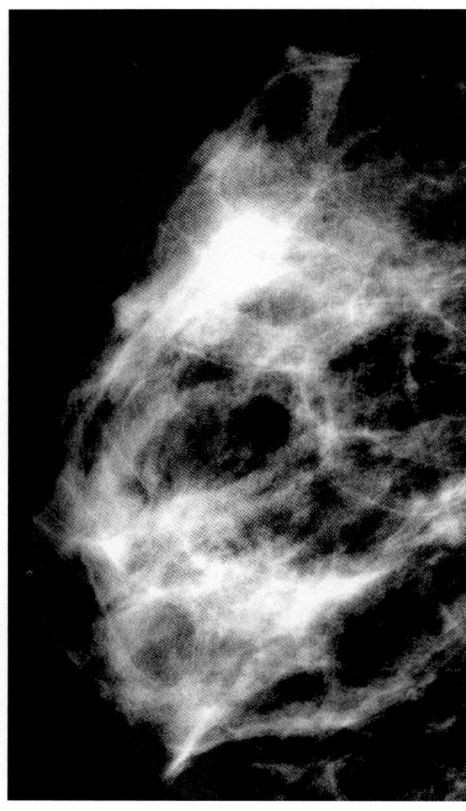

**c** *Oblique mammogram of the right breast* (microspot view) shows the retroareolar region and right upper quadrant as far as the pectoral muscle.

**Fig. 5.36 Mammographic case presentation for training in interpretation. Case 11:** Screening and follow-up in a 45-year-old woman.

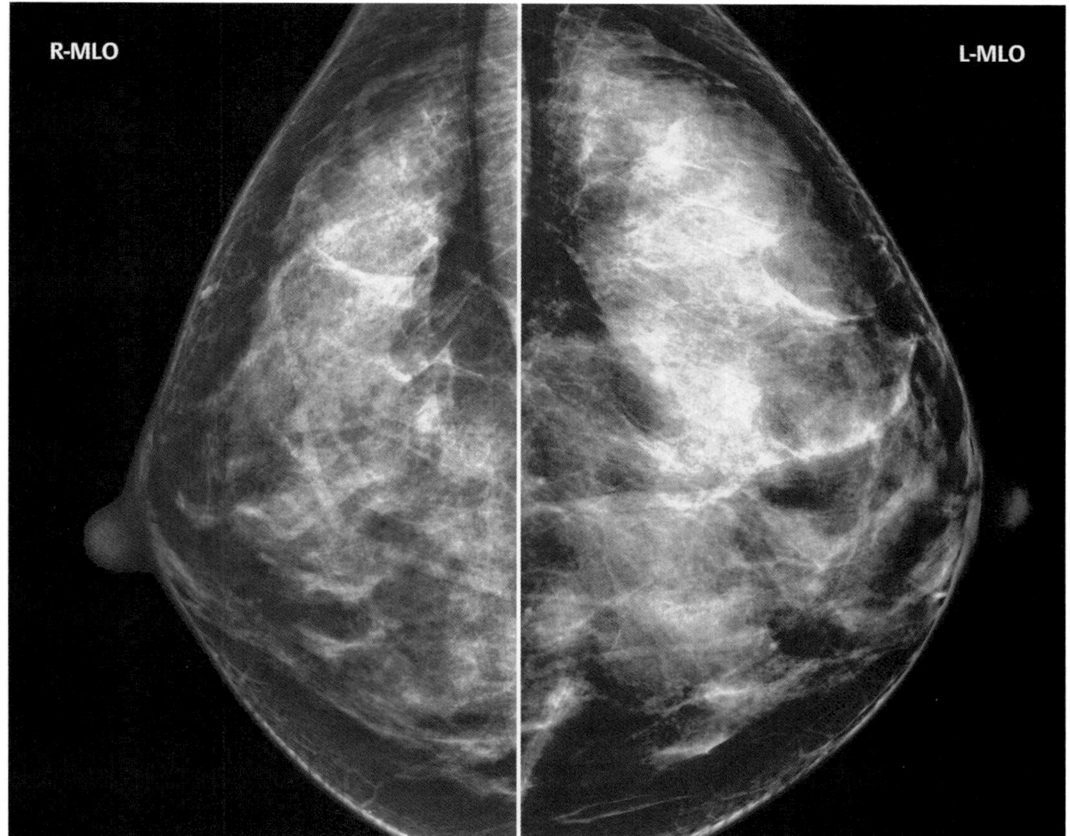


**a** *Bilateral craniocaudal mammograms.*

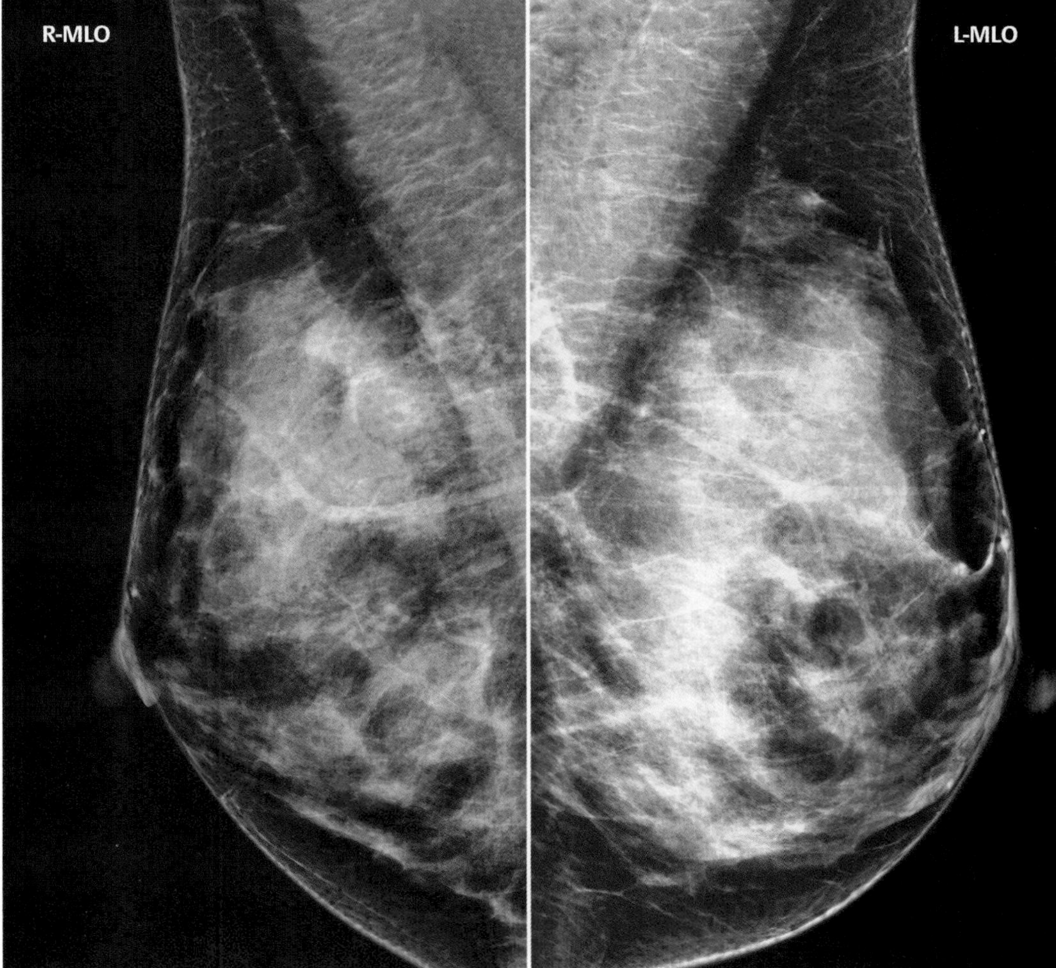


**b** *Bilateral oblique mammograms.*

**Question on Fig. 5.36**

(**a**) PGMI?
(**b**) ACR?
(**c**) BIRADS?
(**d**) Recall?

→ **Answer on p. 357**

**Fig. 5.37 Case presentation for training mammographic interpretation. Case 12:** A 63-year-old woman with a family history of breast cancer presents for screening. Images document the course from **2002 to 2004.**

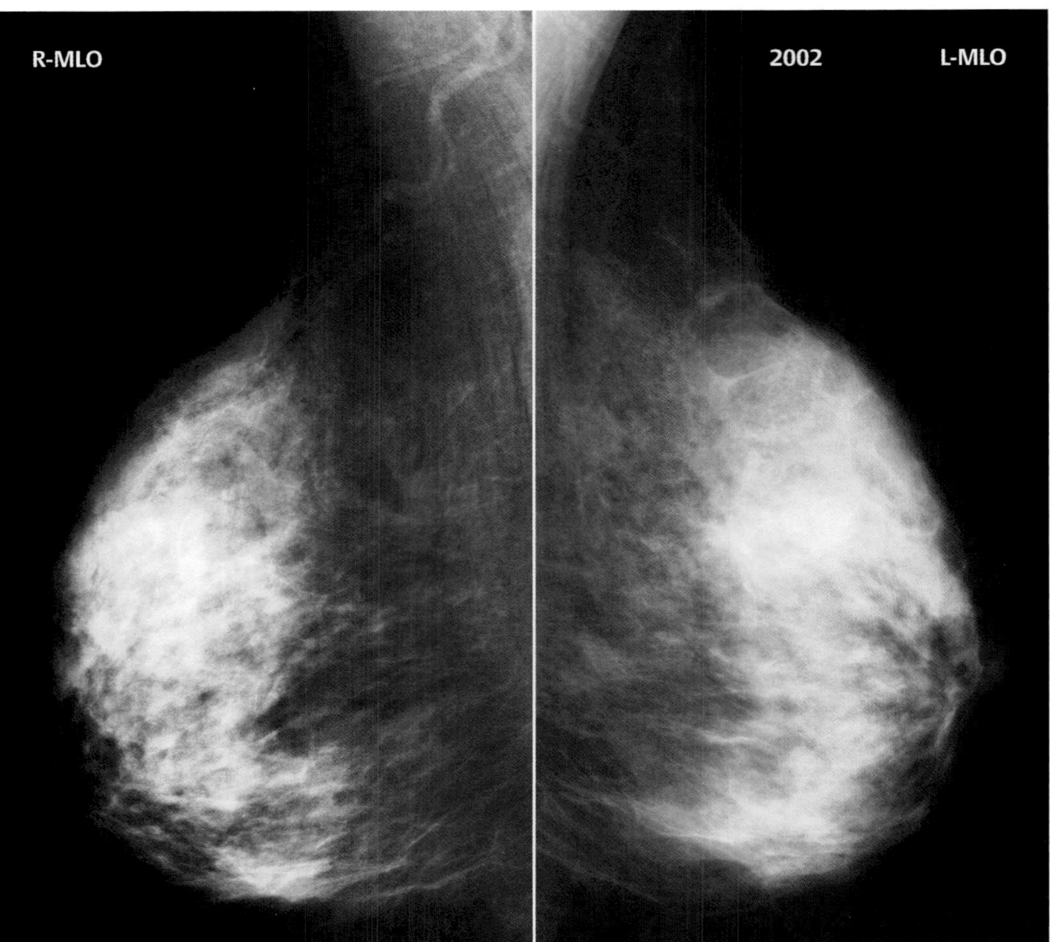


**a** *Bilateral oblique mammograms* in 2002. The craniocaudal view does not add information to the oblique view.

**Question on Fig. 5.37**

(**a**) PGMI in 2002, 2003, 2004?
(**b**) ACR?
(**c**) BIRADS in 2002, 2003, 2004?
(**d**) Recall in 2002, 2003, 2004?

→ **Answer on p. 358**

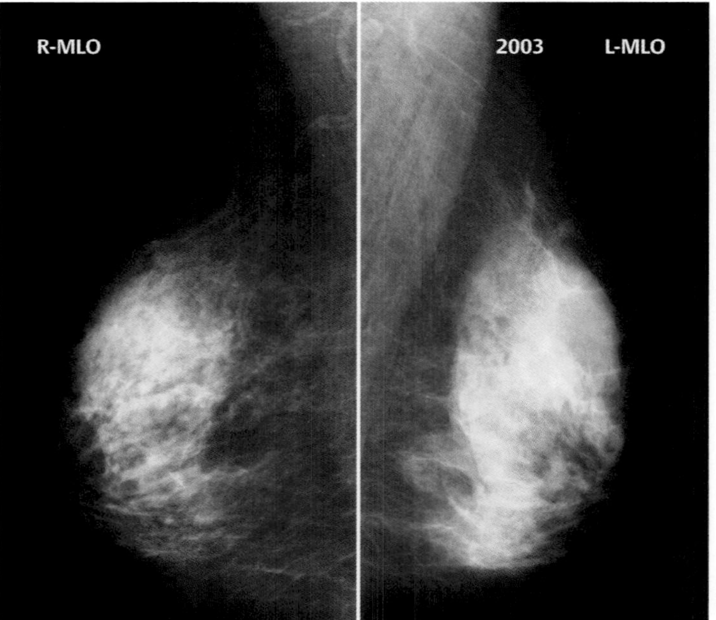


**b** *Bilateral oblique mammograms* in 2003.

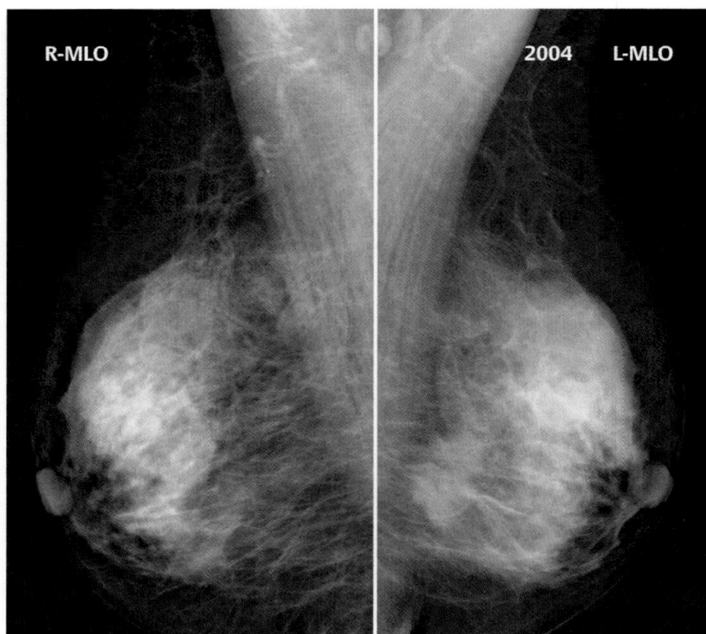


**c** *Bilateral oblique mammograms* in 2004.

**Fig. 5.38 Case presentation for training mammographic interpretation. Case 13:** A 60-year-old woman presents for mammographic screening.

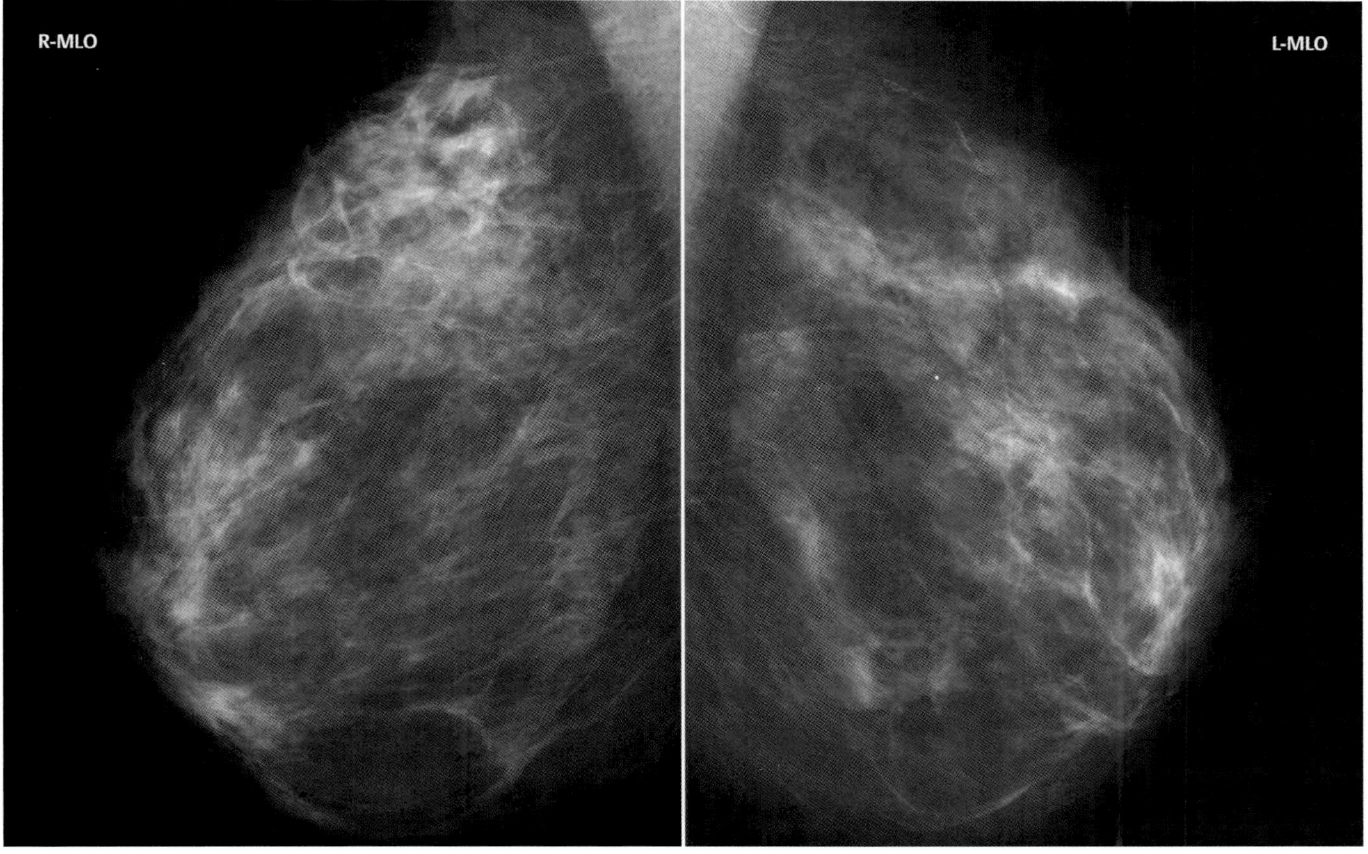


**a** *Bilateral oblique mammograms.*

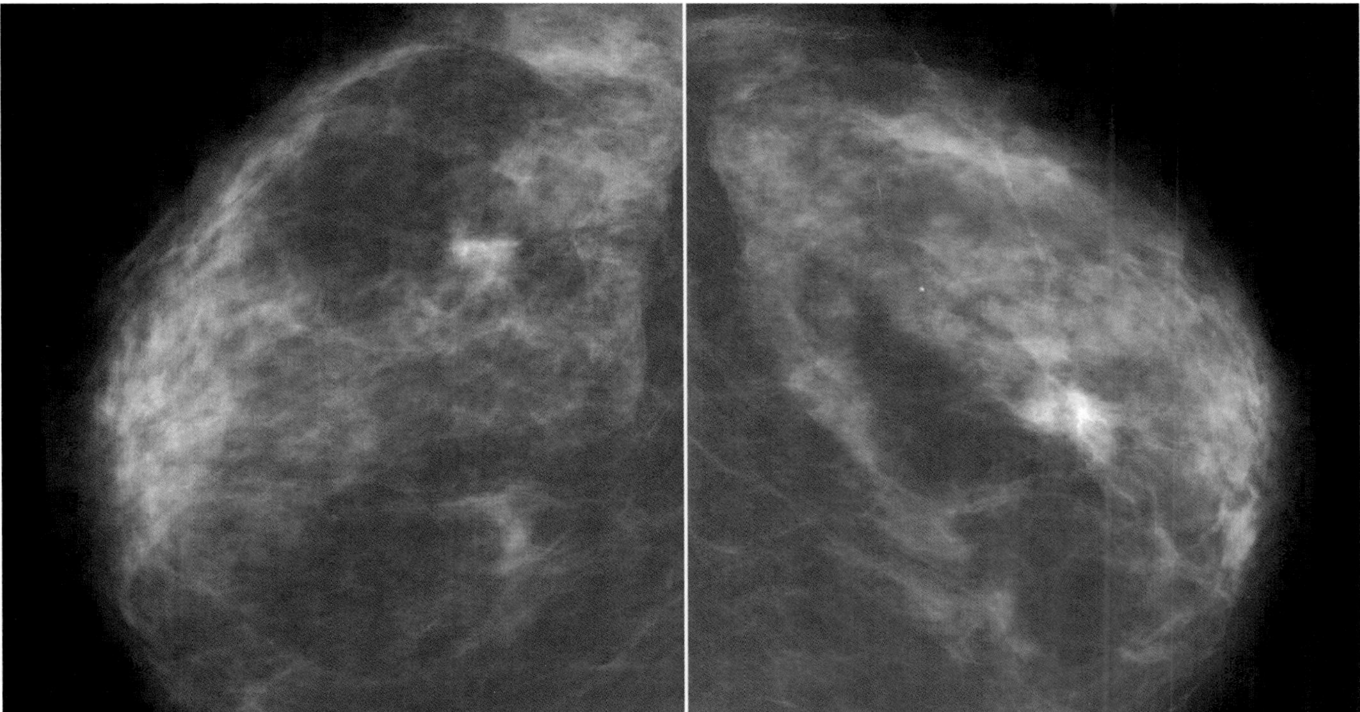

**b** *Bilateral craniocaudal mammograms.*

**Question on Fig. 5.38**

(**a**) PGMI?
(**b**) ACR?
(**c**) BIRADS?
(**d**) Recall?

→ **Answer on p. 358**

**Fig. 5.39 Mammographic case presentation for training in interpretation. Case 14:** A 42-year-old woman with **serous nipple discharge** from a single duct in the right breast (not previously noticed by the patient and detected at mammography).

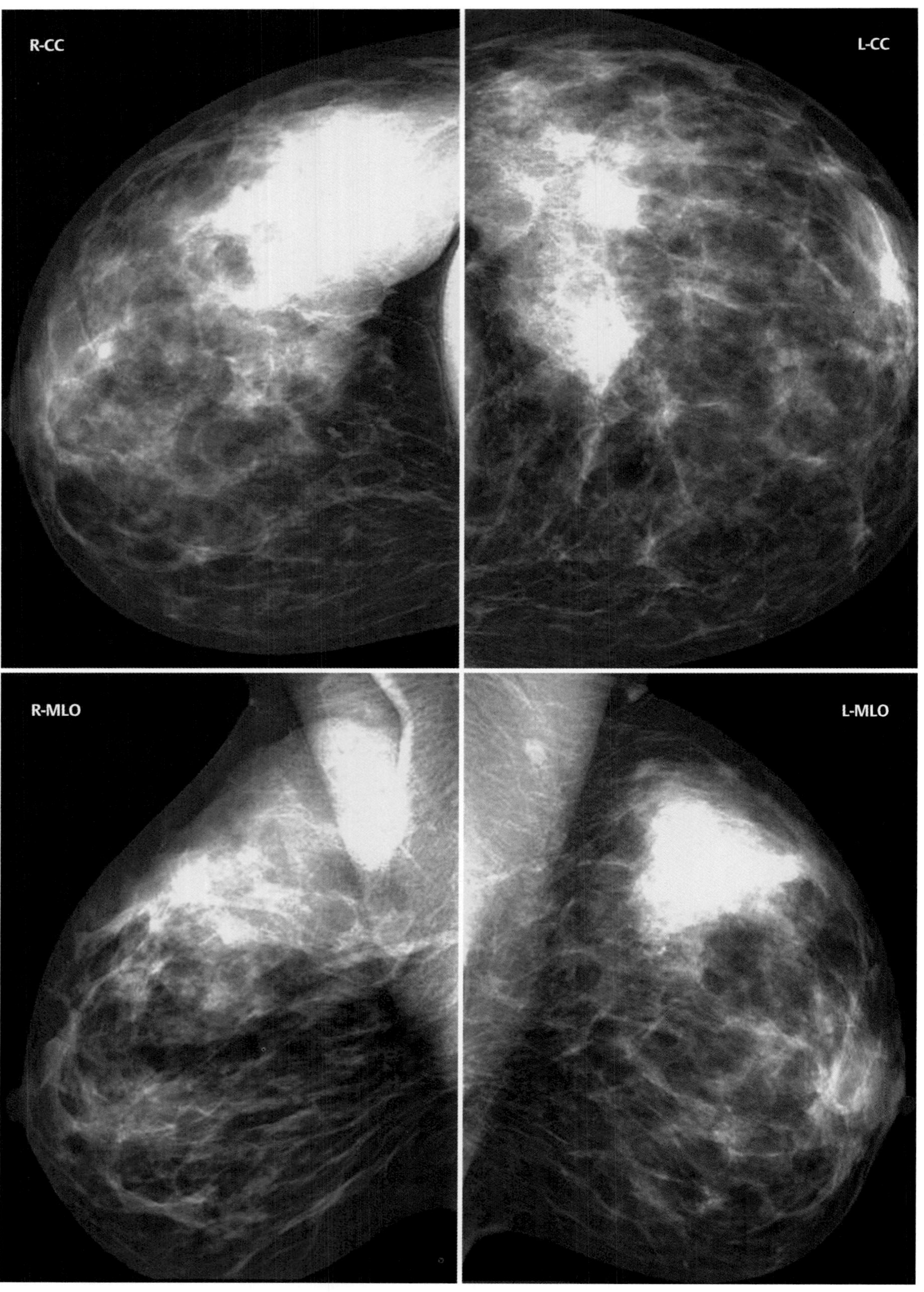


**a, b** *Bilateral mammograms, oblique* (lower images) and *craniocaudal* (upper images). Inhomogenous densities in both breasts in the outer upper quadrants (right: **b–d/23–26** cc; **b–d/12–15** oblique; left: **e–f/21–26** cc; **G–H/12–14** oblique).

**Question on Fig. 5.39**

(**a**) PGMI?
(**b**) ACR?
(**c**) BIRADS?
(**d**) Recall?

→ **Answer on p. 358**

(continued from p. 110)

### Screening

The advantages and disadvantages of pure mammographic screening have already been discussed elsewhere in this book (see pp. 105, 109).

The advantages of general population-wide screening are as follows:

- Coverage of large segments of the population (70%)
- Systematic examinations scheduled at designated time intervals
- Motivation of the female population to participate in screening examinations
- Reduction of breast cancer mortality by 10–30%

However, since breast cancer is less common for women in their 40s compared to those in their 50s or 60s, it would take 1904 women 39 to 49 years of age being invited to annual screening to prevent one breast cancer death. The overall reduction in mortality is about 15%. For women aged 50 to 59 it would take 1339 women being screened to save one life, the reduction in mortality being also 15%. For women aged 60 to 69, 377 women need to be invited to screening to save one life, but the overall reduction of mortality is about 32% (American Cancer Society 2009: www.cancer.org).

National screening programs have existed for decades in Great Britain, France, Holland, and Sweden, and nationwide screening was instituted in Germany in 2005–2006. Regional screening programs have been established in Belgium, Canada (NBSS1 + 2), Greece, Ireland, Italy, Portugal, Spain, and the United States (HIP-study, BCDDP).

There is considerable variation in the screening methods used in different programs (mammograms only, single-view vs. two-view mammograms, mammograms plus physical examination). The selected modality or modalities affect both sensitivity and screening intervals. Currently there is no program that combines single-view mammography, ultrasound, and physical examination. In one regional program, mammography was supplemented by ultrasound in 27825 women, which resulted in the detection of 42 cancers (Kolb et al. 2002)—not an insignificant number!

The efficacy of a screening program depends strongly on participation rates. At least 70% of women who are candidates for screening should participate.

- Nine randomized studies have been conducted throughout the world since the early 1960s. They have shown that the mortality rate for women between the ages of 40 and 50 who have regular mammograms is the same as in women who begin mammographic screening at a later age. The various studies (HIP, Swedish study, Malmö study, Two-County study, Stockholm study, Goteborg study, Uppsala study, Edinburgh study, Canadian study) show an overall **benefit** for women 50–69 years of age (Schreer and Engel 2004).

A significant disadvantage of mammogram-only screening is the number of interval cancers, although it is important to distinguish between missed cancers and actual new tumors. Younger women (under 50 years of age) in particular have a high rate of interval carcinomas screened with mammography alone. From the Two-County study, Tabar et al. (2000) reported an interval cancer rate of 38% in the first year and 68% in the second year for the age-group 40–49 (the 50–59 years group had 13% interval cancers in the first year and 29% in the second).

Analysis of the Nottingham Breast Screening Unit (1988–1993) showed an average participation rate of 73%. Two-view mammography was used in the initial screening round, followed by single-view mammography in the next screening round (2 years later). In the 72 773 women who were screened, 267 carcinomas and 87 interval carcinomas were detected after 2 years. This corresponds to 12 interval carcinomas for every 10000 women screened. The results of other studies are shown for comparison:

- *Swedish Two-County study*: 9 interval carcinomas per 10000 women
- Study covering 8 *northwestern counties in England*: 16 interval carcinomas per 10000 women
- *Nijmegen study*: 16 interval carcinomas per 10000 women
- *Göteborg-Study* only 2 interval cancers per 10000 women.

The interval carcinomas were at an unfavorable prognostic stage (in terms of tumor size, grade, and lymph node involvement). Lymph node metastases were found in association with 60% of the interval cancers. This prognosis is comparable to that of tumors discovered in women who did not participate in mammographic screening.

A relatively large number of the interval cancers were lobular neoplasms. In retrospect, the most commonly missed tumors and interval cancers were detected on the basis of architectural distortion in the breast. Seventy-seven percent of all interval carcinomas were found in dense breasts (Dy = 47%, P2 = 30% in the Wolfe classification). Only 21 of the women had radiolucent breasts (P1 = 3%, N1 = 20%).

The interval cancers in the Malmö study were predominantly of the comedo, medullary, and mucinous types with a markedly short tumor doubling time. Only 15% of interval cancers were of the lobular type, and 21% were in-situ carcinomas (Ikeda et al. 1992).

The number of missed tumors can be reduced by double reading. Nevertheless, the Nijmegen study found almost as many detected and undetected cancers in women 35–40 years of age—54 carcinomas detected at screening versus 51 interval cancers (relative incidence: 48.6%). The relative incidence was 34.5% for women 50–64 years of age (1 in 3 carcinomas was undetected) and 22% for woman 65 or older (1 in 5 carcinomas was undetected).

In the DOM study as well, the number of screening-detected carcinomas and the number of interval carcinomas after 1.5 years were found to be equal in women 40–49 years of age. In women 50–64 years of age, the screening-detected carcinomas outnumbered the interval carcinomas by 4 : 1. In the youngest age group, more interval carcinomas were found 2 years later than were detected in screening (33 vs. 25), while women in the 50–64 age group benefited much more from screening (26 vs. 67).

In the British national program, which has 3-year screening intervals, the incidence of interval carcinomas rose from 31% after the first year to 42% after the second year and 52% in the third year (Schreer and Engel 2004). This is particularly noteworthy, as this study apparently formed the basis for the Million Women Study on hormone replacement therapy.

The various mammographic screening studies are summarized in **Tables 5.10** and **5.11**. The screening model projects have led to a 20–40% reduction of long-term mortality in Germany. It remains to be seen to what extent these successful statistics will be duplicated in the German national screening program launched in 2005. It

**Table 5.10 Mammographic screening studies (Schreer and Engel 2004, S-3 Guidelines for Early Breast Cancer Detection in Germany)**

| Study | Start | Patient age (years) | Screening modality | Interval (months) | Participation (%) | Follow-up (years) | Relative risk (95% confidence interval) All | Age < 50 |
|---|---|---|---|---|---|---|---|---|
| HIP | 1963 | 40–64 | 2-view Mx + PE | 12 | 67 | 10 | 0.71 (0.55–0.93) | 0.77 (0.50–1.16) |
| Two-County | 1977 | 40–74 | 1-view Mx | 24 (age < 50) or 33 (age > 50) | 89 | Kopparberg: 15.2<br>Östergötland: 14.2 | Kopparberg: 0.68 (0.52–0.98)<br>Östergötland: 0.82 (0.64–1.05) | Kopparberg: 0.73 (0.37–1.4)<br>Östergötland: 1.02 (0.52–1.99) |
| Malmö | 1976 | 45–69 | 2-view Mx | 18–24 | 74 | 12 | 0.81 (0.62–1.07) | 0.64 (0.45–0.89) |
| Stockholm | 1981 | 40–64 | 1-view Mx | 24 | 81 | 11.4 | 0.80 (0.53–1.22) | 1.08 (0.54–2.17) |
| Gothenburg | 1982 | 40–59 | 2-view Mx | 18 | 84 | 12 | 0.86 | 0.56 (0.31–0.99) |
| All Swedish studies (1977 update) | | 40–49 | | 18–24 | | 12.8 (median) | | 0.71 (0.57–1.89) |
| Edinburgh | 1978 | 45–64 | 2-view Mx + PE (later 1-view Mx) | 12 (PE) 24 (Mx) | 61 | 14 | 0.79 (0.60–1.02) | 0.756 (0.48–1.18) |
| Canada | 1980 | 40–49 | 2-view Mx + PE | 12 | 100 | 10.5 | | 1.14 (0.83–1.56) |

1-view = single-view mammography; 2-view = 2-view mammography; Mx = mammography; PE = physical examination.

**Table 5.11 Cancer detection rates (cases per 1000 women) in mammographic screening at UCSF (University of California, San Francisco) and MGH (Massachusetts General Hospital), broken down by age (after Feig 2000)**

| Screening | Age (years) 30–39 | (years) 40–49 | (years) 50–59 | (years) 60–69 | (years) 70–79 |
|---|---|---|---|---|---|
| UCSF (initial screening)[a] | 1.3 | 2.7 | 6.0 | 13.1 | 14.2 |
| MGH (initial and subsequent screenings)[b,c] | No data | 2.4 | 3.0 | 3.9 | 5.0 |
| UCSF (second screening)[a] | 1.4 | 1.3 | 2.9 | 1.3 | 3.0 |
| UCSF (initial and subsequent screenings)[b,d] | 1.9 | 3.4 | 5.4 | 7.5 | 9.5 |

[a] Women without a personal or prior family history of breast cancer; calculated from data in Kerlikowske et al. (1996).
[b] Women with and without a prior family history of breast cancer.
[c] Data taken from Kopans et al. (1996), Kopans and Feig (1998).
[d] Calculated from data in Sickles (1995).

should not be forgotten that the 5 million mammograms obtained by traditional "opportunistic" screening led to a yearly breast cancer mortality rate in Germany that was significantly lower than in the UK and Holland, countries with well-established screening programs, although it was somewhat higher than in Sweden, the no. 1 screening country.

How effective could a screening program be if women were screened at 1.5-year intervals instead of 2-year intervals and two-view mammograms were replaced by single-view mammograms plus high-resolution ultrasound? Future screening models are certain to be modified in this direction. The screening program instituted in Germany is a step in the right direction. Since the German mammographic study in 1989, in which Esslingen participated, not much has happened in Germany aside from three model projects that were instituted in Bremen, Wiesbaden, and Weser-Ems. It is difficult for any European countries to withdraw from the European Screening Project and go their own way.

Missed cancers and interval cancers stand at one end of the screening spectrum. At the other end are unnecessary additional tests that are prompted by screening results. These additional, neg-

**Table 5.12 Estimate of the risk-benefit ratio for various ages at initial mammographic screening (from Jung 2001)**

| Age at initial screening (years) | Mortality D 1995 | | Benefit (deaths prevented/100 000) | | | | | Risk (deaths per 100 000) | Risk/benefit ratio |
|---|---|---|---|---|---|---|---|---|---|
| | Age (years) | Deaths per 100 000 | Per age group | | | | Total | | |
| – | 67.5 | 12.2 | – | – | – | – | – | – | – |
| 37.5 | 42.5 | 24.3 | 2.4 | – | – | – | 22.2 | 13.3 | 1.7 |
| 42.5 | 47.5 | 38.0 | 7.6 | 3.8 | – | – | 30.6 | 7.4 | 4.1 |
| 47.5 | 52.5 | 61.0 | 12.2 | 12.2 | 6.1 | – | 37.6 | 5.1 | 7.4 |
| 52.5 | 57.5 | 73.1 | – | 14.6 | 14.6 | 7.3 | 43.8 | 1.9 | 23 |
| 57.5 | 62.5 | 84.4 | 8.4 | – | 16.9 | 16.9 | 51.9 | 1.0 | 52 |
| 62.5 | 67.5 | 98.2 | 19.6 | 9.8 | – | 19.6 | 62.6 | 0 | Very high |
| – | 72.5 | 119.5 | 23.9 | 23.9 | – | – | – | – | – |
| – | 77.5 | 144.3 | – | 28.9 | – | – | – | – | – |
| – | 82.5 | 181.3 | – | – | – | – | – | – | – |

ative tests increase costs and may cause significant physical and emotional distress for the women who are recalled. A reported mammographic sensitivity of 70%, for example, means that 33 of 109 women with breast cancer are given a false-negative report. A reported specificity of 95% means that 5000 of 99 891 women without breast cancer are given a false-positive report (Koubenec 2000).

These statistics, while intriguing, are not very helpful to women individually. We know that women tolerate false-positive findings better than false-negative findings (Schwartz et al. 2000). Despite the possibility of a false-positive report, most women believe that screening is worthwhile and continue to participate in it. Most women know very little about the efficacy of screening or how it might be improved.

In analyzing the risks and benefits of mammographic screening, it is important to consider aspects of radiation biology. Based on an effective radiation dose of 8 mSv per examination (2 mGy per image, two images per side), Jung (2001) states that screening between 40 and 50 years of age (six examinations at 2-year intervals) is associated with a poorer risk–benefit ratio than screening between 50 and 60 years of age (**Table 5.12**) Radiation risk is not a major concern in programs that begin screening women at age 50. When screening is begun at age 40, however, the radiation risk should definitely be considered. Halving the radiation dose would be sensible for all ages, especially in women under age 50, and this can be accomplished with single-view mammography plus ultrasound (see p. 105).

In the British breast screening program (NHSBSB) in 1997–1998, an average parenchymal dose of 2.03 mGy was delivered in the oblique view and 1.65 mGy in the craniocaudal view in a total of 23 752 mammograms. The doses were less in breasts with a smaller compression thickness and correspondingly higher as the compression thickness increased. Current mammographic systems have an automatic parameter optimization mode that does not exceed a mean parenchymal dose of 2.5 mGy per image, even with a large compression thickness. This results in an average dose of 2.07 mGy (oblique) and 1.59 mGy (cc) for the respective views (in full-field-digital-systems about 10% less). There could be a reduction of the dose when using a tungsten anode with rhodium filter, as IMS (Italy) incorporates in their equipment. The life span of these tungsten anode tubes is clearly shorter than that of molybdenum anodes. The average glandular dose (AGD) with a tungsten anode and 50 µm rhodium filter would be very low:

- Less than half of the maximum required by EUREF (and British NHSBSP)
- 40% less than the achievable AGD suggested by the European guidelines EUREF (and British NHSBSP)
- 30% less than the dose released by the equivalent molybdenum anode x-ray tube utilized with the Giotto IMAGE SD & SDL

Let us see what happens with these reduced x-ray-doses.

When a film–screen system with grid technique (sensitivity: 25) is used with a modern mammographic unit with a molybdenum anode and a selective molybdenum filter, it is reasonable to assume that the average parenchymal dose per image would be approximately 2 mGy in an average breast with a mean compression thickness of 50–55 mm. **Table 5.12** shows the risk–benefit ratios for various age groups from the standpoint of radiation biology. According to these figures, single-view mammography using digital technology would lend itself exceptionally well to optimizing the risk–benefit ratio, regardless of the use of molybdenum or tungsten tubes (in every case as low as possible!), even when the x-ray dose of the oblique view is slightly higher than that of craniocaudal view. But remember that the oblique-mammogram shows more detail than the craniocaudal view (see pp. 92, 105).

Becker and Junkermann (2008) published the following computer projections based on the interim results of screening examinations: Thirty-one of every 100 women with breast cancer will die of their disease without screening, as opposed to 20 (35% less) who participate in screening. This fact could explain why women choose to obtain screening even when they consider themselves to be at low personal risk. They recognize that the disease would have profound effects on themselves and their surroundings. If mammographic screening alone has such a positive impact, how much greater would be the benefit (especially when projected to 10 years or more) if the incidence of interval cancers could be reduced from the current 30% to approximately 5% by combining single-view mammograms with ultrasound and physical examination, and if this protocol were offered to younger women at half the usual radiation dose (women under age 50 account for 35% of the malignant diagnoses in our practice!). It is time, therefore, to educate women about screening. They should know that we have the means to bring screening up to date, making it significantly more effective while reducing radiation exposure and discomfort (only one compression per breast). We have stated several times in this book that fully digital mammography has revolutionized mammographic screening. There is no longer a need for the costly developing and archiving of films. Within seconds, the digital images are available for display and interpretation on-site or at remote terminals, and it can be determined very quickly whether a patient should be referred for breast ultrasound or biopsy. Of course, this requires a change of thinking in traditional screening protocols. The time is ripe for such a change. The new German S3 Guidelines recommend that all breasts with a radiographic density of ACR 3 or 4 be additionally examined with ultrasound. This accounts for a full 60% of cases. If this recommendation were enacted, it would be necessary to modify the entire screening process, which currently provides for a maximum recall rate of 6%. The new protocol would be limited to single-view mammograms, and ultrasound would be a cost-neutral adjunct for women with radiodense breasts. Fully digital technology and automated full-field breast ultrasound (AFBUS) make it possible (see also the Preface).

By its nature, screening should at least guarantee that a maximum number of disease cases are reliably detected (Becker 2008). A 30% incidence of "interval cancers" can no longer be tolerated. A 5% incidence is barely acceptable.

It is equally important to create a nationwide cancer registry in Germany (and other countries, of course) that would transcend internal boundaries. This calls for political action.

Mammographic screening is a costly venture. In Germany, screening costs for the next 10 years will be approximately 2.5 billion euro distributed among 100 screening units (Diekmann and Diekmann 2008). While this places a significant burden on the health care system, it is also money well spent and an excellent opportunity for implementing new concepts with greater efficacy and less radiation exposure. But as mammography continues to be the only evidence-based method for early cancer detection, screening in all countries is frozen at the level of the past 30 years, i.e., mammograms only. During that time, ultrasound technology has advanced to such a degree that modern high-resolution scanners can diagnose more early invasive carcinomas than can mammography. Mammograms are superior to ultrasound only in the detection of early calcifying lesions. So why not use a cost-neutral combination of both modalities?

There is already a shortage of new doctors for mammographic screening. In the Netherlands, for example, where screening has been offered for many years, efforts are being made to train radiology technologists in the double reading of mammograms—apparently with some success (Duijm et al. 2007). While this may be a cause for concern, we must ask: if the difficult task of mammographic second readings can be delegated to nonphysicians, why not ultrasound and physical examination as well? Everything can be learned, and the end justifies the means. The ideal solution, of course, would be to keep the review of screening mammograms in physicians' hands.

Additionally, initial studies have been done on the automated combination of ultrasound and mammography in which a physician need not be present for ultrasound image acquisition (the usual practice in screening) (Kapur et al. 2007; Richter et al. 1998). It remains to be seen how such procedures will be implemented as an adjunct to the traditional screening protocol. It is also time to modify the traditional screening protocol by running parallel model projects like those described above.

**Up-to-date, effective, worldwide screening of all woman 40 to 75 years of age would be a welcome alternative to traditional, outmoded screening programs.**

The unquestioned advantages of general breast cancer screening must be weighed against the significant risks, and it is important that we consider these risks despite the soundness of the screening concept. We end this section with a quote from Teboul and Halliwell from as early as 1995: "When *safety and accuracy*, rather than *time and money*, become the main consideration in screening, then every breast with firmness, nodules or other complaints, women in high-risk groups, women with dense breasts, and women with mammographic abnormalities should be examined by ultrasound. Duct-oriented ultrasound will replace mammography as the gold standard for early detection."

## Digital Model of a Screening Unit

*O. Wild*

Every physician involved in screening must perform approximately 2000–3000 *additional* examinations per year. The main difference from "curative" breast imaging is that the women undergo mammography without contact with the physician, who then systematically evaluates the mammograms and passes on the images and findings to a colleague for a second reading. This physician interprets the images without regard for the opinion of the first reader, whose identity should be unknown, although this is impractical since the name of the initial reader is usually annotated on conventional mammograms. Both interpretations are then compared by the physician supervising the program. If they agree, the patient receives a report summarizing the findings. If the interpretations do not agree, the program supervisor evaluates the images and orders additional diagnostic tests as needed (**Fig. 5.40**).

### *Problems in Screening without a Data Network*

We assume that four screening units are needed to cover an area with 1 million inhabitants, 160 000 of whom are women 50–69 years of age, and that ideally 70% of these women will participate in breast cancer screening. This means that a total of 112 000 women will present for screening, and that each of the four screening units will provide 28 000 examinations. If each unit has four physicians, each physician must perform 7000 examinations.

Screening should be scheduled at 2-year intervals, which means that each screening physician must do approximately 3500 examinations per year. When we add to this an equal number of second readings, each physician has to interpret 7000 extra cases per year in addition to "curative" mammograms.

The Union of Health Insurance Fund Physicians (KV) in Baden-Würtemberg, Germany recommends that these additional examinations be done on two workdays per week. During the rest of the week, the screening physicians perform their regular mammograms and conduct the routine activities of their practice. When the 7000 cases are distributed over 88 workdays (based on 220 workdays per year), the physician would have to interpret 80 examinations per day!

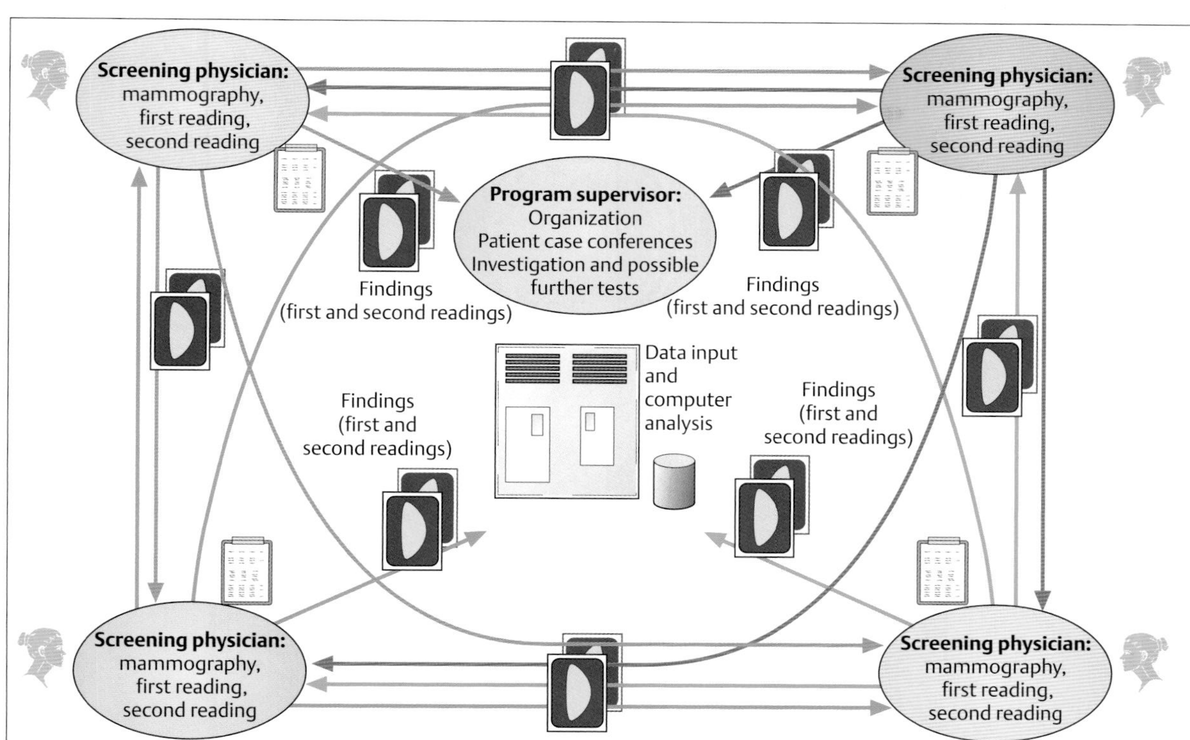


**Fig. 5.40** **Screening workflow without a data network.**

Eighty examinations per day means that 320 mammograms must be placed on a view box and read, the findings recorded, and the films returned to their jackets for further handling and distribution. The physician would have a maximum of 6 minutes for each reading. Meanwhile the radiology technologists must position and x-ray 40 women each day. Given these conditions, the logistics of image acquisition, handling, and reading create a staggering workload with many potential sources of error.

#### *Digital Networking*

It is a logical step, then, to consider digital mammography in setting up a mammographic screening program. Originally (2004), the cooperative group responsible for organizing the screening modalities in Germany planned to allow digital mammography only on a very selective basis. Today (2009), however, most units in Germany employ digital screening, though mainly in the form of storage plate technology. When the screening scenario is changed to include digital mammography, all participating offices should be fully networked to allow for digital information transfer. In this type of system, all mammograms can be digitally processed and stored in a central archive. This can be accomplished by using fully digital mammographic imagers or by digitizing conventional mammograms. The latter can be done locally by the screening physician (if a scanner is available) or centrally as a service of the program supervisor. A screening workflow model with a data network is shown in **Fig. 5.41**.

Image distribution is performed automatically and anonymously based on a specified algorithm. The first reader uploads his or her data and images to the central archive, which is managed by the program supervisor. From there the images are sent via data link or virtual private network (VPN) to another screening physician for a second reading. To ensure confidentiality, the second physician does not know the identity of the physician or of the patient.

All the images are linked to an acquisition template to permit a structured evaluation. The second reading is also uploaded to the central archive, where the software compares both sets of findings and generates worklists for all cases that require further assessment. If both sets of findings agree, reports are automatically printed out for the reader and patient and are distributed via e-mail or postal delivery. All discrepant findings and all BIRADS 4 or BIRADS 5 cases are selected for further assessment (follow-up, interventional procedure such as CNB, or surgery).

In comparing conventional and digital screening modalities it is easy to appreciate that the use of digital equipment is the right way today, and that digital screening saves a lot of time (and money?). Both modalities should be reinvestigated in screening modifications and model projects with single-view digital mammography, high-resolution ultrasound, and physical examination. The goal is to make mass-screening as comfortable, safe, and effective as possible, while limiting radiation exposure to a minimum.

### Capabilities and Limitations of Screening (Pitfalls)

The cases shown in this section illustrate both the capabilities and the limitations of pure mammographic screening. The information content of mammograms is particularly limited in radiographically dense breasts (ACR 2 or higher), even when the images are perfectly exposed and interpreted by highly trained first and second readers. Noncalcifying carcinomas and their precursors as well as lobular carcinomas (approx. 20%) are not the domain of mammography and thus cannot be detected by screening (see **Fig. 5.118**, p. 342) unless the tumor is so extensive that it has produced atypical densities and architectural distortion on mammograms. Interval cancers are most common in radiographically dense breasts and in patients with noncalcifying or lobular neoplasms (see **Figs. 5.42–5.54**).

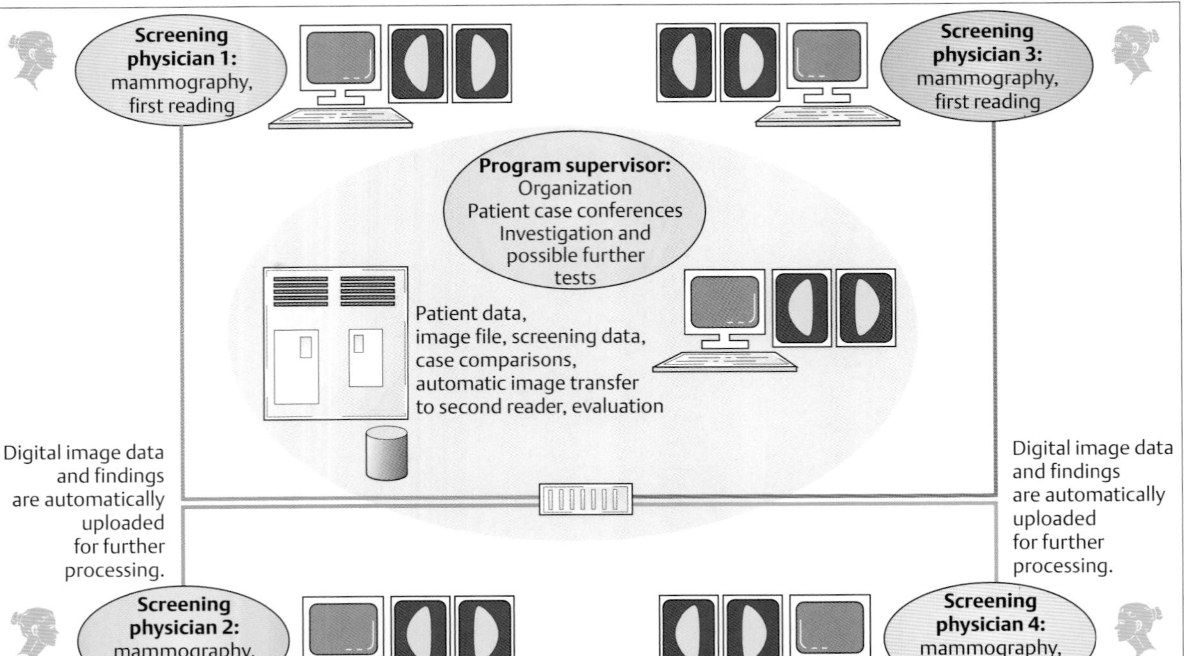


**Fig. 5.41 Screening workflow with a data network.**

**Fig. 5.42 A 69-year-old woman presents for mammographic screening** with no palpable abnormalities. Her mother was diagnosed with breast cancer at age 51, her sister at age 68.

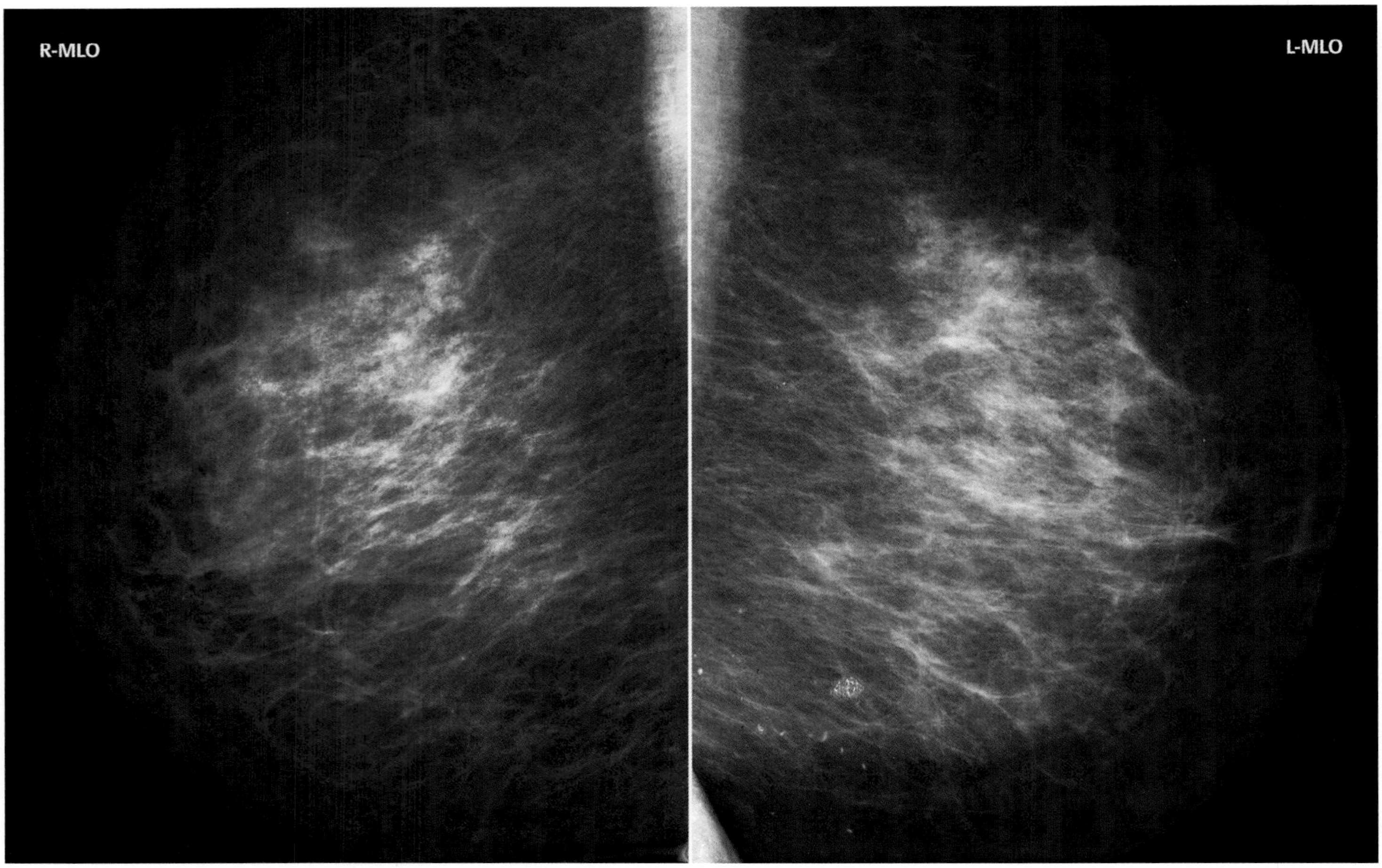

R-MLO

L-MLO

**a** *Bilateral oblique mammograms* (digital full-field mammography) show radiolucent breast parenchyma with microcalcifications in the lower inner quadrant of the left breast (ACR 2, BIRADS?, PG**M**I) (**f–G/5–6**). These findings were not visible in prior mammograms taken 2 years before.

All the mammograms presented in this chapter were produced with the IMS Giotto Image full-field digital mammography system (**Fig. 5.18**) using standard screening protocols. That means that the image data can be compressed with wavelet technology (Image-Diagnost-International, Munich), transmitted via a data link (see **Fig. 5.41**), and decompressed in full quality at a remote workstation for anonymous interpretation (first- and second-reading users, see pp. 100, 107).

**Fig. 5.42 A 69-year-old woman presents for mammographic screening.** *(continued)*

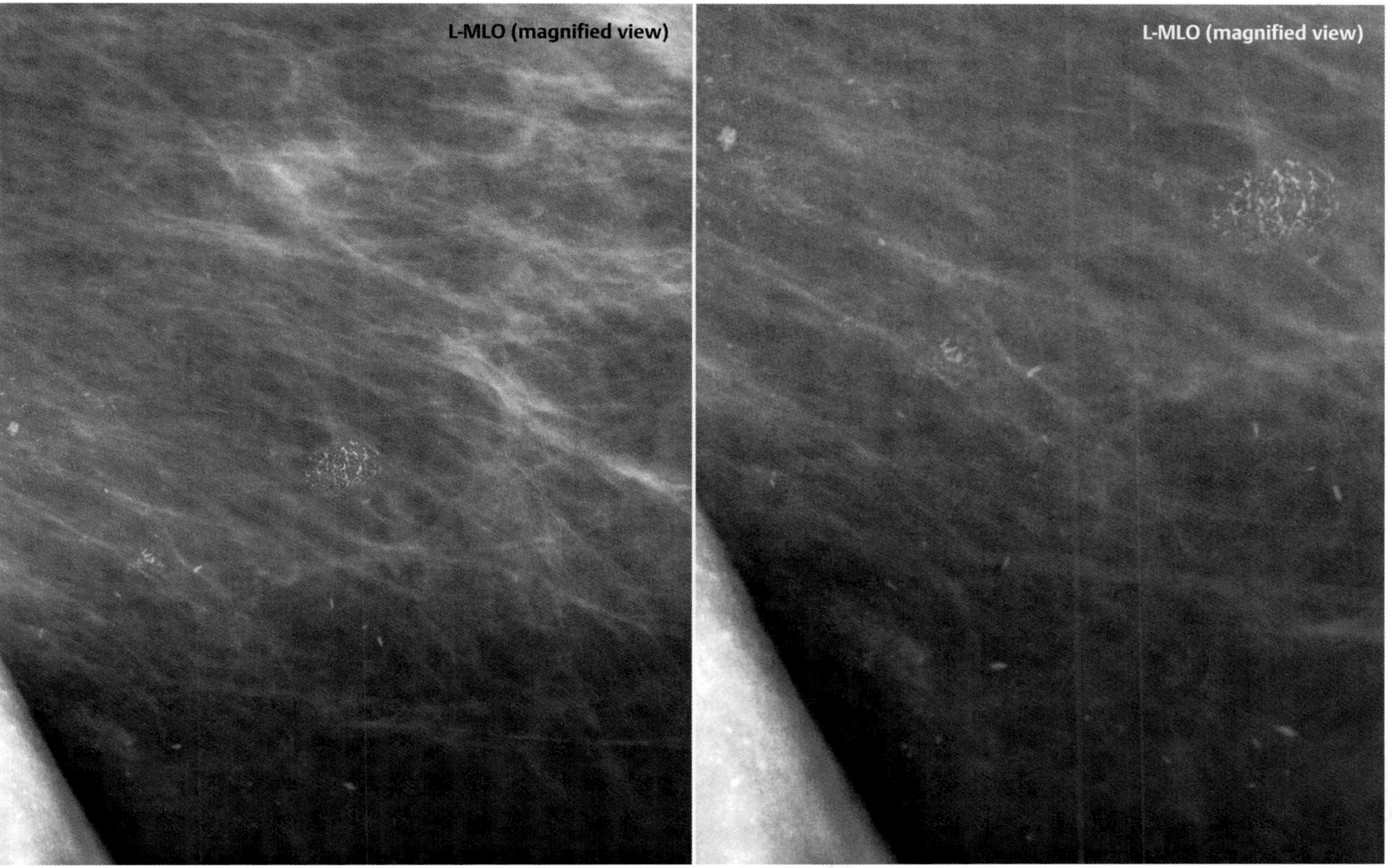


**b** *Mammogram of the left breast* (magnified view, digital full-field mammography). New microcalcifications have appeared in the 2 years since the prior examination.

**Question on Fig. 5.42**

*How would you interpret the calcifications?*

(**a**) Benign
(**b**) Malignant
(**c**) Artifacts

→ **Answer on p. 359**

**Fig. 5.43** **Bilateral oblique mammograms in a patient with no palpable abnormalities.**

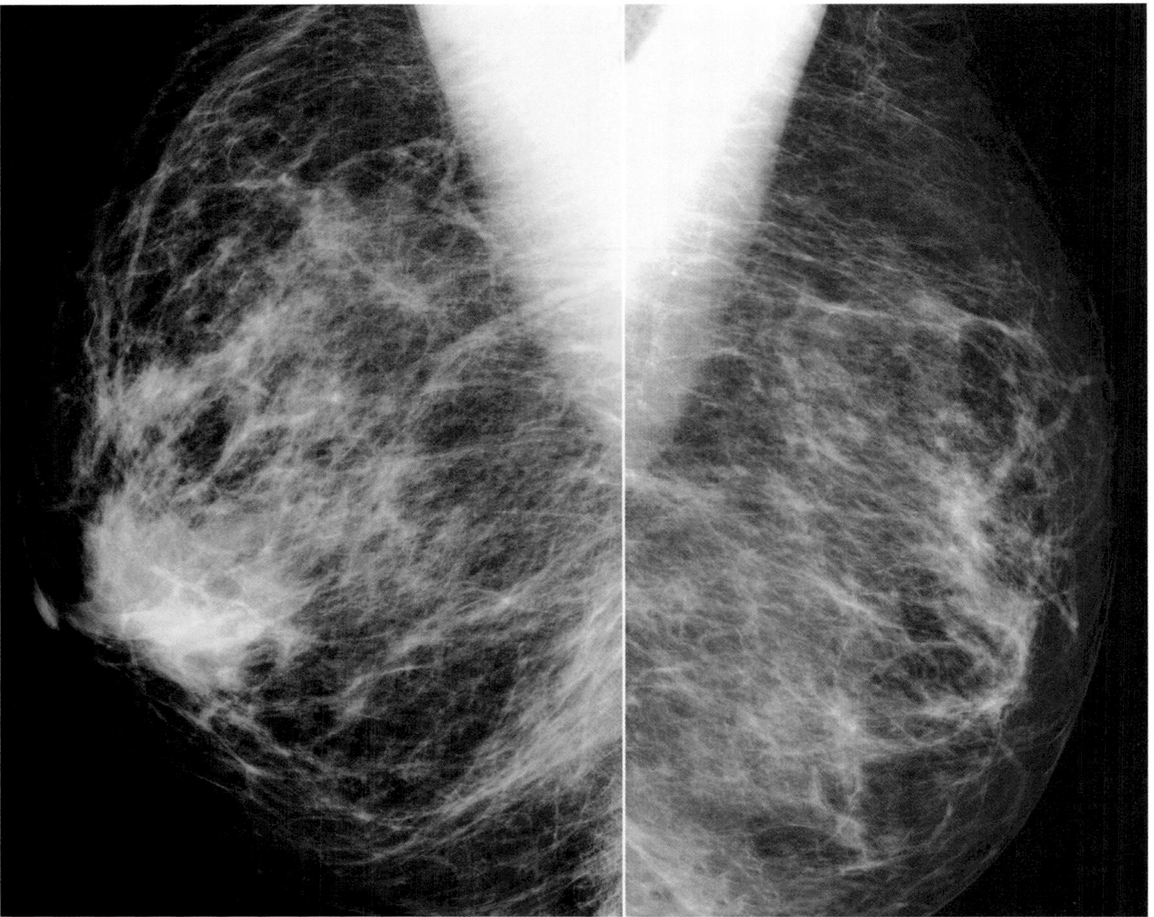

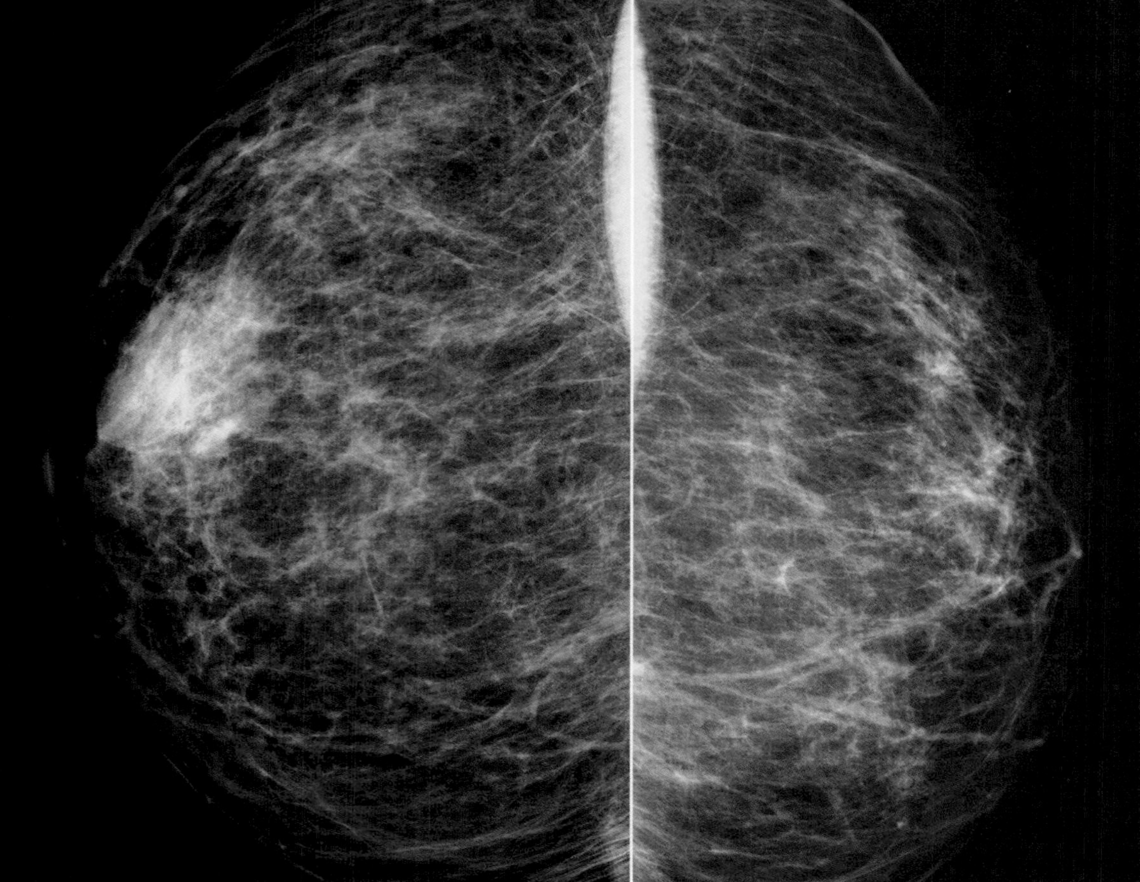

**a, b** *Bilateral craniocaudal mammograms.*

**Question on Fig. 5.43**

*Recall?*

(**a**) No

(**b**) Yes

(**c**) Routine follow-up in 2 years

→ **Answer on p. 360**

**Fig. 5.44** **A 42-year-old woman presents for mammographic screening.**

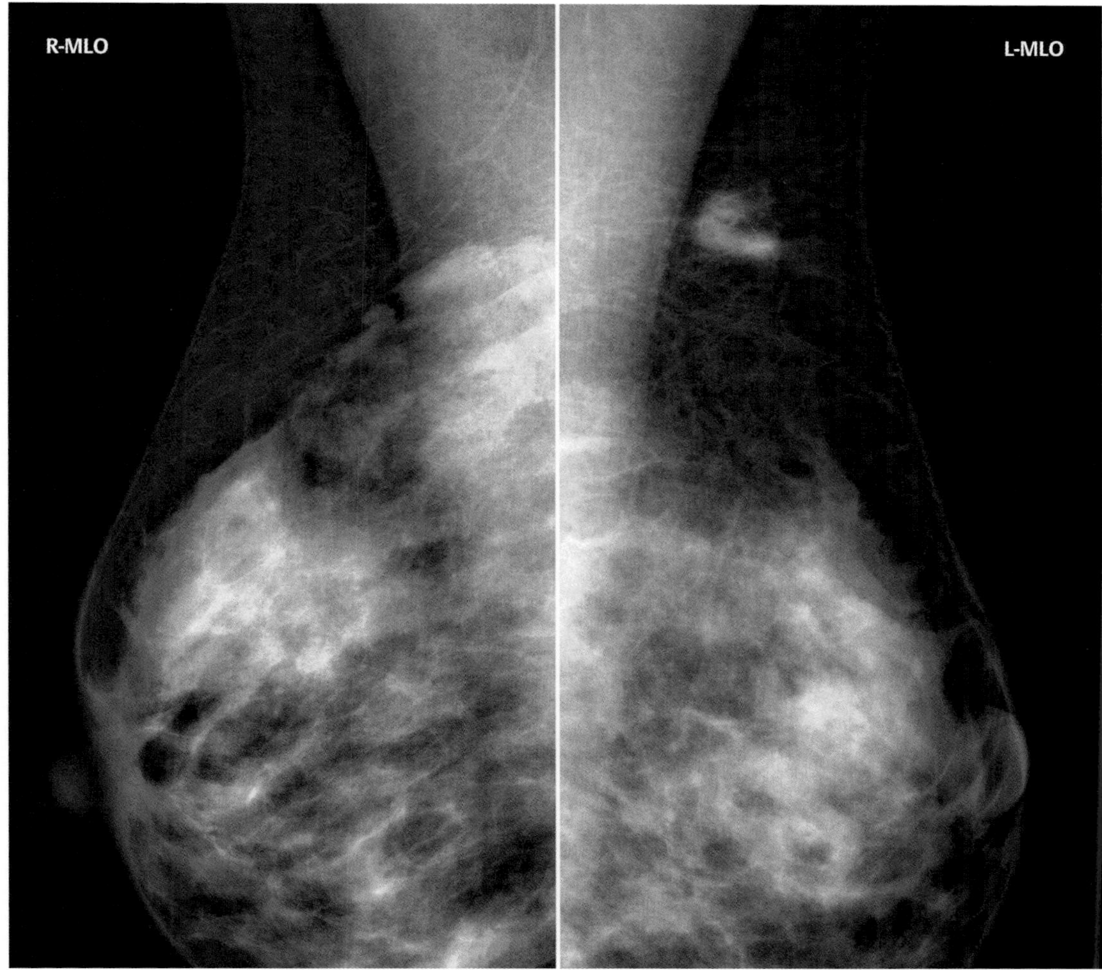


**a** *Bilateral oblique mammograms* show dense, inhomogeneous breast parenchyma (ACR 3, **P**GMI).

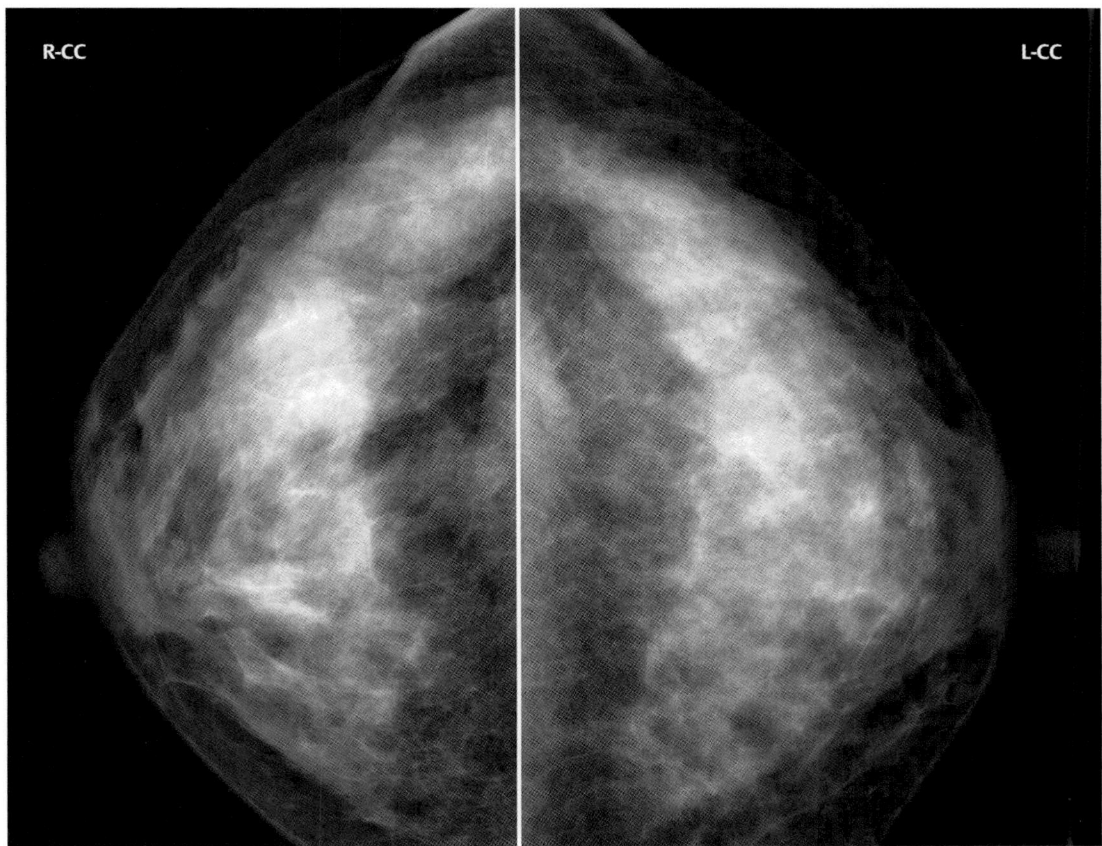


**b** *Bilateral craniocaudal mammograms* show relatively dense, inhomogeneous parenchyma. The right craniocaudal view cuts off some of the lateral portion of the right breast (ACR 3, P**G**MI).

**Question on Fig. 5.44**

*Should this patient be recalled?*

(**a**) No

(**b**) Recall

(**c**) Routine follow-up in 2 years

→ **Answer on p. 360**

**Fig. 5.45** **A 53-year-old woman presents for mammographic screening.** She has no palpable lymph node enlargement.

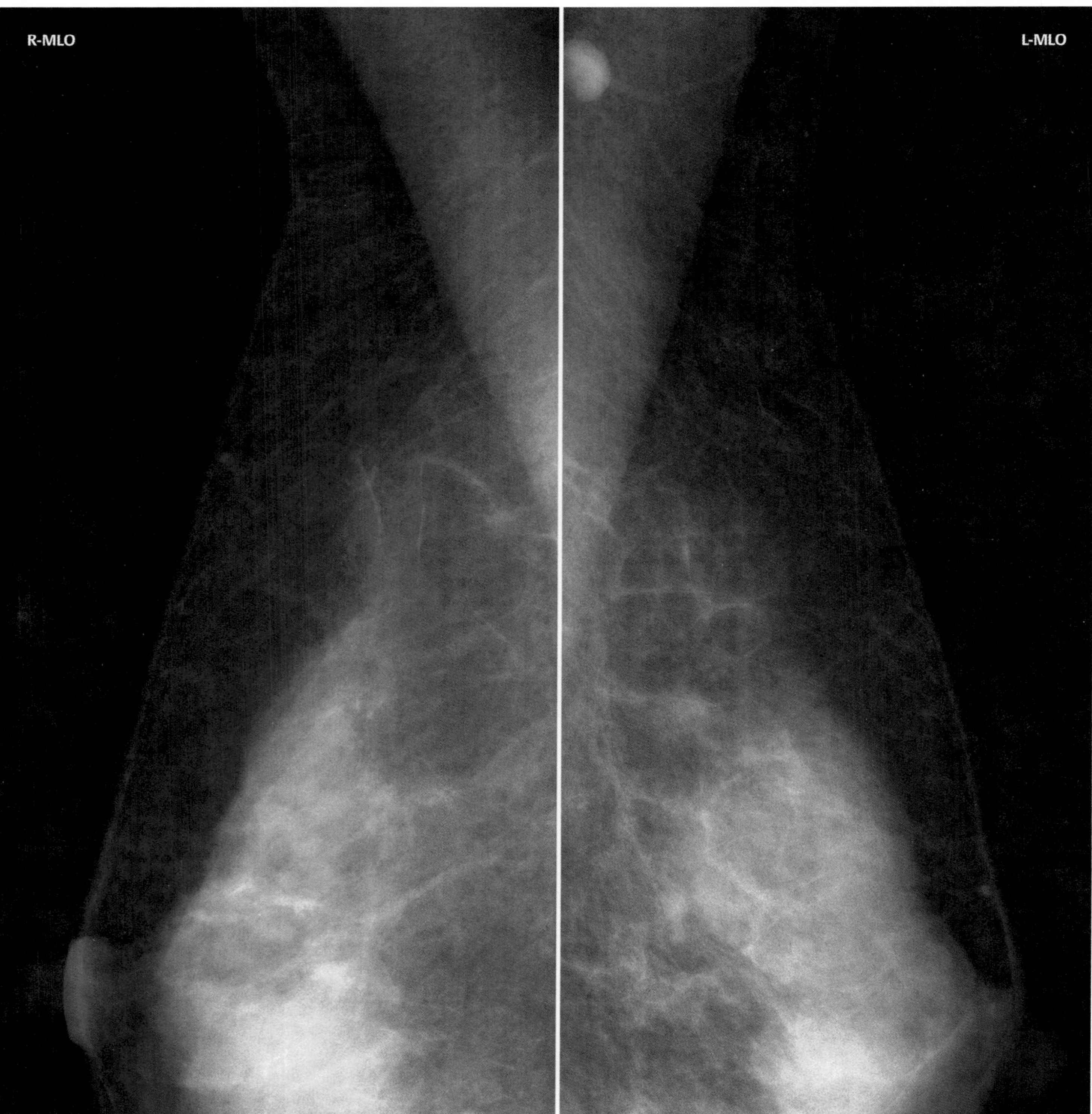


**a** *Bilateral oblique mammograms* (magnified views of the upper quadrants and axilla). The glandular tissue of both breasts is normal but relatively dense (ACR 3). A small nodule is visible in the left axilla (**F/26–27**) (P**G**MI).

**Question on Fig. 5.45**

*How would you interpret the findings?*

(**a**) Pathologic process in the left breast with lymph node metastasis (coordinates?)
(**b**) Normal breast parenchyma with normal lymph nodes
(**c**) Skin wart

→ **Answer on p. 360**

**Fig. 5.46** **A 69-year-old woman presents for screening with a prior history of trauma to the right breast.**

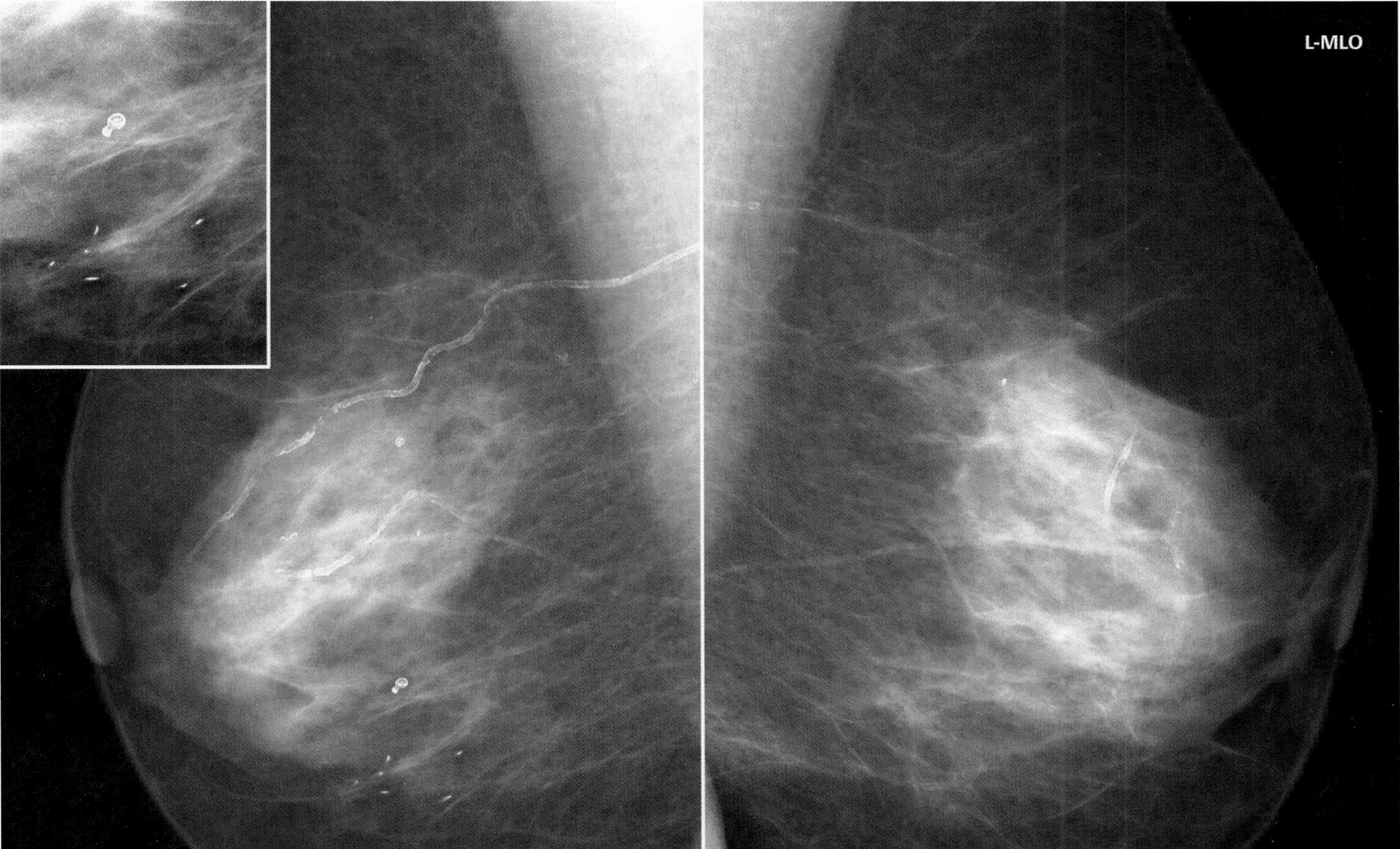


**a** *Oblique mammogram of the right breast* shows radiodense breast parenchyma with extensive vascular calcifications (ACR 3, **P**GMI). The inset at upper left is a spot view of the calcifications (**M–n/17**).

**b** *Oblique mammogram of the left breast* shows radiodense breast with isolated vascular calcifications (ACR 2, **P**GMI). As there were no abnormalities in the oblique view, the craniocaudal view was omitted.

**Question on Fig. 5.46**

*What course of action would you recommend?*

(**a**) Routine follow-up in two years

(**b**) Recall due to findings in the left breast (coordinates?)

(**c**) Recall due to findings in the right breast (coordinates?)

→ **Answer on p. 361**

**Fig. 5.47** **A 32-year-old woman presents for screening.**

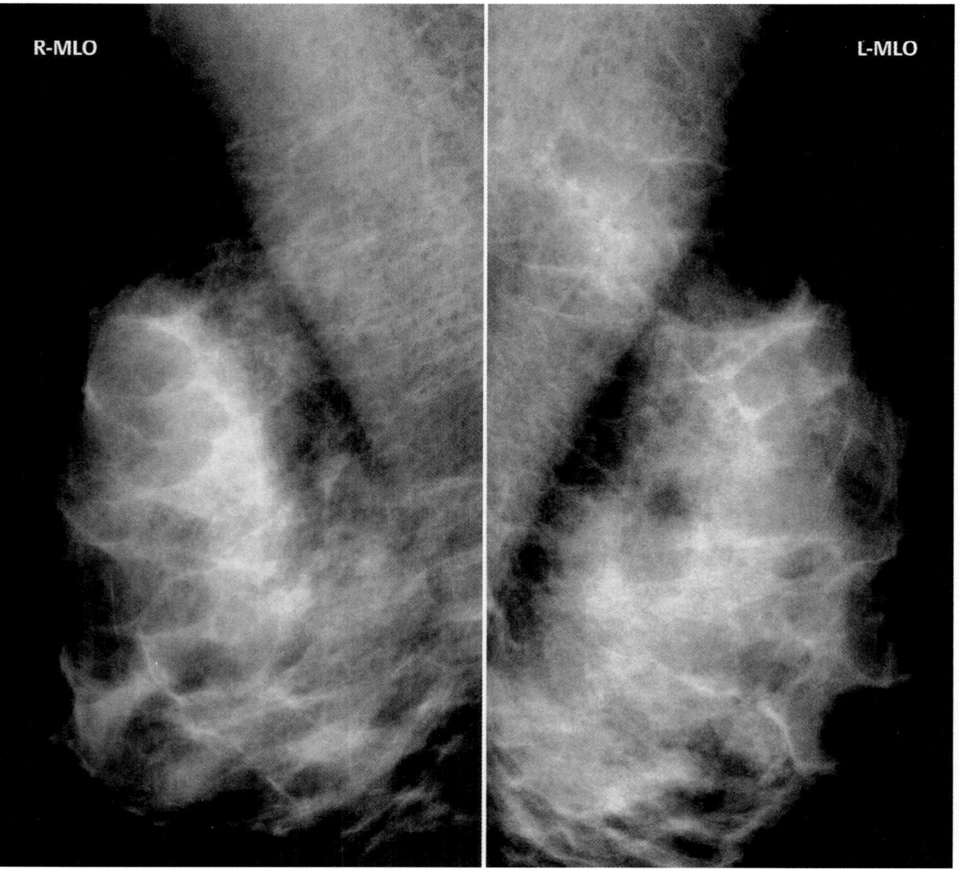


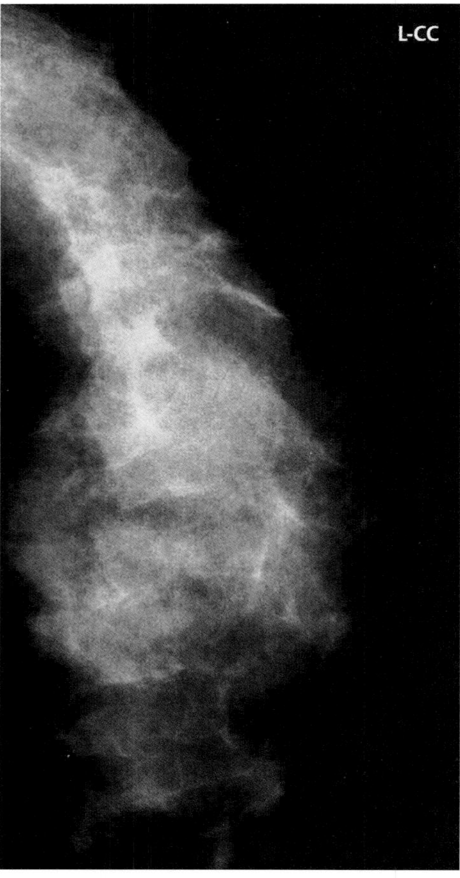


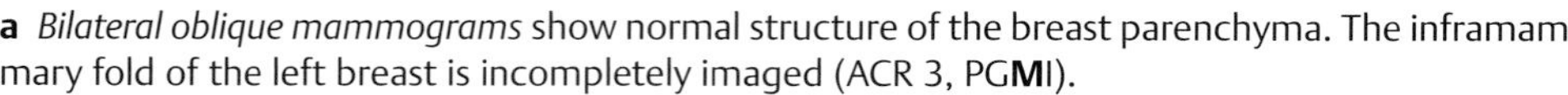

**a** *Bilateral oblique mammograms* show normal structure of the breast parenchyma. The inframammary fold of the left breast is incompletely imaged (ACR 3, PG**M**I).

**b** *Craniocaudal mammogram* of the left breast shows relatively dense breast parenchyma. A portion of the lateral region (**H/27**) is incompletely imaged (ACR 2, PGM**I**).

**Question on Fig. 5.47**

*What is the level of suspicion in this case?*

(**a**) BIRADS 2
(**b**) BIRADS 3 (4 a) (coordinates?)
(**c**) BIRADS 4 (4 b) (coordinates?)

→ **Answer on p. 361**

**Fig. 5.48 A 62-year-old woman presents for screening. She has neoplasms in both breasts.** The tumor in one breast is a well-differentiated (G1) carcinoma in situ (DCIS). The tumor in the opposite breast is a poorly differentiated (G3) invasive ductal carcinoma. There are no palpable abnormalities in either breast, and there is no skin or nipple retraction.

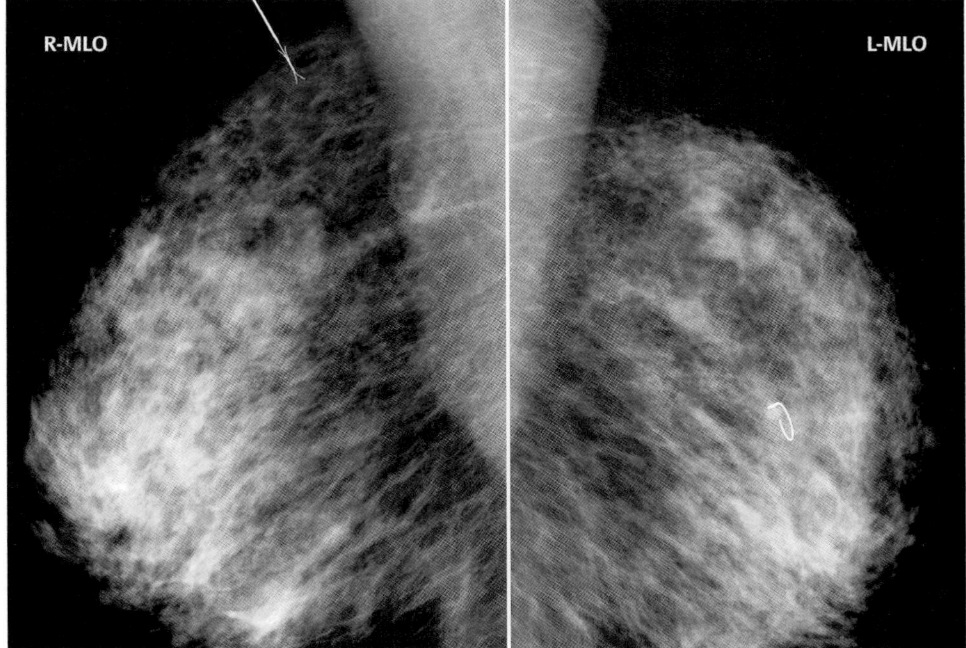


**a** *Bilateral oblique mammograms* (localization films). The calcifications in the right breast are located directly below the localization wire and are not visible (see (**c**). The left mammogram shows normal breast parenchyma with a wire marker at **P/21** (ACR 3, **P**GMI; right BIRADS 4, left BIRADS 1).

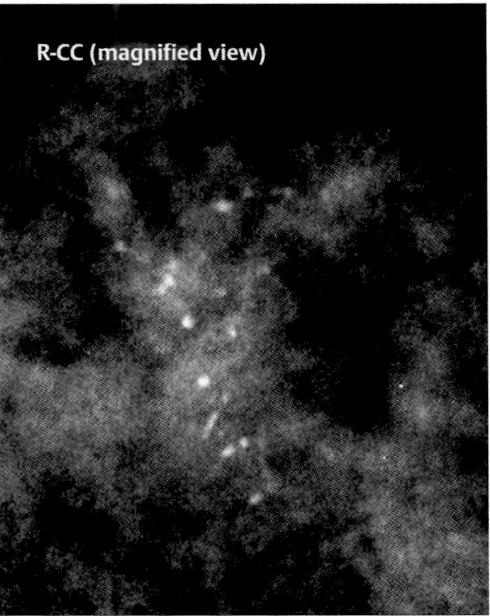


**c** *Craniocaudal mammogram* of the right breast. Magnification view shows relatively pleomorphic microcalcifications in the upper outer quadrant (BIRADS 4).

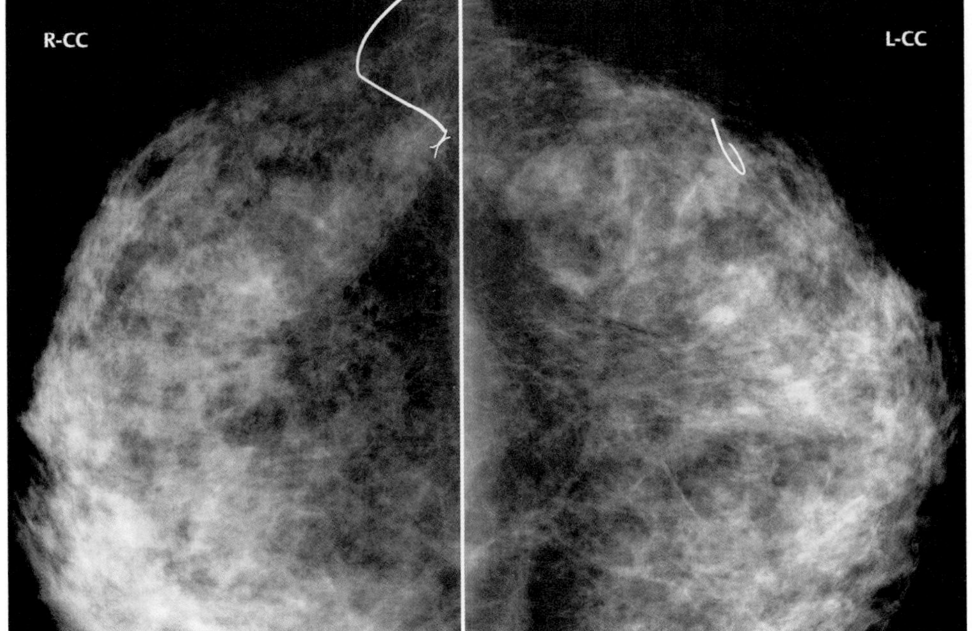


**b** *Bilateral craniocaudal mammograms* (localization films). The localization wire is incorrectly positioned behind the calcifications (see p. 299). The left mammogram shows fairly radiodense breast parenchyma with a nonspecific density near the localization wire (ACR 3, right BIRADS 4, left BIRADS 1, P**G**MI).

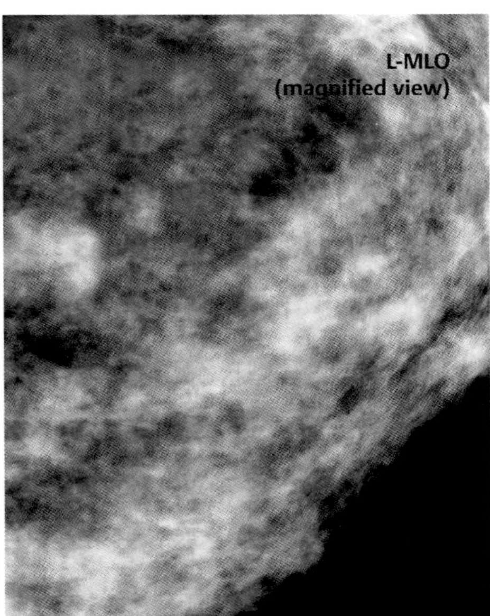


**d** *Mediolateral oblique mammogram* of the left breast, magnified view of the lower quadrant in the localization area. The mammogram appears normal, showing no suspicious focal densities and no microcalcifications.

▶ Fig. 5.48 e–g

**Fig. 5.48** **A 62-year-old woman presents for screening. She has neoplasms in both breasts.** *(continued)*

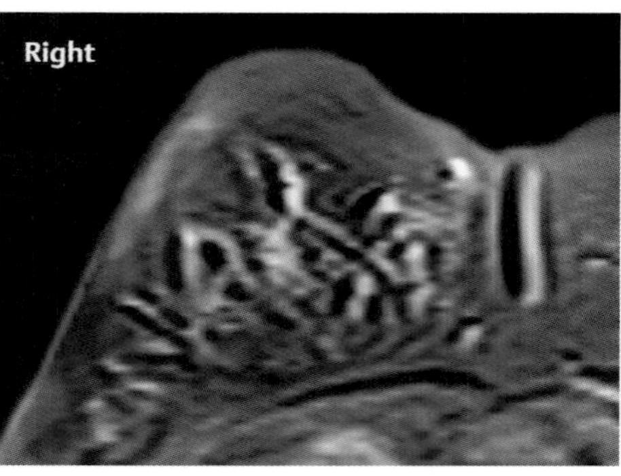


**e** *MR subtraction* image of the upper quadrant of the right breast. Gadolinium enhancement does not occur in the area of the microcalcifications (**B/24–25**).

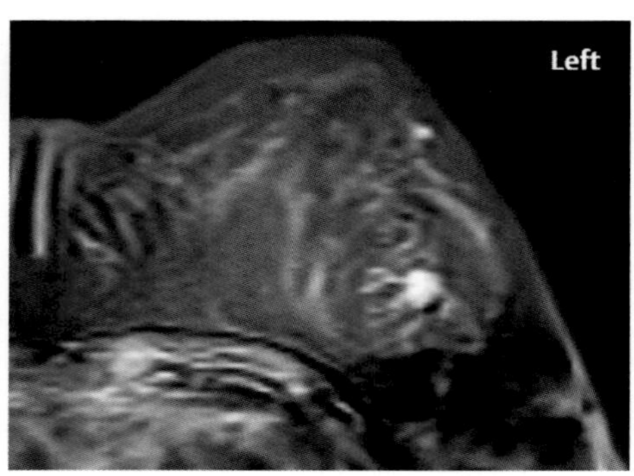


**f** *MR subtraction* image of the lower outer quadrant of the left breast shows an intensely enhancing 1 cm × 1.2 cm×1 cm nodule with ill-defined margins and an atypical time–density curve.

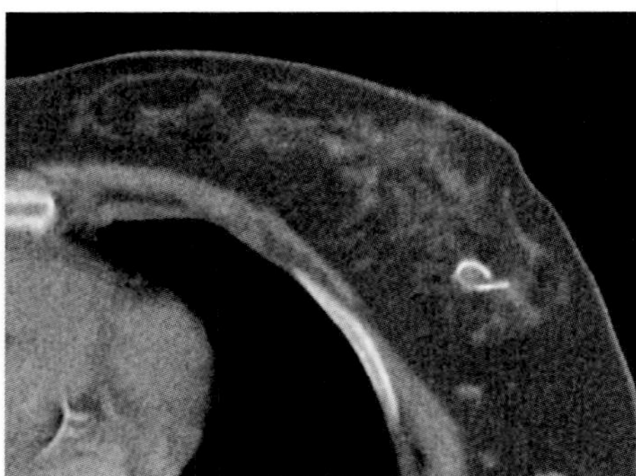

**g** *CT scan* of the lower outer quadrant of the left breast. Localization film after bolus contrast injection shows the curved localizing needle, but the enhancing nodule is obscured by the metal.

**Question on Fig. 5.48**

*In which breast does the invasive ductal G3 carcinoma appear to be located?*

(**a**) Left
(**b**) Right
(**c**) May be in either breast

→ **Answer on p. 362**

**Fig. 5.49** **A 62-year-old woman presents for mammography** because of elevated ferritin levels in her blood (which may occur in malignant diseases such as pancreatic, liver or lung cancer). She has no palpable breast abnormalities.

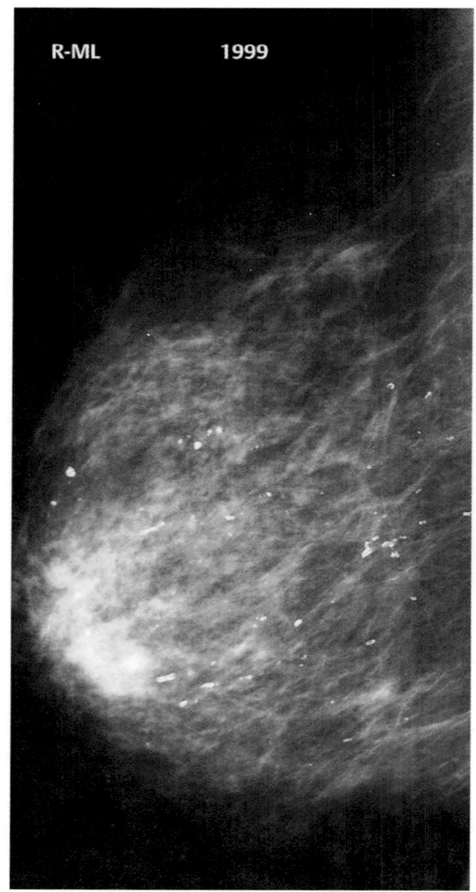


**a** *Mediolateral mammogram* of the right breast in 1999 shows coarse calcifications similar to those in plasma cell mastitis, but no lesions are detected (ACR 3, BIRADS 2, PGMI).

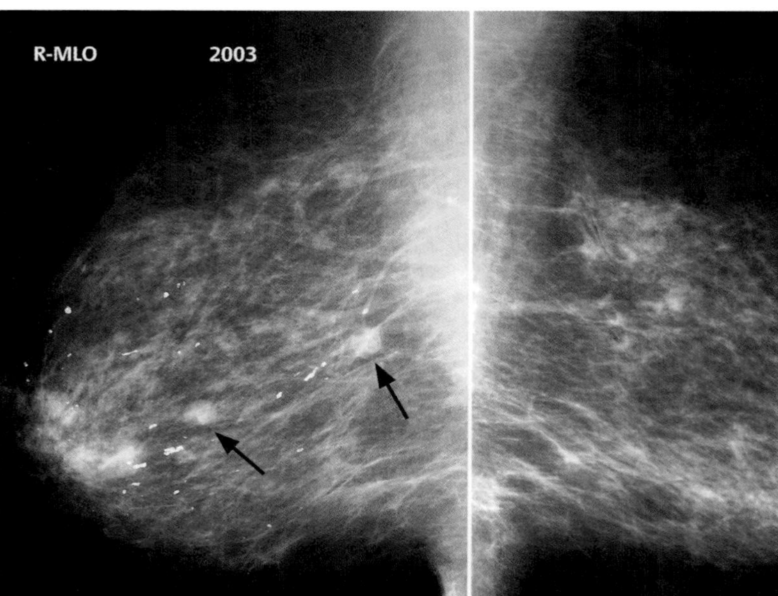


**b** *Bilateral oblique mammograms* in 2003 show increasingly lucent breast parenchyma with two new cystlike opacities (arrows) und unchanged calcifications in the right breast. The left breast appears normal and unchanged relative to the previous examination (ACR 2, BIRADS 3, **P**GMI).

**Fig. 5.49** **A 62-year-old woman presents for mammography.** *(continued)*

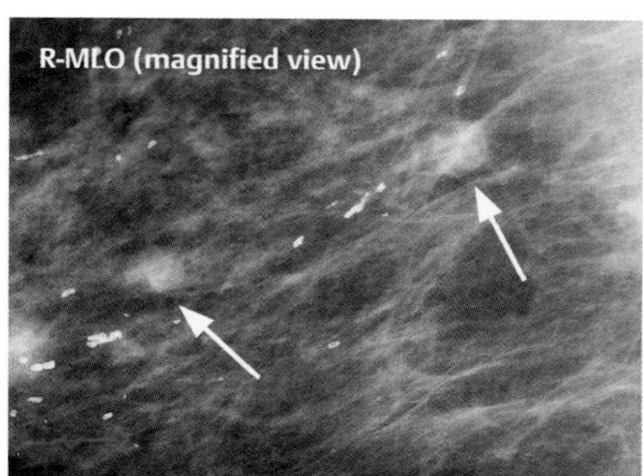


**c** *Oblique mammogram* of the right breast. Spot view of both opacities (indicated by arrows).

**Question on Fig. 5.49**

*What course of action would you recommend?*

(**a**) Follow-up in 12 months

(**b**) Follow-up in 6 months

(**c**) Histologic evaluation (FNA, CNB) of the right breast

→ **Answer on p. 362**

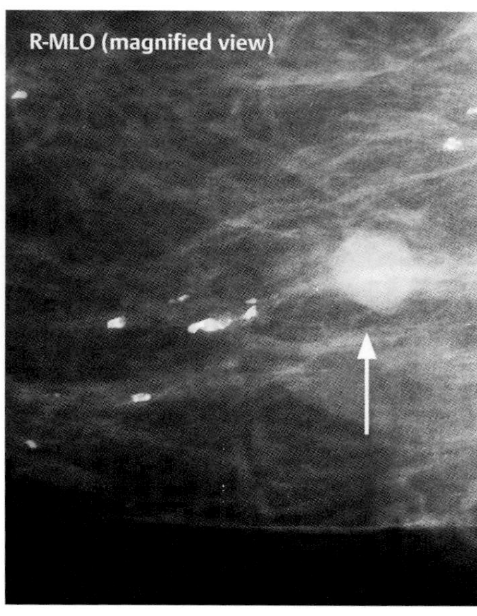


**d** *Craniocaudal mammogram* of the right breast, spot view. The lesion near the chest wall appears as a well-circumscribed nodule with no calcifications (obscured by fibrous septa within the breast parenchyma).

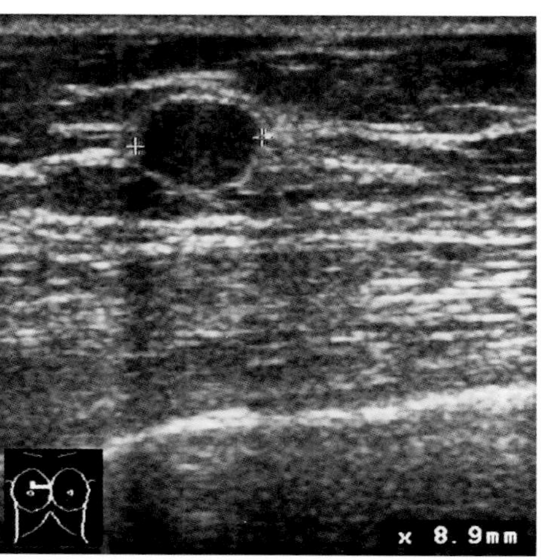


**e** *Sonogram* of the nodule near the chest wall shows a 9.5 mm × 8.9 mm focus with smooth margins, faint internal echoes, and apparently faint posterior acoustic enhancement or lateral edge shadows behind the tangentially scanned wall segments (**R/22–26** and **S/22–26**).

**Fig. 5.50** **A 50-year-old woman presents for screening** with visible pigmentation changes but no palpable breast abnormalities.

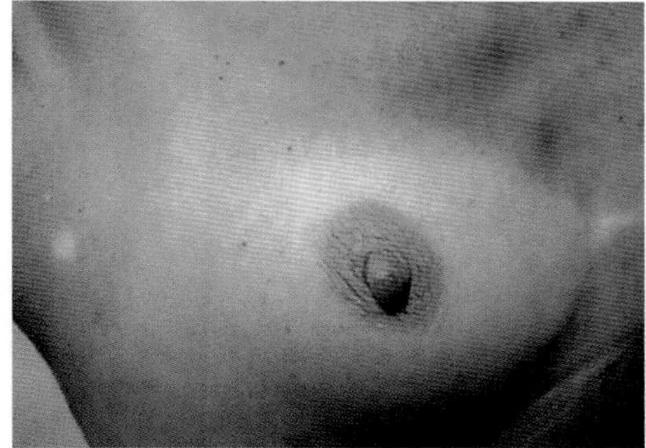

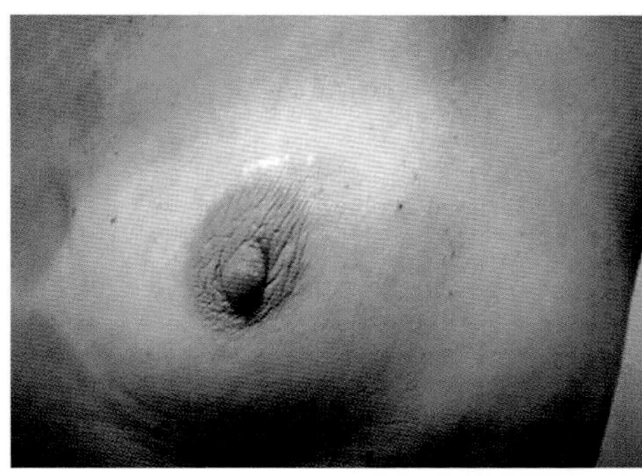

**a** *Clinical inspection* of the left and right breasts reveals slight deviation of the left nipple toward the lower outer quadrant. Pigmentation changes are visible at **K/13, m/12–13** and **l/8**.

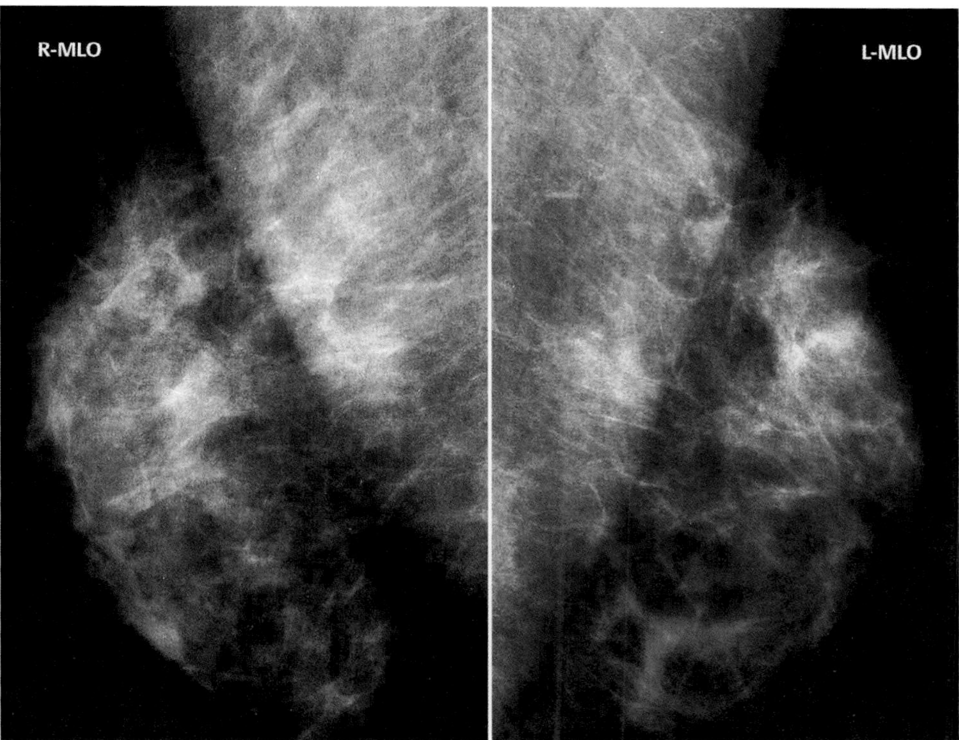


**b** *Bilateral oblique mammograms* show relatively radiodense breasts with focal densities (ACR 3, BIRADS 1, **P**GMI).

▶ **Fig. 5.50 c**

**Fig. 5.50** **A 50-year-old woman presents for screening.** *(continued)*

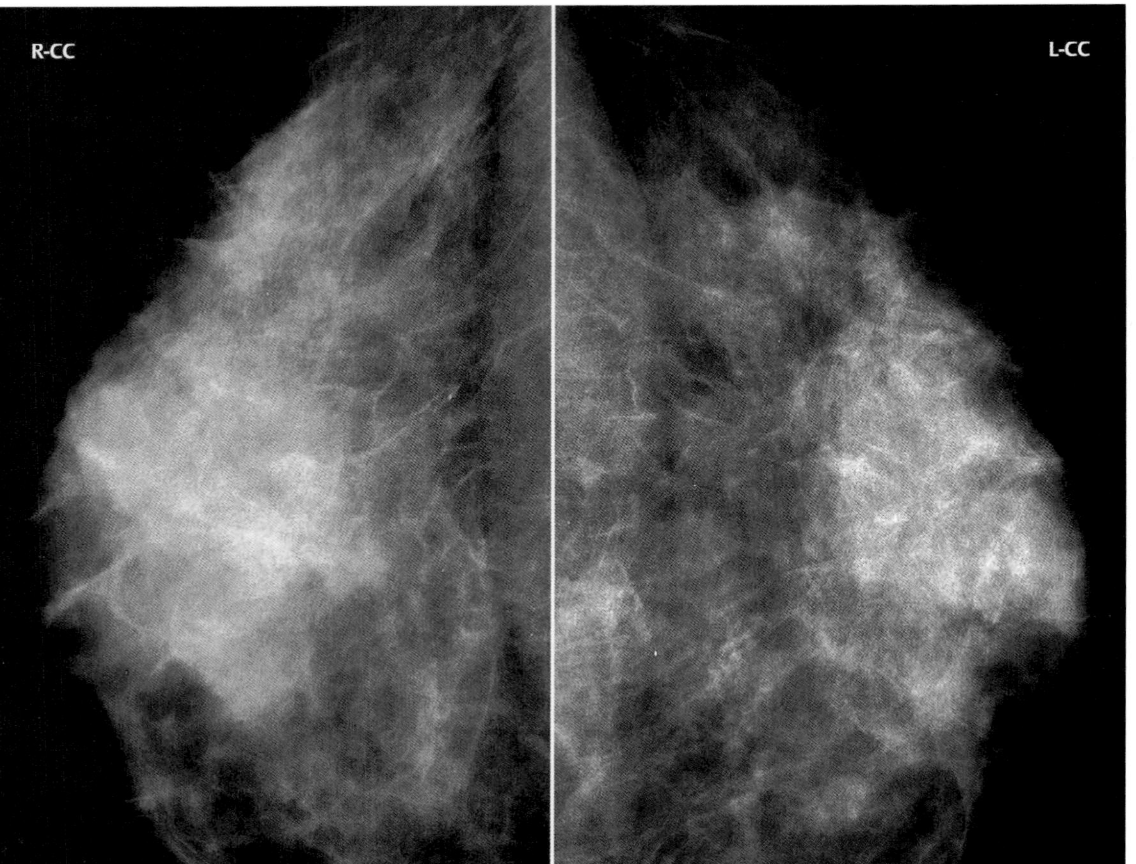


**c** *Bilateral craniocaudal mammograms* show radiodense parenchyma in the retroareolar region on both sides. The pectoral muscle is clearly visualized (ACR 3, BIRADS 1, **P**GMI).

**Question 1 on Fig. 5.50**

*The skin changes are due to*

(**a**) Vitiligo
(**b**) Pigmented nevi
(**c**) Both

→ **Answer on p. 363**

**Question 2 on Fig. 5.50**

*Should this patient be recalled? (More than one answer is possible.)*

(**a**) No
(**b**) Yes, because of a focal lesion (give craniocaudal and oblique coordinates)
(**c**) Yes, because of the ACR 3 density

→ **Answer on p. 363**

**Fig. 5.51** **A 35-year-old woman presents for screening due to a positive family history.** Mammograms were taken in March, 2001, and July, 2002 (abnormalities were noted in 2002).

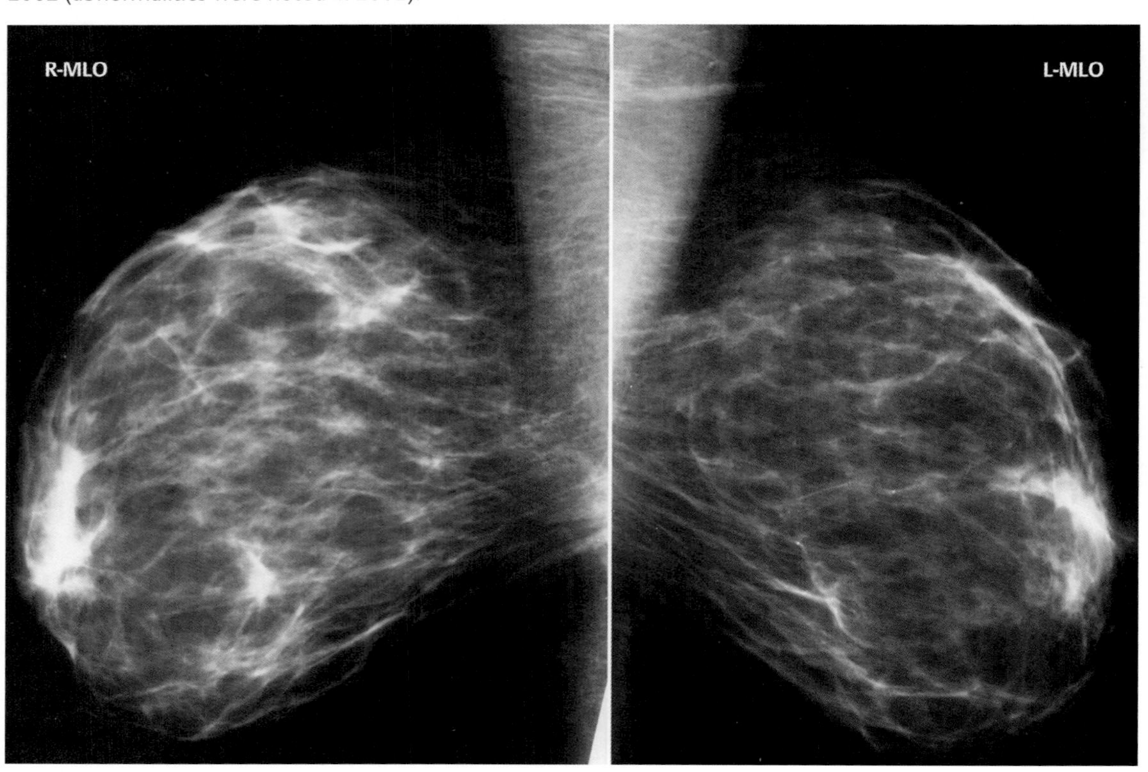


**a** *Bilateral oblique mammograms* in 200**?** show radiolucent breast parenchyma. Both breasts are perfectly positioned (ACR 2, BIRADS 1, **P**GMI).

**Fig. 5.51** **A 35-year-old woman presents for screening due to a positive family history.** *(continued)*

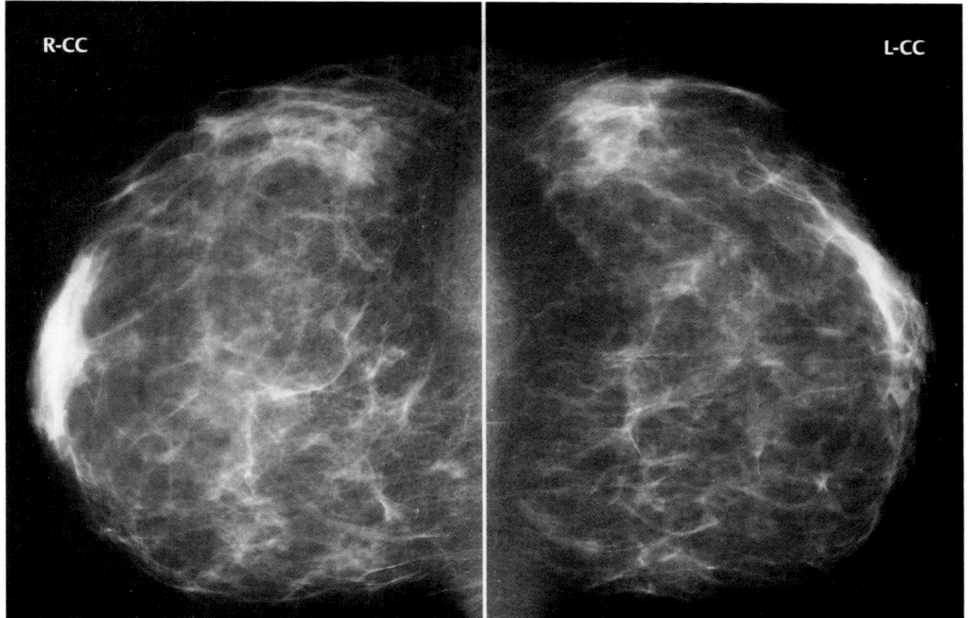


**b** *Bilateral craniocaudal mammograms* in 200? show radiolucent breasts, which again are perfectly positioned (ACR 2, BIRADS 1, **P**GMI).

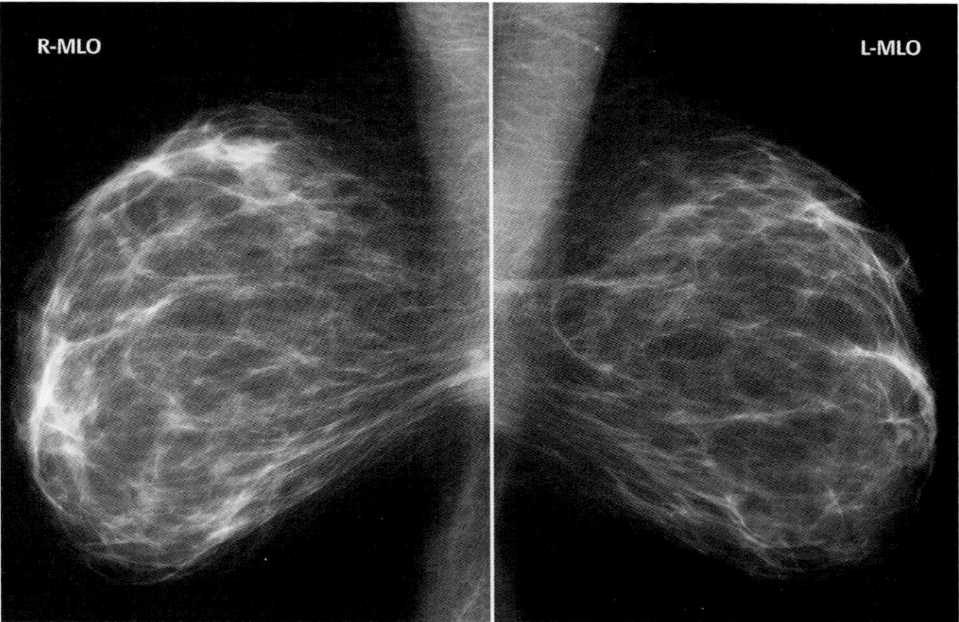


**c** *Bilateral oblique mammograms* in 200? show radiolucent breasts (ACR 2, BIRADS 1, **P**GMI).

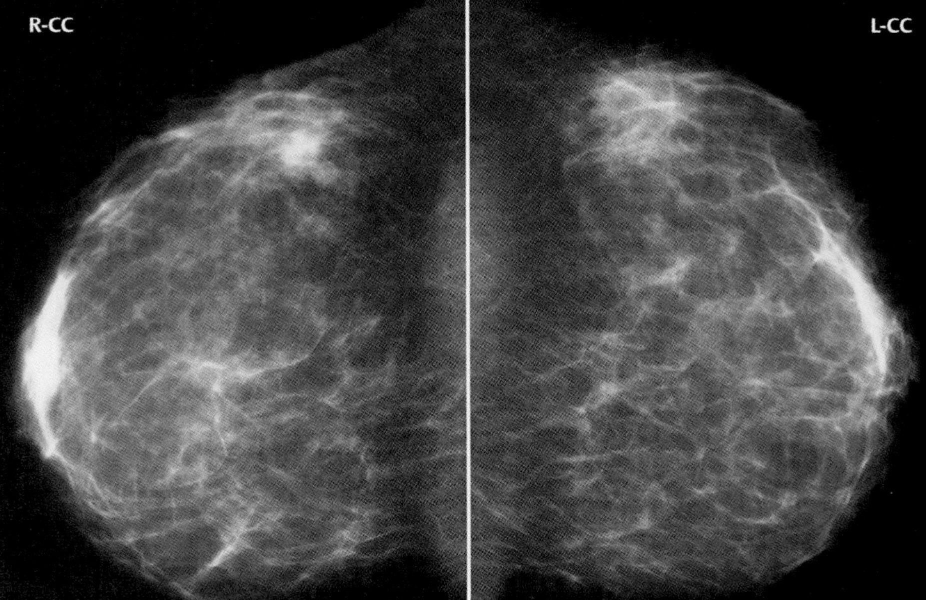


**d** *Bilateral craniocaudal mammograms* in 200?. Status is identical to the findings in **c** (ACR 2, BIRADS 1, **P**GMI).

**Question 1 on Fig. 5.51**

*Which pairs of images are from 2002?*

(**a**) **a, b**
(**b**) **c, d**
(**c**) Cannot be determined

→ **Answer on p. 363**

**Question 2 on Fig. 5.51**

*What action was taken in 2002?*

(**a**) Follow-up in 2 years (screening interval)
(**b**) Recall due to a focal lesion
(**c**) Recall due to radiographic breast density (ACR 2)

→ **Answer on p. 364**

**Fig. 5.52** **An 80-year-old woman presents for screening.**

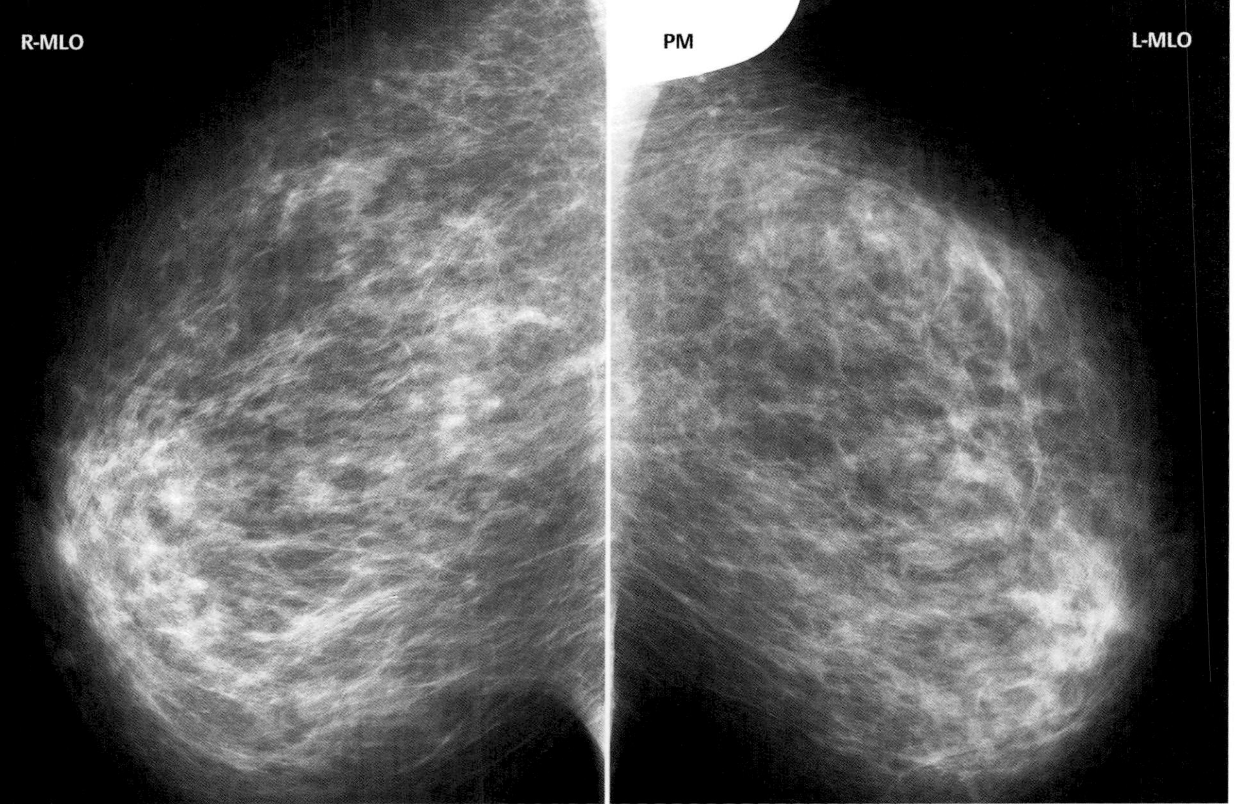


**a** *Bilateral oblique mammograms* show radiodense breasts with no apparent abnormalities (ACR 3, BIRADS 1, PG**M**I). A pacemaker (PM) is visible above the left breast (**e–f/27–28**).

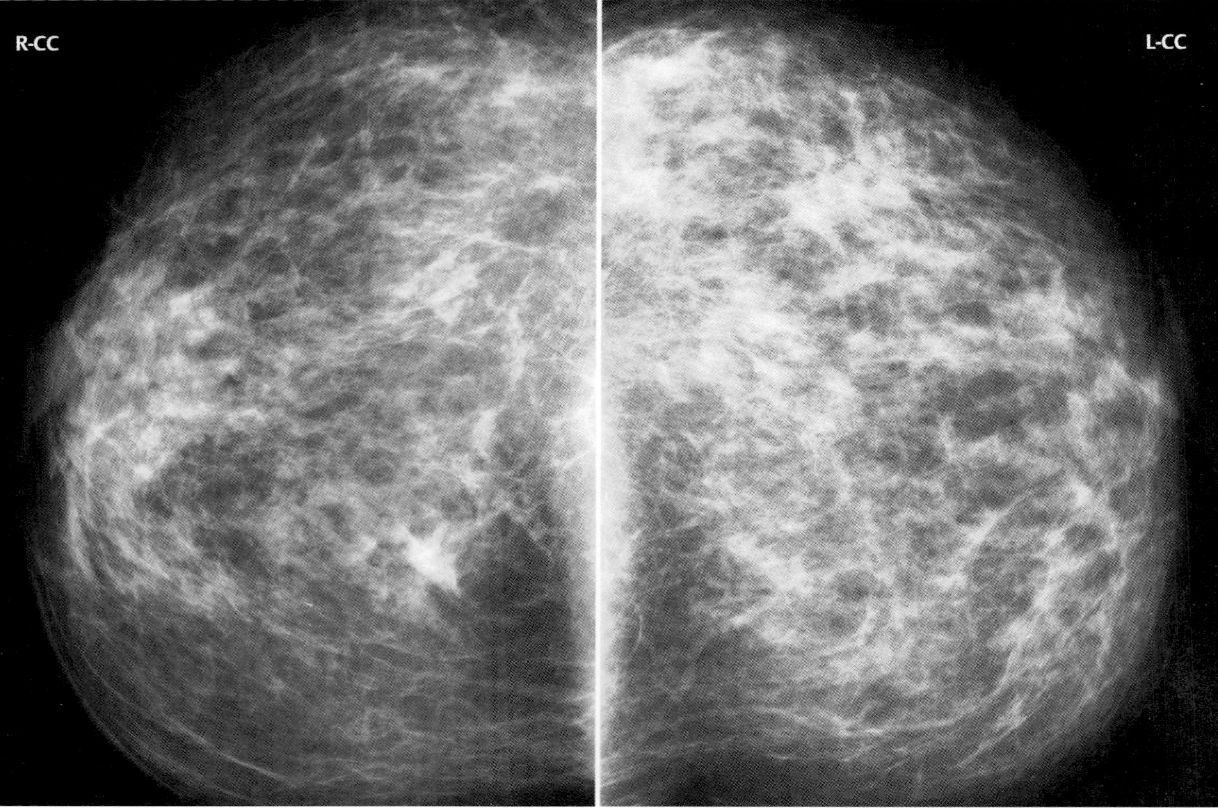


**b** *Bilateral craniocaudal mammograms* show radiodense breasts (ACR 3, BIRADS 1, **P**GMI). The lateral portion of the left breast is particularly dense because of the pacemaker (fibrous encapsulation?).

**Question on Fig. 5.52**

*What course of action would you recommend?*

(**a**) Routine follow-up in two years (screening interval)
(**b**) Recall due to a focal lesion
(**c**) Recall due to radiographic breast density

→ **Answer on p. 364**

**Fig. 5.53 A 77-year-old woman presents for screening** with relative macromastia. The breasts are very nodular, but there are no suspicious palpable findings.

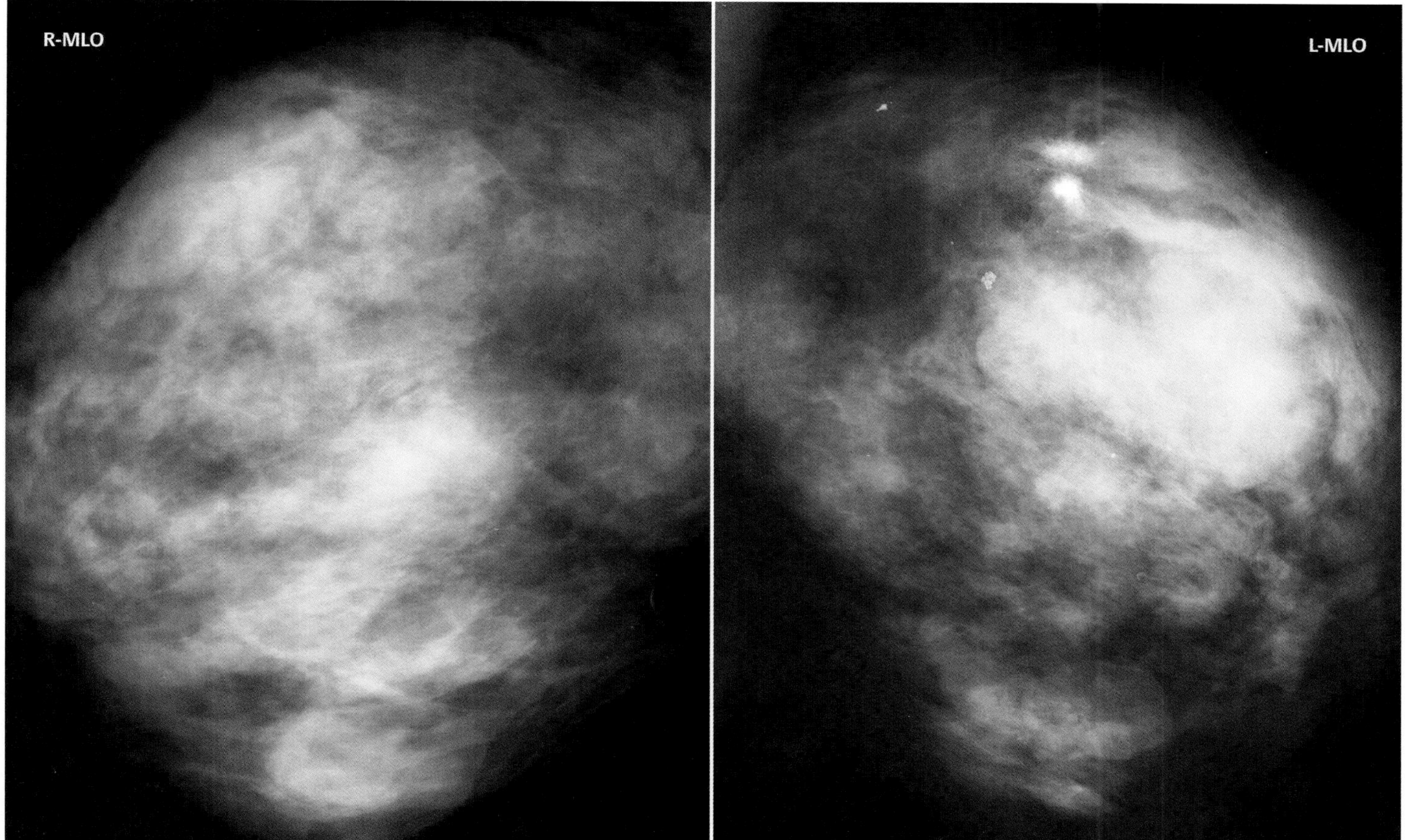


**a** *Bilateral mediolateral mammograms* show dense breasts with numerous confluent homogeneous and inhomogeneous, partly well-defined and partly ill-defined densities as in fibrocystic disease. Because of the breast size, the pectoral muscle is not visible and the posterior breast tissue is incompletely imaged (ACR 4, BIRADS?, PGMI). Craniocaudal mammograms are not suspicious and therefore are not shown.

**Question on Fig. 5.53**

*What course of action would you recommend?*

(**a**) Routine follow-up in two years (screening interval)
(**b**) Recall due strictly to high radiographic density
(**c**) Recall due to a suspected tumor (give coordinates)

→ **Answer on p. 365**

28 27 26 25 24 23 22 21 20 19 18 17 16 15 14 13 12 11 10 9 8 7 6 5 4 3 2 1

K k L l M m N n O o P p Q q R r S s T t

**Fig. 5.54 A 38-year-old woman recently noticed a nonspecific firmness in the pectoral muscle above the left breast (a).** Mammography shows a relatively dense breast (**b**) while ultrasound shows a nodule with smooth margins (**c**). No suspicious lesions are found at subsequent MRI (**d**). Histologic examination reveals a poorly differentiated (G3) invasive ductal neoplasm with a minimal stromal component. The nodule is ultimately removed with clear margins.

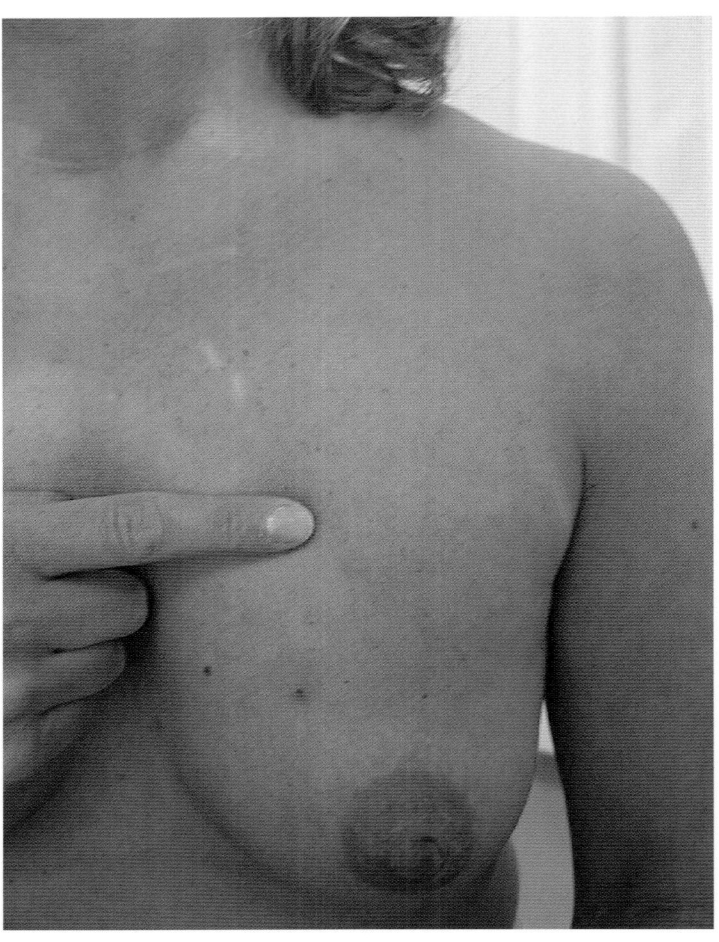

**a** *Physical examination* of the left breast reveals a nonspecific firmness above the breast in the pectoral muscle region (**C/19**). A scar following removal of a mole several years ago is visible at **b/21–22**.

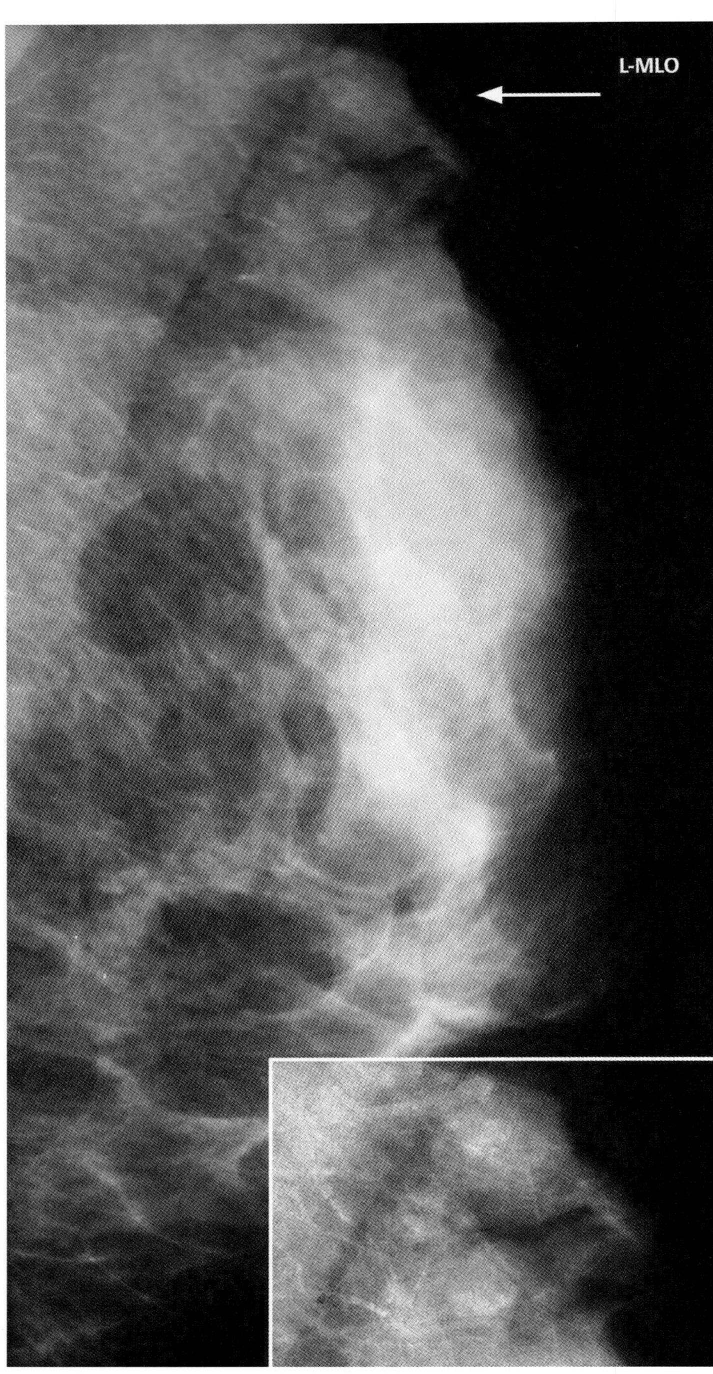


**b** *Oblique mammogram* of the left breast reveals stroma-rich parenchyma. Nonspecific densities are visible at the upper border of the breast (arrow) (ACR 3, BIRADS 2, PGMI). Spot film at lower right shows the palpable mass as a round opacity on the pectoral muscle, devoid of microcalcifications (mass not visible in the craniocaudal view).

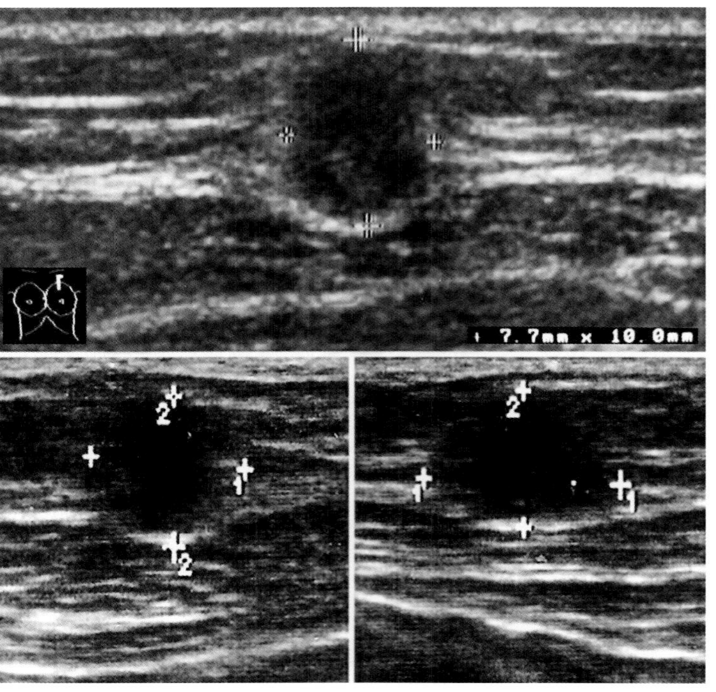


**c** *Sonograms* of the left chest wall. *Upper image* shows a 10.0 mm × 7.7 mm nodule with relatively smooth margins and questionable infiltration of the pectoral fascia and muscle (11 MHz transducer). *Lower images* with a 7.5 MHz transducer demonstrate the smooth margins but give markedly poorer resolution of tumor details.

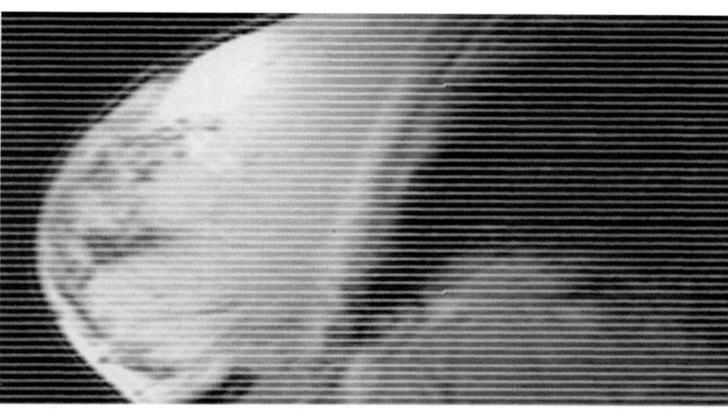

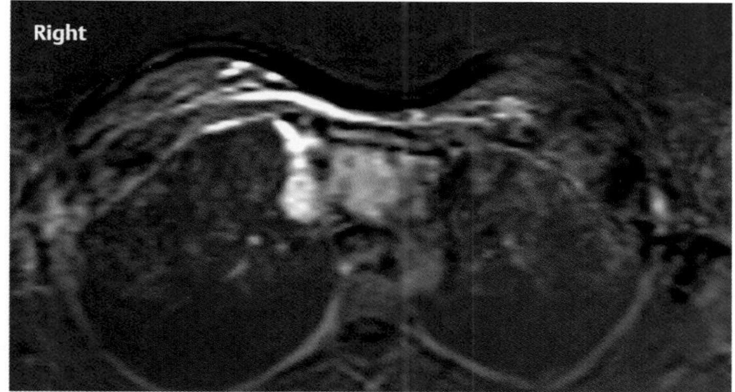


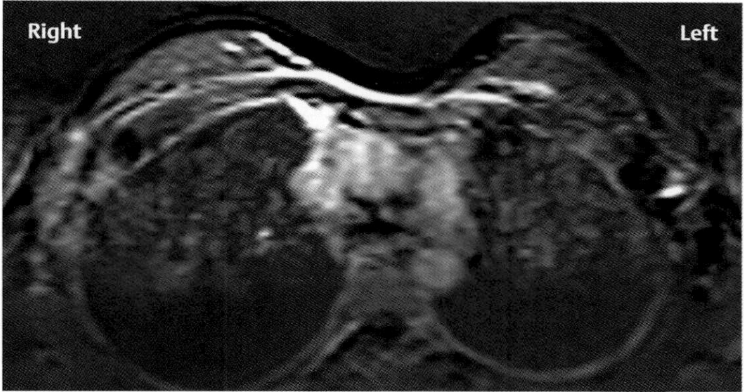


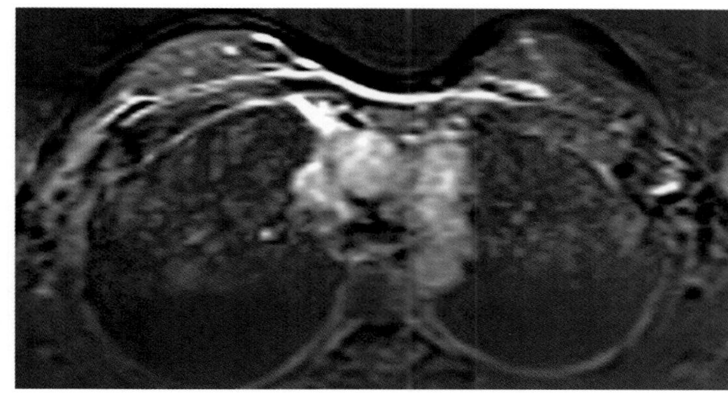

**d** *Bilateral MR images*. The subtraction images show no gadolinium enhancement in the upper quadrants. An enhancing axillary lymph node is visible on the left side (**O/20**).

**Question 1 on Fig. 5.54**

*The tumor cannot be identified on MRI because:*

(**a**) The stroma-rich tumor tissue is poorly vascularized
(**b**) The tumor is located outside the image planes
(**c**) The fascia and muscle are diffusely infiltrated by tumor tissue

→ **Answer on p. 365**

**Question 2 on Fig. 5.54**

*Where did the tumor originate?*

(**a**) In the subcutaneous fat of the chest wall
(**b**) In the clavicular recess of the breast
(**c**) In the axillary recess of the breast

→ **Answer on p. 365**

### *Screening Cases and So-Called Interval Cancers*

Interval cancers are neoplasms that were missed in previous breast examinations (mammography and complementary procedures) and are detected between two routine examinations. Interval cancers are a common occurrence in breast screening (see p. 126). In fact, they are taken into account when programs are set up, and large numbers of women are screened in an attempt to compensate for the phenomenon. This is no comfort for women who develop interval cancers, as most women assume they are in no danger if they have already been screened. When a woman later notices a firmness or even a nodule in her breast, she is not alarmed and often ignores the "lump" because her mammograms and other tests were normal. This results in missed neoplasms, and it is common for diagnoses to be delayed by more than 6 months.

In cases where a neoplasm has been missed, it is very instructive for the breast diagnostician to know how the changes appeared on previous mammograms. This section includes images of lesions that were difficult to detect initially and were later diagnosed as interval cancers. Diagnosticians must constantly hone their intuitive sixth sense so that they can detect even tiny lesions on screening mammograms. Some tumors can be seen only in hindsight, while others are conspicuous. Sometimes it is difficult to understand how a tumor was not detected earlier. It may be that examiners' attention flags during the course of a regular workday, with the result that missed diagnoses are virtually inevitable. Double reading and CAD (see p. 40) are helpful tools that should not be discounted, even in curative mammography (Ikeda et al. 2004). Missed diagnoses and undetected tumors mainly result from the inadequate use of breast ultrasound in screening. A 7% recall rate is too low for effective screening!

In the mammograms that follow (**Figs. 5.55–5.59**), determine where a malignant process is most likely to be located. The answers can be found in the Answers section on pp. 365–370. In the cases shown in the figures, a tumor was noted on later routine mammograms or was detected during the interval as a palpable nodule. In retrospect, this tumor most likely could have been detected in previous examinations. Try to locate it. The figures include only views in which the lesion can be seen.

**Fig. 5.55 A 60-year-old woman underwent breast-conserving surgery of the right breast in 1995.** She presents with no palpable abnormalities. She received 4 years of "follow-up care."

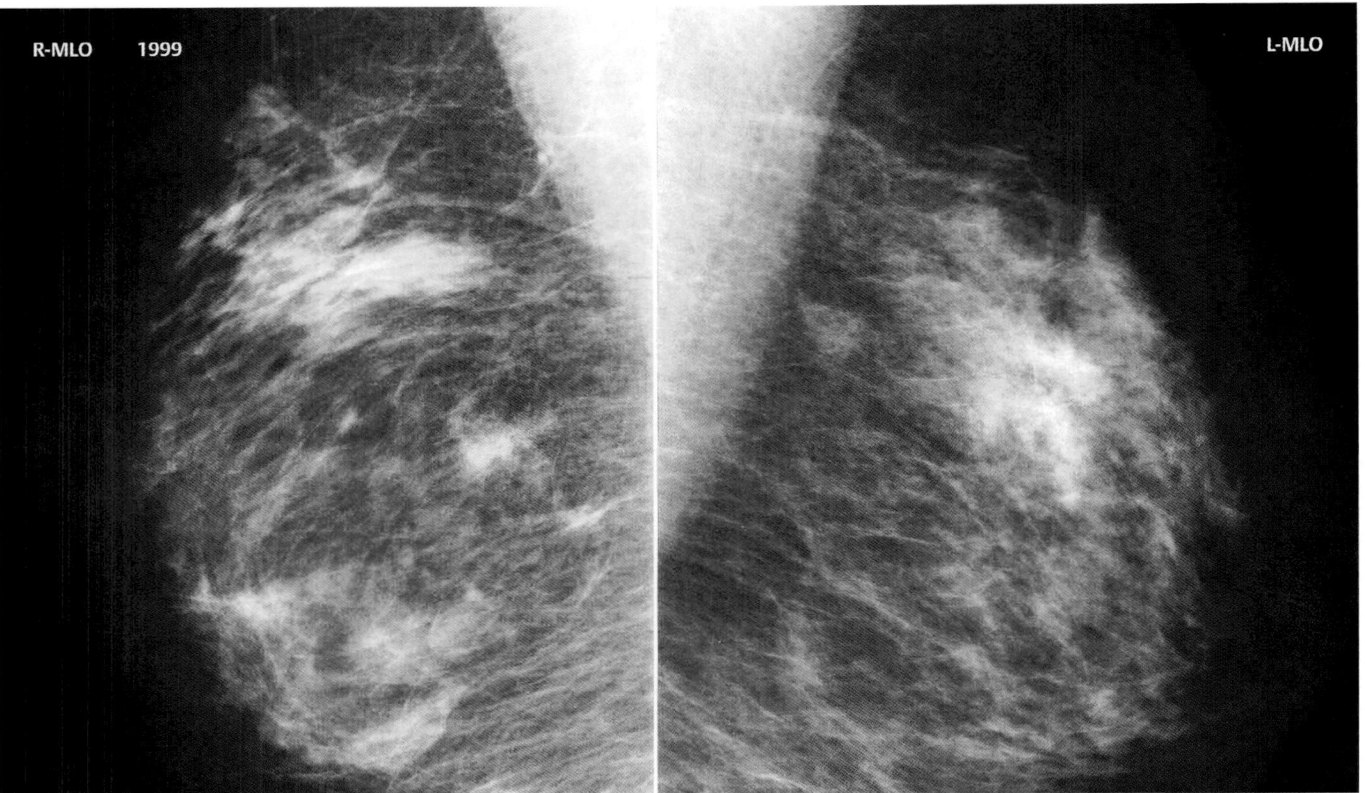


**a** *Bilateral oblique mammograms* in 1999 show involuted breasts. The nipples are at different levels due to previous breast-conserving surgery of the right breast (ACR 2, BIRADS?, PG**M**I).

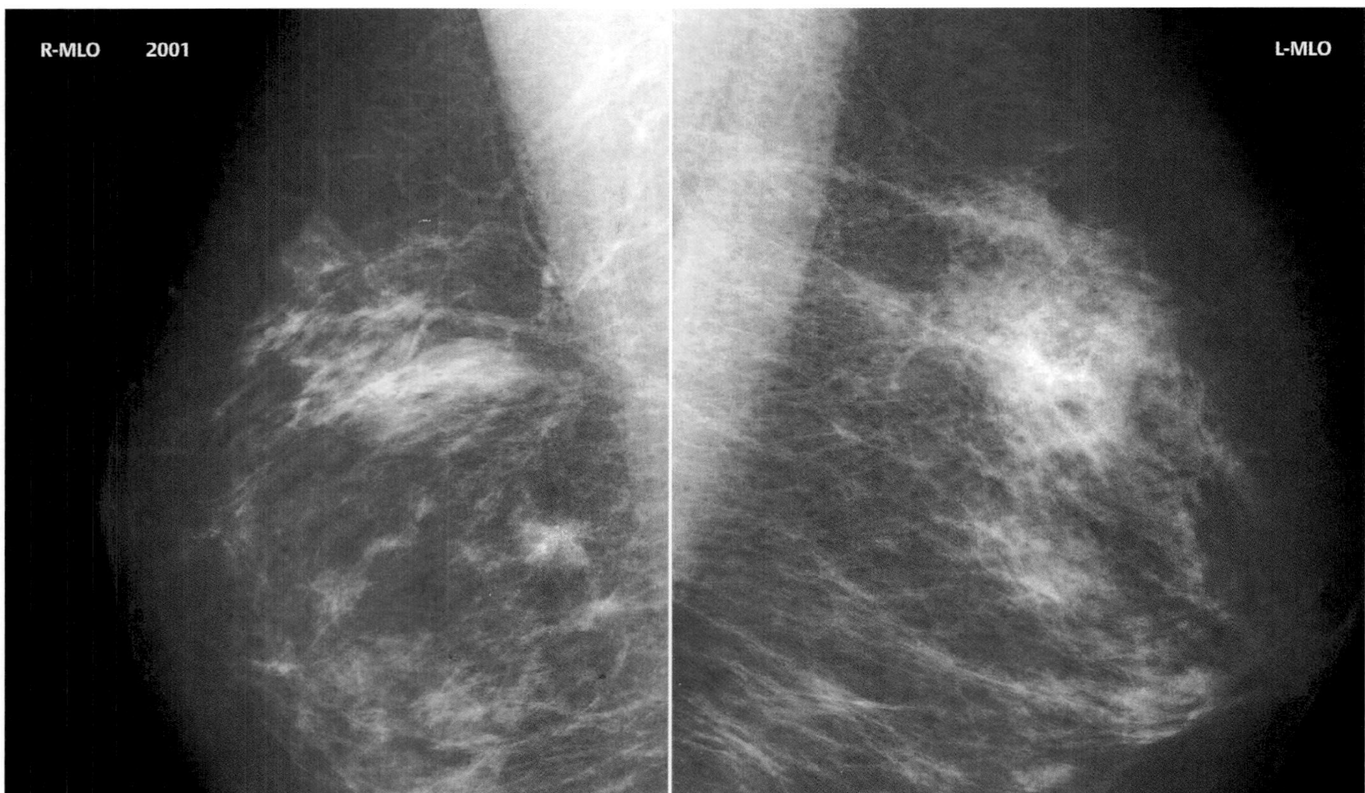


**b** *Bilateral oblique mammograms* (magnified views) in 2001 document the development of atypical changes over time. The decreased breast density relative to the previous examination is a result of antiestrogen treatment with tamoxifen (ACR 2, BIRADS?, **P**GMI).

**Fig. 5.55** **A 60-year-old woman underwent breast-conserving surgery of the right breast in 1995.** *(continued)*

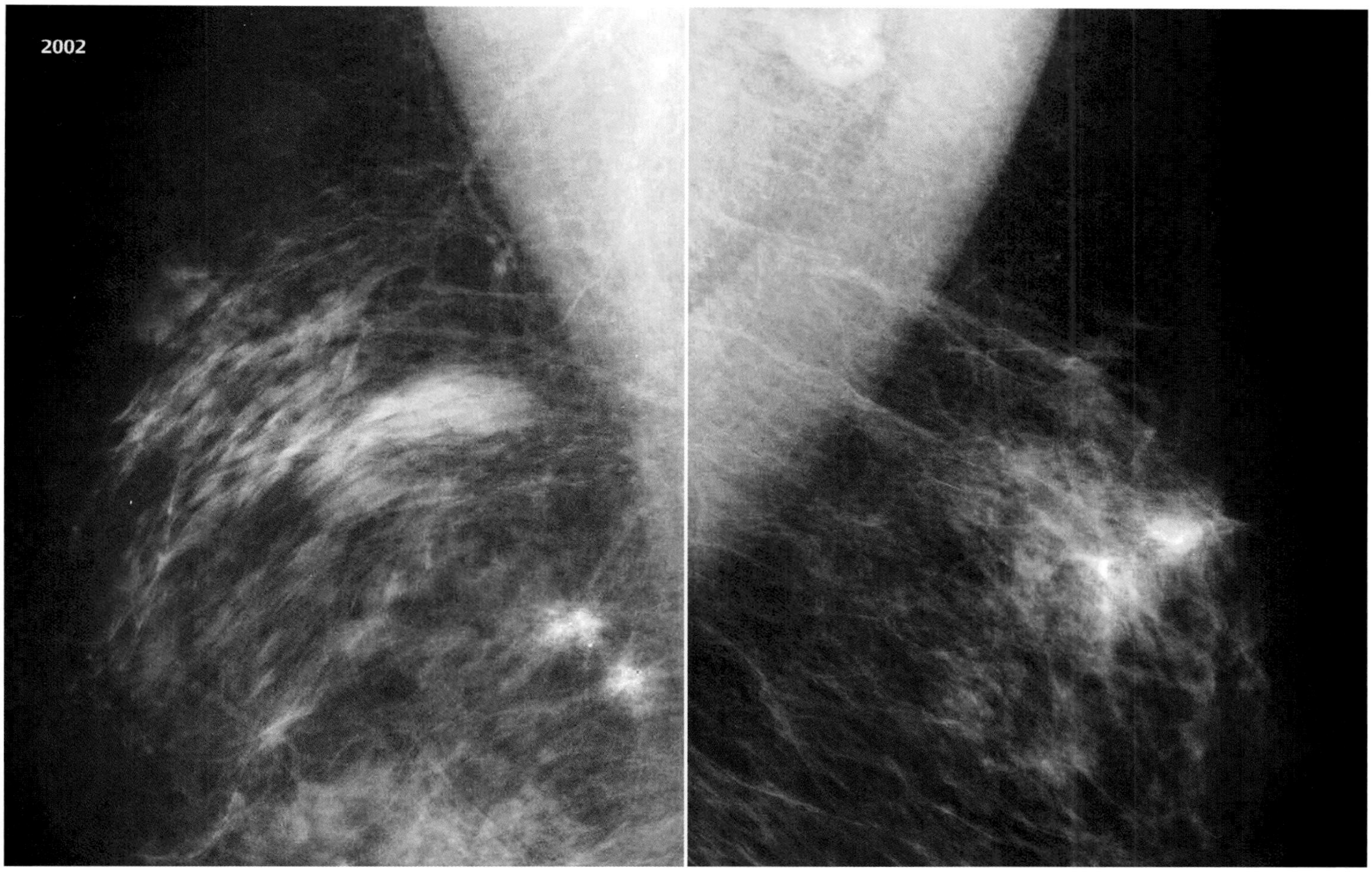

2002

**c** *Bilateral oblique mammograms* (magnified views) in September, 2002.

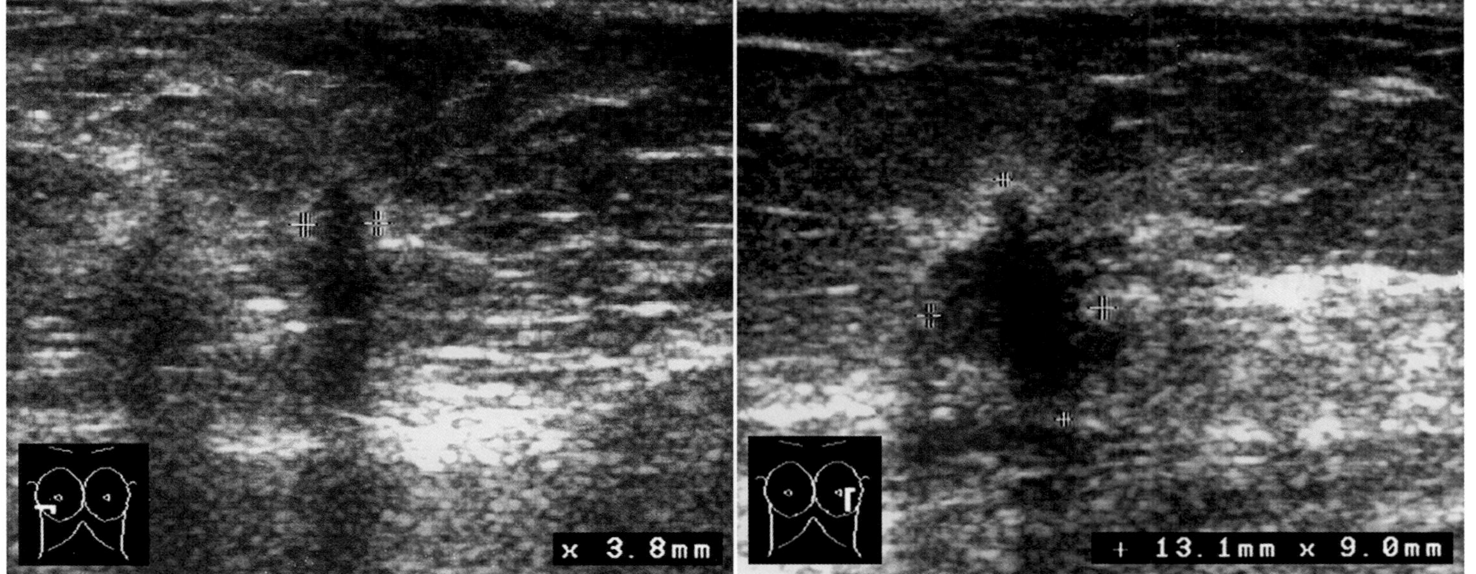


**d** *Bilateral sonograms.*

**Question on Fig. 5.55**

*Where is the tumor located in the mammogram of September, 2002? (Give coordinates)*

→ **Answer on p. 365**

**Fig. 5.56** **A 54-year-old woman presents for screening.**

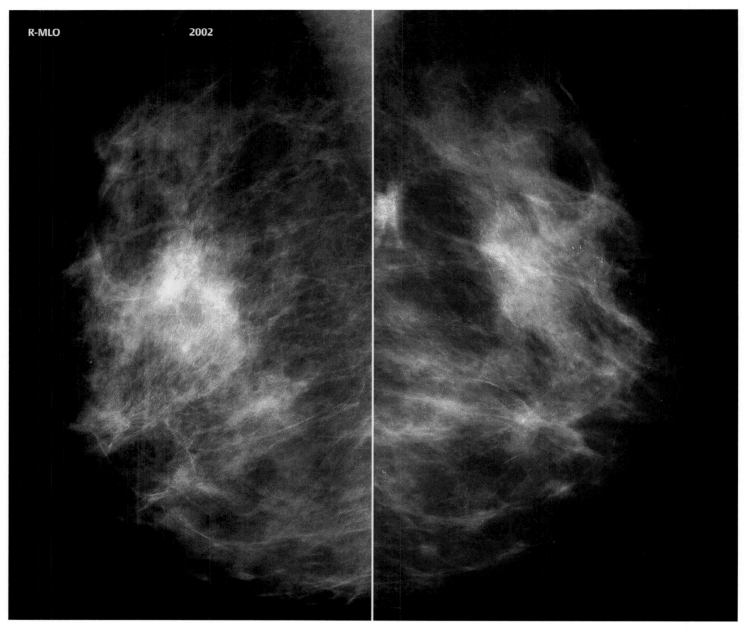

**a** *Bilateral oblique mammograms* in 2002.

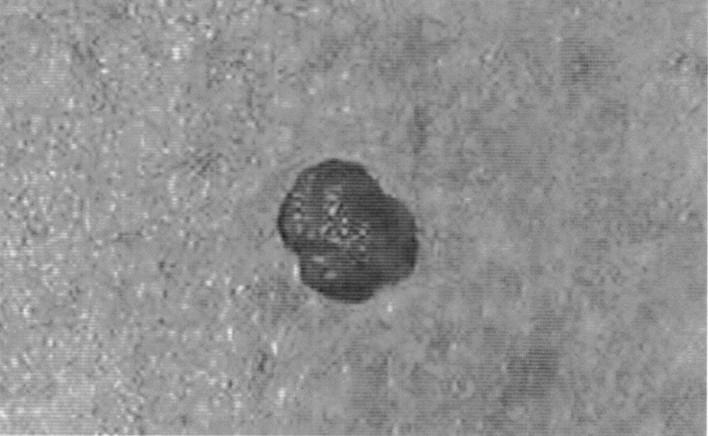

**b** Visual inspection of the upper chest (presternal) reveals a small skin tumor.

**Question 1 on Fig. 5.56**

*How would you interpret the skin tumor in* ***b****?*

(**a**) Amelanotic melanoma
(**b**) Benign papillomatous nevus cell nevus
(**c**) Skin wart

→ **Answer on p. 366**

**Question 2 on Fig. 5.56**

*What is the presumed breast tumor location? (Give coordinates.)*

→ **Answer on p. 366**

**Fig. 5.57** **A 63-year-old woman presents for screening.**

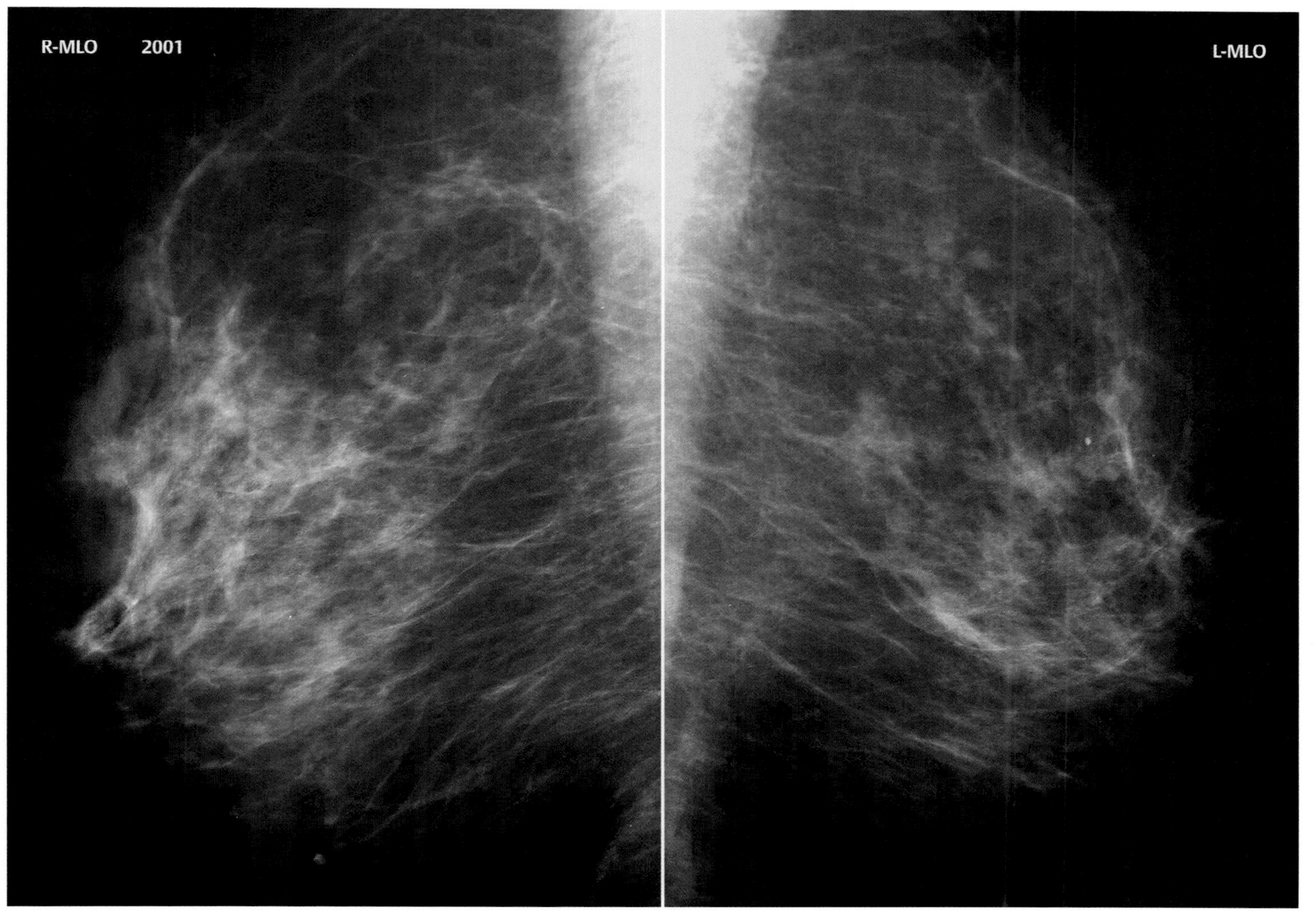


**a** *Bilateral oblique mammograms* in May, 2001 show moderately dense breasts with greater periductal markings on the right side than on the left (**k–N/17–23**) (ACR2, **P**GMI).

**Question on Fig. 5.57**

*Where might the tumor be located?*
*(Give coordinates.)*

→ **Answer on p. 367**

**Fig. 5.58** **A 76-year-old woman presents for screening.**

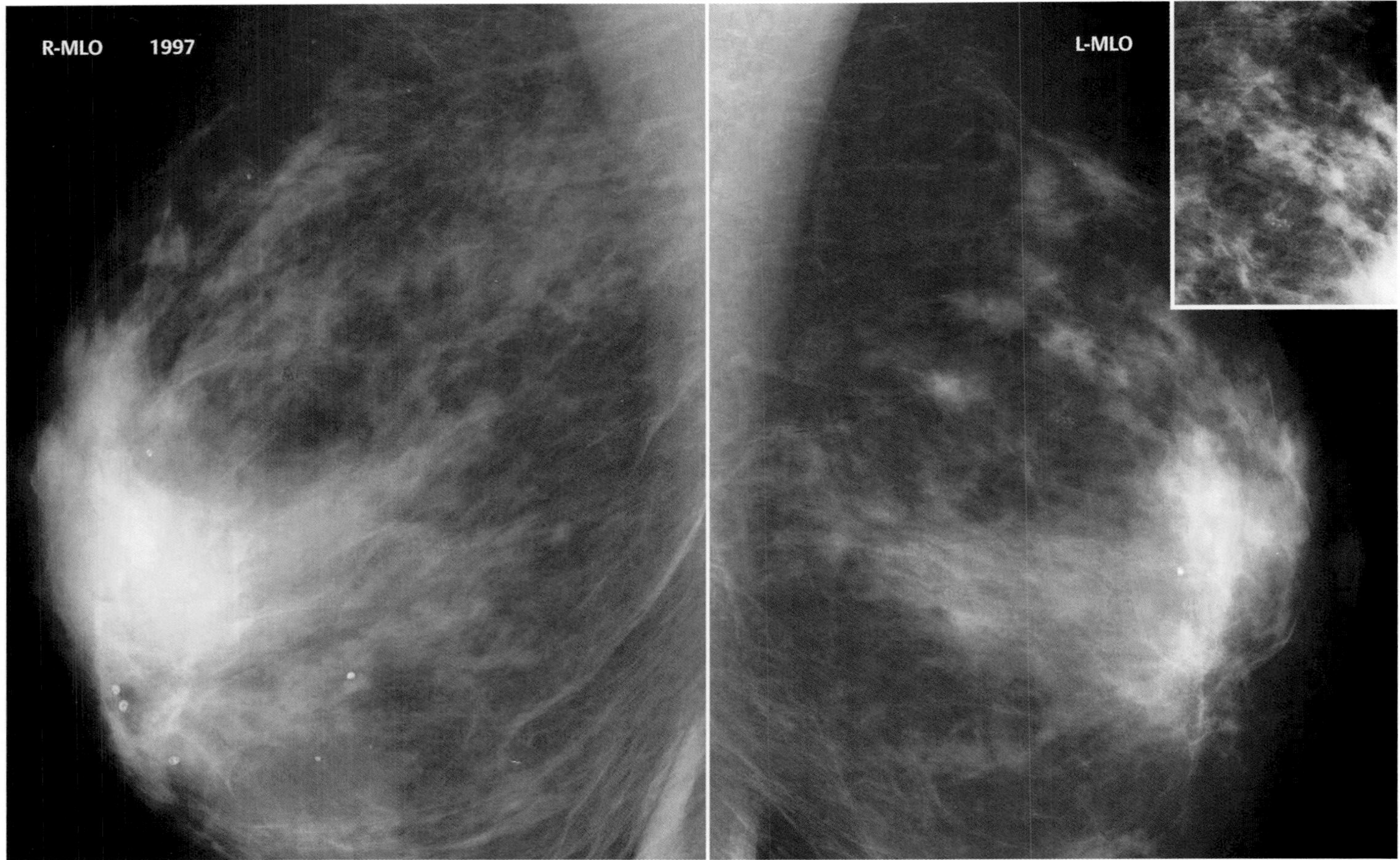


**a** *Bilateral oblique mammograms* in November, **1997** show very dense retroareolar breast parenchyma in both breasts with fading density toward the chest wall (ACR 3, P**G**MI). Magnified view at upper right shows the retroareolar region at **g–I/20–22** of the left breast to aid in evaluating the fine structures (use a magnifying glass!).

**Question on Fig. 5.58**

*Where might the tumor be located?*
*(Give coordinates.)*

→ **Answer on p. 368**

**Fig. 5.59 A 49-year-old woman with a 6-year history of recurrent bilateral axillary lymph node swelling.** She presented in **1989** with severe itching and pronounced scratch marks on the skin. Slight skin retraction was noted over the lower inner quadrant of the left breast in 1991 (**b, c**). A nonspecific mass is palpable over the lower portion of the right breast.

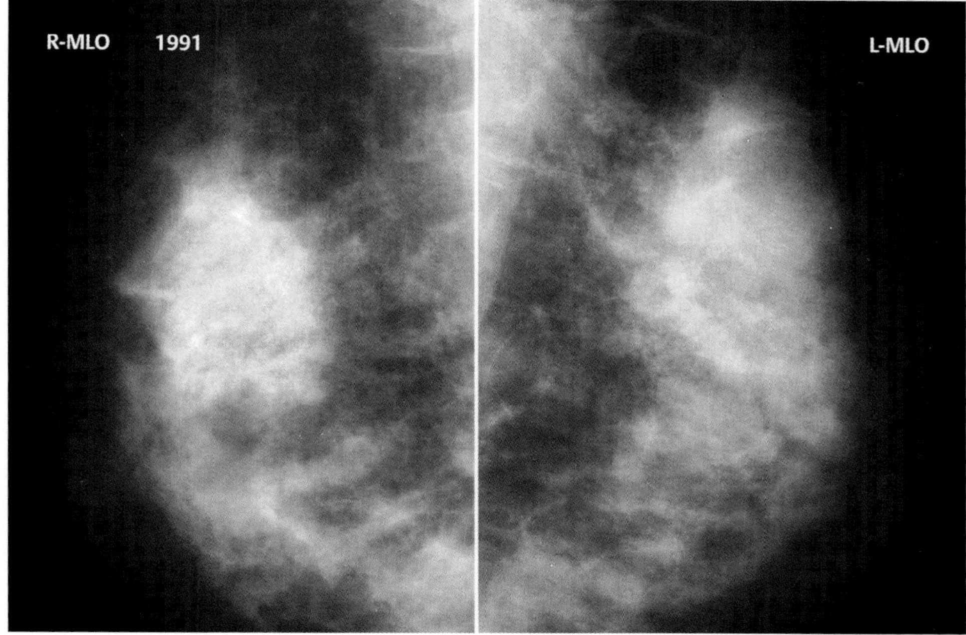


**a** *Bilateral oblique mammograms* in July, 1991 show radiographically dense breast parenchyma with nonspecific bilateral opacities (ACR 3, **P**GMI).

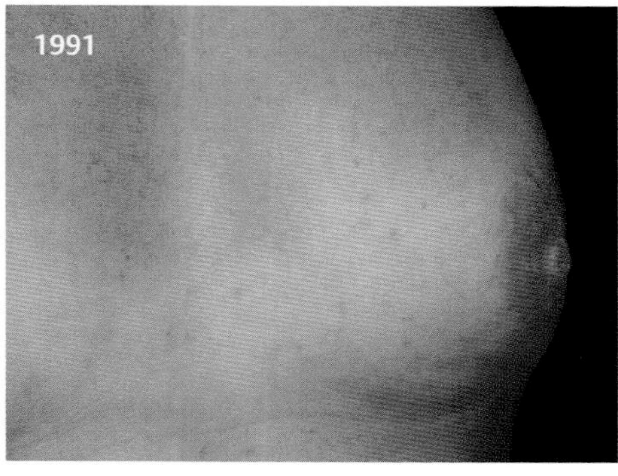


**b** *Clinical appearance* of the left breast in 1991. Slight skin retraction is noted over the lower inner quadrant.

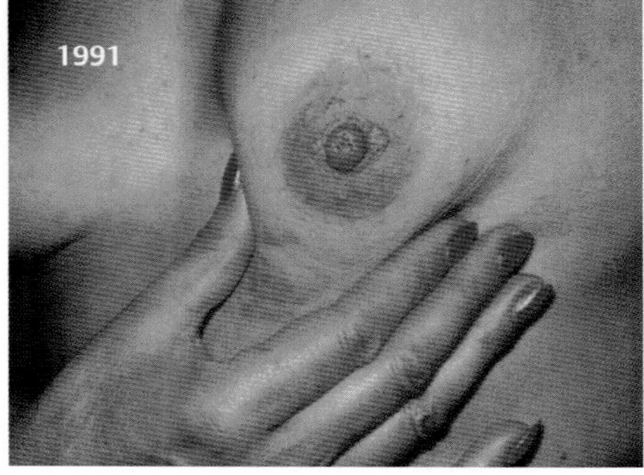


**c** *Clinical appearance* of the breast in 1991. Nonspecific skin retraction is present and enlarges slightly when the lower portion of the breast is squeezed between the thumb and index finger (**r/17**).

**Question on Fig. 5.59**

*Indicate the presumed tumor location (give coordinates).*

→ **Answer on p. 370**

## Ultrasound

**Tip**

**Ten percent of all palpable malignancies and approximately the same percentage of all neoplasms up to 1 cm in size are not mammographically visible because of radiographic breast density or an unfavorable site of the lesion within the breast. Consequently, ultrasound should be mandatory for every asymptomatic woman with a mammographic density between ACR 2 and ACR 4 in cases where breast cancer must be detected or excluded with reasonable confidence.**

Even asymptomatic women with BIRADS 3–5 mammographic lesions, and selected cases classified as BIRADS 2, should be evaluated by ultrasound (see **Fig. 5.51**, p. 142 f).

The use of ultrasound without mammography is handled differently in asymptomatic women and in symptomatic patients. Breast ultrasound in asymptomatic women is not a targeted scan but involves a systematic, time-consuming survey of the entire breast without benefit of mammographic clues. High examiner proficiency and optimal quality equipment are essential in these preventive health services. Hille et al. (2004 b) note that ultrasound is not an *adjunctive* study in patients with equivocal x-ray findings but a *complementary* study that can detect up to 40% of mammographically occult malignancies.

Ultrasound with a high-resolution transducer (11–13 MHz) is not only the procedure of choice for the early detection of noncalcifying breast cancer. It is also a good method for detecting and monitoring physiological and cyclical changes in the breast, which can aid in the interpretation of physical and mammographic findings.

In a 1998 retrospective study by Teh and Wilson of 12 706 ultrasound examinations performed in asymptomatic women (Consensus Conference of the European Group for Breast Cancer Screening in Cyprus), ultrasound detected a total of 1557 clinically and mammographically occult lesions, only 44 of which (2.8%) were malignant. Ultrasound technology has advanced considerably since that time. Modern scanners provide excellent visualization of fine details far beyond the capabilities of equipment in the 1980s and 1990s. It is time, therefore, to conduct randomized prospective studies on the combination of *single-view mammography and high-resolution ultrasound*, recognizing that neither ultrasound nor mammography is effective enough to serve as a stand-alone screening test. It is also clear that breast ultrasound has an approximately 5% rate of false-positive findings (Buchberger 2005).

Thus, ultrasound joins mammography as a first-line method for the early detection and evaluation of cyclical and postmenopausal changes in the breast. But early detection cannot be accomplished with either ultrasound or mammography *alone*, and both tests should be performed by the same physician whenever possible. Diagnostically relevant regions of the breast should be scanned and x-rayed in the same session and evaluated by the same eye. It is inefficient for a gynecologist to perform ultrasound while a radiologist takes the x-rays at a different time and location.

The **indications** for breast ultrasound are as follows:

- Investigation of palpable abnormalities
- Investigation of clinically occult mammographic findings (focal densities with smooth or ill-defined margins, circumscribed asymmetries)
- Radiographic breast density of ACR 2–4
- Previous silicone implantation, reconstruction, or augmentation
- Regular screening examinations in high-risk patients age 25 years or older, supported by mammography and magnetic resonance imaging
- Imaging guidance of diagnostic and therapeutic interventional procedures in the breast
- Questions relating to hormone replacement therapy in menopausal women

The physician who performs mammography—whether a radiologist or gynecologist—should have the option of performing both mammography and ultrasound and to order any necessary interventional procedures without delay.

### Examination Technique

Generally the examiner should scan both breasts while applying carefully controlled transducer pressure. The examination should include both axillae, and the infraclavicular fossae should be scanned in follow-up examinations to rule out malignancy in the clavicular recess (see **Fig. 5.61**, p. 157 and **Fig. 5.54 a**, p. 146), and the other recess (see **Fig. 4.24 k**, p. 347).

The patient is usually positioned supine with the arms clasped behind the head. A semilateral or wedge-supported position may be helpful for evaluating the outer quadrants, especially in patients with large breasts.

With an oblique supine position, the breast is optimally flattened against the chest wall and even peripheral nodules will not slip out of the scanning plane beneath the transducer. The patient should not be examined in a standing or sitting posture unless she has noticed something peculiar in a certain position that is not reproducible in the supine position.

Contact pressure during the examination should be sufficient to provide clear differentiation of intramammary structures (fat, connective tissue, glandular parenchyma), but pressure should not be so high as to induce any pain. During scanning, the transducer should always be held perpendicular to the breast parenchyma as oblique scanning will cause artifacts.

The field of view should maximally occupy the width of the monitor screen. The pectoral fascia should form the lower (far) boundary of the scan and should be clearly defined. If the pectoral fascia cannot be clearly identified, the breast should be scanned at a lower frequency to allow deeper sound penetration.

Uniform focusing should be achieved between the skin and pectoral fascia, preferably through the use of multiple focal zones.

Scanning should be performed in overlapping planes to ensure complete coverage of the breast. Attention is given to the shape of the breast parenchyma. It is best to use a radial scanning pattern, taking as a reference point the retroareolar region and the terminal duct lobular units of a particular mammary lobe. This is particularly important in the investigation of physiologic changes. The transducer is positioned radially for the analysis of individual lobes. From that position the transducer is angled and rotated to locate the principal duct of interest, which provides a landmark for anatomic orientation (**Fig. 5.60**). The breast is scanned primarily in horizontal and vertical planes, however, for the detection or exclusion of suspicious lesions.

The scan planes should be reproducible both in the documentation of abnormalities (scan plane centered over the tumor) and in the visualization of focal lesions. Reproducibility is aided by the body markers that are available in every system.

> ***Tip***
>
> **The documentation of an abnormal finding should at least cover a representative parenchymal region in each breast and should include the nipple region. The abnormality should be visualized and measured in two planes. The axillary region should also be documented if it has been scanned.**

The **documentation of a focal lesion** should include the following data on lesion location:

- Affected side (right/left)
- Clock-face position of the lesion relative to the nipple
- Distance from the center of the nipple to the closest lesion margin (in mm or cm)
- Lesion depth = distance from the skin to the closest lesion margin (in mm or cm)
- Size of the lesion in three dimensions measured in two mutually perpendicular scan planes

The major tumor axis should also be indicated. In addition to purely metric data, the lesion should be characterized in terms of its echogenicity (e.g., a hypoechoic or hyperechoic core with an echogenic rim).

The following features are used to describe the **sonographic morphology** of a lesion:

- **Echogenicity** relative to surrounding tissues: anechoic, hypoechoic, isoechoic, or hyperechoic
- **Shape:** round, oval, complex, patchy
- **Margins:** smooth, lobulated, irregular, ill-defined
- **Internal echo pattern:** homogeneous, inhomogeneous, heterogeneous
- **Sound transmission:** shadowing, indifferent, enhancement
- **Surroundings:** satellite or second lesions, contralateral lesions
- **Axillary lymph nodes:** fatty, indifferent, suspicious, enlarged

The **breast ultrasound report** should include the following data and information:

- Patient identity
- Date of examination
- Essential information on the current and prior history (previous findings!)
- Indication for breast ultrasound
- Visual and palpable findings
- Sonographic findings
- Relationship to mammogram or magnetic resonance image (if available)

**Fig. 5.60 Anatomy of the mammary lobes and scanning technique during breast ultrasound** (from Teboul and Halliwell 1995).

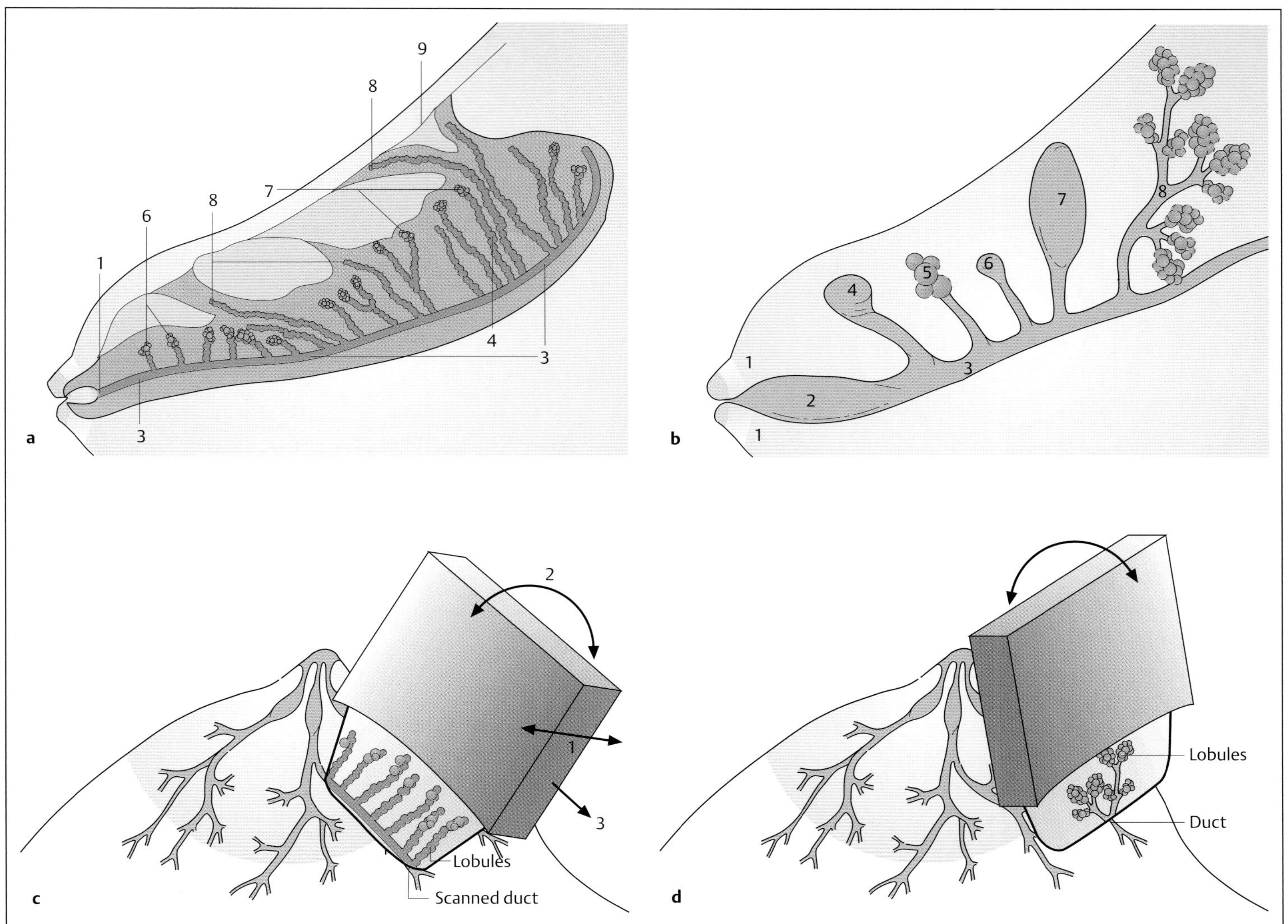


**a** *Diagrammatic representation of a mammary* lobe in the retroareolar region (1). The lobules near the nipple (6) tend to be shorter and thicker than the peripheral lobules (4). Some lobules (7) run perpendicular to the main duct (3) (see also **Fig. 2.1a**) and overlap the anterior edge of the lobe, creating a cobblestone appearance (see **Fig. 5.70 d**). Others (8) extend into the Cooper ligaments and pass with them into the cutaneous fascia (9).

**b** Anatomy of the terminal duct lobular unit: nipple and retroareolar region (1), lactiferous sinus (2), lactiferous duct (3), and the most common types of lobule (4–7): short, thick lobule close to the nipple (4), lobule with microcystic degeneration (5), atrophic lobule (6), cystic enlargement of a lobule (7), and multiple lobules with branched connections (8). Lobules usually exhibit a cloverleaf shape in the periphery.

The *terminal duct lobular unit* of Wellings (1972) is a complex formed by the ductolobular and tubular units and containing acini and terminal ducts. The terminal duct lobular units (TDLUs) are the basic milk-producing units of the breast.

Most carcinomas originate in the TDLU and are basically ductolobular carcinomas (see also **Figs. 4.12, 4.13**, p. 31). During *maturation* of the breast, the lobules sprout from the surface of the main ducts and extend toward the skin, emphasizing the importance of maintaining firm transducer contact during ultrasound scanning.

**c** *Axial (radial) scan* along a milk duct. Scanning in this plane most clearly defines the lobules in relation to their surroundings. Ideally, each individual lobe should be analyzed separately, but in practice this is necessary only if an atypical lesion is found.

The most important sonographic criterion for lobular stimulation is lobar prominence. Radial scanning of the lobes (1) provides the best overview of ductolobular structures and most clearly depicts their pathology and physiology. Some lobules may extend a distance from the main duct and project into the skin or angle back toward the duct.

Transducer position should be tailored to individual anatomy. The probe can be angled from its radial placement along the duct (2) to compensate for the variable position of the TDLUs. Normally the ducts can be traced to the periphery of the lobe by radial advancement of the probe.

**d** *Transverse scans* are directed at right angles to the main duct, providing cross-sectional views of the duct and afferent ductules. The lobules that connect with the terminal duct may occasionally form a stellate arrangement. Sometimes these anatomic patterns are definable, but only with a 13–18 MHz probe.

The ultrasound report should consist of several parts:

- A description of the parenchymal structure to determine assessability
- Localization
- Biometry and sonographic morphology of focal lesions
- Associated findings

Finally, a BIRADS score is determined to express the overall **level of suspicion** for a given lesion (ACR BIRADS):

- **Category S1:** negative
- **Category S2:** benign finding (e.g., cyst)
- **Category S3:** probably benign (follow-up in 6 months)
- **Category S4:** suspicious abnormality (4A, low; 4B intermediate; 4C moderate suspicious)
- **Category S5:** highly suspicious of malignancy
- **Category S6:** histologically confirmed malignancy

Each category is associated with a **recommended action** that includes follow-up intervals and the possible need for further diagnostic or interventional measures.

### Schematic Protocol of Ultrasound Examination

The traditional analysis of malignant structures in breast ultrasound is based almost entirely on the geometry of the lesion while ignoring basic anatomic structures—the ductal and lobular parenchyma.

Teboul and Halliwell (1995) defined benign and malignant criteria for the *terminal duct lobular unit (TDLU)* that are not widely known or utilized. In this approach it is not enough to scan the breast in horizontal and vertical planes to look for atypical lesions; it must also be scanned radially along the course of the duct and documented (**Fig. 5.61 c**), especially for the investigation of tumors or changes during the course of the menstrual cycle. Follow-up examinations should be interpreted with reference to this baseline documentation so that the same segments can be comparatively analyzed. This is the only way to evaluate changes in the TDLUs over time, and it facilitates the detection of new lesions. It also ensures an overlapping examination of all breast segments, which is of forensic importance (**Fig. 5.61 c**).

This examination, then, includes evaluation of the lactiferous ducts, mammary lobes, and lobules. There are many cases in which this analysis can give form and meaning to apparent architectural disarray in a breast sonogram. To make a sonographic analysis of this kind, examiners must have a thorough knowledge of the pathoanatomy of the breast so that they can localize changes to specific anatomic structures (ducts, connective tissue, Cooper ligaments, skin, muscular fascia, pectoral muscles). The diagnosis should be a descriptive one that is stated in relation to these anatomic structures (see p. 23 ff).

Increasingly, breast ultrasound should come to rely more on morphology as a basis for diagnostic analysis. The geometry and margins of a lesion must be placed within an anatomic context.

Teboul and Halliwell (1995) draw the following conclusions:

- A meticulous, duct-oriented sonographic analysis of the breast parenchyma is essential for planning cancer treatment and detecting abnormal parenchymal responses to hormonal stimuli, for example.
- The key to this analysis lies in identifying the terminal duct lobular units (TDLUs) within the breast and determining their relationship to pathologic changes.
- Duct-oriented ultrasound is the only sure way to establish anatomic orientation in the breast and define the relationship between the breast parenchyma and the structures around it.

This kind of localization and identification can often, though not always, be accomplished with a high-resolution transducer (11–18 MHz). Structural analysis of the lobules and TDLUs in response to hormone replacement therapy or contraceptive use, for example, has the potential to become an important and previously unutilized approach in modern diagnostic ultrasound.

It would be desirable for manufacturers to produce higher-frequency transducers as well as ultrasound systems in which the last examination could be automatically displayed on a separate screen for reference, similarly to **Fig. 5.61 d**. The examiner should always work in the same direction, beginning in the axilla and ending at a 6 o'clock position with each breast (see **Fig. 5.61 c**). He/she can thus be sure that each breast quadrant is examined twice and that comparable documents are available for future examinations. The examiner should always follow the same systematic sequence when performing breast ultrasound in order to obtain comparable results (see **Fig. 5.61 d**).

### Basic Structures of the Breast and their Variants on Ultrasound, with Mammographic Correlation

The basic structures of the breast can be analyzed reasonably well with high-resolution transducers. Fat and glandular tissue show contrasting echogenicities. Fatty tissue is dark (hypoechoic), while the glandular tissue, consisting of lobular parenchyma and the intra- and interlobular stroma, appears bright (hyperechoic) (see **Fig. 5.75 e, f**, p. 177). Within the breast parenchyma, the lobes are difficult to distinguish from one another, although this can be done indirectly by visualizing the major ducts. The lobules and TDLUs appear as small, dark (hypoechoic) round to oval structures that are clearly distinguishable from the hyperechoic fibrous septa (see **Fig. 5.65**, p. 163). This requires that the TDLUs are in a proliferative state and are not atrophic (see Chapter 4, p. 23).

The breast consists of up to 12 lobes, each based on a major duct that runs a straight or tortuous course (especially in the retroareolar region) from the nipple to the periphery of the breast. Only radial scanning can define all or part of the main duct, which appears as a hypoechoic channel. The TDLUs (lobules with acini and functional intralobular stroma) are found in proximity to the ducts. The TDLUs are not very well developed before 18 years of age. If they are detectable at all, they appear as focal hypoechoic areas during the second half of the menstrual cycle or the premenstrual phase. Fat and connective tissue (interlobular fibrosis) predominate normally in the adolescent breast (see **Figs. 5.63**, p. 160). Exceptions are possible especially some weeks before menarche (see **Fig. 5.62 a–d**, p. 159) and in cases of malignancy (see **Fig. 5.64**, p. 161).

More lobule-bearing areas can be found in the postpubescent breast. Lobules may be seen in various areas up until the first pregnancy, usually in the relatively long lateral superior lobes in the upper outer quadrants. The lobules become larger and more dense shortly before and during menstruation. Afterward they regress until ovulation, then enlarge again during the second half of the cycle until the next period (see **Figs. 5.65–5.67**, p. 163 ff). The TDLUs are very prominent and easily visualized (often right after ovulation) in women with severe premenstrual complaints, although premenstrual syndrome may occur in the absence of lobular proliferation. The reason for this is unknown.

The lobules are most abundant during pregnancy and lactation, when the breast consists predominantly of milk-producing glandular parenchyma while fat and connective tissue are displaced to the margins of the greatly enlarged TDLUs. The main ducts are dilated, and their fluctuating milk contents can be clearly visualized (see **Figs. 5.68–5.70**, p. 168 ff).

After lactation is completed, focal enlargement of the lobules persists for a period of several months to years (see **Fig. 5.69**, p. 170). After that time the lobules gradually regress to a normal state. Maturation of the breast is complete following the first pregnancy (see p. 7).

Starting at about age 40 years and after menopause, the TDLUs continuously regress from the periphery of the breast toward the nipple, again resulting in a predominance of fat and connective tissue. For unknown reasons, some women retain a substantial volume of lobular tissue after age 40. As a result, approximately 30% of menopausal women have relatively dense mammograms, also due in part to an increase in connective tissue (see p. 98). Researchers should investigate whether these breasts are responding to endogenous or exogenous hormonal stimulation and whether this may increase the risk of breast cancer (especially lobular neoplasms). The *changing* radiodensity of the mammogram depends on the proliferation of TDLUs and not on the interlobular stroma (see p. 23). In any case it could be extremely useful for gynecologists to detect cyclic and atypical lobular proliferation in the breast in order to evaluate hormonal responses. Menopausal women with proliferating TDLUs who are on hormone replacement therapy could be prescribed a different hormone (e.g., an estrogen-only product, especially after hysterectomy) or might discontinue HRT if a different hormone is found to have no effect on lobular regression. Women who do not show significant lobular proliferation at ultrasound presumably would not have an increased breast cancer risk with HRT. Women who do show TDLU proliferation in response to tamoxifen, for example, should be tested for paradoxical hyperestrogenemia, which may require the discontinuation of tamoxifen.

These and other facts have not yet been scientifically investigated but could become important in gynecologic consultations. Ultrasound has yet to fulfill its potential. There are still unsuspected possibilities in the assessment of patients on HRT, perhaps including the use of higher-resolution transducers or even probes that could be "tuned" to the hormone status of individual patients.

**Figs. 5.71–5.83** (p. 172 ff) illustrate numerous cases with mammography and ultrasound imaging which may be diagnostically misleading but which can be considered to be within the realm of normal, non-malignant variants.

**Fig. 5.61 Protocol for breast ultrasound.** The examiner should always follow the same routine when performing breast ultrasound in order to obtain comparable results. In particular, the scans should cover breast regions that are not depicted in mammograms–most notably the recesses (axillary, clavicular, sternal, abdominal, and lateral) (**a**). Sonographic coverage considerably therefore exceeds mammographic coverage (**b**). Starting from the right axilla, the scans should proceed to the lateral, upper, medial, and lower quadrants in an overlapping pattern, and the ducts associated with each quadrant should be documented at approximately the 9-, 12-, 3-, and 6-o'clock positions. The same procedure is followed in the left breast, providing mirror-image information on the breast parenchyma and ensuring that all quadrants are examined twice. This consistent routine has forensic importance as well (**c**). Previous sonograms should be available for follow-ups to facilitate the prompt detection of pathologic changes and physiologic variations in the glandular tissue (**d**). This is effectively accomplished in the digital age by using worklists supplied by equipment manufacturers.

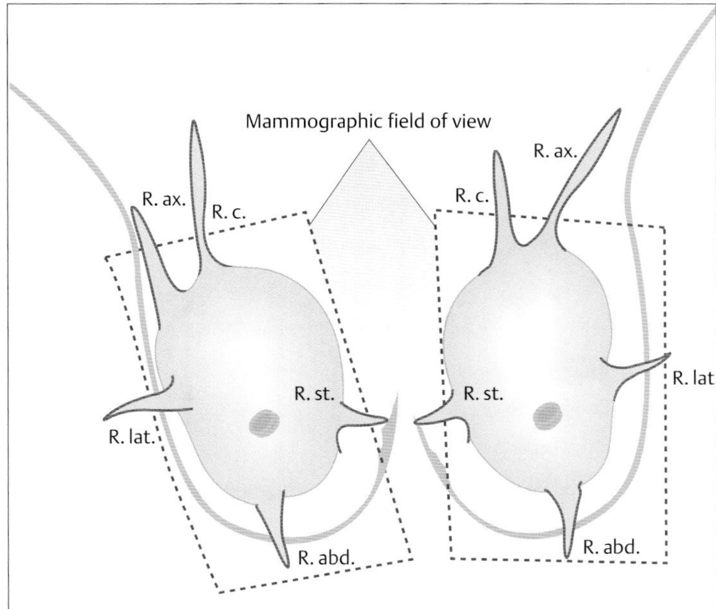


**a** *Diagram* of the recesses and the area covered by mammography (brown shading). Mammograms cannot fully cover the axillary recess (R. ax.), clavicular recess (R. c.), sternal recess (R. st.), abdominal recess (R. abd.), or lateral recess (R. lat.). Some changes, especially in the sternal recess, are not mammographically detectable in obese women (see **Fig. 4.24 e**, p. 50, **Fig. 4.24 j, k**, p. 347).

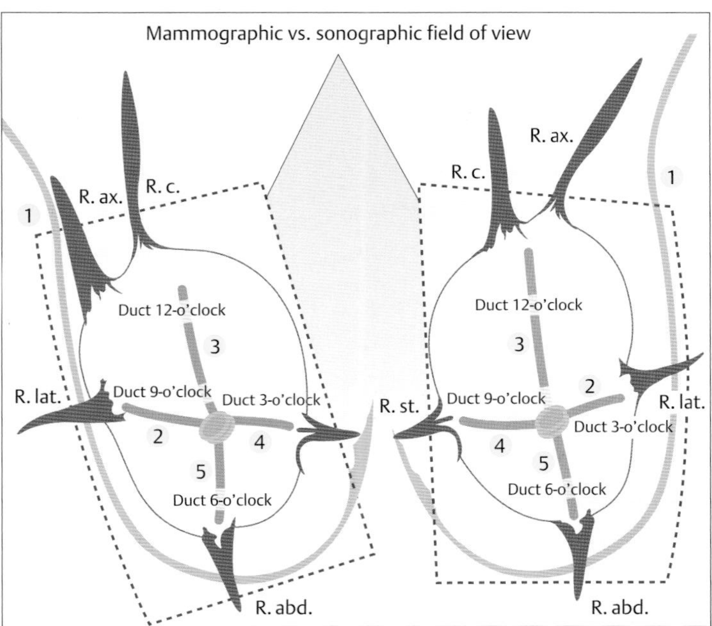


**b** *Ultrasound* coverage of the breast parenchyma. The yellow-shaded area represents the area accessible to ultrasound scanning. The ducts (2, 3, 4, 5) and axilla (1) are indicated in red. These duct-oriented scan planes through the breast parenchyma permit an accurate assessment of physiologic responses to hormonal stimuli, etc.

**Fig. 5.61 Protocol for breast ultrasound.** *(continued)*

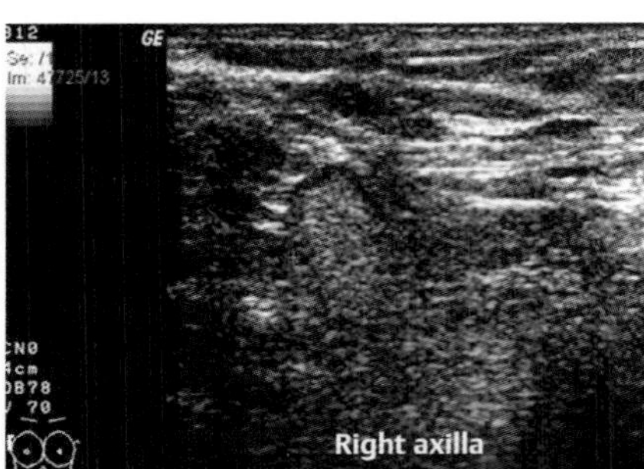


**c** Schematic protocol to illustrate the areas accessible to ultrasound. Coverage should include all breast regions including recess (see **Fig. 5.61 a**) and the axilla.

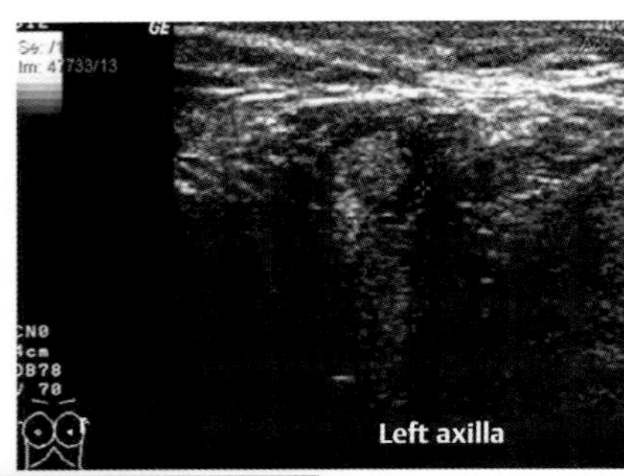


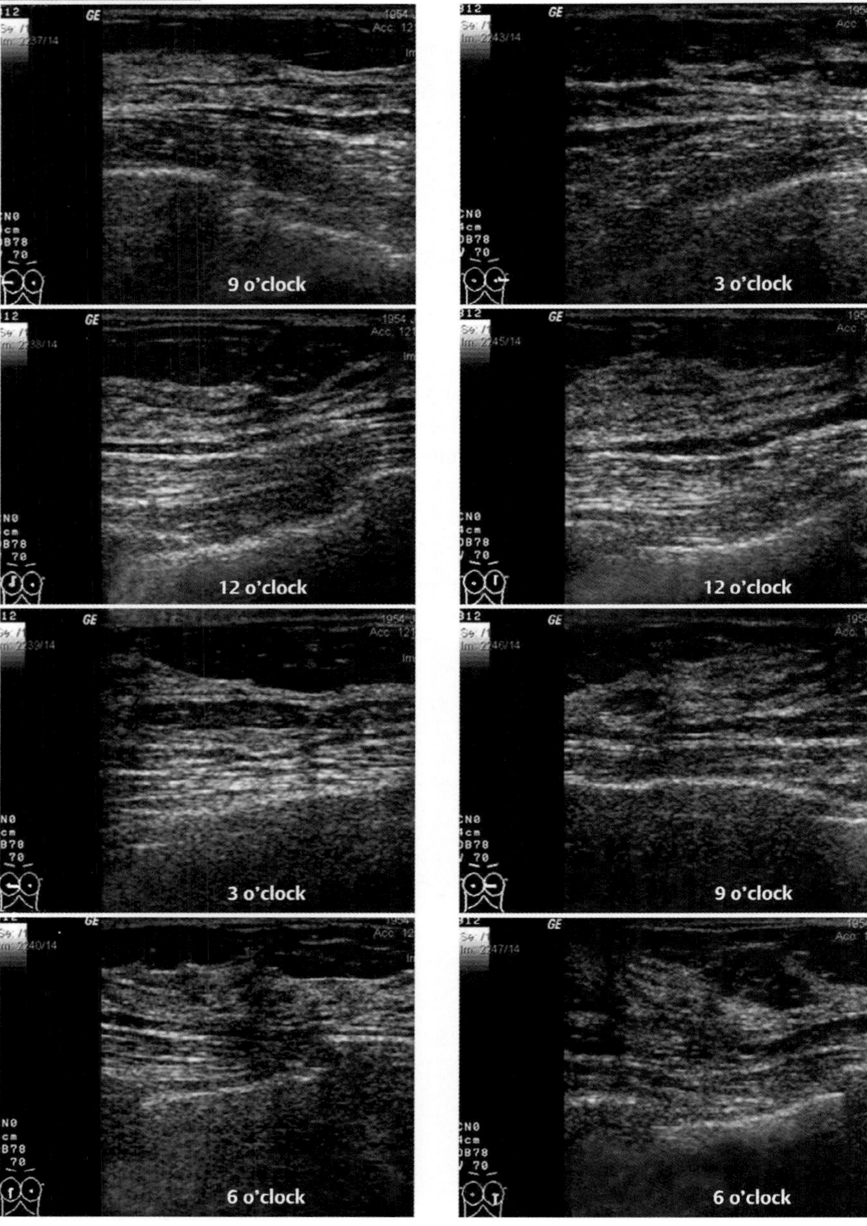


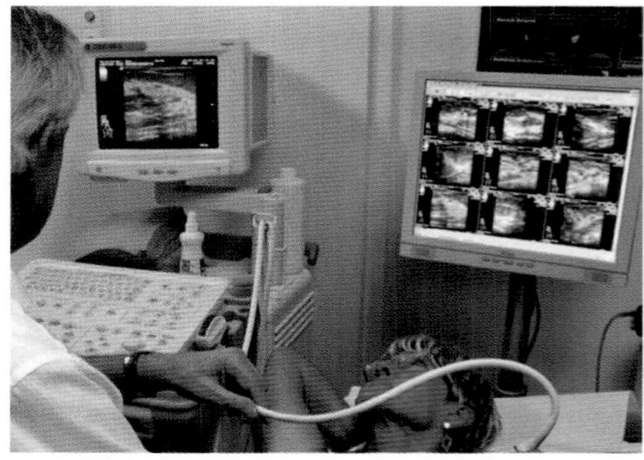

**d** *Previous images* are available for follow-up in a digital tableau and serve as guides for the identification of possible abnormalities (monitors display previous images on the right, current ultrasound image on the left). Ultrasound scanners should be equipped with two monitors—one for previous images and one for current images. A worklist is used for accessing patient data.

**Fig. 5.62 a–d A 13-year-old patient with sudden bilateral breast swelling**, proliferating TDLUs and periductal intralobular stroma, ductectasia, and cysts (**a–c**). The cause of the sudden changes is uncertain. Presumably they relate to a strong progesterone effect or pituitary stimulation, but hormone analysis showed no abnormalities. Several weeks later the patient experienced menarche and the changes regressed (**d**). Similar findings are occasionally seen in women of childbearing age who have been treated with gonadotropins for infertility (see **e–g**).

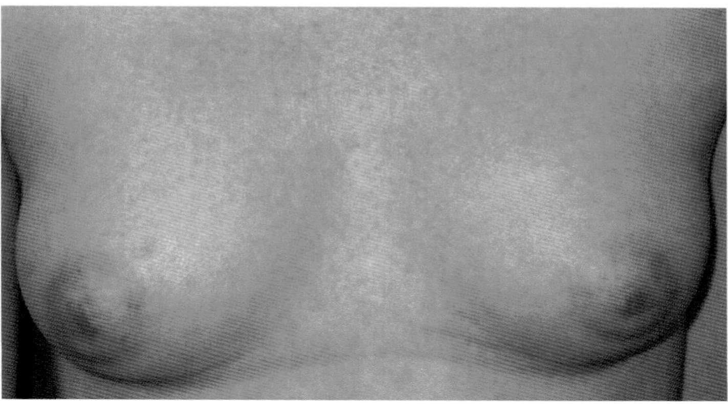

**a** *Clinical aspect*: Bilateral swelling of the breasts several weeks before menarche with a small hemangioma at the 1-o'clock position in the right areola.

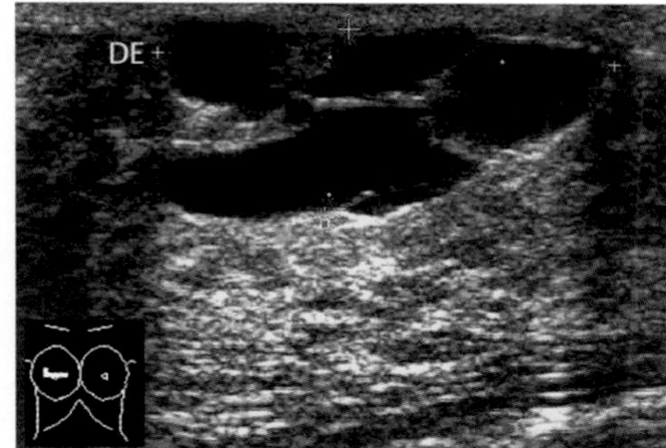


**b** *Sonography:* Marked retroareolar ductectasia. The milk ducts have smooth margins and cytology showed no abnormalities.
De = ductectasia

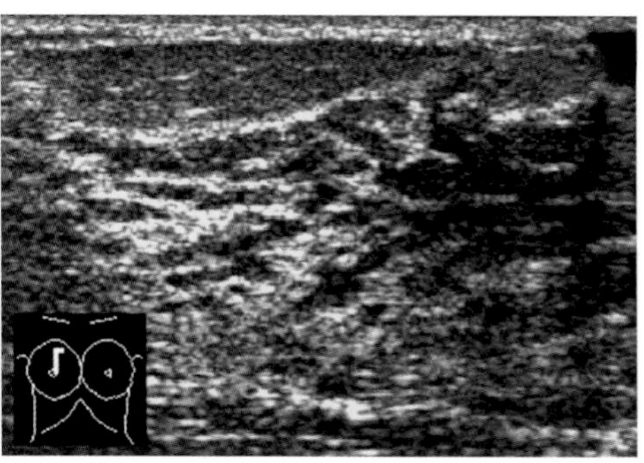

**c** *Sonography:* Heavy proliferation of periductal intralobular stroma arising from the retroareolar region (right).

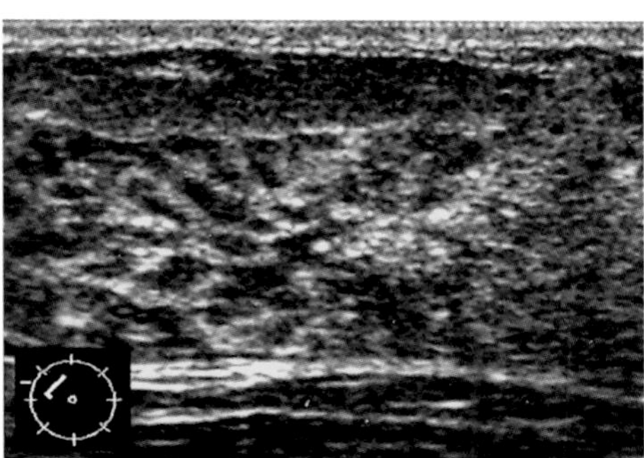

**d** *Sonography:* Heavy proliferation of TDLUs.

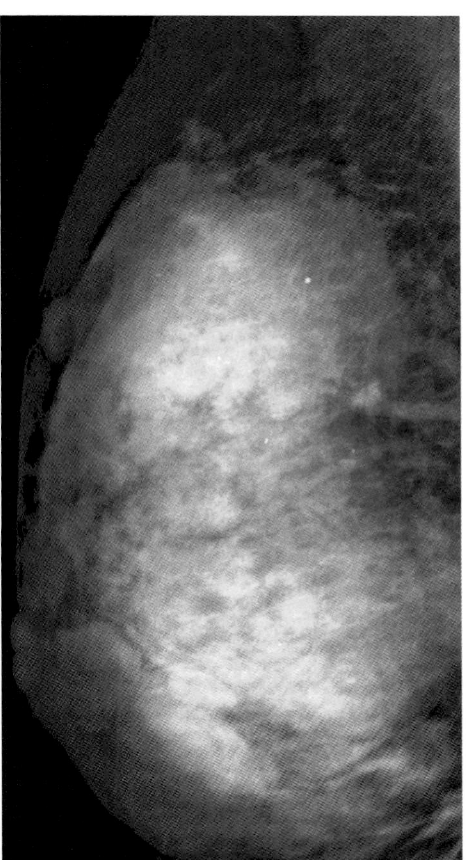

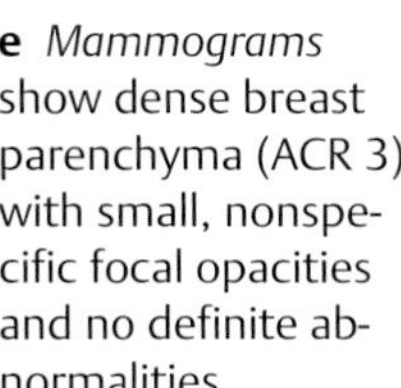

**e–g A 39-year-old woman 5 years after treatment with high doses of gonadotropins for infertility.**

**e** *Mammograms* show dense breast parenchyma (ACR 3) with small, nonspecific focal opacities and no definite abnormalities.

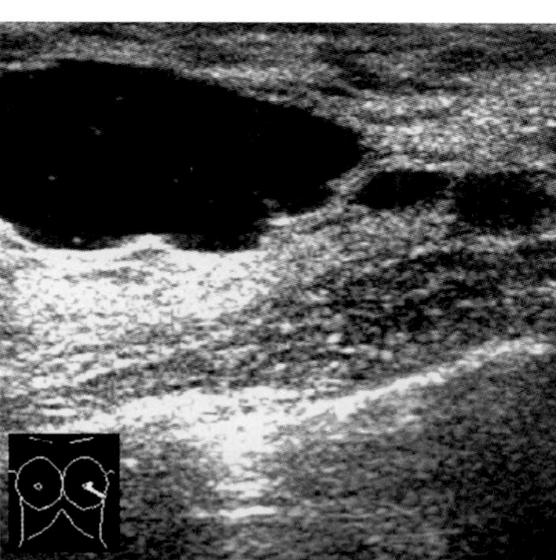

**f** *Ultrasound* shows markedly ectatic retroareolar ducts and cysts.

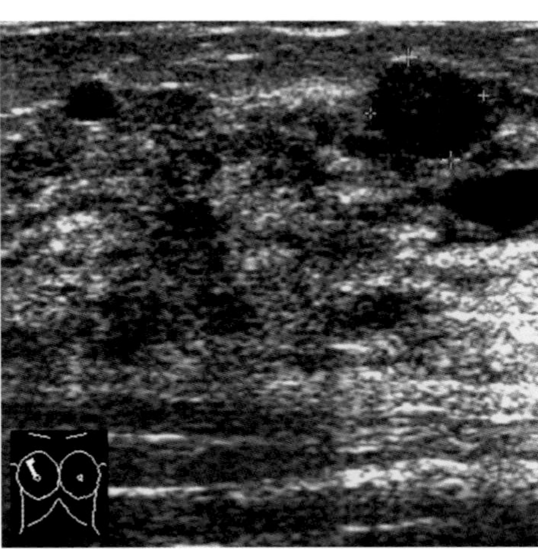

**g** *Ultrasound* shows cysts and proliferated TDLUs.

**Fig. 5.63 Normal-appearing breasts with abundant stroma and bilateral fibroadenomas in a 15-year-old girl.** The breast parenchyma contains abundant interlobular stroma with few definable TDLUs.

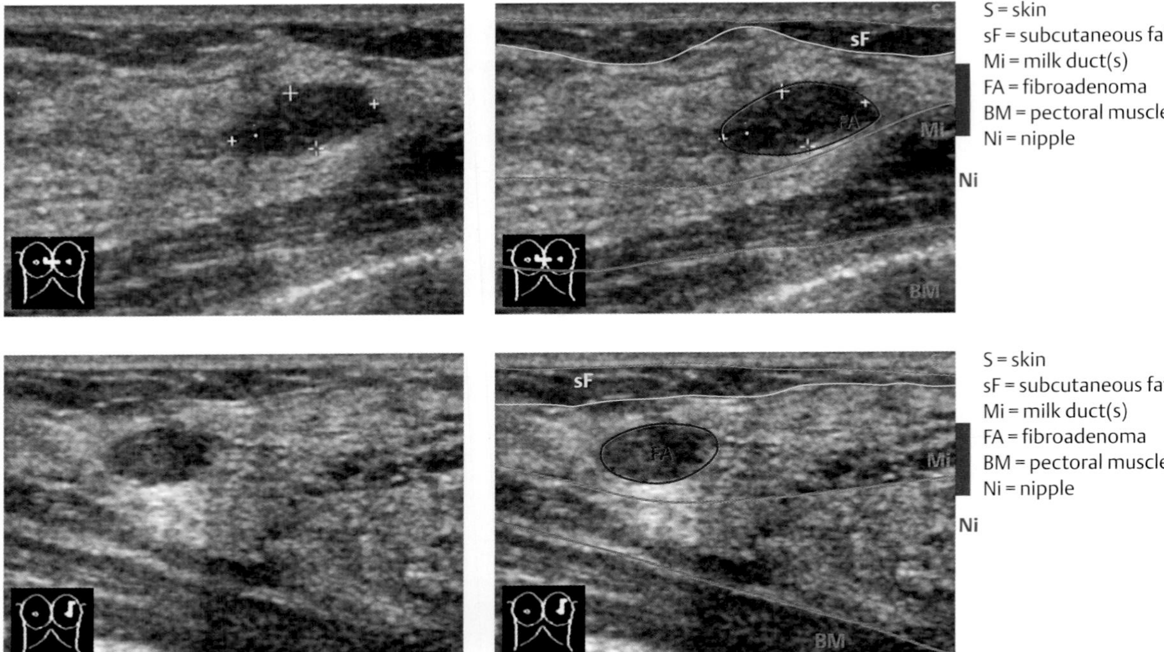


**a, b** *Sonography*: The right breast (**a**, above) and left breast (**b**, below) each contain a well-circumscribed fibroadenoma with internal echoes and posterior acoustic enhancement (diagnosis confirmed by core-needle biopsy). The decreased lobular markings are typical at this age. Interlobular stroma (light) predominates in both breasts.

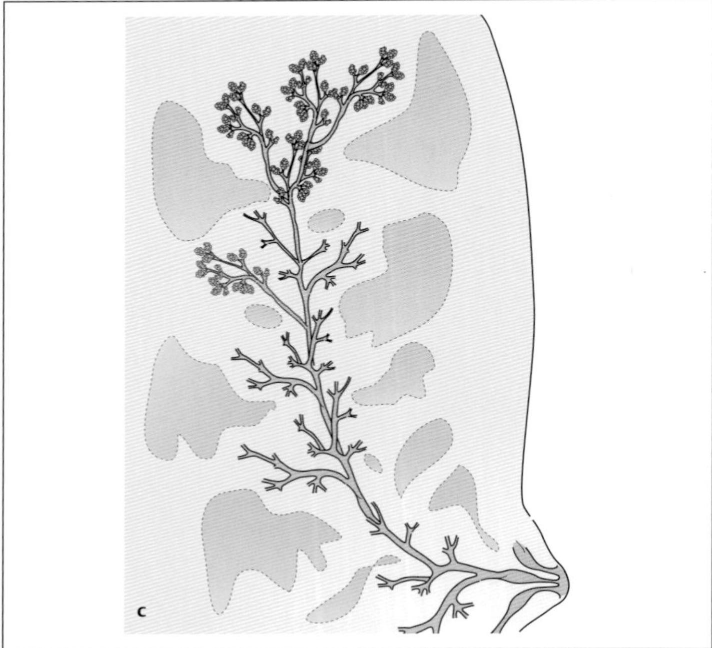


**c** *Anatomical drawing* of the lobular system in one lobe of a 15-year-old girl (after Dabelow and Baessler). Development of the TDLUs begins in the peripheral lobules and progresses toward the nipple. Regression of the TDLUs occurs with aging and spreads toward the periphery.

**Fig. 5.64 Mammography and ultrasound in an 18-year-old woman with left-sided breast cancer.** The tumor is a 2.6 cm × 2.5 cm × 1.1 cm ductal carcinoma with microcalcifications. The patient had no family history of breast cancer, experienced menarche before age 11, and was nulliparous. She had been on oral contraceptives for several years. *Histology:* poorly differentiated invasive ductal carcinoma (G3) with a medullary component, lymphatic invasion, an extensive intraductal component (EIC), and foci of comedonecrosis. The breast has a **normal parenchymal structure with ducts, lobules, and normal TDLU formation.** Estrogen receptor status positive, progesterone receptor status negative, HER-2 status triple positive.

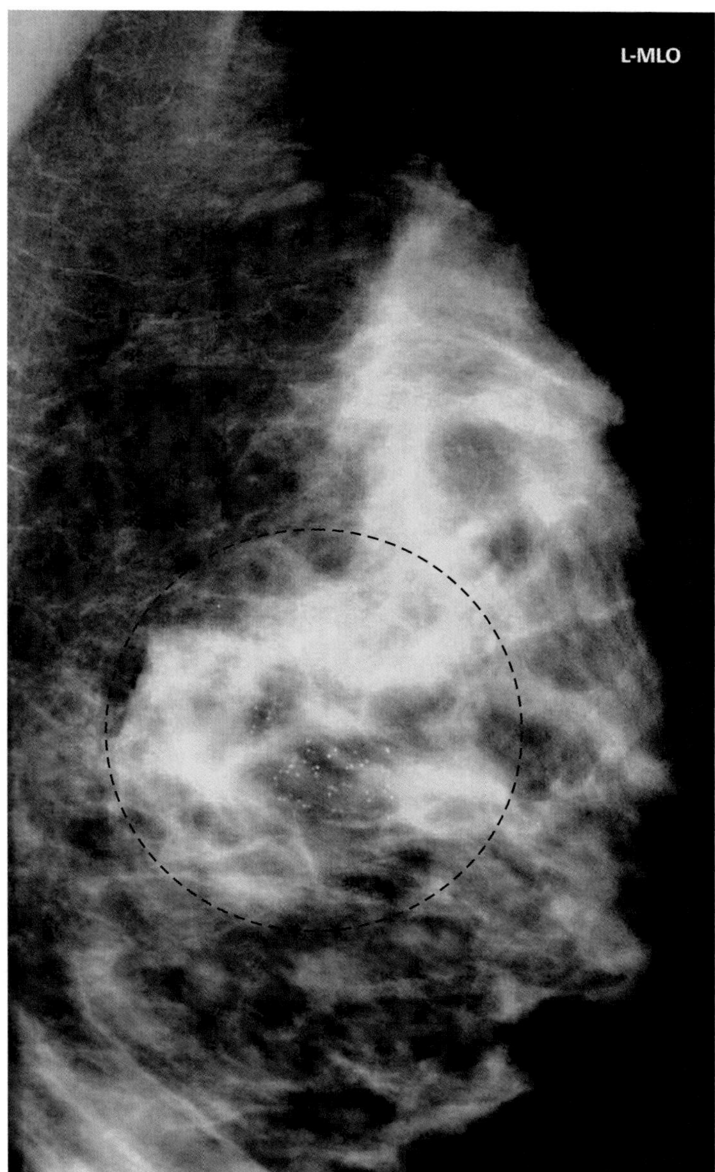


**a** *Oblique mammogram* of the left breast shows a normal parenchymal structure with an irregular, inhomogeneous, 2–3 cm architectural distortion and associated microcalcifications.

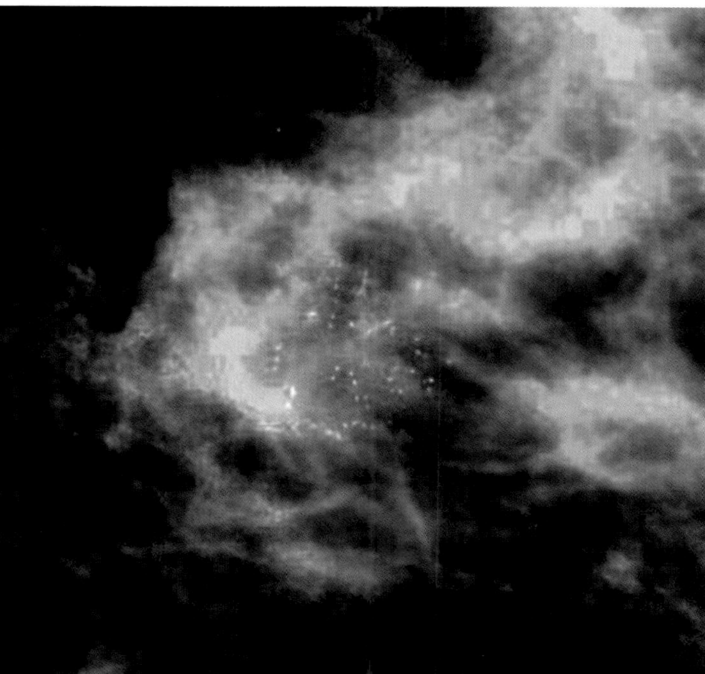

**b** *Magnified view* shows that the tumor is not demarcated from the surrounding glandular tissue. Coarse calcifications are visible at the center and periphery of the lesion. An oblique mammogram of the left breast was ordered *after* the histologic result was known. Mammography would ordinarily be contraindicated in an 18-year-old.

▶ Fig. 5.64 c, d

**Fig. 5.64 Mammography and ultrasound in an 18-year-old woman with left-sided breast cancer.** *(continued)*

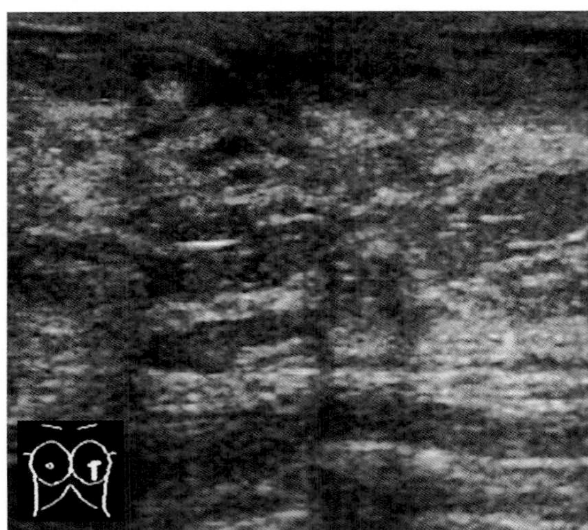

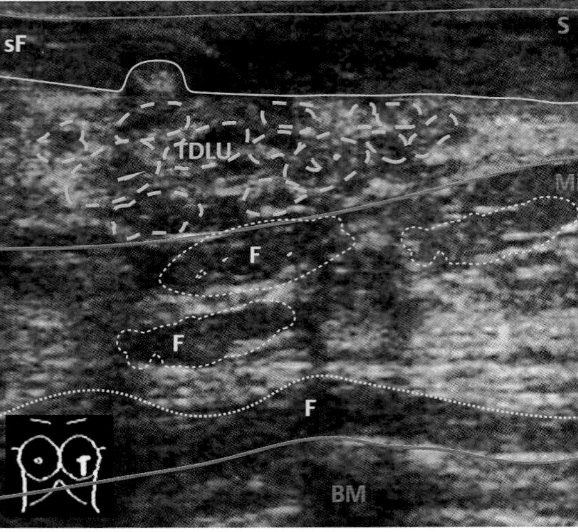


S = skin
sF = subcutaneous fat
Mi = milk duct(s)
F = fat
FA = fibroadenoma
BM = pectoral muscle

**c** *Sonogram* of the lower outer quadrant of the left breast. The breast parenchyma has a spongy texture with areas rich in interlobular stroma and TDLUs (compare with histologic diagnosis).

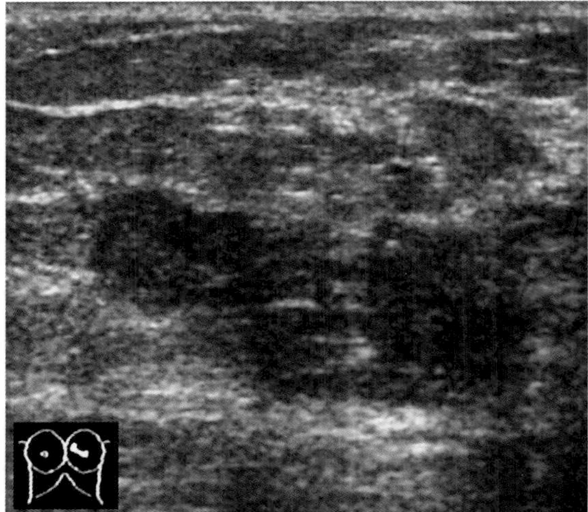

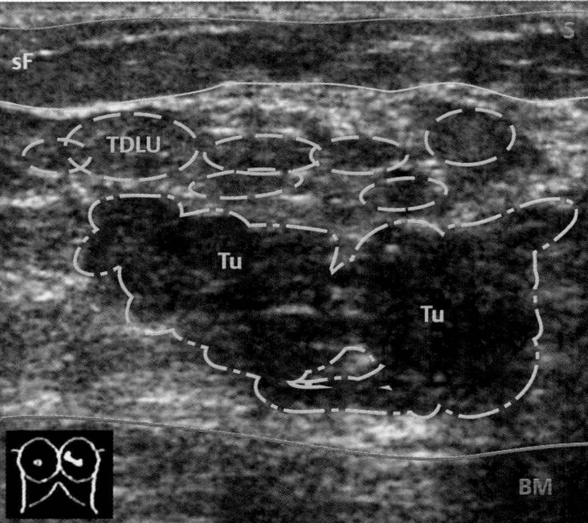


S = skin
sF = subcutaneous fat
TDLU = terminal duct lobular unit
Tu = tumor
BM = pectoral muscle

**d** *Sonogram* of the upper outer quadrant shows an ill-defined tumor nodule surrounded by numerous TDLUs. The TDLUs at the periphery of the tumor are in a strongly proliferative state (compare with basic pattern in (**c**).

**Treatment:** The patient underwent breast-conserving surgery without axillary dissection (sentinel nodes were clear, tumor marker CA 15–3 was normal). She underwent six chemotherapy cycles with the EC regimen while also taking Zoladex. Chemotherapy was followed by radiation to the breast. Given the positive estrogen receptor status, she was placed on antihormonal therapy with tamoxifen and Zoladex (information about treatment with kind permission of Professor H. J. Herschlein, Marienhospital Stuttgart, Germany).

**Fig. 5.65 Breast parenchyma at midcycle in a 19-year-old with fibroadenomas and adenosis.** The patient complained of premenstrual syndrome and had no history of oral contraceptive use. Fibroadenoma was confirmed by core-needle biopsy. Her grandmother had been diagnosed with breast cancer at age 45. Vacuum biopsy was proposed. The TDLUs were prominent and enlarged, coalescing to adenosis and fibroadenomas (see **Fig. 4.4 e**, p. 26).

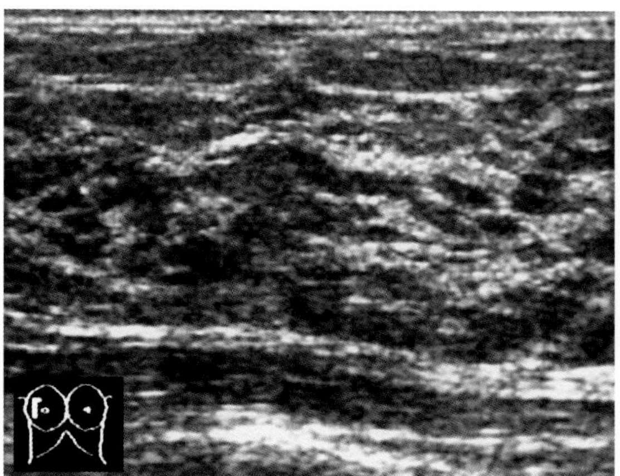

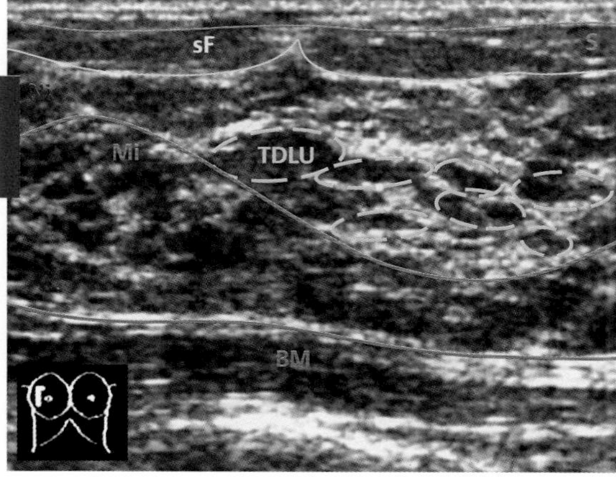


S = skin
sF = subcutaneous fat
TDLU = terminal duct lobular unit
Ni = nipple
BM = pectoral muscle

**a** *Sonogram* of a lobe in the right breast demonstrates a slender milk duct running obliquely through the field. Connective tissue in the breast parenchyma is accompanied by areas with a spongy texture due to proliferating TDLUs.

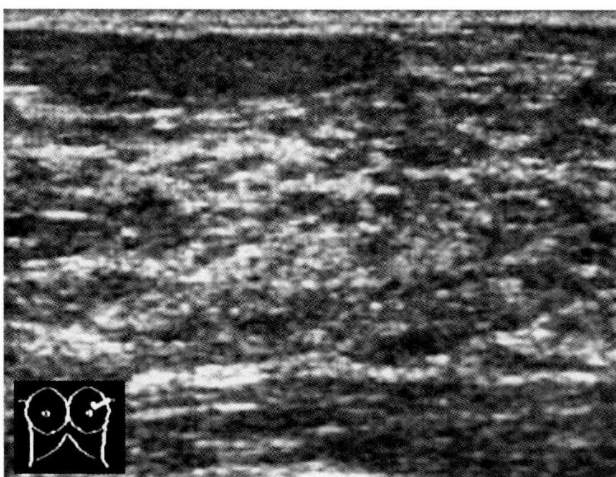

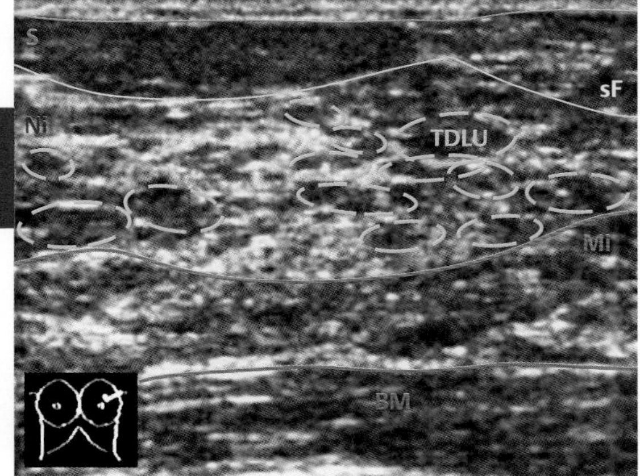


S = skin
sF = subcutaneous fat
TDLU = terminal duct lobular unit
Ni = nipple
BM = pectoral muscle

**b** *Sonogram* of a lobe in the left breast does not show a clearly visible duct. The normal-appearing glandular tissue has a spongy texture with areas of connective tissue alternating with enlarged TDLUs.

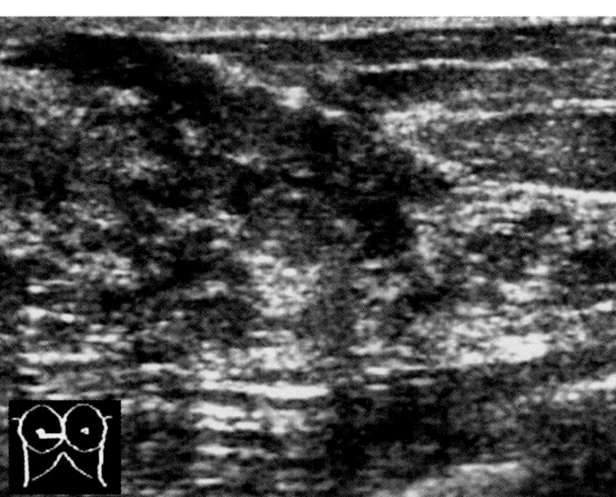

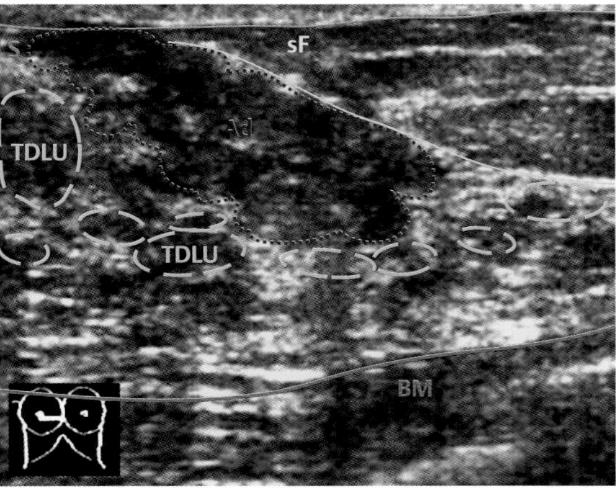


S = skin
sF = subcutaneous fat
TDLU = terminal duct lobular unit
Ad = adenosis
BM = pectoral muscle

**c** *Scan* of a lobe in the lower inner quadrant of the right breast shows confluent proliferating TDLUs consistent with adenosis. This area is surrounded by additional proliferating TDLUs. The adenosis was not visible on mammograms.

▶ **Fig. 5.65 d–g**

**Fig. 5.65 Breast parenchyma at midcycle in a 19-year-old with fibroadenomas and adenosis.** *(continued)*

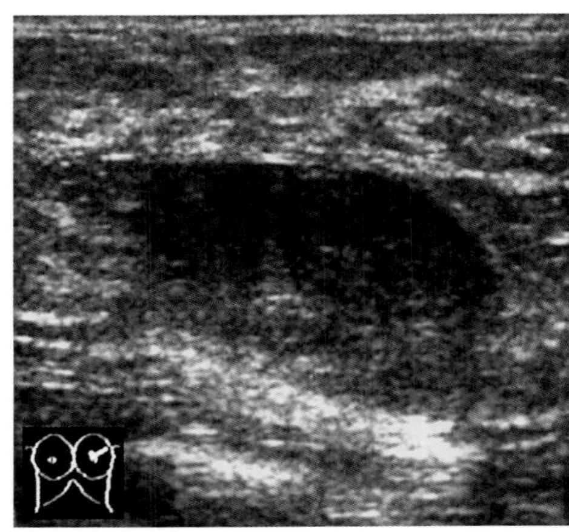

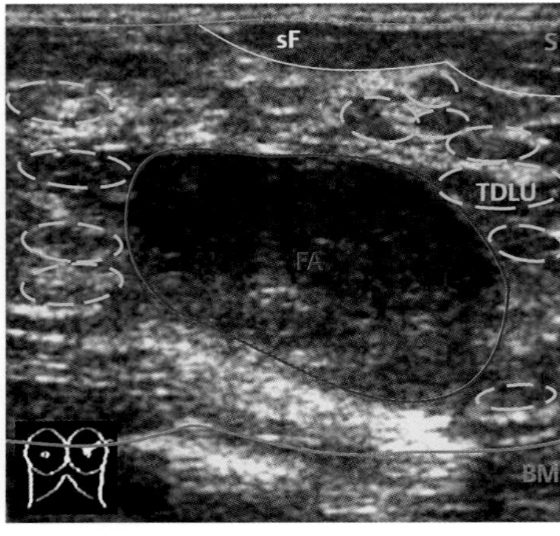


S = skin
sF = subcutaneous fat
TDLU = terminal duct lobular unit
FA = fibroadenoma
BM = pectoral muscle

**d** *Scan* through the upper outer quadrant of the left breast. A fibroadenoma appears as a 2.5 cm × 1.6 cm nodule with smooth margins, internal echoes, and slight posterior acoustic enhancement (not visible on mammograms). The parenchyma around the tumor has a somewhat spongy texture and contains prominent TDLUs.

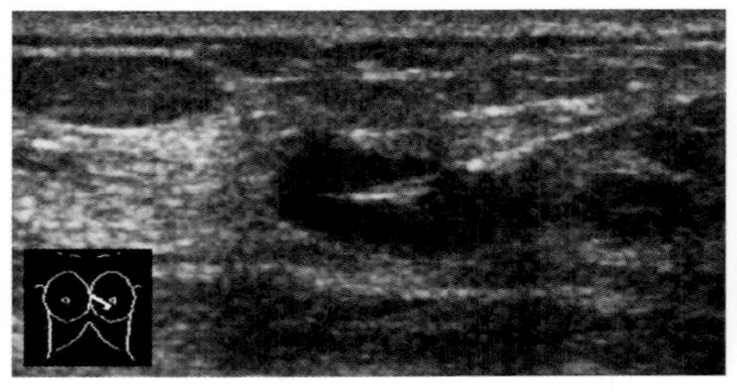

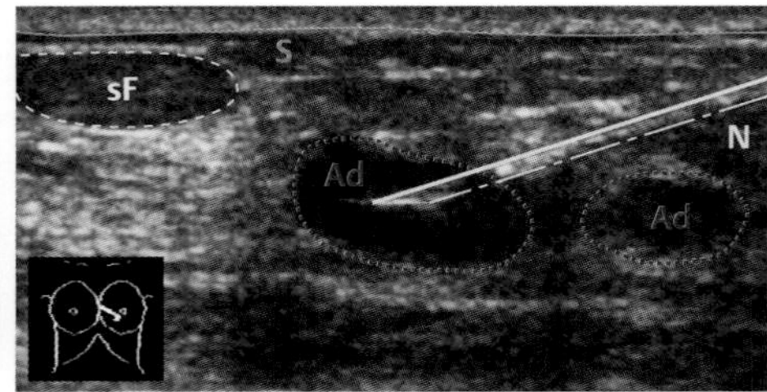


S = skin
sF = subcutaneous fat
Ad = adenosis
N = Needle

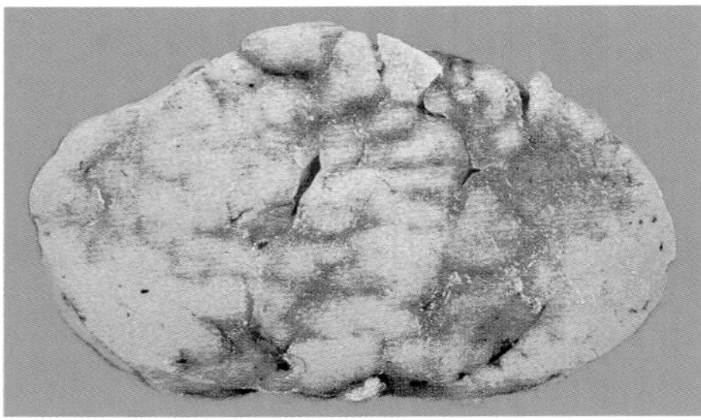

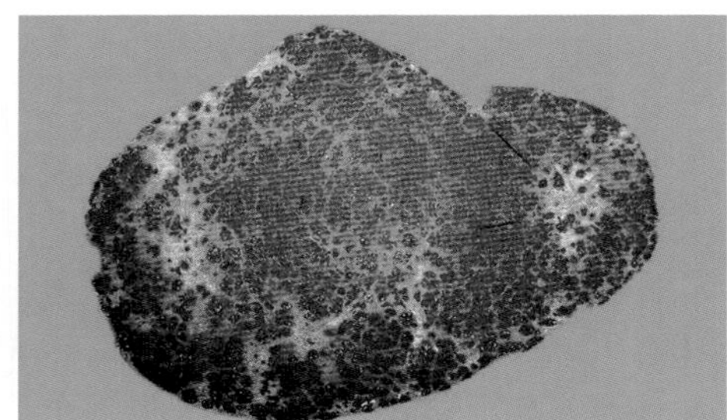

**e** *Comparison scan* in a different, 27-year-old, woman with a pure tubular adenoma. The lesion has smooth margins, no internal echoes, and posterior acoustic enhancement. A biopsy needle is visible in the nodule. The tumor resembles adenosis and fibroadenoma in its sonographic features. The different sonodensities result from differences in the interlobular stromal content of the different lesions. The adenoma was not visible on mammograms.
**Macroanatomy and microanatomy of a pure adenoma.**
**e1** *Macroanatomy:* Cut surface of an adenoma with marked proliferation of lobules, some white and bandlike and others salmon-colored as in a pregnant breast.
**e2** *Histology* of a pure adenoma shows multiple confluent lobules (dark purple) with scant interlobular stroma (light) (courtesy of Roland Bässler, Fulda). The massive accumulation of lobules and TDLUs accounts for the low echogenicity of the nodule at ultrasound.

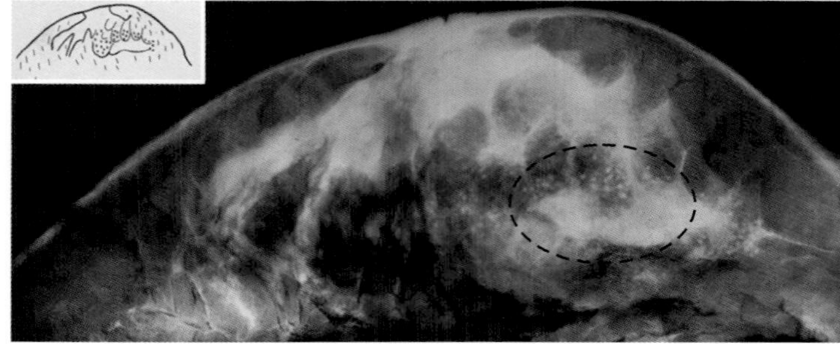

**f** *Specimen radiograph* of a 1 cm-thick slice of breast tissue. The lobes appear as inhomogeneous bandlike densities. The stippled opacities within the lobes are caused by TDLUs (lobules and terminal ducts with intralobular stroma; outlined area) (see also **Fig. 5.67**).

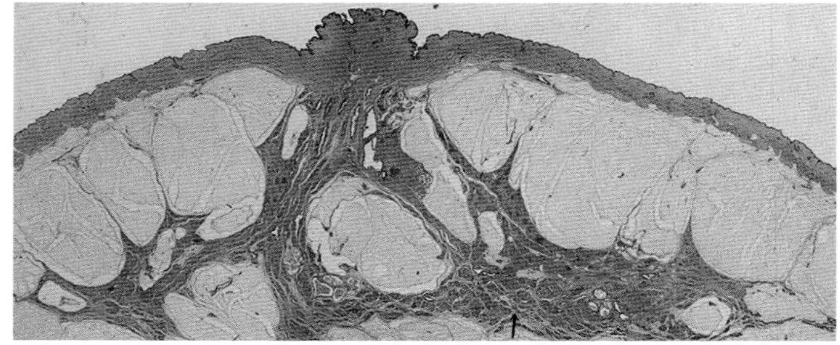

**g** *Gross tissue section* shows the interlobular stroma with ducts (most prominent in the retroareolar region) and numerous small TDLUs (arrow, stained purple).

**Fig. 5.66 Normal breast parenchyma. Case comparison.** The first case is a 25-year-old woman (**a, b**) who had taken oral contraceptives for years and did not suffer premenstrual syndrome. She was scanned during the premenstrual phase at the end of her cycle. Compare with another 25-year-old woman in the same cycle phase who had not taken oral contraceptives (**c**).

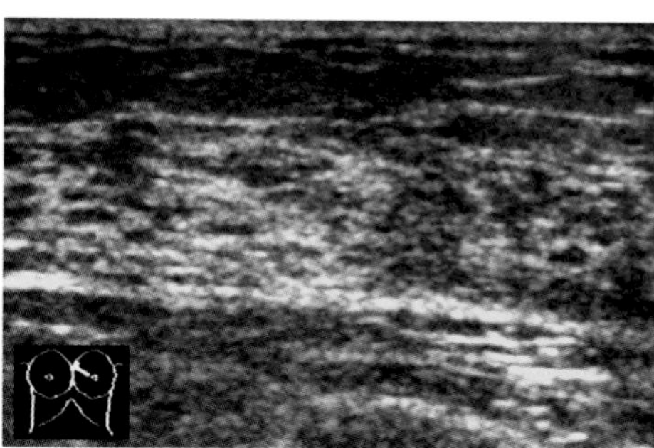

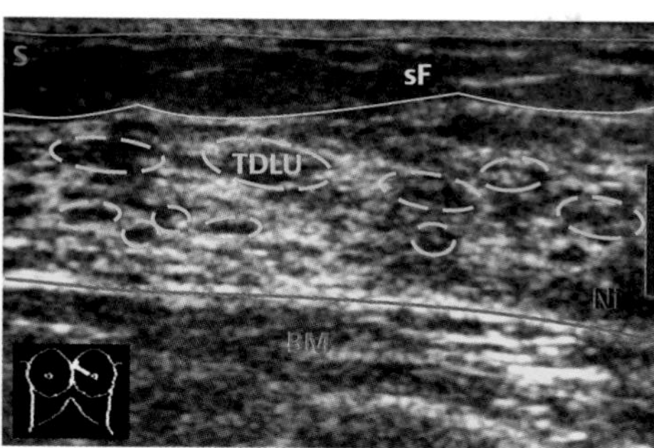


S = skin
sF = subcutaneous fat
TDLU = terminal duct lobular unit
Ni = nipple
BM = pectoral muscle

**a** *Sonogram* of the upper inner quadrant of the left breast shows a lobe with stroma-rich glandular areas and numerous small, elliptical TDLUs.

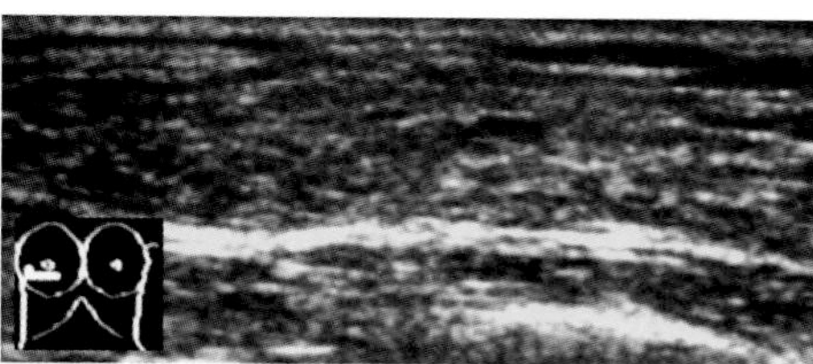

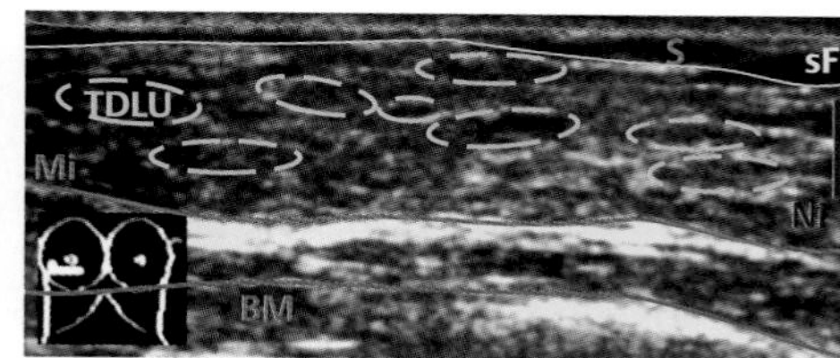


S = skin
sF = subcutaneous fat
TDLU = terminal duct lobular unit
Mi = milk duct(s)
Ni = nipple
BM = pectoral muscle

**b** *Sonogram* of the upper outer quadrant of the right breast shows a glandular area rich in TDLUs. The duct is not visualized. Isolated septa are composed of interlobular stroma.

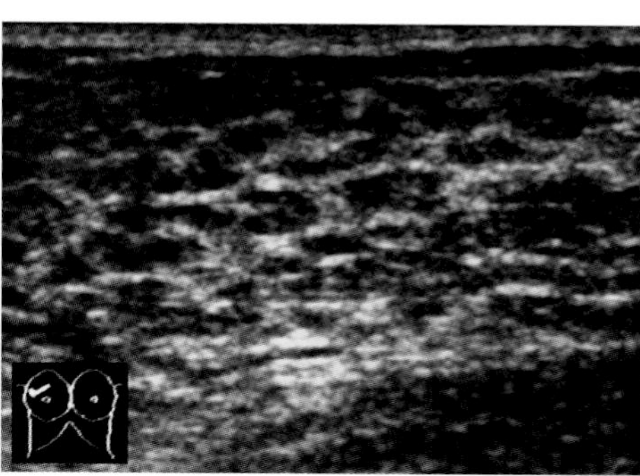

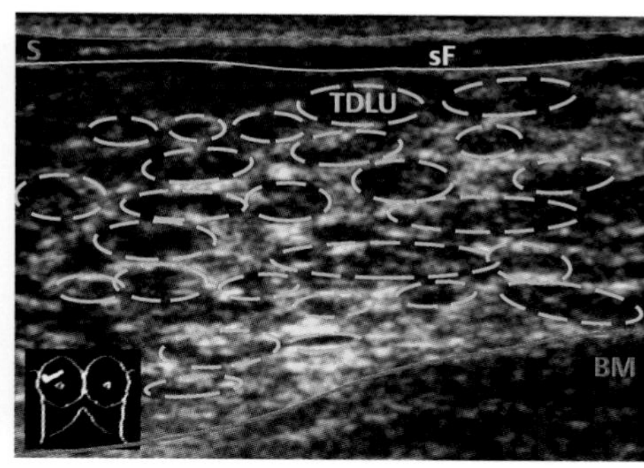


S = skin
sF = subcutaneous fat
TDLU = terminal duct lobular unit
BM = pectoral muscle

**c** *Sonogram* in a different patient of the same age who has not taken oral contraceptives shows greater premenstrual enlargement of the TDLUs along with echogenic septa composed of interlobular stroma.

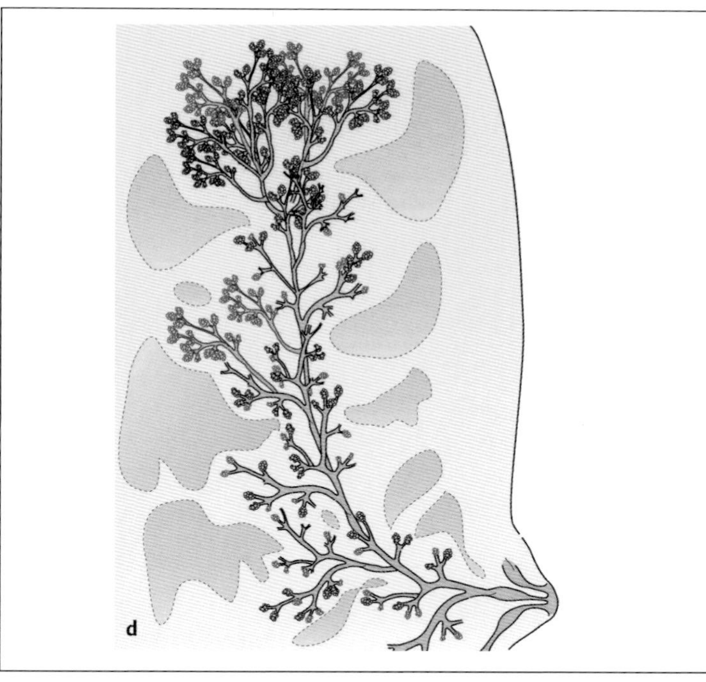


**d** *Anatomical drawing* of the lobular system in one lobe of a sexually mature woman. Note that the TDLUs are fully mature in the periphery of the lobe and less so toward the nipple. Full maturation of all lobules does not occur until the first pregnancy (diagram courtesy of Dabelow and Bässler, Fulda). At any age the lobular parenchyma is most fully developed in the periphery of the lobe, which is where most tumors originate (see also Screening: "no man's land" region between the pectoral muscle and breast parenchyma).

***The TDLUs in women on oral contraceptives show less enlargement during the second half of the cycle than in women not taking the pill. As a result, premenstrual syndrome is often absent.***

**Fig. 5.67 A 29-year-old woman with severe premenstrual syndrome**. The breast parenchyma contains abundant stroma with isolated cysts and moderate lobular proliferation. The patient tried various contraceptives in an effort to relieve premenstrual breast pain and tenderness, but even Progestogel was of no benefit. She had bilateral nipple inversion since puberty and no family history of breast cancer. She reported an occasional discharge of whitish debris [TN4].

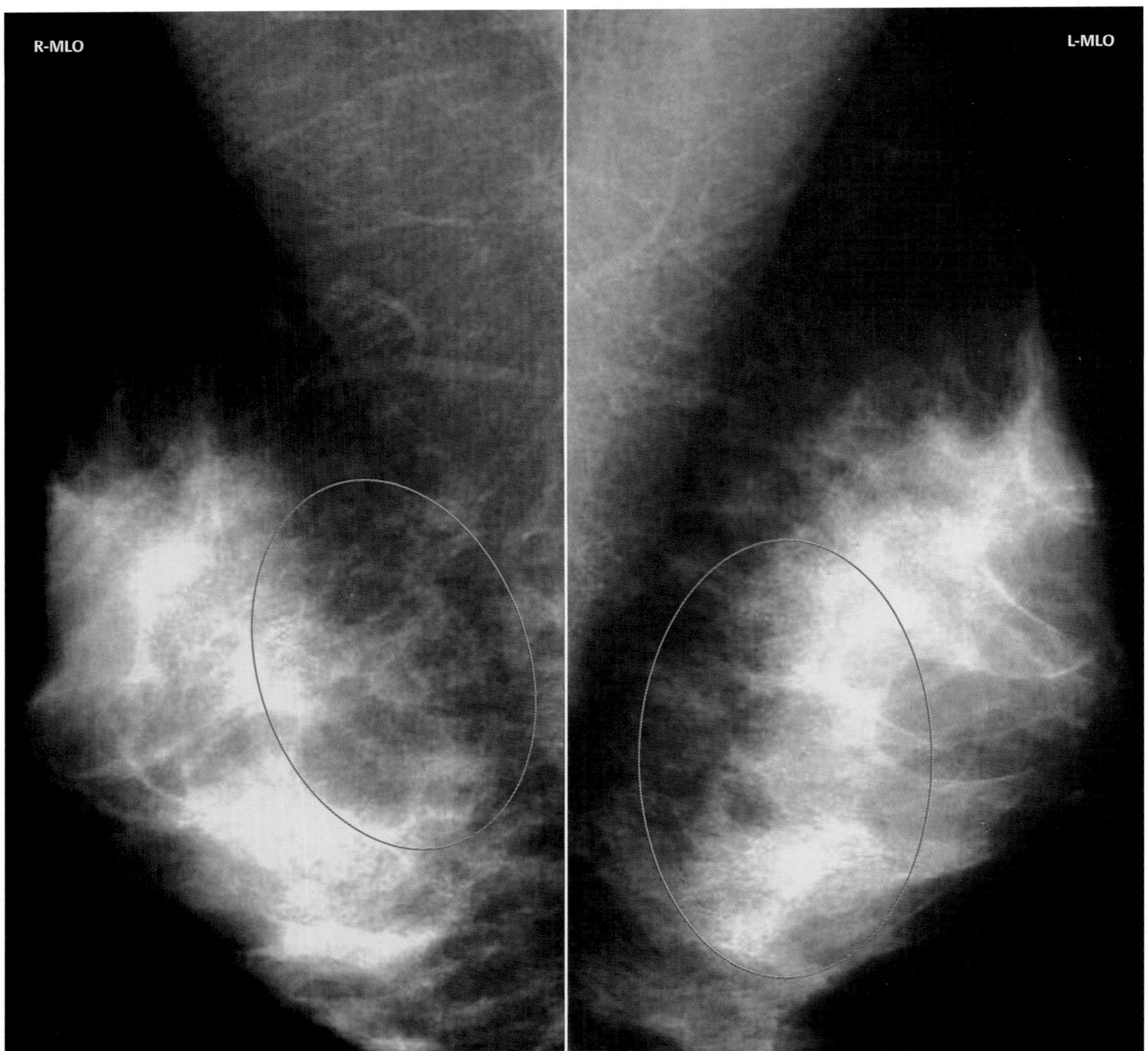


**a** *Bilateral oblique mammograms* show very radiodense breast parenchyma with no visible abnormalities (ACR 3, **P**GMI).
*The ACR 3 mammographic density is caused mainly by interlobular stroma (approximately 70%) despite the patient's youthful age. Increased proliferation of TDLUs cannot account for premenstrual complaints in this patients. The breast is permeated by areas of adenosis, small cysts, and TDLUs encased in connective tissue (approximately 20%). It is unclear which of these structures is the cause of mastodynia.*

**Fig. 5.67 A 29-year-old woman with severe premenstrual syndrome.** *(continued)*

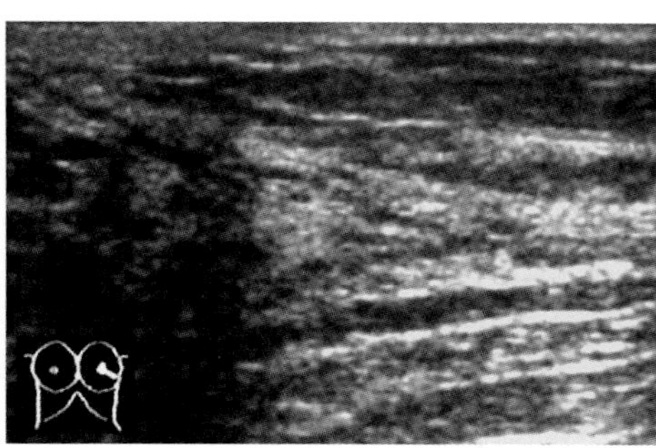

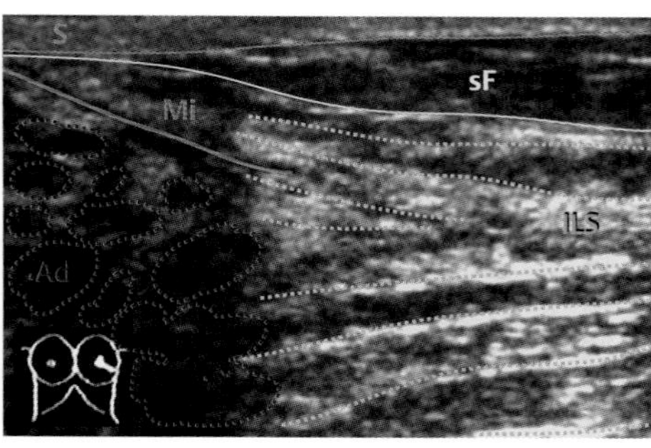


S = skin
sF = subcutaneous fat
Mi = milk duct(s)
ILS = interlobular stroma
Ad = adenosis

**b** *Retroareolar sonogram* of a lobe (enlarged view) in the left breast with a slightly dilated duct. Proliferating, confluent TDLUs form areas of adenosis below the duct. The rest of the parenchymal region is rich is interlobular stroma.

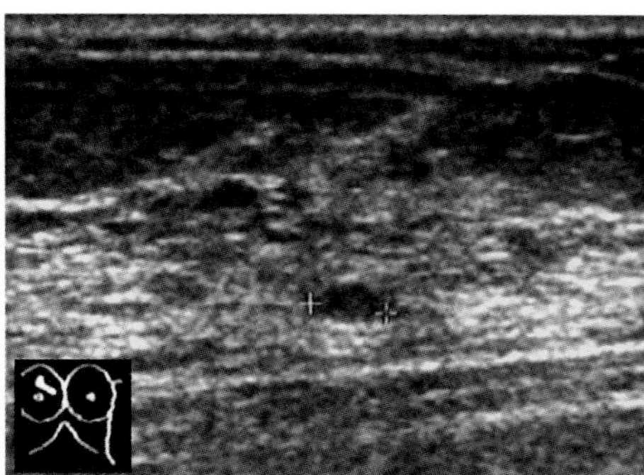

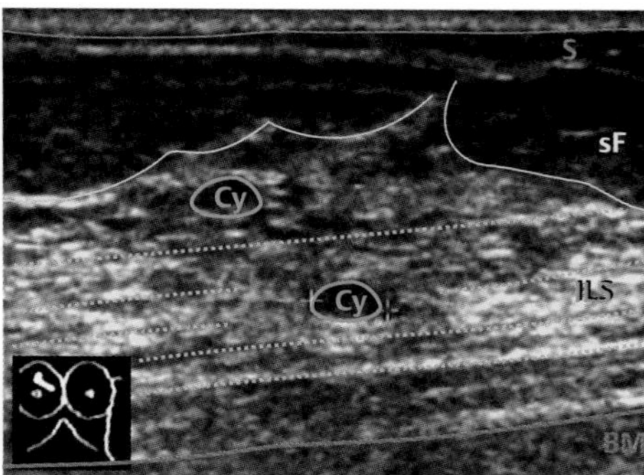


S = skin
sF = subcutaneous fat
ILS = interlobular stroma
Cy = cyst

**c** *Sonogram* of the upper inner quadrant of the right breast displays a lobe in cross section. The breast parenchyma contains abundant interlobular stroma along with small cysts and tiny hypoechoic areas formed by nonproliferating TDLUs.

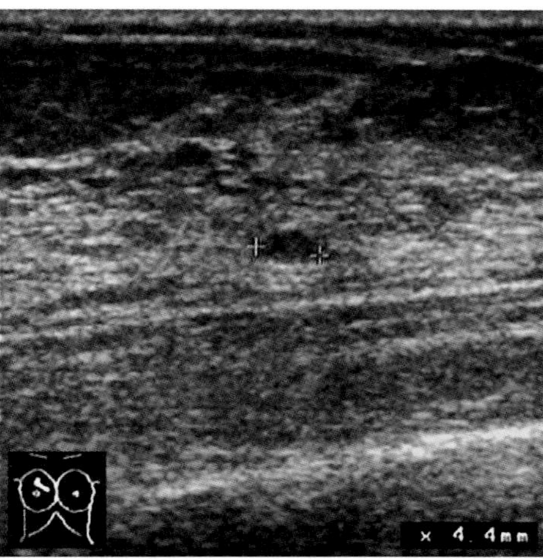


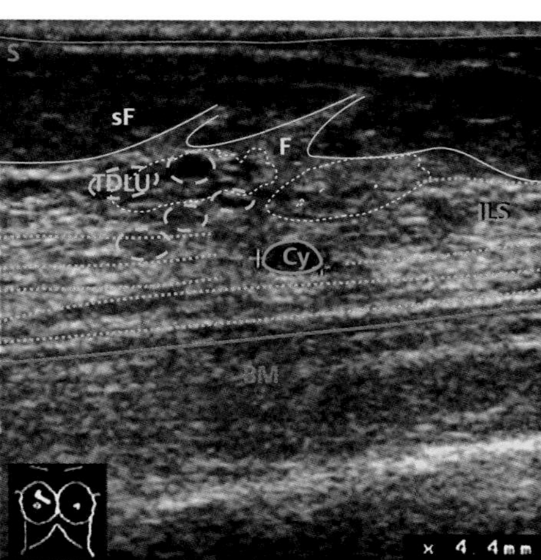


S = skin
sF = subcutaneous fat
F = fat
ILS = interlobular stroma
TDLU = terminal duct lobular unit
Cy = cyst

**d** *Sonogram* at a different site in the upper inner quadrant of the right breast shows glandular areas rich in interlobular stroma, a small cyst, and isolated TDLUs.

**Fig. 5.68 A 33-year-old woman in the seventh month of pregnancy.** The TDLUs are greatly enlarged and confluent, with associated regression of interlobular stroma and fat. Because of the proliferating TDLUs, the cut surface of the breast parenchyma appears salmon-colored rather than white (see **Fig. 5.69 a**). The breast becomes heavy and the skin become thickened and edematous (water retention). Nodular masses are palpable within the breast. This patient had a palpable mass in the upper outer quadrant of her left breast (marked by the fingers in (**a**), which was caused simply by the nodular proliferation of breast parenchyma. The patient was examined in the seventh month of pregnancy (**a–c**) and 3 months after the end of lactation (**d–f**). The mammographic density of this breast (ACR 4) results from approximately 25% interlobular stroma and 70% TDLUs.

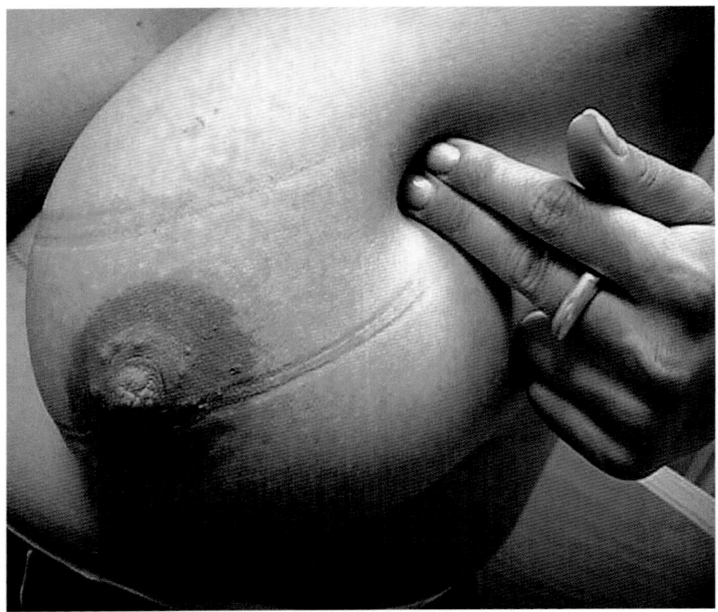

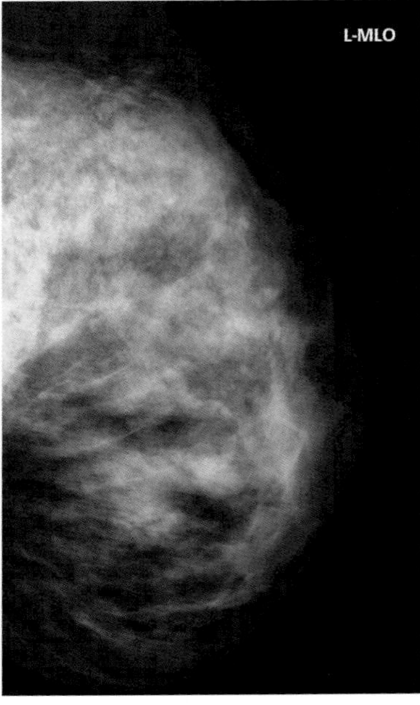


**a** *Physical examination* of the left breast shows typical cutaneous edema with pressure marks, hyperpigmentation of the areola, and a palpable mass in the upper outer quadrant. *Oblique mammogram* of the left breast during pregnancy to exclude microcalcifications shows a dense, inhomogeneous breast (ACR 4). Approximately 70% of the mammographic density results from proliferating TDLUs.

***The ACR 4 density of this mammogram results from abundant interlobular stroma and fat, and approximately 60% results from proliferating TDLUs and fibrocystic nodules in the upper outer quadrant of the left breast.***

**Tip:** Unlike *craniocaudal* mammograms (oblique mammograms direct the x-ray beam away from the pelvis), minimizing radiation exposure to the fetus. For this reason, craniocaudal mammograms are contraindicated in pregnant (and young) women.

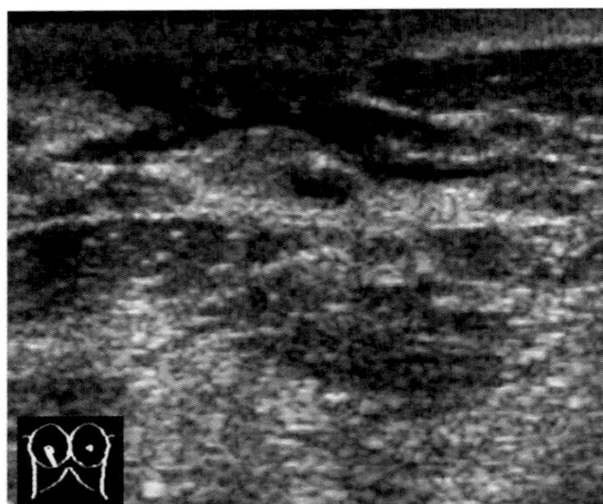

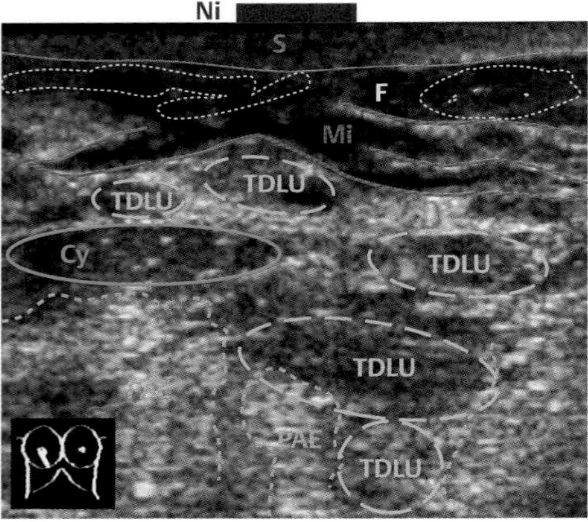


S = skin (thickened)
F = fat
Mi = dilated milk ducts
TDLU = greatly enlarged proliferating terminal duct lobular unit
Cy = cyst with debris
Ni = nipple
PAE = posterior acoustic enhancement

**b** *Retroareolar sonogram* of the right breast shows dilated milk ducts and proliferating TDLUs.

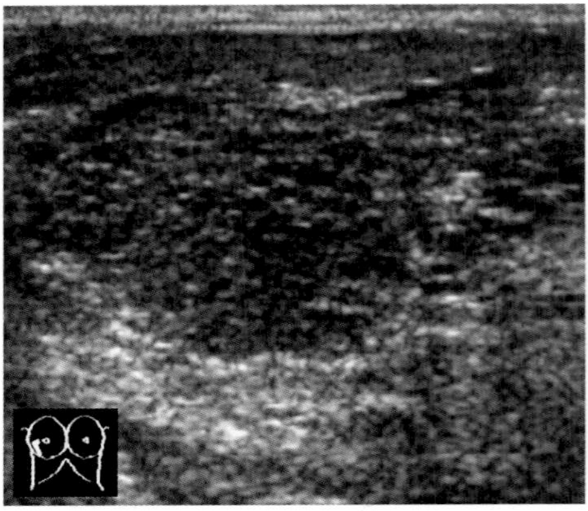

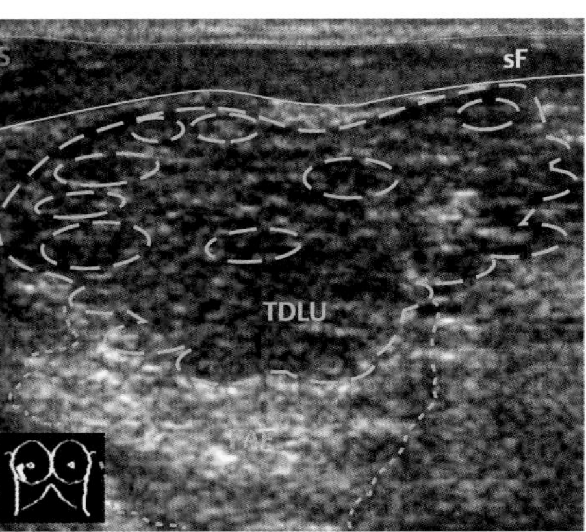


S = skin (thickened)
sF = subcutaneous fat
TDLU = terminal duct lobular unit (adenosis-like)
PAE = posterior acoustic enhancement

**c** *Sonogram* of the lower outer quadrant of the right breast displays a typical cross section of a lobe with multiple confluent TDLUs that show varying degrees of enlargement (compare **Fig. 5.69 f**, p. 170).

**Fig. 5.68 A 33-year-old woman in the seventh month of pregnancy.** *(continued)*

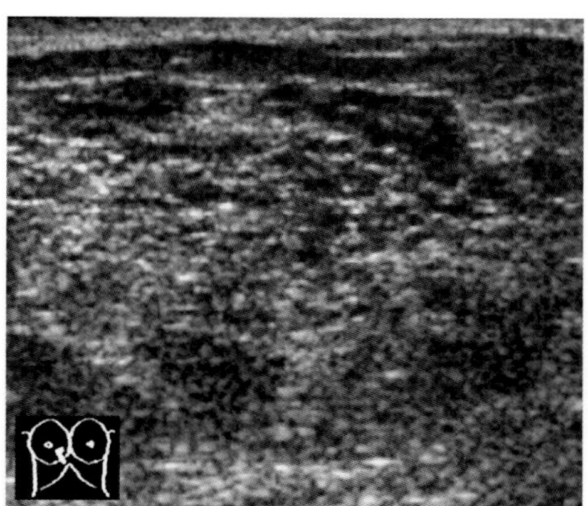

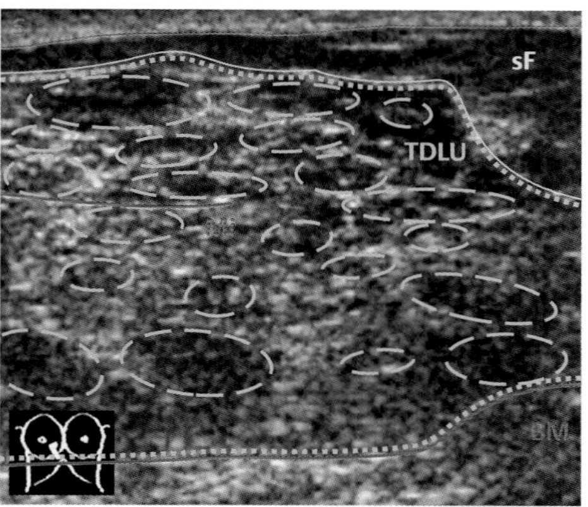


S = skin
sF = subcutaneous fat
TDLU = proliferating terminal duct lobular units throughout the breast
Mi = milk duct
BM = pectoral muscle

**d** *Sonogram* of the lower inner quadrant of the right breast 3 months after the end of lactation shows residual proliferation (forming a nonspecific palpable mass) with otherwise normal basic structures. Postpartum regression of the TDLUs may last for up to 2 years (see **Fig. 5.70 b**).

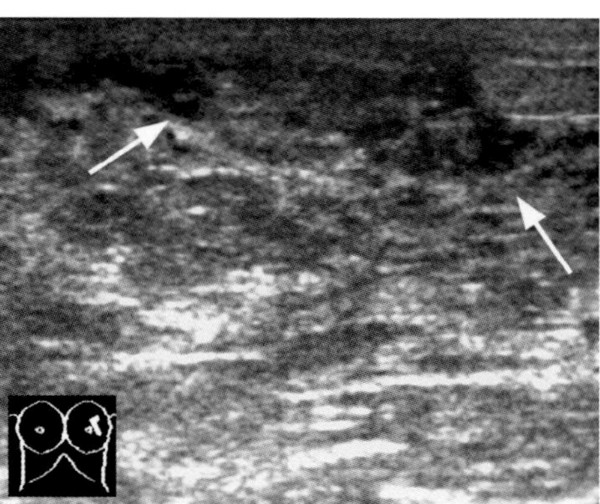

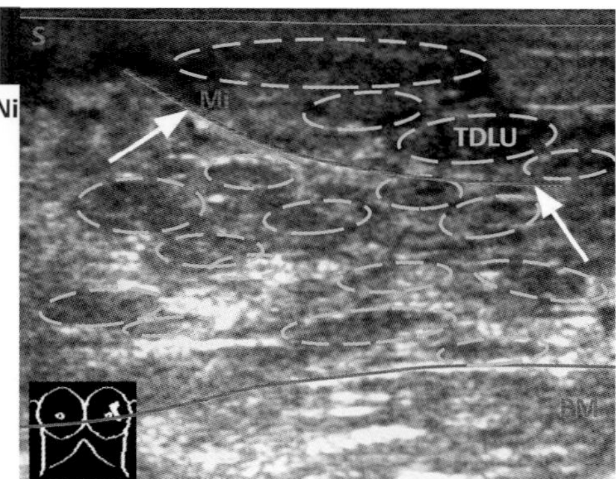


S = skin
TDLU = terminal duct lobular unit
Mi = milk duct (arrow)
Ni = nipple region
BM = pectoral muscle

**e** *Sonogram* of a palpable mass in the upper outer quadrant of the left breast shows residual enlargement of confluent TDLUs (lobules) with no evidence of a discrete tumor.

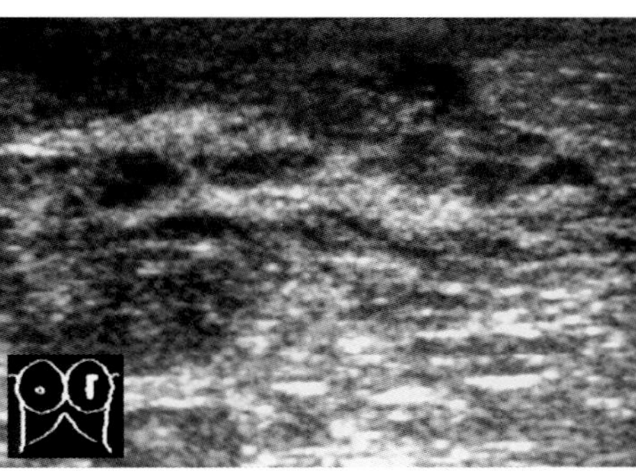

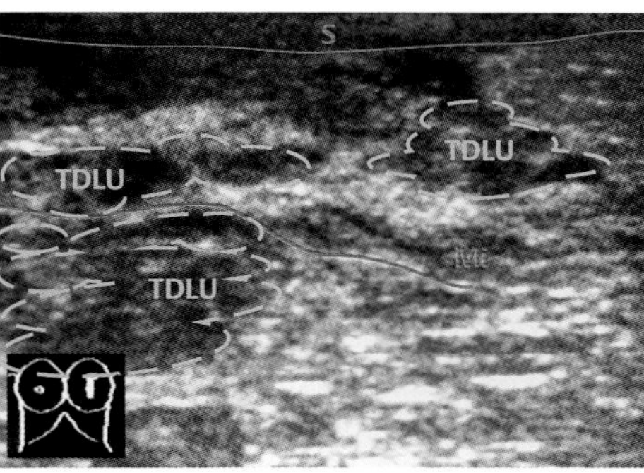


S = skin
sF = subcutaneous fat
TDLU = terminal duct lobular unit
Mi = milk duct

**f** *Follow-up retroareolar sonogram* 3 months after the end of lactation shows residual enlargement of TDLUs accompanied by general regression of glandular tissue with broad septa composed of interlobular stroma. Pressure on the proliferative areas still elicits a milky discharge.

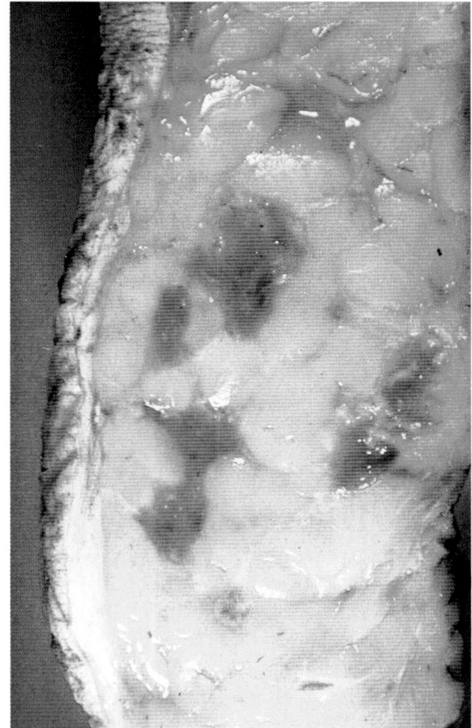

**g** *Macroanatomy* in early pregnancy. The cut surface exhibits yellow fat, grayish-white areas of fibrosis, and small salmon-colored foci of proliferating TDLUs in preparation for pregnancy and lactation.

**Fig. 5.69 Macro- and microanatomic changes during pregnancy (radiographic/anatomical comparison).** Breast of a 35-year-old woman who died of pulmonary embolism in the eighth month of pregnancy.

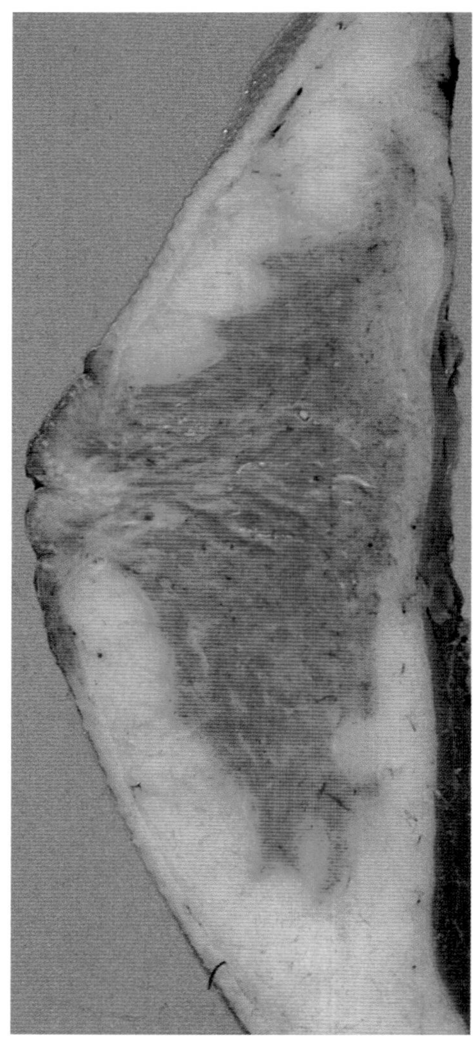

**a** *Gross anatomic section.* The breast parenchyma appears salmon-colored due to proliferating TDLUs with dense lobular development and increased blood flow. The breast parenchyma is surrounded by fat, and deep to the parenchyma (right side of photograph) is the brown-colored pectoral muscle (compare with color of normal breast parenchyma in **Fig. 5.81 h.**

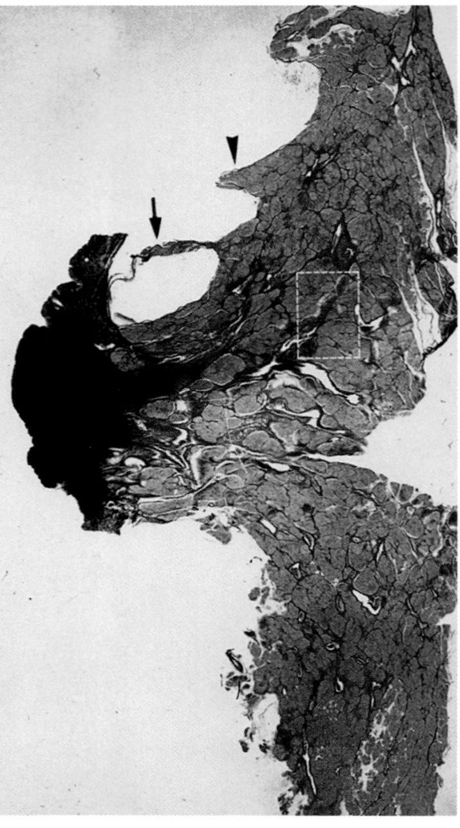

**b** *Microradiograph* (radiograph of a 50 µm-thick tissue slice). The enlarged TDLUs (lobules, gray) are surrounded by a fine rim of interlobular stroma (black). The nipple and retroareolar region appear dark due to connective tissue.

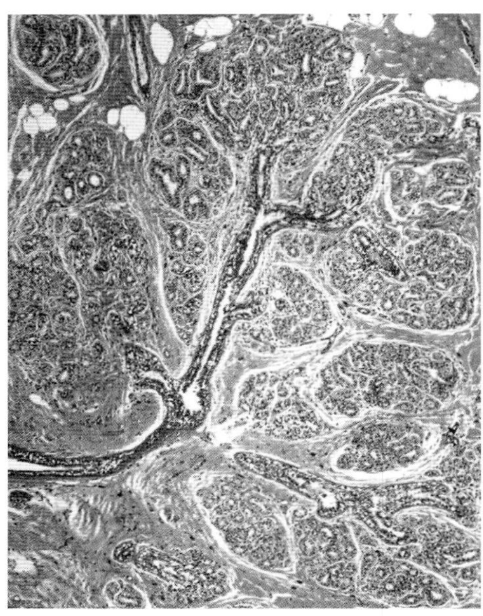

**c** *Histologic section* (approximately 20×, outlined in (**b**) of TDLUs with dense lobular proliferation in late pregnancy. A long milk duct is displayed in longitudinal section, and surrounding lobules show marked proliferation and enlargement.
The radiodensity of the pregnant breast is caused not by connective tissue but by a massive increase in lobular parenchyma. Even the Cooper ligaments are permeated by lobules, which form small nodular surface projections and cause some Cooper ligaments to become palpable as firm, cordlike structures.

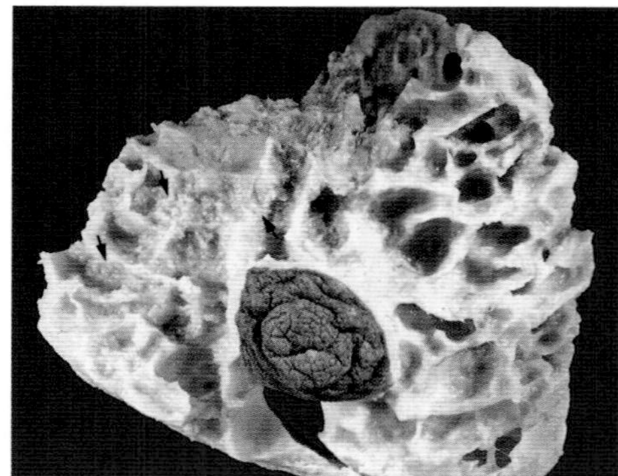

**d** *Breast parenchyma* in pregnancy with the skin, Cooper ligaments, and subcutaneous fat removed. The ends of the lobes are broadened, and enlarged TDLUs appear as small nodular protrusions in the fissures between the lobes (arrows on left side of photograph).

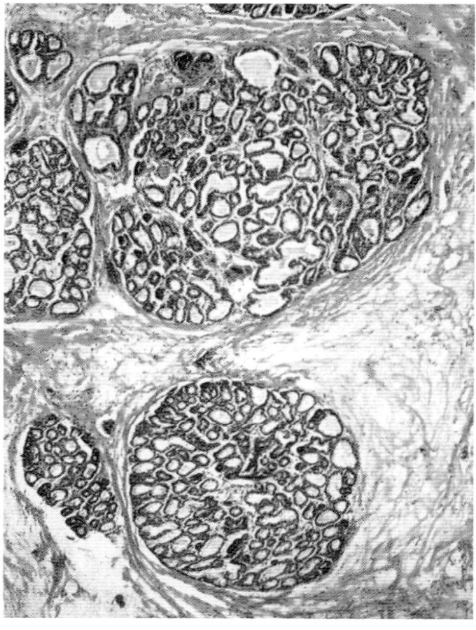

**e** *Histologic section* (approximately 80×) of lactating breast parenchyma shows large TDLUs with acinar differentiation of the tuberoalveolar gland. Interlobular stroma is present between the TDLUs.

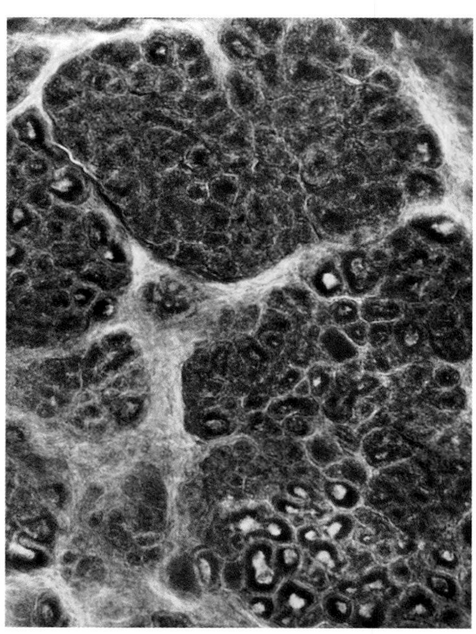

**f** *Microradiograph* (approximately 200×). The TDLUs (lobules) absorb less x-ray dose than the bright surrounding interlobular stroma. The acini are distended and filled with milk of calcium (bright spots especially prominent at lower right). The TDLUs have a similar appearance when imaged by ultrasound. A narrow band of interlobular stroma (white) is visible between the enlarged lobules (dark).

**Fig. 5.70 Mature breast with proliferating lobules and enlarged lobes in a very thin 37-year-old woman.** The patient had two children and was breastfeeding until a year ago, producing large amounts of milk. Pressure on the nipples still elicited discharge of colostrum. The patient was not taking hormones and was examined on the ninth day of the cycle.

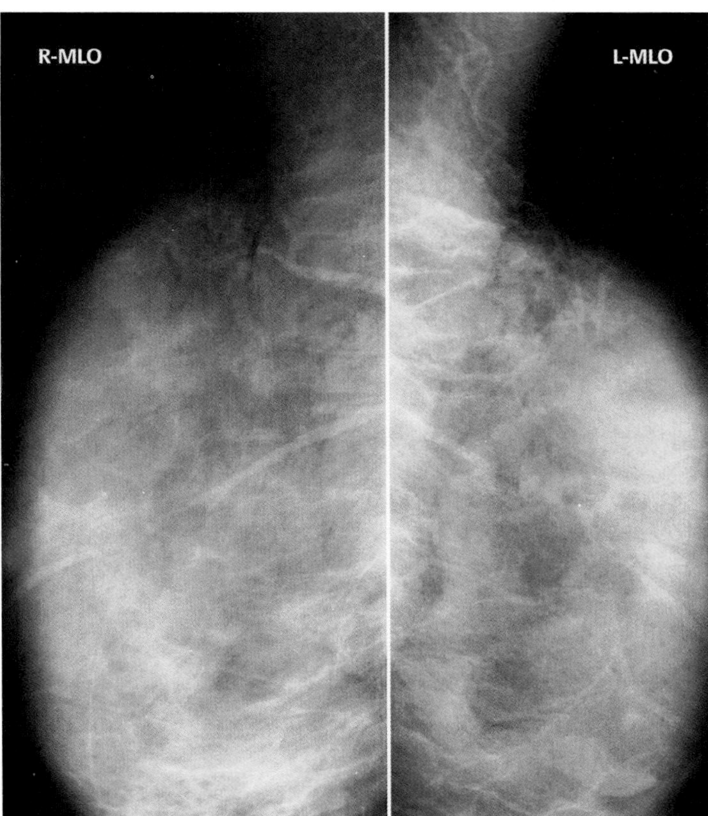


**a** *Bilateral oblique mammograms* show radiographically dense breasts (ACR 4, P**G**MI).

***The density is caused mainly by proliferating TDLUs, with approximately 40% due to interlobular stroma and fat. There is no evidence of neoplasia (classification Dy after Wolfe 1976, see p. 98).***

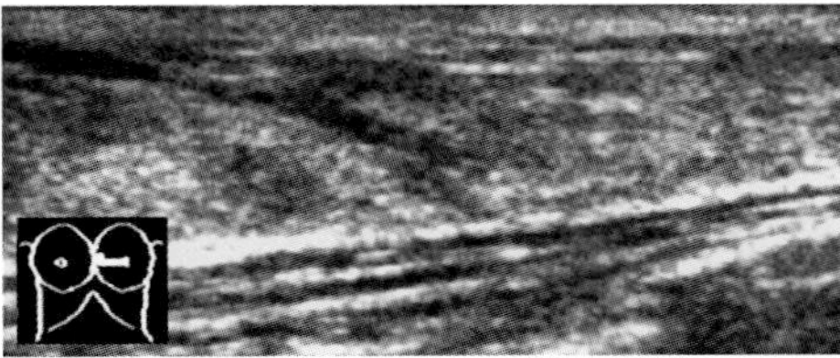

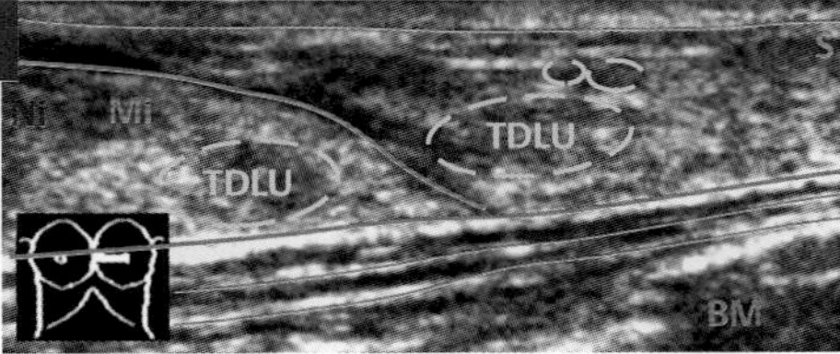


S = skin
TDLU = terminal duct lobular unit
Ni = nipple
Mi = milk duct
BM = pectoral muscle

**b** *Sonogramm* of the left breast shows a slightly dilated duct with abundant lobular parenchyma.

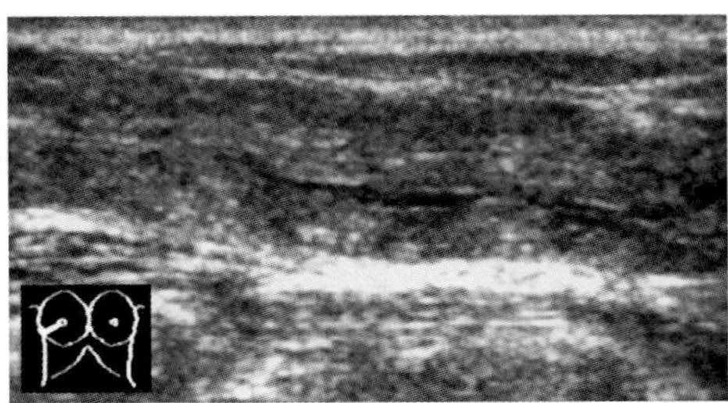

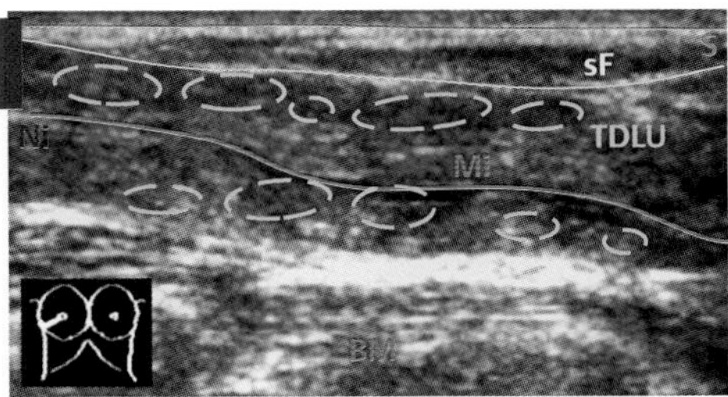


S = skin
sF = subcutaneous fat
Ni = nipple
Mi = milk duct
TDLU = terminal duct lobular unit
BM = pectoral muscle

**c** *Ultrasound-Scan of a peripheral lobe* in the lower outer quadrant of the right breast shows segments of a dilated duct surrounded by heavy lobular proliferation.

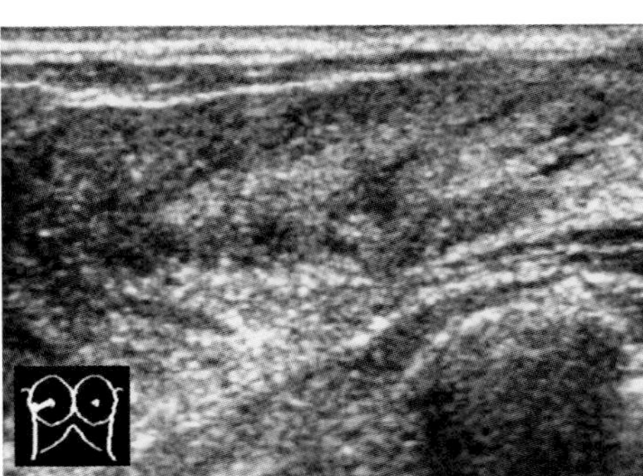

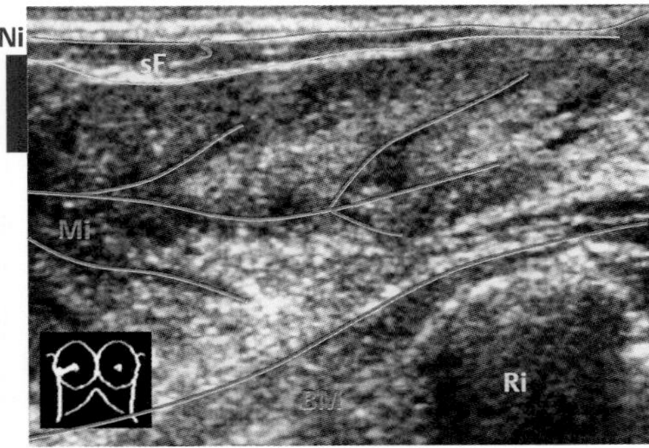


S = skin
sF = subcutaneous fat
Ni = nipple
Mi = milk duct
BM = pectoral muscle
Ri = rib

**d** *An enlarged lobe* scanned in longitudinal section shows peripheral dilatation of the ducts. The TDLUs have coalesced to form a dark, inhomogeneous area and are no longer definable as separate structures. It is unclear whether this is due to the proliferation of lobular tissue and/or intralobular stroma. The breast contains abundant parenchymal tissue (hormone sensitive) and little interlobular stroma (hormonal inactive).

**Fig. 5.71 Nonspecific bilateral nipple discharge in a 39-year-old woman.** Proliferating periductal and intralobular stroma are hypoechoic at ultrasound while the lumina of the bandlike ducts, which usually appear dark, show high echogenicity (**c, d**). The patient had normal hormone levels and was not taking oral contraceptives. Apparent lobular proliferation with unexplained discharge prompted a core-needle biopsy, which showed normal glandular tissue. *Histology:* loose periductular intralobular stroma, slightly edematous (**e**), with no increase in lobular proliferation.

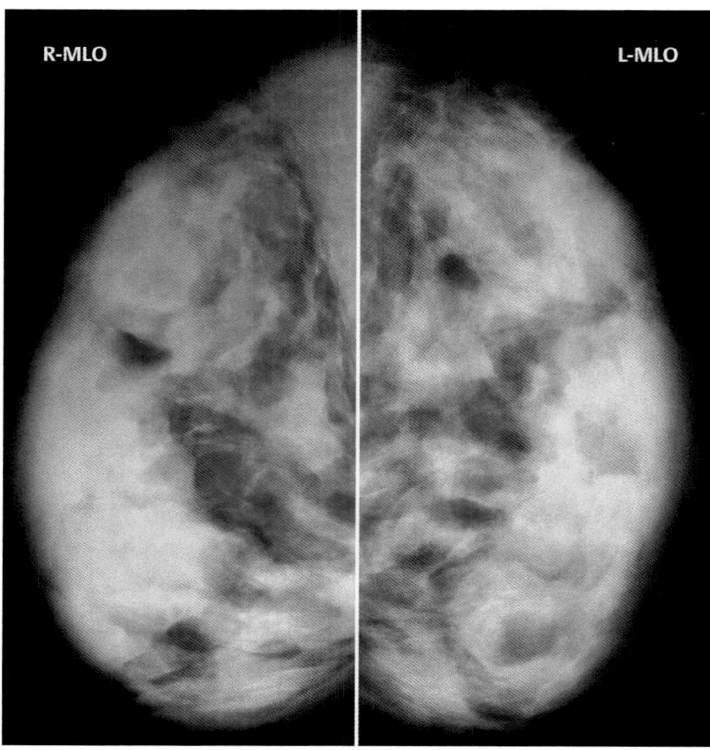


**a** *Bilateral oblique mammograms:* The parenchyma in each breast is inhomogeneous and very radiodense (ACR 3, P**G**MI), and the breasts show increased fatty permeation from the posterior side. There are no microcalcifications or other findings to suggest a malignant process (BIRADS 1).

*Given the breast composition, the ACR 3 density of the mammogram results largely (approximately 80%) from connective tissue (interlobular and intralobular stroma) permeated by fat.*

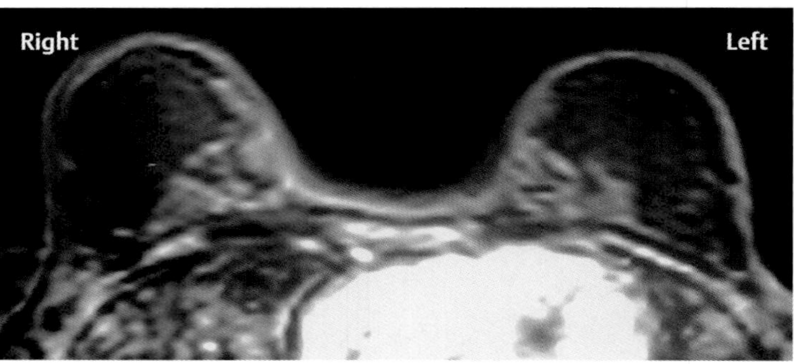


**b** *MRI:* Subtraction image after gadolinium injection shows slight, nonspecific enhancement over the inner quadrants with no other evidence of increased vascularity in the breasts. There appear to be few acini within the TDLUs, with inter- and intralobular stroma predominating. (The patient was examined on the 10th day of her cycle.)

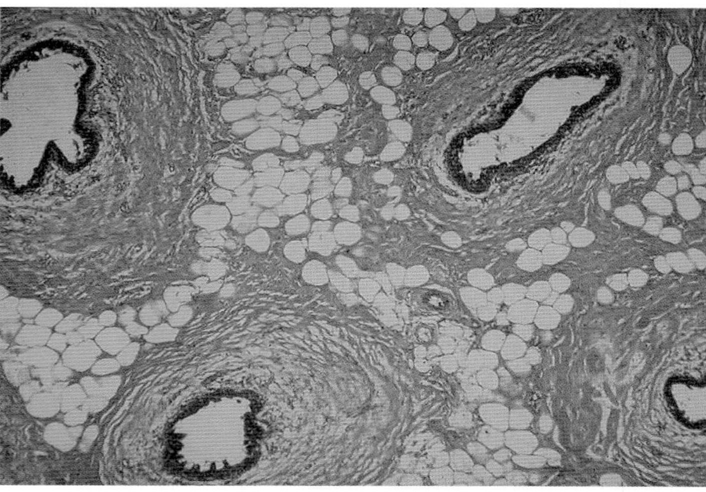

**e** *Histology*: Lactiferous ducts surrounded by loose intralobular stroma (see **Fig. 5.149 i, j**, p. 395) with interspersed fat. Interlobular stroma is stained a deeper pink.

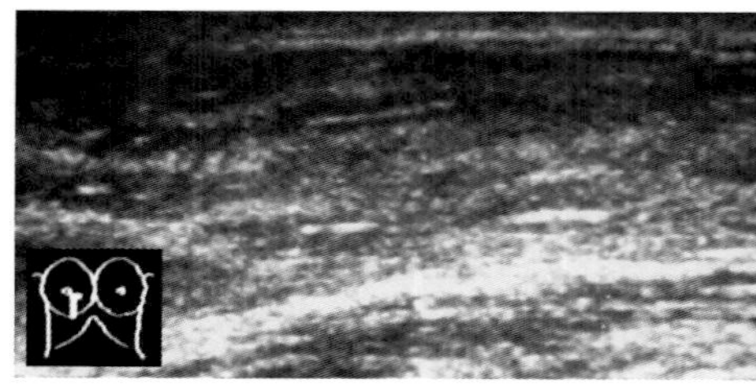

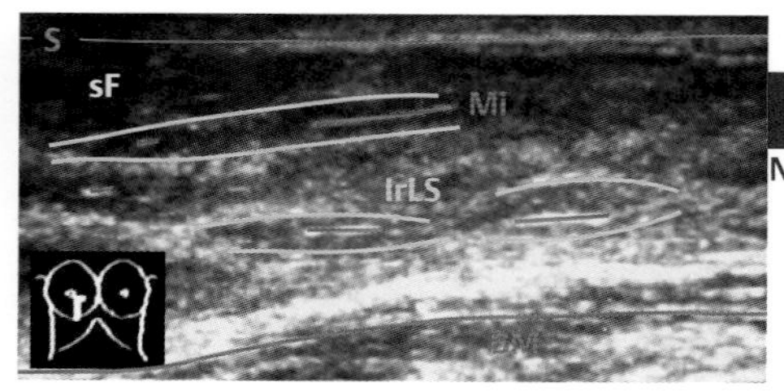


S = skin
sF = subcutaneous fat
Mi = milk duct(s)
Ni = nipple
IrLS = interlobular stroma
BM = pectoral muscle

**c** *Sonogram* of the lower inner quadrant of the right breast shows a lobe with bright linear ducts surrounded by darker, hypoechoic intralobular stroma, which extends into the subcutaneous space.

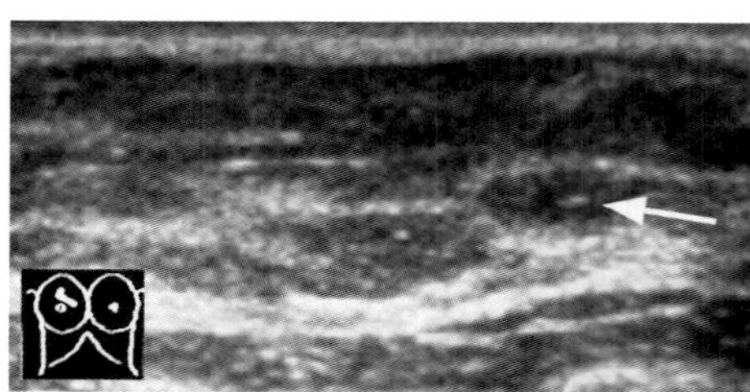

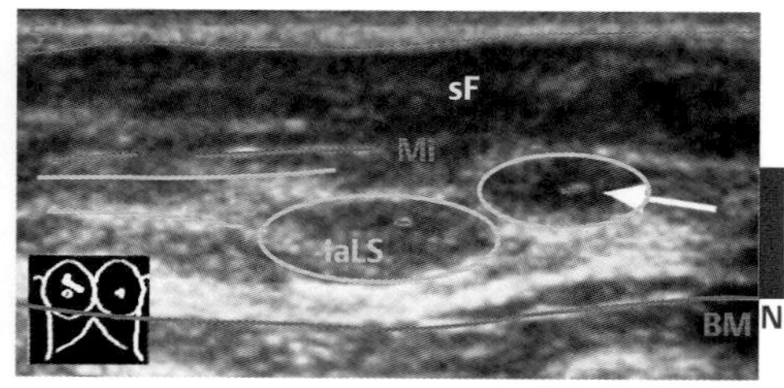


S = skin
Mi = milk duct(s) (arrow)
IaLS = intralobular stroma
BM = pectoral muscle
sF = subcutaneous fat
Ni = nipple

**d** *Sonogram* of the upper inner quadrant of the right breast displays a lobe in cross-section. The bright ducts (arrow) are viewed end-on and are surrounded by well-circumscribed, hypoechoic intralobular stroma. Ducts at left and center are viewed in longitudinal section.

**Fig. 5.72 A 36-year-old woman has worn a hormone-releasing IUD (Mirena) for 2 years.** The patient stopped taking oral contraceptives due to pigmentary changes (facial brown spots). At presentation, both breasts are firm with small palpable nodules. Her grandmother had breast cancer at age 30. The increased mammographic density 2002 (in comparison with 2000) is consistent with the proliferation and enlargement of TDLUs seen on ultrasound.

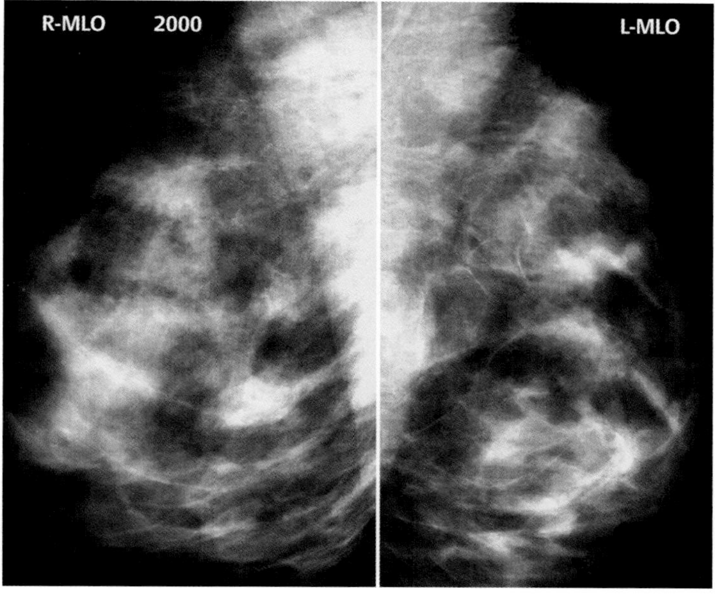


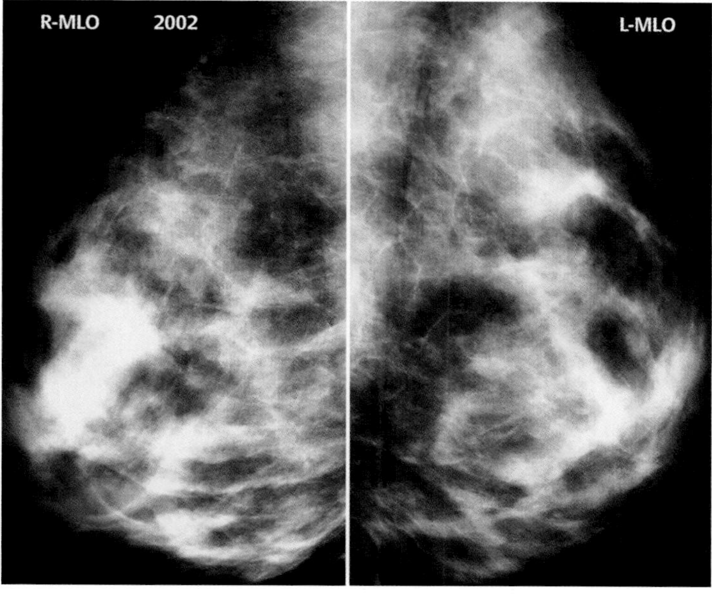


**a** *Bilateral oblique mammograms* in 2000 show normal-appearing, radiolucent breast parenchyma (ACR 2, P**G**MI).

**b** *Bilateral oblique mammograms* in 2002. Breast density is markedly increased due to the proliferation of TDLUs (ACR 3, P**G**MI). Hormonal stimulation by progestin (Mirena)?

*The higher radiodensity of the 2002 mammograms (ACR 3) compared with 2000 (ACR 2) results from an increase in TDLUs with no change in the interlobular stroma.*

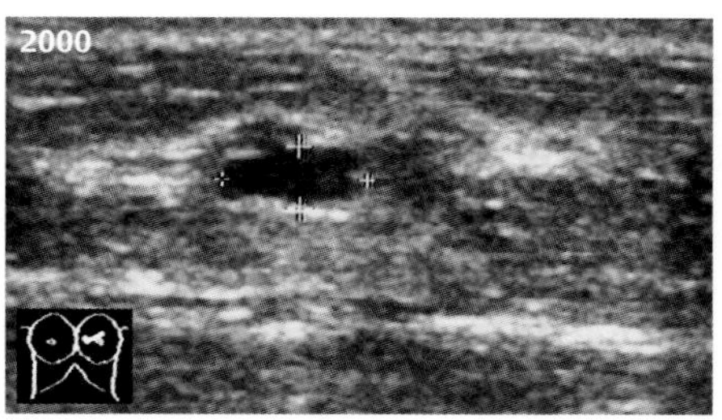


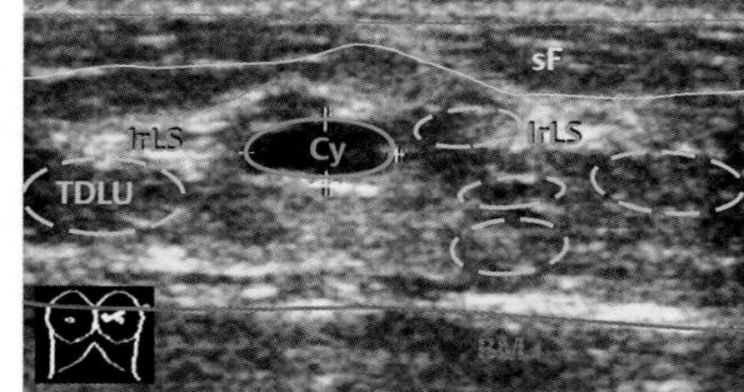


**c** *Sonogram (2000) of the upper inner quadrant of the left breast* shows a small cyst at the 12-o'clock position. Proliferating glandular tissue (dark) is visible next to connective tissue rich in stroma (light).
S = skin
sF = subcutaneous fat
Cy = cyst
IrLS = interlobular stroma
TDLU = terminal duct lobular unit
BM = pectoral muscle

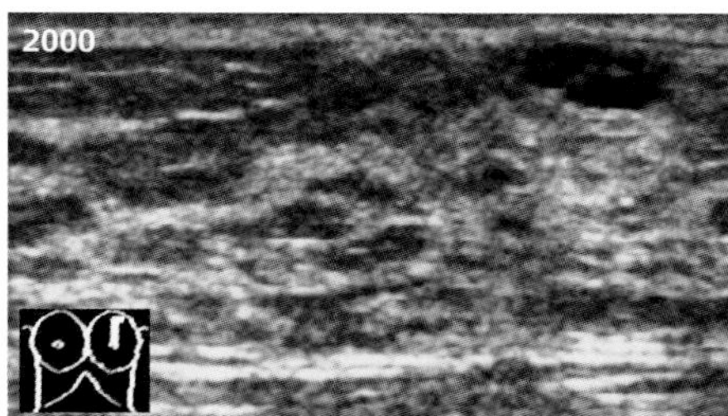


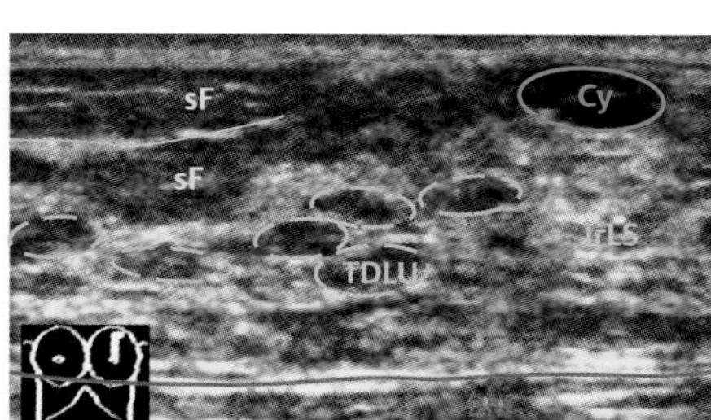


**d** *Sonogram of the supra-areolar left breast* in 2000 demonstrates a small cyst surrounded by proliferating TDLUs.

S = skin
sF = subcutaneous fat
Cy = cyst
IrLS = interlobular stroma
TDLU = terminal duct lobular unit
BM = pectoral muscle

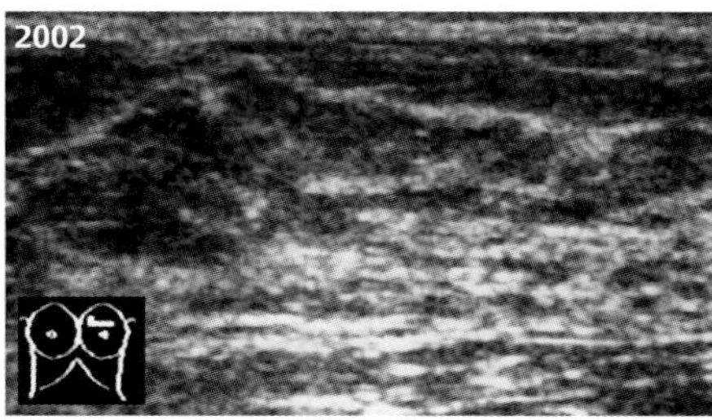


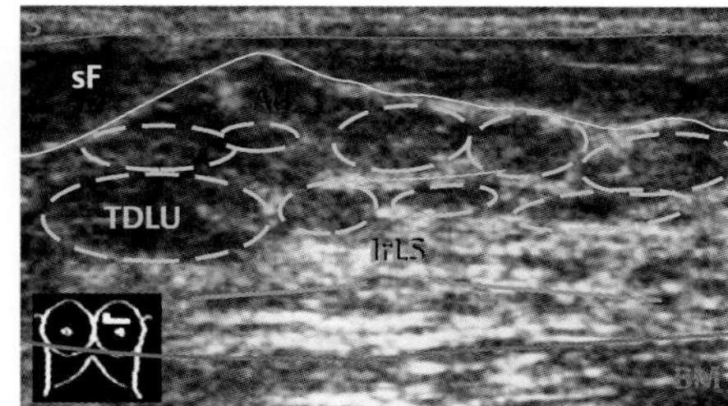


**e** *Sonogram* of the supra-areolar left breast in 2002 shows greater proliferation of TDLUs compared with 2000 along with more stroma-rich areas, especially at the prepectoral level.
S = skin
sF = subcutaneous fat
IrLS = interlobular stroma
TDLU = terminal duct lobular unit
Ad = adenosis
BM = pectoral muscle

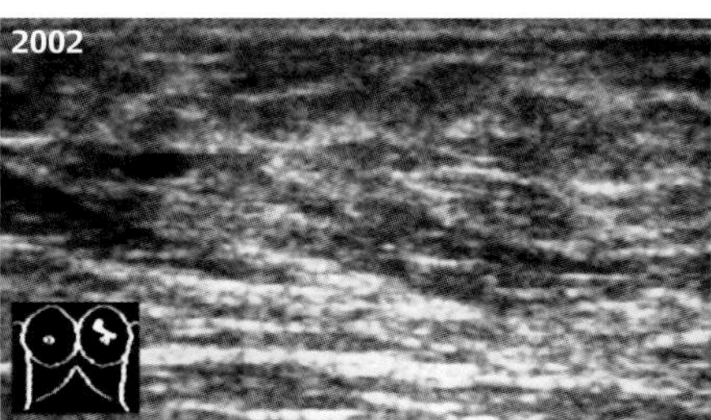


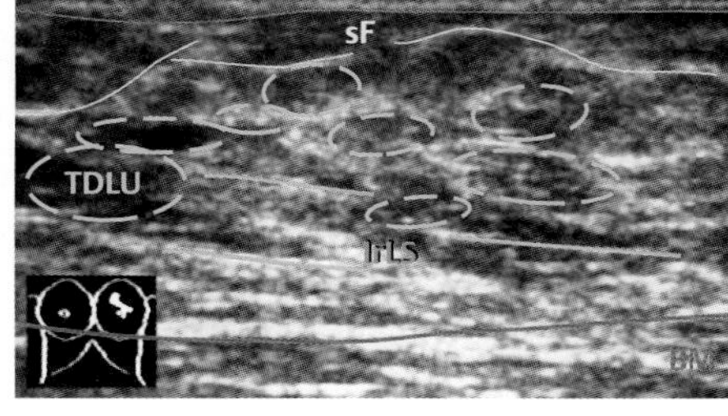


**f** *Sonogram* of the upper inner quadrant of the left breast in 2002 shows a small focus of proliferating TDLUs at the 11-o'clock position, increased relative to the findings in 2000.

S = skin
sF = subcutaneous fat
IrLS = interlobular stroma
TDLU = terminal duct lobular unit
BM = pectoral muscle

**Fig. 5.73 A 52-year-old woman has been on hormone replacement therapy with Lesfemmes for 3 years, following previous HRT with Climodien and estrogen gel.** The breasts were dense due to pronounced ductectasia, cysts, and proliferating TDLUs. The extent to which the breast changes were caused or modified by HRT is unknown.

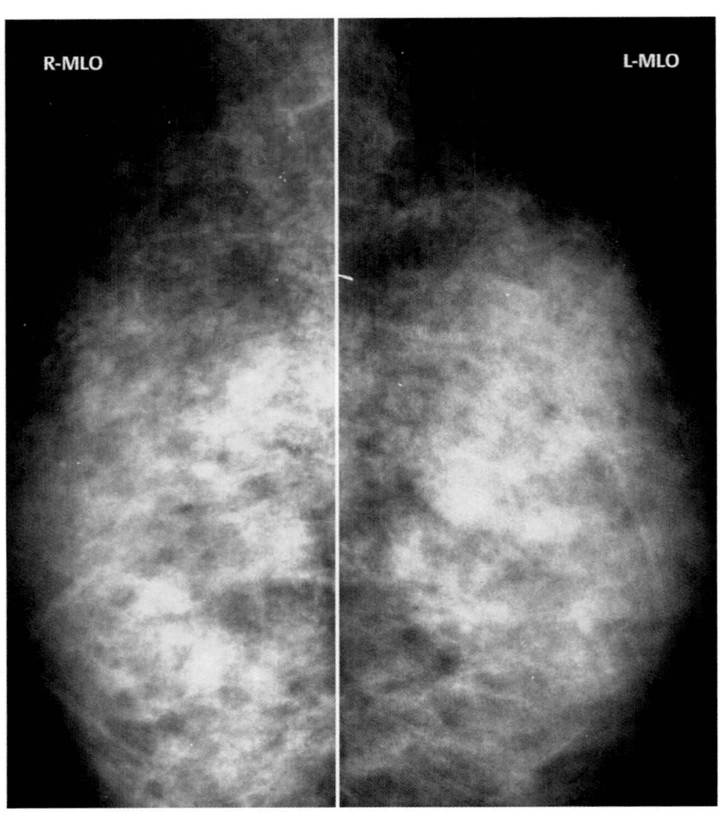


**a** *Bilateral oblique mammograms* show very dense, inhomogeneous breasts with a patchy structure (ACR 4, BIRDAS 1, PGMI). Glandular tissue obscures the pectoral muscle on each side.

*The ACR 4 density of this mammogram is due approximately equally to that of glandular tissue proliferation and ductectasia, with interlobular stroma accounting for approximately 40% of the overall density.*

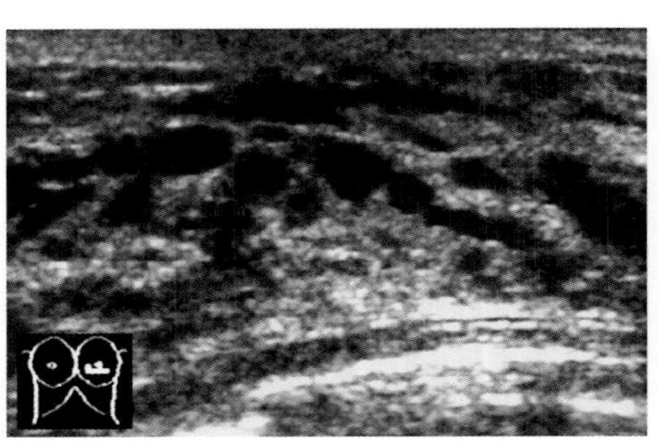

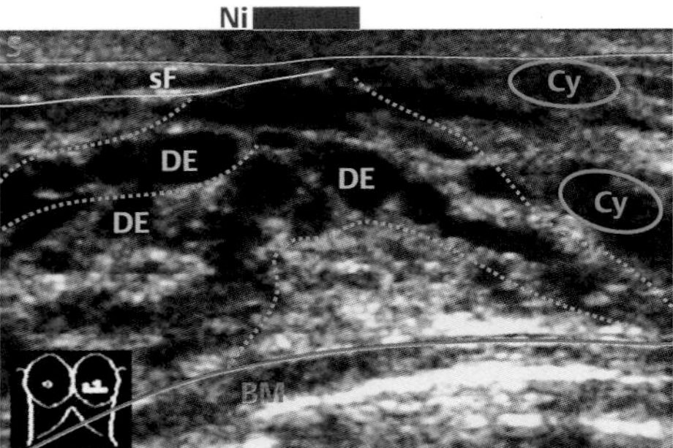


**b** *Sonogram of the infra-areolar left breast* (transverse scan) shows enlarged retroareolar ducts filled with secretions (dark).

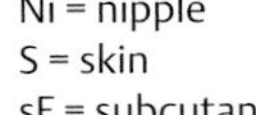

Ni = nipple
S = skin
sF = subcutaneous fat
Cy = cyst
DE = ductectasia
BM = pectoral muscle

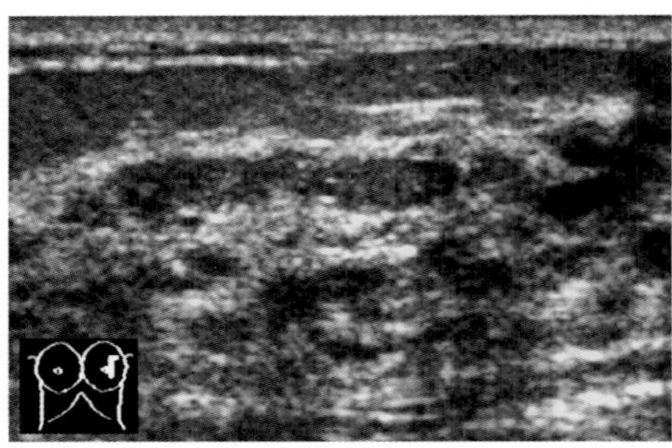

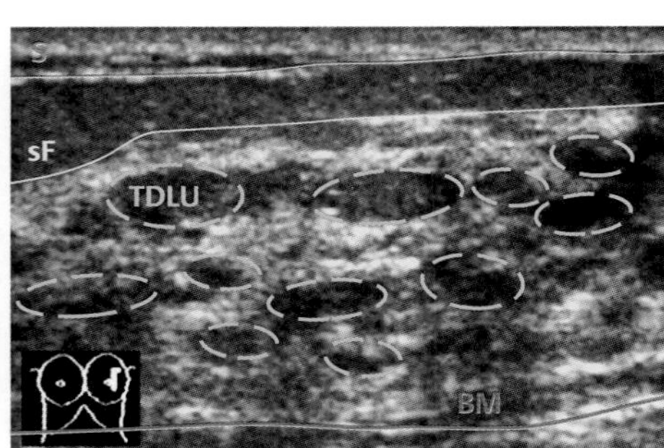


**c** *Sonogram of the upper outer quadrant* of the left breast demonstrates enlarged TDLUs.

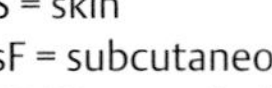

S = skin
sF = subcutaneous fat
TDLU = terminal duct lobular unit
BM = pectoral muscle

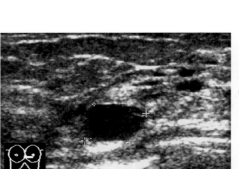

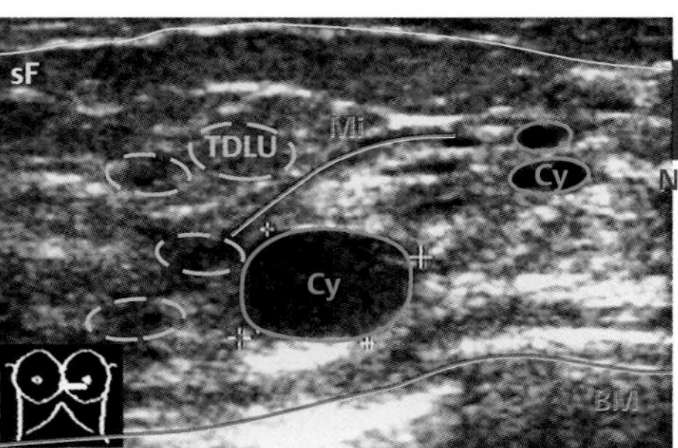


**d** *Sonogram of the lower inner quadrant* of the left breast shows proliferating TDLUs and a prepectoral cyst.

sF = subcutaneous fat
TDLU = terminal duct lobular unit
Cy = cyst
Mi = milk duct
Ni = nipple
BM = pectoral muscle

**Fig. 5.74 A 53-year-old woman presents with bilateral breast firmness and a nodular mass in the left axillary recess** (see the diagram in **c**). Both breasts show very high mammographic density caused by proliferating TDLUs and interlobular stroma.

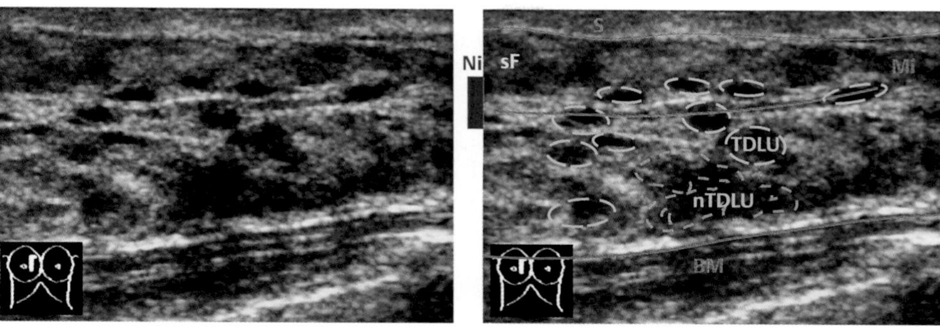


S = skin
sF = subcutaneous fat
Mi = milk duct
Ni = nipple
TDLU = terminal duct lobular unit
nTDLU = nodular TDLU (adenosis?)
BM = pectoral muscle

**a** *Sonogram* of the upper inner quadrant of the right breast shows heavy proliferation of TDLUs and mild ductectasia.

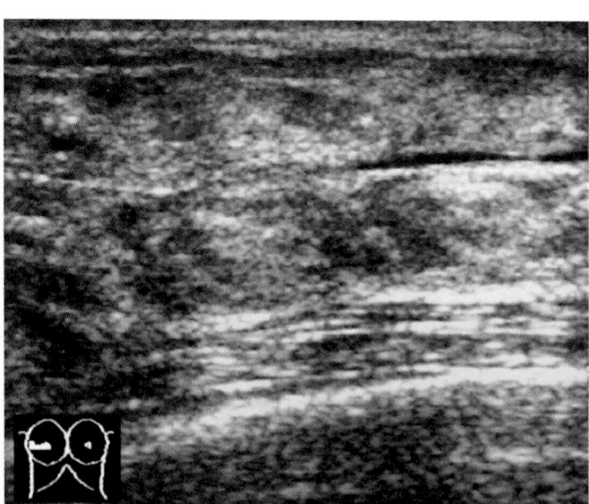

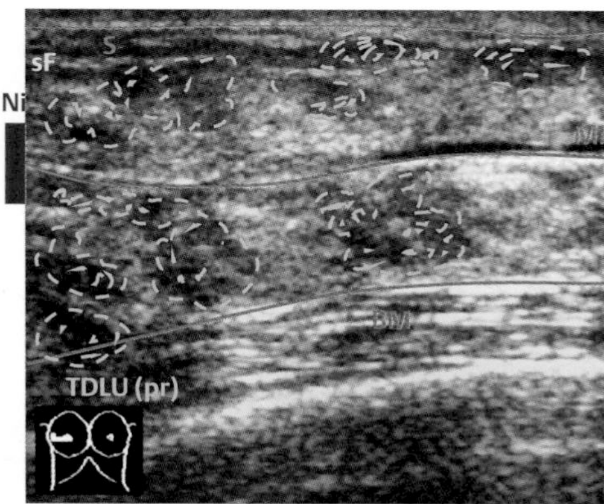


S = skin
sF = subcutaneous fat
Ni = nipple
Mi = milk duct
TDLU (pr) = proliferating terminal duct lobular units
BM = pectoral muscle

**b** *Sonogram* of the upper outer quadrant of the right breast shows ductectasia and marked proliferation of TDLUs (hypoechoic) next to copious interlobular stroma (more echogenic).

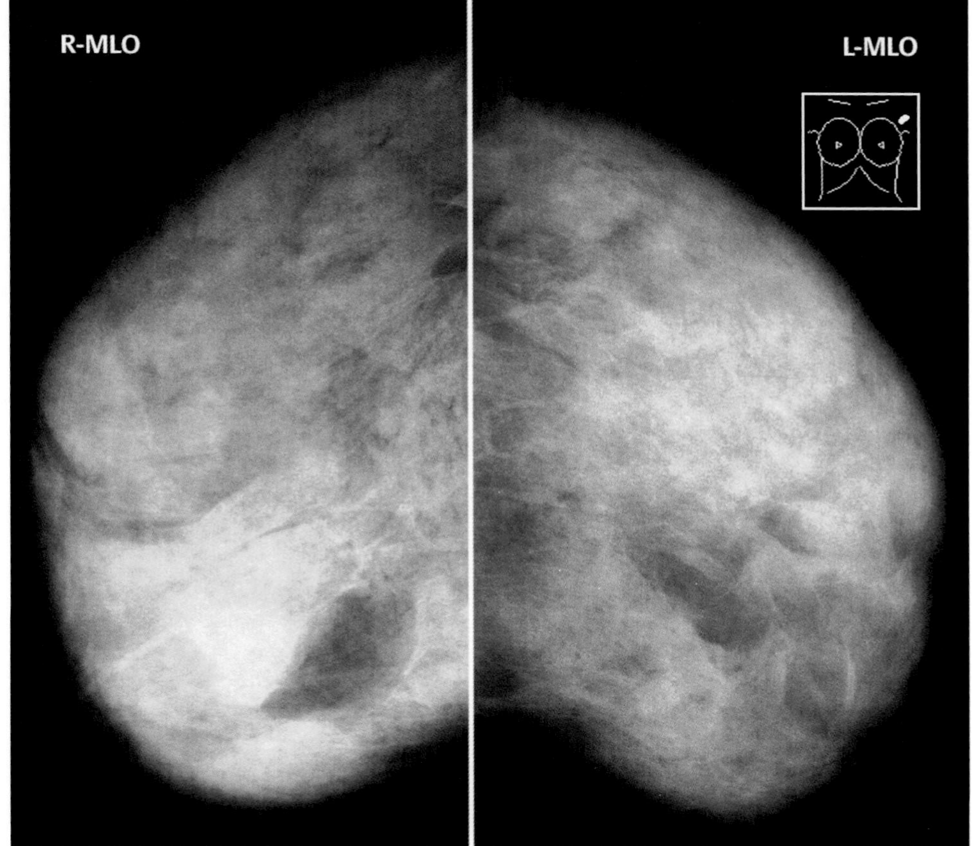


**c** *Bilateral oblique mediolateral mammograms* show very radiodense breasts (ACR 4, PG**MI**).

*The ACR 4 density of the mammograms results from copious interlobular stroma, fat, and approximately 50% proliferating TDLUs and fibrocystic nodules in the upper outer quadrant of the left breast.*

▶ **Fig. 5.74 d, e**

**Fig. 5.74 A 53-year-old woman presents with bilateral breast firmness and a nodular mass in the left axillary recess.** *(continued)*

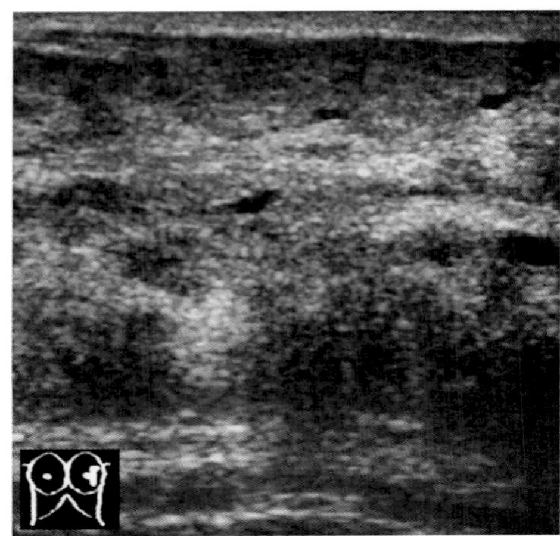

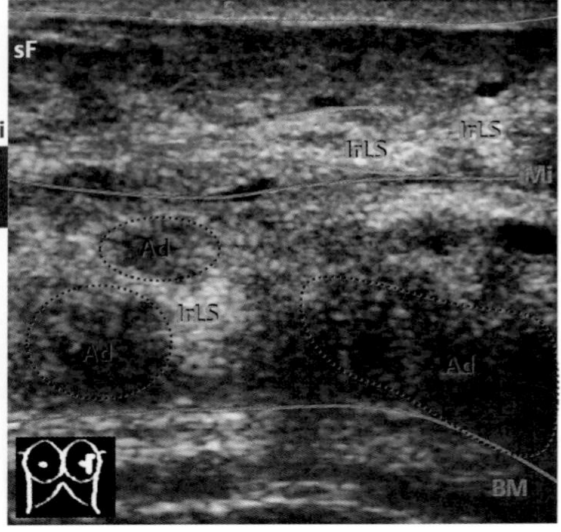


S = skin
sF = subcutaneous fat
Mi = milk duct
Ni = nipple
IrLS = interlobular stroma
Ad = adenosis
BM = pectoral muscle

**d** *Sonogram* of the outer portion of the left breast shows heavy proliferation of TDLUs, which are especially prominent at the prepectoral level.

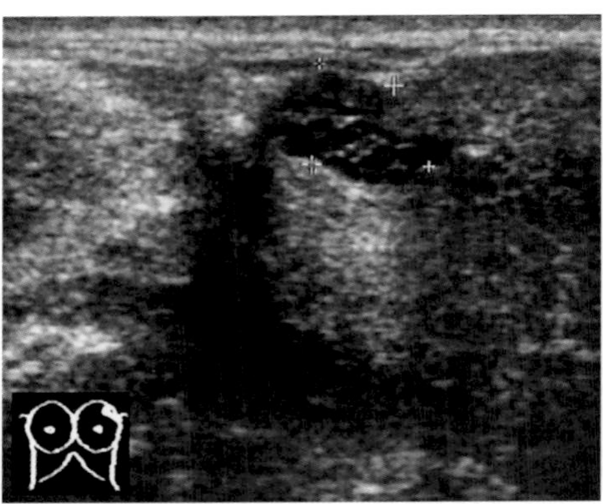

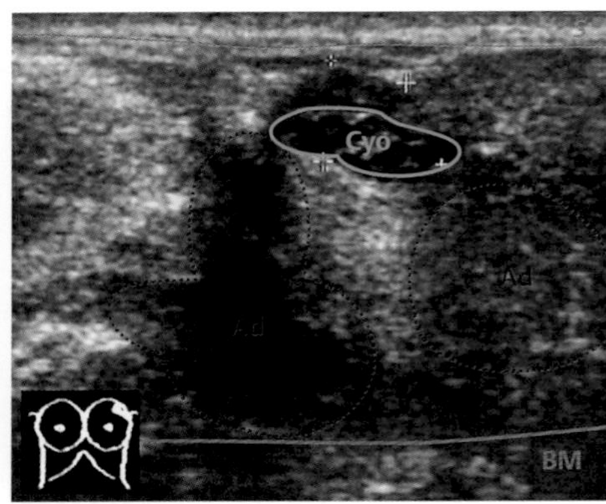


S = skin
Cyo = cystoid (cyst with debris)
Ad = adenosis
BM = pectoral muscle

**e** *Sonogram* of the upper outer quadrant of the left breast in the area of the palpable mass (see the diagram in **c**) shows adenosis-like proliferation of TDLUs along with cystlike structures. An early malignant process cannot be excluded, but a fibrocystic nodule is present.

**Fig. 5.75 A 59-year-old woman has worn an Estraderm patch for years, tapering its use for approximately the past year** (from 2 pads a week 2002 to 1 pad every 2 weeks 2004). Images taken in 2004 (**d–f**) show a marked regression of proliferating TDLUs compared with the previous examination in 2002 (**a–c**). Mammograms show an inhomogeneous breast with areas of copious fat and connective tissue (ACR 4). Aging is another factor that causes regression of TDLUs.

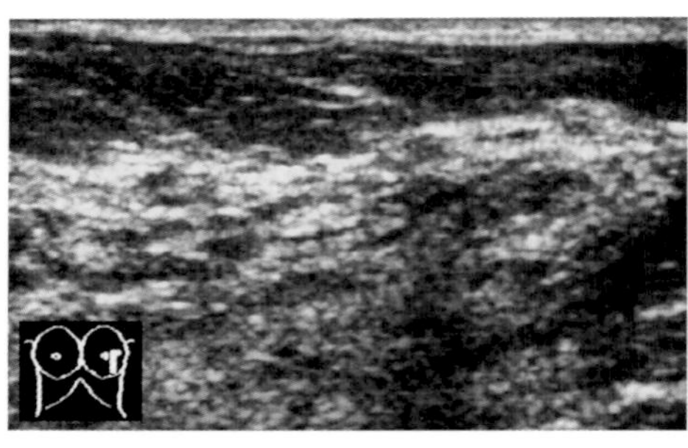

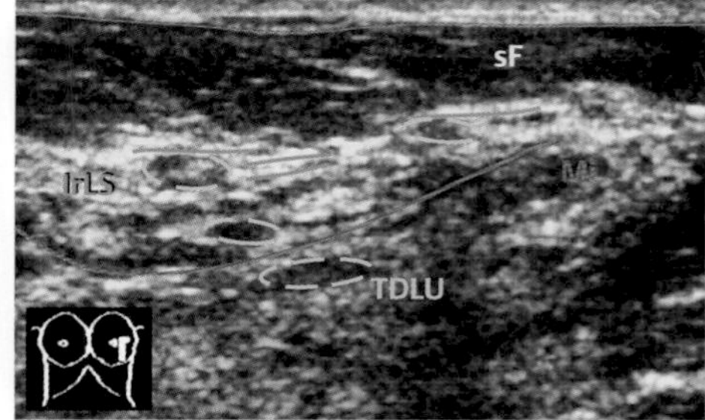


**a** *Sonogram* of the left breast in 2002 during Estraderm patch use shows small foci of TDLU proliferation in a lobe in the lower outer quadrant.

S = skin
sF = subcutaneous fat
Mi = milk duct
Ni = nipple
IrLS = interlobular stroma
TDLU = terminal duct lobular unit

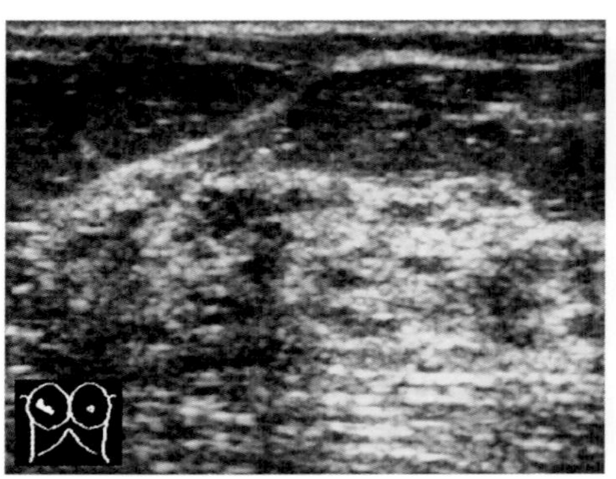

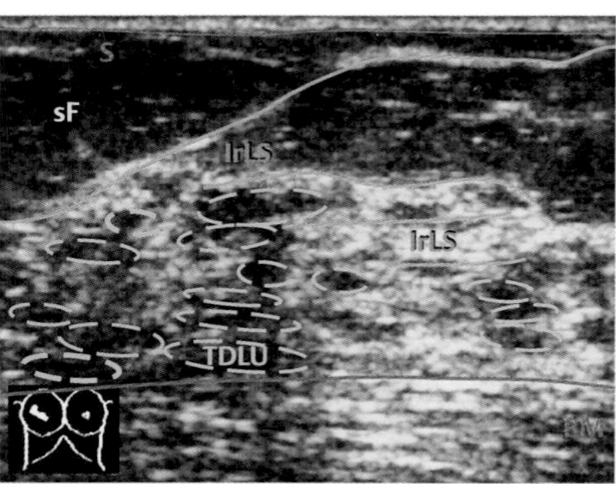


**b** *Sonogram* of the right breast in 2002 shows spongy lobes permeated by enlarged TDLUs.

S = skin
sF = subcutaneous fat
IrLS = interlobular stroma
TDLU = terminal duct lobular unit
BM = pectoral muscle

**Fig. 5.75** **A 59-year-old woman has worn an Estraderm patch for years, tapering its use for approximately the past year.** *(continued)*

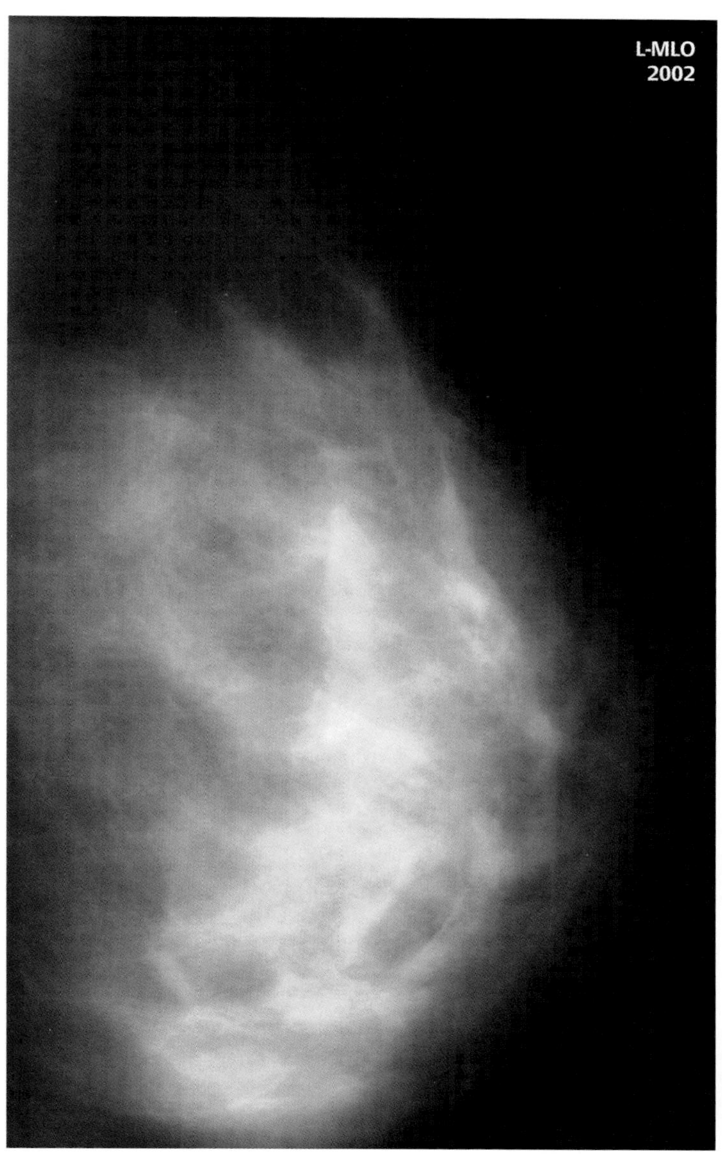


**c** *Oblique mammogram* of the left breast in 2002 shows a homogeneously dense breast (ACR 4, P**G**MI).

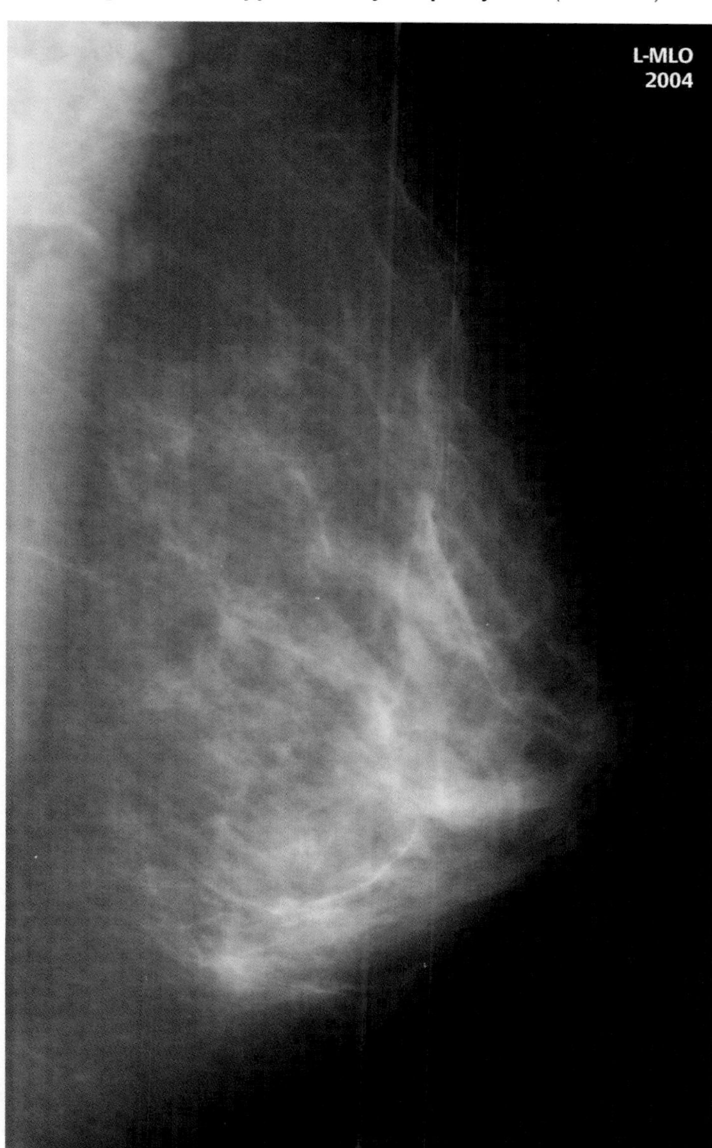


**d** *Oblique mammogram* of the same breast in 2004. Radiographic breast density is considerably less than in 2002 (ACR 2, **P**GMI) due to regression of TDLUs after discontinuation of the Estraderm patch.

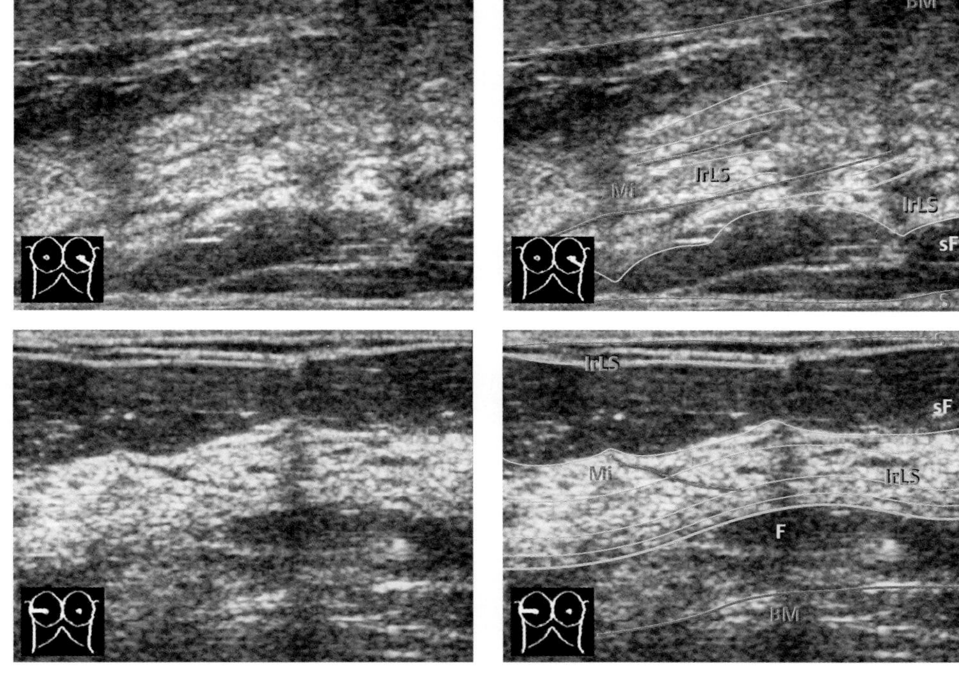


Ni

S = skin
sF = subcutaneous fat
IrLS = interlobular stroma
Mi = milk duct
BM = pectoral muscle

S = skin
sF = subcutaneous fat
IrLS = interlobular stroma
Mi = milk duct
F = fat
BM = pectoral muscle

**e, f** *Sonograms* of the left breast (**e**, above) and right breast (**f**, below) in 2004 show quiescent lobes with regression of the TDLUs and abundant interlobular stroma (see p. 25).

> *The decrease in mammographic density from 2002 to 2004 results from regression of the TDLUs from approximately 40 % to 25 % with an unchanged volume of interlobular stroma and fat.*

**Fig. 5.76 A 62-year-old woman has taken oral contraceptives for many years and is not currently on hormone replacement therapy. She presents now with skeletal complaints.** The images show normal glandular structures and age-appropriate stroma with no lobular proliferation.

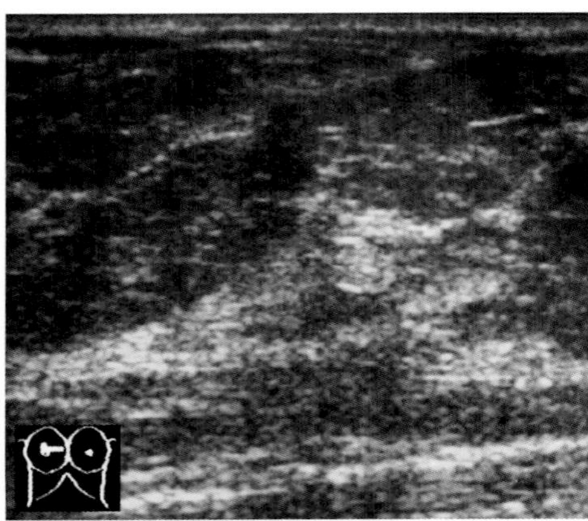

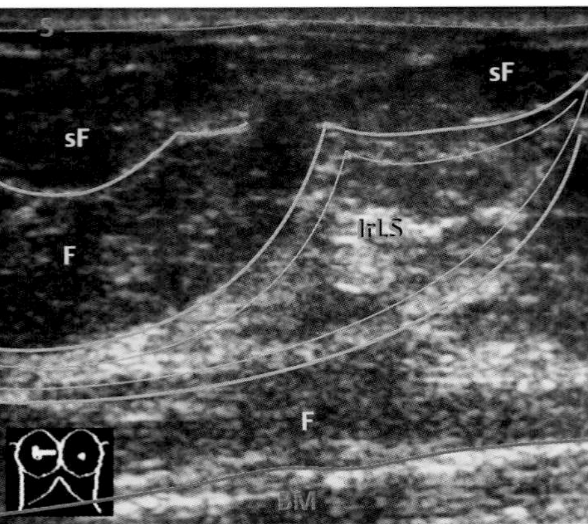


S = skin
sF = subcutaneous fat
IrLS = interlobular stroma
F = fat
BM = pectoral muscle

**a** *Sonogram* of the right breast shows stroma-rich breast parenchyma with numerous septa composed of interlobular stroma and no significant proliferation of TDLUs.

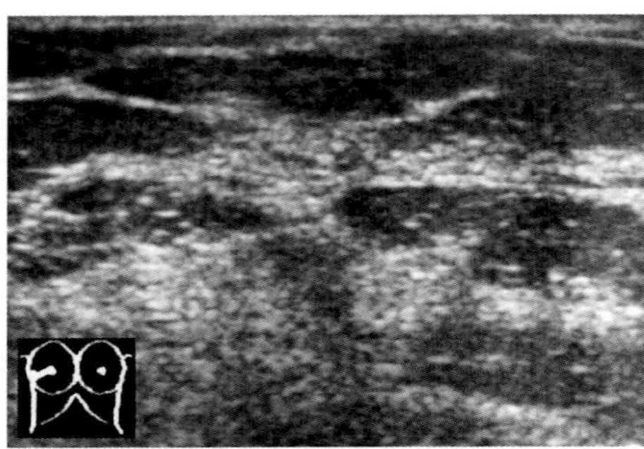

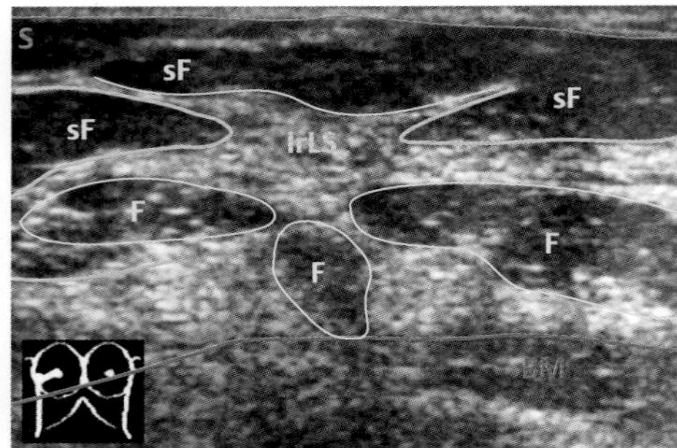


S = skin
sF = subcutaneous fat
IrLS = interlobular stroma
F = fat
BM = pectoral muscle

**b** *Sonogram* of the right breast shows fibrosis of the breast parenchyma with no significant TDLU proliferation.

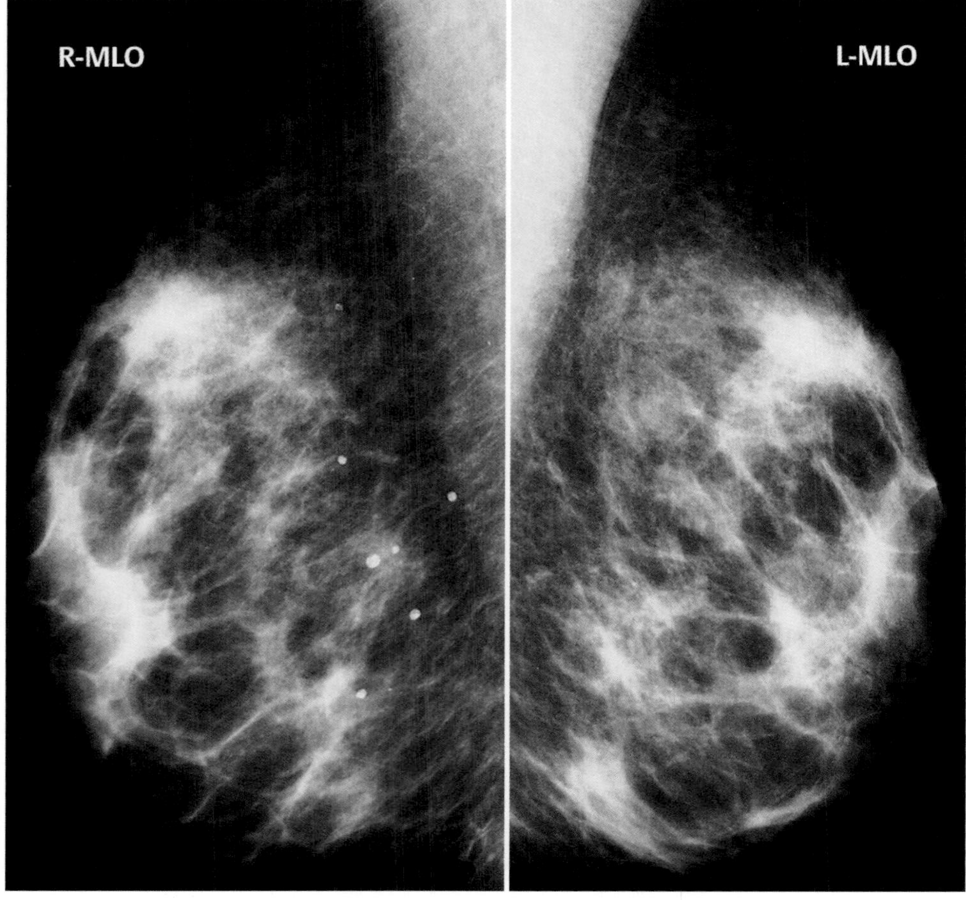


**c** Bilateral oblique mammograms show dense, inhomogeneous breasts (ACR 3, P**G**MI) with calcified cysts in the right breast.

***The density of ACR 3 results largely from interlobular stroma and fat (80 %) and a few TDLUs.***

**Fig. 5.76 A 62-year-old woman has taken oral contraceptives for many years.** *(continued)*

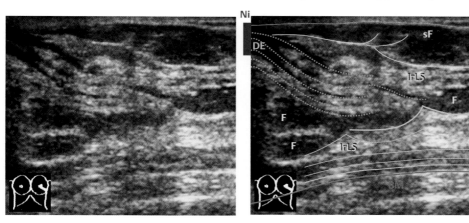

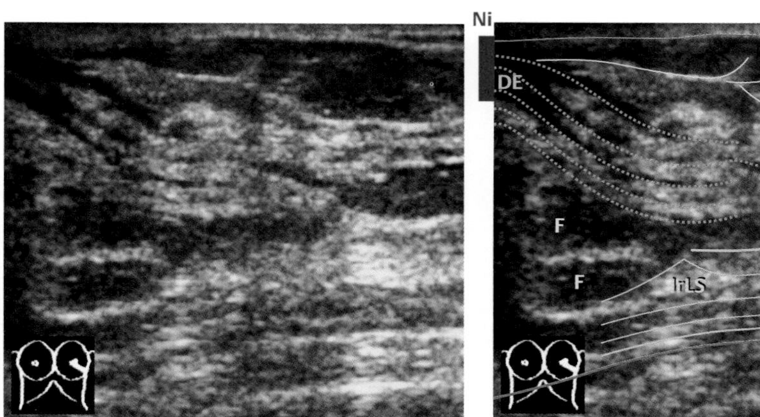


S = skin
sF = subcutaneous fat
IrLS = interlobular stroma
DE = ductectasia
Ni = nipple
F = fat
BM = pectoral muscle

**d** *Sonogram* of the left breast shows abundant interlobular stroma with no sonographically visible TDLU proliferation. Moderate retroareolar ductectasia permeates the entire lobe.

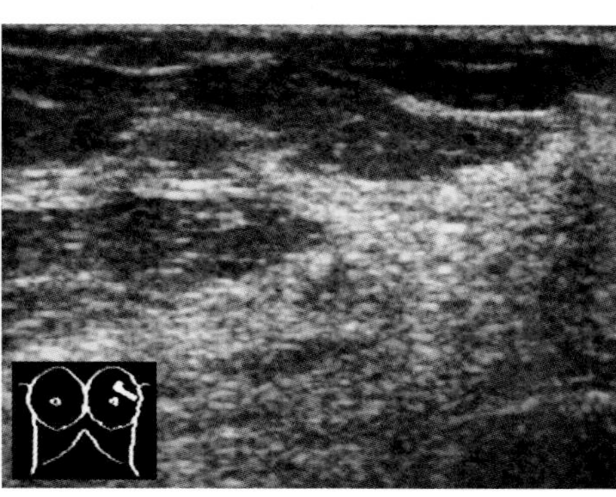

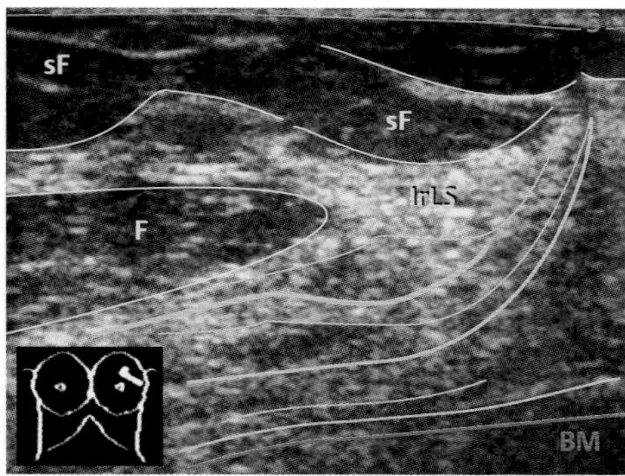


S = skin
sF = subcutaneous fat
IrLS = interlobular stroma
F = fat
BM = pectoral muscle

**e** *Sonogram* of the left breast (transverse scan). The upper outer quadrant contains abundant interlobular stroma with no sonographically visible TDLUs.

**Fig. 5.77 A 45-year-old woman in menopause.** The patient was not on hormone replacement therapy and had involuted breasts with no lobular proliferation. The mammographically visible structures in the right breast consist mainly of connective tissue. The patient was taking oral contraceptives until 2 years before the examination.

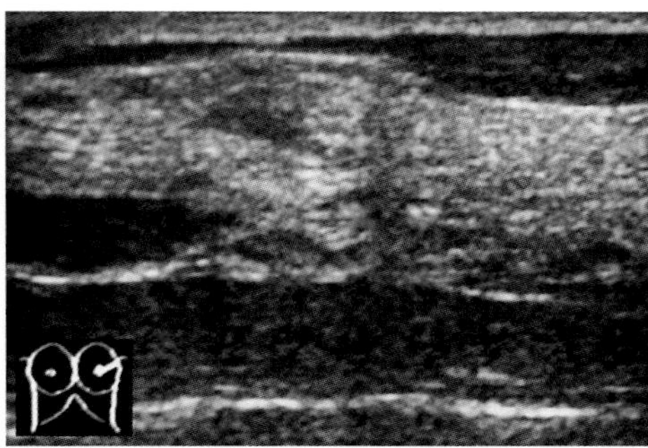

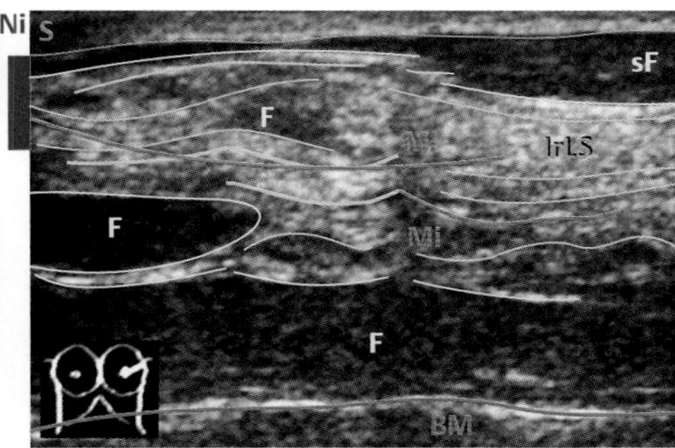


S = skin
sF = subcutaneous fat
IrLS = interlobular stroma
Ni = nipple
Mi = milk duct
F = fat
BM = pectoral muscle

**a** *Sonogram* of the upper outer quadrant of the left breast. The retroareolar region contains abundant stroma and small cysts with no signs of TDLU proliferation.

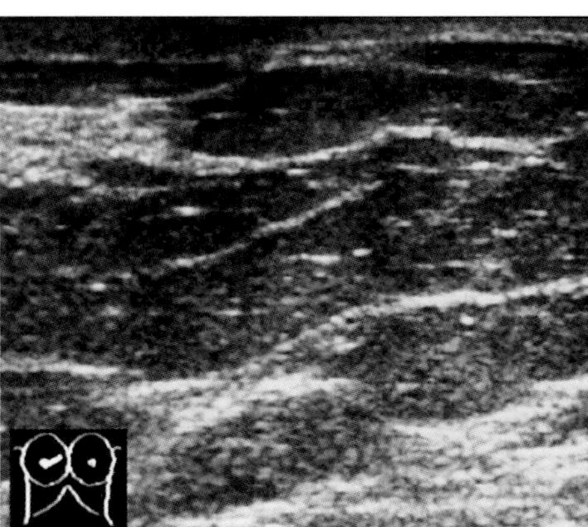

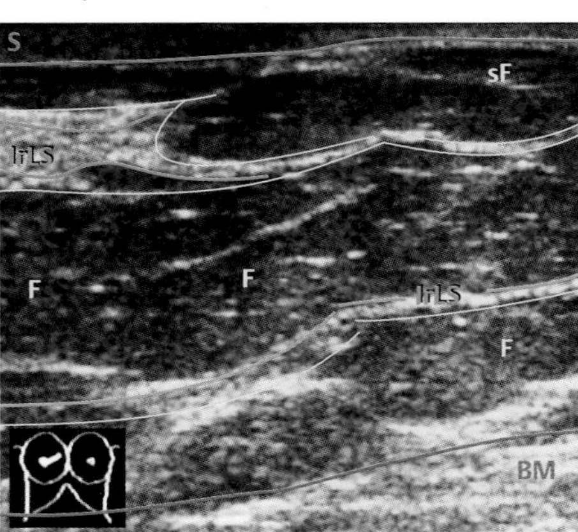


S = skin
sF = subcutaneous fat
IrLS = interlobular stroma
F = fat
BM = pectoral muscle

**b** *Sonogram* of the upper inner quadrant of the right breast shows intramammary connective-tissue septa with no TDLU proliferation.

▶ **Fig. 5.77 c–e**

**Fig. 5.77 A 45-year-old woman in menopause.** *(continued)*

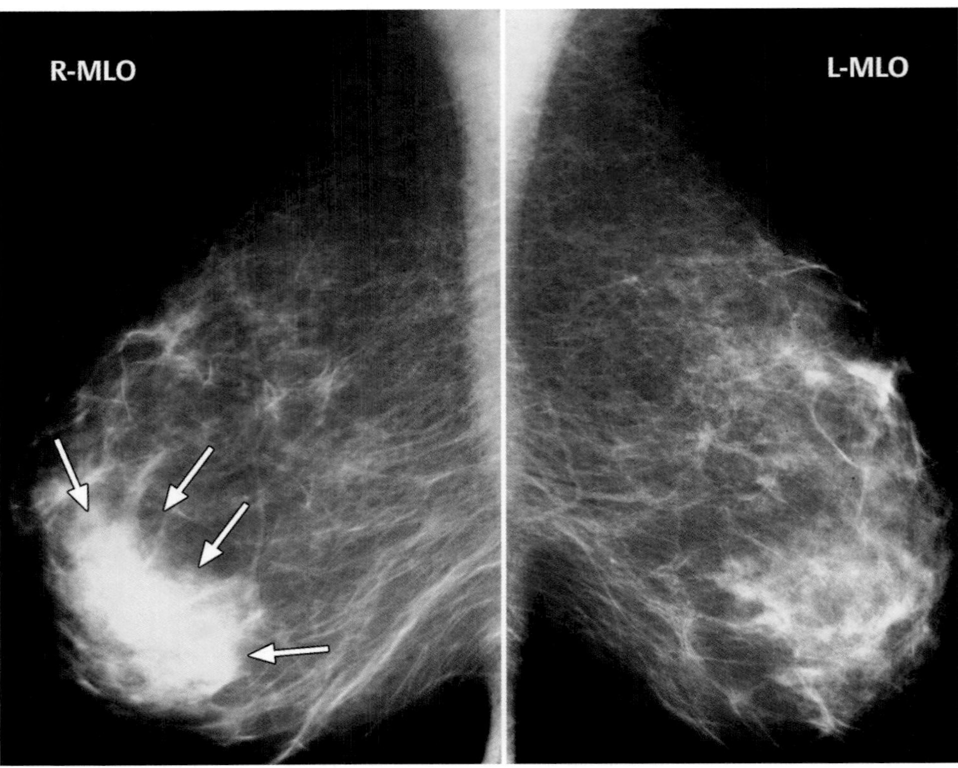


**c** *Bilateral oblique mammograms*. Mammogram of the right breast shows a circumscribed, homogeneous, retroareolar opacity that is concave posteriorly (ACR 2, P**G**MI). Ultrasound identifies this area as fibrosis without lobular proliferation. The other image documents partial involution of the left breast.

*The ACR 2 density of these mammograms results mainly from interlobular stroma (80%), which forms a nodular mass in the lower outer quadrant of the right breast (not a tumor!).*

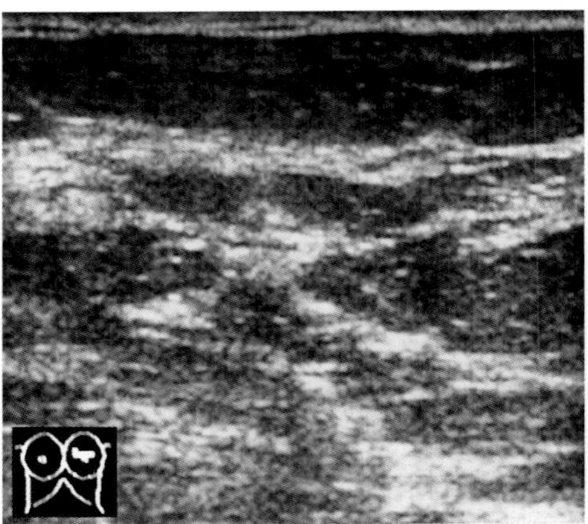

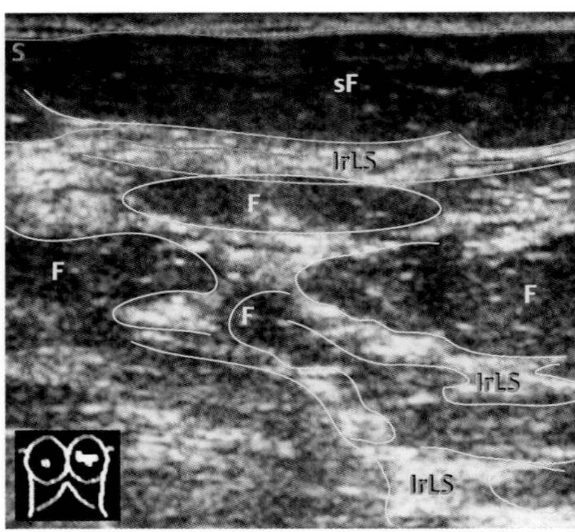


S = skin
sF = subcutaneous fat
IrLS = interlobular stroma
F = fat

**d** *Left supra-areolar sonogram* (transverse scan) shows an involuted breast with connective-tissue bands and no significant lobular proliferation.

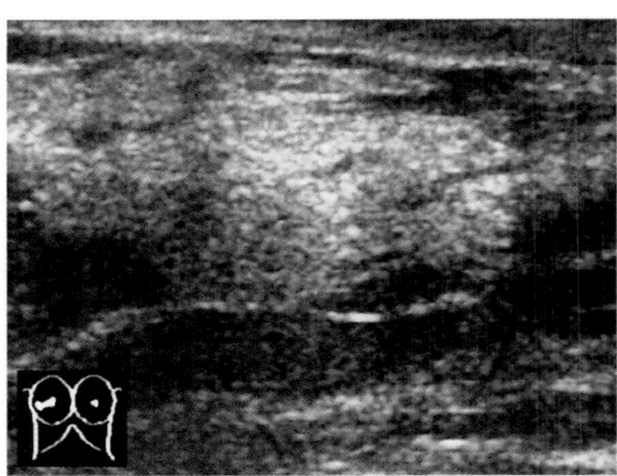

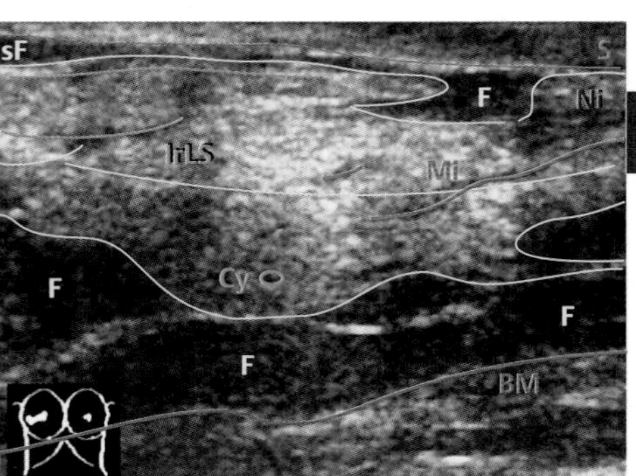


S = skin
sF = subcutaneous fat
IrLS = interlobular stroma
Mi = milk duct
Ni = nipple
F = fat
Cy = cyst
BM = pectoral muscle

**e** *Sonogram* of the lower outer quadrant of the right breast at the site of a mammographic nodular density (**c**). Connective tissue proliferation accounts for the infra-areolar island of parenchyma in the right mammogram (arrows) (not a tumor!). The circumscribed area consists of patchy interlobular stroma with no visible TDLUs.

**Note**: A malignant mass would present a convex posterior border in the mammogram (**c**).

**Fig. 5.78 A 57-year-old postmenopausal women with no palpable breast abnormalities.** The patient had no family history of breast cancer and was not on hormone replacement therapy. Mammograms show an involuted breast with fine stromal septa. Ultrasound shows corresponding septa composed of interlobular stroma with no visible TDLUs (see **Fig. 4.4 c**, p. 26). Is HRT an option for treatment of deficit symptoms?

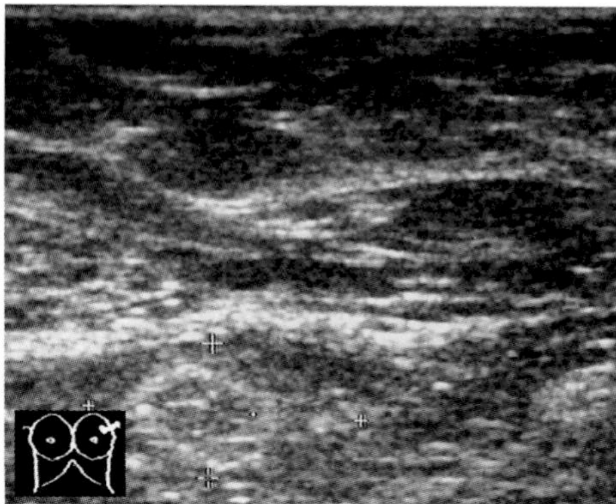

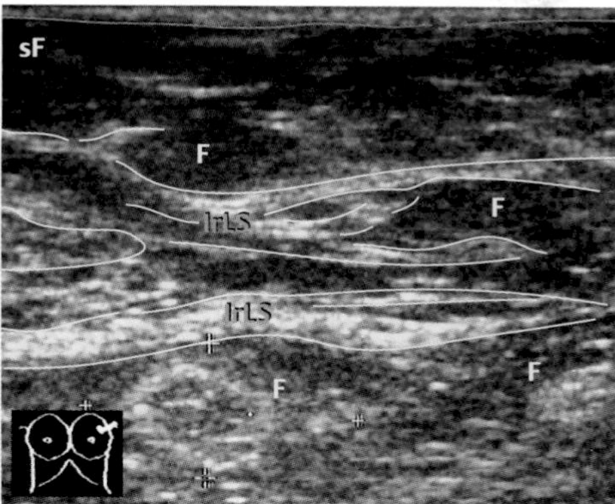


S = skin
sF = subcutaneous fat
IrLS = interlobular stroma
F = fat

**a** *Peripheral sonogram* of the upper outer quadrant of the left breast shows fatty tissue with fine septa composed of interlobular stroma and no visible TDLUs.

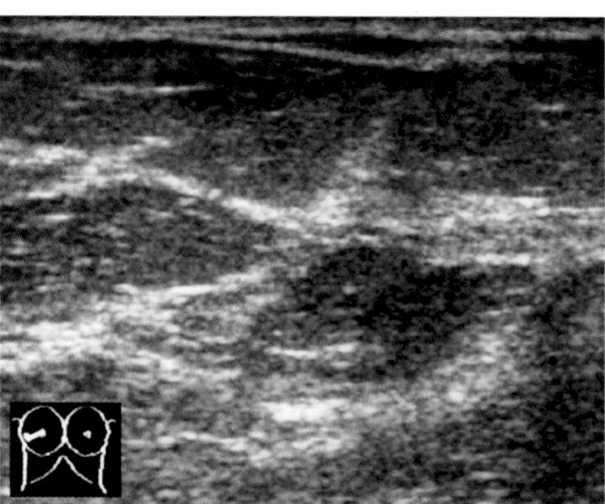

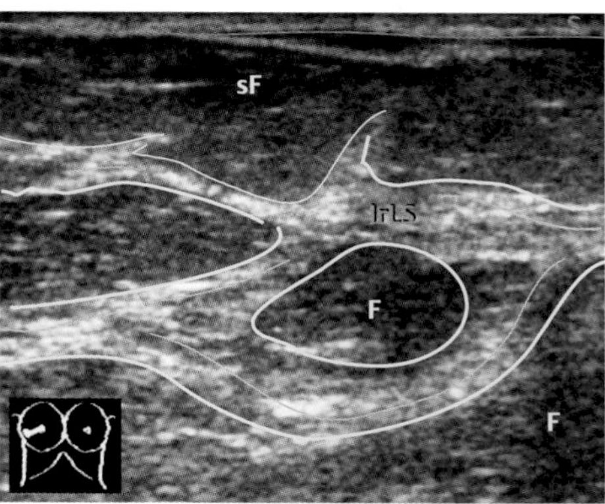


S = skin
sF = subcutaneous fat
IrLS = interlobular stroma
F = fat

**b** *Sonogram* of the lower outer quadrant of the right breast shows septa of interlobular stroma in fatty surroundings. There are no visible TDLUs.

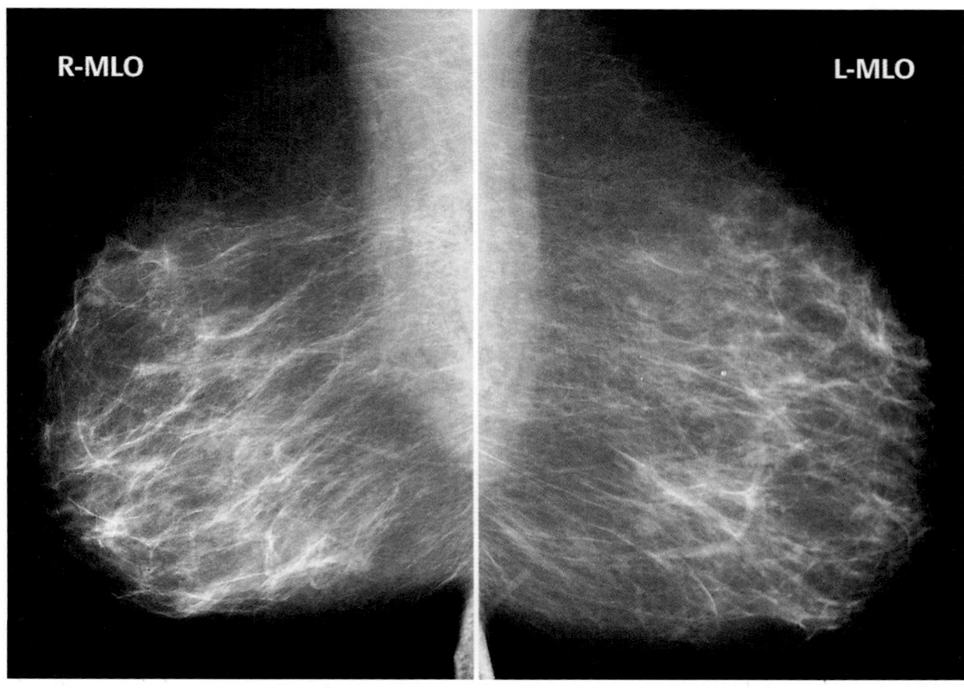


**c** *Bilateral oblique mammograms* show involuted breasts with fine parenchymal septa (ACR 1, PGMI, BIRADS 1).

*Interlobular stroma and fat account for approximately 90% of the ACR 1 density. There should be no concerns about prescribing HRT.*

▶ **Fig. 5.78 d, e**

**Fig. 5.78 A 57-year-old postmenopausal women with no palpable breast abnormalities.** *(continued)*

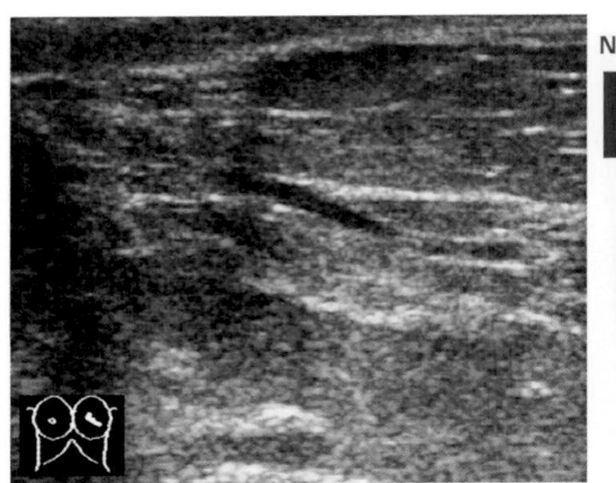

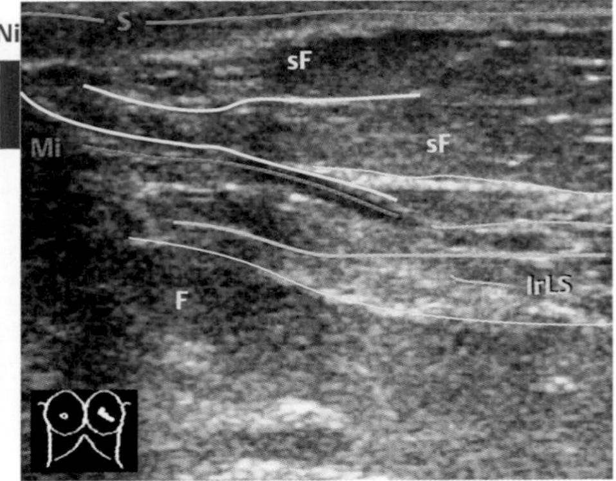


S = skin
sF = subcutaneous fat
Mi = milk duct
Ni = Nipple
F = fat
IrLS = interlobular stroma

**d** *Retroareolar sonogram* of the left breast shows a slightly dilated duct surrounded by fat with fine connective-tissue septa. **Note:** The absence of sonographically visible TDLUs does not preclude the development of cancer. It means only that there is no detectable hormonal stimulus.

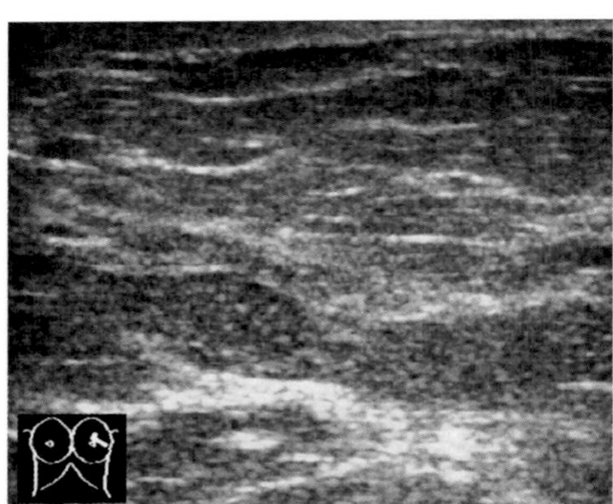

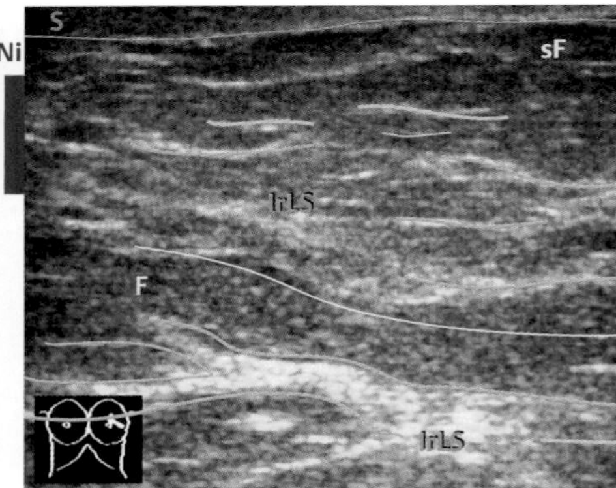


S = skin
sF = subcutaneous fat
Ni = nipple
F = fat
IrLS = interlobular stroma

**e** *Lateral sonogram* of the left breast shows fine septa composed of interlobular stroma and complete involution of the breast parenchyma with no detectable TDLUs.

**Fig. 5.79 A 65-year-old woman had been on hormone replacement therapy until August, 2003.** A CNB of the left breast in 2002 indicated adenosis. Foci of adenosis with blunt duct changes were also present in the right breast at that time. For 6 months prior to examination, the patient had taken only soy tablets. The breast parenchyma showed sonographic improvement in 2003 and was normal by 2004. Adenosis was no longer detectable, and the only residual finding was a hypoechoic area in the lower outer quadrant of the right breast (**j**). Mammograms taken in 2004 (**b**) were more lucent than in 2002 (**a**).

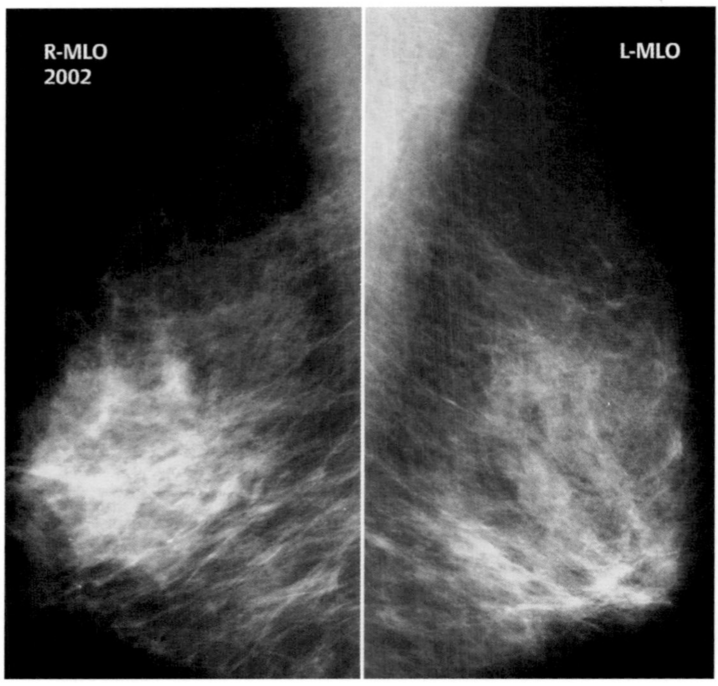


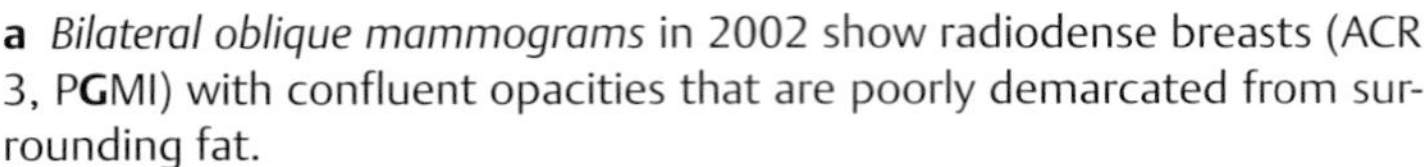

**a** *Bilateral oblique mammograms* in 2002 show radiodense breasts (ACR 3, P**G**MI) with confluent opacities that are poorly demarcated from surrounding fat.

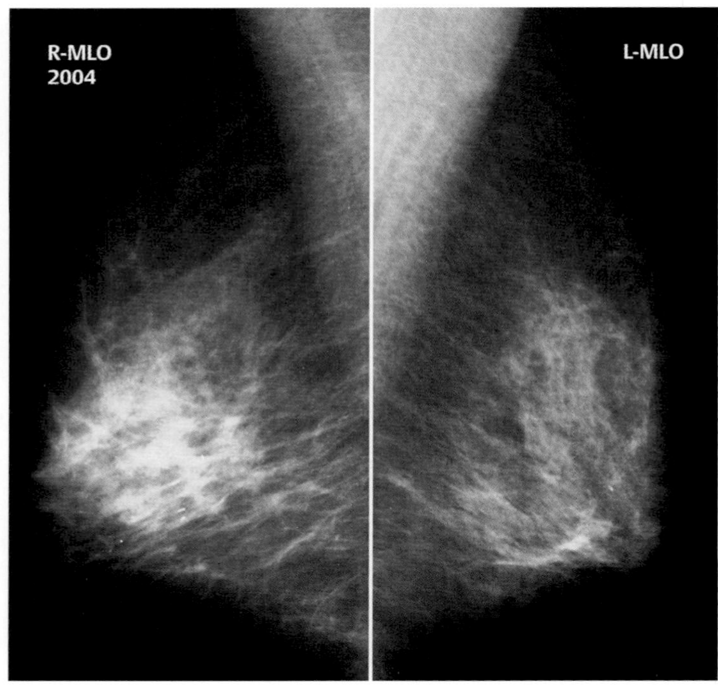


**b** *Bilateral oblique mammograms* in 2004. The breast parenchyma is more lucent than in 2002, especially on the left side (ACR 2). Parenchymal opacities are still present on the right side (ACR 3, **P**GMI).

**Fig. 5.79 A 65-year-old woman had been on hormone replacement therapy until August, 2003.** *(continued)*

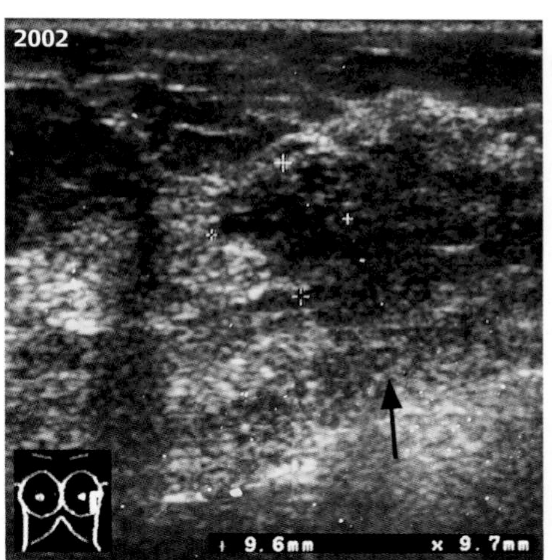


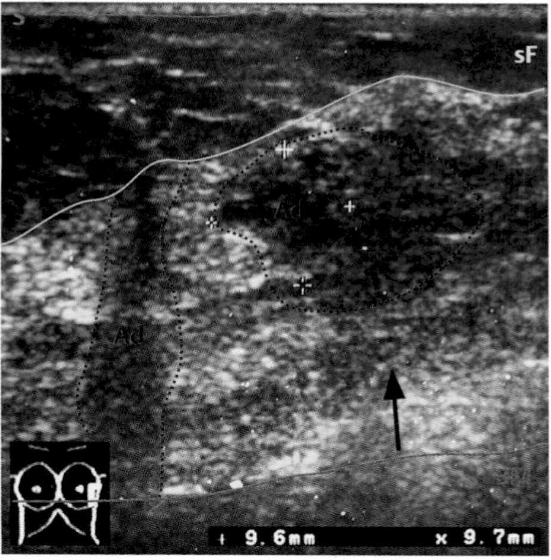


S = skin
sF = subcutaneous fat
Ad = adenosis
BM = pectoral muscle

**c** *Sonogram of the lower outer quadrant of the left breast* in 2002 shows a large area of adenosis with irregular margins relative to the adjacent breast parenchyma, which has a higher stromal content.

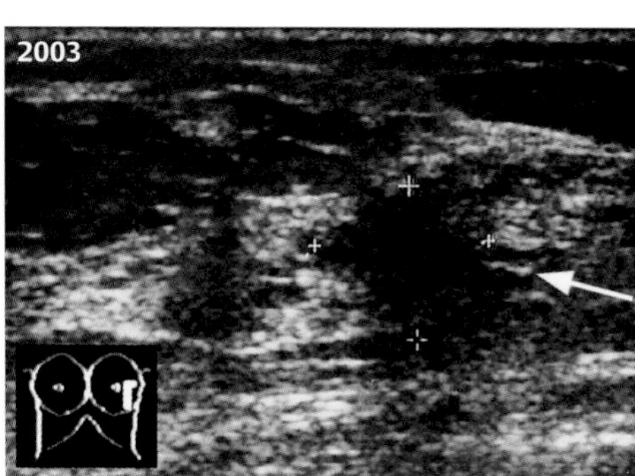


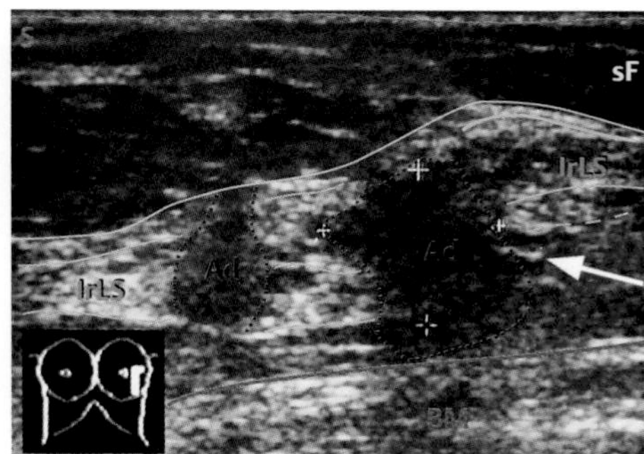


S = skin
sF = subcutaneous fat
Ad = adenosis
IrLS = interlobular stroma
BM = pectoral muscle

**d** *Sonogram* in 2003. The two areas of adenosis in the lateral portion of the left breast have ill-defined margins relative to the more stroma-rich regions of the breast. They are markedly smaller than in the previous examination (**c**) but have irregular margins, presumably because the interlobular stroma also shows higher echogenicity.

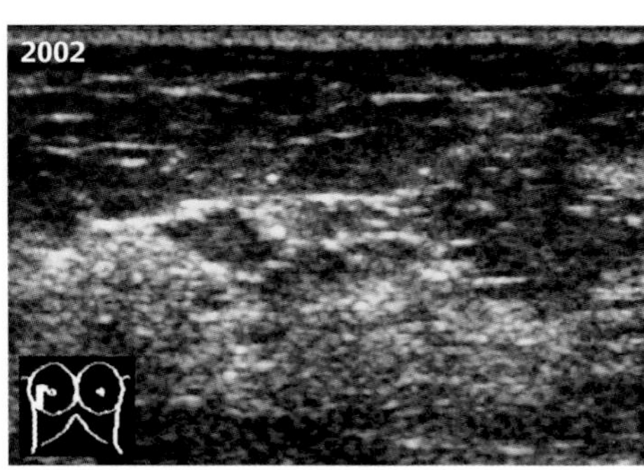


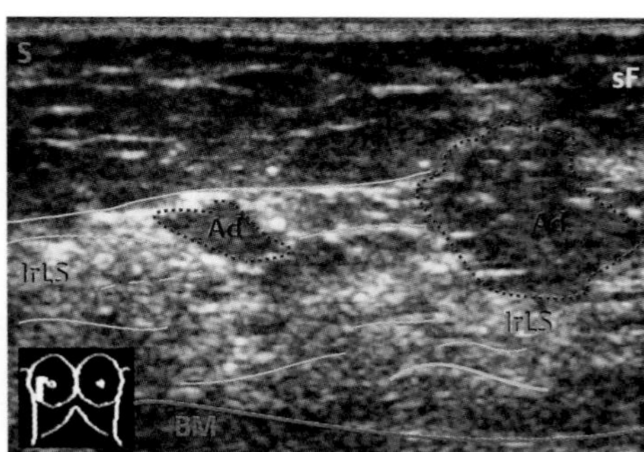


S = skin
sF = subcutaneous fat
Ad = adenosis
IrLS = interlobular stroma
BM = pectoral muscle

**e** *Lateral sonogram* of the lower outer quadrant of the right breast in 2002 shows two foci of adenosis within the spongy breast parenchyma.

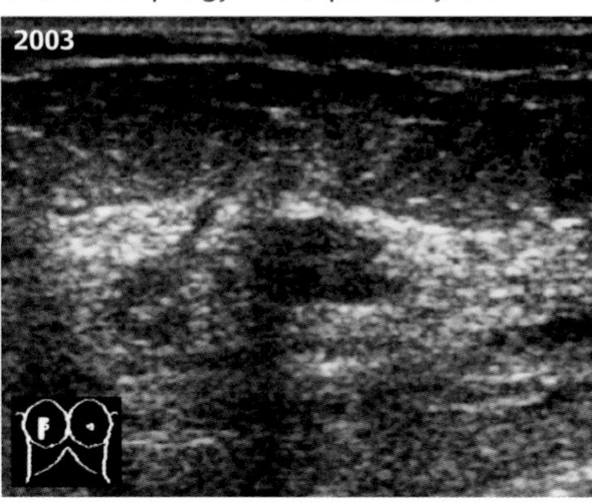


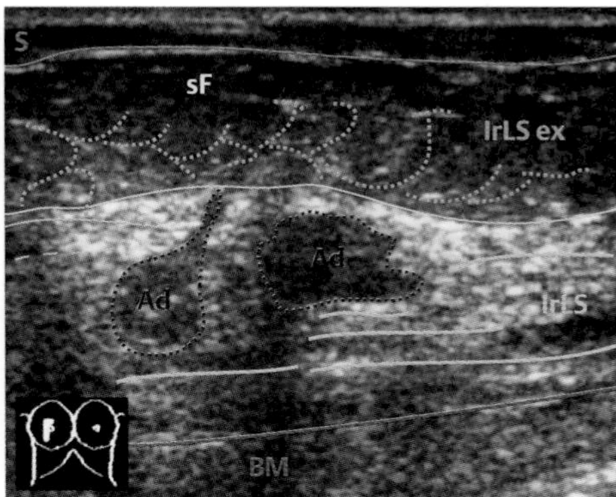


S = skin
sF = subcutaneous fat
Ad = adenosis
IrLS = interlobular stroma
IrLS ex = extensions of interlobular stroma into the fatty tissue
BM = pectoral muscle

**f** *Lateral sonogram* of the right breast in 2003. The larger and smaller foci of adenosis in the central portion of the spongy glandular region are smaller and more clearly defined than in 2002 (**e**). Note the ill-defined margins of the connective-tissue area relative to subcutaneous fat. This may account for the persistence of increased interstitial density in the right breast despite supplemental soy ingestion.

▶ **Fig. 5.79 g–k**

**Fig. 5.79 A 65-year-old woman had been on hormone replacement therapy until August, 2003.** *(continued)*

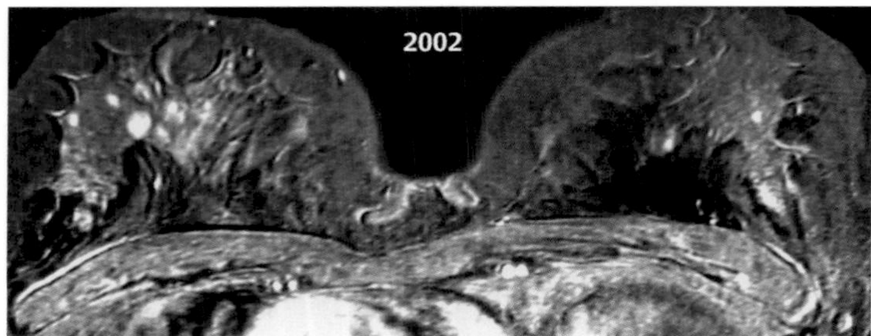


**g** *MRI* in 2002. Subtraction image shows small foci of gadolinium enhancement, presumably representing areas of adenosis, papillomas or DCIS (right breast). But no malignancy was found!

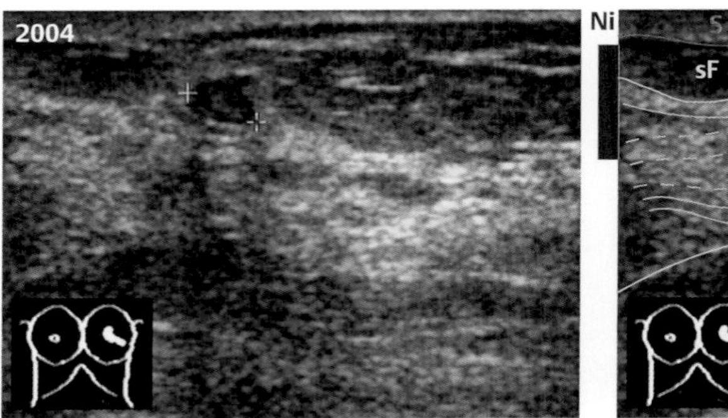


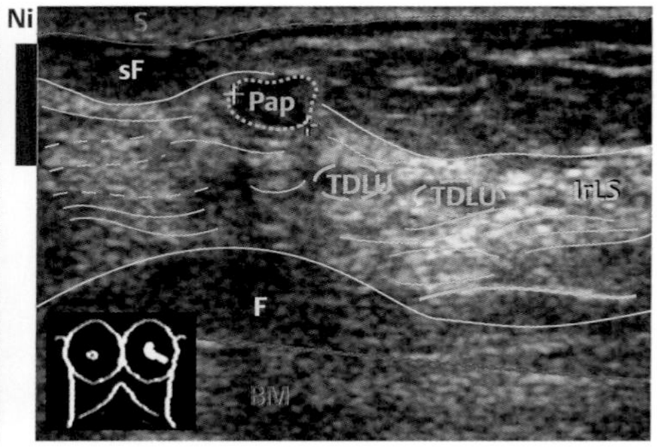


S = skin
sF = subcutaneous fat
Pap = papilloma?
IrLS = interlobular stroma
BM = pectoral muscle
Ni = nipple
TDLU = terminal duct lobular unit
F = fat

**h** *Sonogram* of the lower outer quadrant of the left breast in 2004. The glandular structure is generally quieter and contains more interlobular stroma through the regression of hypertrophic TDLUs. The scan also shows a well-circumscribed focus with posterior acoustic enhancement (papilloma? fibroadenoma? cyst with debris?).

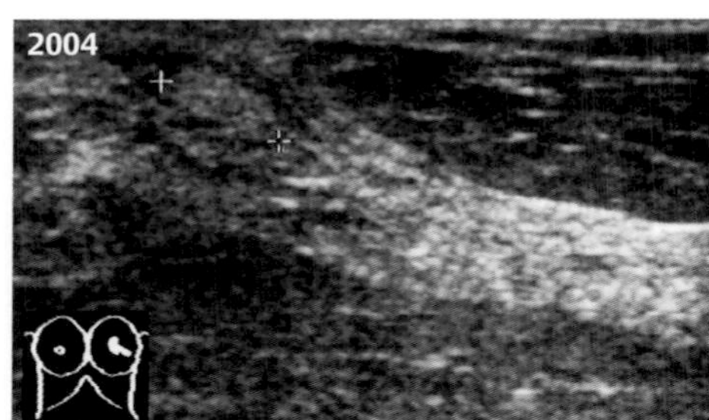


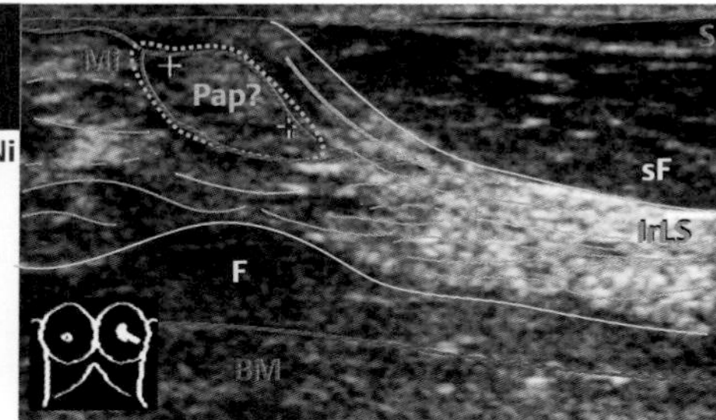


S = skin
sF = subcutaneous fat
Pap? = papilloma?
IrLS = interlobular stroma
F = fat
Mi = milk duct
Ni = nipple
BM = pectoral muscle

**i** *Sonogram* at a different site in the lower outer quadrant of the left breast in 2004 shows a questionable retroareolar papilloma (differential diagnosis: intraductal debris). The breast parenchyma shows a bandlike zone of increased echogenicity and is more homogeneous than in 2002 and 2003 due to more interlobular stroma with an absence of TDLUs and adenosis.

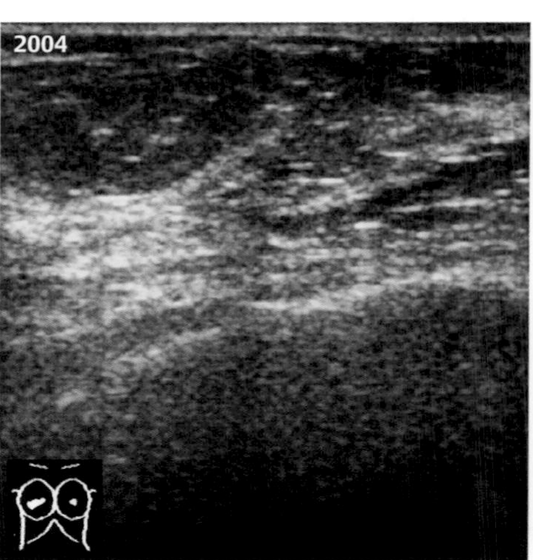


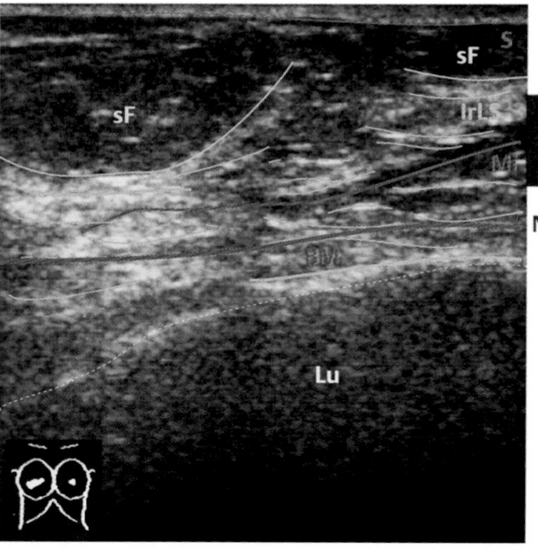


S = skin
sF = subcutaneous fat
IrLS = interlobular stroma
Ni = nipple
Mi = milk duct
BM = pectoral muscle
Lu = lung

**j** *Sonogram* of the lower outer quadrant of the right breast in 2004 documents regression of adenosis with persistence of spongy structures in the breast parenchyma, which is rich in interlobular stroma.

**Fig. 5.79 A 65-year-old woman had been on hormone replacement therapy until August, 2003.** *(continued)*

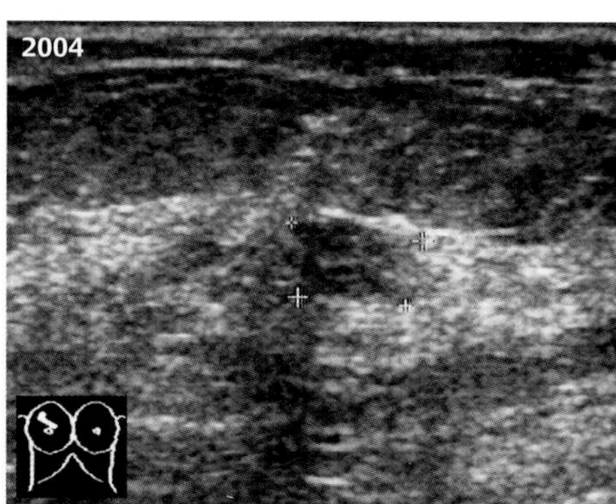


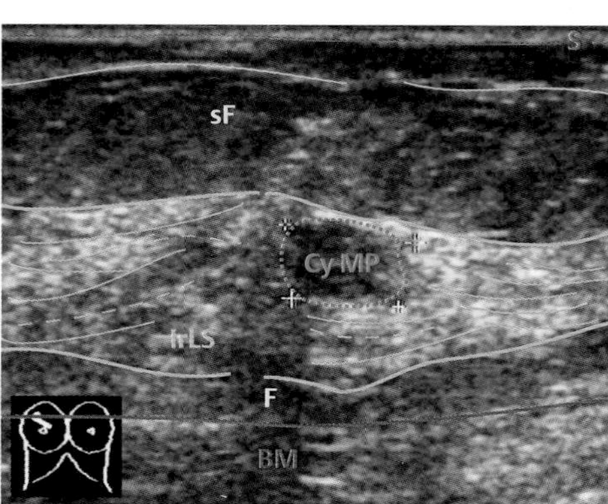


S = skin
sF = subcutaneous fat
IrLS = interlobular stroma
Cy MP = area of cystic metaplasia or residual adenosis
F = fat
BM = pectoral muscle

**k** *Sonogram* of the upper outer quadrant of the right breast in 2004. Compared with 2003 (**f**), the focus of adenosis is markedly smaller (slightly different projection). The focus may also be an area of cystic metaplasia. The surrounding breast parenchyma contains more interlobular stroma (more echogenic).

*From 2002 to 2004, the proportion of TDLUs and adenosis in this patient dwindled from 50% to approximately 20% while the volume of interlobular stroma remained the same. This regression of adenosis and TDLUs explains the decline in mammographic density from ACR 3 (2002) to ACR 2 (2004). The discontinuation of HRT apparently had a positive effect on the breast parenchyma, perhaps with an associated decline in cancer risk!*

**Fig. 5.80 A 56-year-old woman with a painful mass in the upper outer quadrant of the right breast.** The patient had been on hormone replacement therapy (Sisare) for 5 years. CNB confirmed adenosis in the upper outer quadrant with increased parenchymal density relative to 1998 (glandular tissue shows greater development in the right breast than in the left breast). Complaints improved after the patient was switched to phytoestrogens, but some tenderness persisted in the upper outer quadrant with ultrasound showing proliferating TDLUs. The left breast was sonographically normal.

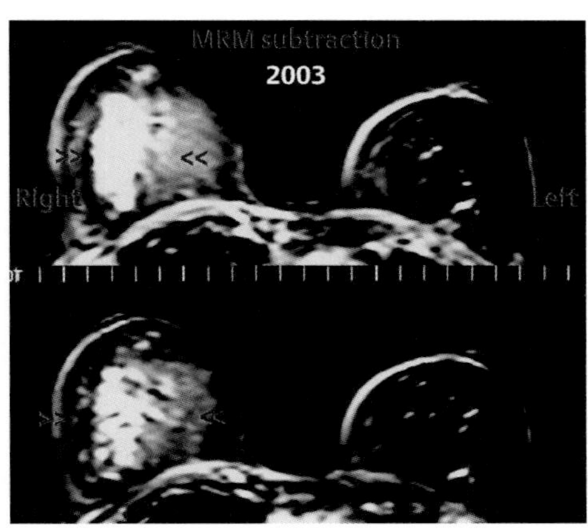


**a** *MRI* in May, 2003. The dense structures seen on mammograms correspond to adenosis with marked lobular proliferation on sonograms and to intense gadolinium enhancement throughout the right upper outer quadrant on MRI.

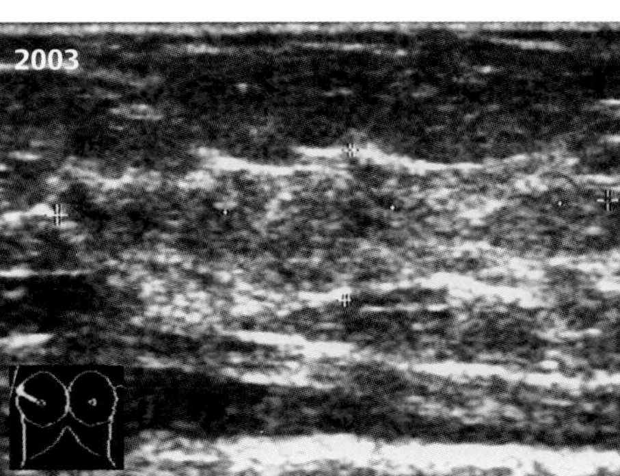


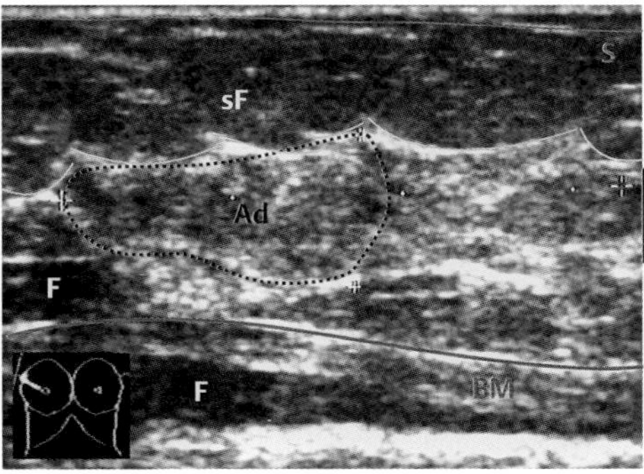


S = skin
sF = subcutaneous fat
Ad = adenosis
F = fat
Ni = nipple
BM = pectoral muscle

**b** *Sonogram* of the upper outer quadrant of the right breast in May, 2003 shows an enlarged lobe with intense proliferation of TDLUs corresponding to the MRI enhancement pattern and the increased mammographic density visible in the upper outer quadrant (**e**).

▶ Fig. 5.80 c–h

**Fig. 5.80** **A 56-year-old woman with a painful mass in the upper outer quadrant of the right breast.** *(continued)*

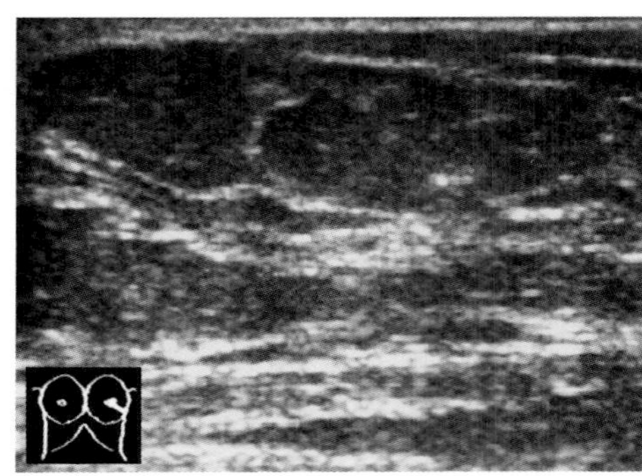

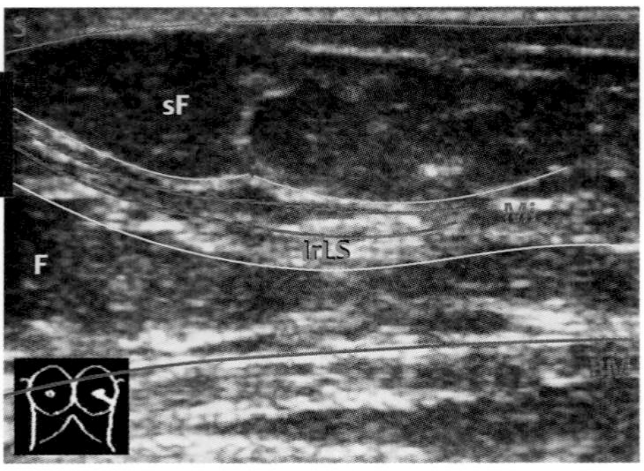


S = skin
sF = subcutaneous fat
F = fat
Mi = milk duct
IrLS = interlobular stroma
BM = pectoral muscle

**c** *Sonogram* of the left breast in May, 2003 shows involuted breast parenchyma with ductectasia in the interlobular stroma. The scan does not show significant proliferation of TDLUs.

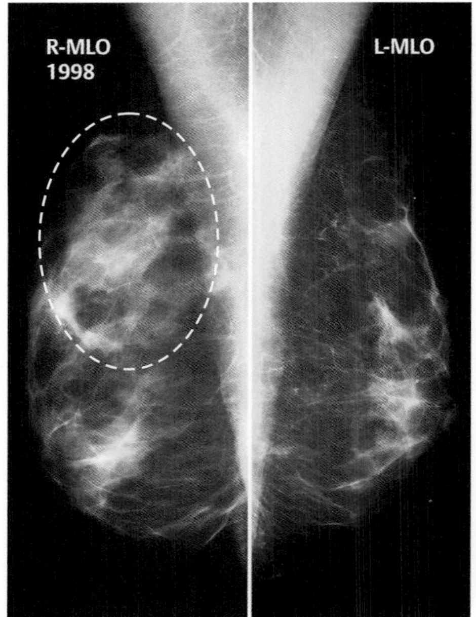


**d** *Bilateral oblique mammograms* in 1998 show asymmetrical breast development with more radiodense areas on the right side, especially in the upper hemisphere (ACR 2, BIRADS 2, **P**GMI).

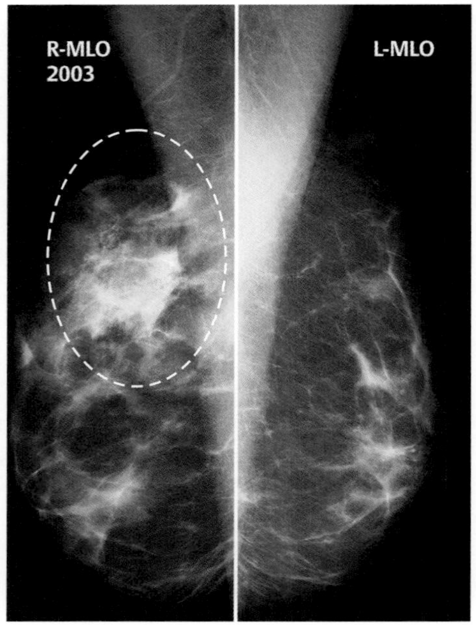


**e** *Bilateral oblique mammograms* in May, 2003 show slight regression of left breast parenchyma compared with the previous mammogram and increased parenchymal density in the upper portion of the right breast (ACR 2).

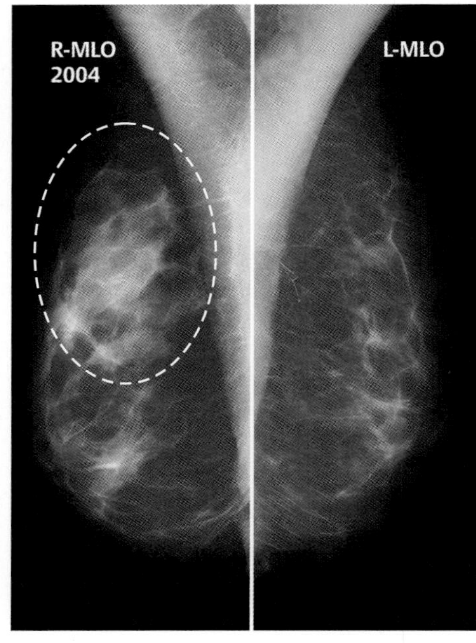


**f** *Bilateral oblique mammograms* in 2004 show a normalization of parenchymal markings with asymmetry favoring the right breast (**P**GMI).

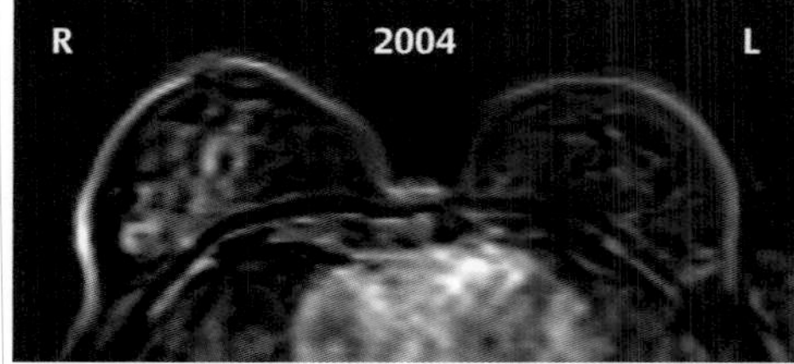


**g** *MRI* in February, 2004. Regression of intense gadolinium enhancement is noted in the right breast (compare with (**a**), which still shows increased diffuse vascularity.

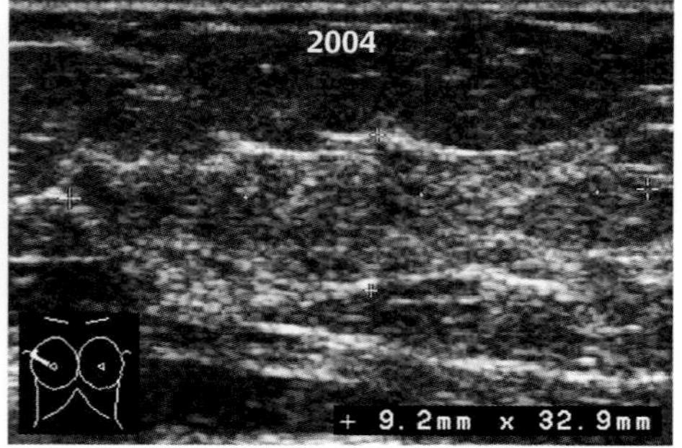


**h** *Sonogram* of the upper outer quadrant of the right breast in February, 2004 still shows lobar enlargement with prominent TDLUs. Ultrasound cannot distinguish between lobules (acini) and intralobular stroma (see p. 23 ff). There is no essential difference between ultrasound findings in 2003 (**b**) and 2004 (**h**) despite the slight change in MRI, mammographic and physical findings (regression of proliferating lobules without regression of the intralobular stroma).

***The transient higher radiodensity of the upper outer quadrant of the right breast (marked area) resulted from a transient proliferation of TDLUs and returned to normal after the discontinuation of HRT, though sonographically there was no change.***

**Fig. 5.81** **A 60-year-old woman with fibrocystic changes.** For years the patient had taken tibolone (Liviella). HRT was discontinued in 2002, followed by the regression of glandular structures and cysts. Proliferating TDLUs are clearly documented in 2002 and 2003 (see also **Fig. 4.4**, p. 26).

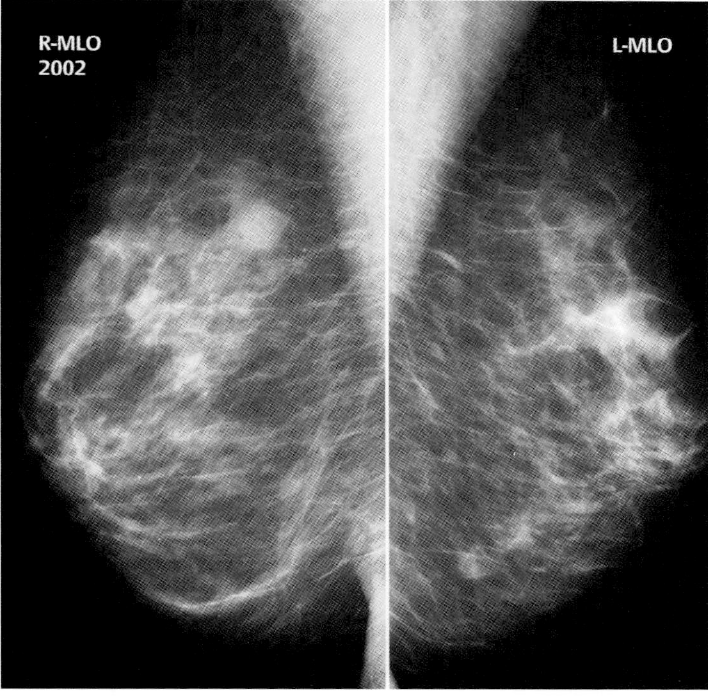


**a** *Bilateral oblique mammograms* in May, 2002 show patchy, moderately dense breast parenchyma. The right breast has higher mammographic density than the left (ACR 3, P**G**MI, BIRADS 2). Cysts appear as small focal opacities in both breasts.

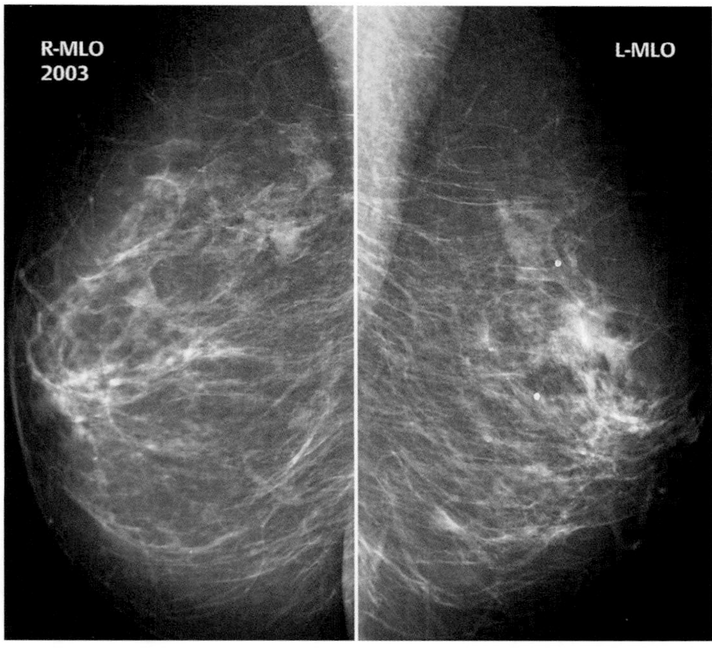


**b** *Bilateral oblique mammograms* in December, 2003–7 months after the patient stopped taking tibolone–show regression of glandular structures and cysts with obvious signs of involution (ACR 2, PG**M**I).

> *The decrease in mammographic density from ACR 3 to ACR 2 after the withdrawal of tibolone is due to the regression of proliferating TDLUs. Increased parenchymal density occurs in 10 % of patients on tibolone (see p. 11) and may be associated with an increased risk of breast cancer.*

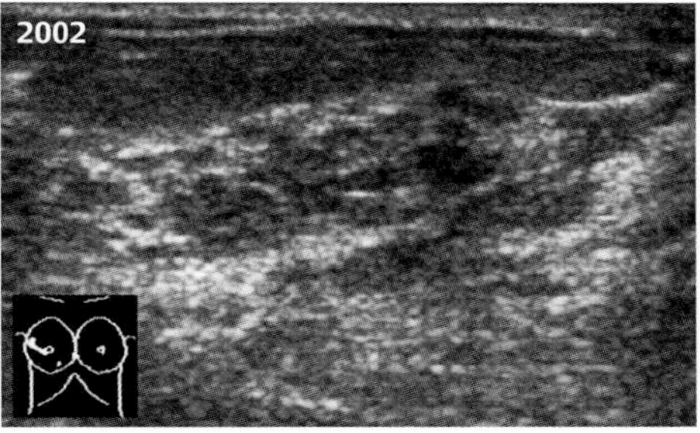


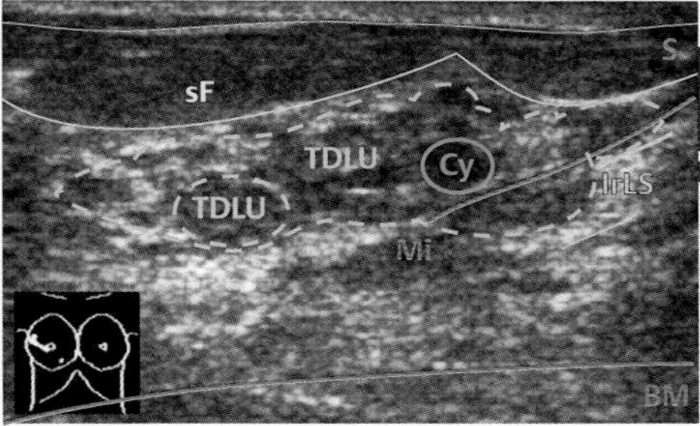


S = skin
sF = subcutaneous fat
Mi = milk duct
Ni = nipple
IrLS = interlobular stroma
TDLU = terminal duct lobular unit (adenosis?)
Cy = cyst
BM = pectoral muscle

**c** *Sonogram* of the upper outer quadrant of the right breast in May, **2002**, shows ductectasia, small cysts, and proliferating TDLUs.

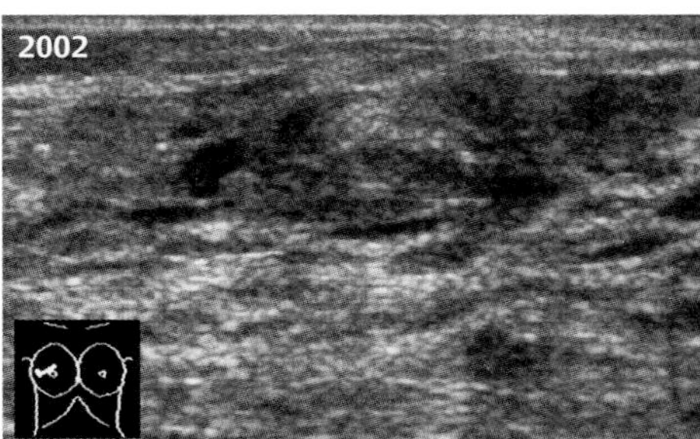


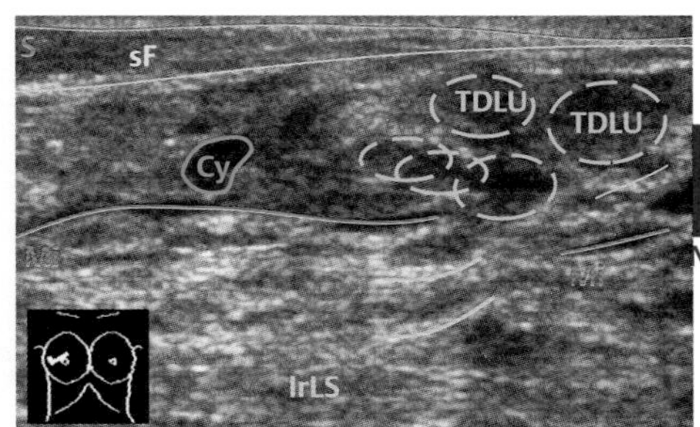


S = skin
sF = subcutaneous fat
Mi = milk duct
Cy = cyst
Ni = nipple
IrLS = interlobular stroma
TDLU = terminal duct lobular unit

**d** *Sonogram* in May, 2002 shows proliferating TDLUs and small cysts, causing the lobe to acquire a spongy, inhomogeneous texture.

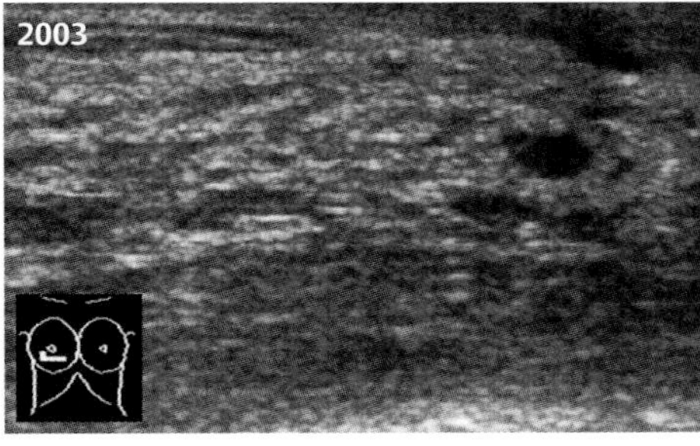


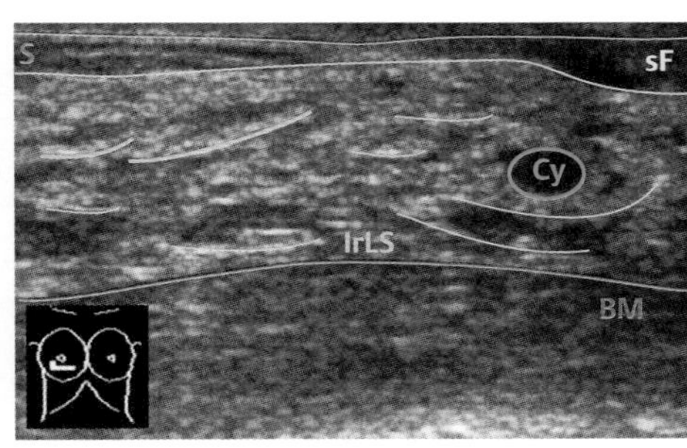


S = skin
sF = subcutaneous fat
IrLS = interlobular stroma
Cy = cyst
BM = pectoral muscle

▶ Fig. 5.81 f–h

**e** *Transverse sonogram* through the lower portion of the right breast. The breast parenchyma is rich in interlobular stroma (echogenic) and contains cysts. The scan also documents regression of proliferating TDLUs.

**Fig. 5.81 A 60-year-old woman with fibrocystic changes.** *(continued)*

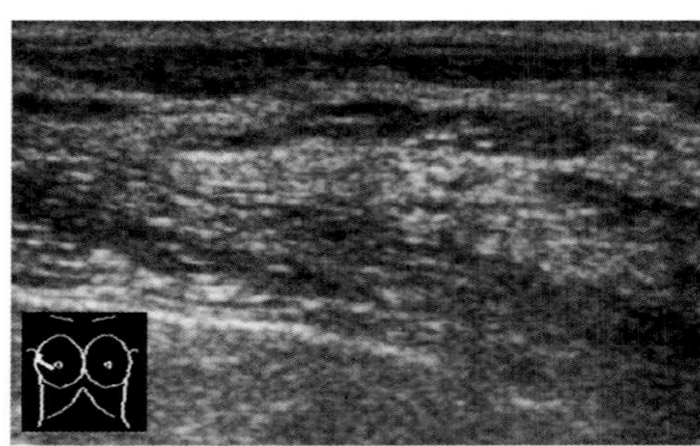

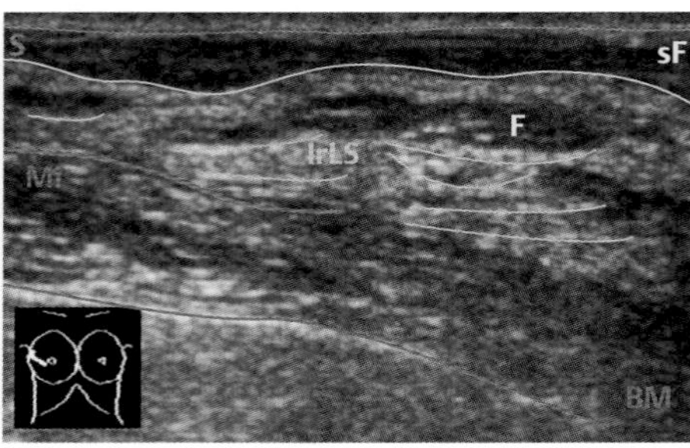


S = skin
sF = subcutaneous fat
IrLS = interlobular stroma
Mi = milk duct
F = fat
Ni = nipple
BM = pectoral muscle

**f** *Sonogram* of the right upper outer quadrant in 2003 (same plane as in **c**) shows an involuted breast with microcystic fibrosis and regression of TDLUs compared with 2002. The glandular structures are more homogeneous and less active than in 2002.

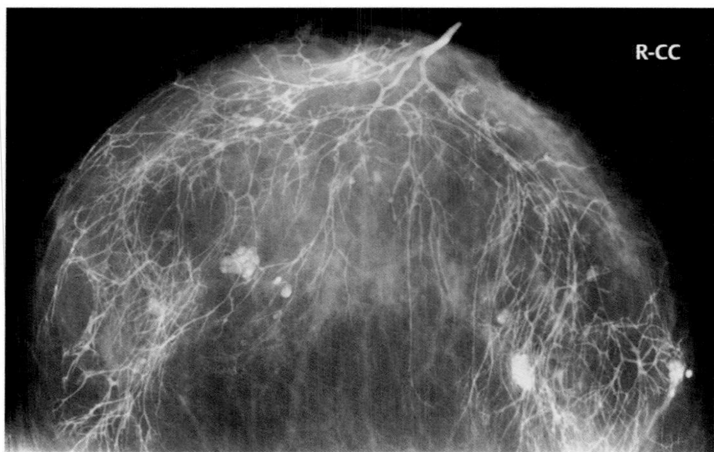


**g** *Craniocaudal ductogram* in **a different, 58-year-old woman** with cystic mammary fibrosis and a light serous nipple discharge. The contrast medium reveals a fine, richly arborized duct system with four visible lobes that are poorly demarcated from one another. Peripheral lobules show cystic dilatation, and some are mulberry-shaped.

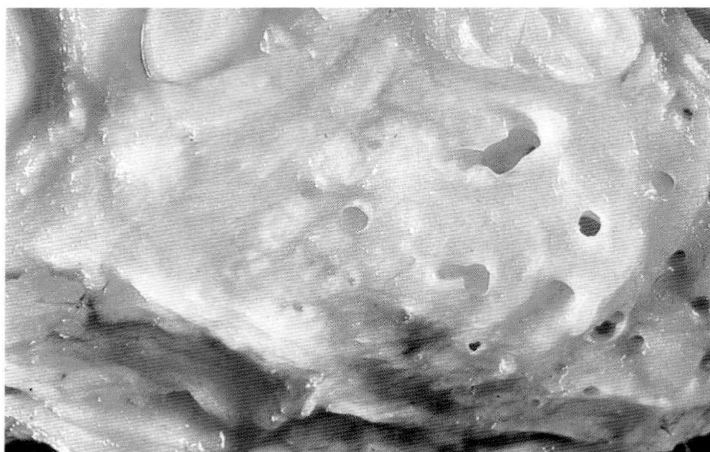

**h** *Gross specimen* of an involuted breast (magnification 5×) displays enlarged ducts and lobules (indistinguishable from each other) and heavy fat permeation of the remaining breast parenchyma (light areas in yellow fat). Portions of the brownish pectoral muscle are visible at the bottom of the specimen.

**Fig. 5.82 44-year-old woman with macromastia.** The essential pathology is fibrocystic change, which is more pronounced on the right side than on the left. Areas of glandular proliferation are more prominent in the left breast. The right breast also contains foci of adenosis (**g**) and ductectasia. But the macromastia and increased mammographic density result mainly from connective tissue, cysts, and relatively scant lobular proliferation–perhaps contributing to an inability to produce sufficient milk during lactation (see **e** and **f**).

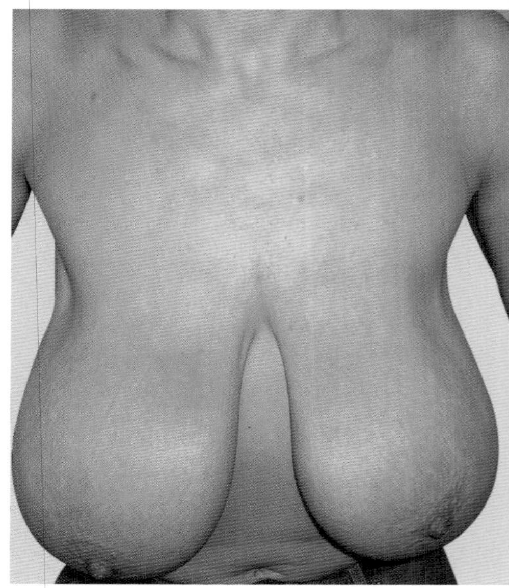

**a** *Macromastia* (with arms lowered).

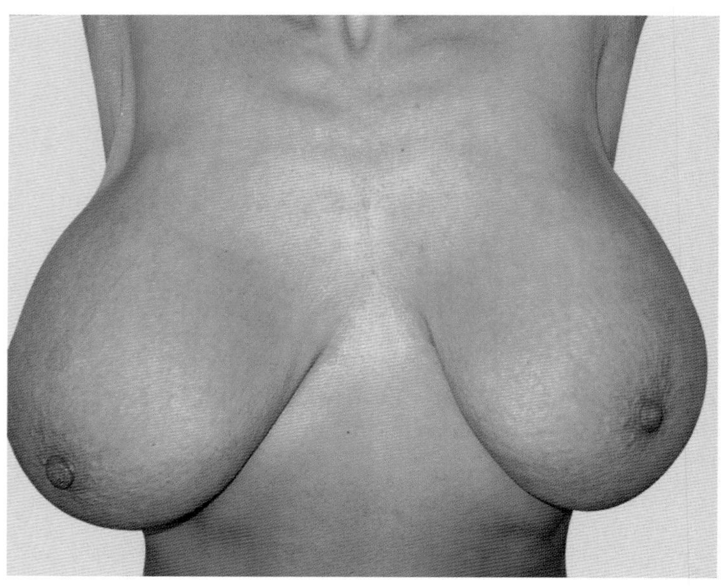

**b** *Macromastia* with arms raised. The breasts are large and pendulous and show no nipple inversion. Status after reduction mammoplasty see **i**, p. 190.

**Fig. 5.82 44-year-old woman with macromastia.** *(continued)*

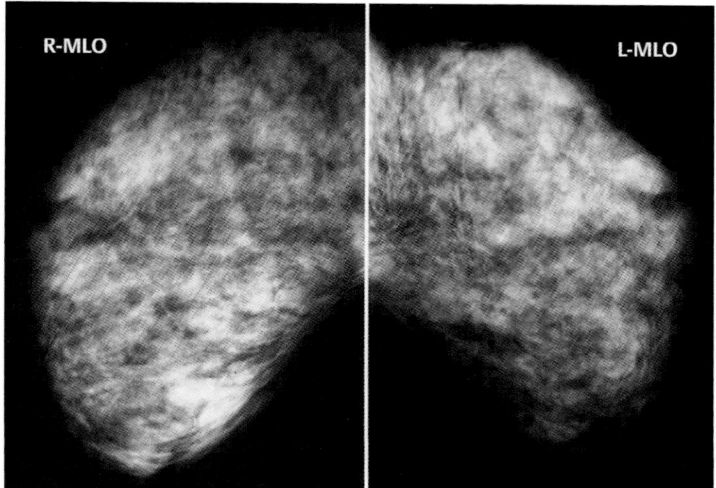


**c** *Bilateral oblique mammograms* show fibrocystic breasts with numerous, confluent stippled and patchy opacities (ACR 3, BIRADS 2, P**G**MI).

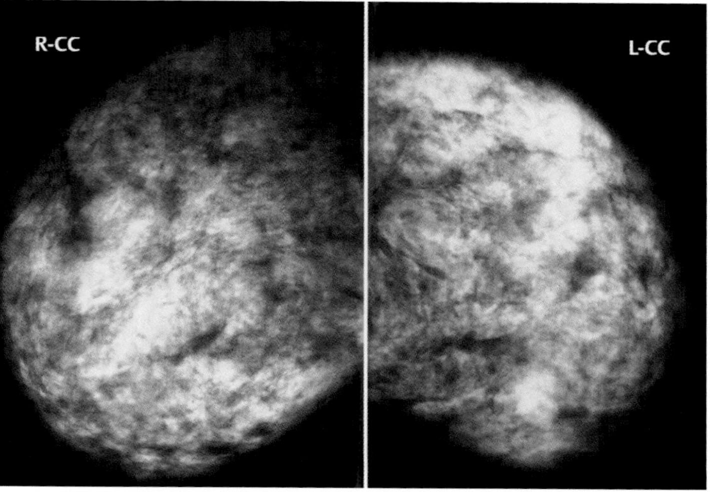


**d** *Bilateral craniocaudal mammograms* show fibrocystic changes with patchy, confluent opacities (ACR 3, P**G**MI). The entire breast is fully imaged with the 24 cm × 30 cm detector of a Giotto digital mammographic system.

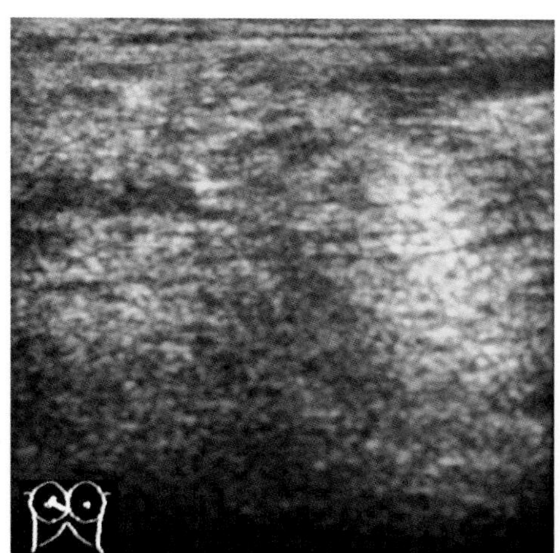

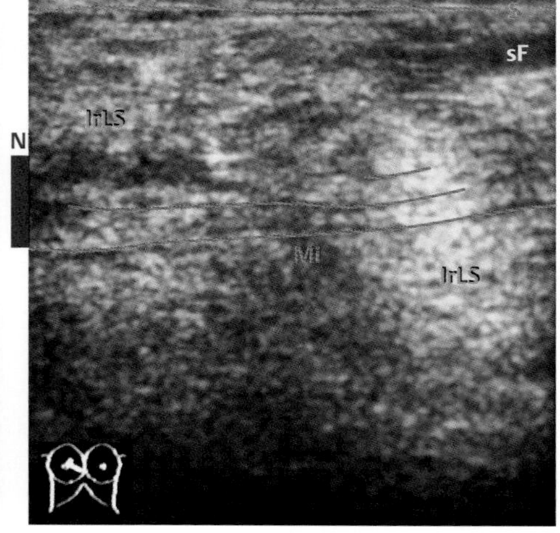


S = skin
sF = subcutaneous fat
Ni = nipple
Mi = milk duct(s)
IrLS = interlobular stroma

**e** *Sonogram* of the lower inner quadrant of the right breast. The breast parenchyma is rich in interlobular stroma, which predominates over the TDLUs. Ducts appear as fine linear features.

*The ACR 3 mammographic density of the hypertrophic breast (c, d) stems mainly from interlobular stroma (approximately 70%) and less from proliferating TDLUs, aside from individual areas of adenosis in each breast.*

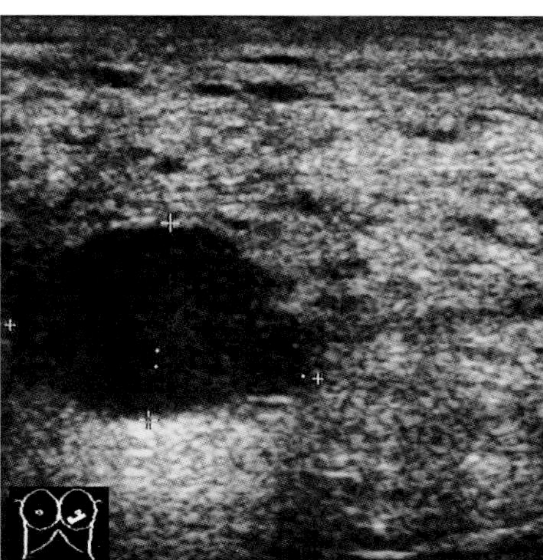

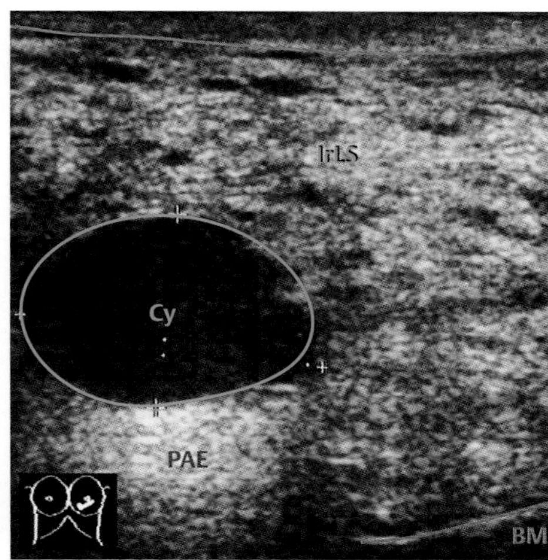


S = skin
Cy = cyst
IrLS = interlobular stroma
PAE = posterior acoustic enhancement
BM = pectoral muscle

**f** *Sonogram* of the infra-areolar left breast shows a 2 cm × 1.3 cm cyst with posterior acoustic enhancement caused by the cyst contents. The cyst is surrounded by breast parenchyma rich in interlobular stroma without prominent TDLU proliferation. There is no visible subcutaneous fat.

▶ **Fig. 5.82 g–i**

**Fig. 5.82 44-year-old woman with macromastia.** *(continued)*

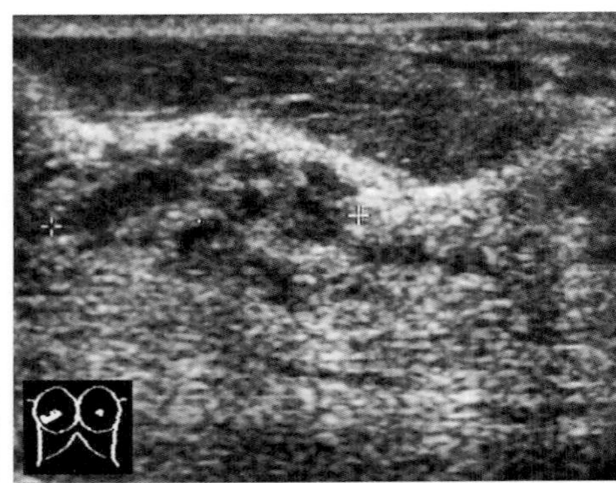

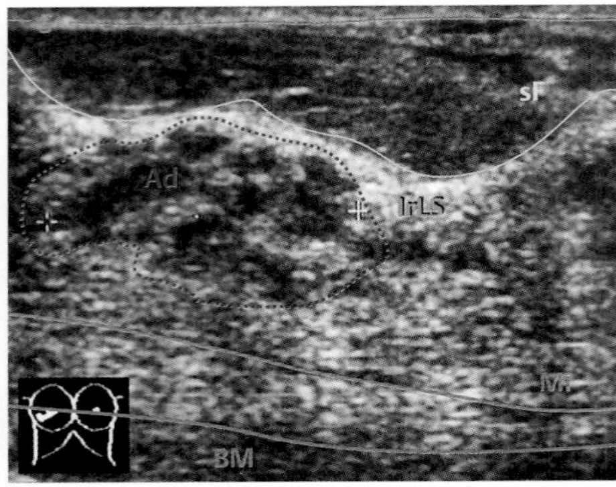


S = skin
sF = subcutaneous fat
Mi = milk duct
Ad = adenosis
IrLS = interlobular stroma
BM = pectoral muscle

**g** *Sonogram* of the lower outer quadrant of the right breast. A dilated duct is visible at the center of the lobe. It is surrounded by adenosis-like areas of confluent, proliferating TDLUs.

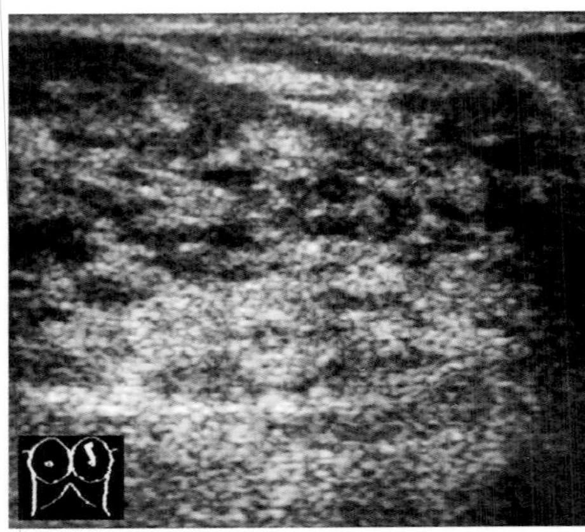

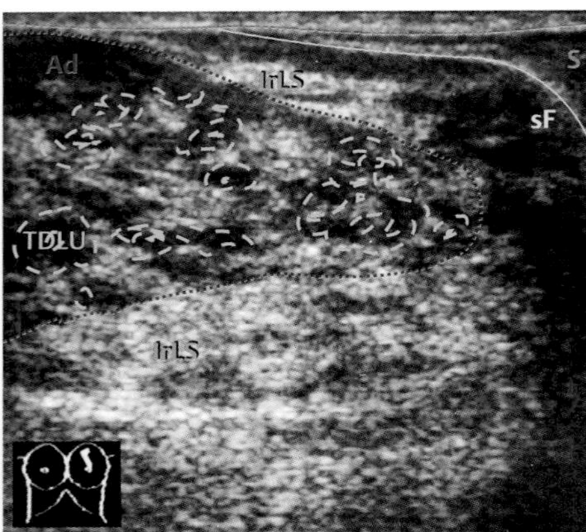


S = skin
sF = subcutaneous fat
Ad = adenosis
IrLS = interlobular stroma
TDLU = terminal duct lobular unit

**h** *Sonogram* of the upper portion of the left breast shows adenosis-like proliferation of TDLUs in one lobe, surrounded by parenchyma that is rich in interlobular stroma.

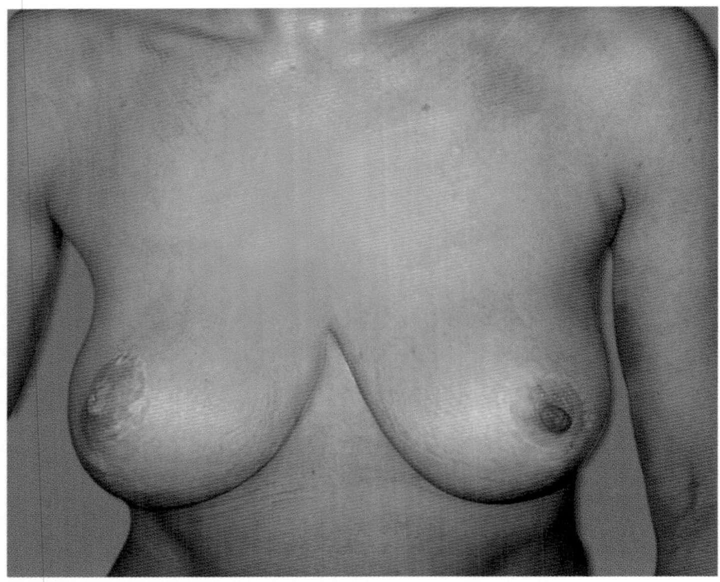

**i** Clinical appearance of the patient in **a** and **b**, 3 years after reduction mammoplasty. The cosmetic result is excellent with a healthy-looking periareolar scar. (Michael Greulich, Breast Surgeon, Stuttgart.)

**Fig. 5.83 35-year-old woman without hormone-therapy presents with significant premenstrual complaints following ovulation.** She has very radiodense breasts. Ultrasound shows very heavy proliferation of TDLUs, multiple cysts, and multiple sites of ductectasia.

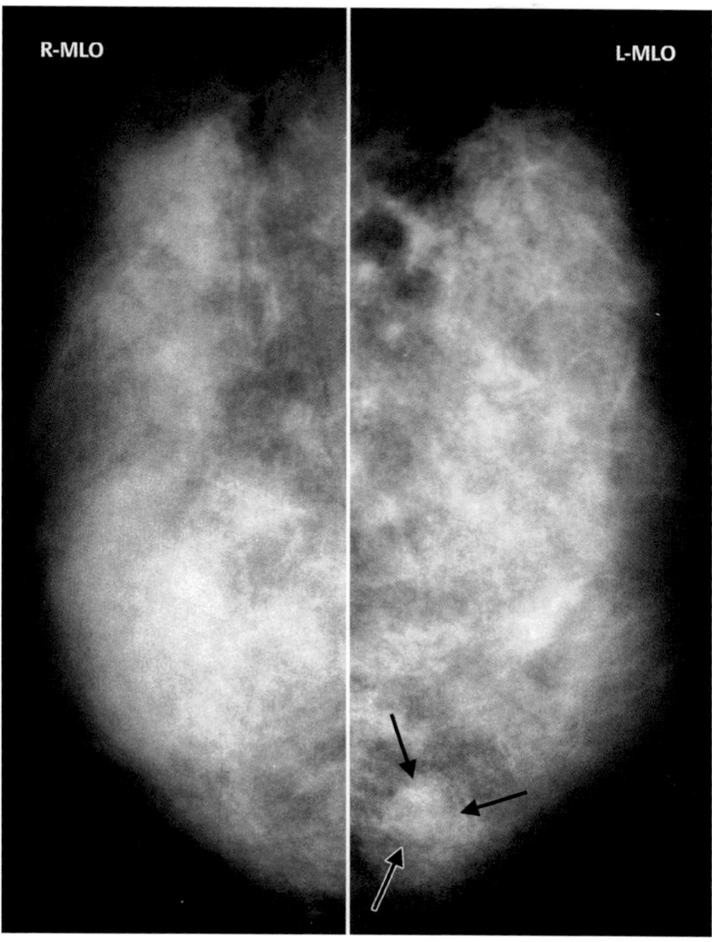


**a** *Bilateral oblique mammograms* show very radiodense breasts with a nonspecific round opacity in the lower portion of the left breast (arrows) and no microcalcifications (ACR 4, PGMI, BIRADS 2).

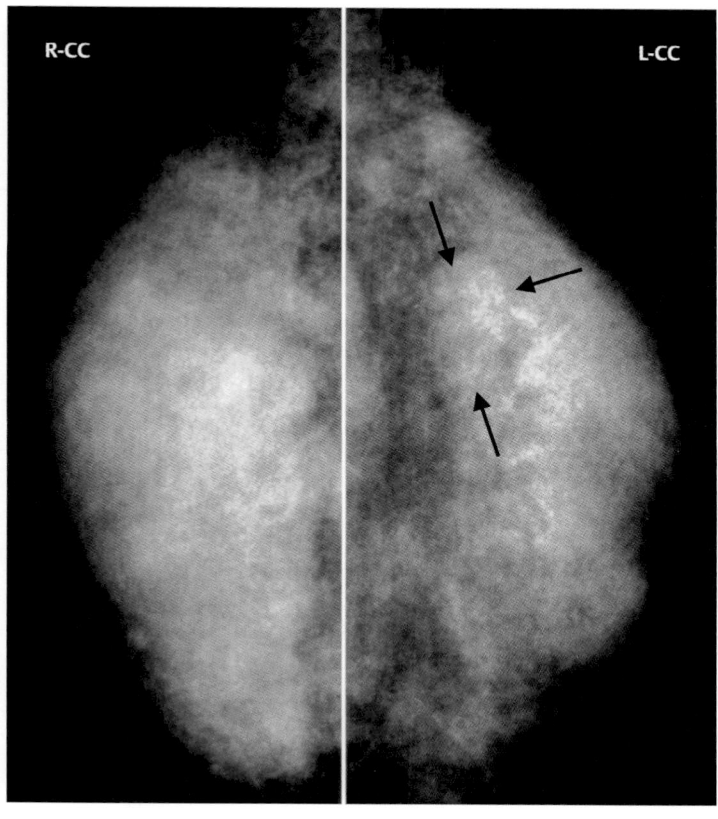


**b** *Bilateral craniocaudal mammograms* show very radiodense glandular tissue (ACR 4, PGMI, BIRADS 2).

***The high mammographic density of the breasts (ACR 4) is caused mainly by proliferating TDLUs, cysts, and ductectasia (approximately 70%) with premenstrual complaints triggered by pressure exerted by the proliferating, hormonally active parenchyma on cysts and enlarged, fluid-filled ducts. In our experience, an oral contraceptive or hormone-releasing IUD will often stop TDLU proliferation, relieving premenstrual mastodynia.***

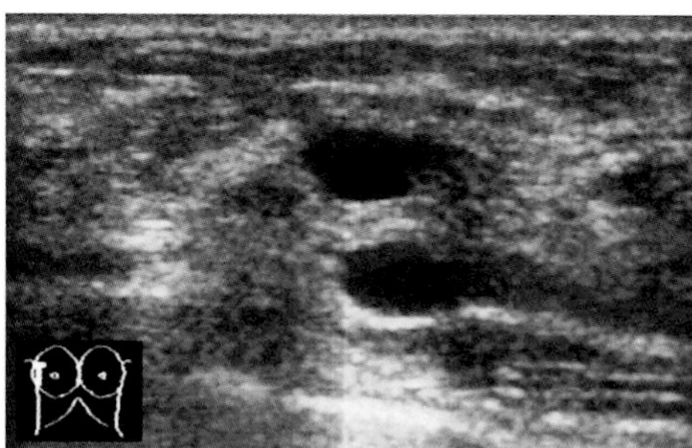

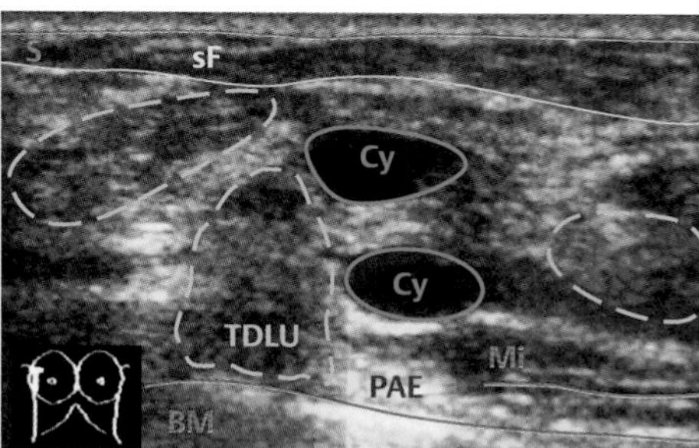


S = skin
sF = subcutaneous fat
Cy = cyst
Mi = milk duct
TDLU = terminal duct lobular unit
PAE = posterior acoustic enhancement
BM = pectoral muscle

**c** *Sonogram* of the upper outer quadrant of the right breast shows small cysts next to strongly proliferating TDLUs.

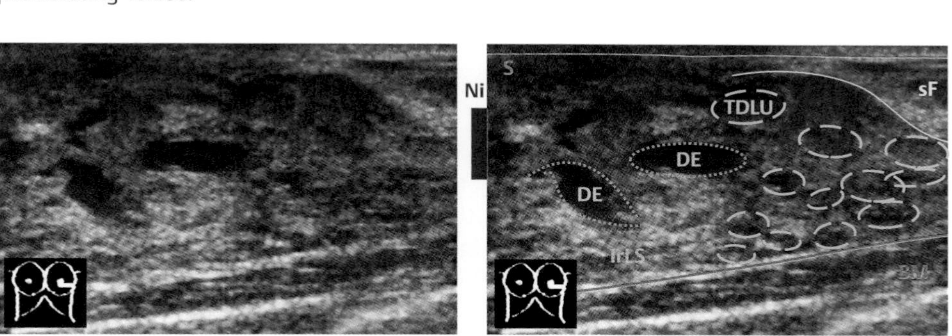


S = skin
sF = subcutaneous fat
TDLU = terminal duct lobular unit
DE = ductectasia
BM = pectoral muscle
IrLS = interlobular stroma

**d** *Sonogram* of the lower outer quadrant of the left breast (marked area) shows foci of ductectasia. Lateral to the dilated ducts are strongly proliferating TDLUs, and below them is prepectoral parenchyma rich in interlobular stroma.

▶ **Fig. 5.83 e, f**

**Fig. 5.83 35-year-old woman not on HRT presents with significant premenstrual complaints following ovulation.** *(continued)*

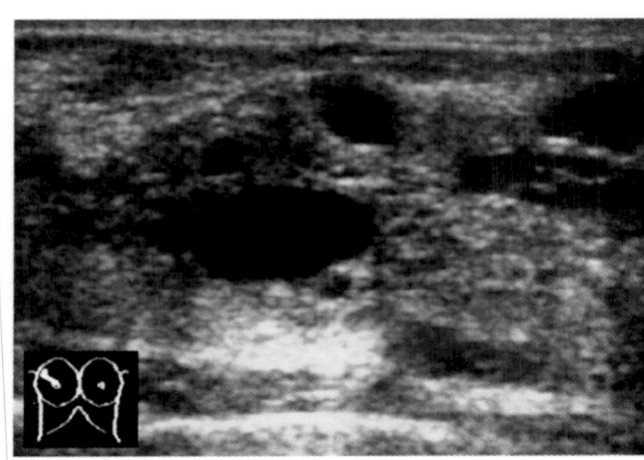

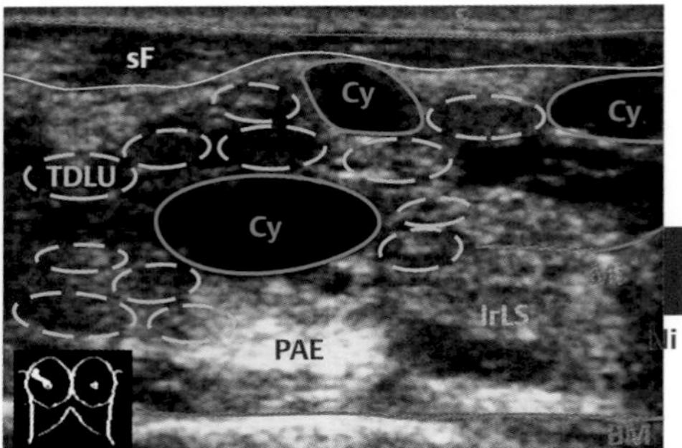


S = skin
sF = subcutaneous fat
Cy = cyst
Mi = milk duct
Ni = nipple
PAE = posterior acoustic enhancement
IrLS = interlobular stroma
TDLU = terminal duct lobular unit
BM = pectoral muscle

**e** *Sonogram* of upper outer quadrant of the right breast shows multiple cysts surrounded by proliferating TDLUs.

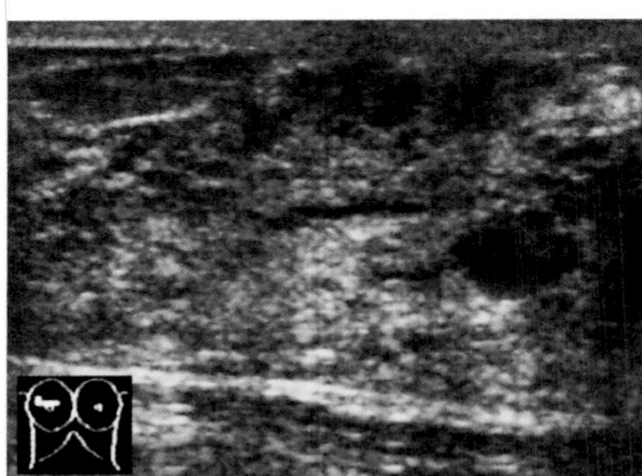

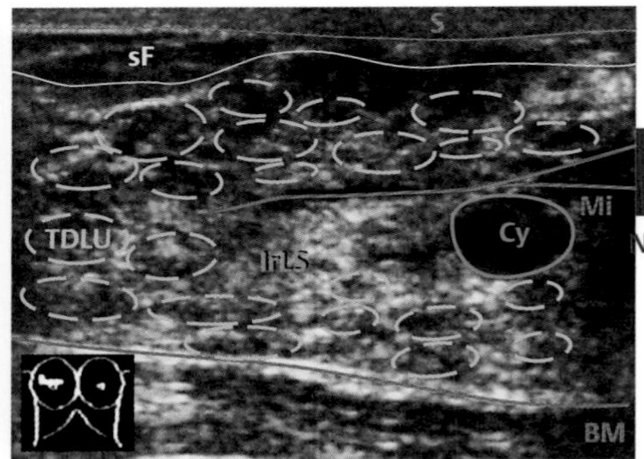


S = skin
sF = subcutaneous fat
Cy = cyst
Mi = milk duct
Ni = nipple
IrLS = interlobular stroma
TDLU = terminal duct lobular unit
BM = pectoral muscle

**f** *Sonogram* of the upper outer quadrant of the right breast shows a strongly proliferating area with numerous enlarged TDLUs. Small sections of a duct and cyst are visible on the right side of the scan.

> ***Ultrasound is useful for investigating mammographically dense regions and identifying them as harmless connective tissue or, in some cases, as proliferating anatomic structures at risk for malignant change. This information is useful in planning adjunctive therapies (e.g., HRT); this cannot be done with mammograms alone.***

Of course, a continuum of findings is seen in the sonographic evaluation of TDLUs, and circumscribed lobular proliferation cannot be accurately classified as "physiologic" or "proliferative" (e.g., adenosis). Further studies are needed in order to make this determination, and analysis of the sonograms should be aided by mammography and, if necessary, by magnetic resonance imaging. A dense mammogram may result from excessive *inter*lobular stroma or the proliferation of TDLUs, but these causes are not mammographically distinguishable. Wolfe and collegues noted that the risk of breast cancer was increased in radiographically dense breasts (Dy/P2 parenchymal structure, see p. 98) but they could only speculate as to the cause of the increased density (Wolfe et al. 1976). Thanks to ultrasound, we now know that the variable density is caused in large part by the proliferation of TDLUs. Assuming that the interlobular stroma in the breast is static, density variations are generally a result of lobular proliferation and/or a cyclic increase in loose intralobular stroma. TDLUs and interlobular stroma can be distinguished from each other by ultrasound. One day, digital mammography may also be able to document density variations in the breast and attribute them to lobule-bearing parenchyma rather than interlobular stroma—a distinction that has therapeutic implications.

Dense mammograms are not always caused by connective tissue and/or proliferating TDLUs. Heavy fibrosis, ductectasia, angiofibrolipomatosis, cysts, and other conditions may also increase the radiographic density of the breast (see **Fig. 5.83**, p. 191). The proliferation of intralobular stroma along the ducts can be recognized by a reversed echo pattern in which the ducts appear as bright linear echoes while loose intralobular stroma appears hypoechoic and dark. Proliferating lobules and proliferating intralobular stroma are generally indistinguishable by ultrasound, though in some cases they may be distinguished by the presence of accentuated, echogenic ducts (see **Fig. 5.71**, p. 172). Both types of proliferation lead to increased mammographic density. But while proliferating TDLUs require critical analysis, proliferating intralobular stroma is essentially harmless. In every breast a continuum exists between the structures described, but the general direction is clear.

The degree of proliferation of the breast parenchyma may be defined as follows:

- **P0:** no detectable TDLUs (at high resolution ultrasound)
- **P1:** proliferating TDLUs account for up to 25% of the volume of both breasts
- **P2:** proliferating TDLUs account for up to 50% of bilateral breast volume
- **P3:** proliferating TDLUs comprise much more than 50% of bilateral breast volume (e.g., in pregnancy)

Further investigations and prospective studies are needed before the P categories can be developed into a risk classification. Higher-resolution ultrasound scanners would be desirable and extremely helpful in advancing the analysis of cyclical and hormonal breast changes. The statements made in this section are more assumptions than hard facts. They are based on numerous biopsies in which the findings were compared with radiographic anatomy and sonograms. In presenting these findings, the author hopes to provide an impetus for further research.

### Combined Sonographic and Mammographic Screening

The World Health Organization (WHO) has listed the criteria that make a breast cancer screening program feasible (Wilson and Junger 1968):

- The condition should be an important public health problem.
- The disease should be detectable at an early stage.
- The screening test should be suitable and should be acceptable to the screened population.
- There should be an accepted treatment for patients with recognized disease.
- The benefits should outweigh possible harm.

These criteria apply to both ultrasound and mammography. An optimum program would be to screen women between 40 and 75 years of age at 18-month intervals with both single-view mammograms and ultrasound (ACR 2–4). This would not have to cost any more than two-view mammographic screening without ultrasound (see pp. 95, 105), even when screening includes breast palpation (see p. 90).

If this type of program cannot be widely implemented (and all signs indicate that it cannot), every woman who presents for mammographic screening should be advised to see her gynecologist for an ultrasound and physical examination as well—despite the practical difficulty of correlating the findings with the patient's mammograms. It remains to be seen whether this multitrack approach is the best economic and diagnostic solution. It is likely that women would flock to a screening program that exposes them to half the usual radiation dose, requires a single breast compression, and increases diagnostic certainty.

Physicians who are concerned with radiation safety must justify the indication for radiography, giving due consideration to all the other alternatives. Given what is known about the capabilities and safety aspects of mammography and ultrasound, how can they justify two-view mammography as opposed to single-view mammography plus ultrasound? Either they do not believe the results of single-view mammography and sonography presented here (which is their right), or they must accept our data and set policy accordingly. But they can act only if payors are willing to provide reasonable reimbursements for this more time-consuming screening combination. But the organization of screening is not in the hands of physicians; it is up to government or a government-appointed commission to establish indications and fee schedules.

### Outlook for Breast Ultrasound

In theory, ultrasound imaging of the breast with a high-frequency transducer can detect cancers as small as 4–5 mm in diameter. But not every 5 mm tumor can be detected. Resolution may be degraded due to cysts, adenosis, cystic metaplasia, ductectasia, or other conditions. In particular, ultrasound cannot detect atypical microcalcifications unless they are grouped into clusters larger than 10 mm (Moon et al. 2000). Ultimately, x-ray mammography and ultrasound are complementary modalities for breast cancer diagnosis. In settings where they cannot be satisfactorily combined, the examiner must resort to MRI (see p. 201) and interventional procedures (see p. 230).

The value of mammography is beyond dispute. The only questions are the number of mammograms per breast and the optimum screening intervals.

Suspicious lesions (including calcifications) that can be visualized with ultrasound should be biopsied under sonographic guidance. This is the surest way to determine whether a tumor has an invasive component. Another advantage of ultrasound is that it is less costly than digital stereotactic core-needle biopsy and MRI-guided interventional procedures.

It is not our intention to sing the praises of breast ultrasound without cause. But at the same time, it is difficult to understand why such an effective modality has become lost in the shadow of conventional mammography. Even today, it is impossible to conceive of breast cancer screening without ultrasound. Women favor the combination of single-view mammography and ultrasound because it reduces their radiation exposure and is less painful than standard craniocaudal and oblique compression views together. This modification of traditional screening mammography is the *optimum* approach to early breast cancer detection. It is hoped that ultrasound manufacturers will be able to supply even higher-resolution transducers in the future. The new automated full-field breast ultrasound (AFBUS, as described by Richter et al. [1998] and Wenkel et al. [2008]) is the way ahead in the digital direction. Now the technical assistant can produce ultrasonograms under standardized conditions and physicians study them on their workstations together with mammograms from a digital PACS.

## Axillary Mammography and Ultrasound

The axilla cannot be adequately evaluated on mammograms. A good oblique projection can demonstrate the level 1 lymph nodes (see **Fig. 5.88**, p. 200), but other axillary processes are not detectable on radiographs (see **Fig. 5.84 a–d** and **Fig. 5.86**). Even magnetic resonance imaging often cannot accurately evaluate axillary structures due to artifacts from the chest cavity, although modern scanners are providing new diagnostic capabilities also in that region (see **Fig. 5.94 e**, p. 211).

Positron emission tomography (PET) can sometimes detect axillary, supraclavicular, and infraclavicular lymph node metastases as small as 5 mm (see p. 227) if the tumor has sufficient tracer uptake, which is not always the case. Ultrasound can demonstrate level 1 axillary lymph nodes as well as level 2 lymph nodes that are enlarged. Level 2 lymph node enlargement most commonly results from fatty infiltration of the nodal parenchyma, which often but not always is detectable by mammography as well. Supra- and infraclavicular lymph node metastases can be detected if they are at least 1 cm in diameter and occur at a peripheral location. The ultrasound appearance of lymph node metastases is quite variable initially, and it is even likely that an early nodal metastasis will cause no visible abnormalities. Other axillary structures, particularly the blood vessels (veins, arteries), are usually given scant attention during ultrasound scanning of the axilla, even though this would be very important in patients with arm edema (may be seen rarely with an axillary recurrence). Venous stenosis may also lead to swelling of the arm (see **Fig. 5.85**). Lymphatic enlargement secondary to postoperative seroma formation is detectable by ultrasound.

*(continued on p. 198)*

**Fig. 5.84 Four women (patients A–D) present with normal lymph nodes or lymphadenopathy.**
**Patient A:** A 53-year-old woman with no palpable abnormalities. Slightly enlarged lymph nodes were palpable in both axillae in 2004.

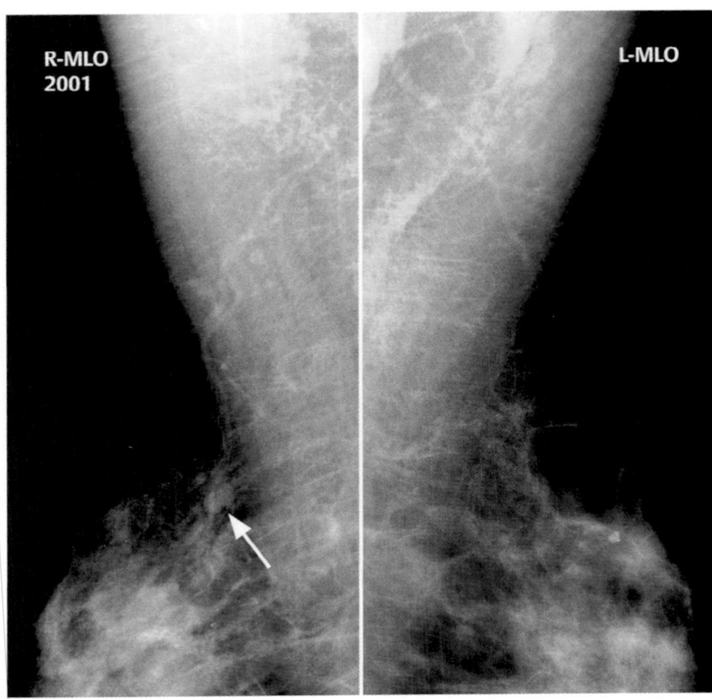


**a** *Mammograms* in December, 2001 (close-up of the axilla) show a small round opacity in the right breast (**b/20**). The axillae appear normal.

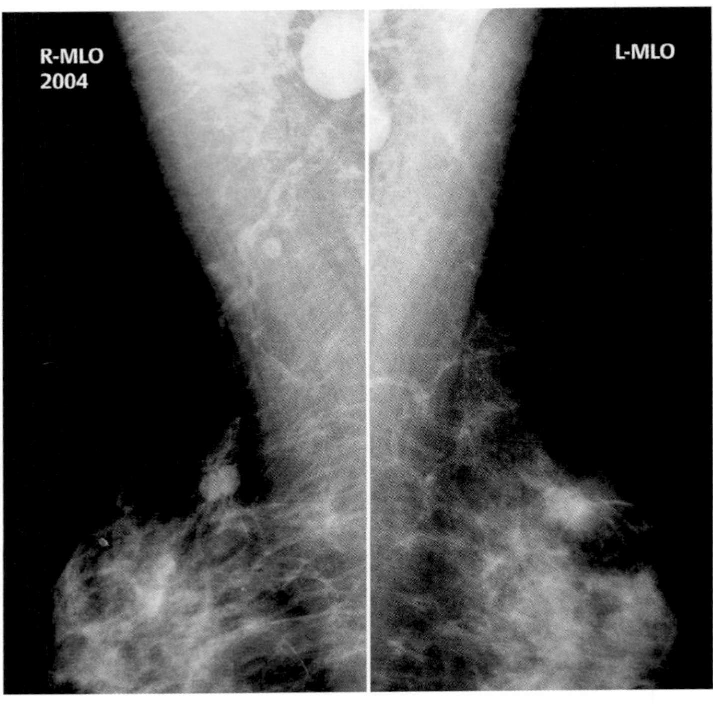


**b** *Bilateral oblique mammograms* in March, 2004 (close-up of the axilla) show slight enlargement of the round opacity in the axillary recess (**g/20**) and enlarged, homogeneously dense lymph nodes (right **h/26–27**, left **I/25–26**) in both axillae.

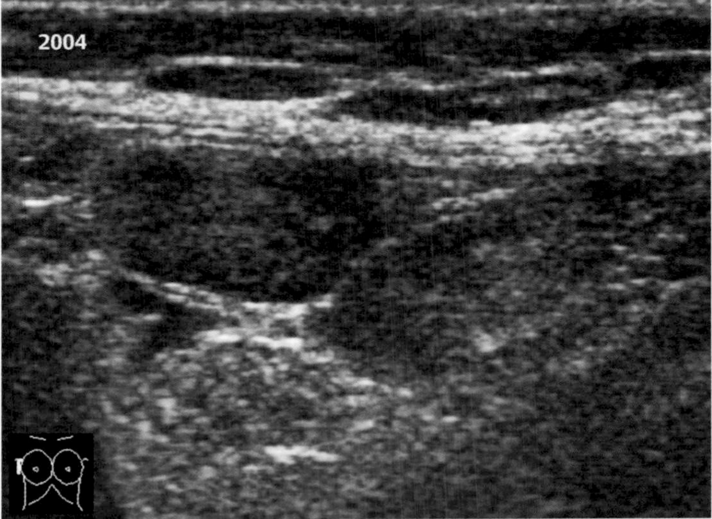


**c** *Sonogram* of the right axilla in March, 2004 demonstrates two enlarged, hypoechoic lymph nodes without central hilar fat.

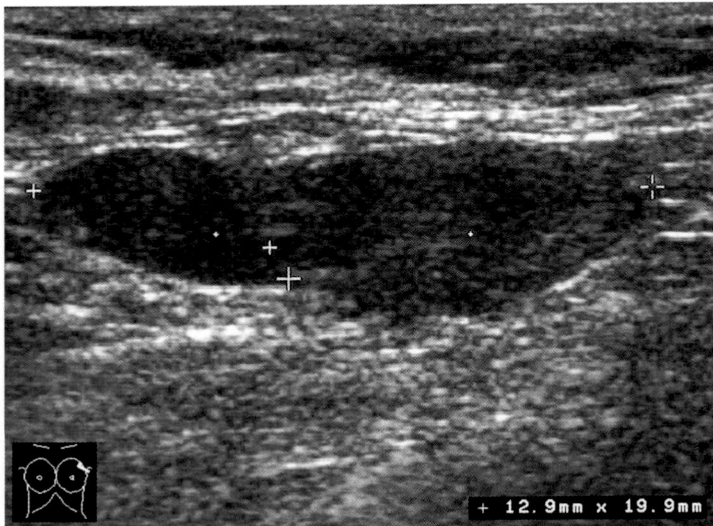


**d** *Sonogram* of the left axilla in March, 2004 shows an enlarged, hypoechoic lymph node without a definable central hilum (see marker).

**Fig. 5.84** *(continued)* **Patient B:** A 64-year-old woman underwent diagnostic excision of an atypical retroareolar density in the right breast, followed by the formation of a healthy-appearing scar from the 9 to 11-o'clock positions (histology was not suspicious at that time). She presented now with a palpable mass in the right axilla.

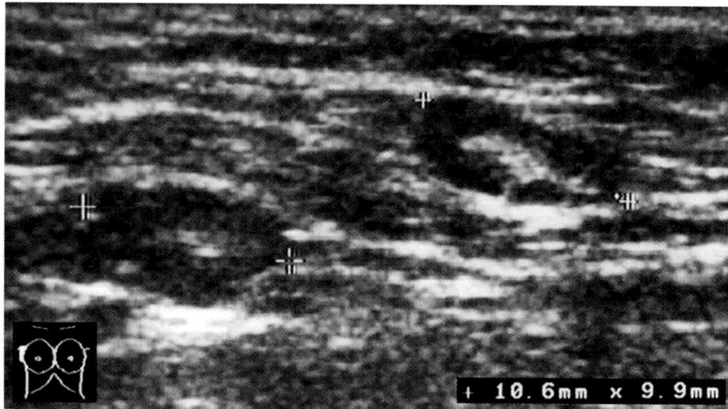


**e** *Sonogram* of the right axilla shows an enlarged lymph node with a compressed central fatty hilum (**L/24** and **N/25**) (see also marker) and broadened lymphatic parenchyma.

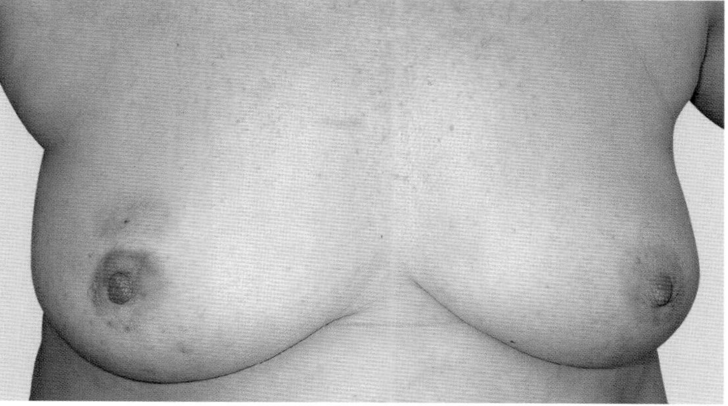

**f** *Clinical appearance* in March, 2002 following an open biopsy of the right breast 2 years before (scar at p/23). A small hematoma is present at **p/24** following core-needle biopsy (CNB).

**Patient C:** A 35-year-old woman with no palpable breast abnormalities and no palpable enlargement of the axillary lymph nodes.

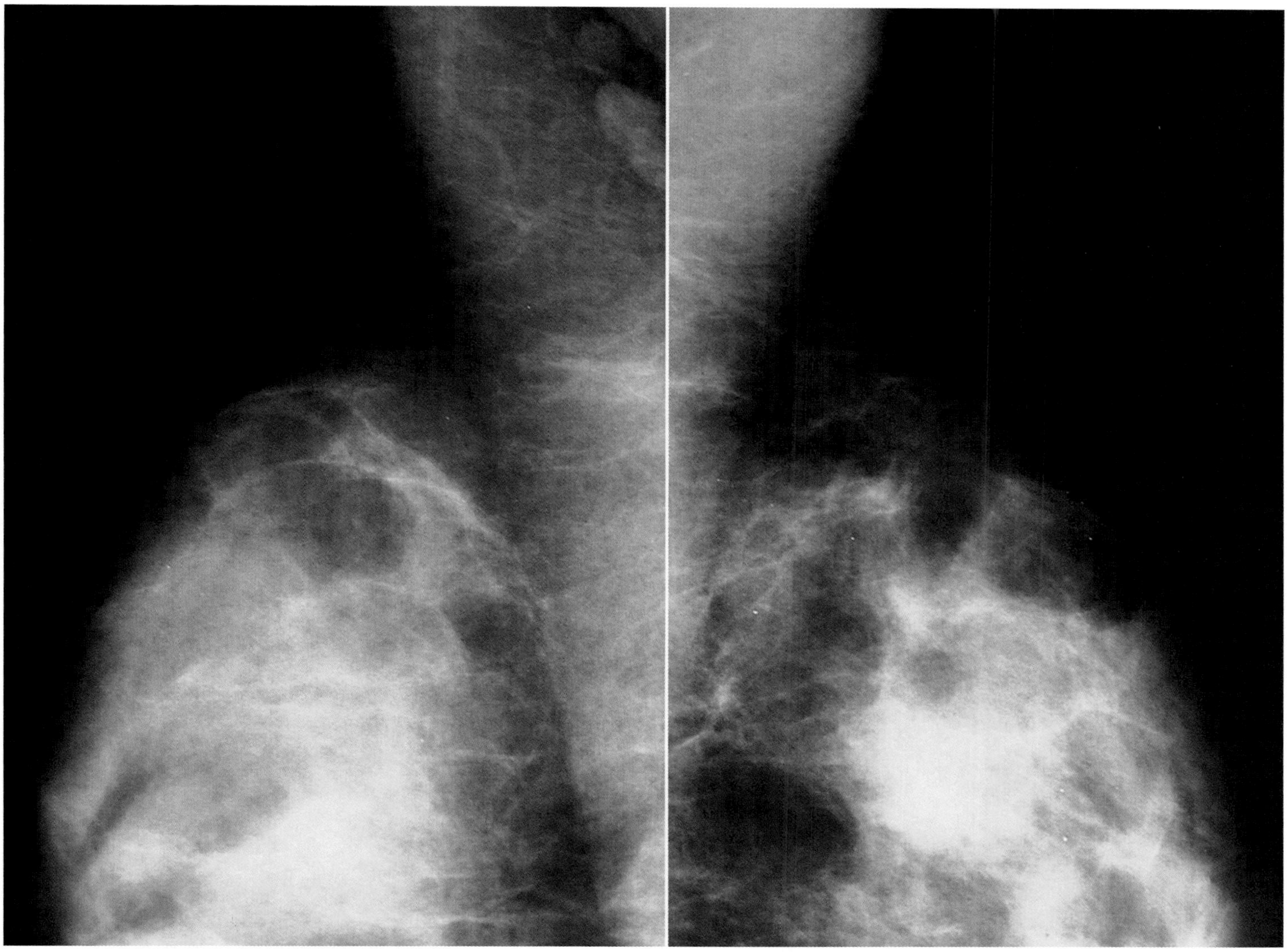

**g** *Bilateral oblique mammograms* (close-up of the axilla and axillary recess) show enlarged axillary lymph nodes on the right side (**O/17**). The breasts are very radiodense and inhomogeneous (ACR 3).

▶ **Fig. 5.84 h–m**

**Fig. 5.84** *(continued)* **Patient D:** A 46-year-old woman with a bulging mass in the right axillary recess (**i**) that was present for 1–2 years. A subcutaneous nodule has been present on the right elbow for several years (**j**). Both breasts appear clinically normal, and there are no mammographic or sonographic abnormalities.

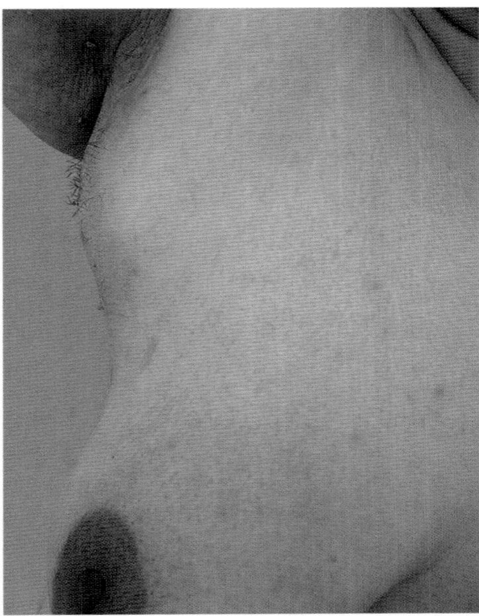

**h** *Clinical appearance* of the right breast and axilla. There is a palpable and visible bulge in the axillary recess (**B/23–26**) and anterior axillary fold.

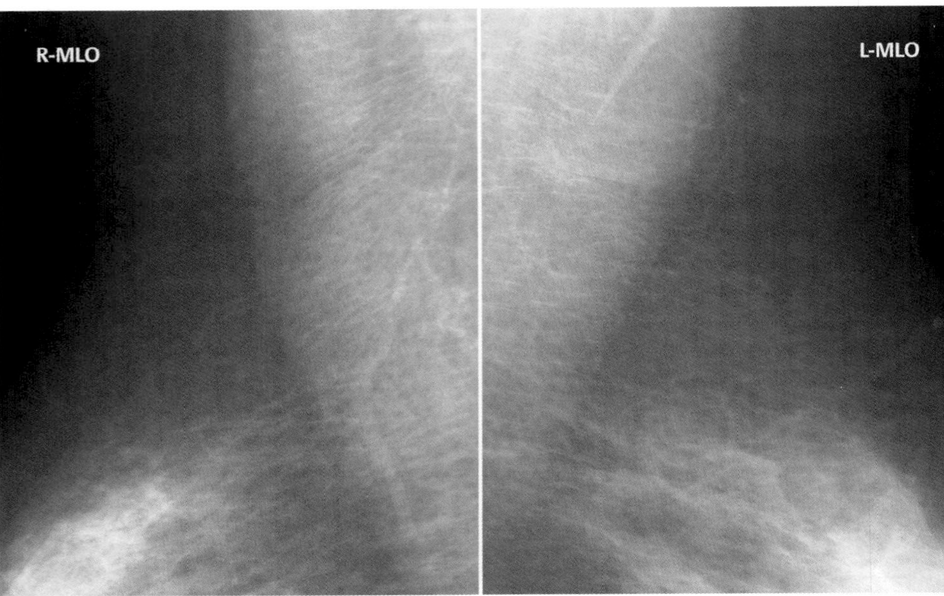


**i** *Bilateral oblique mammograms* (close-up of the axillary recess and both axillae) show no abnormalities aside from a nonspecific faint opacity on the right side (**f/26**).

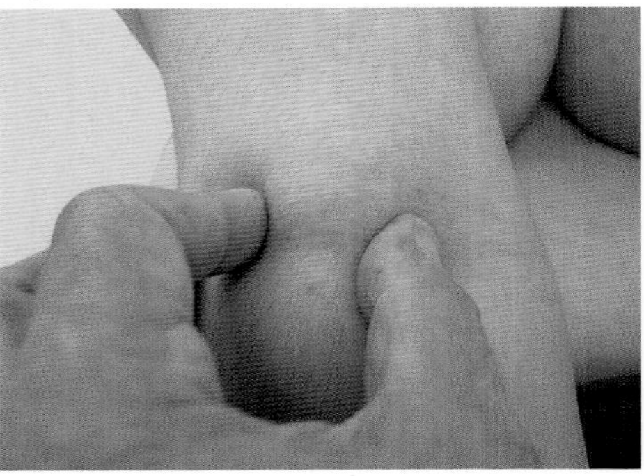

**j** *Physical examination* of the right elbow reveals a soft, mobile subcutaneous nodule (between the fingers), noticed by the patient several years before.

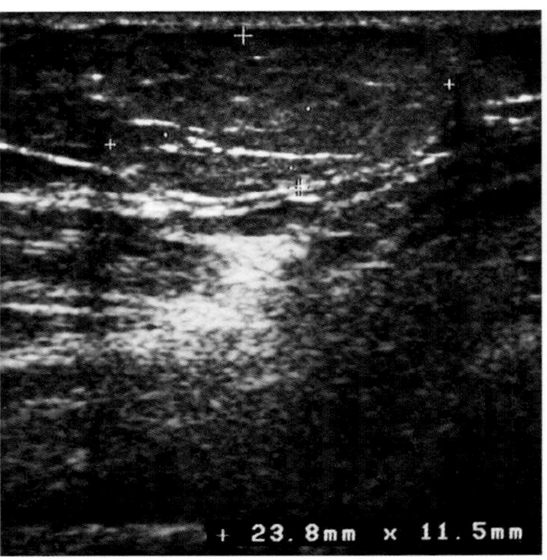


**k** *Sonogram* of the right elbow shows a 2.3 cm × 1.1 cm nodule (**d–g/15–16**, see marker).

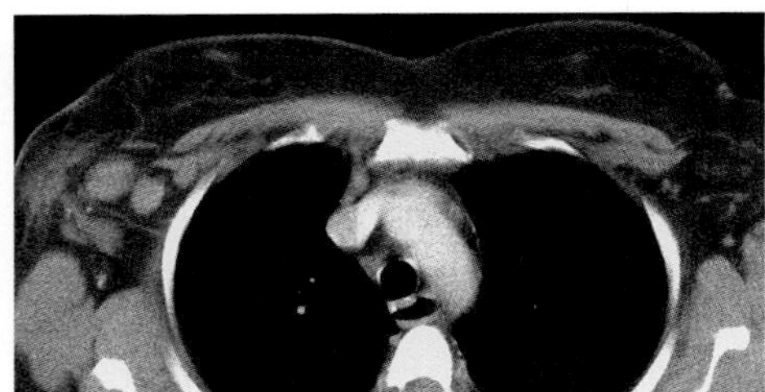

**l** *Axial CT* scan of the right and left axillae, obtained during examination of the stomach for tuberculosis. Enlarged lymph nodes (**H/15**) are noted as an incidental finding.

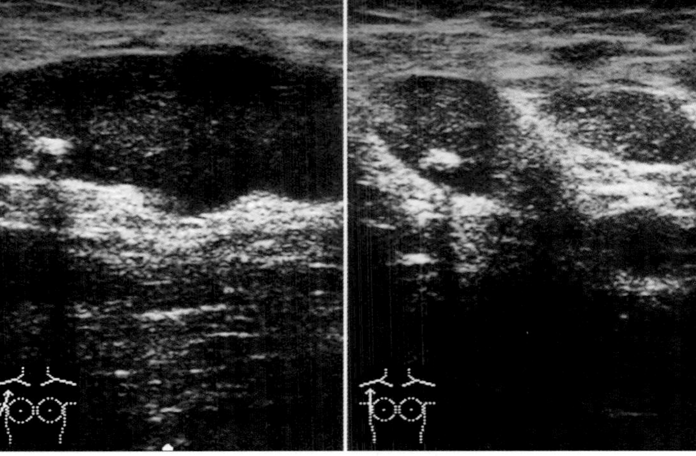

**m** *Sonograms* of the right axilla demonstrate enlarged lymph nodes.

**Question 1 on Fig. 5.84**

*The following diagnoses were made:*

(**a**) Normal axillary lymph node
(**b**) Chronic lymphocytic leukemia
(**c**) Axillary lymph node metastases from breast carcinoma
(**d**) Sarcoidosis

*Which diagnosis goes with which patient (A–D)?*

→ **Answer on p. 371**

**Question 2 on Fig. 5.84**

*On the basis of its clinical and ultrasound appearance, how would you interpret the nodule on the right elbow of patient D (**j**)?*

(**a**) Sarcoidosis
(**b**) Lipoma
(**c**) Myothelioma

→ **Answer on p. 371**

**Fig. 5.85 A 68-year-old woman underwent breast-conserving surgery 5 years before.** She presents with chronic right-sided arm edema and wears a fitted elastic stocking on the affected arm (**a**). Mammograms show no evidence of a local recurrence, and sonograms show no abnormalities in either breast. She states that arm edema is most pronounced and troublesome during the warm months of the year.

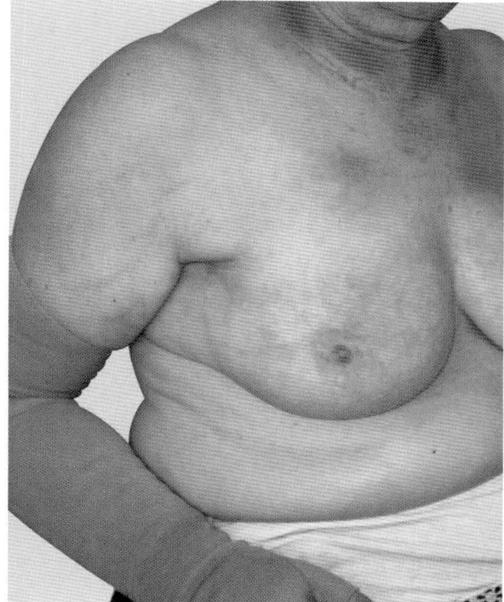

**a** *Clinical appearance*, status post breast-conserving therapy on the right side. The patient has a healthy-looking periareolar scar with mild, therapy-induced skin retraction about the nipple. Livid discoloration is due to mild trophic disturbances in the skin. An elastic stocking is worn on the right arm for edema.

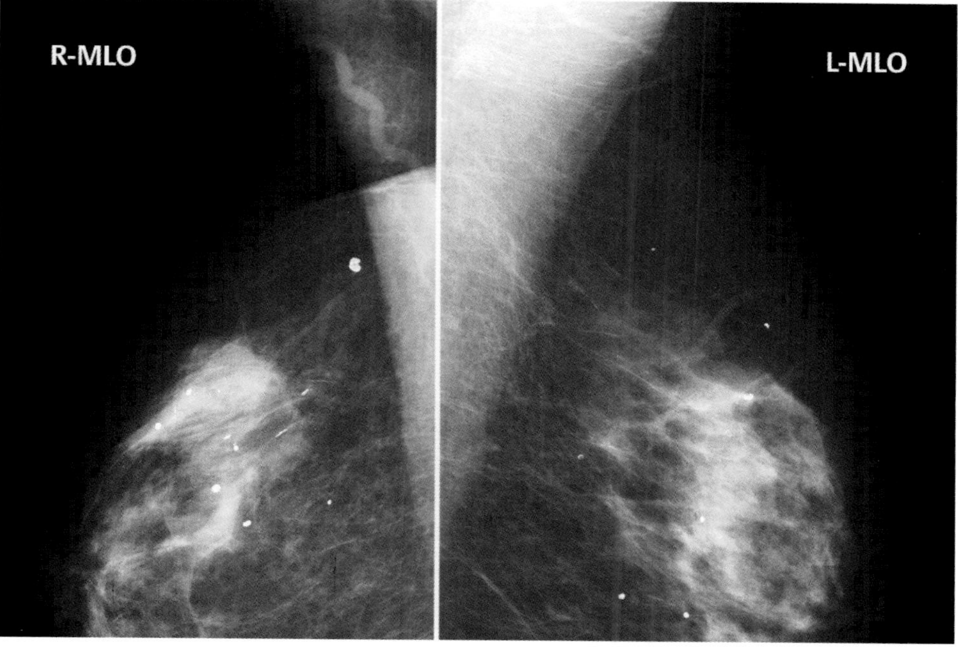


**b** *Bilateral oblique mammograms* 5 years after breast-conserving therapy on the right side show a patchy surgical scar and coarse calcifications (ACR 2, BIRADS 2, P**G**MI). Because of the surgery, the right pectoral muscle is not projected as far into the image plane as the left pectoral muscle.

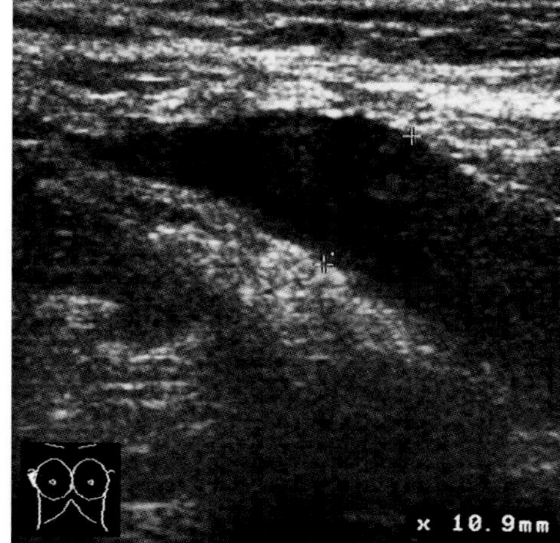


**c** *Sonogram* of the right axilla demonstrates a relatively large vein.

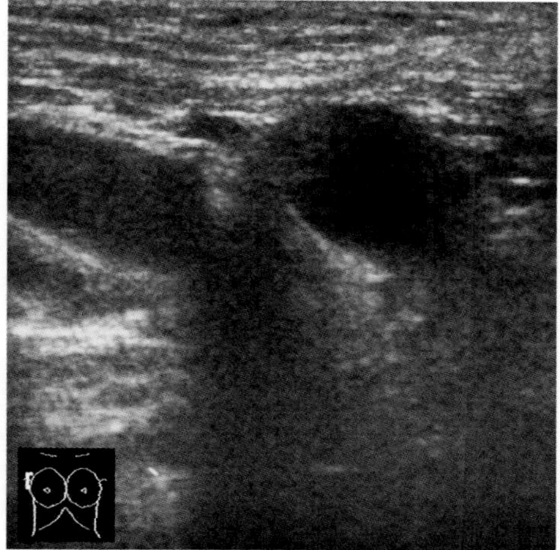

**d** *Sonogram* of the right axilla shows dilated vessels.

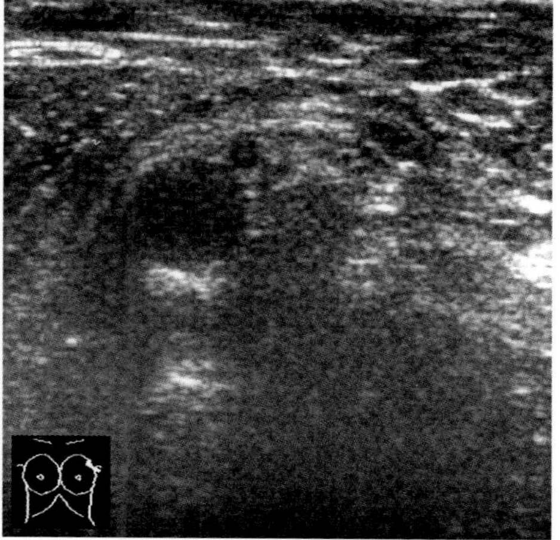

**e** *Sonogram* of the left axilla. Vascular dimensions are normal compared with the right side, and there is no evidence of lymphadenopathy.

**Question on Fig. 5.85**

*What is the principal cause of arm edema in this patient?*

(**a**) Obstruction of venous drainage

(**b**) Obstruction of venous and lymphatic drainage

(**c**) Axillary lymph node metastasis

→ **Answer on p. 371**

*(continued from p. 193)*

It is not uncommon for benign and malignant tumors to develop in heterotopic breast tissue. These malignant and benign processes have much the same ultrasound appearance as intramammary lesions. Axillary lymph node metastases are sometimes difficult to detect and may be recognized only by enlarged, hypoechoic lymph nodes with blurring, *compression*, or absence of the central fatty hilum (see **Fig. 5.87 b**). This contrasts with the ultrasound appearance of inflammatory or systemic lymphadenopathy, which typically shows homogeneous low echogenicity—a pattern that is occasionally seen with metastases as well. Since few lower-level nodes are usually removed in cases with a negative sentinel node biopsy, it may become more common in the future to encounter infra- and supraclavicular lymph node metastases in cases where disseminated tumor cells have bypassed the sentinel node. This problem calls for a properly trained clinical eye (see **Fig. 5.184**). If metastasis is suspected in these areas, sonographic detection and ultrasound-guided FNA can be performed without complications. Ultrasound-guided CNB is more problematic due to the potential for injury to the neurovascular sheath (nerve injuries), pleura (pneumothorax), and arteries (hematomas), although it is feasible if the biopsy needle is inserted to a minimal depth. Thus, ultrasound-guided FNA is the procedure of first choice in the infra- and supraclavicular regions and axilla, but only as a screening test for metastatic disease. Metastases are easily identified by their cytologic features (except for lobular carcinoma). With systemic diseases (Hodgkin disease, non-Hodgkin lymphoma), it is difficult to make a specific cytologic diagnosis. If systemic lymphadenopathy is suspected, CNB should be done only if an effort is made to limit the depth of needle penetration (15 mm instead of 22 mm).

**Tip**

**All breast examinations, including follow-ups, should routinely include palpation of the axilla with the arm at the side and the shoulder muscles relaxed, along with palpation of the cervical lymph nodes. The thyroid gland should also be examined, as it is common to find previously undetected thyroid nodules.**

**Fig. 5.86 A 45-year-old woman presents with an aching pain in the left axilla radiating to the arm and slightly to the breast.** She has no palpable abnormalities and a negative trauma history.

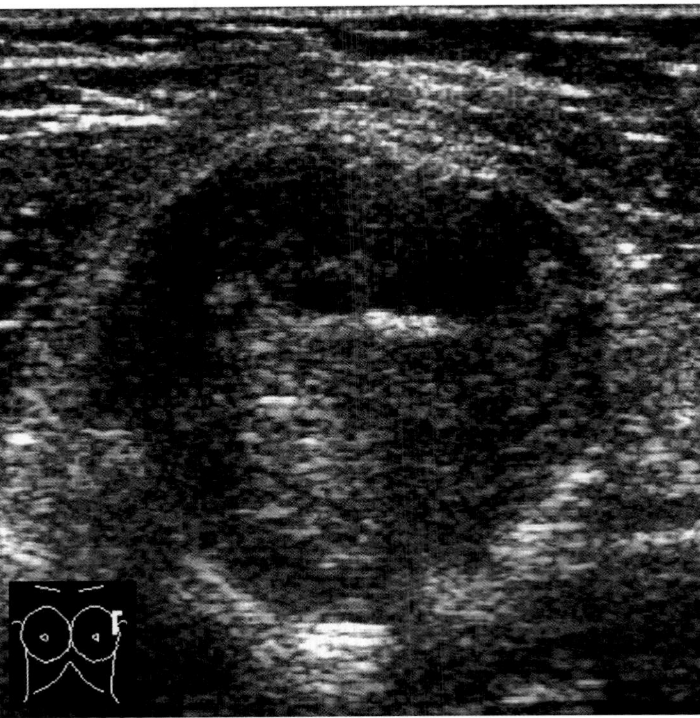

**a** *Sonogram* of the left axilla shows a well-circumscribed, slightly pulsating nodule with high-level anterior echoes and posterior acoustic enhancement.

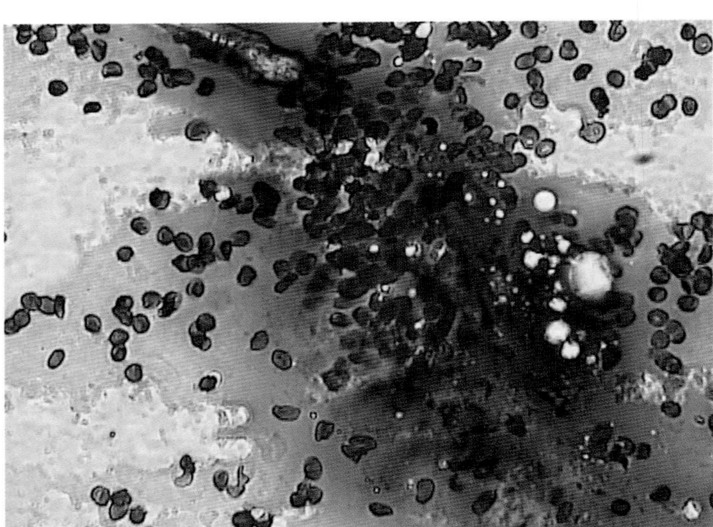

**b** *Fine-needle aspiration* from the periphery of the nodule yields erythrocytes and connective-tissue particles.

**Question on Fig. 5.86**

*How would you interpret the nodule?*

(**a**) Lymph node
(**b**) Vascular aneurysm or neurinoma
(**c**) Medullary carcinoma in heterotopic breast tissue

→ **Answer on p. 371**

**Fig. 5.87 Change in the axilla.** There has been palpable nodule in the right axilla of a 72-year-old woman for 2 years (**a**). The breast appeared normal on physical examination. Ultrasound shows an enlarged lymph node (**b**), which was investigated by FNA (**c**).

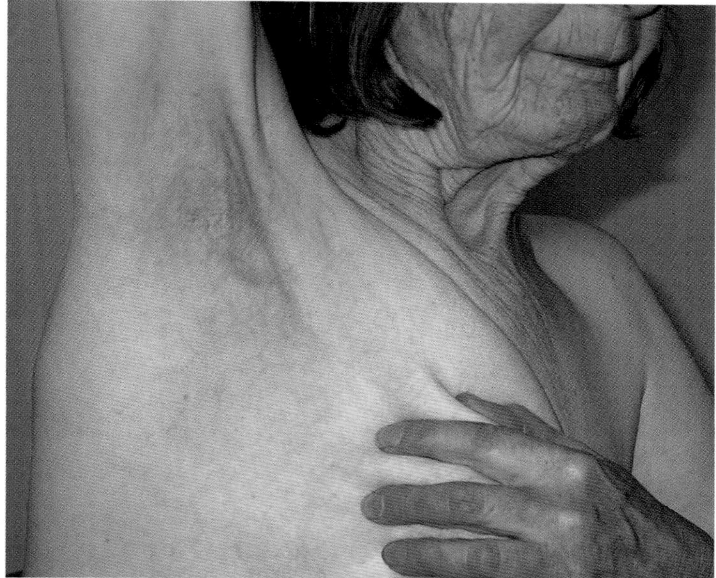

**a** *Clinical appearance* of the right axilla, which bears a palpable nodule (**L/23**).

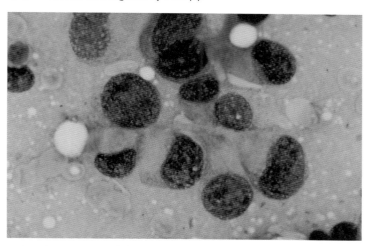

**c** *FNA* shows scattered dissociated cells with varying nuclear sizes and a loose chromatin structure beside some fat cells.

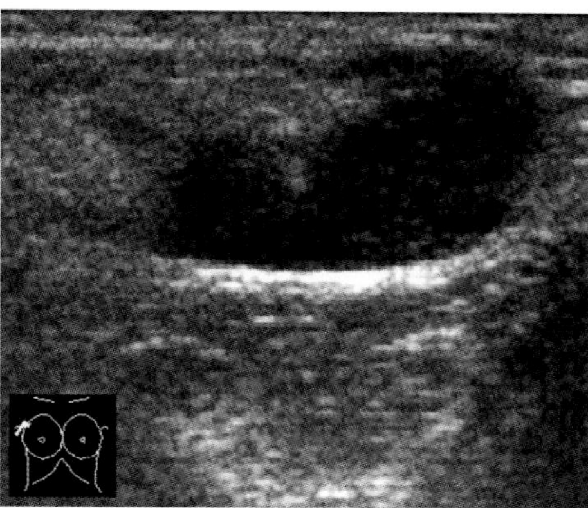

**b** *Ultrasound* reveals an enlarged lymph node with a hypoechoic (dark) component and a hyperechoic (bright) component.

**Question on Fig. 5.87**

*How would you interpret the nodule in the right axilla?*

(**a**) Lymph node metastasis

(**b**) Partial fatty infiltration of a lymph node

(**c**) Fibroadenoma

→ **Answer on p. 372**

***Pathologic changes may be found not just in the axilla but also elsewhere in the body where ectopic glandular tissue is located (d), including the inframammary region and, very rarely, even in the thigh (e). In extreme cases, ectopic glandular tissue may develop into an accessory breast (f).***

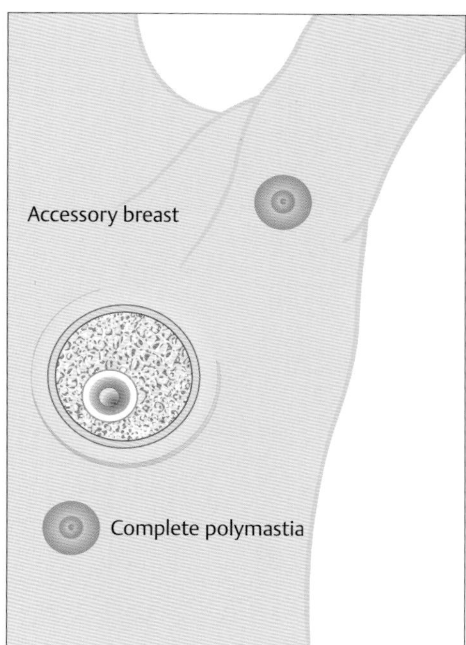


**d** *Diagram* of polythelia in the axillary and inframammary regions (polymastia completa). For the mammographic aspect of heterotopic breast tissue in the axillae see **Fig. 5.91 j**, p. 207.

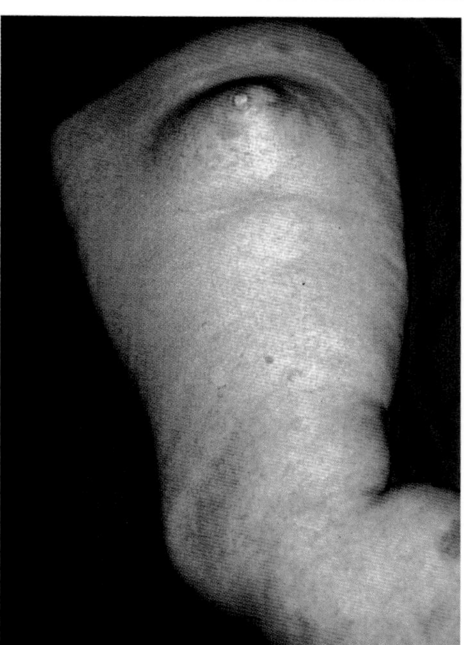

**e** *Clinical appearance* of the right thigh: polythelia with polymastia completa on the inside of the thigh.

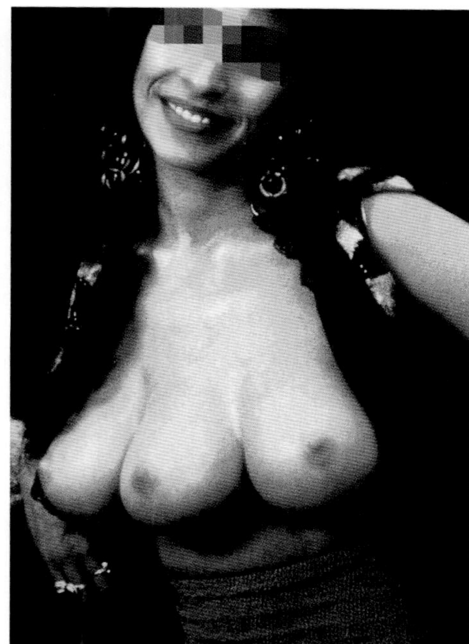

**f** *One complete accessory breast.* (**d–f** courtesy of Prof. Roland Bässler, Fulda).

**Fig. 5.88 A 37-year-old woman with no palpable abnormalities presents for screening mammography.** She has no skin or nipple changes and no regional lymph node enlargement.

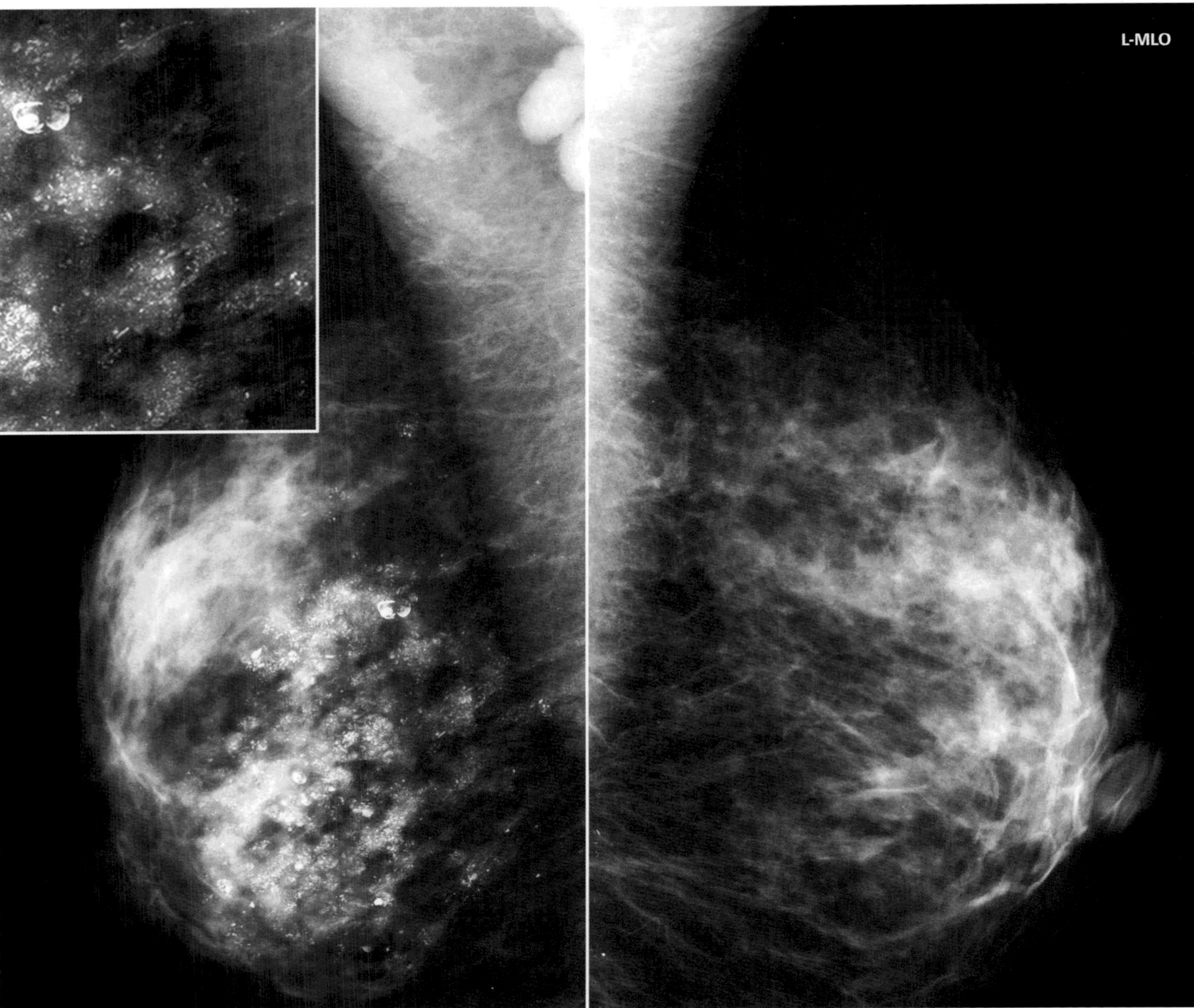


Bilateral oblique mammograms show multiple small clustered calcifications, some flocculent, in the lower outer quadrant of the right breast (**b–e/11–17**). The inset at upper left is a magnified view of some peripheral calcifications. The left breast is moderately radiodense (ACR 2, P**G**MI).

**Question on Fig. 5.88**

*How would you interpret these findings?*

(**a**) Extensive sclerosing adenosis
(**b**) Extensive DCIS
(**c**) Invasive ductal carcinoma with an extensive intraductal component (EIC)

→ **Answer on p. 372**

## Magnetic Resonance Imaging

The prognosis of breast cancer depends partly on the local extent of the tumor, the associated lymph node status, and distant metastasis. It is generally agreed that every diagnostic option should be utilized to detect the tumor at the earliest possible stage.

Magnetic resonance imaging (MRI) is a relatively young breast imaging modality compared with x-ray mammography and ultrasound. At present it is the latest imaging modality that has evolved to a practical level of clinical application.

Although MRI has been in clinical use for a relatively short time, many groups of researchers have explored this modality and have published a great many works on its potential applications in breast imaging (Heywang-Köbrunner 1990; Huang et al. 2004; Kaiser 1993; Fischer et al. 1993; Kuhl et al. 1995; 2000, 2007; Hall-Craggs 2000; Matsubayashi et al. 2000; Warner et al. 2001; Rosen et al. 2003; Hata et al. 2004; Mark et al. 2008; Solin et al. 2008; and many more).

Since the introduction of magnetic resonance mammography (MRM), there has been a great deal of controversy over its capabilities and limitations. The advocates of MRM point out that it can detect carcinomas that are not accessible to any other established imaging modalities, and that it can exclude malignancies in dense breasts with a high degree of confidence. Proponents also believe that MRM can define the extent of disease in the affected breast (unifocal, multifocal) while simultaneously evaluating the clinically healthy breast.

Opponents of this modality cite its high costs and question whether it can improve the prognosis of breast cancer. They also criticize the high false-positive rates of MRM, which may prompt unnecessary interventions and surgery (Allgayer et al. 1993; Fischer et al. 1993; Kaiser 1993; Heywang-Köbrunner et al. 1994, 1998; Zapf et al. 1991).

A positive statement on the necessity of preoperative MRI for histologically proven neoplasm came recently from Kuhl (2008). This author and his team agree with that paper on every point.

In a dissertation (Buyer 2002), 623 MRM cases from our files (Esslingen Imaging Center) between 1993 and 2001 were retrospectively analyzed in cooperation with the Interdisciplinary Breast Center of Esslingen (IMZE) to determine whether MRM added significantly to the information supplied by mammography and breast ultrasound or whether it was an unnecessary expense. On analyzing the results, Buyer found that there were 566 cases (90%) in which MRM yielded diagnostically relevant information, particularly in tumor staging, in young at-risk women with radiographically dense breasts, in the differentiation of scars and local recurrences (see **Fig. 5.185**), and in the setting of primary (neoadjuvant) chemotherapy. Dynamic MRM achieved a sensitivity of 84.2% and a specificity of 93.8%—a number that must be viewed with some skepticism as it was strongly influenced by the other imaging modalities. On the other hand, MRM should not be evaluated by itself but always within the context of the overall diagnostic work-up of the breast.

Since then, MRI-technique has achieved outstandingly good quality, incomparably better than that of the last century, when most of the existing MRI studies of the diagnostic value of this method originated. MRM is not a screening test but an adjunct to mammography, ultrasound, physical examination, and interventional procedures when these latter modalities have reached their limits. It is useful in staging, in assessing the potential responsiveness of locally advanced tumors to primary chemotherapy, in distinguishing scars from local recurrence after breast-conserving therapy, and in young women with an increased breast cancer risk and/or carcinophobia (see p. 203). **Figure 5.89** shows the age distribution of the 623 women who underwent MR imaging. The women who received MRM were mostly under 60 years of age, and half of those were under age 50. Magnetic resonance, then, is basically a method for the examination of younger women.

**Fig. 5.89 Age distribution of 623 patients who underwent magnetic resonance mammography** (Buyer 2002).

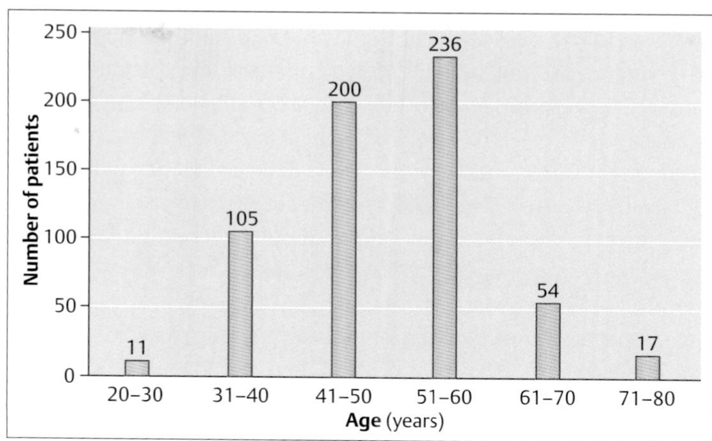


MRM is *not* appropriate for the investigation of circumscribed focal lesions (interventional procedures!) or suspicious microcalcifications.

In summarizing the results of our small study, which are as valid today as they were in 2002, it is helpful to recall the words of Kaiser (1993): "The best diagnosis is the cheapest therapy."

Gatzemeier et al. (1999) conducted a prospective study on the use of MRM for preoperative planning in 125 women with confirmed breast cancer. The patients underwent MRM to check for multifocality, multicentricity (see p. 45), and contralateral lesions. The following *sensitivities* and *specificities* were determined in the work-up of 91 malignancies:

- Physical examination: 73% and 67%, respectively.
- Breast ultrasound: 58% and 86%.
- Mammography: 89% and 20%.
- MRM: 96.7% and 19%.

MRM detected 46 additional lesions—28 malignant and 18 benign. Of the 28 malignancies, 25 were ipsilateral to the known cancer (multifocal or multicentric disease) and 3 were contralateral. The false-positive rate for MRM was 18%. On the strength of the MRM findings, mastectomy was performed in 14.3% of the women instead of the proposed breast-conserving surgery. This led Gatzemeier et al. to conclude that MRM was the procedure of choice for resolving a discrepancy between mammographic and sonographic findings and was an extremely sensitive modality for detecting multifocality and multicentricity in patients with confirmed carcinoma. The authors noted that MRM was instrumental in directing the selection of operative treatment. They also noted that close interdisciplinary cooperation between the radiologist, surgeon, and pathologist was essential for the optimum interpretation of supplementary MRM. Unfortunately, MRM is generally omitted in the preoperative work-up of confirmed breast cancer because it increases costs and because "the diagnosis is already known." For the most part it is used postoperatively and only when absolutely necessary. But postoperative MR images are of limited value, especially when preoperative images are not available for comparison. It is astounding to consider the diseases and complaints (back pain, headache, abdominal pain) that are established indications for MRI and are routinely covered by insurers, and then to observe the stringency with which MRI is utilized and reimbursed in breast cancer—a disease where accurate preoperative planning and a complete resection with clear margins are crucial to the fate of the patient. Clinicians often raise scientific arguments against the use of MRM so that they will not have to perform the examination. It is interesting to note, however, that when the procedure was offered at no cost for a limited time in order to gather study data, the number of examinations skyrocketed.

Particularly in the case of invasive lobular carcinoma, MRM can define the extent of disease with relatively high accuracy (this is not possible with mammography and can only be approximated with ultrasound). Diekmann et al. (2004) report that MRM can also detect 40% of additional satellite lesions and second tumors, doing so with greater accuracy than in the case of invasive ductal carcinoma, for example.

> **!** **Without MRM, preoperative planning for invasive lobular carcinoma is incomplete and increases the likelihood of reexcision, which raises costs and is stressful for patients.**

The analysis of T1-weighted MR images is sometimes hampered by motion artifacts. Various attempts have been made to suppress these artifacts, such as having patients wear tight-fitting T-shirts and packing the breast coil with cotton. The best way to eliminate motion artifacts is to compress both breasts within the coil, which can reduce the incidence of motion artifacts from 11% to 2% (Schorn et al. 1998). In modern MRI systems, the breast coil should be equipped with compression paddles and both breasts should be imaged simultaneously in the sagittal plane.

In patients with histologically confirmed axillary lymph node metastases and patients with an unknown primary tumor **(CUP syndrome: carcinoma of unknown primary)**, MRI is the method of choice for locating the primary breast tumor when mammograms and sonograms are negative (see also PET, p. 227). This cannot always be accomplished, and even malignancies up to 2 cm in size may occasionally escape detection by MRI. Eighty-six percent of tumors 4–30 mm in size are detected, however (Orell et al. 1999).

While some authors caution against the indiscriminate use of MRM in CUP syndrome (Delorme 2004), it is still the procedure of choice and should be used in every case of axillary lymph node metastasis. The only other option for detecting a mammographically and sonographically occult primary tumor would be PET (see p. 227), but this modality is less specific than MRM.

If a primary tumor is not detected in the breast despite the use of MRM, it would not be appropriate to proceed with mastectomy or an untargeted prophylactic quadrantectomy, for example. Follow-up is a better option. When radiotherapy is applied to the axilla, concomitant irradiation of the breast (partial breast irradiation, Görse et al. 2007) may be considered. Not infrequently, the primary tumor may be located in heterotopic breast tissue in the axilla itself, so that the affected and removed lymph node originates from the actual tumor site.

> **Tip**
> **PET is recommended for all unknown primaries with negative MRM findings.**

There are problems associated with the postoperative use of MRM for the detection or exclusion of residual tumor tissue. The overlapping gadolinium enhancement characteristics of malignant lesions and fibrocystic change explains why MRI has only a 33% positive predictive value in distinguishing between residual tumor, postoperative granulation tissue, and benign lesions such as fibroadenoma (Lee et al. 2004). This value could be improved if preoperative MR images were obtained and MRI were repeated in cases where an R0 resection is not achieved. If MRI were employed in this way, additional lesions in proximity to the tumor (Lee et al. 2004: 19 of 82 carcinomas associated with ipsilateral lesions) could be removed in the initial operation and it would be easier to classify ringlike enhancement of the surgical cavity as granulation tissue as opposed to residual tumor. Unfortunately, no one has yet analyzed the costs relating to the diagnosis and treatment of recurrent disease. They should be analyzed and compared with the costs of preoperative MRM. It is likely that this application of MRM would result in a net cost saving.

In cases with an R1 resection (where microscopic residual disease has been left behind), Frei et al. (2000) recommend withholding postoperative MRI for 4 weeks to allow time for all inflammatory reactions to subside. Few doctors and patients are willing to wait that long, however, and we feel that MRI should be performed 2–3 days postoperatively, when inflammatory and reactive changes are still relatively mild. Comparison with preoperative MR images would be helpful in all cases (see Local Recurrences, p. 328).

Rieber et al. (1997) investigated the value of MRM for detecting or excluding local recurrence after breast-conserving therapy. In a series of 140 patients, MRM excluded local recurrence in 82%, detected local recurrence in 14%, and yielded false-positive findings in 5 cases (4%).

Indeterminate mammographic densities are not necessarily an indication for MRI, because digital stereotactic CNB and VB are more accurate than gadolinium enhancement. There may be cases, however, in which the point of maximum contrast enhancement on MRI may indicate the optimum site for an interventional procedure.

We do not advocate the broad, indiscriminate use of MRI. For cost reasons, however, this modality is still underutilized at the present time. The value of MRM may not be appreciated until follow-up visits years later, when knowledge of the initial pre- and postoperative findings may be diagnostically helpful, say, in detecting or excluding a local recurrence or a benign tumor.

Hormone replacement therapy leads to atypical MR images, especially in radiographically dense breasts. Abnormalities seen at MRI should always be viewed critically in patients with normal mammograms and sonograms. Hormone replacement therapy must not be discontinued prior to an MRI examination.

MRI-guided breast interventions are still associated with certain problems. They are practiced at only a few centers because of the additional equipment costs. There are only a few lesions that produce MRI findings in patients with completely normal mammograms and sonograms, do not regress on MRI follow-ups, and can be aspirated or biopsied under MRI guidance (Heywang-Köbrunner et al. 2000; Liberman et al. 2003; Fischer and Baum 2008)

*Caution is advised when MRM is performed in women of childbearing age, because false-positive findings are extremely common during the second half of the cycle and especially in the premenstrual phase.* These findings are easily mistaken for pathology and should never prompt an intervention or operation unless the finding has been rechecked between days 7 and 12 of the cycle. It is unclear whether oral contraceptives should be discontinued during that time. These agents suppress progestational effects during the second half of the cycle and may inhibit the proliferation of breast parenchyma.

Gadolinium-enhancing foci are a normal premenstrual finding in women of childbearing age.

Kuhl detected focal lesions of this kind in 69% of the young female subjects whom she examined by MRI (Kuhl et al. 1995). Lesions with an irregular configuration showed a steadily rising time–density curve that exceeded the malignancy threshold during the initial minutes after contrast administration in half of the women examined. This pattern would have been suspicious for malignancy based on current criteria if individual cycle phase had not been taken into account. The great majority of these lesions are focal, making them difficult to distinguish from tumors that would require biopsy. In women who are inadvertently examined during the second half of their cycle and are found to have this type of focal lesion, breast biopsy should be deferred pending reexamination between days 7 and 12 of the cycle. In patients with diffusely enhancing breast parenchyma, tamoxifen may be safely administered for 2–3 weeks to improve the readability of MR images. Moreover, an atypical MR image in a given patient may return to normal during the next cycle phase or a few months later even though the patient is examined at the same point in the cycle and she has not received any therapy or change in hormone regimen (Kuhl et al. 1995).

The studies by Kuhl also confirm that MRM cannot classify a lesion as benign or malignant based on the shape of its time–density curve. The diagnosis should always be based on a combined evaluation of clinical, mammographic, sonographic, and interventional findings before invasive therapeutic conclusions are drawn from an abnormal finding at MRM (**Figs. 5.90–5.94**).

The American Cancer Society recommends screening MRI for women with an approximately 20–25% or greater lifetime risk of breast cancer, including women with a strong family history of breast or ovarian cancer and women who were treated for Hodgkin disease. There are several risk subgroups for which the available data are insufficient to recommend for or against screening, including women with a personal history of breast cancer, carcinoma in situ, atypical hyperplasia, and extremely dense breasts on mammography (Saslou, et al. 2007).

The possible future role of MRI in minimally invasive surgery remains to be seen. It should be possible to completely remove or thermoablate all enhancing areas in a lesion under MRI guidance, resulting in minimal scarring and less cosmetic deformity (Hall-Craggs 2000). The practical details of this approach are still unclear.

Unquestionably, MRI detects more premalignant lesions (PPV about 80%) than does mammography–ultrasound (PPV about 50%). MRI is therefore the method of choice for breast-examinations in young women from *high-risk families* (Kuhl et al. 2007). Because MRI cannot image microcalcifications of these lesions, mammography cannot be discarded and single-view oblique exposures can reveal them. Accordingly, MRI and single-view mammography—alternating annually—is the best net to catch DCIS as early as possible.

*(continued on p. 212)*

**Fig. 5.90** A 69-year-old woman presents for screening mammography.

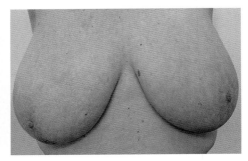

**a** *Inspection* reveals bilateral relative macromastia with pigmented warts over the upper inner quadrant of the left breast (**i/26**).

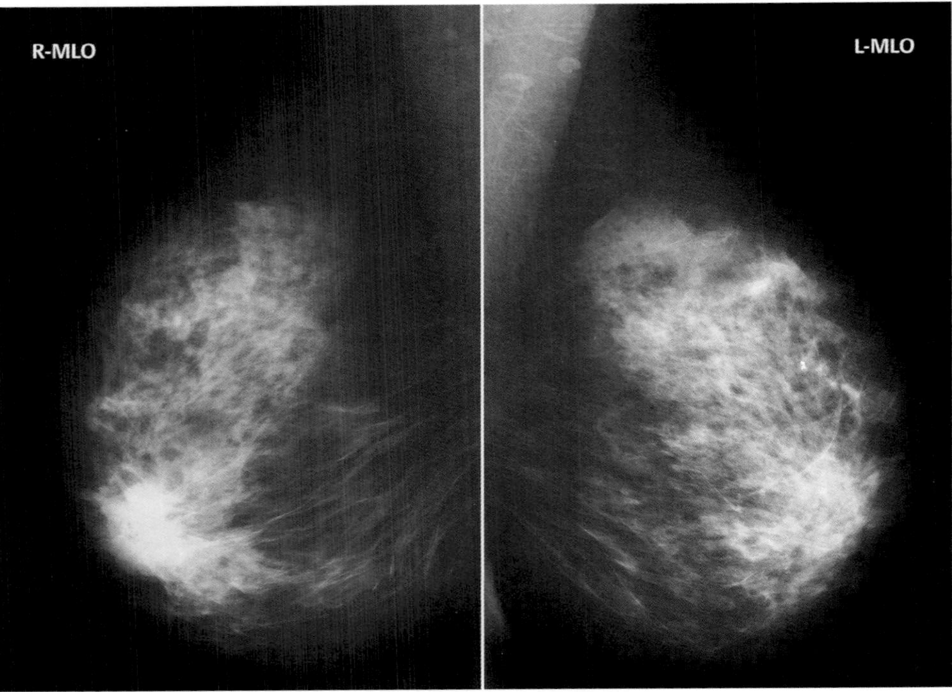


**b** *Bilateral oblique mammograms* show bilateral stroma-rich breasts (ACR 3, **P**GMI).

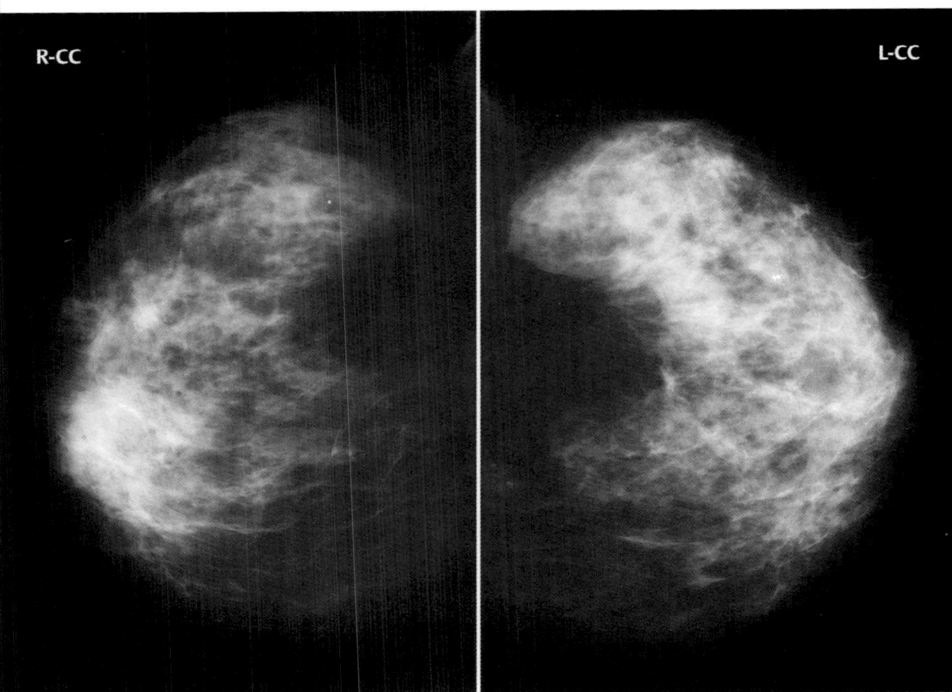


**c** *Bilateral craniocaudal mammograms* show bilateral stroma-rich breasts with inhomogeneities (ACR 3, BIRADS?, **P**GMI).

**Question 1 on Fig. 5.90**

*What course of action would you recommend?*

(**a**) Routine follow-up in 18 months
(**b**) Targeted follow-up of one side in 6 months (coordinates?)
(**c**) Additional tests

→ **Answer on p. 372**

**Question 2 on Fig. 5.90**

*How would you interpret the findings in* **c**?

(**a**) Invasive lobular neoplasm (hypercellular)
(**b**) Fibroadenoma (hypocellular)
(**c**) Papilloma (hypercellular)

→ **Answer on p. 373**

**Fig. 5.91 Evaluate the indications for MRI in the following three patients (A–C), giving particular attention to the time–density curve. Patient A: A 59-year-old woman with a small palpable breast nodule.** Ultrasound findings were equivocal, and (oddly enough) dynamic MRI of the palpable nodule was recommended.

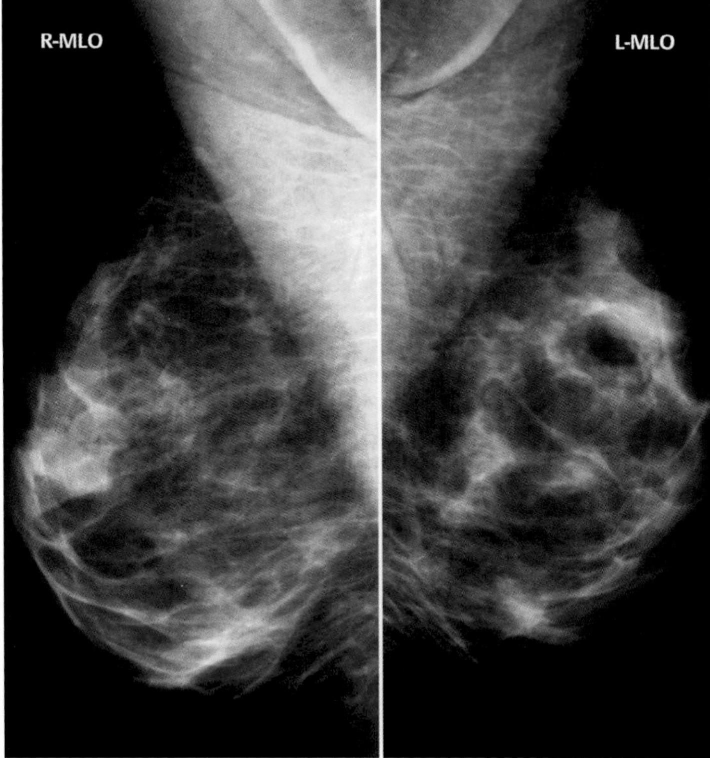


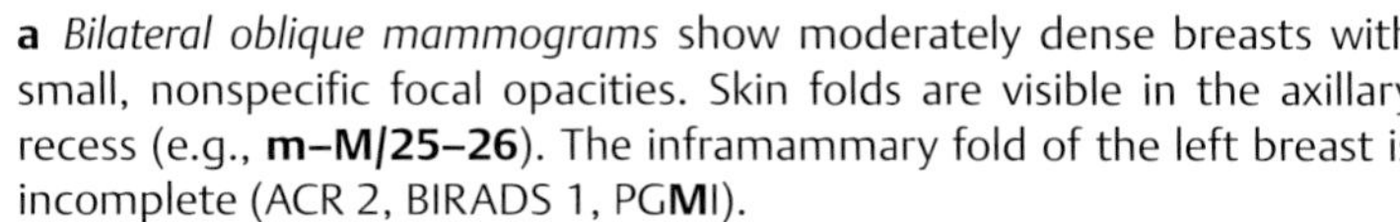

**a** *Bilateral oblique mammograms* show moderately dense breasts with small, nonspecific focal opacities. Skin folds are visible in the axillary recess (e.g., **m–M/25–26**). The inframammary fold of the left breast is incomplete (ACR 2, BIRADS 1, PGM**I**).

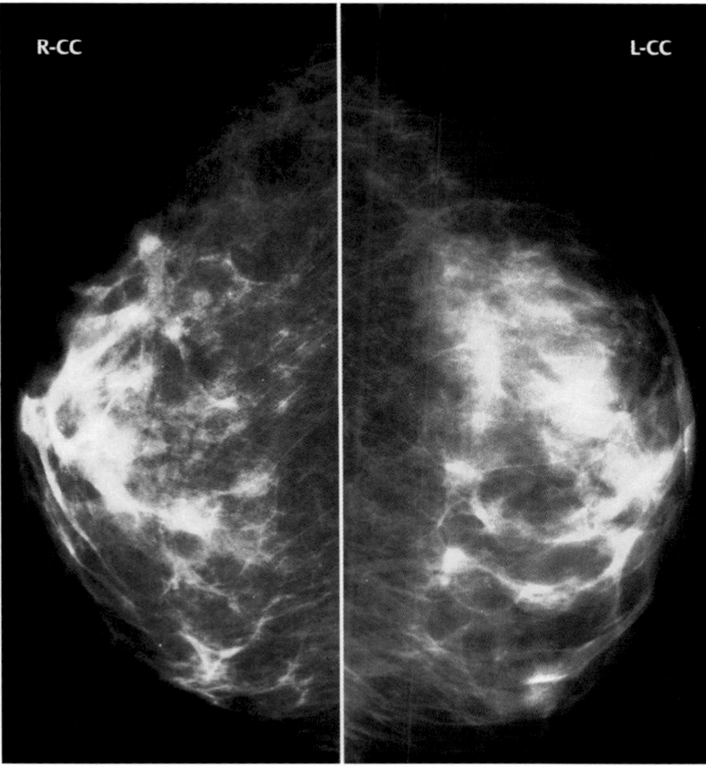


**b** *Bilateral craniocaudal mammograms* show radiodense breasts (the left denser than the right) with good positioning technique. Small opacities are visible in both breasts (ACR 2, BIRADS 1, P**G**MI).

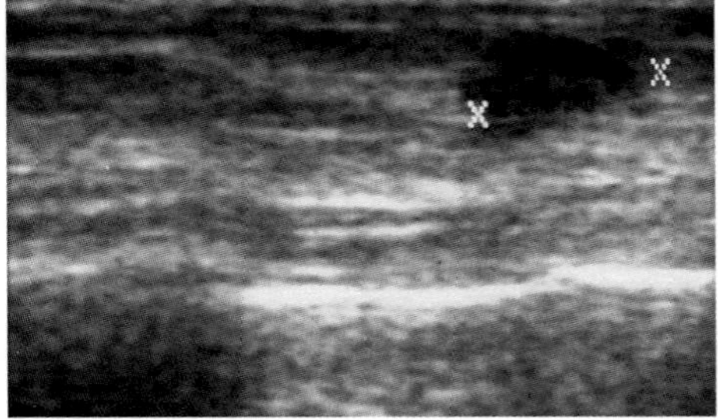

**c** *Ultrasound* demonstrates a 7 mm × 8 mm hypoechoic nodule with smooth margins.

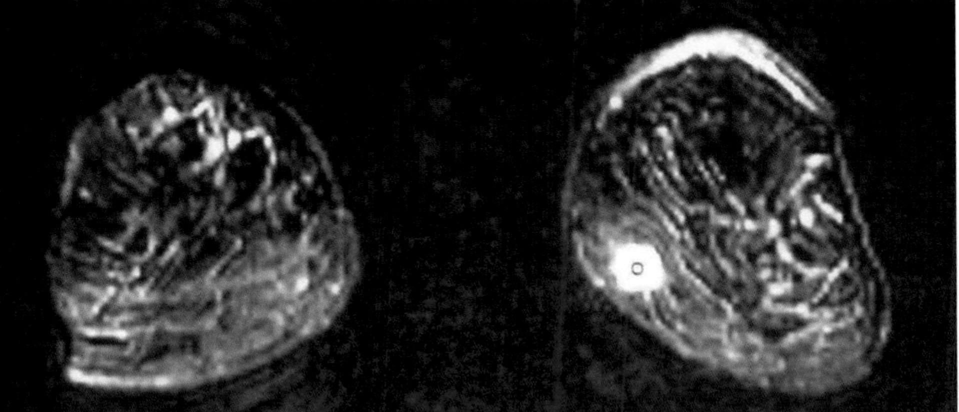

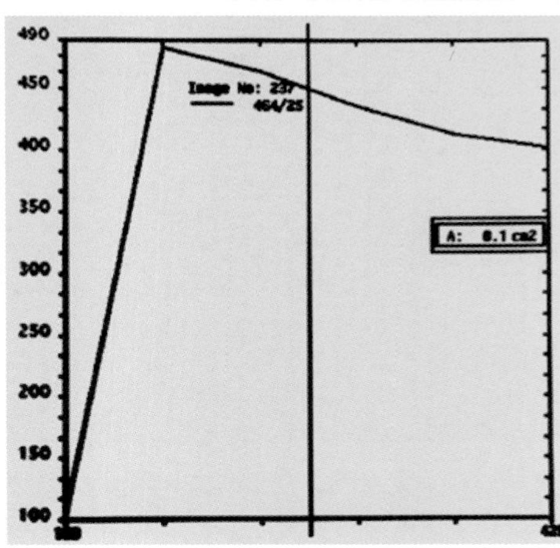


**d** *Coronal MRI* with time–density plot shows an intensely enhancing nodule with a sharply rising curve during the first minute and gradual fading of enhancement thereafter, typical for a carcinoma.

**Question 1 on Fig. 5.91**

*What is the location of the mammographic nodule?*

(**a**) Lower inner quadrant of the left breast (coordinates)

(**b**) Lower outer quadrant of the right breast (coordinates)

(**c**) Neither (**a**) nor (**b**) but at ... (coordinates)

→ **Answer on p. 373**

▶ **Fig. 5.91 e–n**

**Fig. 5.91 Patient B: 39-year-old woman with a strong family history of breast cancer presents for screening mammography.** *(continued)*

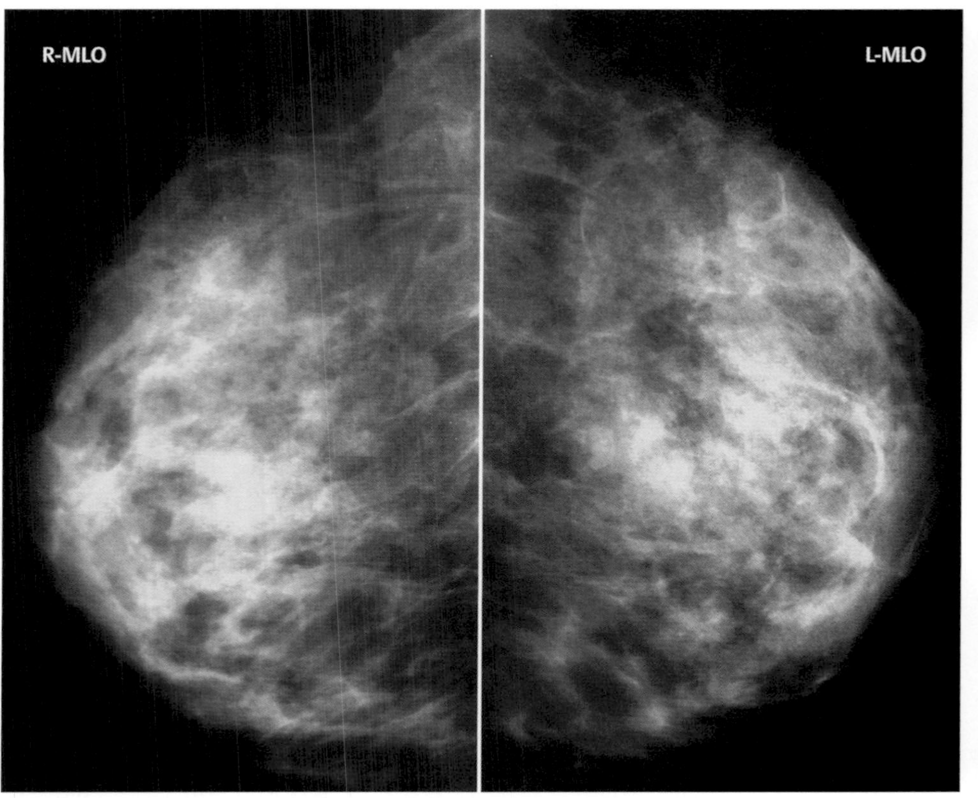


**e** *Bilateral oblique mammograms* show radiodense breasts with nonspecific inhomogeneities. The views are well positioned (ACR 3, P**G**MI).

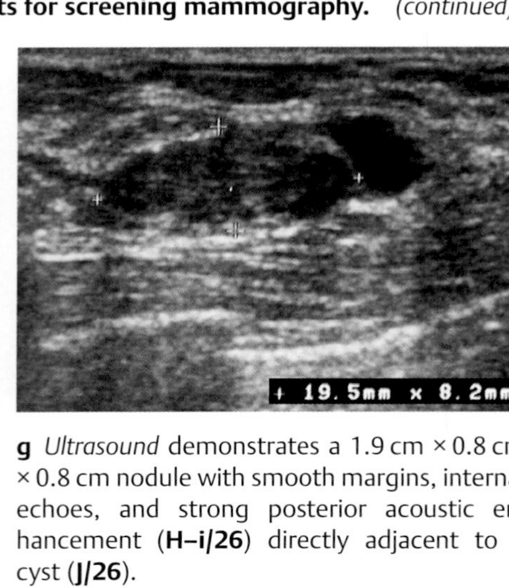


**g** *Ultrasound* demonstrates a 1.9 cm × 0.8 cm × 0.8 cm nodule with smooth margins, internal echoes, and strong posterior acoustic enhancement (**H–i/26**) directly adjacent to a cyst (**J/26**).

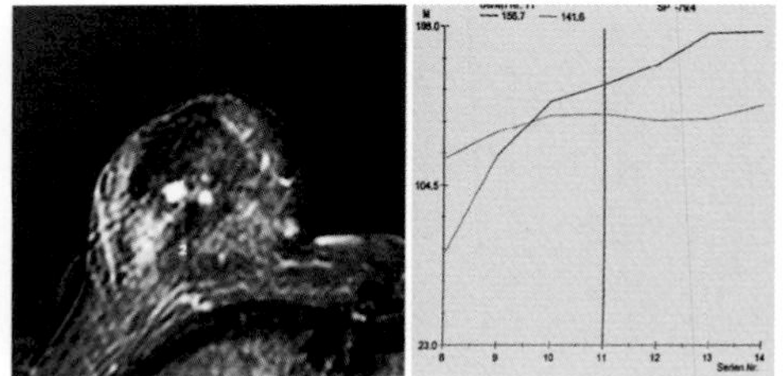

**h** *MRI*. Subtraction image of two enhancing nodules up to 1 cm in diameter, each with a slowly rising time–density curve typical for a fibroadenoma or mastopathy lump.

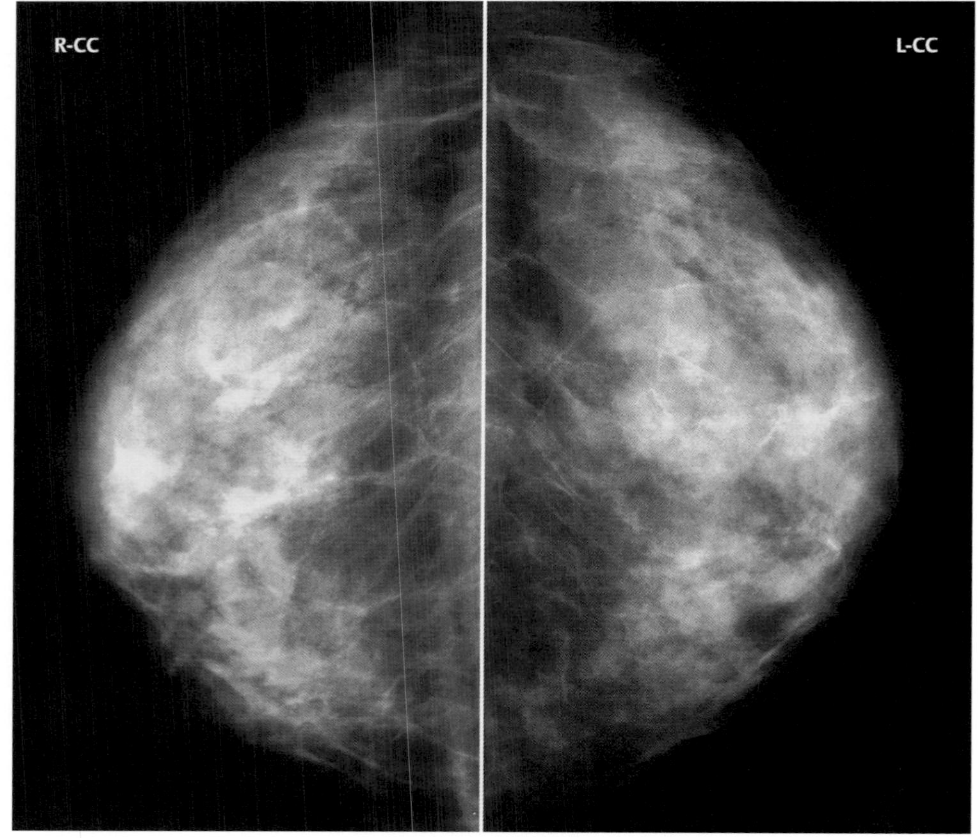


**f** *Bilateral craniocaudal mammograms* show radiodense breasts with inhomogeneities and no evidence of a malignant process (ACR 3, BIRADS 1, **P**GMI).

**Question 2 on Fig. 5.91**

*What is the location of the* mammographic *nodule?*

(**a**) Left breast (coordinates)
(**b**) Right breast (coordinates)
(**c**) Cannot be assessed

→ **Answer on p. 373**

**Fig. 5.91 Patient C: A 58-year-old woman with slight skin retraction over the lower portion of the left breast (i).** Mammography shows an ill-defined density. Diagnosis was established by ultrasound and cytology. Dynamic MRI was performed to exclude additional lesions in the affected breast and clinically healthy breast. *(continued)*

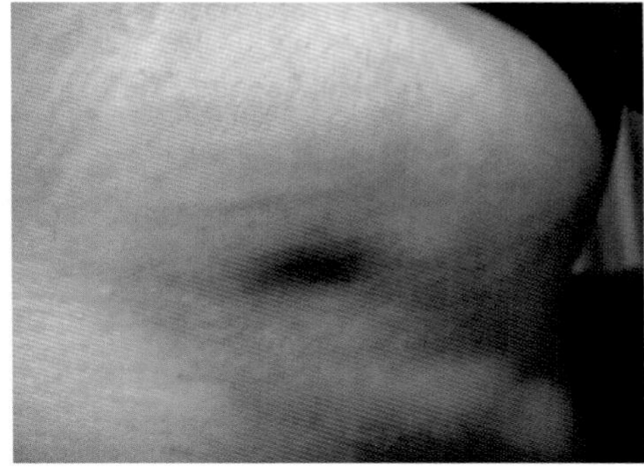

**i** *Inspection* of the left breast shows circumscribed skin retraction in the inframammary fold (**L–l/24**).

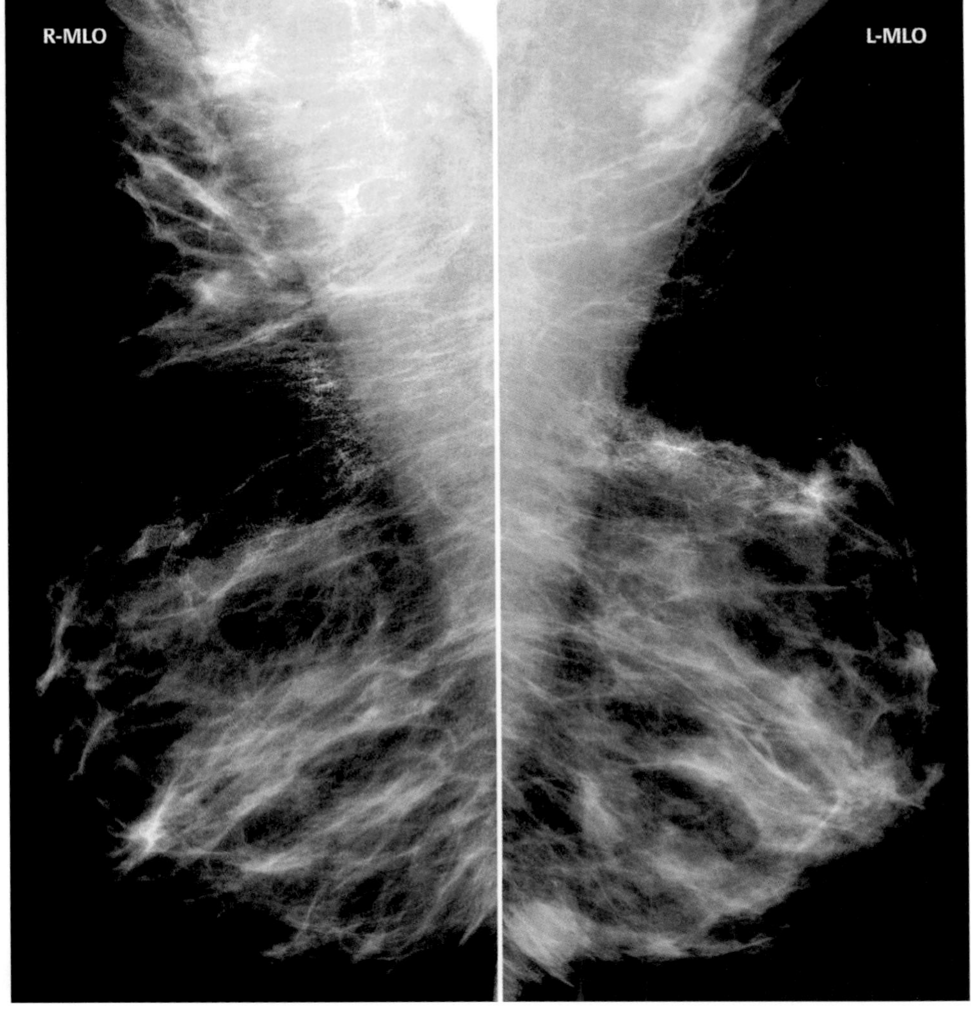


**j** *Bilateral oblique mammograms* show a normal parenchymal breast structure with a nonspecific round, lentil-sized density in the left inframammary crease (**q/13–14**) (ACR 2, **P**GMI) and heterotopic breast tissue in both axillae (**O–Q/22–26** right, **R–s/23–26** left).

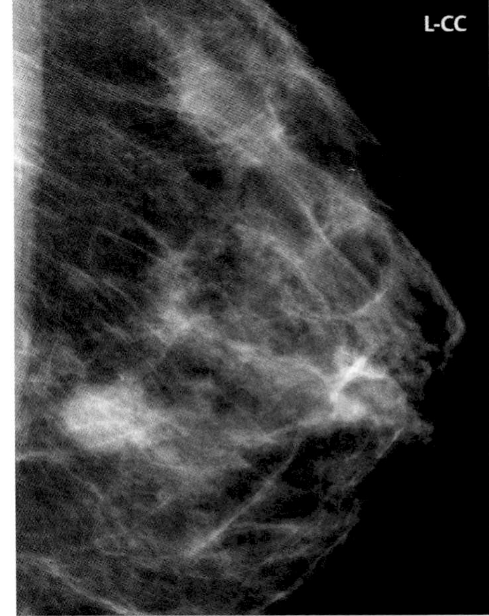


**k** *Left craniocaudal mammogram* shows a generally lucent breast with an ill-defined focal density corresponding to the clinical finding over the lower inner quadrant (**K–k/7–8**) (ACR 1, **P**GMI).

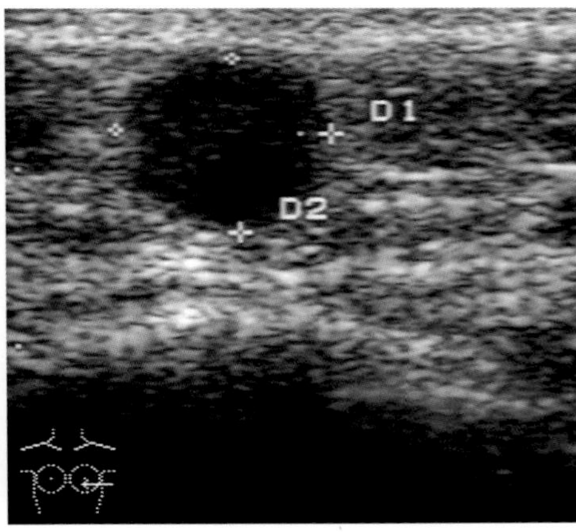


**l** *Sonogram* of the lower left breast at the quadrant boundary shows a 1.1 cm × 0.9 cm × 0.9 cm nodule with relatively smooth margins, internal echoes, and faint posterior acoustic enhancement.

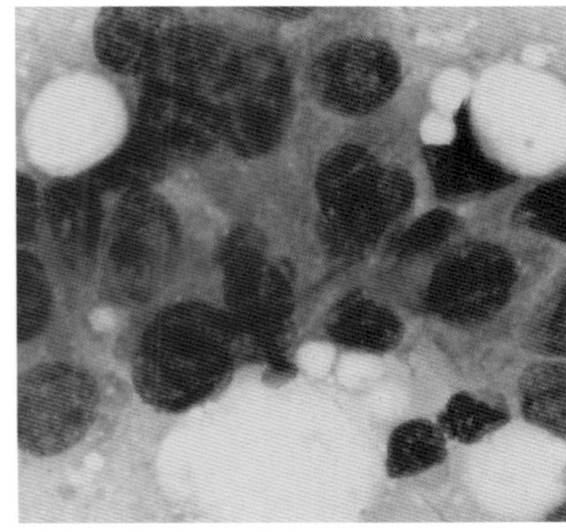

**m** *Fine-needle aspiration cytology* shows a 1- to 3-row aggregate of duct cells with pleomorphic nuclei, enlarged nucleoli, and disintegrated chromatin strands.

▶ Fig. 5.91 n

**Fig. 5.91** **Patient C: A 59-year-old woman with a small palpable breast nodule.** *(continued)*

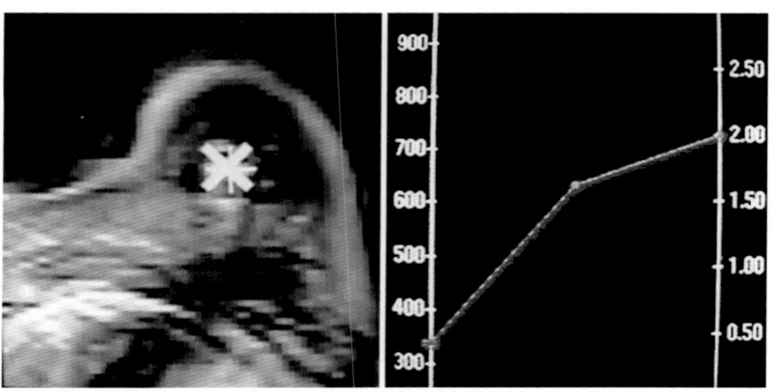


**n** *MR subtraction* image with time–density curve of **patient C** shows a slowly rising enhancement pattern over a 3-minute period typical for a fibroadenoma.

**Question 3 on Fig. 5.91**

*The following histologic diagnoses were made for patients A, B, and C:*

(**a**) Fibroadenoma

(**b**) Ductal carcinoma in situ (DCIS)

(**c**) Well-differentiated invasive ductal carcinoma

*Using only the time–density curves, match each patient to the correct diagnosis.*

→ **Answer on p. 373**

*The time–density curves for patients A and B (**d, h**) are pictured again to help you answer the question.*

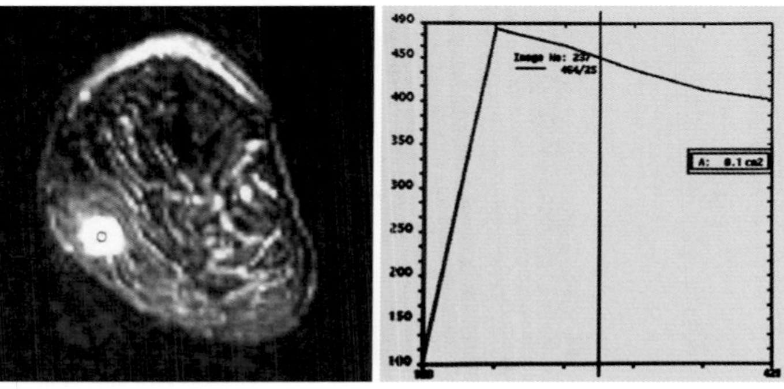


Fig. 5.**91 d** *(Repeated, **patient A**)*

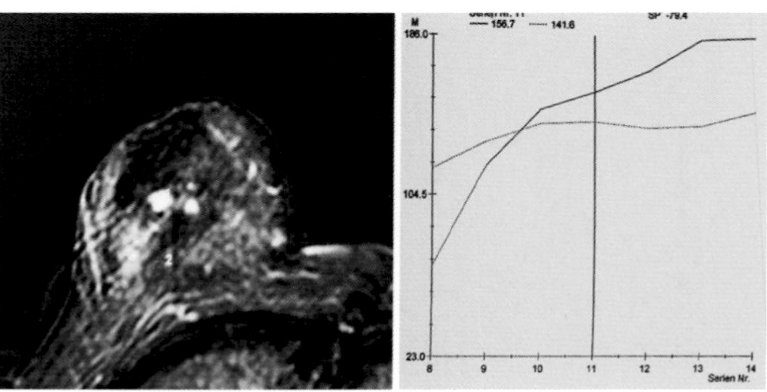


Fig. 5.**91 h** *(Repeated, **patient B**)*

**Fig. 5.92** **A 61-year-old woman presents with a 6-month history** of a slowly enlarging palpable nodule at the 3-o'clock position in the left breast (**a**). A small lymph node is palpable in the axillary recess at presentation. A mammogram taken 6 months before was declared normal (**b**), and the current mammogram (**c**) shows nonspecific changes. Palpation reveals a 1 cm rounded, mobile nodule with no associated skin or nipple retraction and no discharge. The right breast shows no abnormalities.

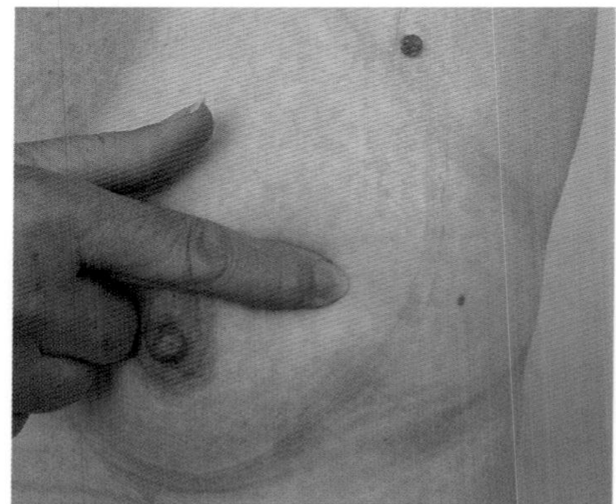

**a** *Nodule* in the left breast. A pigmented seborrheic wart (**C/13**) is visible in the axilla (histologically confirmed).

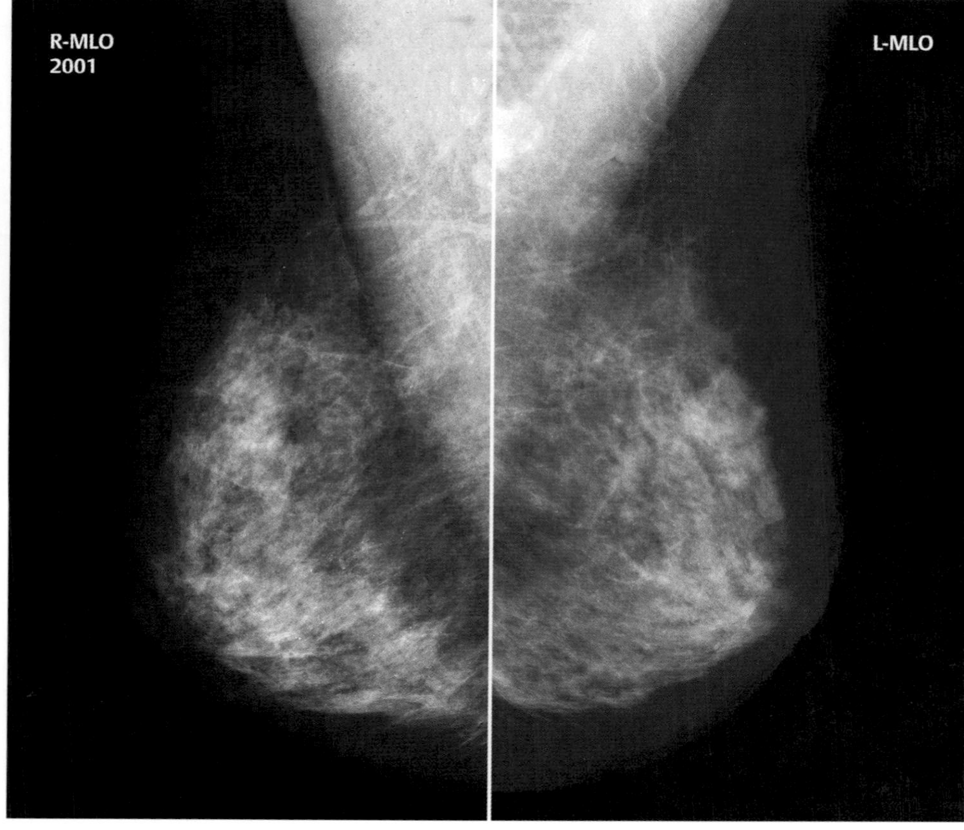


**b** *Bilateral oblique mammograms* in November, 2001 show radiodense breasts with no apparent abnormalities (ACR 2, BIRADS 2, PGMI).

**Fig. 5.92** **A 61-year-old woman presents with a 6-month history.** *(continued)*

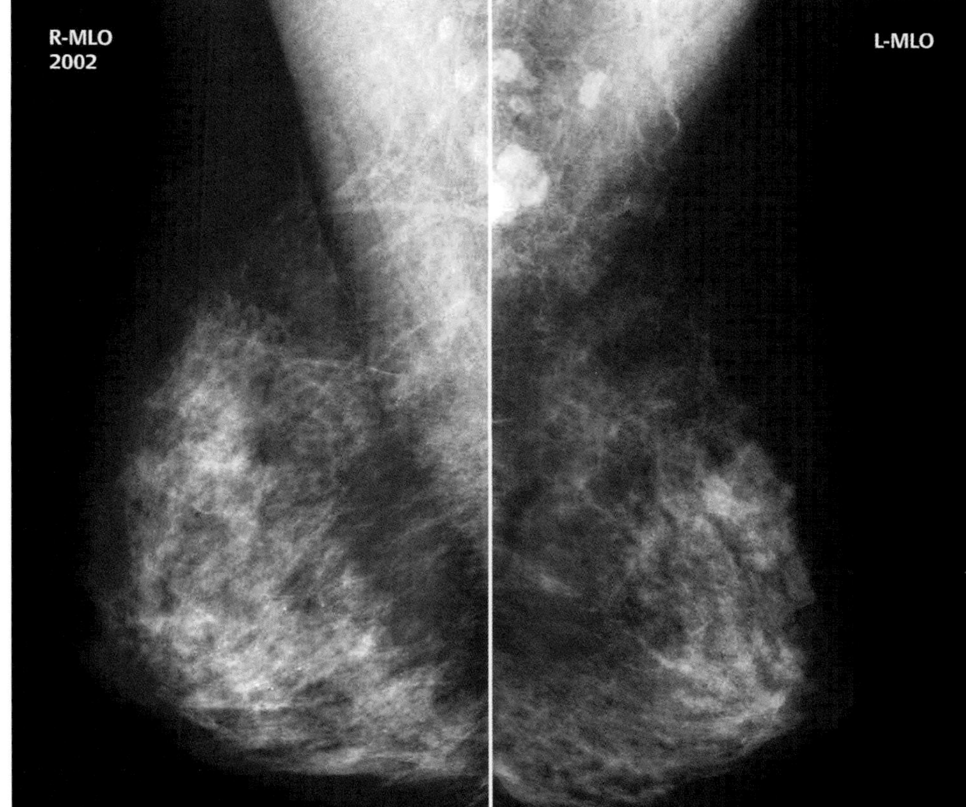


**c** *Bilateral oblique mammograms* in May, 2002 show a nonspecific density in the left breast (ACR 2, BIRADS 2, PGMI).

**d** *Sonograms* of the palpable nodule in the left breast. The nodule measures 1.7 cm × 1.6 cm × 1.2 cm. It is hypoechoic and inhomogeneous (p. 64) and is surrounded by a slightly echogenic rim.

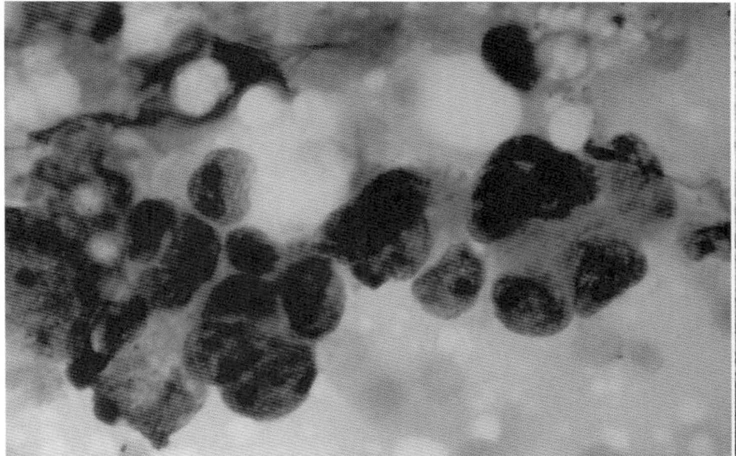

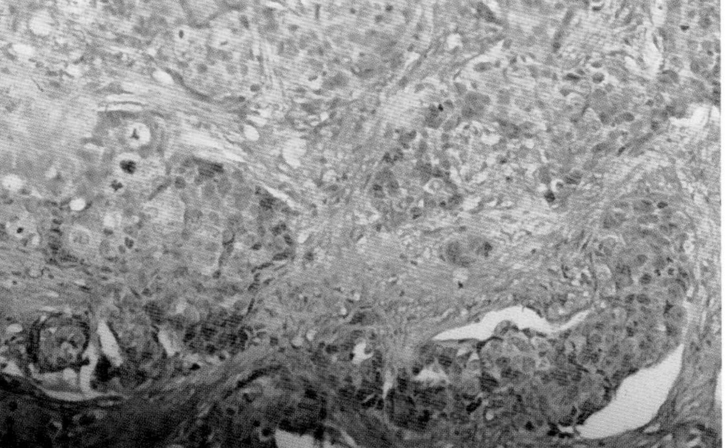

**e** *FNA cytology* shows a microlobular aggregate of cells with hyperchromatic nuclei and prominent nucleoli. *Histology* (right): cellular aggregates infiltrating the glandular tissue.

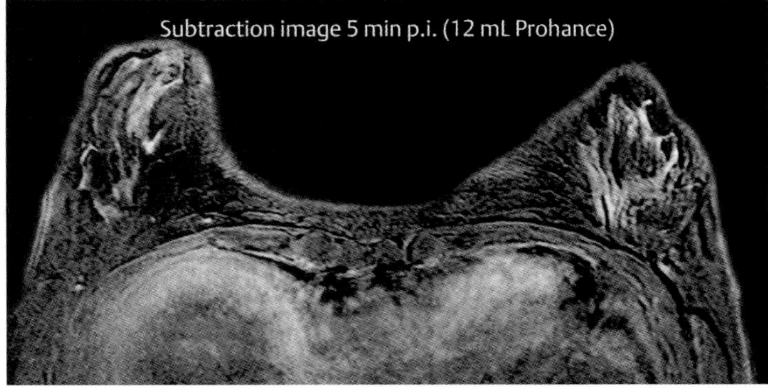


**f** *MR subtraction* image does not show tumor-type gadolinium enhancement at the site of the palpable nodule.

**Question on Fig. 5.92**

*How would you interpret the nodule in the left breast?*

(**a**) Fibroma/fibrosis

(**b**) Fibroadenoma

(**c**) Carcinoma

→ **Answer on p. 374**

**Fig. 5.93 A 41-year-old woman underwent left mastectomy and silicone implantation in 1997 for multifocal invasive ductal carcinoma.** She received adjuvant chemotherapy and postoperative radiation to the left breast. The left nipple was reconstructed in 1998, and a reduction mammoplasty was performed on the right side. Bilateral keloids developed. MRM in 1999 was suspicious for bilateral retroareolar and right periareolar tumors. Additional surgery was proposed, and the patient was referred for ultrasound-guided localization of suspicious foci in her MR images.

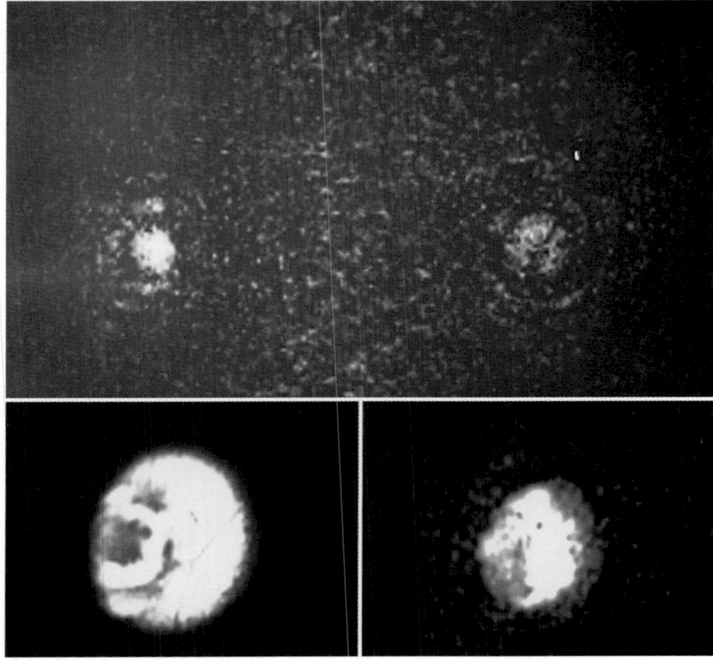

**a** *Subtraction MRI* in 1999. Coronal images shows bilateral retro- and periareolar gadolinium enhancement with a more localized density on the right side (see upper image with a different window).

**Question on Fig. 5.93**

*What has caused the MRI, mammographic, and sonographic changes in both breasts?*

(**a**) Retroareolar tumor in both breasts (recurrence on the left, second tumor on the right)

(**b**) Keloids

(**c**) Fat necrosis

→ **Answer on p. 374**

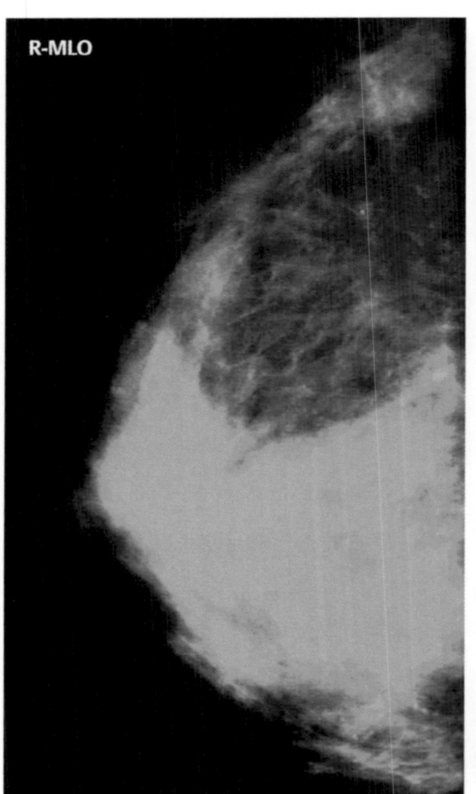


**b** *Oblique mammogram* of the right breast shows very dense, scarred glandular tissue with no recognizable structural details.

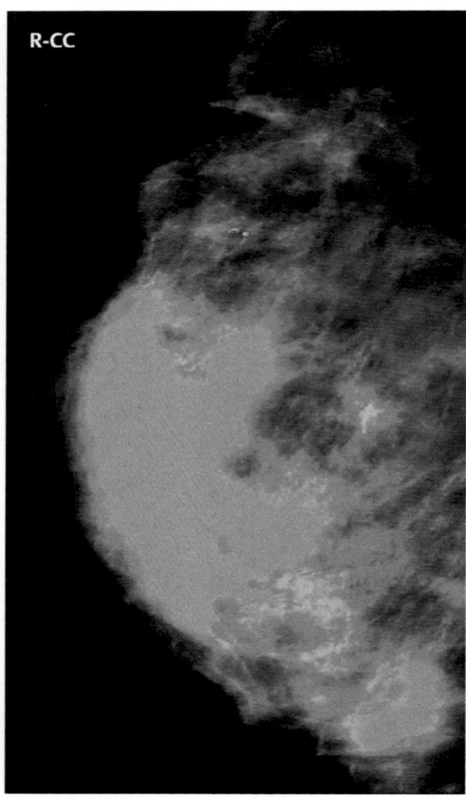


**c** *Right craniocaudal mammogram* shows a very dense, poorly differentiated breast (ACR 3).

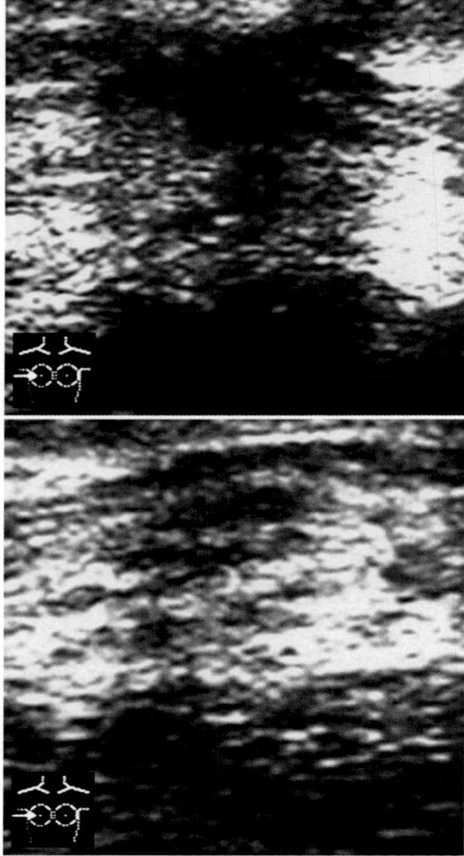

**d** *Sonogram* of the right retroareolar region shows a nonfocal, somewhat patchy area of low echogenicity.

**Fig. 5.94 A 43-year-old woman with redness of sudden onset** on the lateral side of the right breast between the 8 and 11-o'clock positions, associated with a circumscribed mass. She has no nipple discharge and no regional lymph node enlargement.

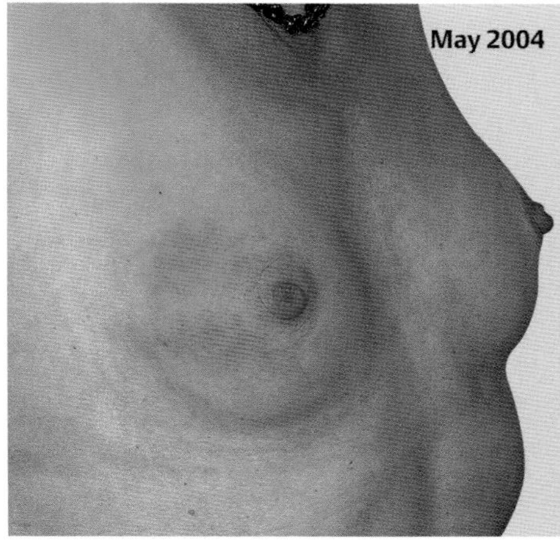


**a** *Clinical appearance* of the right breast in May, 2004. Inspection reveals slightly inhomogeneous redness over the lateral quadrants with no nipple retraction.

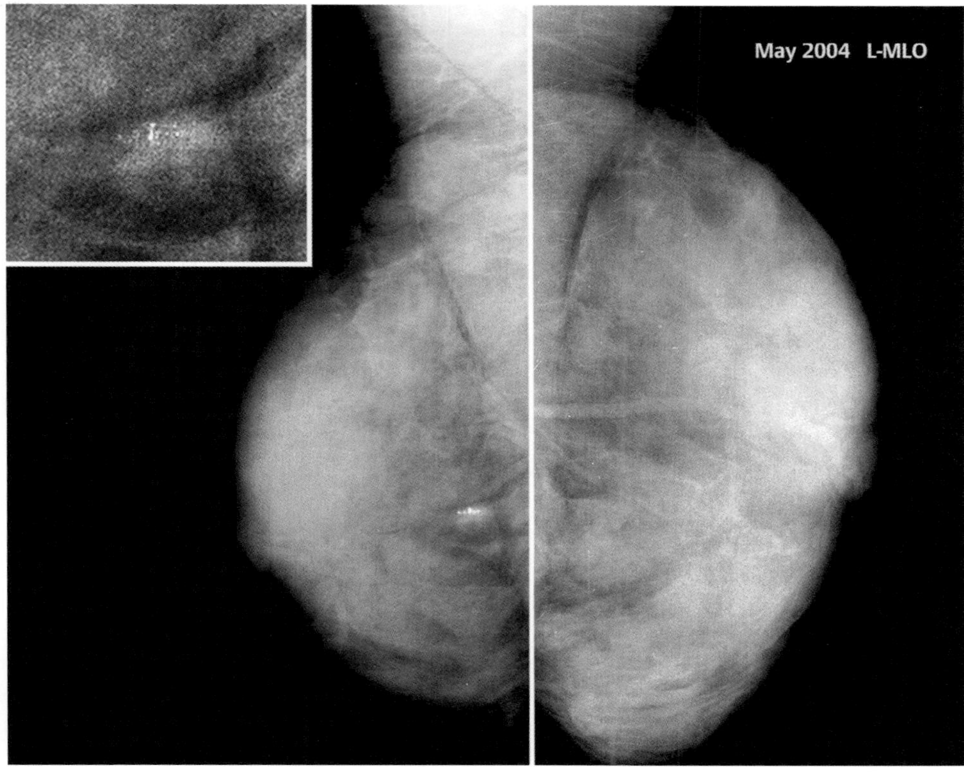


**b** *Bilateral oblique mammograms* in May, 2004, show very radiodense breasts with microcalcifications in the right breast (**Q/20**) (ACR 4, BIRADS 4, P**G**MI).

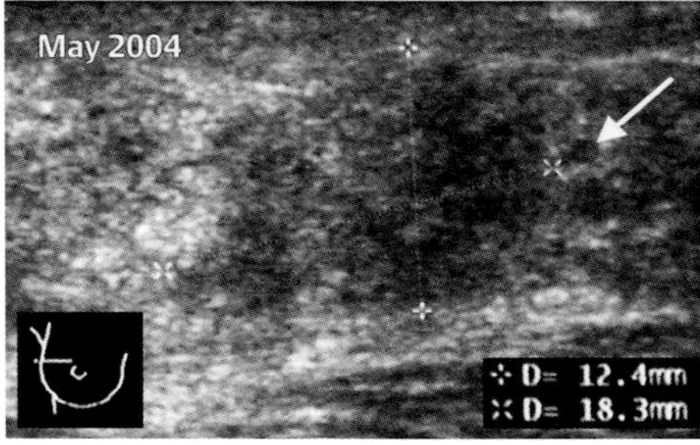


**c** *Sonogram* of the upper outer quadrant of the right breast in May, 2004 (lobar cross-section) shows a hypoechoic, inhomogeneous 1.2 cm × 1.8 cm area without posterior acoustic enhancement or shadowing and a mild degree of ductal dilatation (arrow).

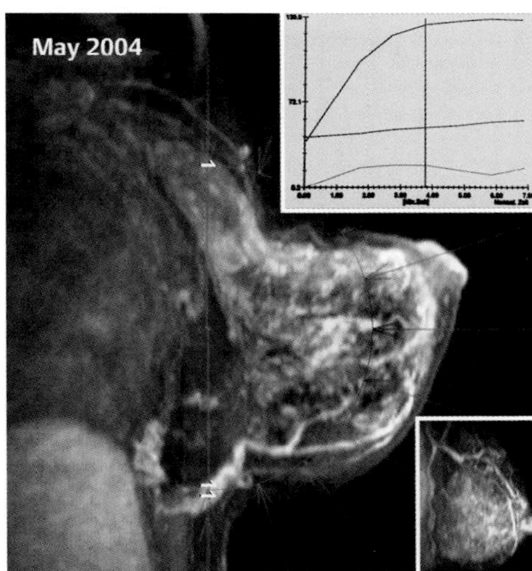


**d** *MRI.* Sagittal postgadolinium T1-weighted image in vascular mode shows intense gadolinium enhancement throughout the upper portion of the right breast with a rich vascular supply (inset at lower right) and draining veins inferiorly. Time–density curve see upper inset.

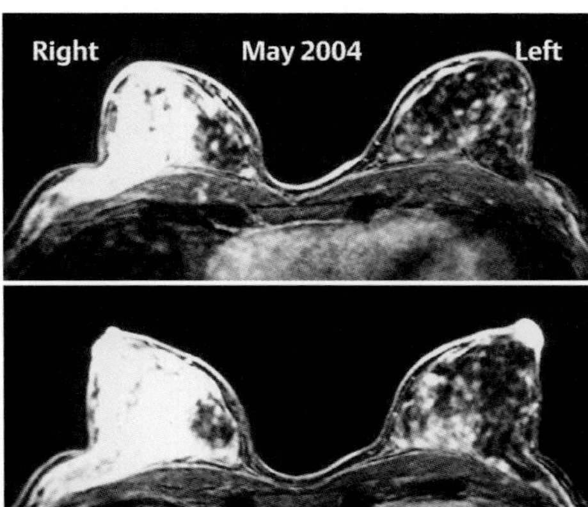


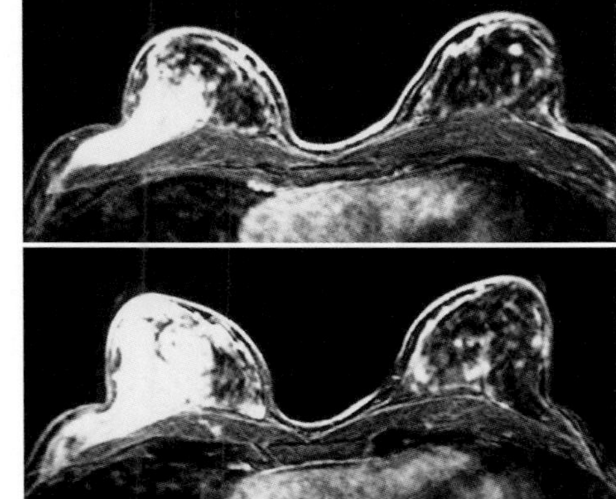

**e** *MRM* in May, 2004 shows intense gadolinium enhancement throughout the breast (e.g., **n–o/12–13**) except for the upper inner quadrant. The axillary recess is also infiltrated (e.g., **n/9**).The time–density curve (inset in **d**) shows a slowly rising pattern. The left breast contains small foci of nonspecific gadolinium enhancement.

**Question on Fig. 5.94**

*How would you interpret these findings?*

(**a**) Inflammatory breast carcinoma
(**b**) Mastitis
(**c**) Ductal breast carcinoma with EIC (microcalcifications)

→ **Answer on p. 375**

### Value of Magnetic Resonance Imaging and Other Modalities in Aesthetic Breast Reconstructions and Implantations

Magnetic resonance images of breasts with implants are sometimes difficult to interpret. More than 700 different types of breast implant have been marketed during the past 35 years, the most common being saline implants and single- and double-lumen devices (Greenstein 2004). Some types, such as soybean oil implants, have been pulled from the market because of toxic side-effects from breakdown products (see **Fig. 5.98**, p. 218).

A **single-lumen silicone implant** consists of viscous silicone gel enclosed within an outer silicone shell (see **Fig. 5.102**). The **double-lumen implant** has an inner lumen filled with viscous silicone gel surrounded by an outer shell filled with physiologic saline solution. Between the inner and outer shell are fine silicone fibers or other elastic fiber structures.

Implants with an outer polyurethane shell often incite a reactive collection of tissue fluid around the implant, but this fluid collection is not considered pathologic.

When the inner shell of a double-lumen implant ruptures (which has no adverse effects for the patient), MRI shows wormlike septations within the silicone called the "linguine sign" of intracapsular rupture. The same applies to ruptured single-lumen implants that have undergone fibrous encapsulation. The fibrous capsule forms an endogenous barrier that prevents silicone leakage into the breast tissue.

The outer shell of the implant consists of a semipermeable membrane of variable thickness that is made of polymerized silicone and forms an elastic unit. The purpose of the outer shell is to contain the silicone gel and convey a natural feel while maintaining the contours of the breast. The most common type of implant rupture involves this outer shell, in which case the silicone is still contained within the fibrous capsule formed by the host. When the linguine sign is present, both MRI and ultrasound show multiple linear intensities surrounded by the high signal intensity or echogenicity of the silicone gel. These curved lines represent the collapsed capsule of the implant, and the linguine sign is the most common sign associated with an intra- or extracapsular implant rupture. The "snowstorm pattern" seen at ultrasound results from silicone particles mixed with endogenous tissue. This characteristic hyperechoic pattern of extracapsular silicone within the breast parenchyma is a specific sign of free silicone surrounded by glandular breast tissue (see **Fig. 5.99 d**, p. 219).

Not all implants collapse when they rupture, so the linguine sign is not always present. The natural folds or wrinkles in the surface of the implant should not be mistaken for a true linguine sign (see **Fig. 5.102 b**, p. 222). It is not yet fully understood why some implants do not collapse. It may be that the relatively stiff and rigid outer shell or the silicone gel itself keeps the implant in an expanded condition. Gorczyca and Brenner (1997) published an excellent review of the many types of breast implant and the complexity of capsule problems.

A breast implant may be placed at the subpectoral level (total mastectomy), the subglandular level (breast augmentation), or the subcutaneous level (subcutaneous mastectomy), depending on anatomic constraints.

Following subcutaneous mastectomy, a thin layer of breast parenchyma and fat remains between the oval-shaped implant and the skin. The implant surface is usually wavy due to fibrous encapsulation, but this is not considered an abnormal finding (see **Fig. 5.102 a**, p. 222).

**Gel bleed** refers to the seepage of silicone into the host capsule through microperforations in the outer shell of the implant. This phenomenon eventually occurs with almost all implants and does not produce a silicone leak that is detectable by mammography or even MRM. Gel bleed may produce a snowstorm pattern at ultrasound, but this does not have immediate implications for implant removal or exchange. Gel bleed is not synonymous with implant rupture (see **Fig. 5.102 a**).

> ***Tip***
>
> **MRI should be used (with mammography and ultrasound) to investigate any nodular change near a breast implant to determine whether it is caused by a tumor or by silicone leak. While contrast administration is usually unnecessary for simple evaluation of the capsule, it is essential for investigating palpable lesions near a breast implant.**

#### *Intracapsular and Extracapsular Ruptures of Silicone Implants*

The most important monographs on this subject (e.g., Gorczyca and Brenner 1997; Gros 1996) stress the importance of MRI in implant ruptures, adding that MRI should be used for this indication only if it will have therapeutic implications. If the patient refuses any kind of surgery in advance, it is unnecessary to proceed with MRI.

Implant ruptures may affect the inner shell (single-lumen implant), the outer shell (double-lumen implant), and/or the fibrous host capsule. Rupture of the inner shell is the most common. It is harmless, as it does not allow silicone to escape through the outer shell into the breast parenchyma. Rupture of the inner membrane leads to a linguine sign within the implant. These wavy lines are produced by the collapsed inner shell floating in the gel. A fat-suppressed (silicone-specific) T2 sequence is best for the MR imaging of these changes, as the silicone has very high signal intensity while the collapsed shell is hypointense. Ultrasound also clearly demonstrates the linguine sign (**Fig. 5.99 d**, p. 219) as well as the snowstorm sign (see **Fig. 5.100 e**, p. 221).

MRI has the highest sensitivity and specificity for detecting ruptures and local recurrences in proximity to breast implants (see **Figs. 5.95** and **5.103**, p. 225). If MRI is contraindicated due to the presence of a cardiac pacemaker, cochlear implants, or severe claustrophobia, computed tomography can also supply valuable information.

Breast ultrasound is very examiner-dependent, and few diagnosticians have adequate experience with implants unless they own an ultrasound scanner. The least rewarding modality is mammography. Eighty percent of all implant ruptures—whether intra- or extracapsular—cannot be detected by mammography.

With any questionable implant rupture, the patient's history should be checked to exclude previous intramammary silicone injection, which was especially common from 1940 to 1960. Free silicone was formerly injected into the breast for augmentation and is manifested by typical light, focal opacities on mammograms. When an implant exchange has been performed, it cannot be determined whether the silicone leaked from the previous implant or was administered by direct injection. In all implant assessments, it is important to know the implant design, i.e., whether it is a single-, double-, or triple-lumen device. Very few patients know what type of implant they have.

It should be noted that breast implants may rupture during compression mammography, especially if they are old and friable (this no longer occurs with newer implants). An intracapsular rupture may easily progress to an extracapsular rupture when breast compression is applied. *Women with implants more than 10 years old should be informed of this risk prior to mammography.* With subpectoral implants that have been placed for cosmetic augmentation in micromastia, the breast tissue in front of the implant may be so compressed that the implant is pushed backward, providing a very clear view of the breast parenchyma. This is not associated with a risk of implant rupture.

In all cases mammography should be performed very carefully, as many women with implants are already fearful about having mammograms. Two views should be obtained in most cases, because in single-view mammography the implant will obscure large portions of the breast parenchyma and may cause microcalcifications or other lesions to be missed. It should be noted that some breasts are easier to palpate after prosthetic implantation, and any firmness or nodularity can be detected at an earlier stage owing to the flattened condition of the breast tissue between the implant and the skin.

The following mammographic changes may signify an implant rupture:

- Visible opacity outside the capsule surface
- Calcifications next to the implant
- Asymmetries of the implant and circumscribed hernias
- Extravasation of silicone

Except for silicone extravasation, none of the above signs are specific for implant rupture.

Mammographically detected changes in the breast should always be correlated with the recent history. Patients with extracapsular ruptures will present with pain or systemic manifestations.

Sonographic changes are more specific than mammographic changes. The most reliable sign of an intact implant is an echo-free interior. All portions of the implant wall are smooth, although some wrinkling is a normal finding.

The sonographic signs of implant rupture are as follows:

- High-level echoes (snowstorm) surrounding and extending into the implant
- Discontinuity in the inner or outer shell
- Multiple parallel lines within the implant (stepladder sign)
- Variable hypoechoic areas within the implant
- Wavy lines inside the implant (linguine sign)

Typical MRI features of implant rupture are as follows (see p. 201):

- Silicone leakage (bleeding) between the implant and fibrous capsule
- Silicone leakage through the outer capsule into the breast parenchyma
- Wavy inner shell (linguine sign)
- "Teardrop sign" within the implant
- Silicone outside the fibrous capsule in the breast parenchyma (differential diagnosis: previous instillation of free silicone; Gorczyca and Brenner 1997).

Aesthetic breast reconstructions may also lead to problems of differential diagnosis. In cases where muscle tissue is transferred to the breast (TRAM flap or latissimus dorsi flap), only small amounts of muscle tissue (20%) are transferred into the augmented breast, together with fatty tissue (80%). Accordingly, one sees mainly fat in the reconstructed breast with mammography, ultrasound, and MRI. The vascular pedicle of the flap appears as a mammographic density and may cause diagnostic confusion. The situation may become quite confusing in cases where a flap transfer to the breast has been augmented by silicone implantation. Even MRI may yield equivocal findings in the presence of scars and granulation tissue.

Very difficult is the diagnosis of a capsulitis of the outer shell (**Figs. 5.95–5.105**).

**Fig. 5.95 A Questionable local recurrence following esthetic breast reconstruction in a 59-year-old woman** who had a previous left mastectomy for multifocal disease. The patient underwent an esthetic reconstruction of the left breast and reduction mammoplasty of the right breast, at which time portions of the right nipple were transplanted to the left breast. She had no other previous surgery. Is there evidence of a local recurrence?

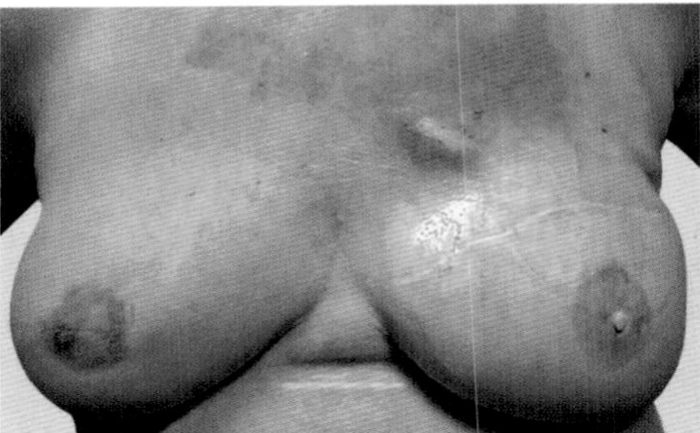

**a** *Inspection* of both breasts with the arms raised shows a good cosmetic result following bilateral esthetic reconstruction. The left nipple has healed well, and scarring is visible in the lower right areola (**b–C/23**). Any other unusual findings?

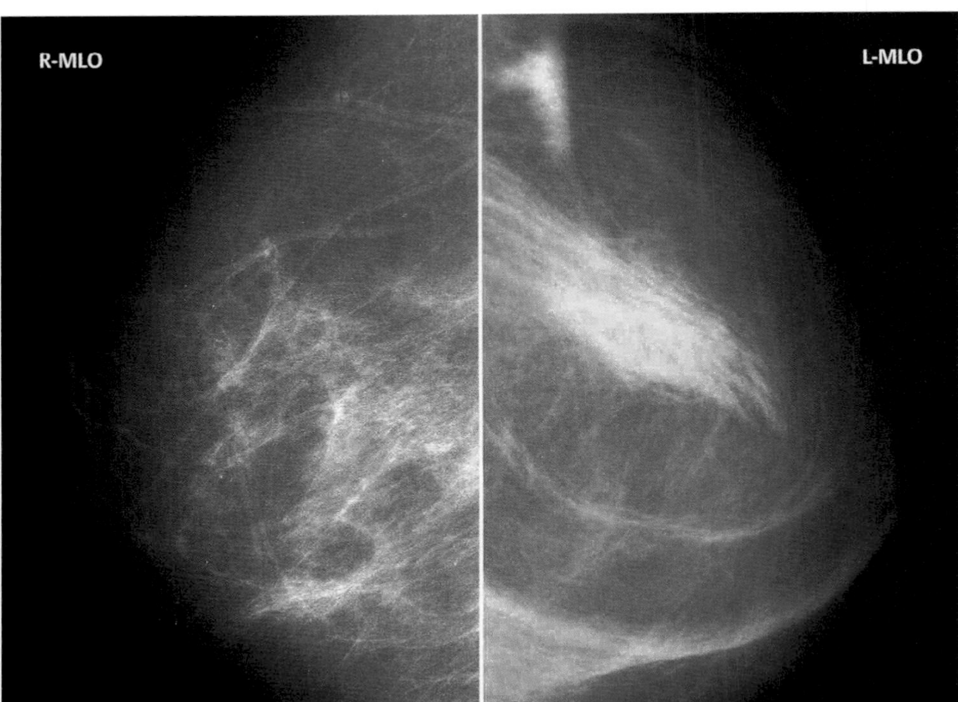


**b** *Bilateral mediolateral mammograms* show a fatty left breast with a vascular pedicle at **H–i/21–24** and an involuted right breast with small focal opacities. Because of the straight mediolateral projection, the pectoral muscle is not seen and the breast parenchyma near the chest wall is only partly visualized (ACR 2, BIRADS?, PGM**I**).

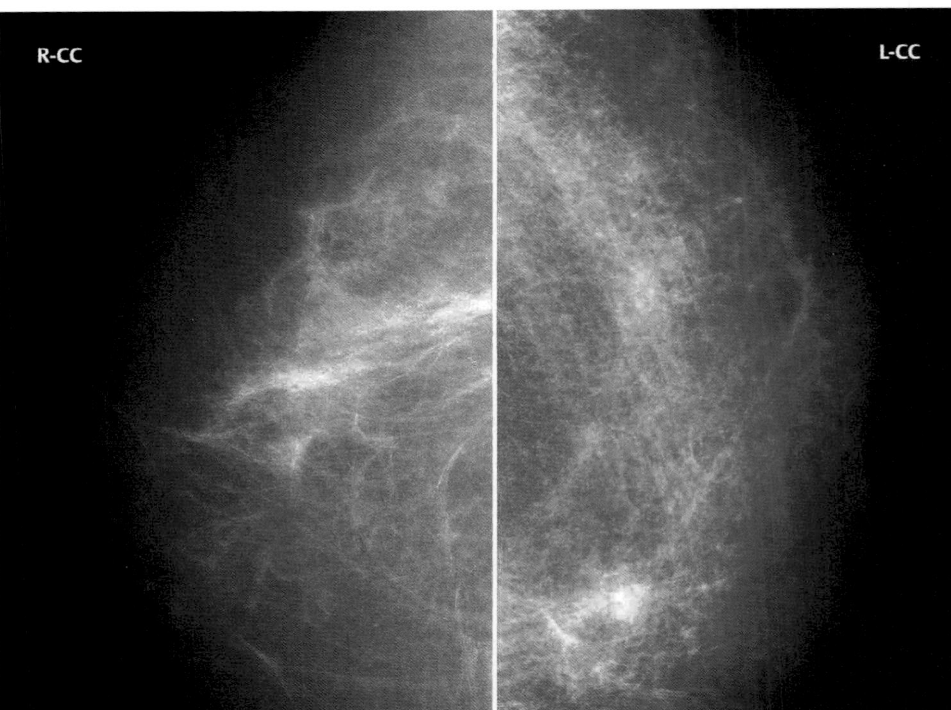


**c** *Bilateral craniocaudal mammograms* show fatty breasts with nonspecific opacities on both sides. The vascular pedicle seen in **b** is not visible in the craniocaudal view. The pectoral muscle is not visualized on either side, probably as a result of the surgery (ACR 2, BIRADS?, PG**M**I).

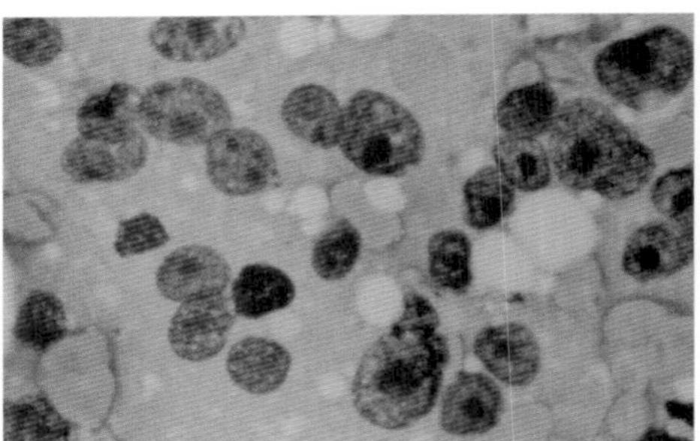

**d** *FNA* reveals multiple cells with bare nuclei, finely clumped cytoplasm, and enlarged nucleoli (Papanicolao 5).

**Question 1 on Fig. 5.95**

*What type of reconstruction was performed?*

(**a**) Latissimus dorsi flap transfer
(**b**) Autologous fat transplantation in the left breast
(**c**) Transverse rectus abdominis myocutaneous flap (TRAM flap)

→ **Answer on p. 376**

**Question 2 on Fig. 5.95**

*What is the location of the cytologically confirmed local recurrence?*

(**a**) Left breast (coordinates)
(**b**) Right breast (coordinates)
(**c**) Both breasts

→ **Answer on p. 376**

**Question 3 on Fig. 5.95**

*Is the recurrence visible on inspection (**a**)?*
*If so, does this correspond to the mammographic location?*

(**a**) Yes (coordinates)
(**b**) No

→ **Answer on p. 376**

**Fig. 5.96 Silicone. A 56-year-old black African woman with nodular breasts presents for screening.** She has considerable difficulty communicating with the technologist. Circumference firmness is noted in the lower portion of the right breast.

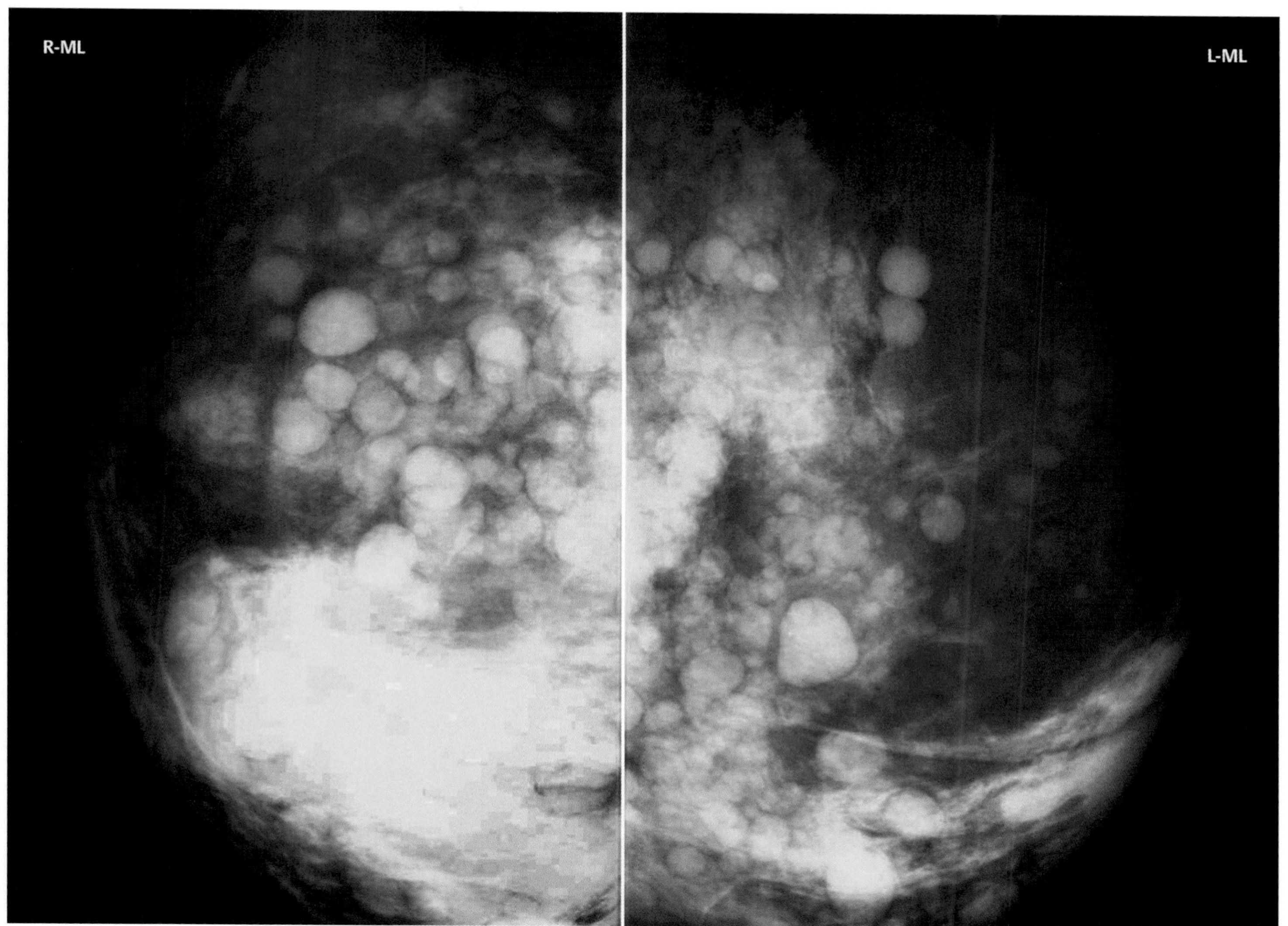


Bilateral mediolateral mammograms show numerous well-circumscribed nodules of homogeneous density that are confluent in the lower portion of the right breast (images courtesy of H. P. Josef, Uedelhoven).

**Question on Fig. 5.96**

*How would you interpret these findings?*

(**a**) Ruptured silicone implants
(**b**) Free silicone injections into the breast parenchyma
(**c**) Hydatid cysts

→ **Answer on p. 376**

**Fig. 5.97 Esthetic breast reconstruction in a 53-year-old woman following a missed diagnosis** (the patient presented in 2001). Progressive nodular firmness was present in the upper outer quadrant of the left breast from 1997 (**a**). Regular clinical, mammographic, and sonographic follow-ups of the left breast were conducted until 2001, and no malignant changes had been diagnosed. Clinical progression prompted excisional biopsy of the nodules in 2001 (recommended by the patient's internist) without new mammograms, and cancer was diagnosed. Several reoperations were unsuccessful in achieving an R0 resection, but esthetic breast reconstruction ultimately yielded an excellent cosmetic result. Surprisingly, the sentinel lymph node and 12 other axillary lymph nodes remained negative despite the 4-year "observation period." One year later (2002), magnetic resonance imaging shows various sites of gadolinium enhancement in the operated left breast and healthy right breast.

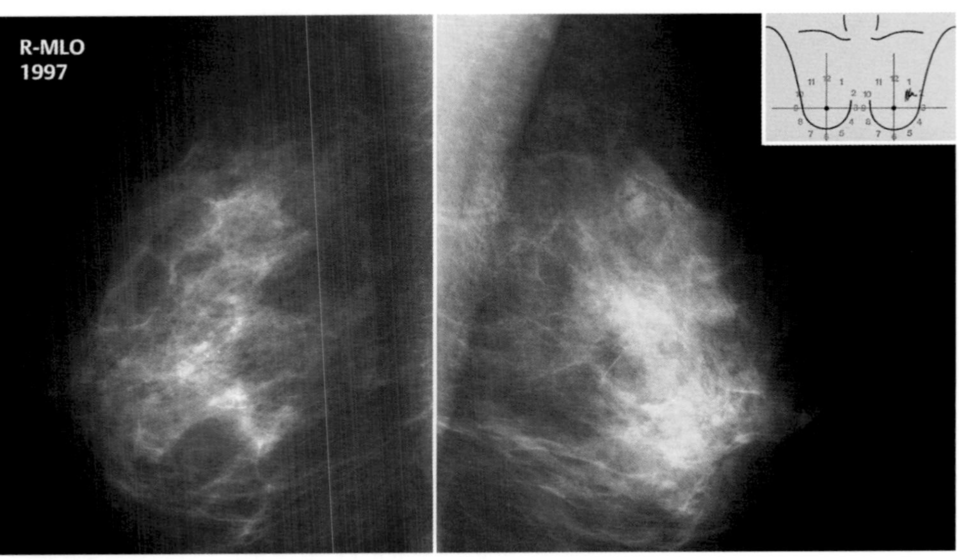


**a** *Bilateral oblique mammograms in* 1997 show dense inhomogeneous breasts, particularly on the left side, with small focal opacities correlating with palpable findings (mass in the upper outer quadrant of the left breast, see inset drawing) (ACR 2 right, ACR 3 left, BIRADS 2, P**G**MI).

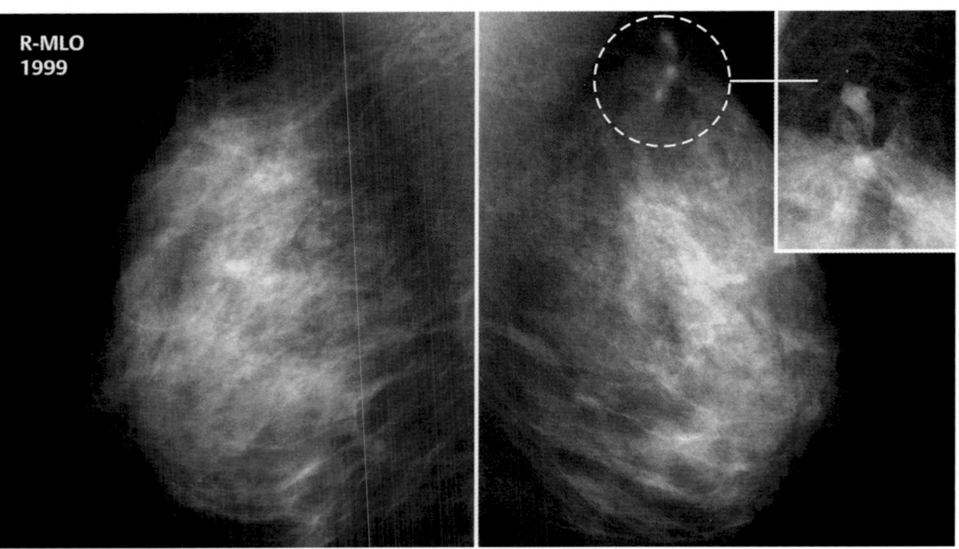


**b** *Bilateral oblique mammograms* in 1999 show dense breasts with nonspecific opacities that are more pronounced in the left breast and no evidence of a circumscribed tumor (ACR 3, BIRADS 3 left, P**G**MI). The inset at upper right is a secondary digital enlargement of the upper outer quadrant of the left breast at **e/14**.

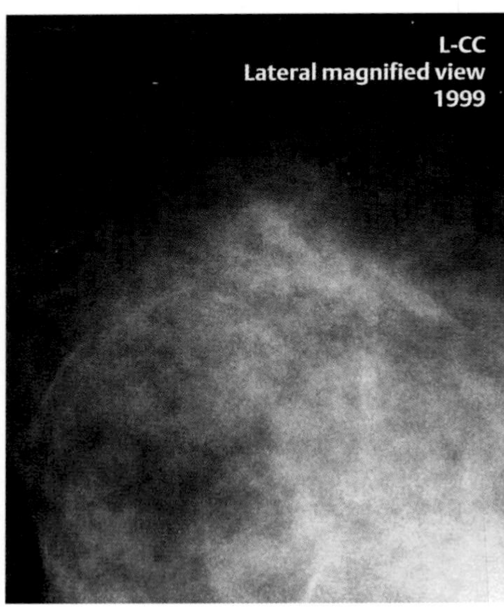


**c** *Left craniocaudal mammogram* in 1999. Secondary digital reconstruction and enlargement of the upper outer quadrant of the left breast in the last preoperative examination. The tumor appears as a spiculated density (**I–J/11–12**).

**Fig. 5.97 Esthetic breast reconstruction in a 53-year-old woman following a missed diagnosis.** *(continued)*

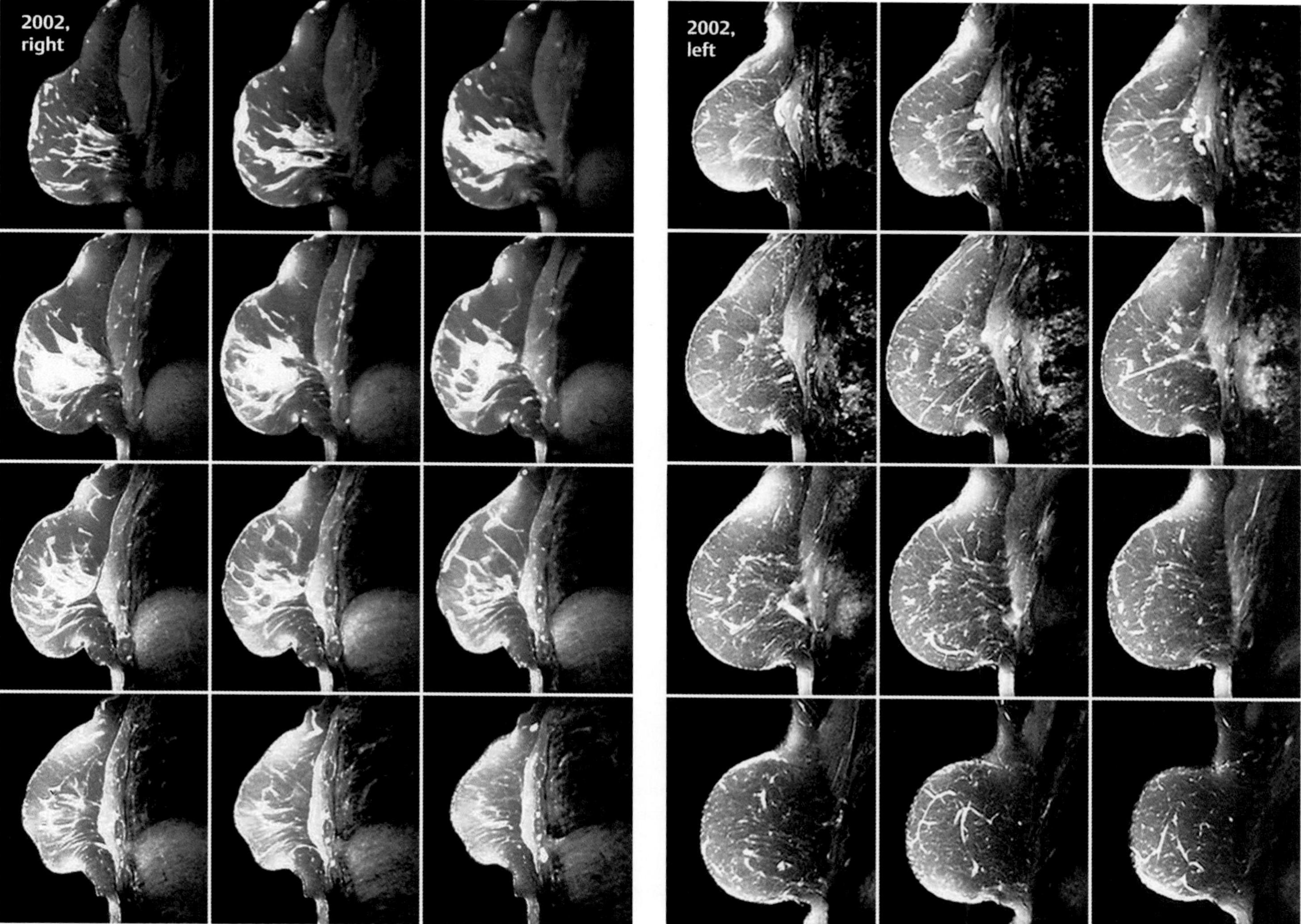


**d** *Sagittal MRI subtraction* images of the right breast in December, 2002 show intense vascularization of the breast parenchyma from the chest wall to the nipple.

**e** *Sagittal MR subtraction* images of the left breast in December, 2002. Vascularity is less pronounced than on the right side and is maximal in the lower part of the pectoral muscle (e.g., **s/25–26**).

**Question 1 on Fig. 5.97**

*What is the most likely classification of the tumor in the left breast?*

(**a**) Unifocal medullary carcinoma (see p. 63)
(**b**) Diffuse comedo-type DCIS (see p. 37)
(**c**) Multifocal tubulolobular carcinoma (see p. 71)

→ **Answer on p. 376**

**Question 2 on Fig. 5.97**

*Based on the MR images in 2002, what kind of procedure was performed on the left breast?*

(**a**) Breast-conserving surgery and postoperative radiotherapy
(**b**) Subcutaneous mastectomy and reconstruction with soybean oil implants
(**c**) TRAM flap

→ **Answer on p. 376**

**Fig. 5.98 Folds and wrinkles in the breast implants of a 48-year-old woman.** The patient underwent bilateral subcutaneous mastectomy and prosthetic implantation for cosmetic reasons.

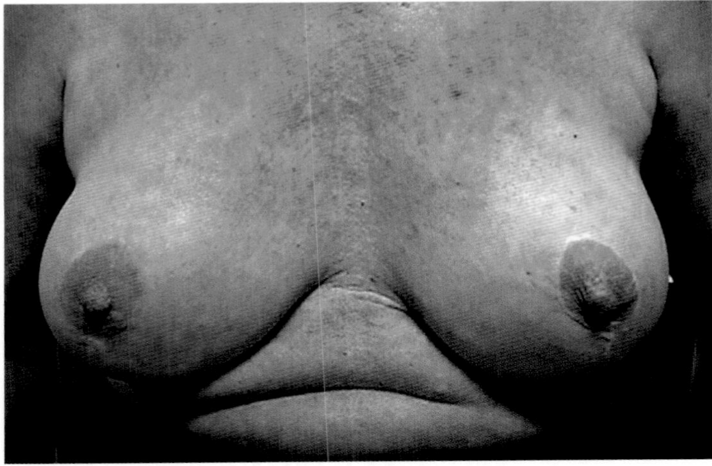

**a** *On clinical inspection*, both breasts show healthy-appearing periareolar scars. The implants create an harmonious transition from the upper to lower quadrants.

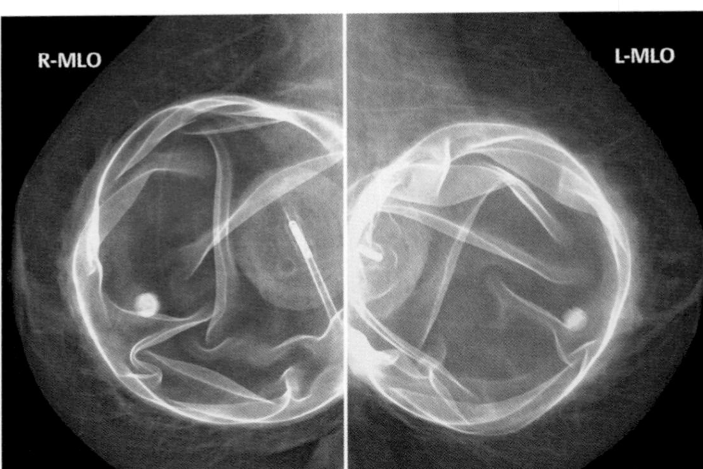


**b** *Bilateral oblique mammograms* demonstrate folds and wrinkles in the implants. The filler port is visible near the nipple on each side (**G/23** right, **J/23** left).

**Question 1 on Fig. 5.98**

*What type of implants are these?*

(**a**) Silicone
(**b**) Saline
(**c**) Soybean oil

→ **Answer on p. 377**

**Question 2 on Fig. 5.98**

*What accounts for the folds and wrinkles in the implants?*

(**a**) Fibrous encapsulation
(**b**) Capsular rupture and deflation
(**c**) Adaptation to the shape of the breasts

→ **Answer on p. 377**

**Fig. 5.99 A 39-year-old woman. Implant rupture or fibrous encapsulation** (?) The patient underwent right mastectomy in 1994 for a neoplasm (T2 N0 M0) and a prophylactic left subcutaneous mastectomy in 1997 (strong family history of breast cancer with two sisters affected at a young age). Both breasts were reconstructed with implants in 1997, at which time the right nipple was reconstructed with tissue from the left nipple (**a**). Surgery was followed by nonspecific inflammation with "bulla formation" in the right breast. Since then the patient has had recurring breast problems, especially on the right side (pain, foreign body sensation, feeling of fluid accumulation). Contraction of the pectoral muscles compresses both implants, producing skin folds and nonspecific nodularity in the lower outer quadrant of the right breast and upper inner quadrant of the left breast (**b**).

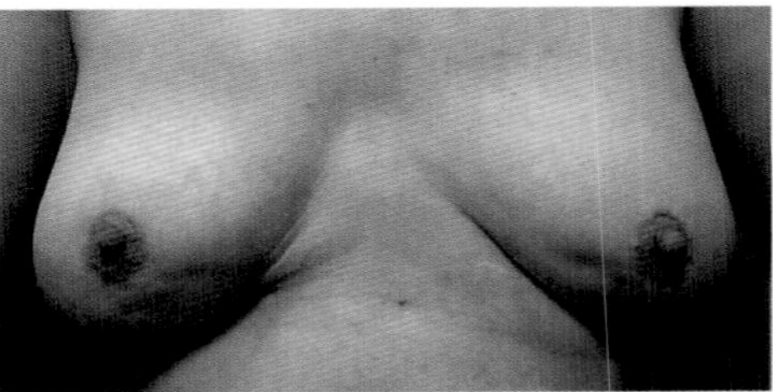

**a** *Clinical inspection* shows slight undulation of the skin surface over the lower inner quadrant of each breast (**c/11** left, **a–B/10–11** right). Otherwise the breasts have a normal shape with well-reconstructed nipples.

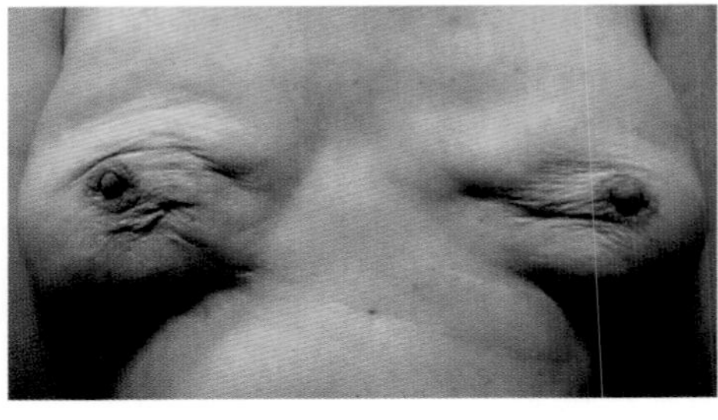

**b** *Clinical aspect:* On active contraction of the pectoral muscles, both breasts move upward and form horizontal creases with circumscribed bulges over the upper inner quadrants. Subcutaneous mastectomy and prosthetic implantation have resulted in a left infra-areolar scar.

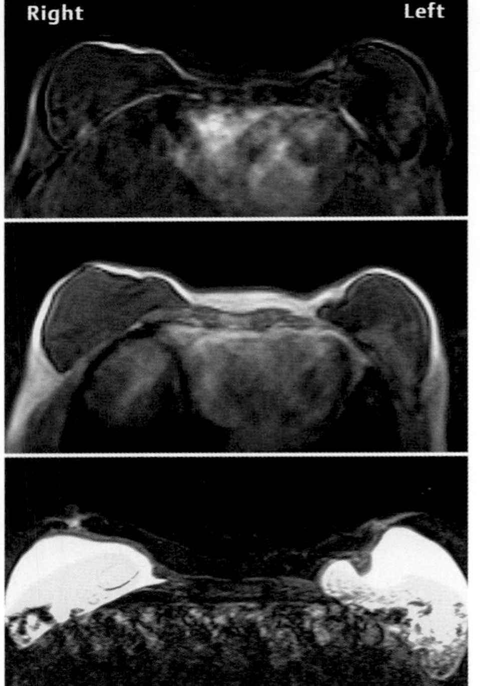

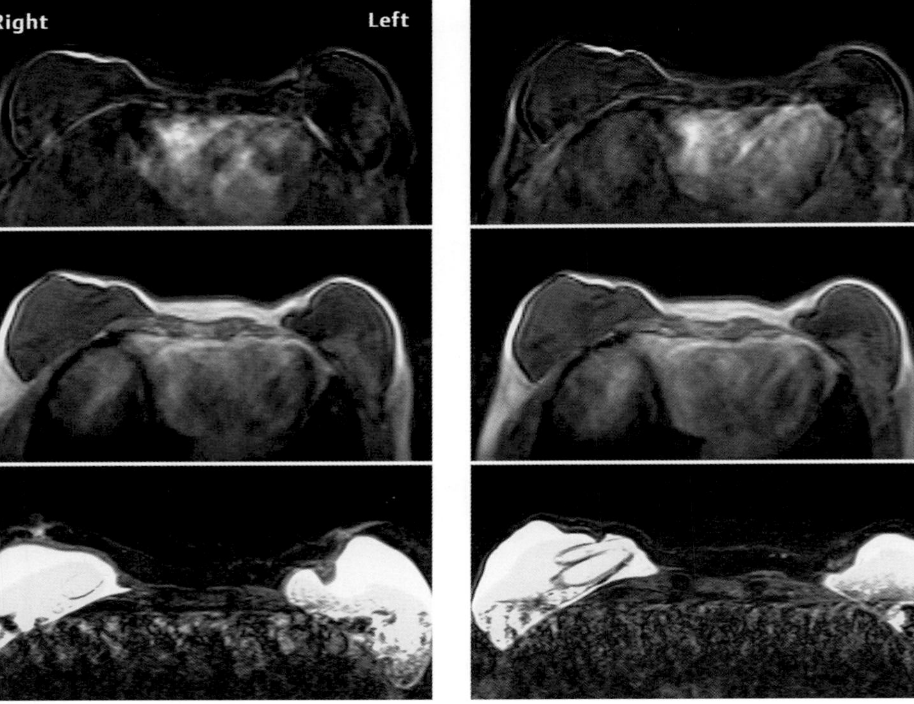


**c** *MR images* (spin-echo, 3D gradient and fat-suppressed IR sequences) show bilateral intracapsular ruptures (**H–i/4–5**, linguine sign, see p. 212) with an intact outer shell.

▶ **Fig. 5.99 d**

**Fig. 5.99** **A 39-year-old woman. Implant rupture or fibrous encapsulation.** *(continued)*

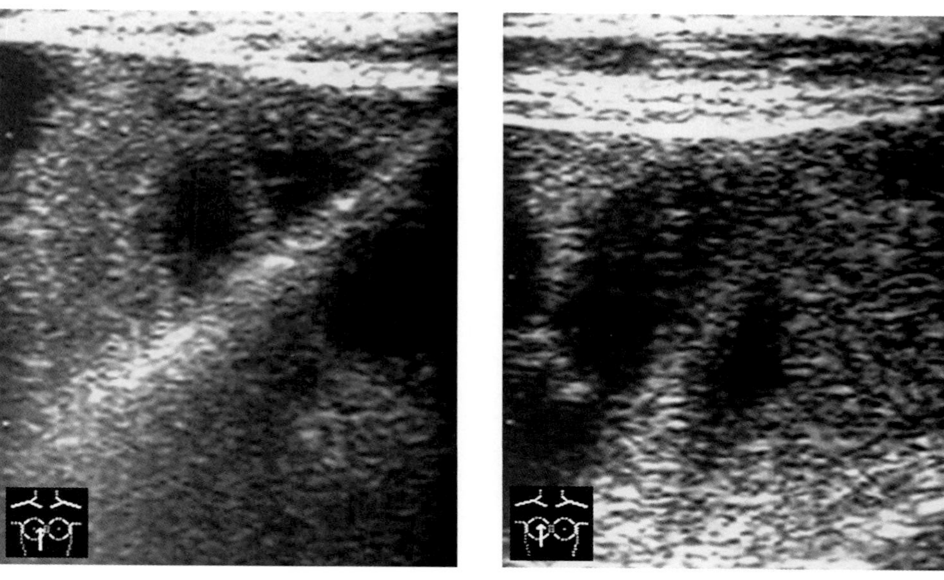

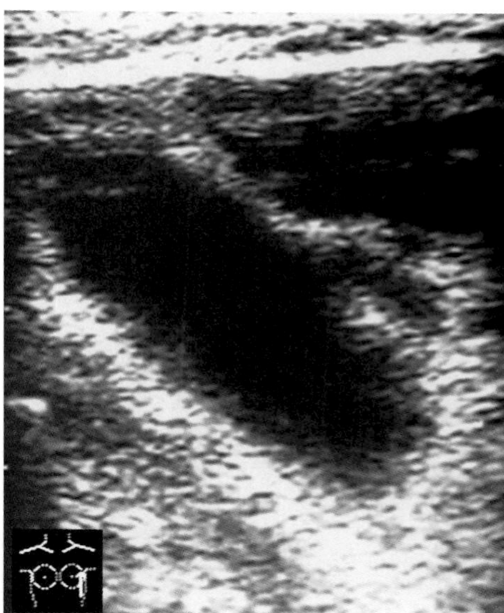

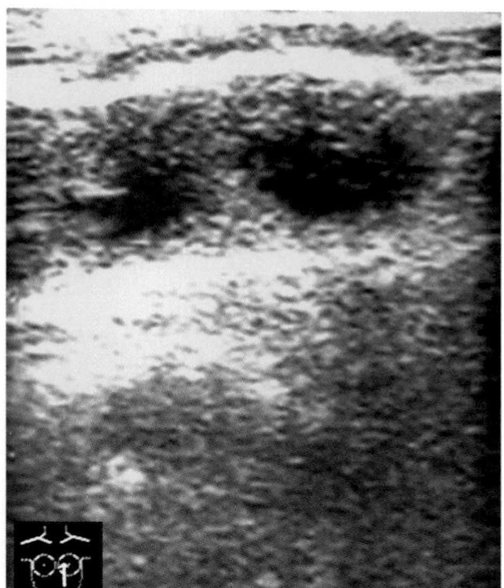

**d** *Bilateral sonograms* show a "snowstorm pattern" (e.g., **K–k/22–27**) in the implants with broad hyperechoic streaks ("linguine sign") separated by irregular hypoechoic areas (dark "holes").

**Question on Fig. 5.99**

*Why does pectoral muscle contraction cause such pronounced deformation of the breasts?*

(**a**) Implant rupture in which the outer shell remains in place and distorts the pectoral muscles

(**b**) Massive bilateral fibrous encapsulation

(**c**) Both

→ **Answer on p. 378**

***Note:*** *The mammographic, sonographic, and MRI findings after esthetic breast reconstructions (with or without silicone implants) are extremely diverse. This variation relates to the type of implant used (single- or double-lumen, etc.) and to the fibrous host capsule that forms around silicone implants. This capsule isolates the implant from the breast parenchyma and pectoral muscle and forms a replacement cavity in the event of an implant rupture.*

**Fig. 5.100 A 57-year-old woman. Gel bleed due to a complete or incomplete implant rupture?** A subpectoral double-lumen silicone implant (*McGhan*) has been placed in each breast; this was done for a tumor excision on the left side and for esthetic reasons on the right side. Both implants are normal to palpation. The patient has a positive family history of breast cancer.

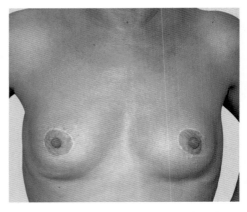

**a** *Visual inspection* following bilateral esthetic breast reconstruction shows healthy-appearing periareolar scars and a slight irregularity of the skin surface in the lower portion of the right breast (**a/22**) that is more pronounced than on the left side.

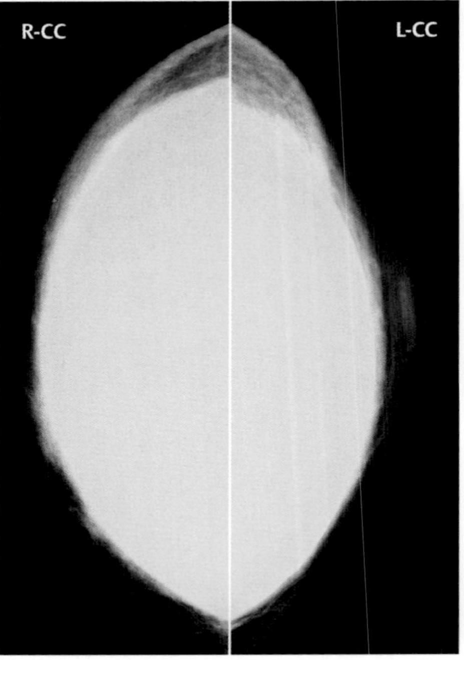


**b** *Bilateral craniocaudal mammograms*. The silicone implants present smooth surface contours and show homogeneous density (no mammographic evidence of water/gel double lumina). Subcutaneous breast parenchyma is no longer visible.

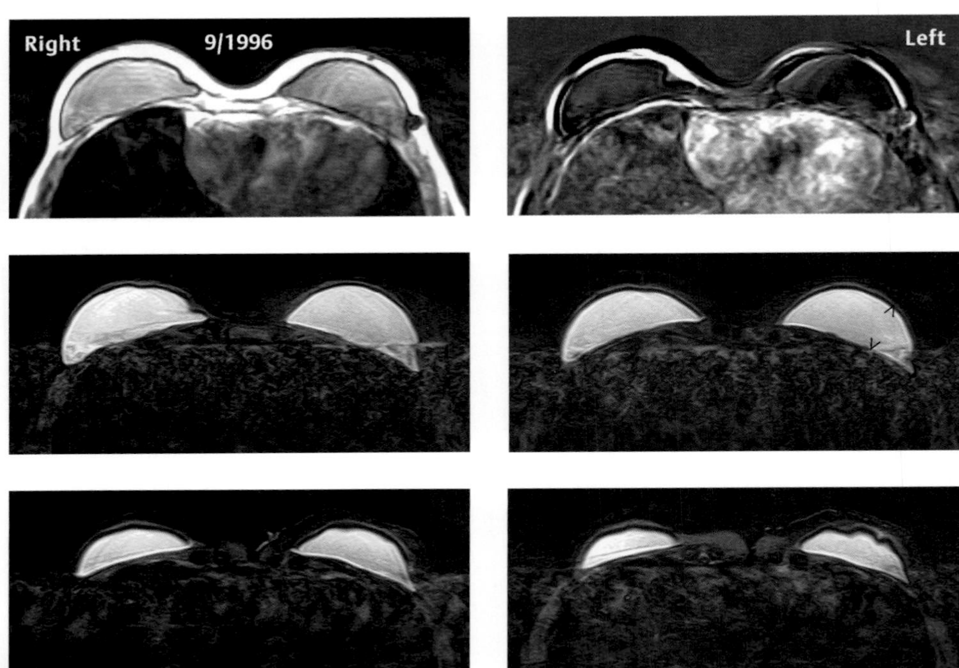


**c** *Fat-suppressed MRI sequences* in September, 1996. The McGhan double-lumen prosthesis is a homogeneous silicone implant surrounded by a thin water-filled chamber (e.g., lower outer quadrant of the right breast). The subpectoral implants are indented posteriorly by parasternal rib cartilage (**e/22**).

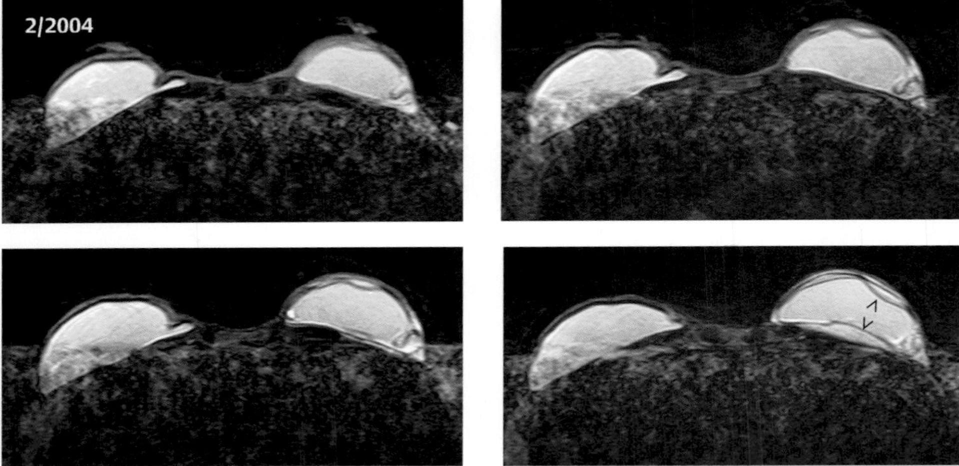


**d** *Fat-suppressed MR sequences* in February, 2004. The double-lumen contour is well preserved on the right side, where findings are unchanged relative to 1996. On the left side, silicone is visible outside the inner shell in the water-filled chamber in the lower outer quadrant, and the implant is deflated (horizontal diameter is decreased compared with 1996, arrows).

**Fig. 5.100** **A 57-year-old woman. Gel bleed due to a complete or incomplete implant rupture?** *(continued)*

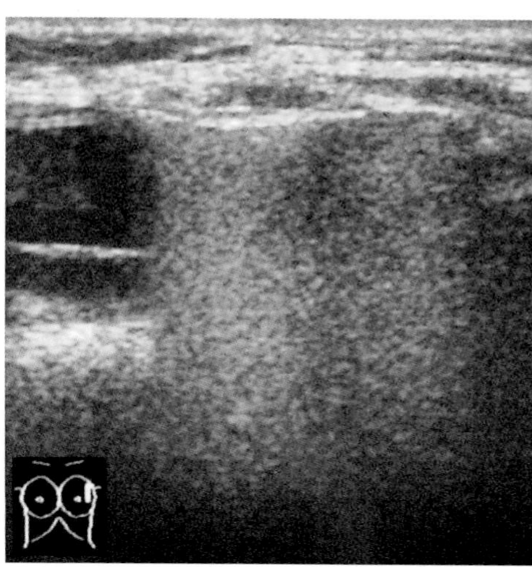

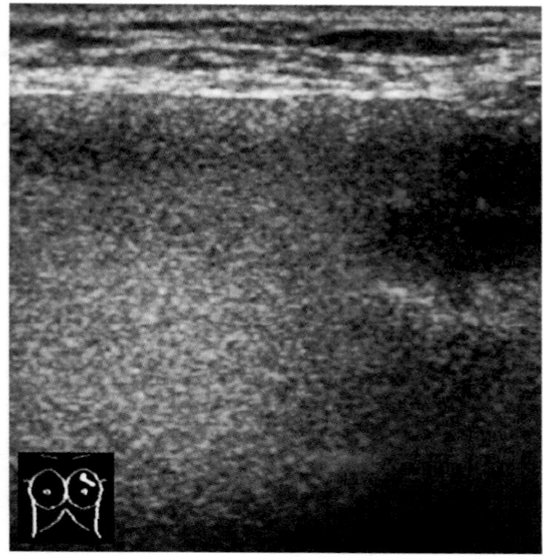

**e** *On ultrasound*, the implant is partially obscured by a "snowstorm" pattern due to extracapsular silicone.

**Question on Fig. 5.100**

*How would you interpret these findings?*

(**a**) Complete rupture (of the inner and outer shells)
(**b**) Incomplete rupture confined to the inner shell
(**c**) Gel bleed

→ **Answer on p. 378**

**Fig. 5.101** **A 47-year-old woman. Bilateral prosthetic implantation in followed by trophic skin changes/mastitis/fibrous encapsulation?** The patient had two previous operations for tumors in the right breast. Bilateral silicone implants have been inserted (on the left after prophylactic subcutaneous mastectomy). The right breast shows inframammary skin discoloration overlying a subcutaneous lentil-sized nodule. The nodule shows no enlargement relative to the previous examination. Severe tenderness is present along the axillary extension of the implant on the right side. The patient has a history of recurrent local and diffuse inflammations in the left breast. The left breast is warm to the touch, while the right breast feels cool.

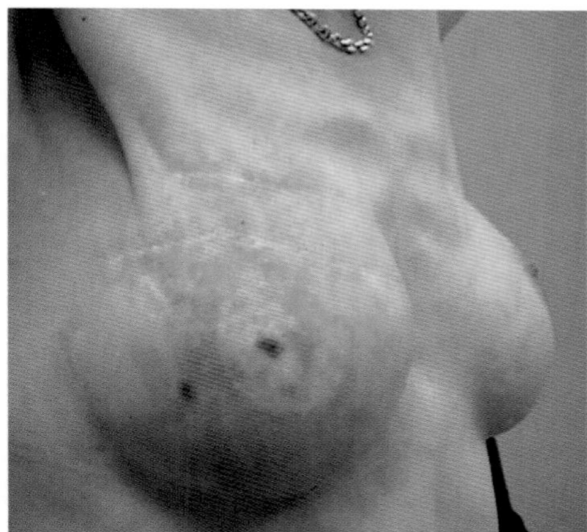

**a** *Visual inspection* of the right breast shows a transverse mastectomy scar with a smaller, parallel scar above it (**L/15**). The right nipple appears pale (reconstructed from vulvar skin) while the skin of the right breast shows reddish-purple discoloration. A small nodule is palpable in the right breast at the 8-o'clock position (**k/13**). The left breast is of normal color.

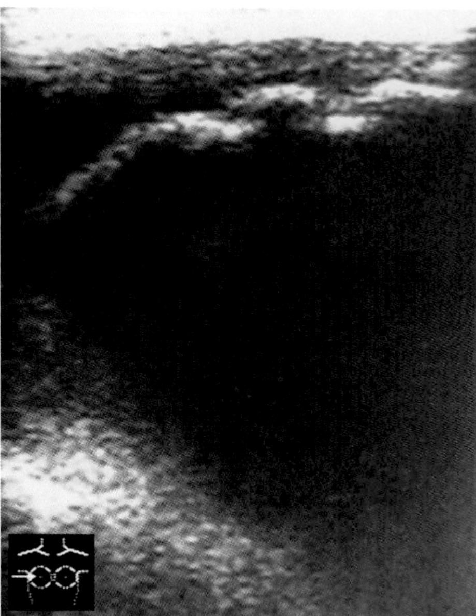

**b** *Sonogram* of the right breast shows an undulating implant wall in the area of the palpable nodule with circumscribed bulging of the implant (**P/16**). Diagonally opposite is a hyperechoic feature at **N–o/9–11** overlying the posterolateral portion of the implant border.

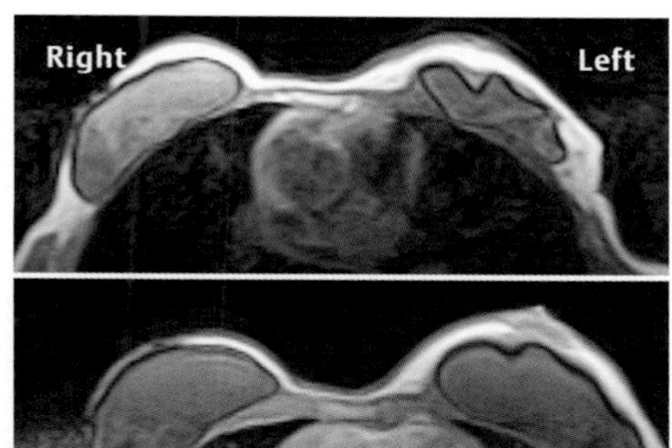


**c** *T1-weighted MR subtraction* image shows circumscribed increased density of the subcutaneous fat with no peri-implant irritation. The left implant shows greater wrinkling due to fibrous encapsulation.

**Question 1 on Fig. 5.101**

*The diffuse skin changes in the right breast are a sign of what?*

(**a**) Trophic disturbance (poor blood supply)
(**b**) Fibrous encapsulation
(**c**) Implant rupture

→ **Answer on p. 378**

**Question 2 on Fig. 5.101**

*Does one of the images show evidence of circumscribed silicone leakage?*

(**a**) The clinical photograph (coordinates)
(**b**) The sonogram (coordinates)
(**c**) The MR images (coordinates)

→ **Answer on p. 378**

**Fig. 5.102** **Gel bleed/implant type/implant rupture** (?) **in a 66-year-old woman.** Both breasts underwent silicone implantation years before for cosmetic reasons. MRI raised suspicion of a left-sided implant rupture due to gel bleed (**a**). The implants were removed and examined.

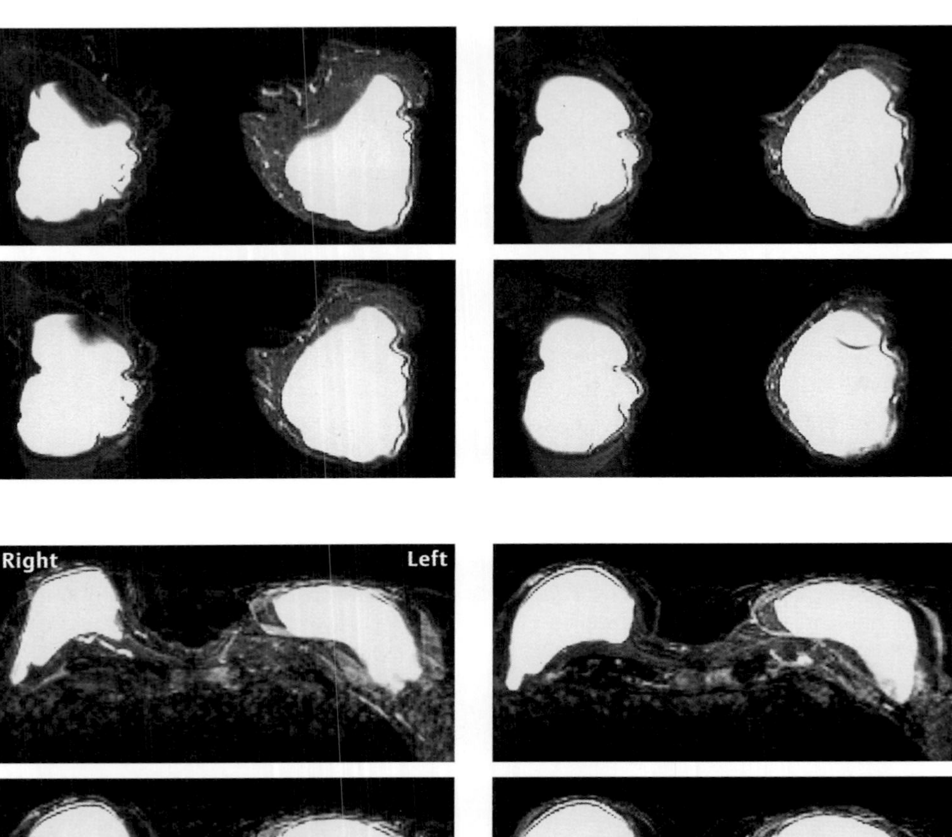


**a** *Fat-suppressed inversion-recovery MR* sequences show deep wrinkling of the implant surfaces with silicone oil outside the implants (e.g., **c–D/21–22**). A linguine sign is not present (upper two pairs of images coronal, lower two pairs transverse).

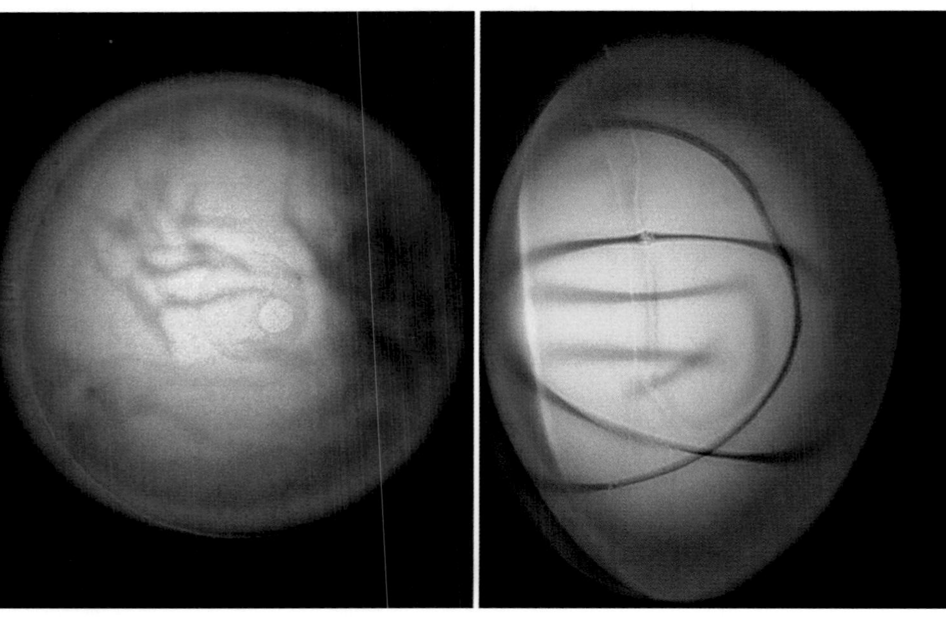

**b** *Mammography* of the right implant under compression shows numerous lines and streaks caused by implant seams and surface wrinkles (compare with **d**). *Left:* The implant was imaged from the front. *Right:* The implant was imaged from the side.

**Fig. 5.102 Gel bleed/implant type/implant rupture.** *(continued)*

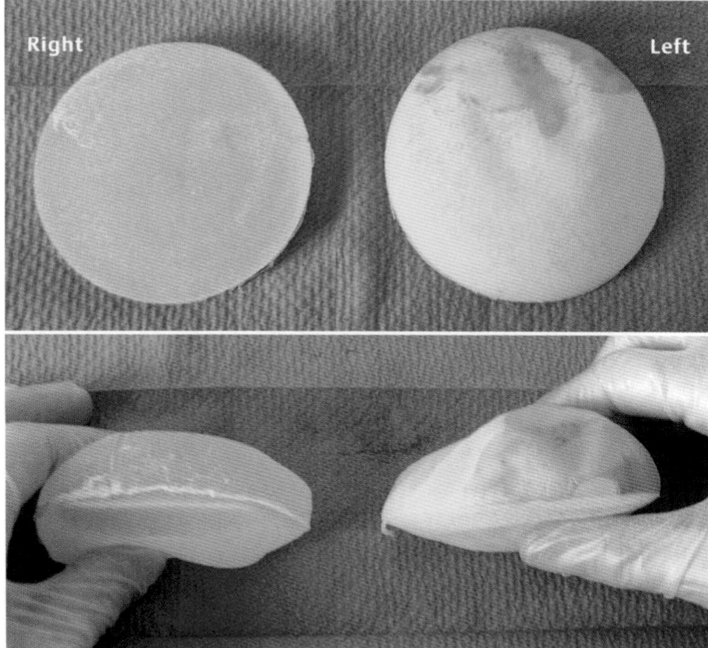


**c** *Appearance of the implants.* Front views (above) show fibrous encapsulation of the left implant (reddish-white coating) while the right implant is clear. Portions of the outer shell are visible on the upper portion of the left implant (**N/26–27**). Side views (below) show the outer shell "baked onto" the left implant (reddish-yellow coating, **N/21**).

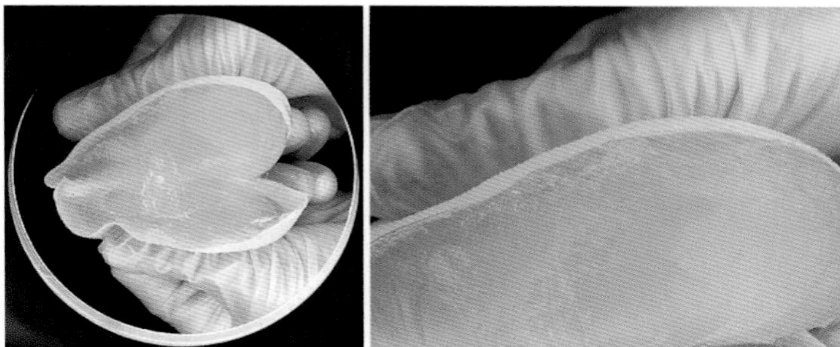

**d** *Cut surface of the right implant* (compare with **c**). Silicone has a uniform greenish-yellow color and a relatively firm, nonfluid consistency. No cavity is present between the silicone and capsule.

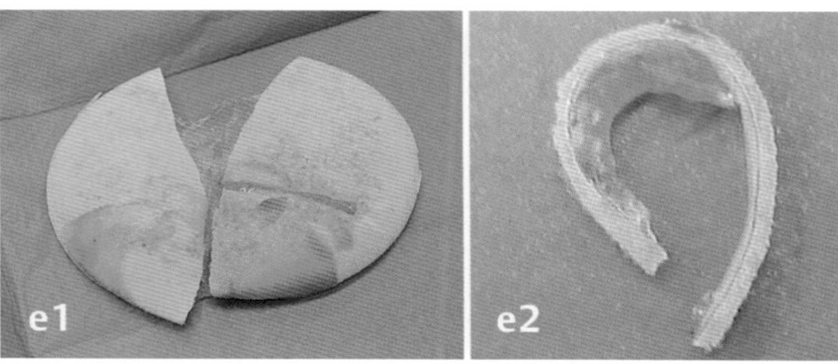


**e1, e2** *View of the left implant.* The pathologist cut a specimen from the reddish portion of the outer shell (fibrous encapsulation at **Q–q/25**).

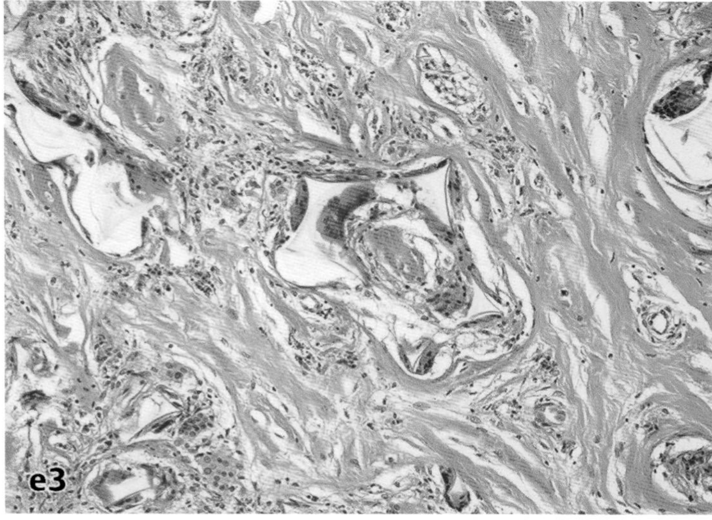


**e3** *Histologic section* from the outer shell (80× magnification) shows a firm, fiber-rich capsule with foreign body granulomas and silicone particles (p. e. **R–S/18**, pink) (image courtesy of Hans-Helmut Dahm, Esslingen).

**Question 1 on Fig. 5.102**

*What type of implants are these?*

(**a**) Single-lumen implants
(**b**) Double-lumen implants
(**c**) Triple-lumen implants (gel/water/gel)

→ **Answer on p. 378**

**Question 2 on Fig. 5.102**

*How would you interpret the MRI changes?*

(**a**) Gel bleed
(**b**) Partial rupture of the outer implant shell
(**c**) Complete rupture of the whole implant

→ **Answer on p. 378**

▶ **Fig. 5.102 f–h**

**Fig. 5.102 Breast implants and fibrous encapsulation (anatomic aspects).** *(continued)*

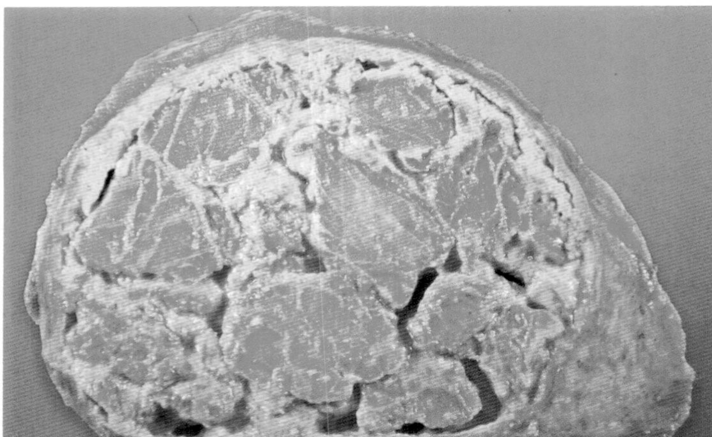

**f** *Breast augmentation* with a *fat allograft*. Old, indurated fatty tissue with calcified areas of fat necrosis (light) and an irregular fibrous capsule.

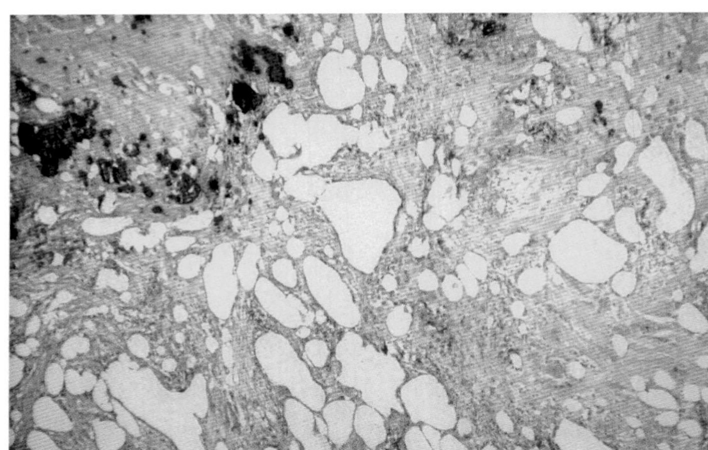

**f1** *Histology:* fat necrosis with abundant connective tissue and interstitial calcifications (upper left).

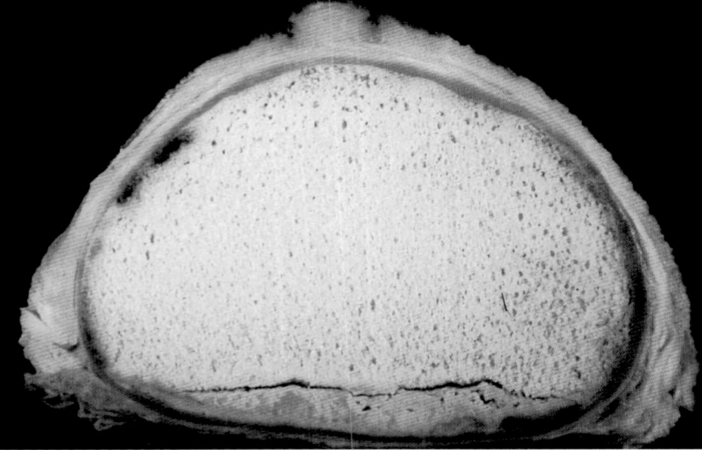

**g** *Soybean oil implant*. Spongy, porous soybean oil. Thin capsule with small hemorrhagic areas at upper left and lower right.

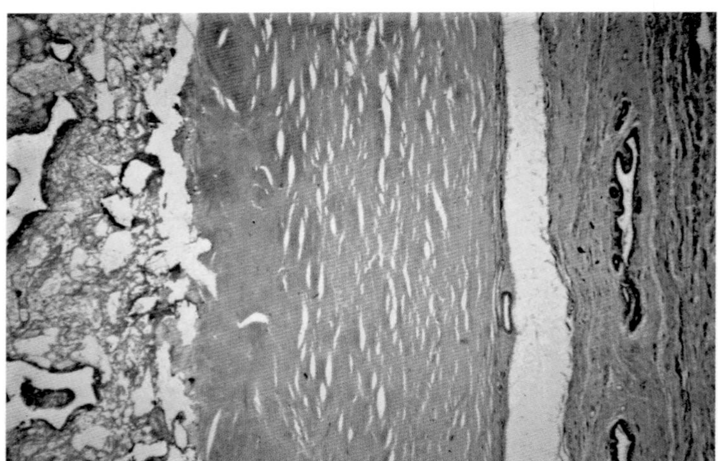

**g1** *Histology:* fibrous encapsulation. Cholesterol crystals and granulation tissue are visible on the left with tough, fibrous capsular tissue at the center. Compressed glandular parenchyma rich in connective tissue is visible on the right (**J–j/14–18**).

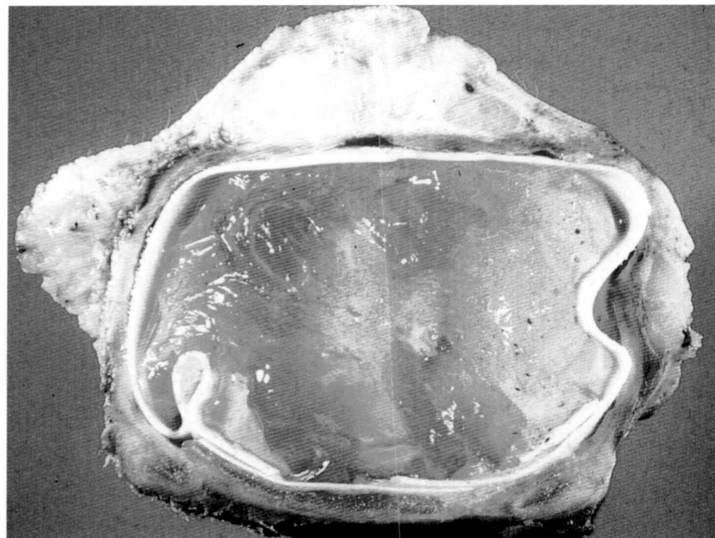

**h** *Implant rupture* following silicone breast augmentation. The fibrous capsule shows surface buckling, particularly at lower left (**B–b/6**). Tears have occurred near the chest wall (below).

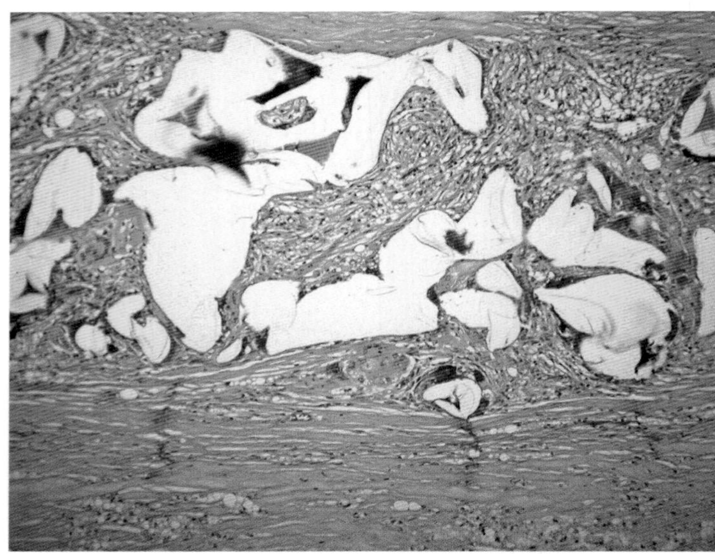

**h1** *Histology:* tough fibrous capsule with silicone inclusions (gel bleeding) (images courtesy of Roland Bässler, Fulda).

**Fig. 5.103 A 63-year-old woman. Implant leak/fat necrosis/DCIS** (?) with pronounced fibrous encapsulation (**a–c**) decades after bilateral silicone implantations. For some time the patient has been aware of a firm, slightly mobile nodule at the 10-o'clock position in the upper outer quadrant of the right breast (**a**). Benign–malignant differentiation is required.

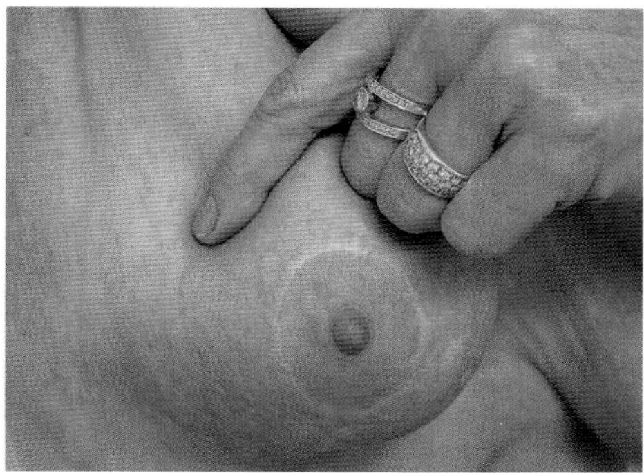

**a** *Clinical appearance* of the right breast. The patient is indicating the site of a relatively fixed nodule that is not associated with skin retraction.

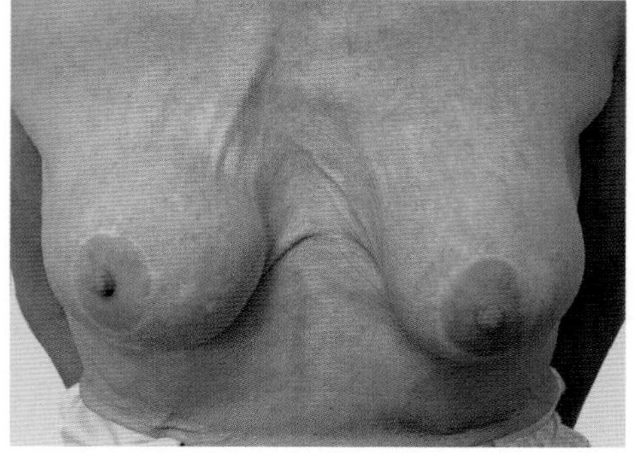

**b** *Clinical appearance* of both breasts with the arms lowered. The right implant has undergone fibrous encapsulation. Despite skin folds above and directly over the sternum (cleavage), the patient is satisfied with the cosmetic result. Normal scars are present on each side.

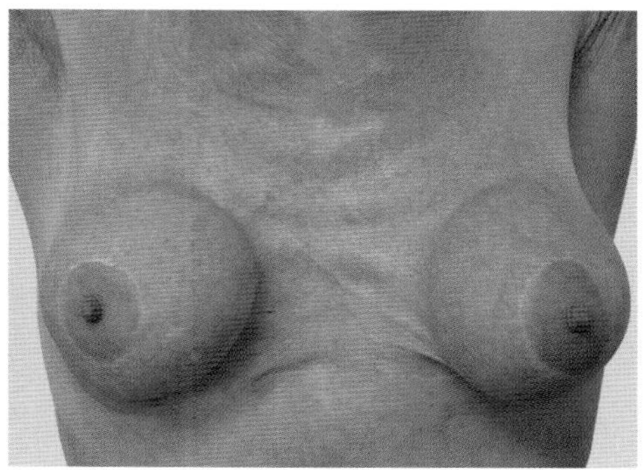

**c** *Clinical appearance* of both breasts with the arms raised. Fibrous encapsulation is visible on both sides. The skin folds are effaced in this arm position.

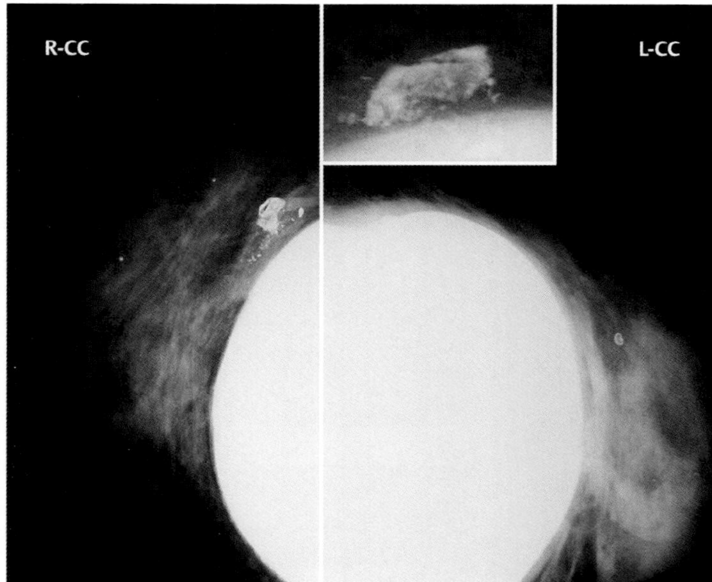


**d** *Bilateral craniocaudal mammograms* show smooth implant borders with a clumped calcification in the area of the right-sided nodule (**l/16**, see inset). Heavy fibrous encapsulation is visible on the left side.

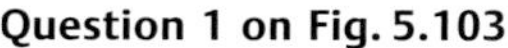

**Question 1 on Fig. 5.103**

*Why did this patient have prosthetic implantations?*

(**a**) Cosmetic reasons
(**b**) Bilateral subcutaneous mastectomies
(**c**) Subcutaneous mastectomy on the right side and cosmetic implantation on the left

→ **Answer on p. 378**

**Question 2 on Fig. 5.103**

*How would you interpret the calcified nodule?*

(**a**) Comedo-type DCIS adjacent to fat necrosis
(**b**) Old implant leak with calcified granulation tissue on silicone particles
(**c**) Fresh implant leak with silicone extravasation

→ **Answer on p. 378**

Right Left

**e** *T1-weighted MR* images show smooth implant borders with slight posterior wrinkling of the right implant and a mushroom-shaped lateral protrusion corresponding to the palpable nodule (**k–L/3+7**). The breast parenchyma is smaller and denser on the left side than on the right.

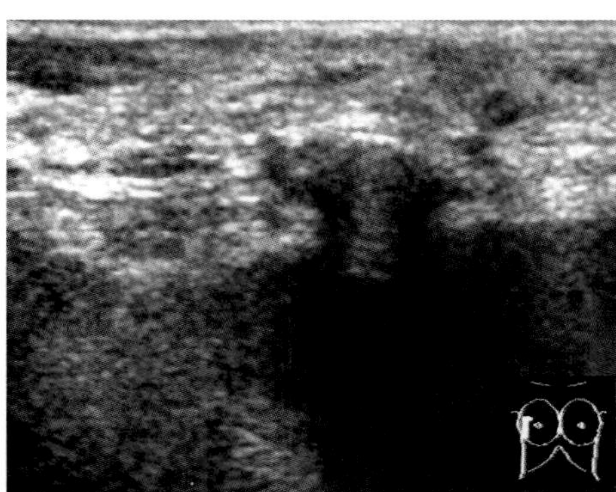

**f** *Sonogram* of the right breast at the level of the nodule. The implant shows a combination of low echogenicity and (at left) a bright snowstorm pattern (**q–S/5–7**) consistent with gel bleed. The upper contour of the implant is interrupted by a diamond-shaped, hypoechoic, inhomogeneous structure with an associated circumscribed "snowstorm" (**r–s/7–8**).

**Fig. 5.104 A 70-year-old woman had a mastectomy in 1986 followed by esthetic breast reconstruction with a silicone implant.** A leak developed in 1998 (**a**), and the implant was exchanged (**a1**). A reasonably good cosmetic result was obtained with a single-lumen silicone implant (**a2**). In 2007, two months after trauma to the left breast (blow from a golf ball), the breast was greatly swollen (**b**) with fluid accumulation around the implant and no evidence of tumor cells or blood in needle aspirate (F in **b1**). The fluid is also well demonstrated by MRI (b2). **Cause?**

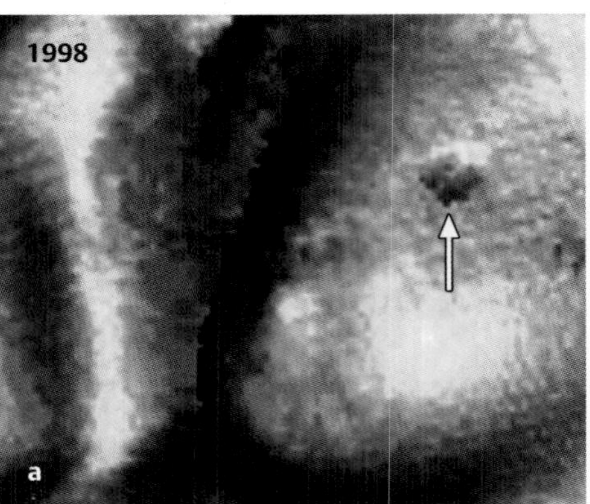


**a** *MRI* (3D reconstruction) of the left implant in 1998 shows a supramamillary defect (arrow).

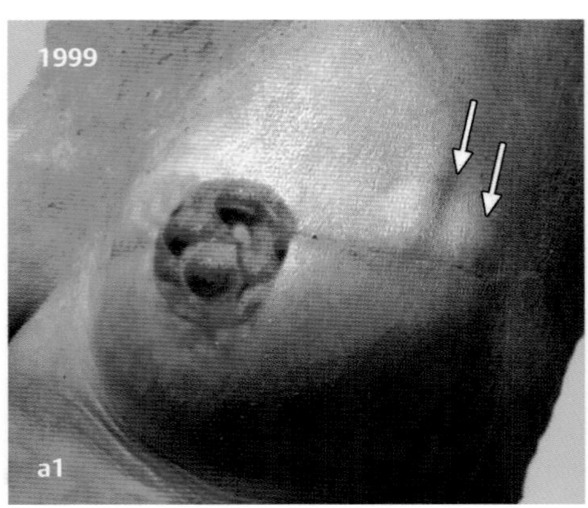


**a1** *Clinical appearance* after the implant was exchanged. Note the slight lateral undulation of the skin (arrows).

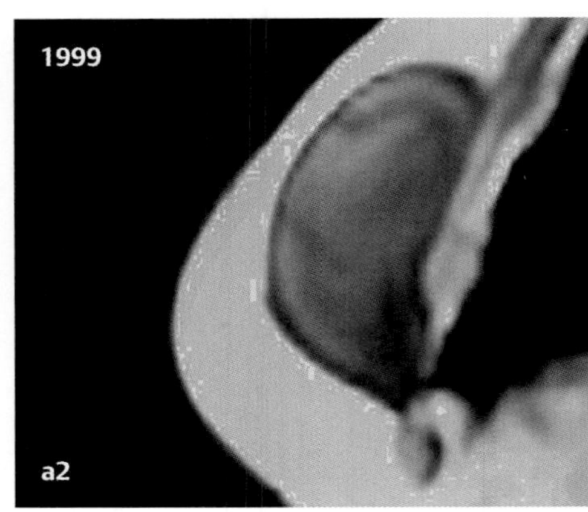


**a2** *MRI*. Sagittal image shows the smooth-walled (single-lumen) implant in longitudinal section.

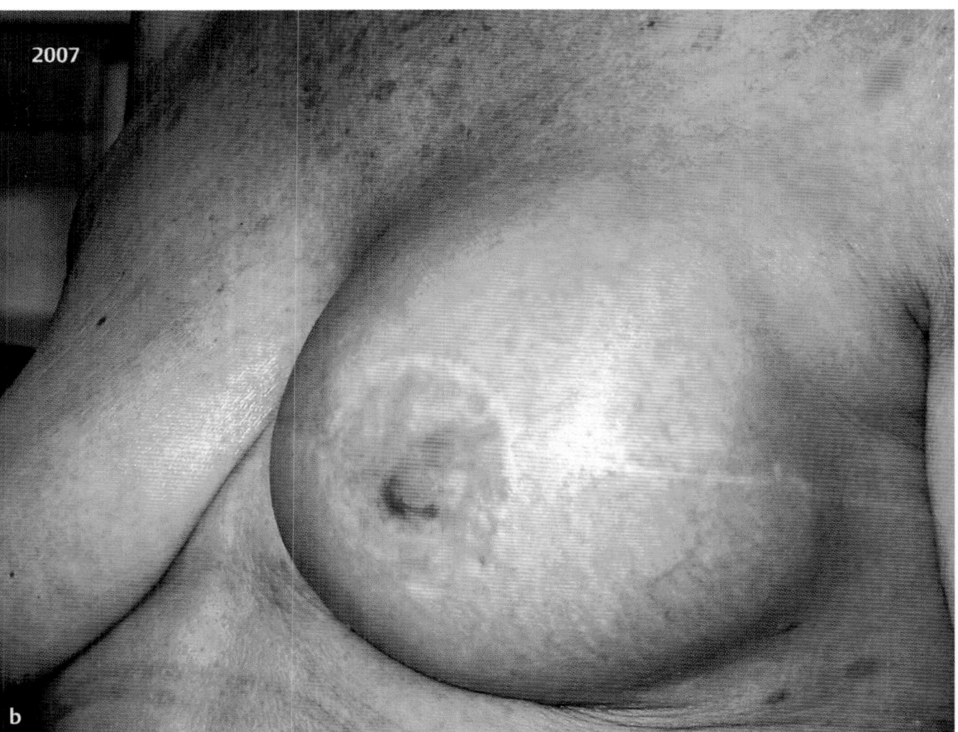


**b** Clinical inspection of the left breast in 2007 shows significant swelling.

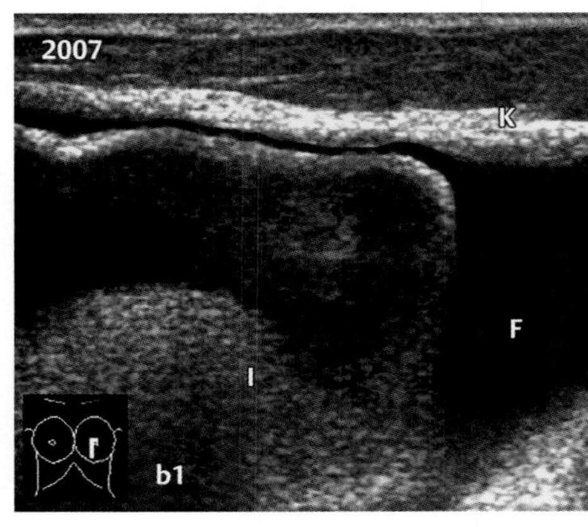


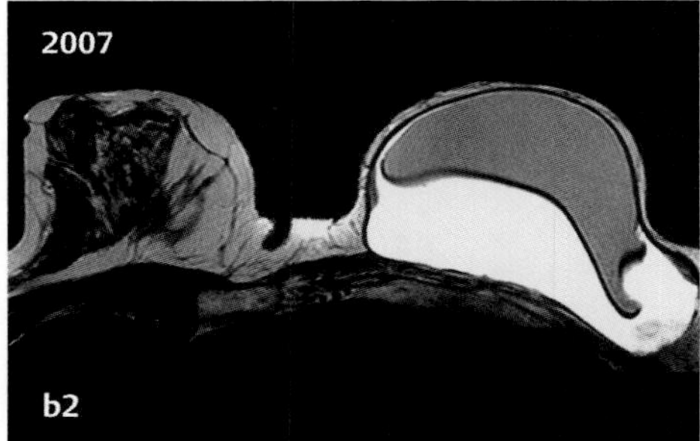


**b1** *Ultrasound* shows copious fluid accumulation between the silicone implant and outer capsule (I = implant, F = fluid, K = capsule).
**b2** *MRI*. T1-weighted image of the right breast appears normal. The implant in the left breast (dark) is separated from the pectoral muscle (dark) by copious fluid (white).

**Question on Fig. 5.104**

*How would you interpret the findings in the left breast 2007?*

(**a**) Inflammatory exudate
(**b**) Neoplastic exudate
(**c**) Implant displacement

→ **Answer on p. 378**

## Positron Emission Tomography with Computed Tomography

Positron emission tomography (PET) is currently the best scintigraphic technique for mapping the three-dimensional distribution of radiotracer activity within the body. PET is up to 50 times more sensitive than conventional nuclear medicine techniques such as single-photon emission computed tomography (SPECT). Today there are three branches of medicine in which PET offers definite advantages over other imaging modalities: oncology, cardiology, and neurology. The indications for PET were established by leading nuclear medicine specialists and clinicians based on recent consensus conferences (Reske et al. 1997).

While PET is a very costly modality, it allows for accurate, comprehensive staging in the diagnosis and treatment of breast cancer. PET examinations are useful in:

- Staging of locally advanced breast cancer for the exclusion of distant metastases (if this would have therapeutic implications)
- Detection of axillary lymph node metastases from an unknown primary tumor (negative mammograms, ultrasound and MRI; CUP syndrome, see p. 202)
- Detection of local axillary recurrence (and exclusion of other metastases in nearby lymph nodes or peripheral tissues)
- Diagnosis of intramammary metastases from an unknown primary tumor (renal, thyroid, etc.)
- Evaluation of treatment response of metastatic breast cancer in symptomatic women who cannot be evaluated by other means (tumor markers, visible and measurable lymph node metastases, etc.)
- Planning the excision of presumed isolated pulmonary or hepatic metastases (metastatic surgery)

PET is a costly and technically complex modality that places stringent demands on patient endurance. When used for the above indications, however, PET is definitely rewarding when we compare its costs with those of many other modalities such as endoscopy, radiography, and other nuclear medicine studies. Unnecessary curative therapies are costly as well, and they can be avoided in patients found to have disseminated disease that would have been missed without PET scanning.

On the other hand, not even PET can detect all neoplasms. Low-grade (G1) tumors are particularly likely to be missed on PET scans, whereas high-grade tumors are generally detected owing to their increased level of glucose metabolism.

Samples of PET (PET-CT, **Fig. 5.109**), especially in the follow-up of breast-cancer-treatment, are shown in **Figs. 5.105–5.109**.

**Fig. 5.105 Rising tumor marker levels after breast-conserving surgery. Local recurrence? Second tumor? Disseminated disease?** This 48-year-old woman underwent breast-conserving surgery of the left breast (**a, b**) because of a G3 neoplasm in 2001. Slight retraction of the medial portion of the scar was noted during the 2 years after surgery (**b, c**). Mammographic follow-up at 11 months shows no abnormalities (**e, f**). Question: What is the cause of the rising tumor markers?

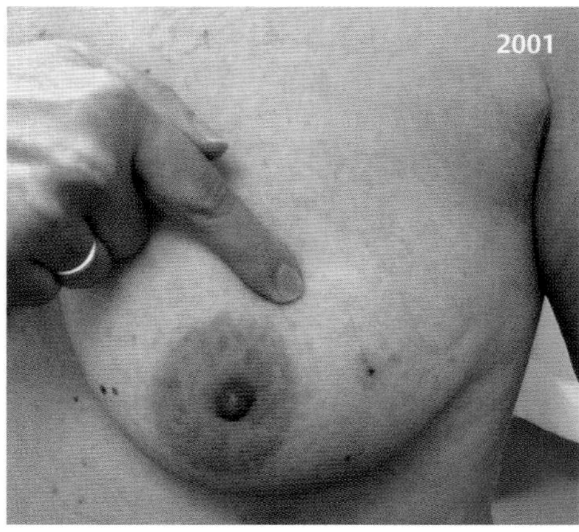


**a** *Clinical appearance* of the left breast on initial presentation. The index finger marks the site of a palpable nodule.

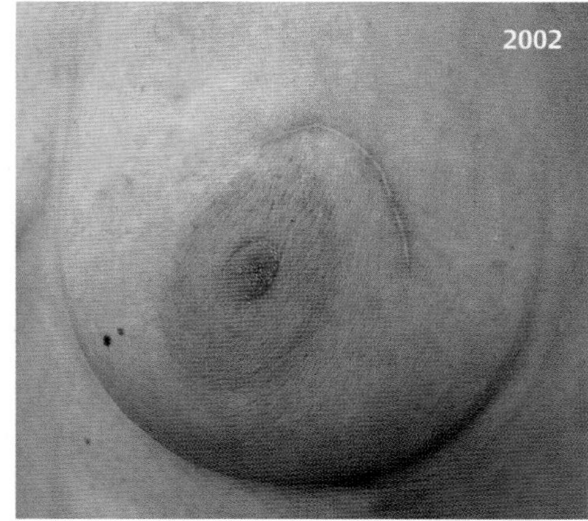


**b** *Clinical inspection* of the left breast 11 months after breast-conserving surgery shows a small cicatricial keloid with normal breast contours and slight supra-areolar skin retraction (**o/8**).

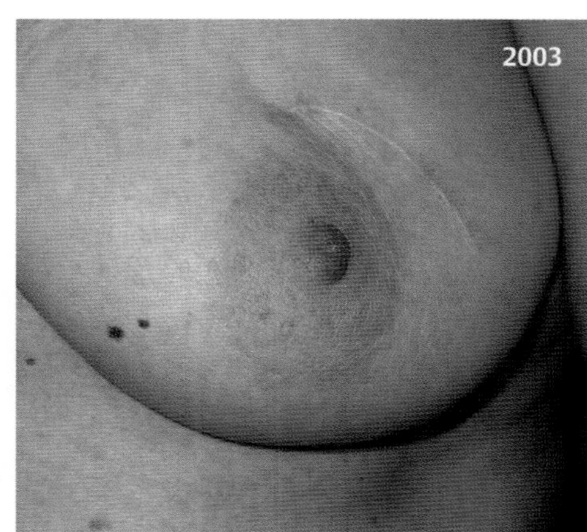


**c** *Clinical inspection* 12 months later shows slight retraction and pallor of the supra-areolar scar (**r–S/9**).

▶ **Fig. 5.105 d–i**

**Fig. 5.105 Rising tumor marker levels after breast-conserving surgery.** *(continued)*

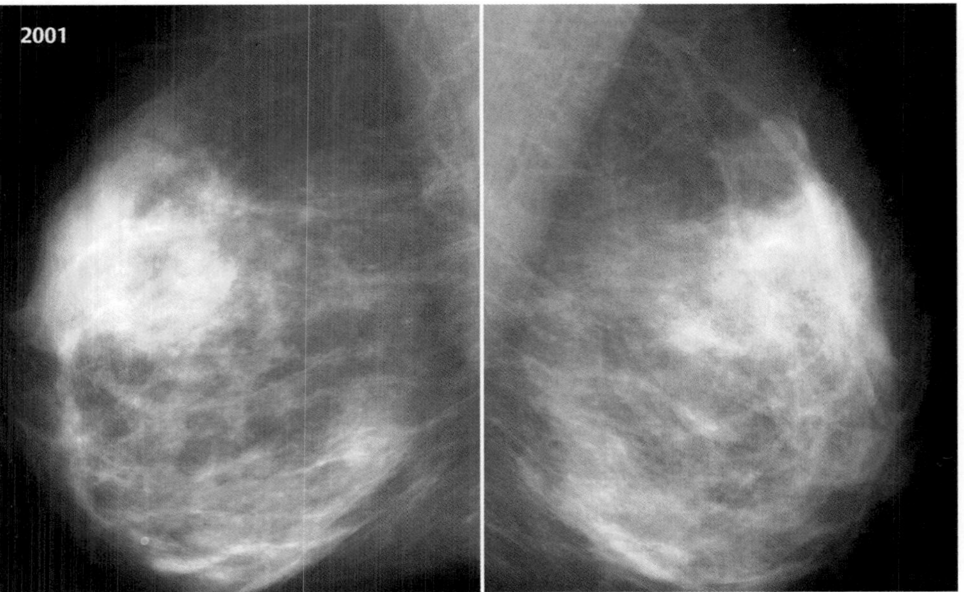


**d** *Initial bilateral oblique mammograms* show radiodense breasts with no detectable tumor (ACR 3, BIRADS 2, **P**GMI). Bilateral craniocaudal mammograms (not shown) were normal.

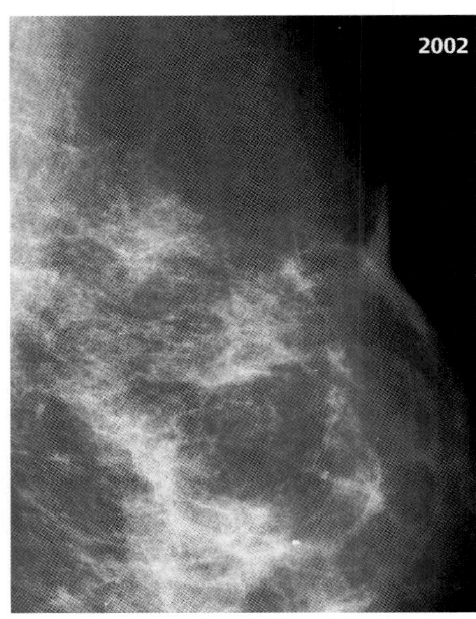


**e** *Oblique mammogram* of the left breast 11 months after therapy (corresponding to (**b**) shows a scar with associated skin retraction and a faint, nonspecific subcutaneous density (**I–i/23–24**).

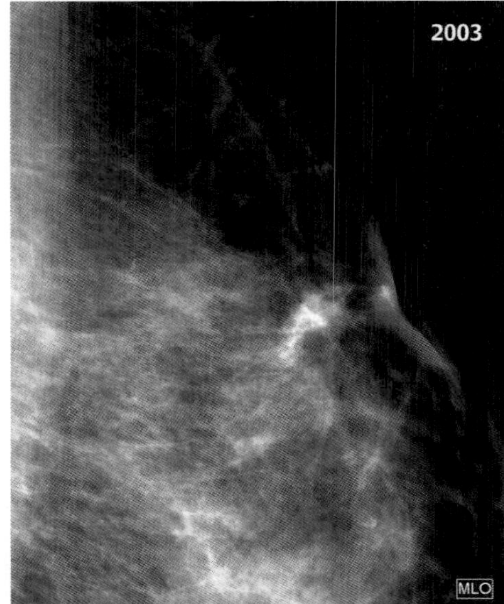


**f** *Oblique mammogram* of the left breast 18 months later shows progressive scarring (**C/13**) with skin retraction but no other changes relative to the previous examination. Increasing radiolucency is noted in mammograms **e** and **f** due to the regression of TDLUs in response to antiestrogen therapy.

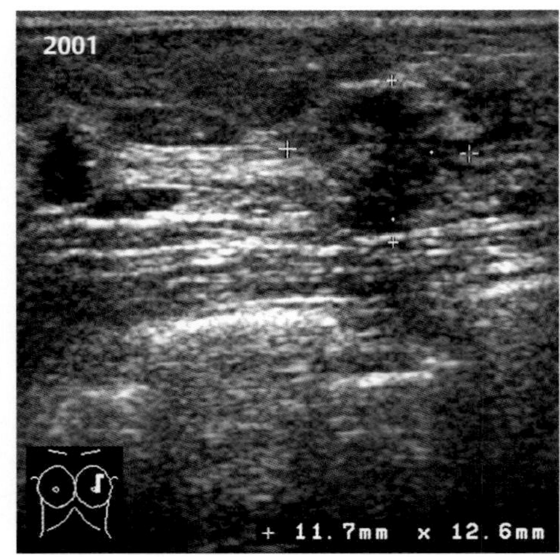


**g** *Initial sonogram* shows two hypoechoic nodules with irregular margins (**d/15, F–G/15–16**).

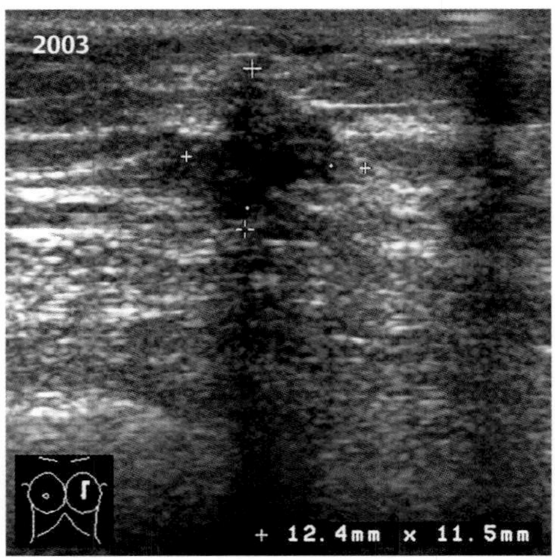


**h** *Sonogram* of the left breast at 18 months shows a hypoechoic zone in the scar area with posterior acoustic shadowing. CNB yielded three cores containing scar tissue but no tumor.

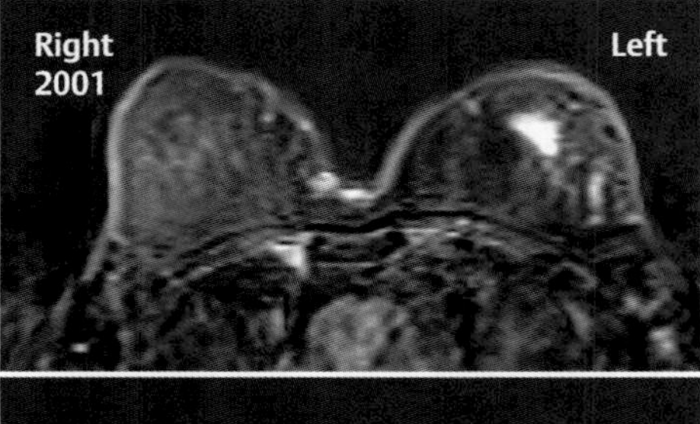


**i** *MR subtraction* images before treatment show multifocal tumor growth with small and large foci of intense gadolinium enhancement in the left breast (**f–G/3** and **f–G/7**) (only the main focus is shown). Moderately diffuse gadolinium enhancement is also noted in the right breast. The enhancing foci in the sternal portion of the right breast (**e–F/2** and **e–F/6**) and retrosternal region are blood vessels.

**Question on Fig. 5.105**

*On the basis of the images, where is the cause of the rising tumor markers located?*

(**a**) Scarred area in the left breast
(**b**) Left axilla
(**c**) Neither (**a**) nor (**b**)

→ **Answer on p. 379**

**Fig. 5.106 Local recurrence, fat necrosis, or mastitis (?) in a 56-year-old woman** 3 years after breast-conserving surgery of the left breast plus whole-breast radiation with a boost. The patient (a health professional) had heard of a new method (positron emission/computed tomography, PET/CT) for excluding local recurrence and metastases and underwent the study. PET/CT shows no suspicious findings elsewhere in the body but does show a hypermetabolic focus in the operated left breast. Mammography shows no abnormalities in this area other than a tissue defect left by breast-conserving surgery. This region is very tender to pressure.

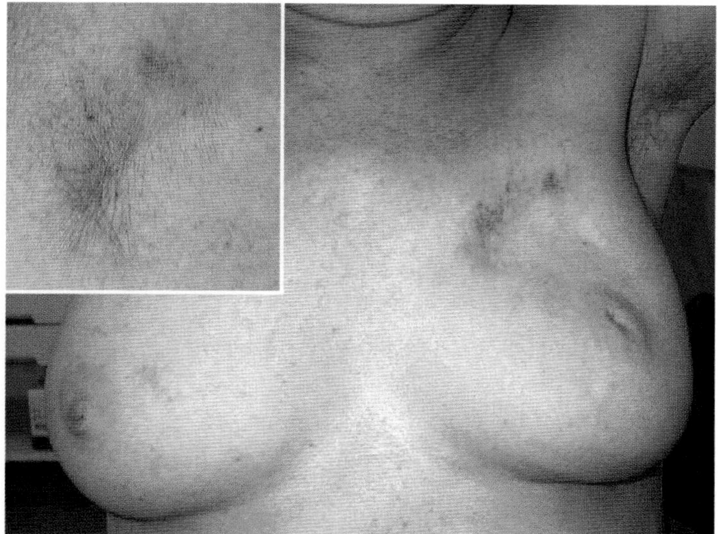

**a** *Clinical inspection* 3 years after breast-conserving therapy shows a circumscribed, tender skin depression and redness (telangiectasis) over the former tumor site (**N/22–24**) (see inset).

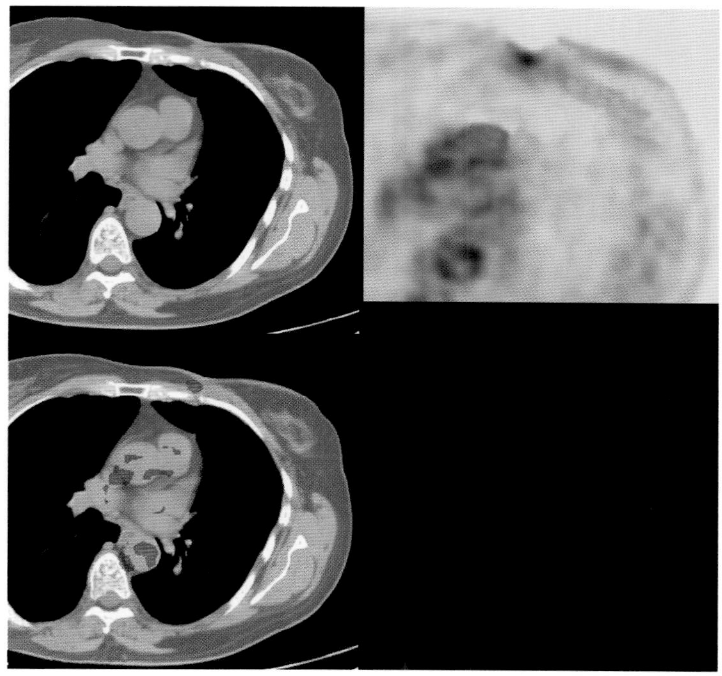

**b** *Positron emission/computed tomography (PET/CT)* shows a circumscribed subcutaneous focus (red on CT [**Q/20**]) over the upper inner quadrant of the left breast (images courtesy of Heiner Bihl, Stuttgart). PET demonstrates a hypermetabolic focus at upper right (**S/25**).

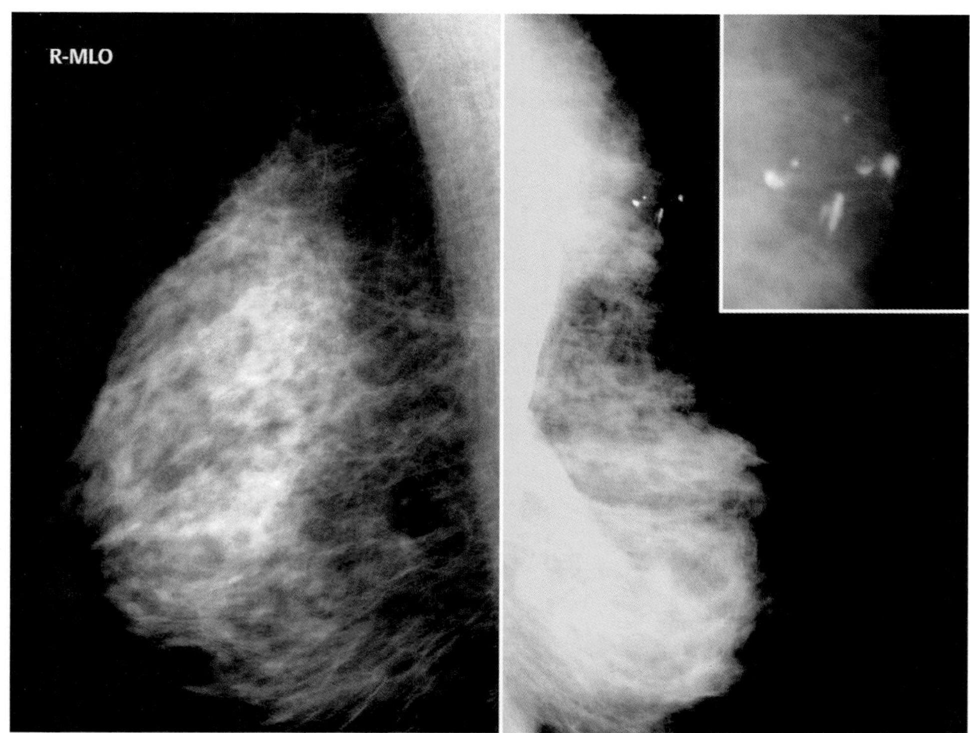


**c** *Bilateral oblique mammograms* show a dense left breast (shown with different windows) and coarse subcutaneous calcifications (**O/11**) (magnified view at upper right), cicatricial changes, and a relatively large tissue defect with no evidence of a tumor (ACR 3 right, **P**GMI, ACR 4 left, BIRADS 2).

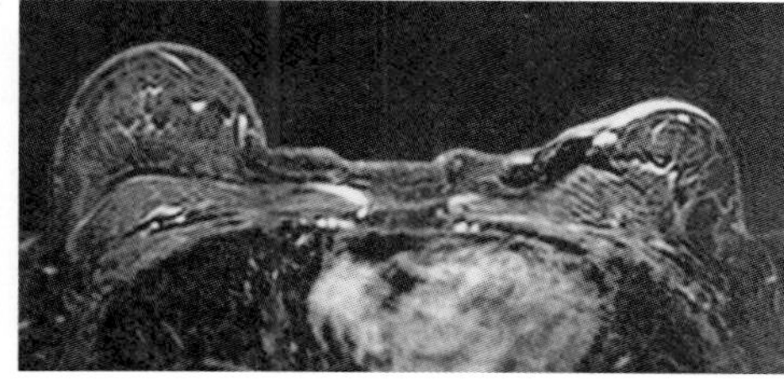

**d** *Craniocaudal MR subtraction* image shows circumscribed gadolinium enhancement over the upper inner quadrant of the left breast (**s/12–13**).

▶ **Fig. 5.106 e–g**

**Fig. 5.106 Local recurrence, fat necrosis, or mastitis.** *(continued)*

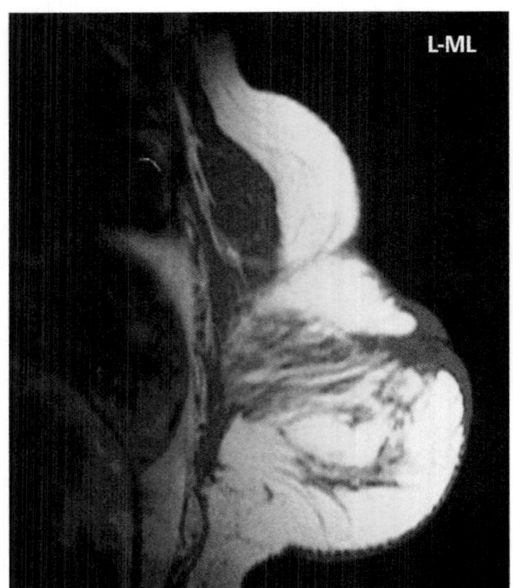


**e** *MR survey image* shows skin deformation with no other abnormalities (**C/24–25**) (MRI-images courtesy of Levente Mitrovics, Ludwigsburg).

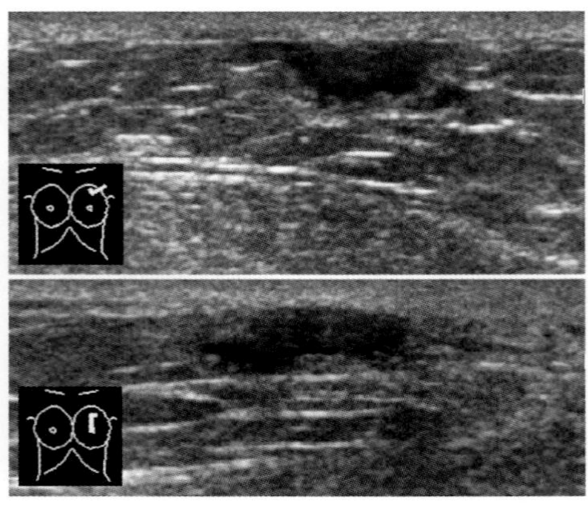

**f** *Sonograms* of the left breast show a defect in the subcutaneous fat with mixed smooth and irregular margins (**F/24 + 27**).

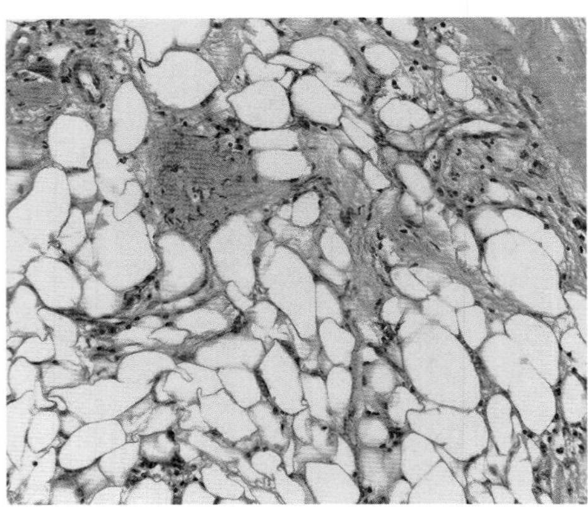

**g** *Histologic section* shows fibrotic fatty tissue with lipophage granulomas (image courtesy of Hans-Helmut Dahm, Esslingen).

**Question on Fig. 5.106**

*How would you interpret the PET/CT focus detected in the left breast?*

(**a**) Fat necrosis

(**b**) Local recurrence

(**c**) Focal mastitis

→ **Answer on p. 380**

## Interventional Procedures: Fine Needle Aspiration (FNA), Core Needle Biopsy (CNB), Vacuum Biopsy (VB), Preoperative Localization, and Specimen Radiography

Interventional procedures are a better option than open surgical biopsy for the investigation of suspicious mammographic, sonographic, and/or MR findings. They can eliminate the need for 25% of open biopsies and the associated burdens on patients (hospital stay, informed consent, general anesthesia, dressing changes, scars, surgical morbidity, etc.) while reducing hospital costs. In 2008 a new *ACR Practice Guideline for the Performance of Screening and Diagnostic Mammography* was adopted. There are other ACR guidelines for the performance of stereotactically (ultrasound guided) interventions from 2006. Similar guidelines are issued in Europe from *EUSOBI* (www.eusobi.org) and *EUSOMA*. ACR guidelines and standards are published annually with an effective date of October 1 in the year in which amended, revised, or approved by the ACR Council.

According to current guidelines in Germany, interventional procedures for a breast abnormality should be scheduled within 5 working days. The procedure that is most cost-effective and best tolerated by the patient should always be selected.

Interventional techniques are used mainly for the investigation of BIRADS 4 and 5 lesions, the goal being to establish a preoperative histopathologic diagnosis so that only patients with breast cancer will be hospitalized while excisional biopsies for benign lesions will be kept to a minimum. The ratio of benign to malignant cases should be at least 1 : 4, which means that 75% of all patients who come to the hospital for breast surgery have a histologically proved diagnosis. The ratio at our center, for example, is 1 : 5. The diagnostician at a breast center should work closely with the pathologist and surgeon and use all available test results to establish an accurate, histologically confirmed diagnosis that will contribute to an optimum treatment outcome.

The decision whether to use fine-needle-aspiration (FNA, see **Fig. 5.108**, p. 236), core-needle biopsy (CNB, see **Fig. 5.107**, p. 232 ff), or vacuum biopsy (VB, see **Fig. 5.109**, p. 240 f) depends on the clinical question and the accessibility of the lesion. CNB is better than FNA for establishing a preoperative cancer diagnosis because tissue cores are better for making a *definitive histologic evaluation* and performing *immunohistochemical tests* (receptor and HER-2/neu status, protease determination, etc.). VB is not always necessary for the investigation of lesions detected by mammography, ultrasound, or MRI, and the need for VB should be critically assessed because it is more costly than CNB and FNA and causes greater trauma, making it more difficult to achieve an R0 resection while providing the same degree of diagnostic accuracy (see p. 250).

CNB, like VB, is a reliable technique for tissue sampling. VB offers significant advantages, particularly its ability to supply more representative tissue. But it should not be used for all calcifications and benign changes and should be reserved basically for the investigation of local recurrences; the removal of fibroadenomas, papillomas, and gynecomastia; and perhaps even for small foci of FEA and ADH (see p. 35) when pathology confirms the presence of a minimal lesion in an otherwise negative sample.

Both digital stereotactic CNB and VB reach their limits in the case of lesions that are subcutaneous, retroareolar, axillary, or located near the chest wall. Subcutaneous lesions may be accessible to punch biopsy. FNA can sample lesions at all of these sites.

In a German multicenter study (Kettritz et al. 2004) only 30% of the VB samples were diagnosed as malignant (7% invasive carcinoma, 15% DCIS, 5% ADH, 0.6% LCIS). Forty-nine of the 2874 vacuum biopsies were failures, meaning that for various reasons a representative histological sample was not obtained. The following problems arose in 72 of these biopsies:

- In 19 patients the suspicious calcifications could not be located by digital palpation because of their minuscule size.
- Twenty-seven lesions were located too close to the skin or chest wall.
- Multiple tissue cores taken from 19 patients contained no calcifications ($n = 8$) or the result was not representative for other reasons.
- In one patient the coordinates were incorrectly defined.
- Vacuum biopsy was discontinued in four patients due to pain.
- In two cases the procedure was terminated due to a technical failure.

With all due respect for the excellent scientific quality of this multicenter study, it should be noted that the results of the vacuum biopsies were not truly optimal when compared with CNB (setting aside FNA for the moment)—though in fairness it should be added that this study had to contend with selection criteria and other indeterminate factors from five different breast centers.

FNA is recommended for lesions so unfavorable that they are not accessible to CNB or VB, provided an experienced cytologist is available to interpret the smear. With the declining trend in the utilization of FNA in Germany, these experts are becoming more difficult to find there; this is less the case in countries like the United States, the United Kingdom, and Sweden, for example.

A patient undergoing digital stereotactic biopsy may be placed in a sitting position (GE, Senovision, Siemens), in the supine position (Fischer, Giotto, Lorat) (see **Fig. 5.22**, p. 104), or in left or right lateral decubitus on a simple height-adjustable table. All sonographically visible lesions can be biopsied (FNA or CNB) under ultrasound guidance to reduce costs, or they can be removed with a hand-held VB system (Atec, Biosys, Coramate, Vacora, and others) since ultrasound-guided biopsy is more economical than digital stereotactic biopsy (see **Table 5.13**, p. 253). The old belief that interventional procedures may promote breast cancer by *inoculation metastasis* at the puncture site has not proven true for benign or malignant lesions despite a worldwide increase in percutaneous biopsies. We have not found a single instance of inoculation metastasis in approximately 120 000 biopsies (FNA, CNB, VB) performed over a 35-year period.

The patient should be told to wear comfortable clothing and that a compression bandage will be applied. Whenever possible, the patient should be accompanied by a friend or family member who can drive her home. This is particularly important following a vacuum biopsy, which requires large amounts of local anesthetic with epinephrine added.

The patient should receive instructions on what to do if the bandage is no longer fitting properly or if postprocedure bleeding occurs. She is told exactly when the bandage will be removed, when she can shower again, and when she can resume athletic activities. The physician or one of the physician's assistants should address these questions prior to the procedure. Information sheets are available (in several languages) from Thieme Compliance GmbH (www.procompliance.de) that cover the principal complications and behavioral measures.

**For more information on interventional procedures, see the ACR guidelines for "Nonoperative Diagnostic Procedures and Reporting in Breast Cancer" of the NHSBSP at www.cancerscreening.nhs.nk/breastscreen/puplications/99-08.html, or in Europe EUSOBI at www.eusobi.org.**

### Tip

**Before every interventional procedure, the patient should attend a general consultation that includes inspection and palpation of the breast. Based on available mammograms and sonograms, it is decided which procedure would be the best for that patient. Possible complications are also disclosed at this time. Standard information sheets should be used.**

Any of the following **complications** may arise:

- Hematoma
- Inflammation
- Pneumothorax during FNA or CNB of lesions located near the pleura
- Choroid plexus lesions during axillary or supraclavicular biopsy
- Allergic reactions to local anesthetics
- The possibility that the biopsy may miss the lesion, yielding a false-negative result

The practice at our center is to perform ultrasound-guided FNA and CNB during the patient's regular breast appointment. This procedure takes approximately 15 minutes and eliminates the need for an additional appointment. This may leave less time for detailed disclosure, but even if time is short the patient should definitely be questioned about any allergies to local anesthetics and a possible bleeding diathesis.

Digital stereotactic interventions take approximately one hour. This includes the interview with the patient and family members, disrobing, the induction and maintenance of brief general anesthesia if required (e.g., with propofol), the biopsy itself, collection of the material, specimen radiography, the explanation of protocols, patient discharge, transfer of the material to pathology, cleaning the equipment, and preparing the room for the next intervention. A hectic atmosphere due to a hurried schedule should be avoided in interventional procedures, as it makes the patient and staff nervous. It is prudent to review the patient's records on the day before the scheduled procedure and discuss the protocol with the technologist.

It is possible during VB or CNB to make a cytologic smear from the last tissue sample and send it together with the biopsy tissue to the pathologist or to a cytologist. This way, one can have the preliminary report for the patient immediately or in a few hours. This **"contact cytology" (CC)** is effective in solid tumors, but not so reliable in biopsies of microcalcifications. The waiting time for histologic results of the intervention (sometimes, in spite of guidelines, 2 weeks and more!) is a considerable psychological burden for the patient. In our center the waiting time is 1–3 days.

It is not our practice to take a mammogram after the completion of an interventional procedure. Either calcifications are visible in the biopsy specimen radiograph (see **Fig. 5.107f**), or the biopsy will have to be repeated if the pathologist does not describe calcifications.

If it is found during the procedure that the lesion is not accessible to CNB due to an unfavorable location (e.g., subcutaneous), FNA should be performed. At our center we immediately stain and examine the aspirated cells and report the result to the patient. The specimens are then sent to the pathologist who will confirm or modify the immediate diagnosis.

**Fig. 5.107 Technique of digital stereotactic core-needle biopsy (D-CNB).**

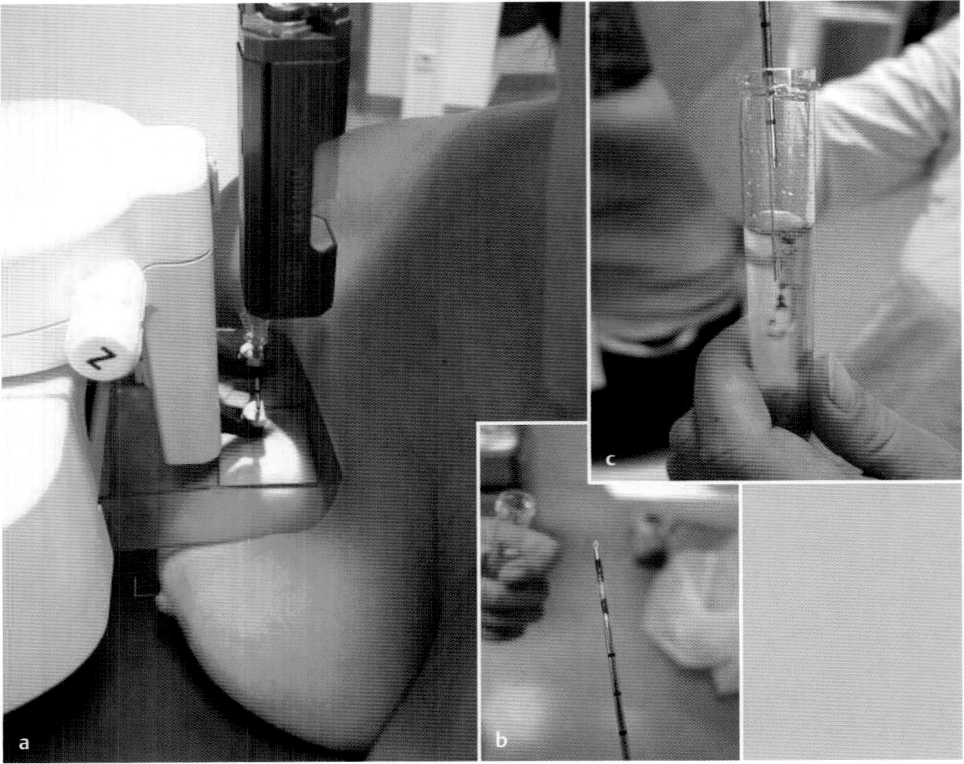

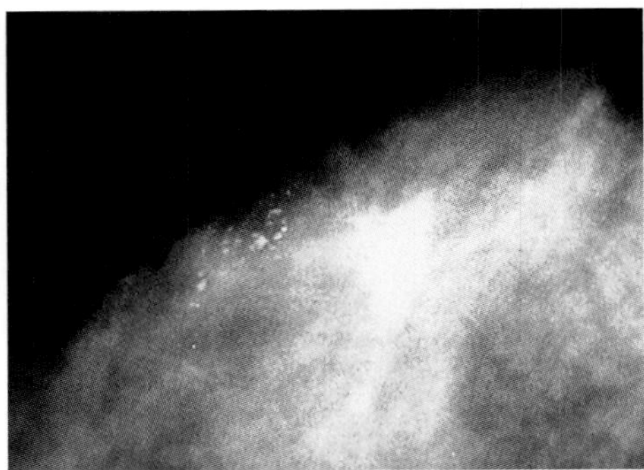

**d** *Craniocaudal spot compression mammogram* of atypical clustered microcalcifications (BIRADS 4).

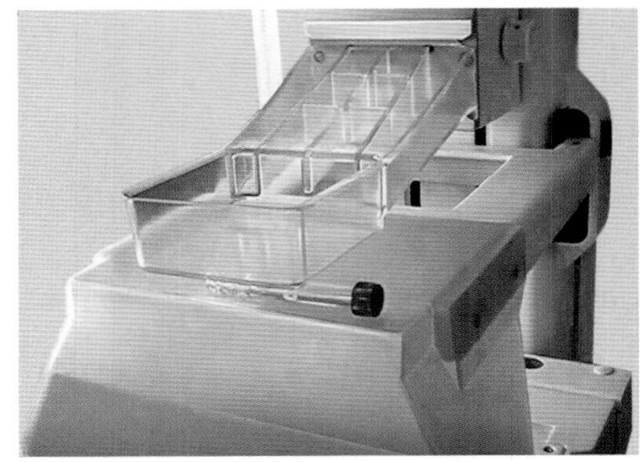

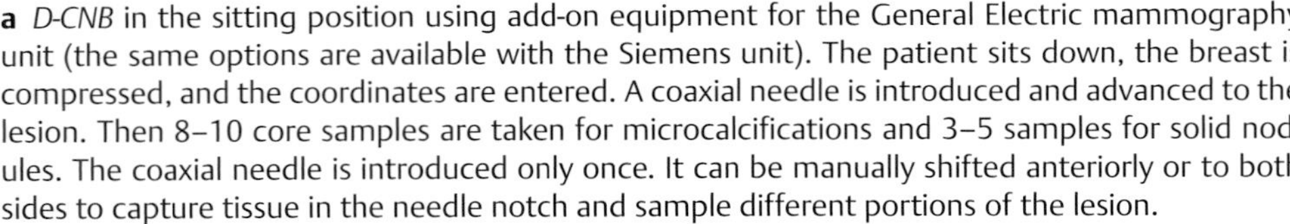

**a** *D-CNB* in the sitting position using add-on equipment for the General Electric mammography unit (the same options are available with the Siemens unit). The patient sits down, the breast is compressed, and the coordinates are entered. A coaxial needle is introduced and advanced to the lesion. Then 8–10 core samples are taken for microcalcifications and 3–5 samples for solid nodules. The coaxial needle is introduced only once. It can be manually shifted anteriorly or to both sides to capture tissue in the needle notch and sample different portions of the lesion.
**b** *Tissue core* in the biopsy needle.
**c** *Tissue core* placed in physiologic saline in a test tube (saline is immediately replaced with formalin at the end of the biopsy) (**f**). Three or four cores are taken from solid nodules, 8–12 from microcalcification clusters. The calcifications are examined in a specimen radiograph (**f1**, **f2**).

**e** *After the sterile saline has been replaced with formalin*, the test tube with the tissue cores is radiographed (it is helpful but not essential to have a second x-ray source parallel to the digital needle guide).

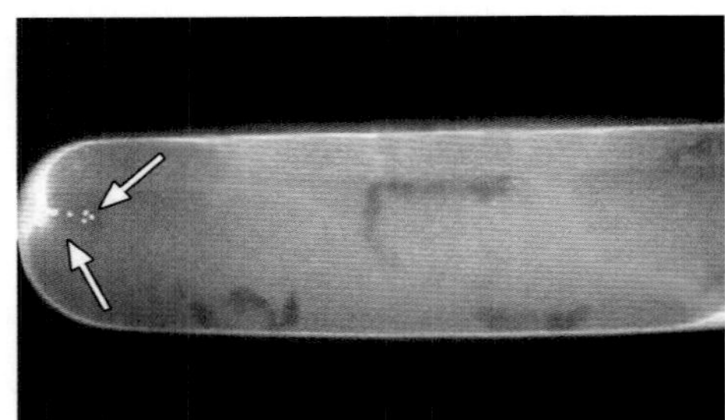

**f** *Specimen radiograph*. Calcifications appear as small white dots in the fatty tissue cores (dark "worms") in the left half of the test tube (arrows). If calcifications are not found, the biopsy should be repeated.

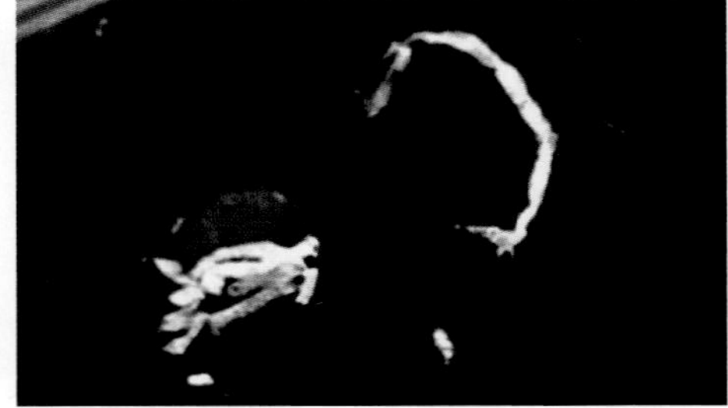

**f1** *Tissue cores* after VB in a Petri dish with saline-impregnated gauze.

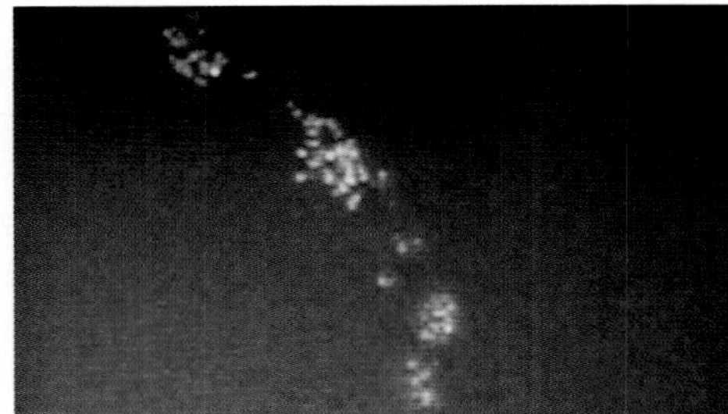

**f2** *Specimen radiograph* of the core biopsies shows numerous clustered microcalcifications in one long core. The calcium particles are isomorphic (histology: adenosis). The other tissue cores (left side of figure) contain fat.

**Fig. 5.107 Technique of digital stereotactic core-needle biopsy (D-CNB).** *(continued)*

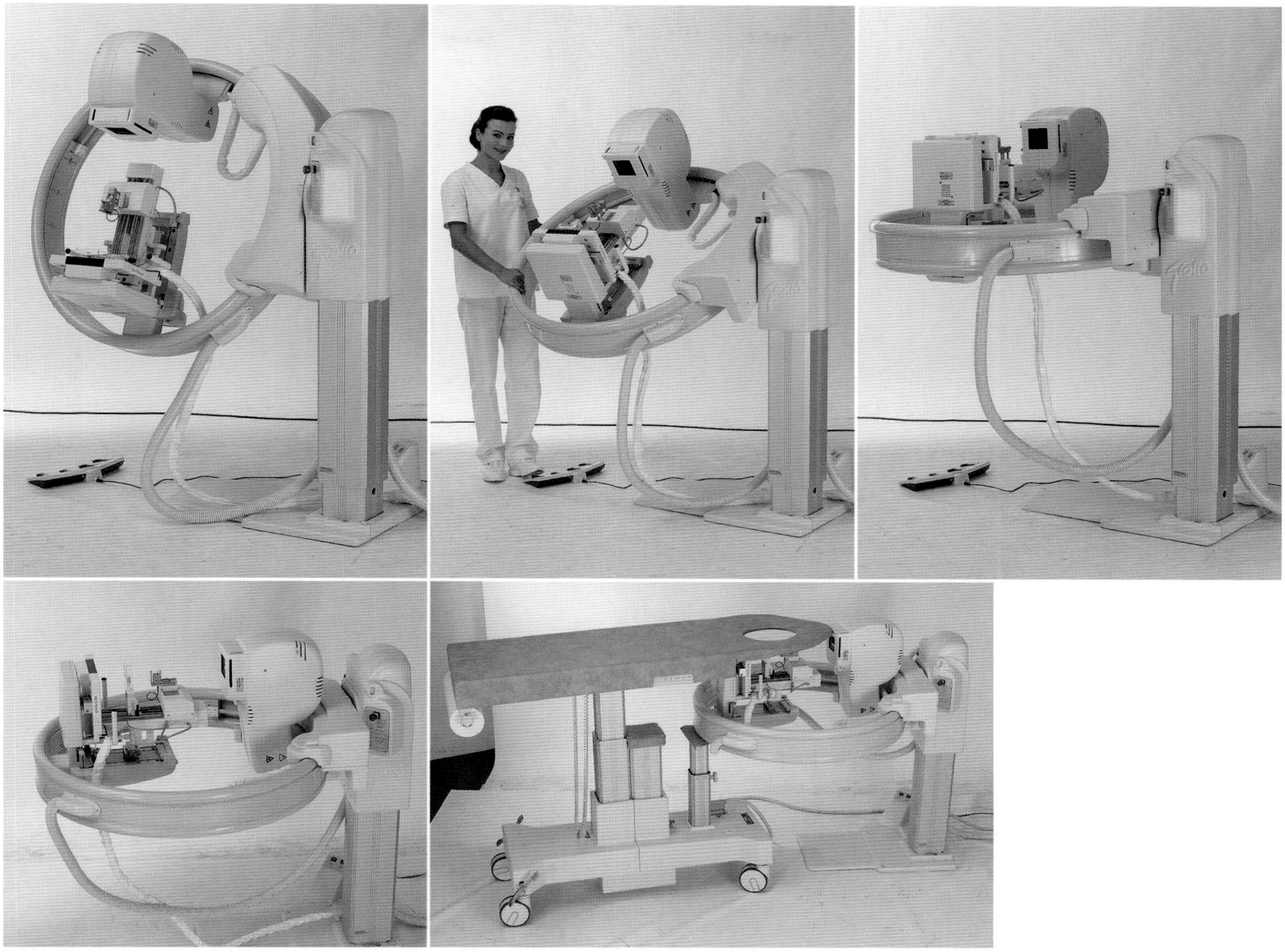

**g** *Digital stereotactic biopsy* with the Giotto table (IMS), which is more elegant and cost-effective than a standard biopsy table. Digital stereotaxy (FNA, CNB, or VB) is performed on a digital mammography system. The x-ray tube is tilted 90°, a digital biopsy unit is attached, and the biopsy is performed in the sitting or prone position (see also **Fig. 5.22**).

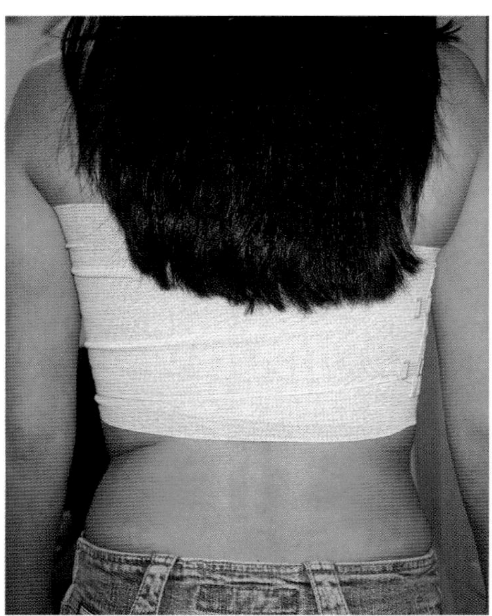

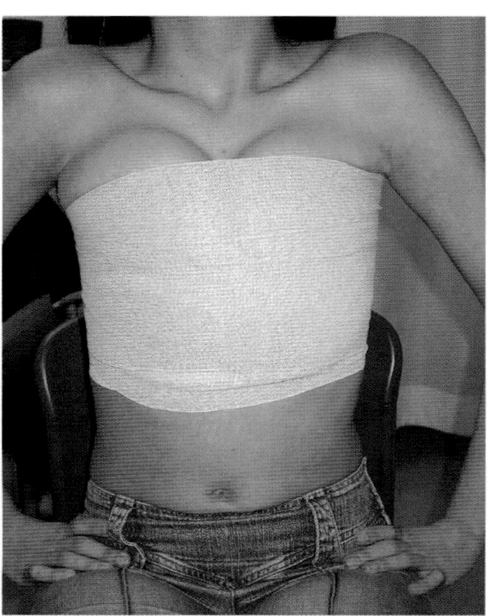

**h** An elastic *pressure bandage* is wrapped around the upper body after a core-needle or vacuum biopsy. It should remain in place for 4 hours after CNB and 12 hours after VB to prevent hematoma formation and postintervention pain (with permanent cooling, beginning immediately after the intervention).

▶ **Fig. 5.107 i–k**

**Fig. 5.107 i–k Various postinterventional defects.** *(continued)*

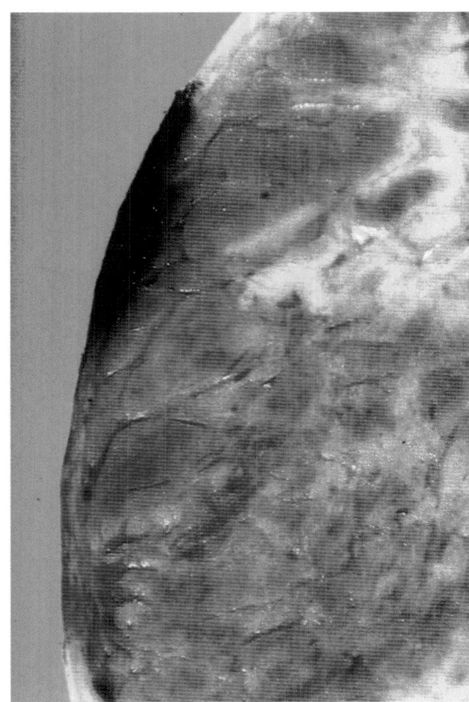

**i** *Macroanatomy:* superficial biopsy (e.g., punch biopsy) with bleeding into the skin (dark area on left side of specimen) and diffuse hematoma in the fatty tissue (red).

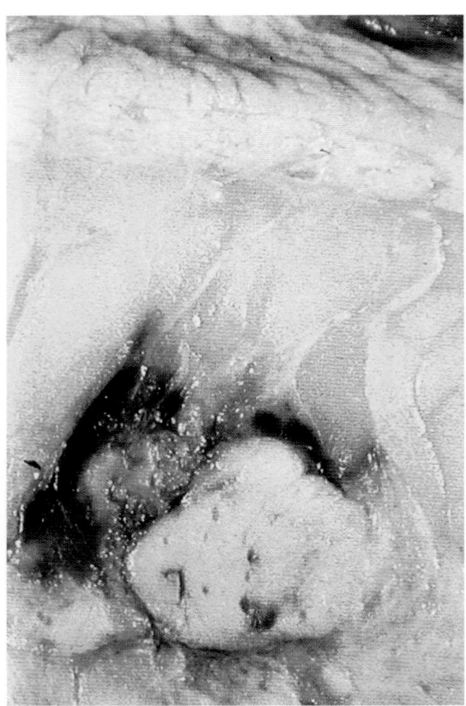

**j** *Macroanatomy:* nodules (pale yellow) caused by multiple needle insertions during core-needle biopsy. Small bleeding left of the nodule.

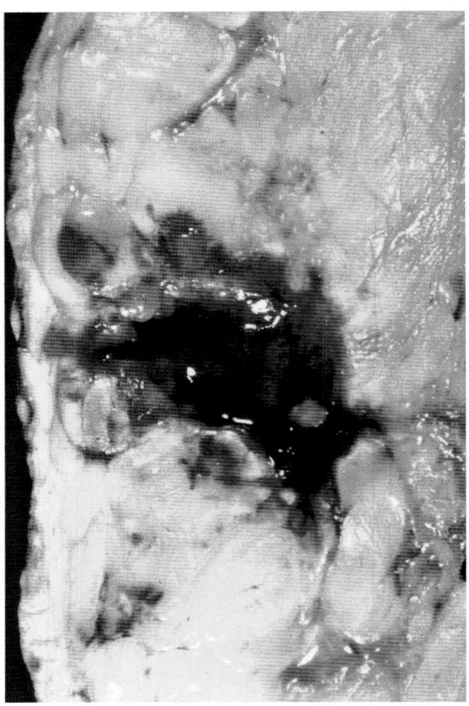

**k** *Macroanatomy:* Vacuum biopsy of microcalcifications left a relatively large defect with perifocal hematoma (image courtesy of Klaus Prechtel, Starnberg).

**Tip**

**Vacuum biopsy is generally more traumatizing than core-needle biopsy. Peripheral hemorrhagic changes can make it difficult for the surgeon to identify tumor remnants at reexcision and remove them with clear margins. (Some operators suture a surgical sponge into the resection cavity to aid orientation.)**

**Tip**

**When an interventional procedure is done in the sitting position, the room should be air-conditioned to minimize the risk of a vasovagal reaction with syncope.**

Every interventional procedure should be conducted in a calm, quiet atmosphere in which the technical and medical staffs communicate with the patient in a way that involves her in the process. Not every patient can be calmed in this manner, and small, thin patients are especially prone to syncope, often because they were too nervous to eat before the examination. All patients should be advised to eat something before coming in for the procedure. Coffee and tea are also recommended as hemodynamic stimulants.

Syncopal attacks are most common in sitting patients and usually have premonitory signs such as cold sweats, slowed reactions, etc. If these signs are noted, an effort should still be made to quickly obtain several tissue cores so that the procedure will not have been in vain. Then the needle should be promptly withdrawn and the patient moved in a flat position on a special fold-out chair or to a nearby couch. General Electric offers such a fold-out biopsy chair that is very practical for this kind of situation and eliminates the need to carry an unconscious patient to a separate couch.

Whenever possible, very anxious or sensitive patients should be placed initially in a recumbent position. Usually the patient can be placed in lateral decubitus on an ordinary adjustable-height table (see **Fig. 5.22 d**).

After the examination is completed, the patient or technologist should compress the biopsy site for 10 minutes with the fist or heel of the hand. An elastic bandage is then wrapped around the chest to maintain compression (**Fig. 5.107 h**). The compression bandage is left in place for the rest of the day, and preferably overnight after a vacuum biopsy, to reduce pain and control hematoma formation.

The patient is released home with a report sheet that has basic information about the examination. She is told to return the form a week later and indicate on the form whether she has noticed any complications such as dark bruising, inflammation, an allergic reaction to the local anesthetic, etc. The form also includes questions on the quality of the patient's experience and the conduct of the procedure. It should give a hotline number for the patient to call in the event that complications arise. Each physicians can find the solution that works best for their own situation.

With this type of feedback and a return rate of approximately 80%, we have gained an accurate picture of the postinterventional complications that are most likely to occur. They have an overall incidence of approximately 10%, are usually harmless, and relate mainly to varying degrees of hematoma formation (see **Fig. 5.119 f**). In over 3000 interventions performed during the past 10 years (620 FNAs, 2510 CNBs, 123 VBs), we have experienced only one infection of a large aspirated cyst and three large post-VB hematomas (especially in one patient with Willebrand–von Jürgens syndrome) that required percutaneous drainage. Willebrand–von Jürgens syndrome is the most common congenital bleeding disorder, with a prevalence of 800 per 100 000 population. It is caused by congenital absence of the von Willebrand factor (factor VIII-associated antigen), which is necessary for coagulation. This condition can be deceptive, as the patient may have a normal blood count, Quick, PT, and bleeding time in laboratory tests. **Never underestimate the importance of Willebrand–von Jürgens syndrome in interventional procedures and surgical operations.**

With our protocol, we have not found it necessary to reexamine the patient the day after undergoing an interventional procedure. Questions on the quality of the patient's experience relate to the procedure itself, the examination suite, the staff, the physician, and the general atmosphere. The examining physician should telephone the patient immediately on receipt of the histologic result. The patient's home telephone number or cellphone number should be on record for this purpose. During the call the physician may ask the patient about any reactions or complications and discuss further options if a malignancy has been found.

### Ultrasound-Guided Interventional Procedures

#### *Fine-Needle Aspiration (FNA)*

**Breast cytology is dead!** Today it is common to hear radiologists and breast experts make this statement at conferences and continuing-education forums (especially in Germany; Decker and Böcker 2008). It is usually made by colleagues who have not personally experienced the evolution of breast cytology, do not appreciate its value, and mainly perform core or vacuum biopsies. FNA is an art whose technical details must be learned and which few physicians actually master. Those who do not master it would rather stay with core biopsy, which is technically familiar and yields a more definitive result.

As valuable as CNB and VB are as modern tools for breast interventions, FNA is still the simplest, fastest, and most economical method (in experienced hands) for making a benign–malignant differentiation and setting the stage for the appropriate treatment.

Enlarged axillary lymph nodes, retroareolar and peripheral breast areas, and subcutaneous breast nodules are easily investigated by aspiration cytology. This cannot always be done by CNB without causing significant trauma or endangering the patient (pneumothorax). It should be added that CNB costs 10 times more than FNA while VB costs 150 times more (see **Table 5.13**, p. 253). The leading pioneer of cytodiagnosis in Europe was J. Zaijcek of the Karolinska Institute in Stockholm (Sweden). He advanced the clinical development of aspiration cytology during the 1970s and early 1980 s and showed that breast nodules could be morphologically evaluated at low cost and by simple means.

Fine-needle aspiration cytology as described by S. R. Orell (1999) is the most widely practiced invasive diagnostic procedure in the breast. An accurate cytologic diagnosis requires that FNAs always be performed in conjunction with physical examination and imaging procedures ("triple test" approach). Guidelines for the practical conduct of FNA and its uniform interpretation were developed at the Bethesda Consensus Conference (Bethesda, Maryland, USA) under the auspices of the National Cancer Institute in 1996, analogous to the Bethesda System for reporting cervical cytology. Numerous prominent medical and scientific societies took part in this conference, and the resulting guidelines were adopted as a worldwide standard (Steinberg et al. 2000).

The following cytologic classification is used for the reporting of FNA findings in the breast:

- **Class I: benign.** There is no cytologic evidence of malignancy. Nevertheless, the findings should still be described, for example, as an inflammatory process, fat necrosis, nonproliferative breast disease such as cysts, apocrine metaplasia, proliferative breast disease without atypical cells, fibroadenoma, pregnancy-associated changes, or pharmacologically induced changes.
- **Class II: atypical cells that cannot be definitely classified (indeterminate cells).** The cellular constituents in the specimen cannot be definitely evaluated. Again, the findings should always be described, especially in a proliferative disease with atypical cytology that would raise issues of differential diagnosis (atypical hyperplasia versus well-differentiated carcinoma, papilloma versus papillary carcinoma, fibroadenoma versus phylloides tumor, etc.). The imaging results and physical findings should be reviewed in the light of the cytologic result.
- **Class III: suspicious, probably malignant.** The cellular constituents in the material are highly suspicious for malignancy. A definitive diagnosis requires the histologic examination of a tissue sample.
- **Class IV: definitely malignant.** The cellular constituents show definite malignant criteria. The specific type of neoplasm should be identified whenever possible.
- **Class V:** unsatisfactory smear. The smear cannot be adequately evaluated due to an insufficient number of cells, too many artifacts (e.g., findings obscured by blood or inflammatory cells), or other factors.

Today it is still common practice to use the Papanicolao system (Pap I–V) for classifying cytologic findings in the breast.

The **indications** for FNA of the breast are as follows (Steinberg et al. 2000):

- All palpable masses (triple test)
- Nonpalpable masses (with stereotactic guidance)
- Simple smooth-walled cysts (diagnosis the treatment)
- Indeterminate palpable masses during pregnancy
- Confirmation of a locally advanced process
- Postoperative confirmation of clinically suspected malignancy
- Detection of recurrent malignancy (also in scars) or metastases (during follow-up)
- Collecting tumor cells for special tests (DNA analysis, immunocytochemical testing; limited indication)

One objection to this list of indications is that changes during pregnancy are better evaluated by CNB. This is because the marked cellular proliferation that occurs in pregnancy is likely to yield a false-positive cytologic result (see **Fig. 5.146**, p. 286 f). Scars should also be core-biopsied, because experience has shown that a low cell yield is obtained from local recurrences in scars.

In most studies on diagnostic accuracy, FNA has shown a sensitivity of approximately 95%. This is illustrated by the figures from Ketteler Hospital in Offenbach, Germany, where breast cancer was

**Fig. 5.108 Ultrasound-guided fine-needle aspiration (FNA).**

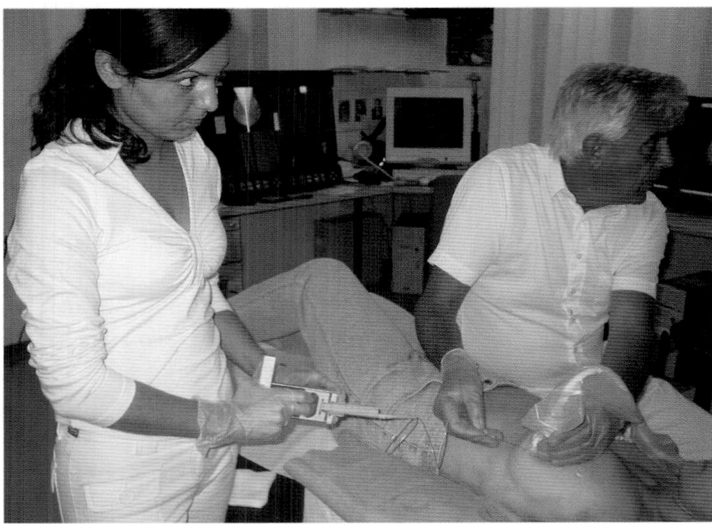

**a** The technologist creates a vacuum by drawing the plunger of a 10 mL syringe to 1–2 mL in a Cameco holder. The syringe is connected by tubing to the aspiration needle.

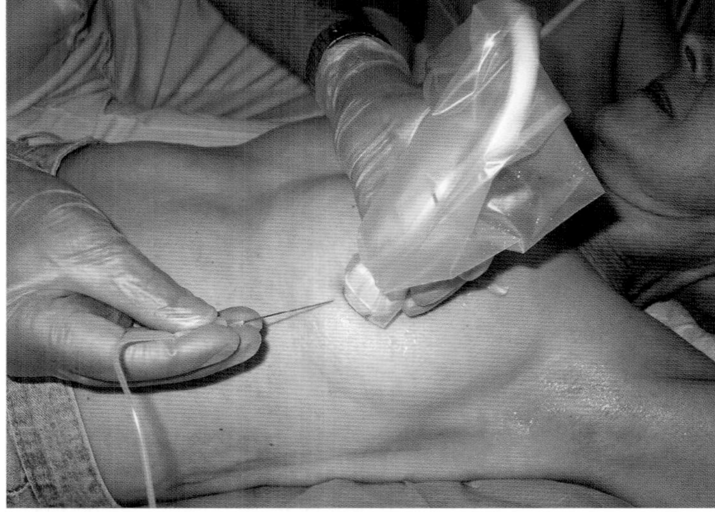

**b** The needle is advanced into the nodule under ultrasound guidance.

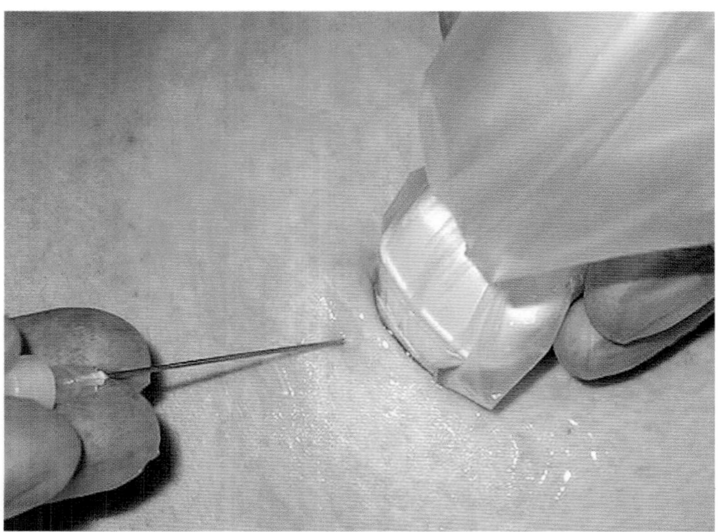

**c** The needle and transducer are in the same plane and should be parallel to each other if possible.

histologically confirmed in 856 women. The cancer was not palpable in 142 cases. The previous cytologic diagnoses based on FNA in 854 cases (two patients refused FNA) were as follows:

- Malignant ($n = 675$)
- Suspicious for malignancy ($n = 111$)
- Equivocal ($n = 35$)
- Not suspicious for malignancy ($n = 12$)
- Material could not be evaluated ($n = 12$)

Based on reports in the literature, the rate of false-negative cytologic findings is between 5% and 10%. This rate can be reduced to less than 1% by the triple-test protocol. The combination of palpation, mammography/ultrasound, and FNA has greater than 99% diagnostic accuracy in cases where all three tests are concordant for benign or malignant disease. With nonpalpable lesions detectable only by mammography or ultrasound, the triple protocol can reduce negative excisional biopsies by 90% (Steinberg et al. 2000).

Freehand needle placement for FNA is appropriate only for clearly palpable cysts and fibroadenomas. It is advisable, however, to use ultrasound guidance for freehand FNA and place a length of tubing between the needle and syringe holder (**Fig. 5.108**). Cysts can be completely evacuated using this technique. Palpable breast nodules and especially the diagnostically important peripheral zones of nodules can be sampled with greater accuracy under sonographic guidance. This is done by *carefully* and repeatedly advancing and retracting the needle through the nodule while simultaneously rotating it. Try to avoid aspirating cells from the center of larger tumors, where necrosis will make analysis difficult. The peripheral zones of a nodule are better for both cytologic and histologic assessment. Ultrasound-guided interventions can be performed rapidly, and an experienced operator can obtain an adequate sample without having to use a special needle guide or 3D ultrasound imaging (Lell, Aichinger, Schultz-Wendtland et al. 2003).

**Technique and accuracy of FNA:** Like freehand FNA, ultrasound-guided FNA is performed with a no. 18, no. 12 or no. 1 needle depending on the accessibility of the lesion, the clinical question, and the sensitivity of the patient to pain. A gentle vacuum is recommended to avoid damaging the cells. Local anesthesia is not necessary.

**To assure successful FNA, directing the needle must be done with great care, and with a minimum of vacuum. Every patient and every examining physician should be proficient in breast inspection and palpation.**

After all needle passes have been made through the lesion, the vacuum is removed, the needle is withdrawn from the nodule, and its contents are *carefully* expelled onto a glass slide with the mounted 10 mL syringe. This should be done immediately, before the blood in the sample can coagulate. Care is taken not to crush the cells. A smear is prepared by spreading the sample out forward with a second slide or coverslip and then lightly dragging the slide or coverslip back over the sample. Special care is required with material that has been aspirated from lymph nodes. It should either not be smeared or smeared with extreme care, as any crush artifacts may prevent evaluation of the sample. See page 231 for contact-cytology (CC).

The air-dried smears are sent to the pathologist or cytologist. The patient should compress the puncture site for 5 minutes following FNA. An adhesive bandage is not required.

Suspected *lobular carcinoma, inflammatory carcinoma*, or *breast cancer during pregnancy* (see above) should never be cytologically evaluated. FNA would probably yield a false-positive diagnosis because even experienced cytologists have difficulty distinguishing the cells in these tumors from normal ductal epithelium. All cases of this kind should be evaluated by CNB. False-positives may also occur in association with certain fibroadenomas, pregnancy, rare *lactating adenomas*, and radiogenic dysplasia following radiotherapy. The cells look malignant but the process itself is not malignant (see **Fig. 5.168 e**, p. 399).

In 620 FNAs performed at our center during the past 10 years, the procedure had an overall positive predictive value of 93% for breast cancer (compared with 93% for ultrasound-guided core-needle biopsy and 97% for stereotactic core-needle biopsy). Five of the false-positive diagnoses were fibroadenomas, one was a lactating adenoma (see **Fig. 5.145**, p. 285), and one was radiogenic dysplasia (**Fig. 5.168 e**, p. 399). These lesions had a benign histology with no evidence of malignant cells in the aspirated sample.

Manual needle placement for FNA allows the operator to "feel" nodules with the needle, especially when aided by ultrasound guidance. Soft nodules (especially lymph nodes) should be aspirated without a vacuum, while firm nodules should be aspirated with just a moderate vacuum (1–2 mL in a 10 mL syringe) to collect cellular material (Lindholm 1999).

**False-positive and false-negative diagnoses:** The following lesions and conditions may yield a **false-positive diagnosis** by FNA:

- **Papillomas:** Intraductal papilloma, papillary carcinoma in situ, and invasive papillary carcinoma are indistinguishable from one another by FNA cytology.
- **ADH:** Ductal hyperplasia (DH) and atypical ductal hyperplasia (ADH) are on a continuum, although DH has a less organized cellular pattern than ADH (see p. 35). The enlarged nuclei in some ADH foci raise undue suspicion of malignancy. The presence of bipolar cells with bare nuclei (myoepithelial cells) in the smear is more suspicious for ADH than carcinoma.
- **Fibroadenoma:** Some fibroadenomas have a "dramatic" cytologic appearance. Again, bipolar myoepithelial cells suggest that the lesion is benign and support (but do not confirm) a diagnosis of fibroadenoma.
- **Inflammatory epithelial reactions:** Leukocytes and lymphocytes in the aspirate prompt a low index of suspicion because inflammatory processes can produce atypical changes in normal epithelial cells. The same applies to nipple smears.
- **Pregnancy and lactation:** The cells in pregnant and lactating breasts can mimic carcinoma as pregnancy-related hormonal stimulation creates a somewhat disordered cell pattern.
- **Lactating adenomas:** These tumors contain atypical cells that may resemble carcinoma. CNB is helpful in making the correct diagnosis.
- **Intraductal and intracystic proliferation:** Epithelial cells of the oxyphilic type (oncocytes), like those occurring in cystic fluid, may appear suspicious. If the fluid is hemorrhagic or if no residual internal echoes are visible after the cyst has been evacuated, it is unlikely that malignant transformation has occurred.
- **Dermal appendages:** Cells from a syringocystadenoma papilliferum can mimic the appearance of breast cancer.

Cases with equivocal or suspicious findings should be investigated by CNB to help establish the diagnosis. The following lesions may yield a **false-negative diagnosis** by FNA:

- **Tumors with central necrosis or sclerosis:** Smears from these zones may be acellular or may contain debris that prevents cytologic evaluation. Scirrhous carcinoma, sclerotic fibroadenoma, necrotic tumor tissue, and ductectasia cannot be distinguished from one another.
- **Carcinoma next to benign lesions:** Lipomas, cysts, or fibroadenomas may overlie malignancies, and a freehand technique may yield benign findings because cells are aspirated from the benign lesion.
- **Complex proliferative lesions:** Epithelial hyperplasia with or without atypias may contain small elements of invasive or in-situ carcinoma but is indistinguishable from a benign lesion. It is essential in these cases to supplement FNA with CB (see **Fig. 5.140**).
- **Well-differentiated carcinomas:** Tubular carcinomas can be particularly difficult to diagnose because they often yield isolated bare nuclei with little or no atypia. Again, the histologic evaluation of a tissue core is essential.
- **Small-cell neoplasms:** Lobular carcinomas in particular often have small, uniform cells that are easily mistaken for normal glandular epithelium. Lobular carcinoma is the most frequent incorrect cytologic diagnosis (Lindholm 1999).
- **Excessive vacuum:** FNA with a sharp needle and too much vacuum will yield only debris, especially when large needle excursions are made.

In experienced hands, FNA is a valuable and extremely precise adjunct that should not be displaced from the diagnostic armamentarium by more costly and invasive procedures.

### *Ultrasound-Guided Core Needle Biopsy*

Also under sonographic guidance and aided by a technologist, the examiner advances a coaxial needle to the target lesion and extracts 3–5 tissue cores from different parts of the nodule, especially the peripheral zones.

The core-biopsy samples are either placed directly into formalin solution with a forceps (better for malignant lesions) or are "shaken" directly from the biopsy needle into sterile physiologic saline solution. After the biopsy is completed, the saline solution is discarded and replaced with formalin. The tissue cores should not remain in saline for more than 1–2 minutes, as this would make them difficult for the pathologist to interpret. See p. 231 for more on contact cytology (CC).

CNB is performed with a 14-gauge core biopsy needle (> 2 mm in diameter) with a sampling window 1.5–2 mm long, depending on the size of the lesion. In dealing with a suspected malignancy, great care should be taken that the needle does not pierce the pectoral muscle. Besides being painful, this could inoculate tumor cells into the muscle tissue. Thus, when dealing with lesions that are suspicious for malignancy, the examiner should select a sampling window that will extract tissue only from the lesion and not its surroundings. Every needle biopsy will cause some local seeding of tumor cells, but experience has shown that these cells are destroyed by host defenses and do not cause inoculation metastasis. Nevertheless, it is still good practice to preserve healthy tissue during the biopsy. Since tumor cells are found to be present within the coaxial needle following 70% of all malignant biopsies, it is reasonable to assume that they are also present in the needle tract. It is best, therefore, to include the needle tract in surgical excisions.

Local anesthetic should be used sparingly in the biopsy of hypoechoic lesions. It is most important to anesthetize the skin and subcutaneous fat (ask about allergy to local anesthetic!). The breast parenchyma itself is not very sensitive to pain. Injection of local anesthetic and intralesional hemorrhage may cause a hypoechoic tumor to become isoechoic so that it is no longer visible with ultrasound. Thus, all manipulations (local anesthesia, coaxial needle placement) should respect the tumor area if at all possible.

As a general rule, microcalcifications are not biopsied under ultrasound guidance unless they are grouped in large clusters that are visible on sonograms. The detection of calcifications is ordinarily the domain of mammography, bearing in mind that the morphology and intramammary extent of calcifications are not useful for determining invasiveness (Stomper et al. 2003) (see **Fig. 5.88**, p. 200). On the other hand, if hypoechoic zones (not to be confused with acoustic shadows!) are found in or adjacent to suspicious calcifications, the calcifications can be biopsied under sonographic guidance. This pattern generally indicates that DCIS is no longer present and the lesion has already progressed to invasive cancer. Thus, ultrasound can help to improve the sensitivity and specificity of mammography in the assessment of microcalcifications, but it cannot displace mammography from its important role in early detection (Yang and Tse 2004). When clustered calcifications are biopsied under sonographic guidance, a specimen radiograph should be taken to demonstrate the calcifications.

After the needle is removed, the patient herself should maintain pressure on the biopsy site for 5–10 minutes. Then a compression bandage (**Fig. 5.107 h**, p. 233) may be applied (not compulsory) and is left in place for 4–5 hours. The patient should place a mild cold pack on the site (through clothing!) to suppress inflammation and prevent hematoma formation. A cooling device may be used to cool the site even before the procedure and then immediately after the biopsy, and the patient may continue to use it at home to prevent hematoma formation. Ice should never be placed directly on the skin, as the frostbite effect could delay healing and hamper evaluation of the site (see **Fig. 5.8**, p. 86).

If an existing hematoma makes the lesion isodense or isoechoic so that it cannot be visualized for biopsy, the procedure should be discontinued and reattempted 3–4 weeks later.

CNB is not used exclusively for BIRADS 4 and 5 lesions but is occasionally used in cases where it is unclear whether the lesion is BIRADS 3 or 4 (BIRADS 4a in screening). The BIRADS classification can then be adjusted on the basis of the histologic findings.

Needle guides that attach to the transducer are available for FNA and CNB. While these devices are practical and allow for relatively precise placement, they are not essential because even small lesions can be accurately biopsied under sonographic guidance using freehand technique. Mechanical guides cannot direct the needle tangentially to the pectoral muscle, and there is always a risk of pleural injury. Three-dimensional ultrasound is unnecessary for CNB (Lell, Aichinger, Schultz-Wendtland et al. 2003).

Whenever FNA, CNB, or VB yields a benign diagnosis, the mammographic and histologic results must be compatible. Follow-up examination of the biopsied breast at 6 months is both prudent and necessary in every patient. This follow-up may be performed by the referring gynecologist or radiologist. If the breast center receives no word to the contrary, it may assume that a malignancy was not missed.

The same considerations apply to vacuum biopsy (VB). In our experience, there is no need to place marker clips at the site of biopsied calcifications to aid localization of the tumor site in the event of surgery. Clips are costly and mostly unnecessary. In some situations it is helpful to insert a clip, coil or radioactive seed (very small lesions, neoadjuvant chemotherapy).

As a rule, not all calcifications are removed by CNB. The biopsy also causes local hematoma formation with associated scarring that visibly marks the "site of action." When necessary, a vascular ligation clip is preferred over a metal coil because it costs much less than a coil and is just as visible on mammograms (Margoli et al. 2003).

In the future, we may be able to place probes in benign as well as malignant tumors under precise sonographic (or digital stereotactic) guidance to thermoablate or cryoablate the lesion. It is known that thermoablation probes placed in small (< 2 cm) malignant tumors (confirmed by CNB) can destroy the lesion by the sustained application of heat or cold (Fornage et al. 2004). The procedure is technically straightforward and safe, especially in women with high surgical risk. Thermoablation has already been successfully used in the treatment of metastases. The main problem with malignant tumors is achieving clear margins. This would have to be confirmed by vacuum biopsy weeks after treatment, and sentinel node biopsy should also be done to determine axillary status.

Thus, interventional procedures are currently in a state of flux, and it is reasonable to expect that the treatment of even small breast cancers will become less and less invasive.

#### *Ultrasound-Guided Vacuum Biopsy*

Following the same principle as ultrasound-guided CNB, ultrasound-guided vacuum biopsy (SO-VB) can also be performed with a hand-held system (see **Fig. 5.109**, p. 240 f). VB should be preceded by FNA or CNB to make a benign–malignant determination. VB is not recommended for malignant lesions because of the higher costs and greater tissue trauma, making it more difficult for the surgeon and pathologist to evaluate tumor margins. We use VB mainly for the removal of fibroadenomas and intraductal or intracystic papillomas. The 11-gauge needle (8-gauge for large nodules) is positioned so that the sampling chamber is beneath the targeted nodule. Local anesthetic (lidocaine with adrenaline) should be injected liberally below and around the nodule to demarcate the nodule from its surroundings, especially with subcutaneous lesions. Tissue samples are extracted under ultrasound guidance until the nodule has been completely removed.

When dealing with subcutaneous nodules, be careful not to injure the skin or nipple with the cutter (visible scar, pain, pitting). Gross visual inspection will usually show whether the tissue samples are from a fibroadenoma (white), surrounding fat (yellow), or a papilloma (blue after staining of the duct with patent blue dye). More local anesthetic should be used for a vacuum-assisted biopsy than for CNB, and there is still a risk that the nodule will be masked by the anesthetic or a hematoma. In a VB, additional local anesthetic can be injected through the needle lumen at any time during the procedure.

With a fibroadenoma, it is not essential to remove the entire nodule. When the complete VB of a fibroadenoma is attempted, remnants of the nodule cannot always be positively identified near the end of the procedure because they are obscured by hematoma. But if 70–80% of the nodule is found to be benign, it is reasonable to conclude that the rest is also benign. In our experience, residual fibroadenoma is often completely absorbed by the body following division of the lesion capsule. To date we have seen no instances of additional growth or recurrence following VB.

If remnants of a benign tumor are left in the breast, they can be completely removed at a later date if this is considered important for the patient. If a palpable nodule cannot be completely removed in one sitting for whatever reason, it should at least be reduced to a size that is no longer palpable by the patient. If there is no guarantee that the nodule is removable by VB (larger than 2 cm, unfavorable location, etc.), it should be removed by primary surgical biopsy or the patient should be advised concerning a possible second procedure.

There is no need for mammography or ultrasound after the completion of VB. Imaging at this time would show only a hematoma, and fine tissue structures could not be identified.

From 20 to 30 tissue samples may be collected in one VB, depending on the size of the nodule. It is very tedious to remove a 2 cm nodule with an 11-gauge needle; an 8-gauge needle is a much better option. Recumbent patients should not experience syncopal episodes during VB. The patient compresses the biopsy site for 10 minutes after the procedure (placing pressure not just on the skin incision but especially on the area of the biopsied nodule). Then a pressure bandage is worn for 24 hours (see **Fig. 5.107 h**, p. 233). We have experienced a hematoma rate of 10% at our center, and none of these cases required surgical evacuation. One relatively large hematoma that formed after papilloma removal was successfully evacuated with a large-bore needle (see **Fig. 5.119**, p. 252 f).

During the past 10 years, 123 vacuum biopsies have been performed at our center under sonographic and digital stereotactic guidance. In all of these cases the lesion was identified as benign by previous FNA or CNB but still had to be removed for special reasons (the patient's aversion to a palpable nodule, cosmetic concerns, proliferative changes, etc.). Malignant lesions were not referred for vacuum biopsy, although VB did identify one ADH, one DCIS, one LCIS, one tubular carcinoma, and one lobular carcinoma—proof that we cannot rely on a negative FNA or CNB when other factors suggest a malignant process. On the other hand, the numbers clearly indicate that CNB is very accurate in identifying benign processes and yields essentially the same results as VB (Weining-Klemm 2004; see p. 251).

#### *Cost-Saving Potential of Needle Biopsy Compared with Open Biopsy*

Needle biopsy (core, punch, or vacuum biopsy) for histology and especially fine-needle aspiration (FNA) for the cytologic examination of a lesion are alternatives to open surgical biopsy that can reduce the diagnostic costs of suspicious breast lesions by up to 96% (depending on the procedure used). In up to 85% of patients, moreover, percutaneous biopsy can eliminate the need for open surgery with all its physical and emotional consequences. The actual cost saving depends on the particular biopsy method and lesion type and varies in different countries (Gruber et al. 2008).

There have been several reports that VB yields better results than CNB with a 14-gauge needle, especially in patients with breast microcalcifications (Liberman et al. 2001). Our own experience does not confirm these reports. Accurate placement of the biopsy needle is essential to ensure that microcalcifications will be visible in the specimen radiograph. In this case the pathologist should have no difficulty in making the correct diagnosis without additional biopsy material, and therefore vacuum biopsy cannot be justified. Vacuum biopsy is ten times more costly than a simple CNB. We can cite the following figures on potential cost savings with interventional procedures based on the first model screening project in Germany. Approximately 10.4 million women are eligible for screening participation. Based on the current 1.8% recall rate for further testing, it is reasonable to predict that approximately 187 000 women per year will require a histologic diagnosis. The primary diagnostic costs for these procedures would be approximately 3.76 million euro for open surgical biopsy versus approximately 1.9 million euro for needle biopsy. According to Gruber et al. (2008), this would yield a potential cost saving of more than 3.57 million euro annually—a considerable sum.

In the United States, the American College of Radiology (ACR) has published uniform guidelines for the coding of percutaneous needle biopsy methods (CBT Code).

Although there are already ample data to show that the needle biopsy of indeterminate breast lesions has a high cost-saving potential, there is an urgent need for survey studies to assess the specific costs in different EU countries given the significant national differences in service reimbursements, patient populations, types of biopsy, and the selection of surgical and interventional procedures (**Figs. 5.110–5.117**).

**Fig. 5.109 Nodule at the 1-o'clock position in the upper outer quadrant of the left breast in a 39-year-old woman (a).** Mammograms show a nonspecific density with irregular, ill-defined margins in this region (**b–d**). Ultrasound shows a 2.5 cm nodule with scalloped margins and internal echoes consistent with a *fibroadenoma* (**e**). Local anesthetic (lidocaine) is injected into the nodule and its surroundings (under ultrasound guidance), and an 8-gauge biopsy needle is placed manually below the nodule. The lesion is then removed from the breast by vacuum biopsy (**f**).

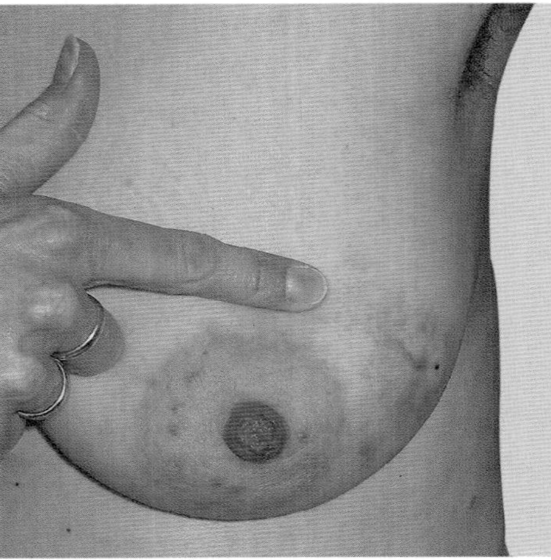

**a** *Physical examination:* A 2 cm nodule is palpable at the 1-o'clock position in the left breast. Bruising is visible over a previous fine-needle core biopsy.

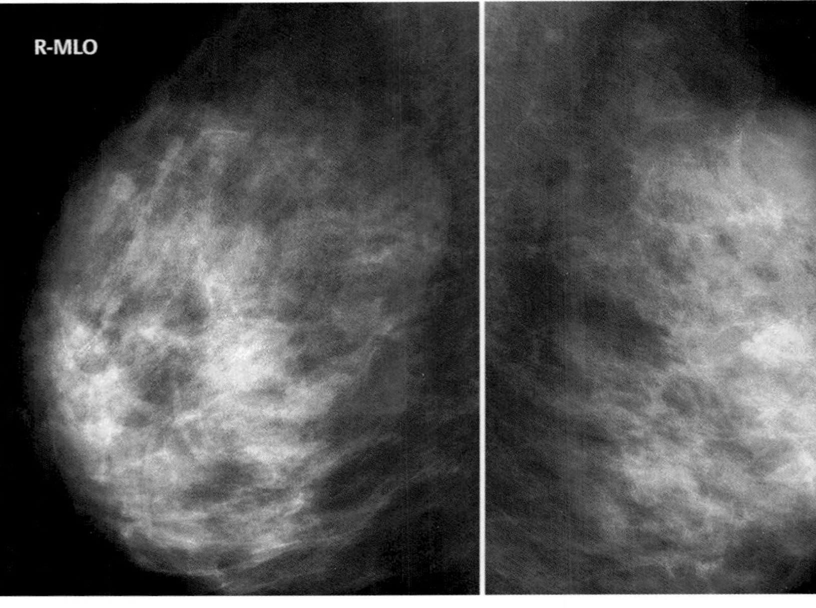


**b** *Bilateral oblique mammograms* show very radiodense breasts with inhomogeneities, especially at the upper border of the left breast (**i–J/23–24**) (ACR 3, BIRADS 4, P**G**MI).

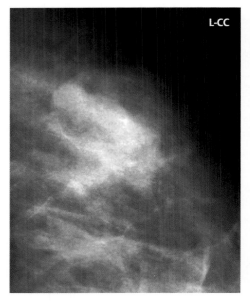


**c** *Craniocaudal mammogram* of the left breast. The nodule appears on a conventional mammogram as a relatively well-circumscribed mass of homogeneous density (**a–B/13–14**)(ACR 3, BIRADS 3).

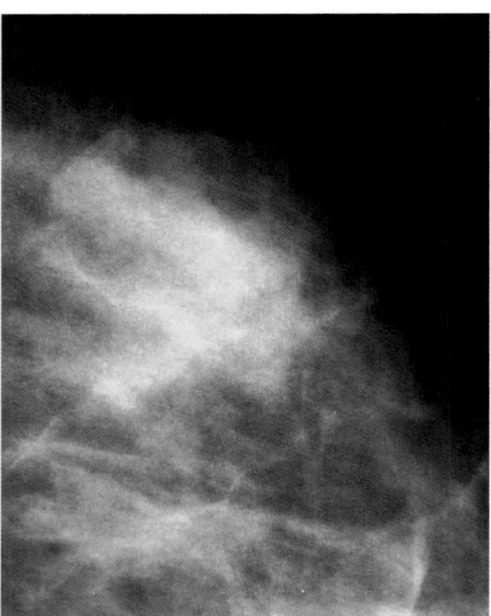

**d** *Digital mammogramm:* No qualitative difference is seen relative to the conventional mammogram (**c**).

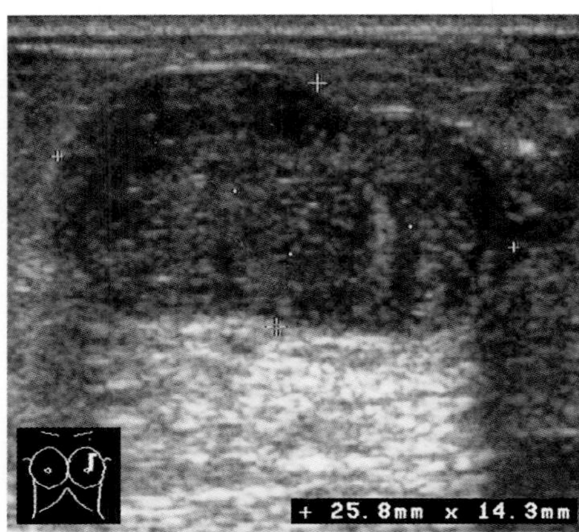


**e** *Sonogram* of the left breast shows a 2.5 cm × 1.4 cm nodule with smooth margins, homogeneous internal echoes (**h–J/11–12**), and slight posterior acoustic enhancement (**H–j/13–15**). CNB confirmed fibroadenoma before vacuum biopsy, accounting for the small hematoma at the biopsy site (compare with **a**).

**Fig. 5.109 Nodule at the 1-o'clock position in the upper outer quadrant of the left breast in a 39-year-old woman.** *(continued)*

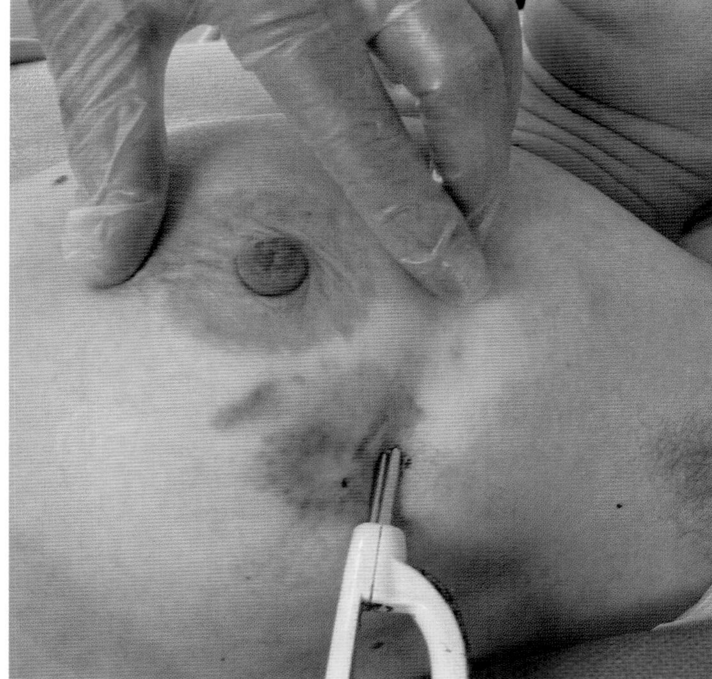

**f** *Clinical view SO-VB.* The fibroadenoma is removed by vacuum (mammotome) biopsy under sonographic guidance.

**Question on Fig. 5.109**

*Up to what size can fibroadenomas or papillomas be removed completely in one sitting with an 8-gauge biopsy needle?*

(**a**) 0.5 cm

(**b**) 1 cm

(**c**) 2 cm

→ **Answer on p. 380**

### *Ductography*

The technique of ductography, in which contrast medium is instilled into a secreting duct, is an art that requires continual training. Local anesthesia of the nipple is generally unnecessary with the ultra-thin cannulas in current use (see **Fig. 5.111 c, d**), but the nipple can be desensitized by applying an anesthetic patch 1 hour before the procedure (**Fig. 5.111 b**). In very sensitive patients, 1% lidocaine injected beneath the areolar margin (not the nipple!) will numb the tissue within seconds.

The secreting duct is slightly dilated with an extremely fine probe before introducing the injection needle, from which all air has been expelled and replaced by contrast medium. As the needle is inserted, the nipple should be slightly elevated to straighten the retroareolar ducts. Then contrast medium is carefully instilled until the patient announces that a dull pain is felt. Contrast instillation should be immediately stopped at this point to prevent extravasation. The nipple should not be compressed during contrast instillation so that the material can drain freely from the nipple as the intraductal pressure rises.

**Fig. 5.110 Papillomatous ductal proliferation.** Macro- and microanatomic features.

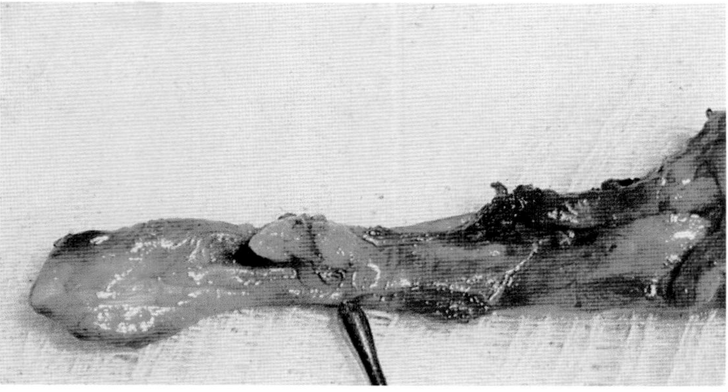

**a** *Anatomic preparation of a papilloma*: The duct has been extirpated and cut open to display a cylindrical intraluminal mass.

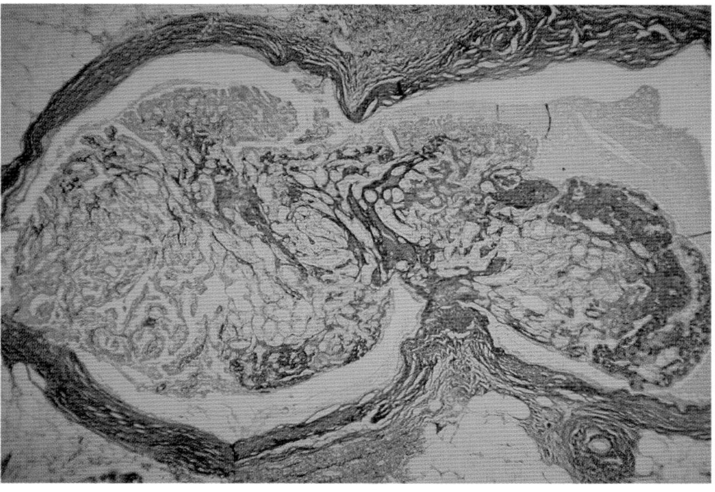

**b** *Histologic section* of intracanalicular ductal papilloma shows thickened, branched, connective-tissue papillary cores lined by hyperplastic epithelium (interlobular stroma appears red with van Gieson stain). In the lower part of the section (**r–S/15–16**) is a narrow papilloma neck with feeding blood vessels.

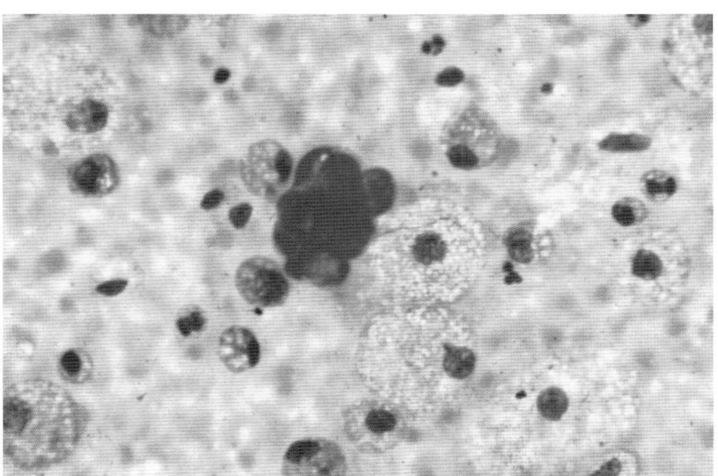

**c** *Cytologic smear* shows a darkly stained, mulberry-like cell cluster in addition to foam cells, granulocytes, and lymphocytes as evidence of an accompanying inflammation.

**Fig. 5.111 Technique of ductography.** The patient was reexamined at 12 months due to a circumferential duct stricture found in initial ductograms (**e**). The patient herself can perform optimum compression of the retroareolar sinuses. This is a more normal finger position than if the physician were to attempt the maneuver while sitting in front of the patient (**a**). Ductography may be done in retrograde fashion with a very thin injection needle (**d**). If this is unsuccessful, antegrade ductography can be performed by injecting contrast medium directly into the dilated ducts under sonographic guidance.

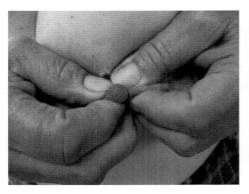

**a** *Clinical appearance* of the left nipple. Many patients already know how to compress the retroareolar sinuses from their experience with breastfeeding. The physician could sit behind the patient and reach around her to compress the nipple, but then he could not see the duct orifices or discharge, and this position might be unpleasant for the patient.

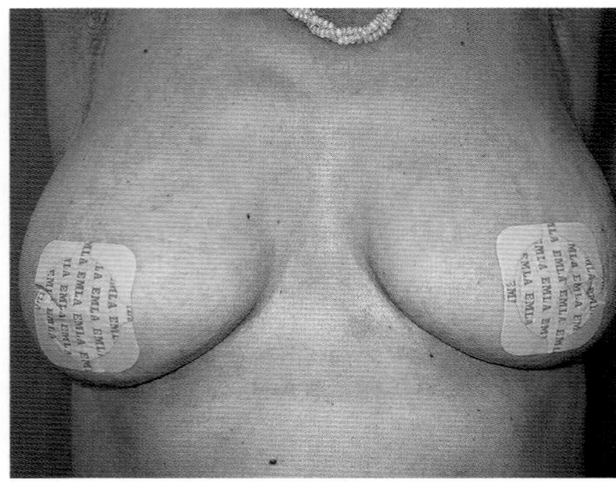

**b** *An adhesive patch* can be placed over each nipple prior to ductography.

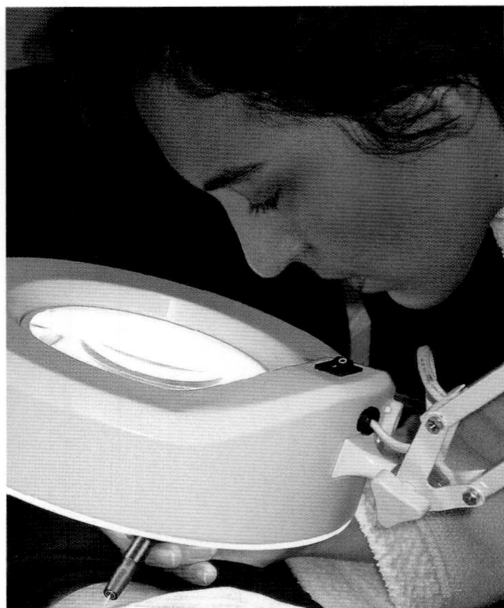

**c** A large *magnifying lamp* facilitates cannula insertion into the secreting duct.

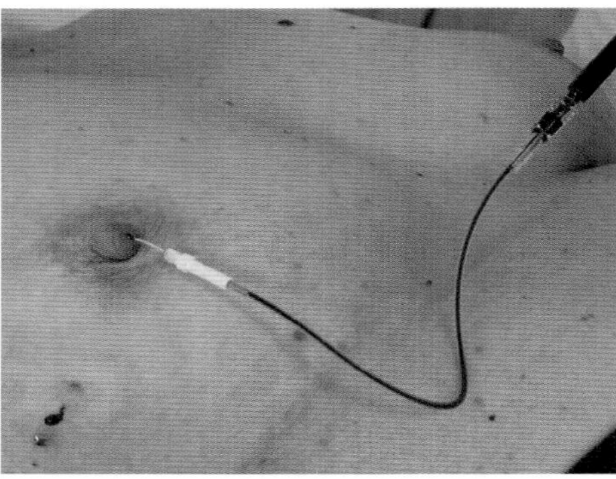

**d** *Technique of retrograde ductography.* An ultra-thin (30-gauge) cannula is used to locate and then slightly dilate the secreting duct, and contrast medium is instilled (in this case 2 parts contrast medium and 1 part patent blue dye to stain the site blue and direct the possible vacuum biopsy of a papilloma). The old practice of dilating the ducts with a tapered dilator is no longer necessary. The current technique of ductography with a 30-gauge cannula is virtually painless.

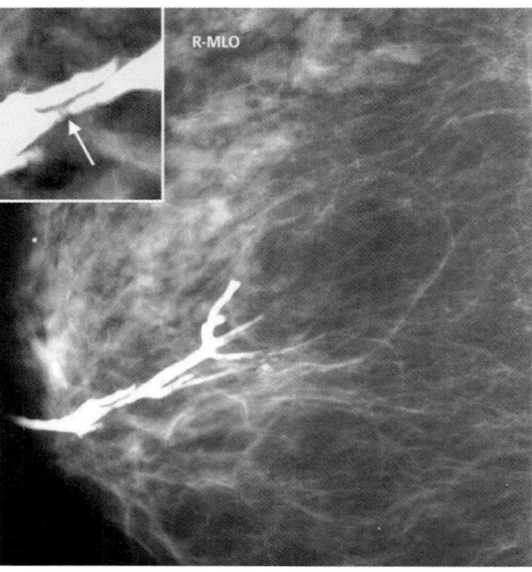


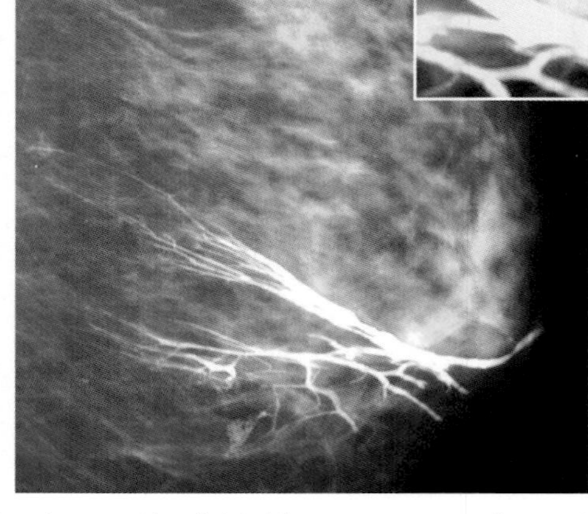


**e** *Ductography* (retrograde technique). The duct system on the right side appears normal except for a discrete stenosis at **E/12** (see arrow in inset). On the left side, the slight circumferential ductal narrowing at **i/12** (see arrows in inset) is presumably a stricture due to scarring. When the patient was reexamined 12 months later, nipple discharge could no longer be elicited.

**Question on Fig. 5.111**

*What is the purpose of the adhesive patches on both nipples?*

(**a**) Soften and clear debris plugging the duct orifices

(**b**) Local anesthesia

(**c**) Seal the ducts after the procedure to prevent contrast leakage

→ **Answer on p. 380**

**Fig. 5.112 Digital imaging of papilloma.**

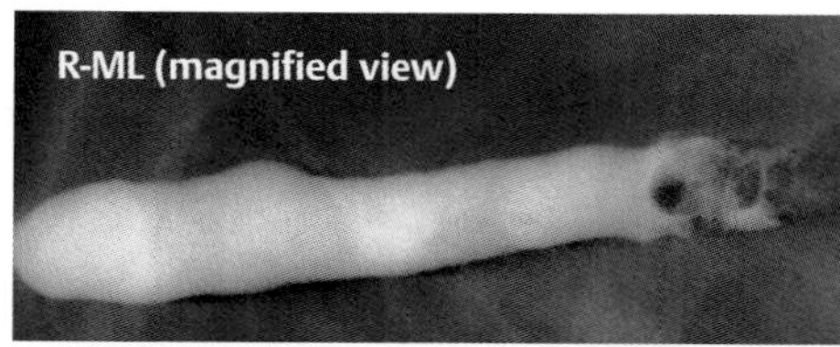


**a** *Conventional ductogram* with filling defects at **m/26**.

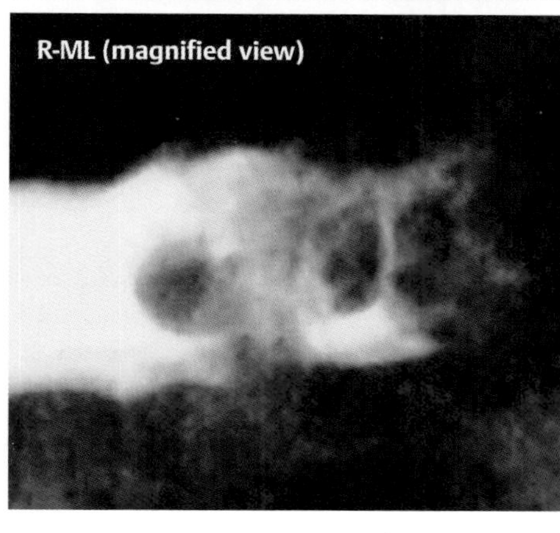


**b** *Digital enlargement* of **a** shows the irregular margins of the papilloma.

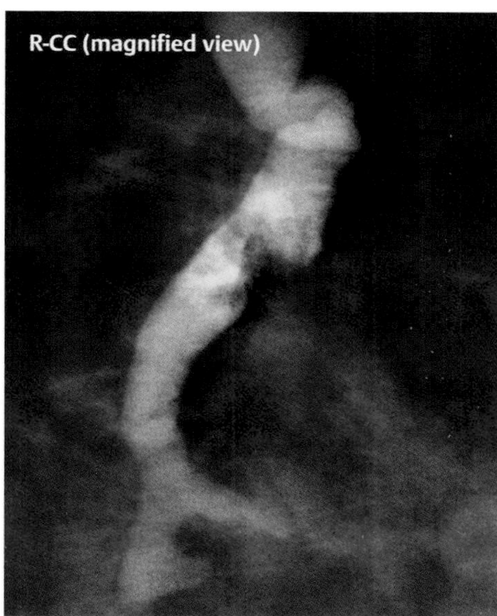


**c** *Conventional ductogram* shows a retroareolar duct with slight wall irregularities at **l/15**.

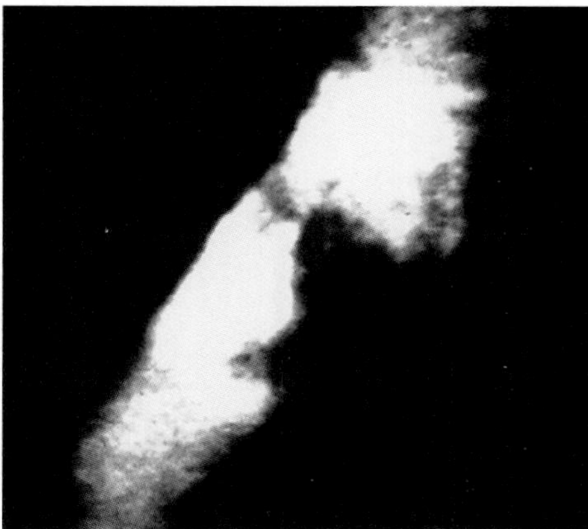

**d** *Digital image* of **c** shows bulging of the duct wall by a mural lesion at **L–M/6–7**.

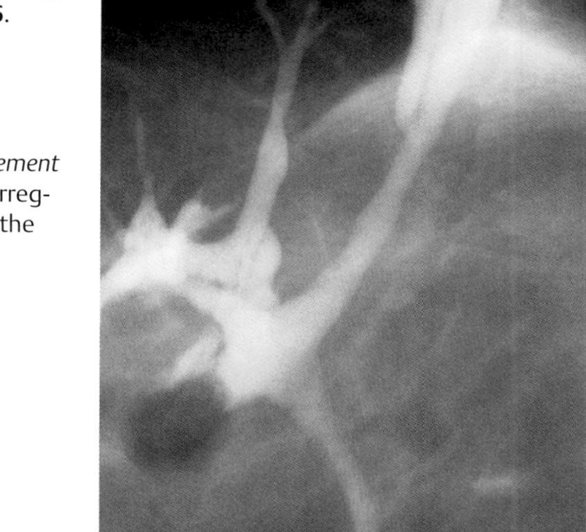


**e** *Conventional ductogram* shows a small filling defect at **P/22**.

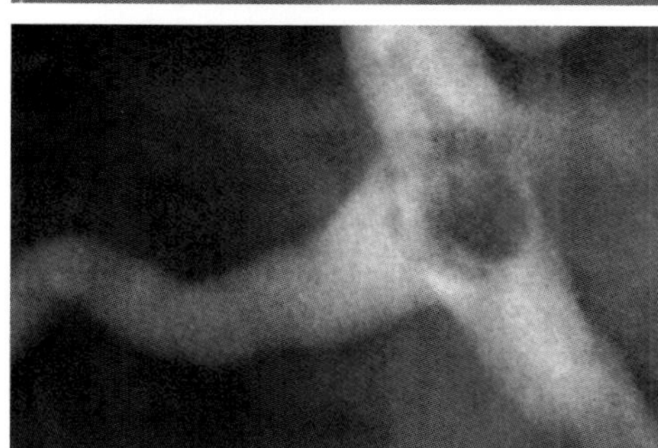

**f** *Digital enlargement* of **e** shows a mural papilloma at **R/18**.

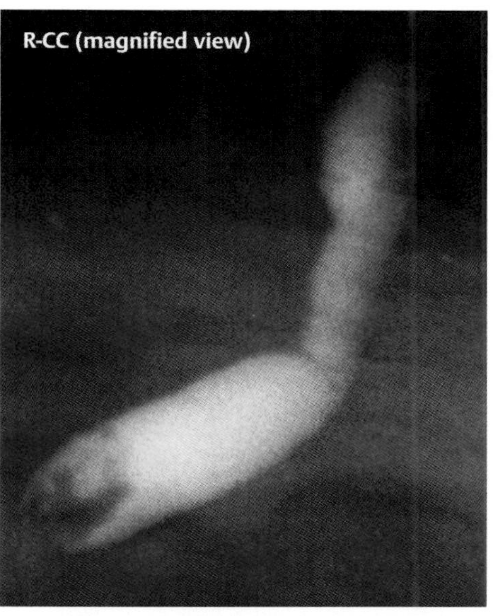


**g** *Conventional ductogram* shows retroareolar cutoff of the contrast column at **P–p/8**.

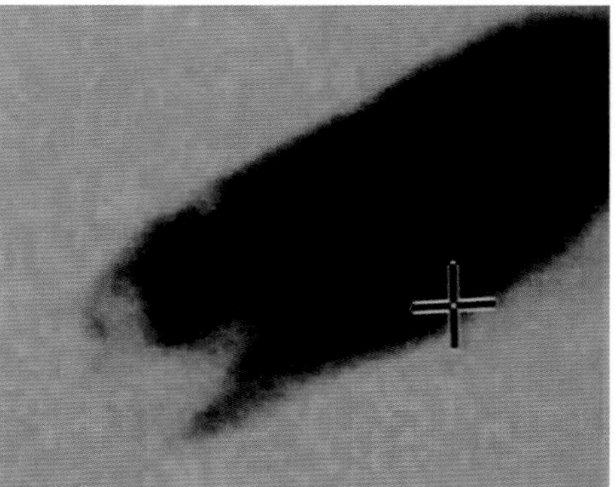

**h** *Digital enlargement* of **g** shows irregular margins of the papilloma protruding into the duct at **p/3** (image reversed).

▶ **Fig. 5.112 i–k**

**Fig. 5.112 Digital imaging of papilloma.** *(continued)*

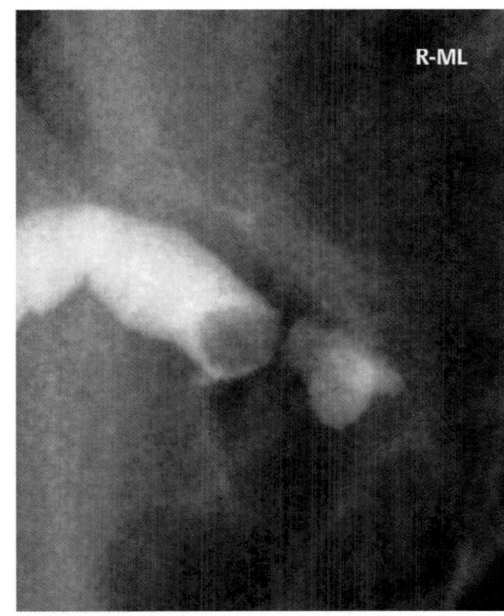


**i** *Conventional ductogram* shows a localized discontinuity in the duct (**b/23**).

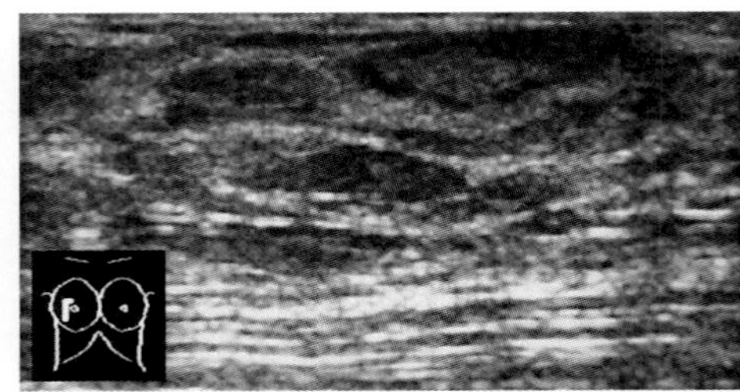

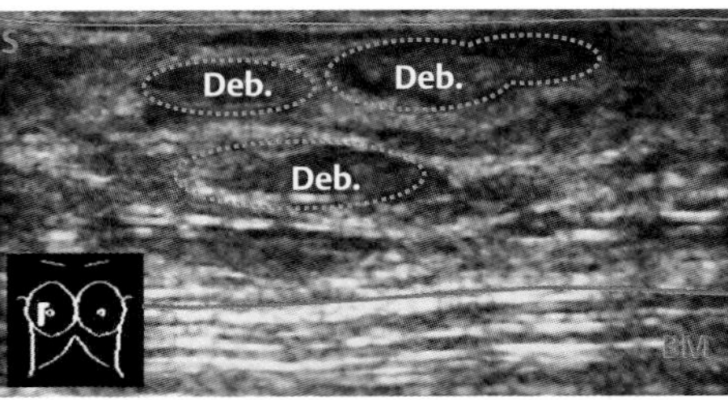


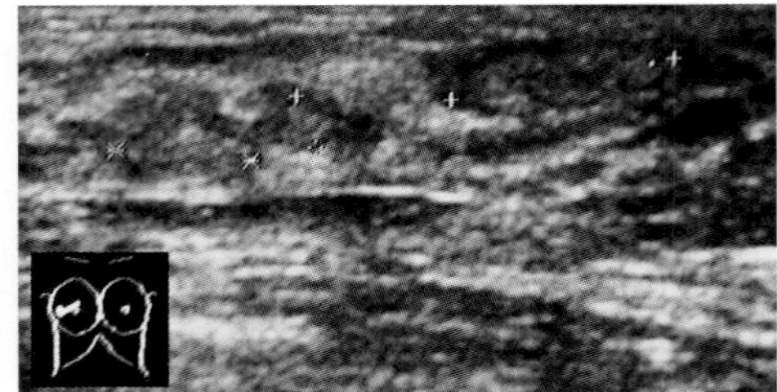

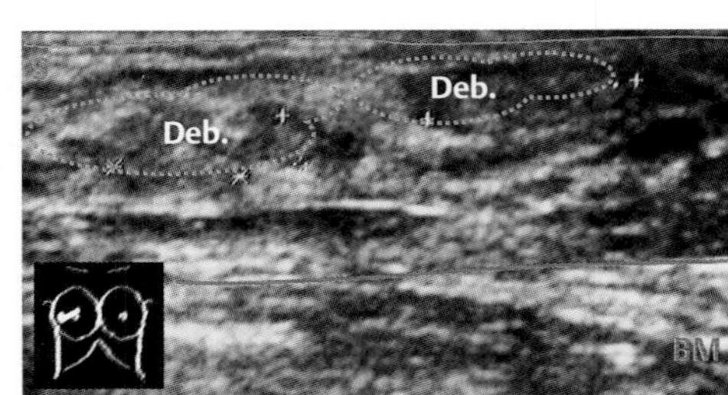


S = skin
Deb. = intraductal debris
BM = pectoral muscle

**k** *Retroareolar sonograms* show dilated milk ducts with intraductal debris (see diagrams; cytologically confirmed by FNA) with no evidence of a papilloma.

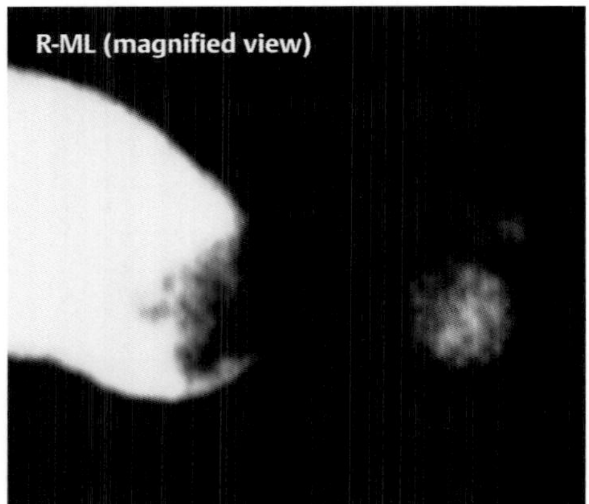


**j** *Digital enlargement* of **i** demonstrates the irregular surface of the papilloma.

**Question on Fig. 5.112**

*What distinguishes intraductal debris from intraductal papilloma?*

(**a**) It is never adherent to the duct wall.

(**b**) It has consistently smooth margins.

(**c**) It is never calcified.

→ **Answer on p. 380**

**Fig. 5.113 Ductographic and anatomic appearance of a papilloma.**

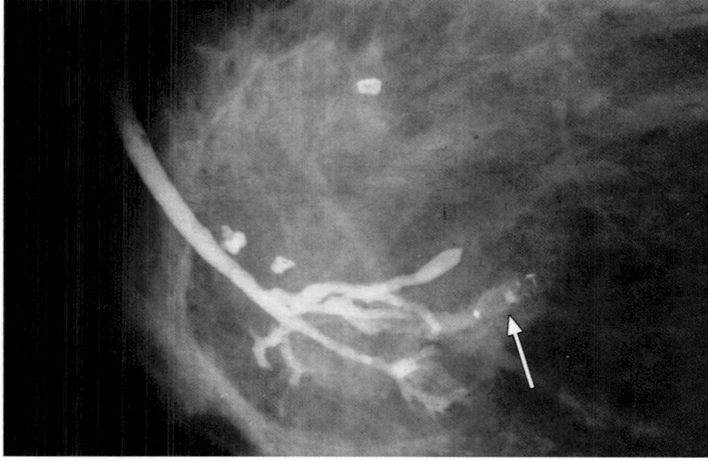

**a** *Conventional ductogram* (magnified view) shows coarse calcifications in the upper part of the breast at **c/9** and **b–C/6** and at the periphery of the opacified duct at **d/5** (arrow), where the contrast column is cut off by intraductal papilloma (arrow).

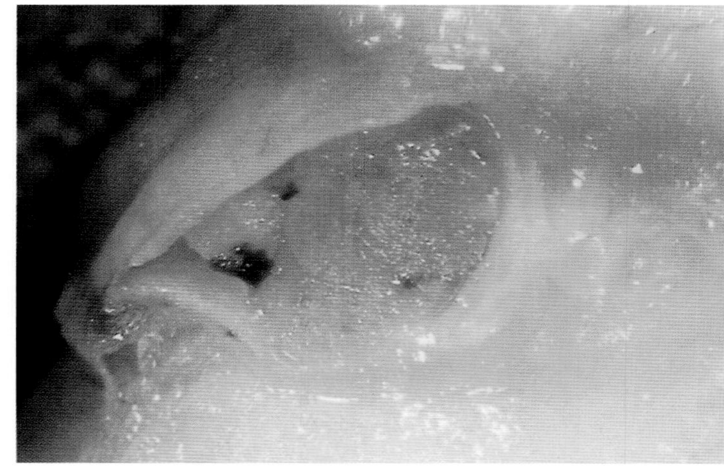

**b** *Anatomical specimen* (magnified 30× relative to (**a**) following injection of the secreting duct with contrast medium and patent blue dye (see **Fig. 5.111 d**, p. 242). The tumor has been extirpated, and the blue-stained duct is visible on the cut surface. **(This is why you should keep cutting in vacuum biopsies until all the blue dye is gone.)** Compare with **Fig. 5.119 e**, p. 252. The brown areas (**g/6**) are foci of calcified necrosis.

**Fig. 5.114 Nipple discharge at fibrocystic nodule and suspected papilloma.** A 43-year-old woman presents with a bloody right nipple discharge of sudden onset (**a**). The discharge contains abundant cellular material (**f**). Ductography reveals a tortuous, moderately ectatic duct with microcystic structures (**b, c**). Ultrasound shows an elliptical nodule with microcystic lucencies (**d, e**). MRI does not show increased gadolinium enhancement (**g**).

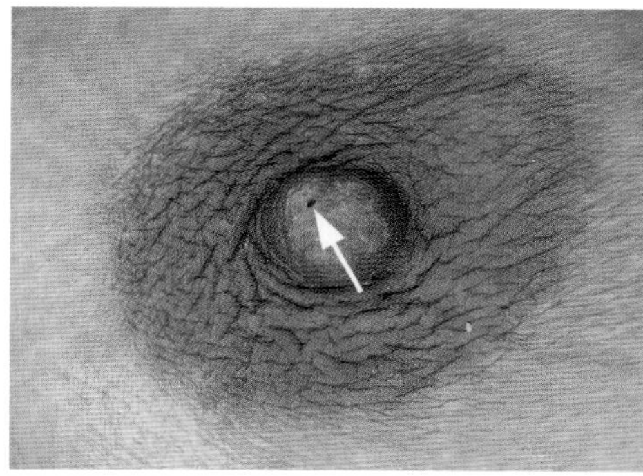

**a** *Clinical inspection* of the right nipple shows bloody discharge from a duct at the 11-o'clock position (arrow).

> ***Note:*** *The location of the bleeding duct is an indication that the affected lobe is also at the 11:00 o'clock position!*

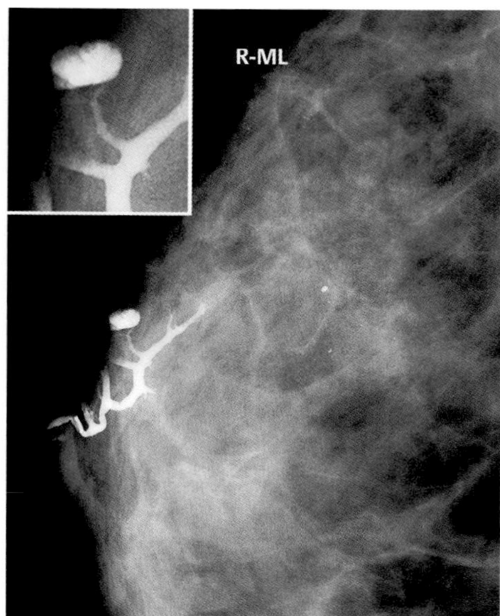


**b** *Mediolateral ductogram* of the right breast shows an ectatic retroareolar duct with subcutaneous cystic areas at **O/22**. There are no circumscribed cutoffs or filling defects.

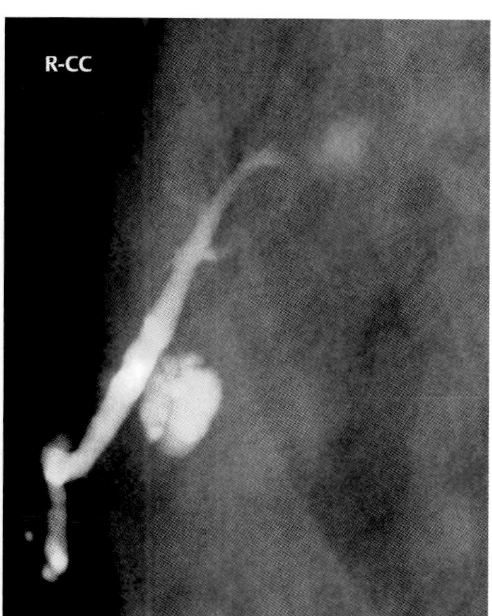


**c** *Craniocaudal ductogram* of the right breast shows an ectatic retroareolar duct with a septated cyst at **r/21**. There is no evidence of a papilloma.

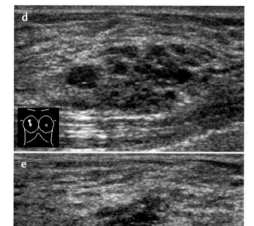

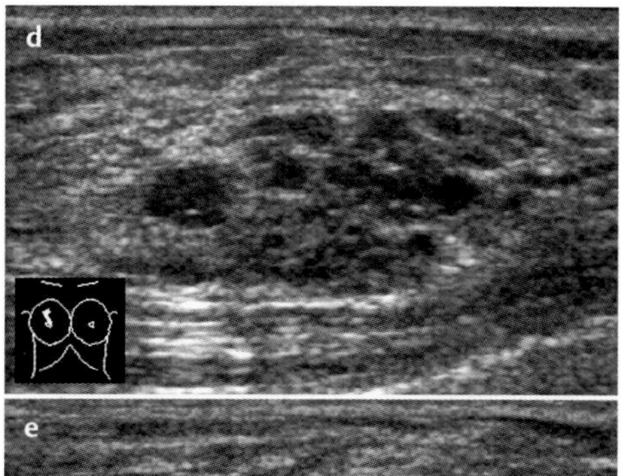


**d** (Above) *Periareolar sonogram* of the right breast at 11-o'clock shows a 2.7 cm × 1.8 cm × 1.6 cm lesion with microcystic changes (compare with **h**, p. 380). There is no definite evidence of posterior acoustic enhancement (except a small cyst left at **k/17**).
**e** (Below) *Scan* of the same region in a different plane.

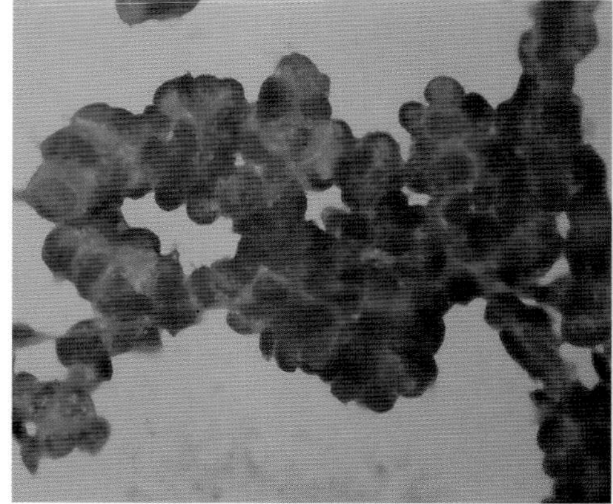

**f** *Cytologic smear* of nipple discharge shows compact aggregates of epithelial cells at different magnifications. Note the micropapillary proliferation of epithelial cells with enlarged, pleomorphic nuclei.

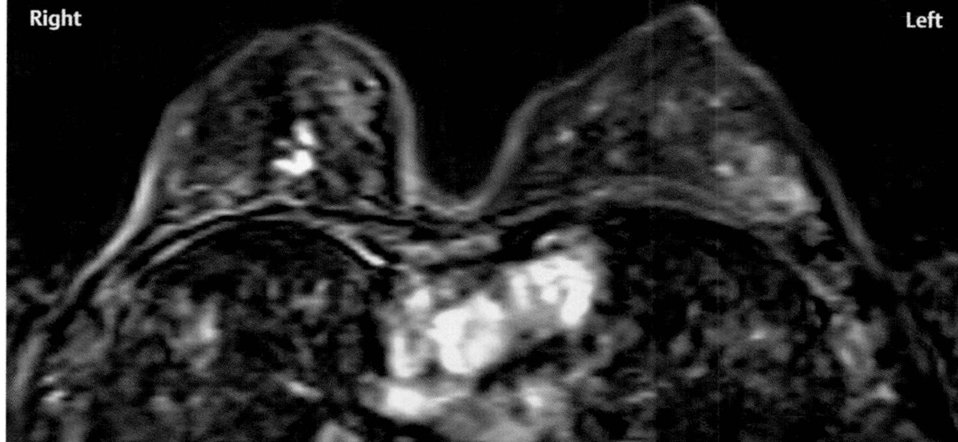


**g** *MR subtraction* image shows small, central foci of gadolinium enhancement (**P/6–7**) that are not identical to the sonographic in **d** and ductographic lesions in **b** and **c**. Fibrocystic nodules were detected at this site 4 years later.

**Question on Fig. 5.114**

*What is the source of the nipple discharge?*

(**a**) Intraductal carcinoma
(**b**) Fibrocystic nodule with a cyst and papillomas
(**c**) Cystic fibroadenoma communicating with the duct system

→ **Answer on p. 380**

### *Ultrasound-guided VB of Papillomas*

Eighty percent of the papillomas detected by ductography (see p. 243 f) are also visible sonographically and can be removed by ultrasound-guided VB. We recommend using an 11-gauge needle for small papillomas located just deep to the areola because it is less traumatizing than the 8-gauge needle. An 8-gauge needle is better for more peripherally located papillomas, as it can remove not just the visible papilloma but also any other ones that may surround the visible lesion. During VB the biopsy needle is positioned below the papilloma, which is resected from below upward. Bleeding may occur from the duct system following VB. While this is harmless, the patient should be advised of possible bleeding so that she will not be alarmed. Nipple discharge should cease after VB if the correct papilloma has been removed. Ductography in patients with abnormal discharge will occasionally show only a *dilated duct* with no visible papilloma. Ultrasound will often demonstrate the papilloma next to or at the end of the dilated duct, enabling it to be removed by ultrasound-guided VB. In the absence of discharge, many papillomas can be detected only sonographically and it may be difficult to distinguish these lesions from intraductal debris or a preinvasive lesion (**Figs. 5.115–5.117**).

*(continued p. 249)*

**Fig. 5.115 A 44-year-old woman presents with unexplained, yellowish watery discharge from her left nipple that has been present for years.** Two ductograms taken 3 years apart (**b** shows the earlier from 2001) and mammograms (**a** shows the most recent from 2004) were normal. The discharge is very troublesome for the patient because it repeatedly stains her blouse and bikini top yellow during the summer.

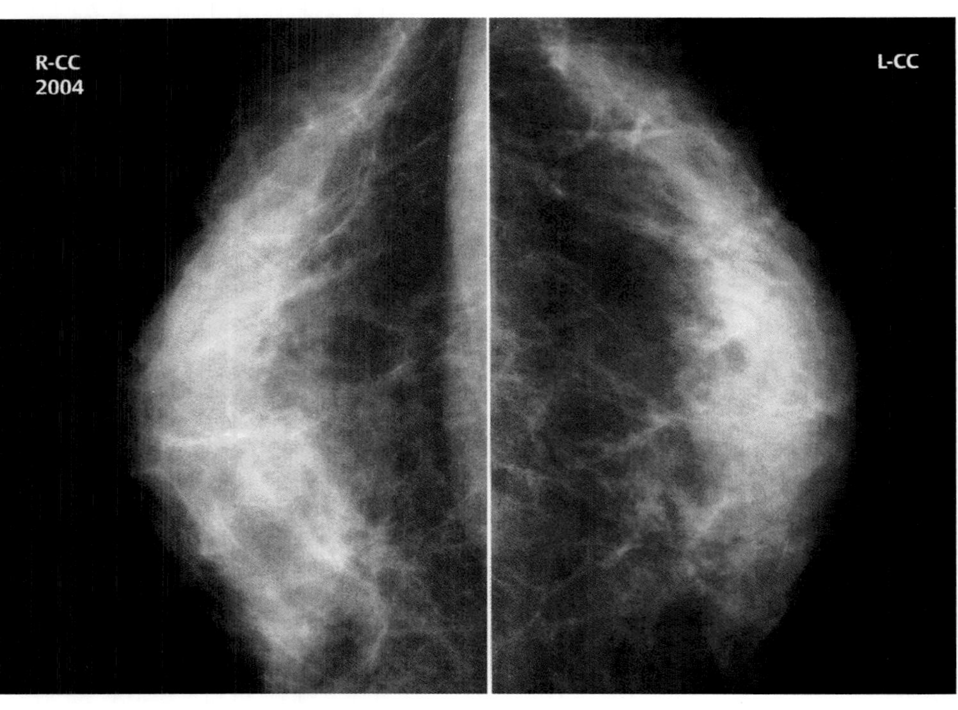


**a** *Bilateral craniocaudal mammograms* in 2004 show radiodense breasts and relative micromastia with no atypical changes or microcalcifications (ACR 3, BIRADS 1, **P**GMI).

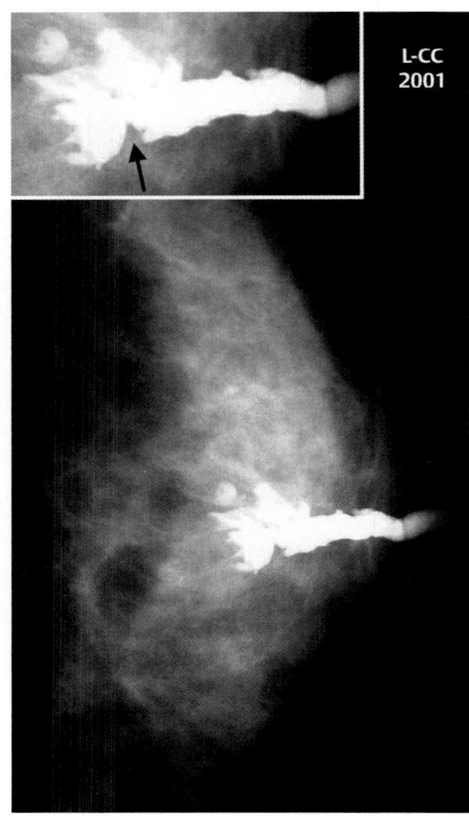


**b** *Craniocaudal ductography* of the left breast in May, 2001. The duct system is markedly dilated from nipple to periphery with a small kink (arrow in inset). The inset at upper left is a 2 × magnified view of the ectatic duct.

**Question on Fig. 5.115**

*In the ductograms, where might the papillomas be located that are perpetuating the ductectasia and nipple discharge?*

(**a**) Retroareolar (give coordinates)
(**b**) In the area of the duct bifurcation (give coordinates)
(**c**) In continuity with the ectatic ducts toward the chest wall (give coordinates)

→ **Answer on p. 381**

**Fig. 5.116 Recurrent bloody nipple discharge in a 58-year-old woman.** Ductography shows a vermiform filling defect in the retroareolar main duct (**b**). This area shows intense gadolinium enhancement on MRI (**c**), and cytology reveals typical changes (**a**).

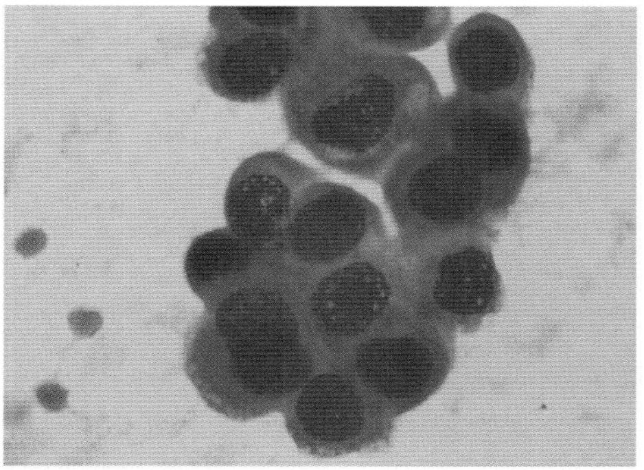

**a** *Cytologic examination* of a nipple smear shows a papillary fragment with low-grade nuclear atypia and prominent nucleoli.

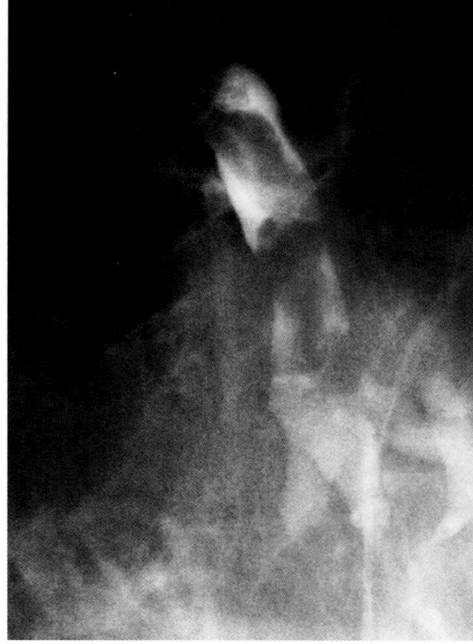

**b** *Ductography.* Instillation of contrast medium into the bleeding duct shows a curvilinear filling defect.

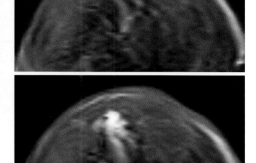

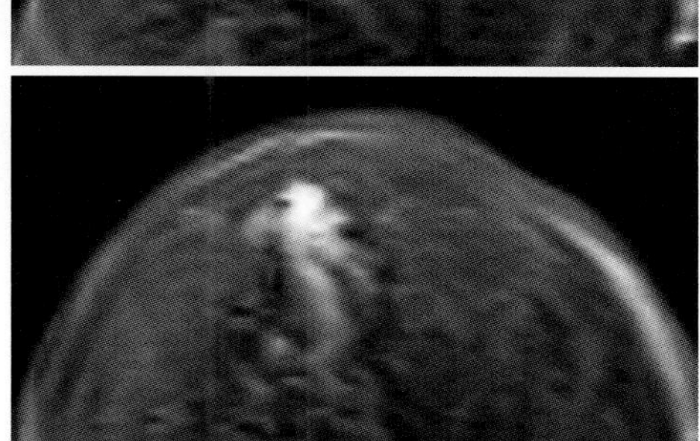

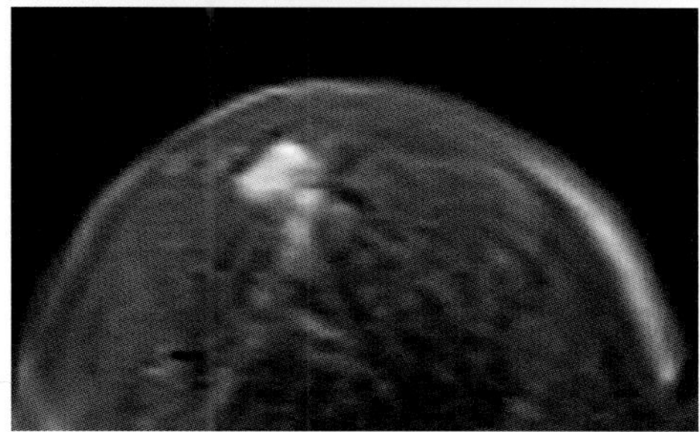

**c** *MR subtraction* image shows intense gadolinium enhancement along the affected duct (e.g., **r/21–22**).

**Question on Fig. 5.116**

*How would you interpret these findings?*

(**a**) Papilloma

(**b**) Papillary carcinoma

(**c**) Ductectasia with debris

→ **Answer on p. 382**

**Fig. 5.117 Palpable 5 cm × 6 cm × 6 cm supra-areolar nodule in the left breast of a 45-year-old woman (a).** Mammograms show fibrocystic changes with coarse nodular densities in both breasts (**b**). Ultrasound demonstrates a cyst with irregular wall deposits (**c**) that enhance on post-gadolinium MRI (**d**). Following needle aspiration of the cyst contents, the collapsed cyst still contains wall irregularities (**f**), which are removed by vacuum biopsy. At 6-month follow-up, ultrasound again demonstrates a cyst with an intraluminal nodule (**g**).

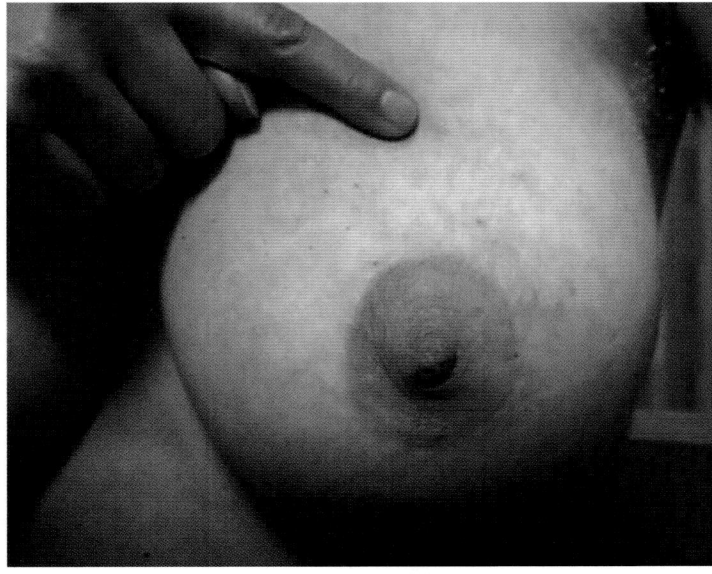

**a** *Physical examination* of the left breast shows a palpable supra-areolar nodule (**M–m/8–9**) not associated with retraction or bulging of the skin. The nipple appears normal.

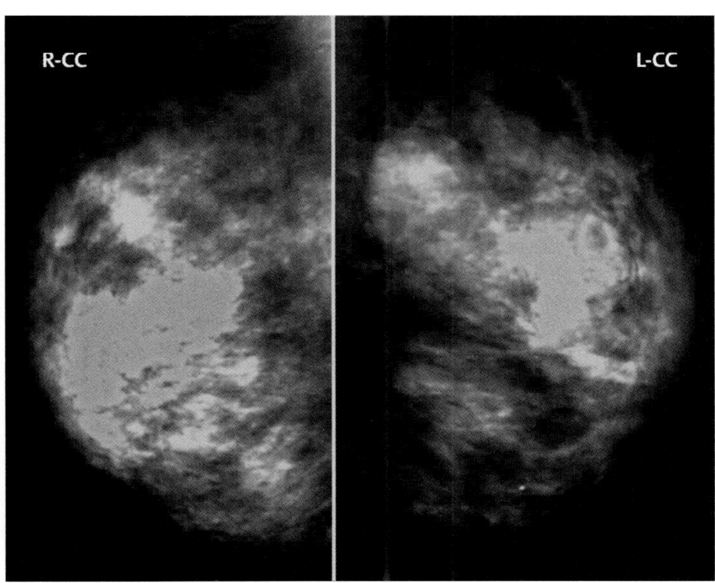


**b** *Bilateral craniocaudal mammograms* show very dense, inhomogeneous breasts with irregular, partially confluent densities predominantly on the right side (ACR 4, BIRADS 1, PGMI).

▶ **Fig. 5.117 c–g**

**Fig. 5.117 Palpable 5 cm × 6 cm × 6 cm supra-areolar nodule in the left breast of a 45-year-old woman.** *(continued)*

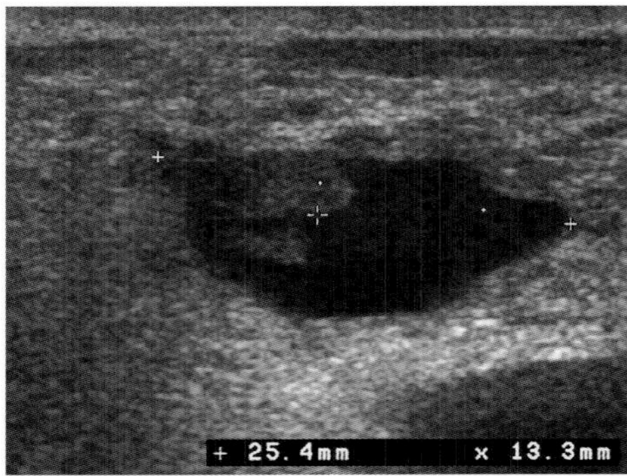

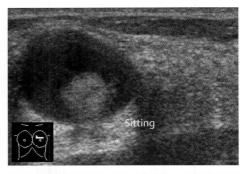

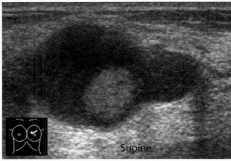

**c** *Sonogram* of the palpable nodule in **a** demonstrates a large cyst with intracystic vegetations.

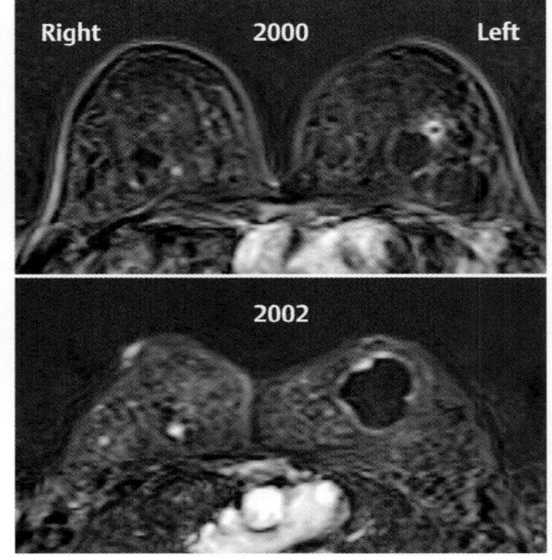


**d** *MR subtraction* images in 2000 (above) and 2002 (below). The 2002 image shows intense, irregular gadolinium enhancement of the cyst wall in the left breast. The same site showed ring enhancement 2 years earlier (**f/23+26**).

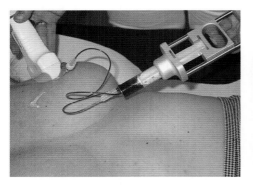

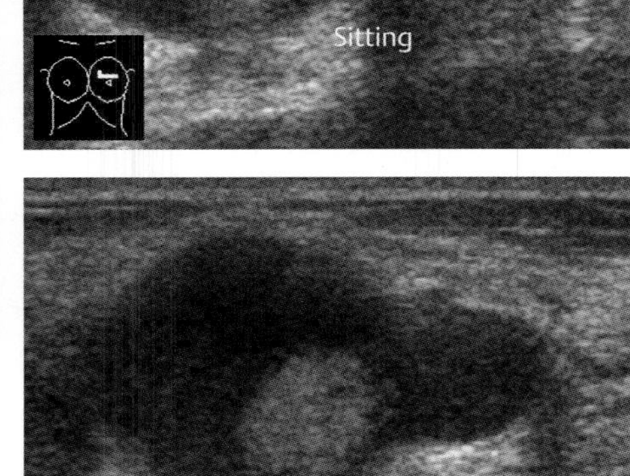

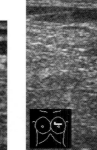

**e** *Fine-needle aspiration.* The cyst contents are evacuated under ultrasound guidance, yielding a bloody aspirate.

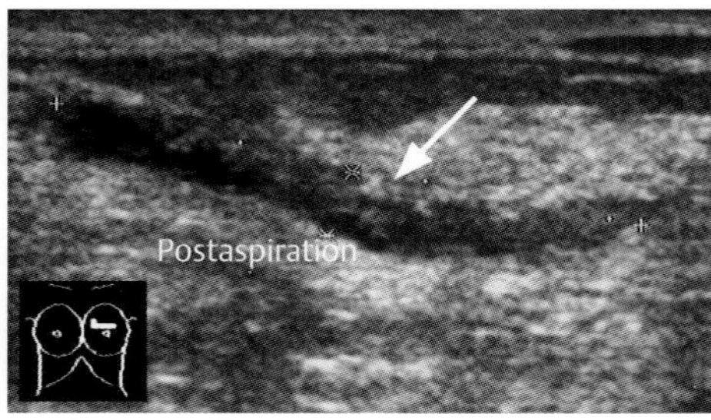


**f** *Ultrasound* after cyst aspiration. The cyst does not collapse completely but shows irregular intracystic wall changes, which were removed by vacuum biopsy.

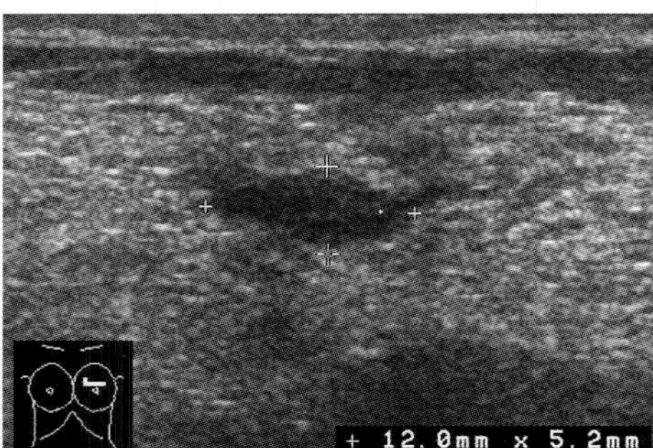


**g** *Ultrasound* 6 months after vacuum biopsy reveals new cysts with an intracystic nodule at **i/25**. The nodule changes its position slightly when the patient moves from a sitting to supine position. As before, *percutaneous aspiration* does not completely evacuate the cyst (**i/16**).

**Question 1 on Fig. 5.117**

*How would you interpret the intracystic wall changes in* ***c–f****?*

(**a**) Intracystic papillomas
(**b**) Intracystic mural debris in ductectasia
(**c**) Papillary cystic carcinoma

→ **Answer on p. 382**

**Question 2 on Fig. 5.117**

*What is on the floor of the new cyst detected 6 months later?*

(**a**) Papillary tumor
(**b**) Blood clot following vacuum biopsy
(**c**) Intracystic nodular, fatty debris as in ductectasia

→ **Answer on p. 382**

### Digital Stereotactic Interventions

Digital stereotactic breast needle biopsies are most commonly performed in patients with atypical microcalcifications that require biopsy to exclude DCIS or comedocarcinoma. Some authors consider this an indication for VB (Kettritz et al. 2004), but we believe that primary CNB is appropriate for all atypical mammographic changes to establish a definitive diagnosis.

> **!** **Fine-needle aspiration (FNA) should not be used to investigate microcalcifications. It is too imprecise and should be used only for subcutaneous or prepectoral calcifications that are not accessible to CNB.**

If the biopsy indicates malignancy, the remaining calcifications should be surgically excised with a healthy tissue margin (R0). If the lesion is benign (sclerosing adenosis, etc.), the remaining calcifications should be left alone. In many cases they will resolve spontaneously over time (see **Fig. 4.20**, p. 41 and p. 345).

There are only a few cases (small-cell ADH) in which the remaining calcifications should be removed by VB in consultation with the pathologist. If the VB shows no additional ADH lesions, there is no need for further interventions. Otherwise the lesion should be surgically removed with clear margins.

#### *Digital Stereotactic Fine-Needle Aspiration (ST-FNA)*

Digital stereotactic fine-needle aspiration (ST-FNA) is used only for subcutaneous or immediate retroareolar lesions that are not accessible to core biopsy. The tissue is biopsied by making careful needle excursions with a mounted vacuum syringe holder or with tubing between the aspiration needle and vacuum syringe (see **Figs. 5.108 a–c**, p. 236) while very gentle suction is applied. The aspirate is handled as described on p. 235. FNA can be completed in a very short time. Vasovagal syncope may still occur, however. A compression bandage is not necessary following FNA.

#### *Digital Stereotactic Core-Needle Biopsy (ST-CNB)*

In digital stereotactic core-needle biopsy (ST-CNB), the skin is anesthetized with a maximum of 1 mL lidocaine solution and the coaxial biopsy needle is introduced under mammographic guidance to a targeted site designated by computer coordinates (see **Fig. 5.107**). The tissue within the breast is not very sensitive to pain. Too much anesthetic will displace the calcifications from the biopsy plane, causing the radiologist to lose sight of the needle and making it necessary to redefine the target coordinates. Initially the patient is placed in a comfortable sitting position in front of the stereotactic unit. To aid patient relaxation, the wheels of the chair should be locked so that the patient does not have to tense the buttocks and spine to keep the chair stationary. The needle can be introduced in the craniocaudal, mediolateral, or lateromedial direction (but not upward), depending on the location of the targeted lesion within the breast. Hemodynamically stable patients should be biopsied in the prone position. There should always be at least 2 cm distance between the lesion and skin; otherwise the outer sheath and core needle will be intracutaneous or just subcutaneous so that any forward or lateral needle movement will include skin in the biopsy, creating relatively large tissue defects (see **Fig. 5.118 b**). At times, then, the biopsy device should be angled in order to achieve the minimum 2 mm distance from the skin. If a large skin defect is created, its edges should be approximated with a wound closure strip (Leukostrip) to avoid unsightly scarring. Generally the defects will heal well with an acceptable cosmetic result.

> **For cosmetic reasons, intramammary lesions located in the cleavage area should be biopsied from the lateral side whenever possible, rather than from above.**

Finally, the breast is positioned on the film holder such that the calcifications or other mammographic lesions are at the approximate center of the 6 × 8 cm detector field indicated by a light beam. The breast is carefully compressed. It is very important in digital CNB to work quickly and calmly, especially when the patient is sitting upright. This may enable the examiner to collect at least some of the necessary 8–13 tissue samples in the event of a syncopal episode. Digital technology is essential for working quickly. Analog stereotactic units and film-screen mammography units without stereotaxy are too slow and too arduous for the patient; today they are considered obsolete (Yang and Tse 2004).

For sampling calcifications, the needle holder is moved manually or with a motor drive (Giotto) several millimeters toward the nipple after each pass. This allows new tissue to enter the notch of the biopsy needle. Several core samples are collected in this way (3–5 for solid lesions, 8–13 for calcifications). Intermittent check images are taken to show the current needle position and remaining calcifications. Tissue cores should be sampled from various regions of the calcification cluster or density and should contain calcifications.

For calcifications, a specimen radiograph may be taken concurrently on a separate unit or the samples may be placed in formalin and x-rayed on the stereotactic unit (see **Fig. 5.107 e**). The ideal solution would be to have a second mammography unit for specimen radiography so that removal of the calcifications could be continuously monitored.

The patient compresses the biopsy site after the needle is withdrawn, taking care to place pressure not just on the skin but especially on the deeper area from which the samples were taken. Afterward a compression bandage is wrapped around the chest and worn for 3–5 hours (see **Fig. 5.107 h**, p. 233) to control hematoma formation and pain.

The following **documentation** is needed for digital stereotactic breast needle biopsies:

- Mammographic views (0°, + 15°, − 15°)
- Two prefire images (to document the coaxial needle at different tube angles)
- Two postfire images (deployed biopsy needle at different tube angles)
- After VB: two images of the biopsy cavity after needle removal (at different tube angles)

The prefire images can be used to adjust the needle position, and the postfire images show the biopsy needle within the lesion. All the images are digitally stored.

If the patient shows signs of faintness during CNB in a sitting position, the operator should continue to take core samples for as long

**Fig. 5.118 Atypical microcalcifications in a 64-year-old woman.** The microcalcifications occupy a high retroareolar site approximately 2 cm beneath the skin (**a**). Digital stereotactic core-needle biopsy yields benign calcifications (sclerosing adenosis). Given the subcutaneous location of the calcifications, the outer sheath of the biopsy needle is placed just within or beneath the skin and easily slips from skin level when the needle is moved along the *x* and *y* axes. This causes the sheath to pierce the skin during the next pass, creating fairly large skin defects (**b**).

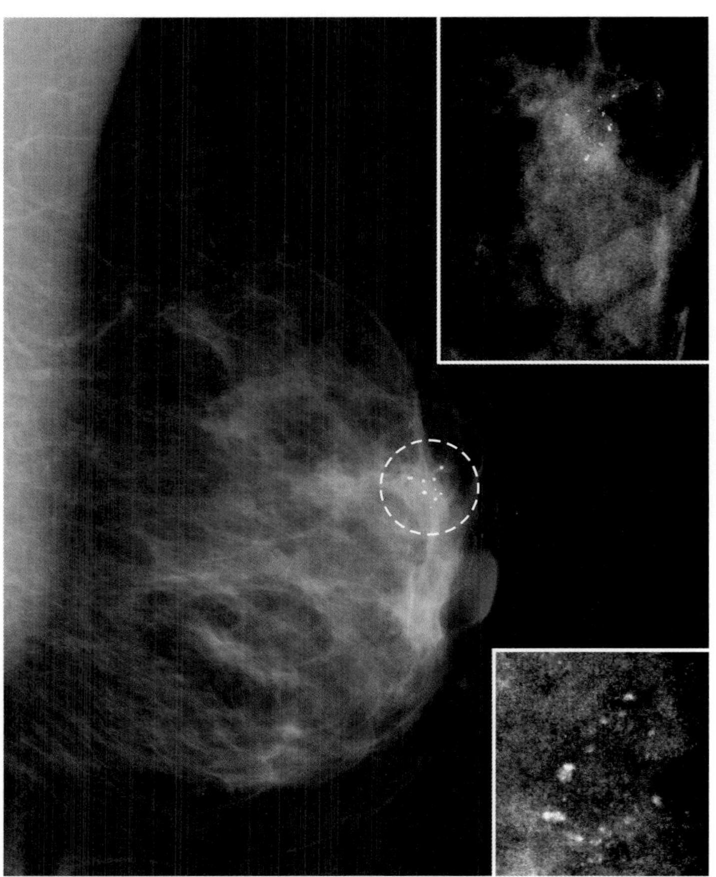

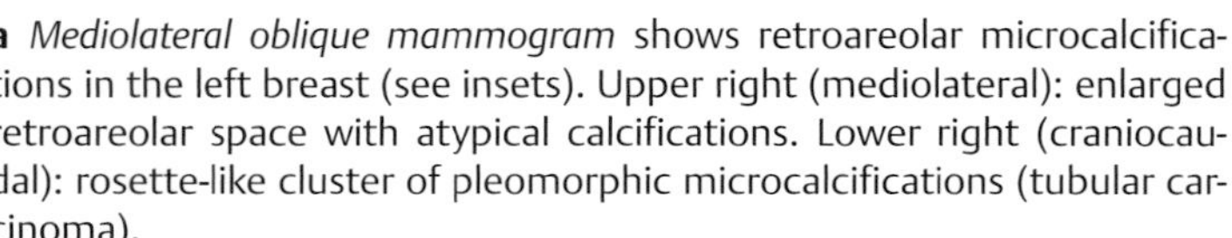

**a** *Mediolateral oblique mammogram* shows retroareolar microcalcifications in the left breast (see insets). Upper right (mediolateral): enlarged retroareolar space with atypical calcifications. Lower right (craniocaudal): rosette-like cluster of pleomorphic microcalcifications (tubular carcinoma).

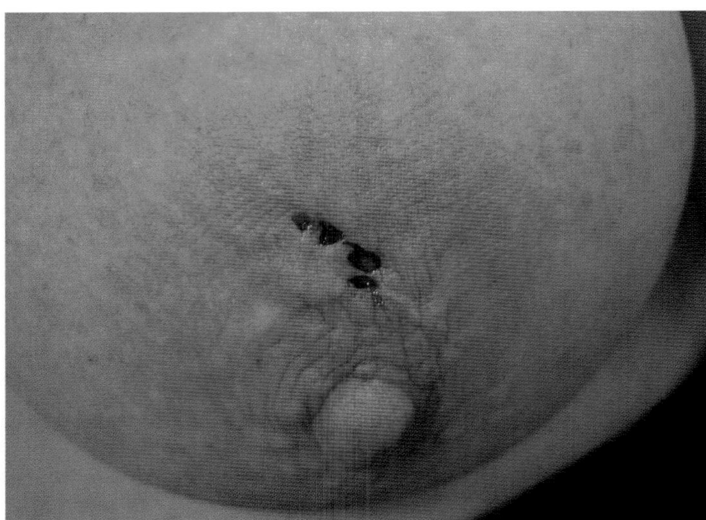

**b** *Physical aspect*: Skin defects following core biopsy. The outer sheath was placed too close to the skin, resulting in multiple adjacent skin defects.

**Question on Fig. 5.118**

*How can these tissue defects be avoided?*

(**a**) Biopsy from the lateral side

(**b**) Use a longer guide sheath

(**c**) Biopsy from the nipple-areola

→ **Answer on p. 382**

as possible so that a diagnosis can be made. If the patient loses consciousness, which should be the exception rather than the rule (this problem is less common with dedicated biopsy tables, see **Fig. 5.107 g**, p. 233), the needle should be quickly withdrawn; breast compression is released, and the patient is placed in a flat recumbent position, either by opening the examination chair to a reclining position or by moving the patient to a separate couch. **When the patient is moved, her head should be supported so that it cannot loll back, causing cervical spine injury.** When her legs have been elevated, a strong pulse should return within a few seconds. If the biopsy needs to be continued, 90% of patients will tolerate it without experiencing another syncopal attack.

When a digital stereotactic biopsy unit is available with a special table (produced by Fisher, Lorad, Giotto, and other manufacturers), the patient lies prone for the procedure. Vasovagal reactions may still occur but will not cause syncope in the prone patient. Other aspects of equipment handling are the same as with upright units.

### *Digital Stereotactic Vacuum Biopsy*

Digital vacuum biopsy (D-VB) can be performed in the sitting or recumbent position. Add-on equipment (Senovision, GE) is available for performing VB in the sitting position (see **Fig. 5.21**, p. 104). With the Senovision system, VB can be performed with the patient sitting or lying down. In the latter case the patient is positioned laterally on a mobile, height-adjustable couch.

Various special tables are available for performing VB in the prone position (Fisher and Giotto, IMS; see **Fig. 5.22**, p. 104).

When a lateral approach is used (mandatory with the GE system, craniocaudal also available with the Siemens and Giotto systems), the breast is compressed in the craniocaudal direction. The approach is tailored to leave a minimum distance of 1 cm between the skin and targeted lesion. When this requirement is met, the VB needle should follow the shortest path between the intramammary lesion and skin. For example, lesions in the inner quadrants are not biopsied from the lateral side.

A survey image is taken of the targeted lesion, which is positioned at the center of the image. Then two oblique images are obtained, and the coordinates are calculated somewhat differently than in CNB.

The biopsy needle is advanced to the lesion in the cocked position. Confirmatory images are taken, and the VB is performed. After each sampling the biopsy needle is rotated 10° and the lesion is progressively removed from the center out to the periphery. When relatively large calcification clusters are removed, we recommend a "second run" in which the surrounding tissue is separately sampled and histologically processed without changing the needle. The calcifications in the first run and the surrounding tissue in the second run are placed in different containers for separate radiographic and histologic evaluation.

We do not routinely obtain a mammogram immediately after VB or on the following day. A mammogram at this time may demonstrate a hematoma but would have no other practical value.

When VB is performed with an 11-gauge needle, at least 20 tissue samples should be collected. Fewer samples are collected with an 8-gauge needle. In all cases, enough tissue samples should be collected to remove the entire lesion (see **Fig. 5.119**).

#### *Papillomas: Digital Imaging and Vacuum Biopsy*

Papillomas appear as circumscribed filling defects in ductograms (see p. 243). When these defects are digitally enlarged, the margins, location, and surface characteristics of the papillomas can be defined and evaluated much better by adjusting the digital window than they can on conventional ductograms. If the papillomas are visible sonographically, they can be removed under ultrasound guidance. Otherwise they are removed by digital stereotactic guidance.

Before digital stereotactic VB (see **Fig. 5.119**) is begun, the secreting duct is visualized with a 2 : 1 mixture of contrast medium and patent blue dye. The nipple is sealed with *liquid collodion* to prevent external leakage of contrast medium and patent blue dye from the duct system (see **Fig. 5.119 a**). The now-visible papilloma is centered in the digital detector field, and moderate compression is applied to the breast. The rest of the procedure corresponds to the technique of digital stereotactic VB described on p. 238.

In removing the papilloma, the biopsy is continued until blue-stained tissue is no longer visible in the sampled material (see **Fig. 5.119 e**).

If pain occurs during the biopsy, additional local anesthetic can be delivered to the tip of the palpable biopsy needle, either through the needle bore itself or by direct percutaneous injection.

> ***Tip***
>
> **As in CNB, only a little local anesthetic should be injected initially before placement of the VB needle to avoid displacing calcifications or other lesions away from the computer coordinates.**

It is sufficient to anesthetize the skin and subcutaneous fat before making the incision with a small scalpel. The incision should be no longer than 5 mm (the tip of the 8-gauge VB needle has a built-in scalpel that must be introduced *parallel* to the incision).

After the biopsy needle has been withdrawn, the patient compresses her breast for 10–15 minutes. Then a compression bandage is applied (see **Fig. 5.107 h**) and worn for 24 hours.

Hematomas are common following the VB of papillomas (see **Fig. 5.119 f**). Often the hematoma looks bad and is alarming for the patient, but usually it will clear spontaneously within a few weeks.

#### *Summary and Evaluation of Various Interventional Procedures in Our Patients*

Please see Weining-Klemm (2004).

Percutaneous biopsy methods such as fine-needle aspiration (FNA) and core-needle biopsy (CNB) with sonographic guidance (SO-CNB) or digital stereotactic guidance (ST-CNB) are well-established procedures. Vacuum biopsy (VB) that can be performed with sonographic guidance (SO-VB) or digital stereotactic guidance (ST-VB). The overall costs of VB are 8 times higher than those of FNA and 3.3 times higher than those of CNB (the difference in material costs is even higher). The costs of different biopsy methods are compared in **Table 5.13**, and a graphic cost comparison is shown in **Fig. 5.120**. VB is increasingly favored in Europe (Kettritz et al. 2004), while FNA in particular is becoming less popular even though it is the most economical choice.

The financial resources of our healthcare system and the costs of mammographic screening force us to consider whether VB is always appropriate for the investigation of indeterminate breast lesions. Our general goal should be to reduce the costs of screening (see p. 126) while keeping the costs of interventional procedures as low as possible.

What has been our experience with FNA, CNB, SO-CNB, ST-CNB, and VB at the *IMZE*? VB has been and is the procedure of choice for benign breast lesions (fibroadenoma, papilloma, etc.). What results have we had with respect to positive predictive value (PPV), false-positive rate, negative predictive value (NPV), false-negative rate, and sensitivity and specificity? How do the complication rates vary among the different procedures?

A total of 1113 biopsies were performed in 771 women at our center between 1993 and 2003. Three hundred eighty-one patients had a suspicious lesion and underwent surgery, and 390 women with benign histologies had an initial follow-up at 6 months and then yearly. To eliminate individual variations due to different examiners, we analyzed only the data from biopsies that were personally performed by the author of this book.

FNA was most commonly done with ultrasound guidance. In 310 cases (151 benign, 159 malignant), **ultrasound-guided FNA** had a sensitivity of 90%, a specificity of 95%, a PPV of 95%, a NPV of 92%, a false-positive rate of 2%, and a false-negative rate of 4.5%.

**SO-CNB, ST-CNB,** and **VB** had sensitivities of 95% (benign) and 94% (malignant), specificities of 98.5% (benign) and 100% (malignant), a PPV of 97% (benign) and 100% (malignant), and a NPV of 97% (benign) and 100% (malignant) (**Fig. 5.123**, p. 254). The false-positive rates were 1% (benign) and 0% (malignant), while the false-negative rates were 2% (benign) and 1% (malignant) (**Figs. 5.121, 5.122**, p. 254).

All the results were comparable to those reported in the literature. FNA and CNB were less specific in the diagnosis of fibrocystic changes, suggesting that VB is a good alternative in these cases. FNA, SO-CNB, and VB were less sensitive in the diagnosis of calcifying DCIS. VB was associated with a higher incidence of postprocedure hematoma (10%) than FNA and CNB (2%).

*(continued on p. 254)*

**Fig. 5.119 A 65-year-old woman has had a bloody right nipple discharge for several months.** Physical examination shows no nodularity and no skin or nipple retraction. Ductography of the right breast (**a**) shows changes suspicious for papilloma in the upper outer quadrant (**b**). The duct system was opacified with a mixture of patent blue dye and contrast medium, and the nipple was sealed with liquid collodion to prevent contrast spillage (**a**). The papilloma was localized in the digital image with the aid of a radiopaque centimeter marker stuck to the skin (**a, b** right) (not mandatory; used only for lesions difficult to locate in a small digital window). Digital stereotactic localization of the papilloma was performed (**c**), and the lesion was removed with visual feedback from the blue-stained tissue cores (**e**). A second run was completed to remove all blue-stained tissue.

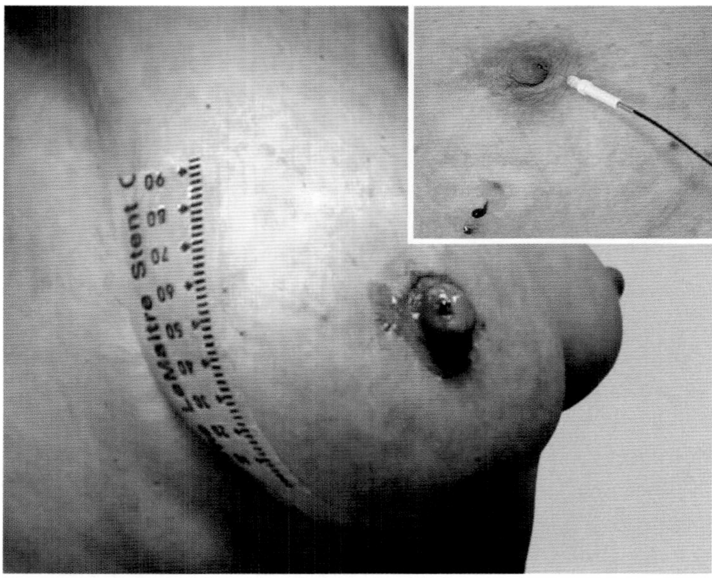

**a** *Clinical appearance* of the right breast after ductography, staining of the duct system with a patent blue dye mixture, and sealing of the nipple with liquid collodion. A radiopaque centimeter marker may aid in locating the papilloma during digital vacuum biopsy. Injection of the patent blue dye and contrast medium through an ultra-thin ductography needle is shown at upper right.

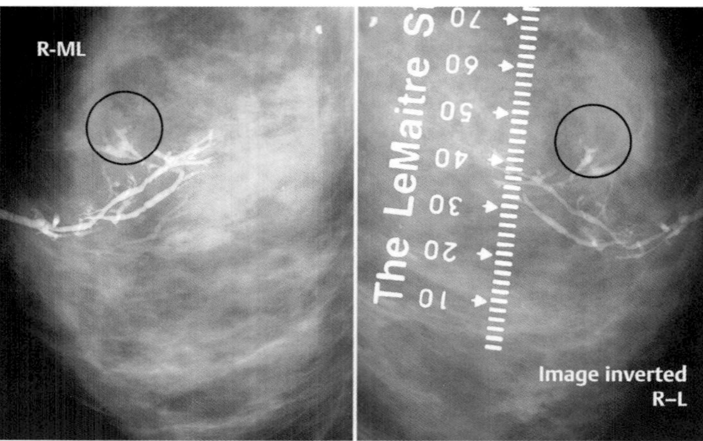


**b** *Ductography* (magnified view). The image at left shows the papilloma (circle) in the upper periphery of the breast. At right is a right/left inverted image showing the illuminated centimeter marker.

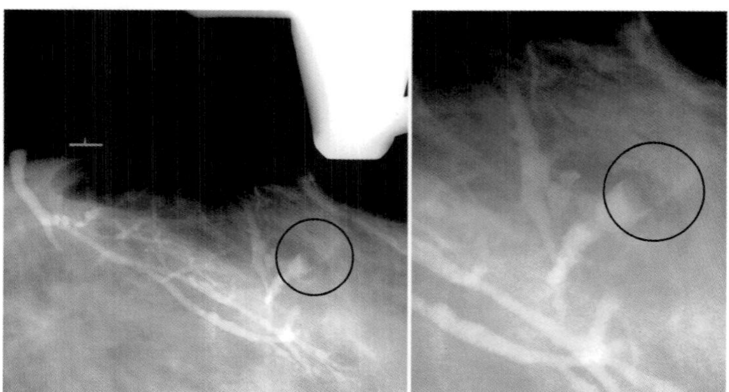

**c** *Prefire digital images*. Each image is a 15° oblique view for localizing the lesion.

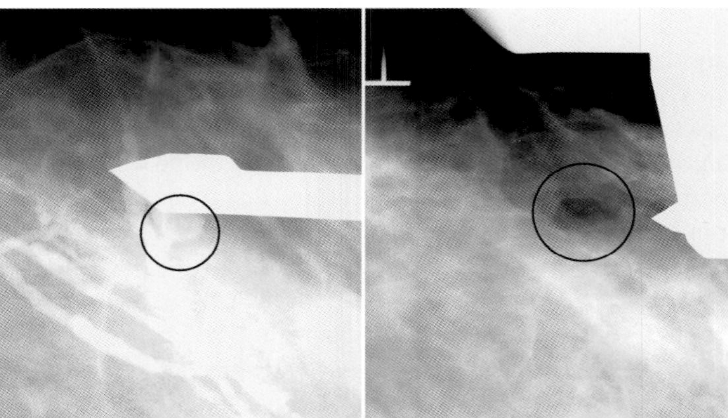

**d** *Digital images*. At left the biopsy needle has been introduced and manually advanced a few millimeters to place the needle notch over the papilloma. At right the biopsy has been performed and the needle removed, leaving a small air-filled tissue defect at the former site of the papilloma.

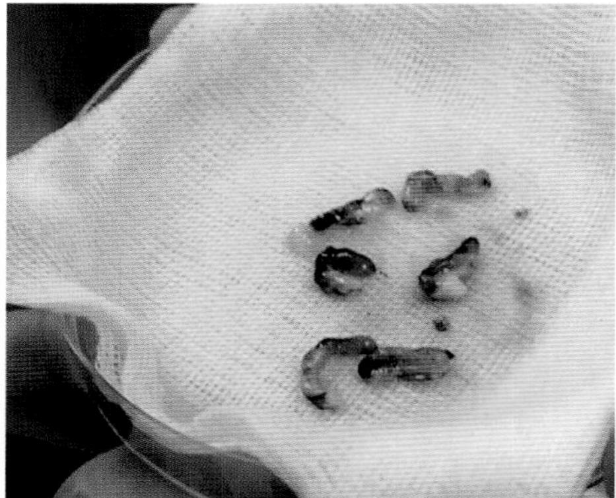

**e** *Biopsy specimens.* The blue-stained tissue fragments represent papilloma.

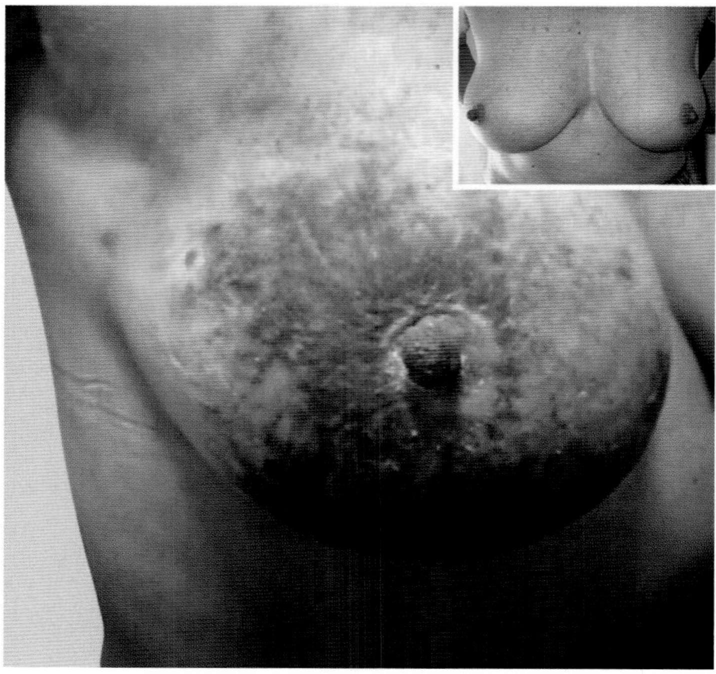

**f** Extensive bruising (large hematoma) is visible 12 days after vacuum biopsy. The inset at upper right shows a normal clinical appearance 6 months later.

**Fig. 5.119** **A 65-year-old woman has had a bloody right nipple discharge for several months.** *(continued)*

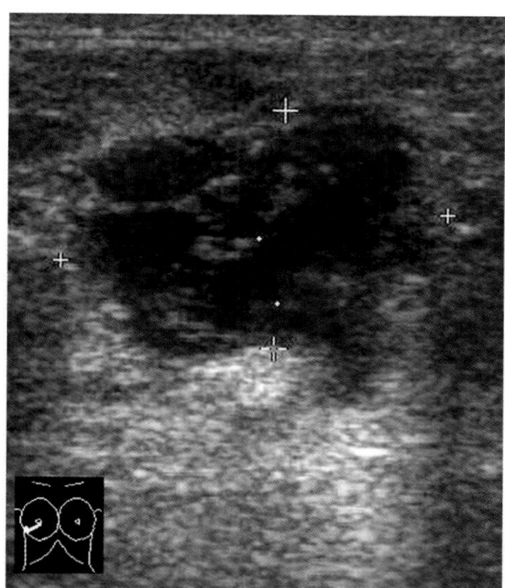

**g** *Sonogram* demonstrates a 5 cm × 2.4 cm × 2.4 cm hematoma with extensive internal echoes due to clotted blood.

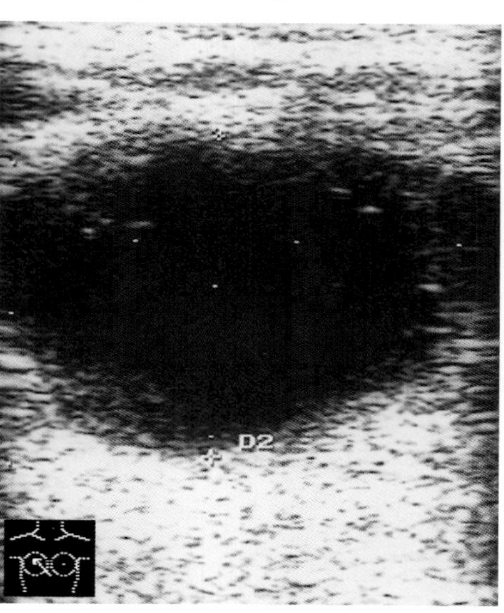



**h** Sonogram 8 days later shows liquefaction of the hematoma after treatment with Hirudoid. Fewer internal echoes are visible.

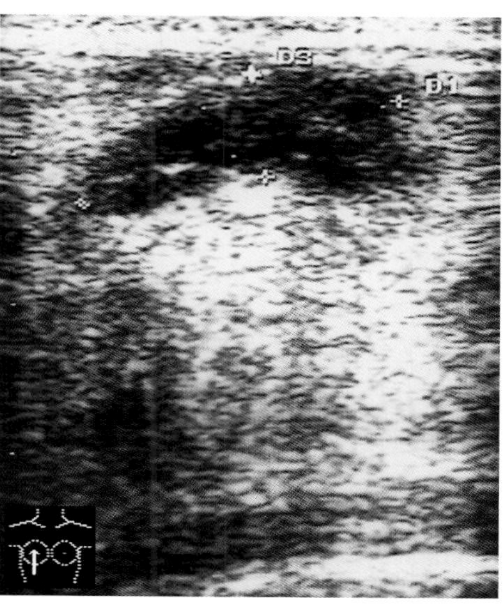



**i** Scan after hematoma evacuation. Residual cavity is present due to clotted blood.

**Question on Fig. 5.119**

*Which would you recommend in this case: vacuum biopsy or excisional biopsy?*

(**a**) Vacuum biopsy is generally adequate for therapeutic papilloma removal.

(**b**) Vacuum biopsy generally does not provide adequate treatment.

(**c**) The procedure of choice depends on clinical response and histologic findings.

→ **Answer on p. 383**

**Table 5.13 Cost comparison of various biopsy methods (German medical fee scale [GOÄ] in Euro*, 2004), disregarding initial expenditures for instruments and equipment**

| GOÄ codes, services and materials | SO-FNA (euro) | SO-CNB (euro) | SO-VB (euro) | ST-FNA (euro) | ST-CNB (euro) | ST-VB (euro) |
|---|---|---|---|---|---|---|
| 1: Conference | 4.66 | 4.66 | 4.66 | 4.66 | 4.66 | 4.66 |
| 5: Examination | 4.66 | 4.66 | 4.66 | 4.66 | 4.66 | 4.66 |
| 418: Breast ultrasound one side | 12.24 | 12.24 | 12.24 | | | |
| 420: Second breast ultrasound | 4.66 | 4.66 | 4.66 | | | |
| 5266: Two-view mammograms one side | | | | 26.23 | 26.23 | 26.23 |
| 5267: Extra mammographic view | | | | 8.74 | 8.74 | 8.74 |
| 5298: Digital radiography surcharge | | | | 13.99 | 13.99 | 13.99 |
| 2402: Excisional biopsy | | 21.57 | 21.57 | | 21.57 | 21.57 |
| 314: Breast needle biopsy | 6.99 | | | 6.99 | | |
| 297 × 5: Five cytology examinations | 13.10 | 13.10 | 13.10 | 13.10 | 13.10 | 13.10 |
| 200: Dressing | 2.62 | 2.62 | 2.62 | 2.62 | 2.62 | 2.62 |
| 75: Report | 7.58 | 7.58 | 7.58 | 7.58 | 7.58 | 7.58 |
| Core-biopsy needle + Truguide (Bard) | | 50.81 | | | 50.81 | |
| VB needle | | | 334.00 | | | 334.00 |
| Needle guide | | | | | | 10.78 |
| Compression wrap | | 7.26 | 7.26 | | 7.26 | 7.26 |
| Total | 56.51 | 129.16 | 412.35 | 88.57 | 161.22 | 444.41 |

FNA = fine-needle aspiration; CNB = core-needle biopsy; SO = sonographic guidance; ST = digital stereotactic guidance; VB = vacuum biopsy;
* 1 Euro = 1.25 US-Dollar = 0.9 £ (2010).

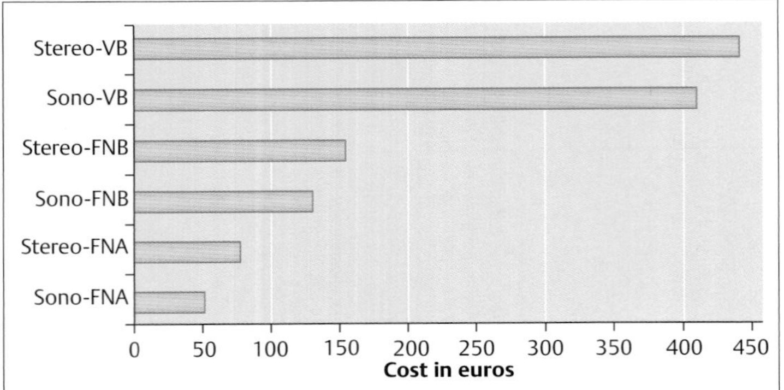


**Fig. 5.120 Graphic cost comparison of different biopsy methods.** FNA = fine-needle aspiration, CNB = core-needle biopsy, Sono = sonographic guidance, Stereo = digital stereotactic guidance, VB = vacuum biopsy without investment costs (as of 2004, see also **Table 5.13**, p. 253).

*(continued from p. 251)*

The study by Weining-Klemm (2004), with its consistently good values for FNA and CNB, shows that it would be worthwhile to utilize these techniques in the future and train personnel for them. This could effectively reduce the costs of rising biopsy rates without risking loss of diagnostic information, making it possible to reserve VB for selected indications. These would consist mainly of benign fibroadenomas or papillomas, gynecomastia in males, and small foci of ADH in consultation with the pathologist. In any case it is unnecessary to investigate all lesions (microcalcifications, suspicious mammographic densities) by VB. This leads to disproportionately high costs without a significant diagnostic gain over CNB (**Fig. 5.120**).

The results reported by Fischmann et al. (2004) in 96 women with 116 lesions who underwent VB are interesting in this regard. The vacuum-assisted biopsies yielded 24 malignant and 92 benign lesions, resulting in a PPV of just 25%. It is virtually certain that these lesions could also have been identified by digital stereotactic CNB at one-third the cost (see also the German multicenter study by Kettritz et al. 2004). The current financial situation in the German healthcare system does not allow us to be too generous with our resources, although sometimes this cannot be avoided within the framework of scientific studies or the introduction of new techniques. But these indications for VB cannot reasonably be applied to routine diagnostic tests and screening examinations.

FNA is still the fastest, cheapest, and least traumatizing procedure for the investigation of palpable and clinically occult lesions.

### MRI-Guided Core Needle Biopsy and Vacuum Biopsy

Suspicious areas of gadolinium enhancement in the breast detectable by MRI can be biopsied using a commercially available breast coil. These special coils are relatively expensive, and only a few breast centers keep them on hand. Lesions localized in this way are biopsied by CNB or VB using the same technique described for the digital stereotactic method (**Fig. 5.124**).

Larger gadolinium-enhancing lesions in the breast can also be biopsied and localized under computed tomographic (CT) guidance. Approximately 80% of gadolinium-enhancing tumors also enhance with ordinary radiographic contrast media and are visible after bolus contrast injection. This makes them relatively easy to biopsy under CT guidance (see **Figs. 5.48 f, g**, p. 140).

**Fig. 5.121 False-positive and false-negative rates of various biopsy methods.** False-positive results in FNA may occur when core biopsy detects preinvasive lesions that are not found on definitive histologic examination (*). FNA = fine-needle aspiration, CNB = core-needle biopsy, SO = sonographic guidance, ST = digital stereotactic guidance, VB = vacuum biopsy (sonographic and digital).

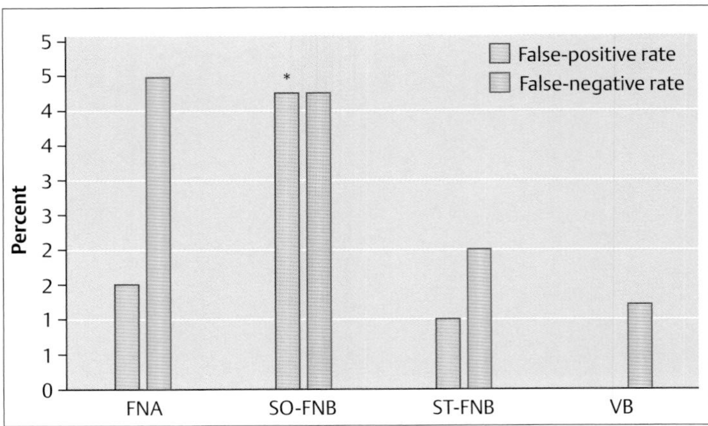


**Fig. 5.122 Sensitivity and specificity of various biopsy methods.** FNA = fine-needle aspiration, CNB = core-needle biopsy, SO = sonographic guidance, ST = digital stereotactic guidance, VB = vacuum biopsy (sonographic and digital).

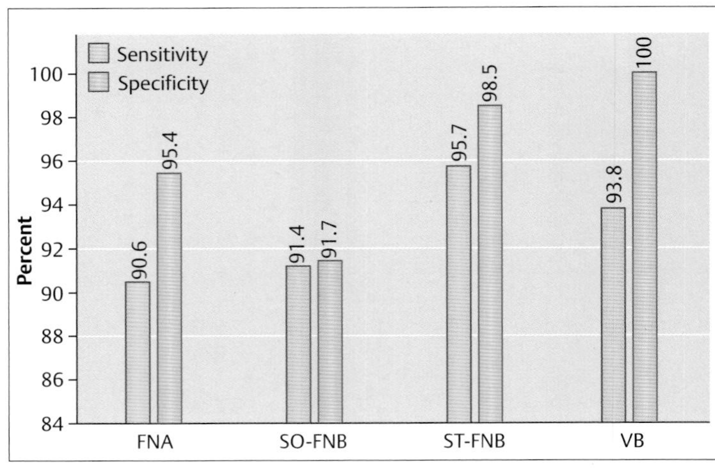


**Fig. 5.123 Positive predictive value (PPV) and negative predictive value (NPV) of various biopsy methods.** FNA = fine-needle aspiration, CNB = core-needle biopsy, SO = sonographic guidance, ST = digital stereotactic guidance, VB = vacuum biopsy.

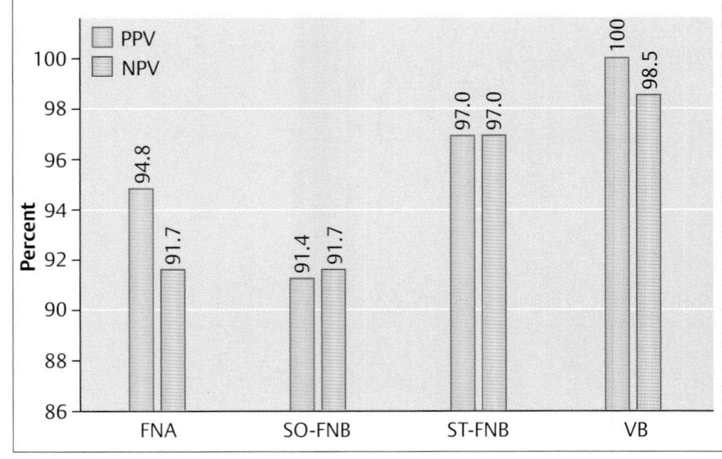

**Fig. 5.124 MRI-guided interventional procedures.**

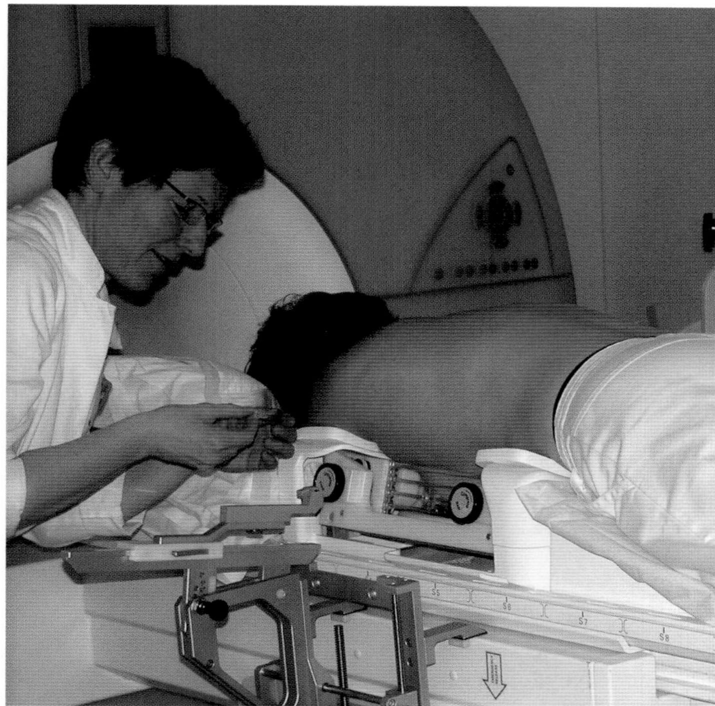

**a** *Overview:* 1.5 T MRI system (Symphony, Siemens) with a special biopsy coil. The coil is used here for localizing a suspicious breast lesion.

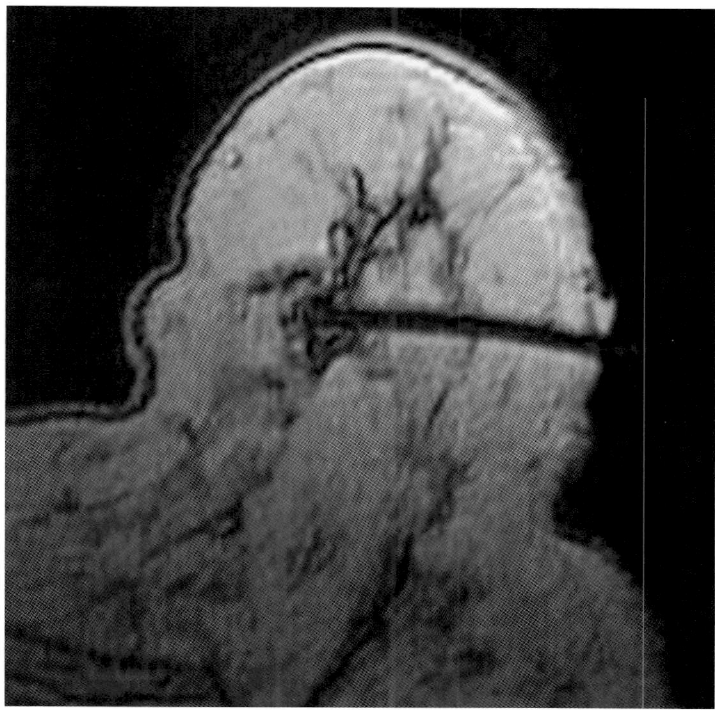

**c** *MRI:* A nonmagnetic needle is advanced to the suspicious focus under MRI guidance for lesion localization (histology: DCIS). (Images courtesy of Stefan Krämer, IMZE Esslingen, Germany)

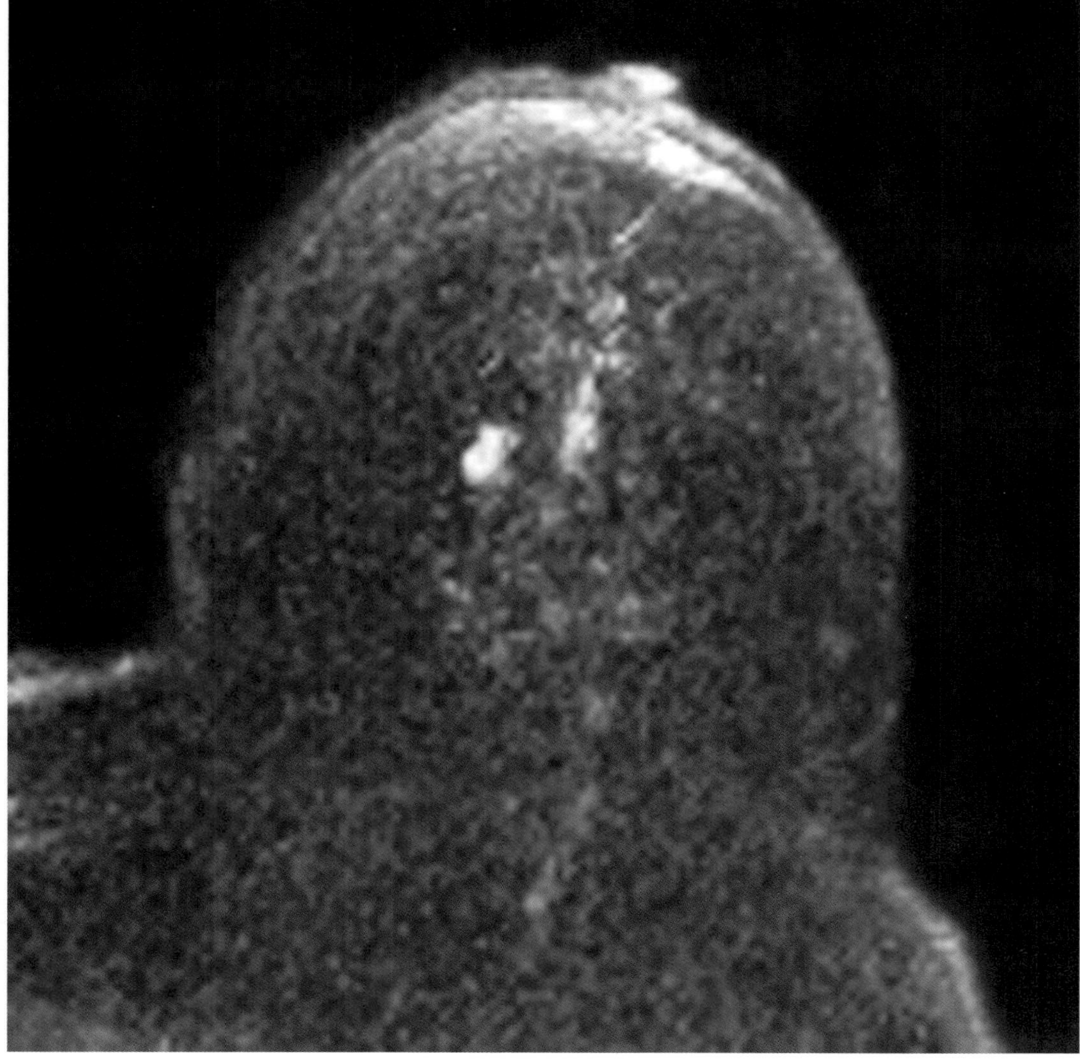

**b** *MRI:* Subtraction image shows circumscribed, atypical gadolinium enhancement at the margin of an invasive lobular carcinoma (focus not visible by mammography or ultrasound).

Ninety percent of atypical gadolinium-enhancing lesions are also seen in ultrasound if the beam is carefully directed to the suspect area seen in MRI.

Details on MRI-guided biopsy can be found in the works of Langen et al. (2000) and Heywang-Köbrunner et al. (2000). Liberman et al. (2003) and Fischer and Baum (2008), describe MRI-guided VB as a fast and safe alternative to open biopsies, which still require localization under MRI guidance. After VB the authors placed metal localizing coils, which they then marked for the surgeon by digital stereotactic localization. MRI-guided VB should be used only in cases where lesions detectable by MRI are mammographically and sonographically occult.

Liberman et al. (2003) premedicate their patients with 5 mg of diazepam on the morning of the examination. They perform MRI-guided biopsy using a compression grid and vitamin E skin marker, which aid in determining the coordinates for biopsy needle placement and the mammotome biopsy following the bolus injection of 1 mmol gadolinium/kg body weight. The biopsy was successful in 95% of the 20 women examined (average lesion size: 0.4–6.4 cm). A malignant lesion was found in 6 of 19 women (32%). The value of MRI-guided VB for mammographically and sonographically occult lesions is illustrated in **Fig. 5.127**.

### Possibilities, Limitations, and Risks of Interventional Procedures

Based on the previous chapters on interventional procedures, we can begin to appreciate the possibilities of the combined use of these minimally invasive procedures as well as their limitations and risks. Interventional procedures can eliminate the need for 25% of recommended excisional biopsies. Besides providing emotional relief for patients, this would mean a substantial cost saving for payors: 740–1000 USD per patient in the United States compared with surgical biopsy (Golub et al. 2004), and 320 000 euro in Germany based on the elimination of 300 recommended surgical biopsies. Surgeons worldwide still perform far too many excisional breast biopsies, yielding an average of two benign diagnoses for every malignancy. A ratio of 4 : 1 (one benign histology for every 4 cancers or preneoplasias) would be desirable. Most benign lesions could be diagnosed without hospitalization, for even papillomas and fibroadenomas as large as 2 cm can be removed from the breast by vacuum biopsy. It is unclear why German guidelines state that only 80% of preoperative diagnoses, rather than 100%, should be histologically confirmed. It may be because a certain number of women prefer primary excisional biopsy under general anesthesia over an interventional procedure with local anesthesia. Otherwise, a lumpectomy should never be performed unless an interventional procedure has already established the diagnosis of a malignant tumor or preinvasive disease. We have had good results with ultrasound-guided VB performed under brief general anesthesia ("twilight sleep") with intravenous propofol.

While interventional procedures have definite potential for reducing healthcare costs, there are also risks to be considered. These are concerned less with complications such as hematomas, inflammation, and allergies to local anesthetics than with the possibility of missing a lesion at biopsy, yielding a false-negative result. In all cases the preinterventional working diagnosis must agree with the histologic or cytologic findings by CNB or FNA. If calcifications have been biopsied, the pathologist must mention them in his report and calcifications must be detectable in the specimen radiograph. If calcifications are visible in the specimen radiograph but the pathologist does not describe them, the paraffin block should be x-rayed (see p. 51). Sometimes calcifications are dislodged from the edges of the tissue cores during histologic processing and are not seen on histologic examination (Fischmann et al. 2004). I have had no instances of inoculation metastasis in any of the biopsies performed by myself or others since 1972 in about 40 000 breast-interventions.

**Tip**

**Six months after any interventional procedure, the breast should be reexamined using the same modality that disclosed the lesion. But attention should not be limited to biopsied calcification clusters, for example; the entire breast should be scrutinized. It would be tragic to focus all our attention on a calcification cluster while a nearby carcinoma is growing unabated (see Fig. 5.128, p. 260).**

The interventional procedures themselves produce changes (hematomas, clotted blood) that should not be mistaken for malignancies (see **Fig. 5.117**, p. 247). Figures **5.125** through **5.128** illustrate the possibilities, limitations, and risks of interventional procedures. You will note that all interventions require a definite indication if they are to yield a definitive result, and that they all have the same goals: *using the most appropriate procedure, investigating suspicious lesions as cost-effectively as possible, and detecting every malignancy.*

**Fig. 5.125 Possibilities, limitations, and risks of interventional procedures,** illustrated in **a 40-year-old woman with a palpable nodule in the upper inner quadrant of the right breast** at the 2-o'clock position (**a**). The nodule is freely movable and is clearly defined mammographically in the stroma-rich breast (**b, c**). It enhances intensely on MRI (**d**), and ultrasound shows a combination of smooth and irregular margins (**e**). The lesion is investigated using FNA cytology (**f**).

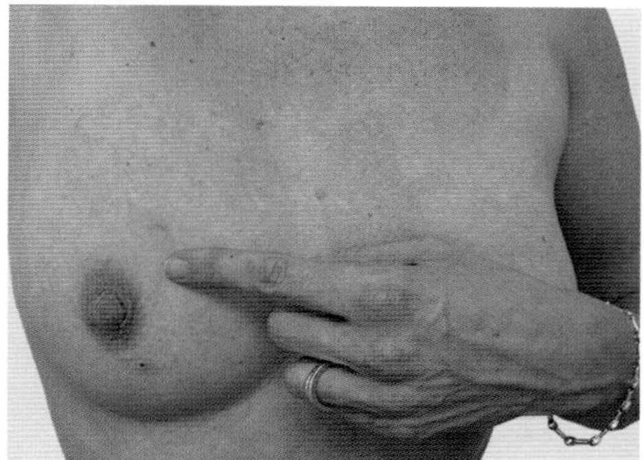

**a** *Physical examination* shows a palpable nodule in the upper inner quadrant of the right breast with no skin or nipple retraction.

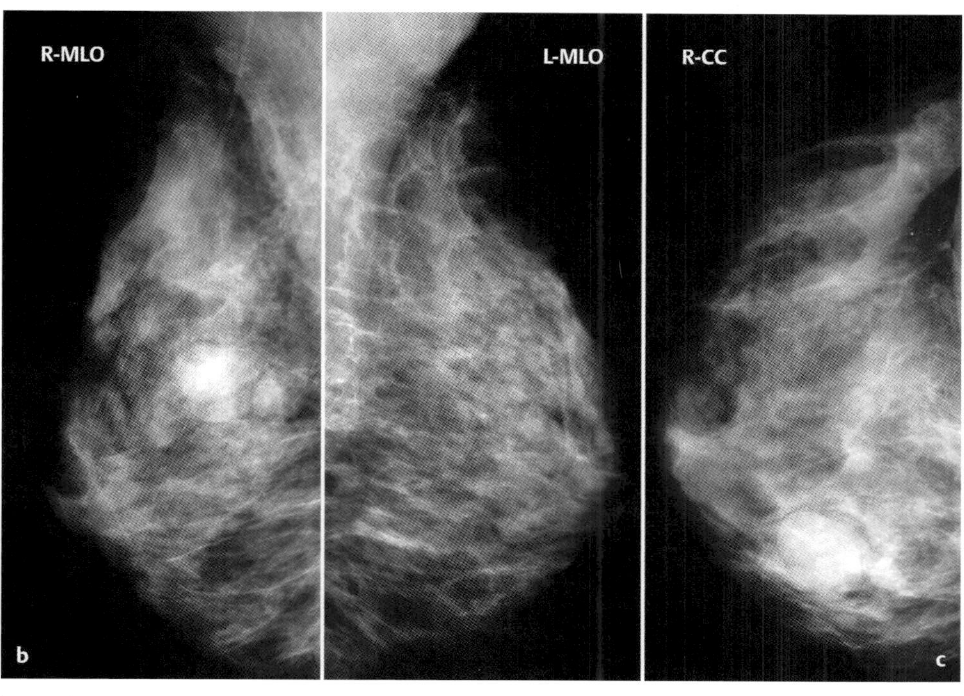


**b, c** *Bilateral oblique mammograms* (**b**) show a stroma-rich breast with two adjacent, well-circumscribed nodules partially surrounded by a lucent halo (**o/21**) (ACR 3, BIRADS 3, PGMI). Right craniocaudal mammogram (**c**) shows a stroma-rich breast with a well-circumscribed nodule in the inner quadrant. The lesion is partially surrounded by a halo (**S–s/18–19**) (ACR 3, BIRADS 2, PGMI).

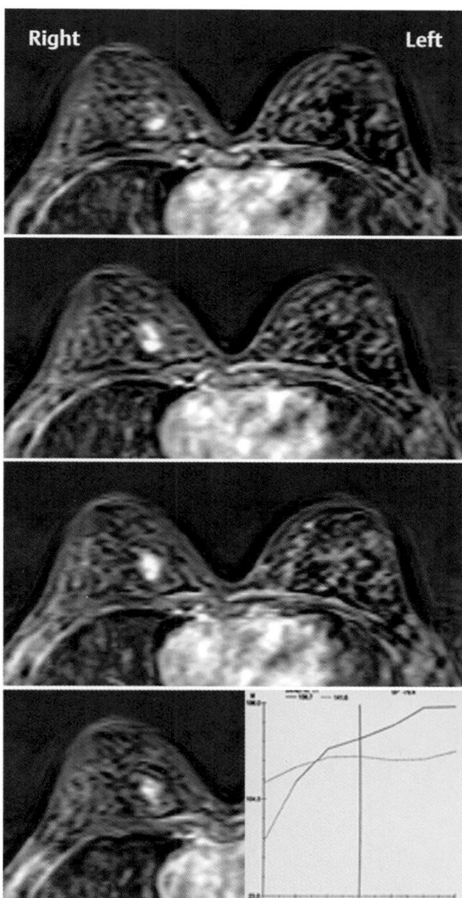


**d** *MRI subtraction* image shows an intensely enhancing nodule with ill-defined margins at the site of the palpable mass in the right breast. The left breast appears normal.

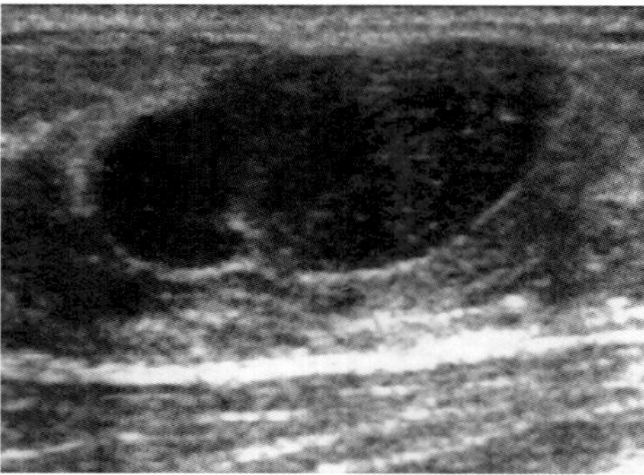

**e** Ultrasound shows an hourglass-shaped lesion with smooth margins, internal echoes, and posterior acoustic enhancement.

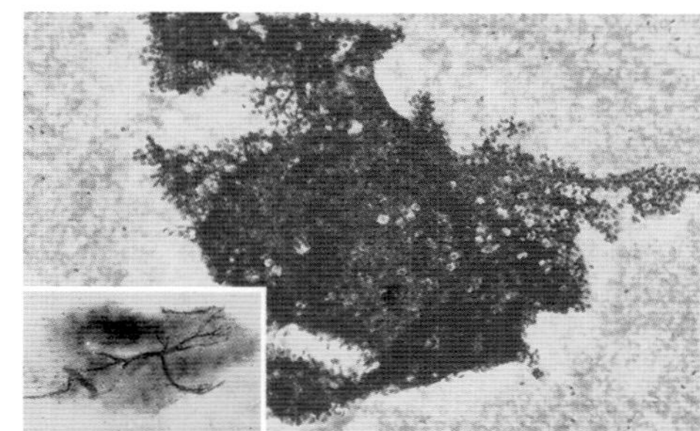

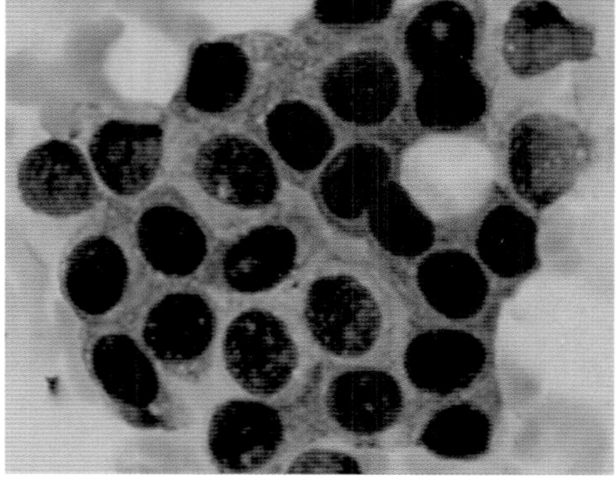

**f** *FNA cytology* (right upper image) shows a typical parenchymal fragment with abundant close-packed cells and a characteristic smooth, *concave* border. *Lower image:* cluster of cells with uniformly enlarged nuclei and a somewhat loose chromatin structure. *Inset:* typical stromal fragment from the nodule.

**Question 1 on Fig. 5.125**

*Is the palpable mass in a identical to the mammographic density (**b, c**)?*

(**a**) Yes
(**b**) No
(**c**) Uncertain

→ **Answer on p. 383**

**Question 2 on Fig. 5.125**

*Would the nodule be more accurately described as cellular or fibrous?*

(**a**) Cellular
(**b**) Fibrous
(**c**) Uncertain

→ **Answer on p. 383**

**Question 3 on Fig. 5.125**

*Is the cytology more consistent with a benign or malignant lesion?*

(**a**) Benign
(**b**) Malignant
(**c**) Uncertain

→ **Answer on p. 383**

**Fig. 5.126 A 48-year-old woman presents with a nodule at the 11-o'clock position in the left breast close to the chest wall (a).** The nodule has been present for years. The lesion is not mammographically visible in the very radiodense breast (ACR 3), so MRI was performed 7 years earlier, yielding no suspicious findings. Mammography shows a nonspecific, inhomogeneous density above the breast parenchyma (**b**). Clustered pleomorphic calcifications are visible at various sites in the center of the density (BIRADS 4). At ultrasound the nodule shows a combination of smooth and slightly irregular margins (**c**), and MRI shows intense gadolinium enhancement at the site of the palpable mass (**d**). Ultrasound-guided CNB indicates stromal hyperplasia with breast lobules showing slight nuclear pleomorphism. The patient is therefore advised to have the nodule removed by vacuum biopsy.

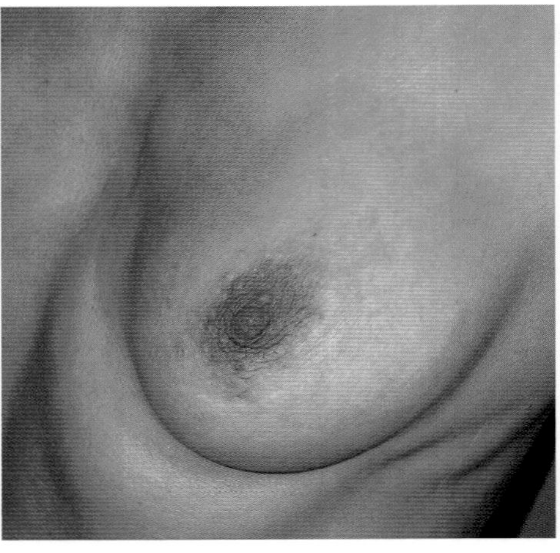

**a** *Clinical appearance* of the left breast with the arm raised. The nodule is clearly visible as a raised area at the 12-o'clock position (**b/23**). It measures 2 cm × 1 cm × 1 cm in size.

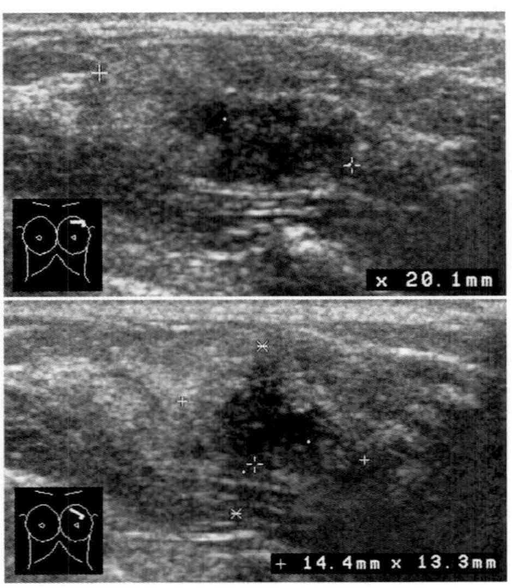


**c** *Sonograms* of the upper left breast. *Above:* a 2 cm smooth-bordered nodule with focal inhomogeneities. *Below (different plane):* 1.4 cm × 1.3 cm nodule with a hypoechoic, inhomogeneous center and a slightly more echogenic rim (see cursors).

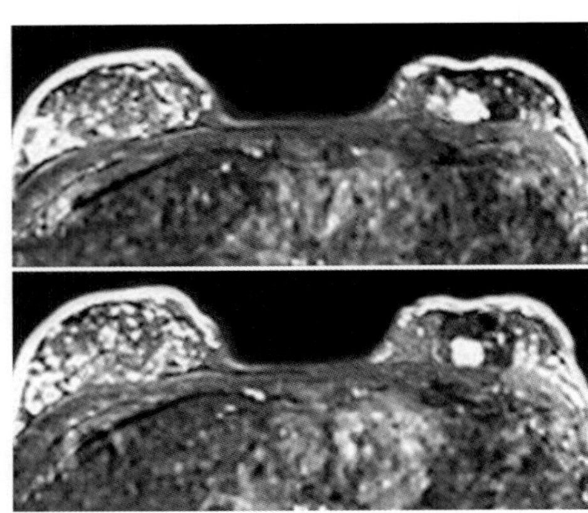

**d** *MR subtraction images*. The nodule has smooth margins and shows intense gadolinium enhancement (**J/21+24**). An approximately 1 cm enhancing area is visible at a corresponding site in the lateral right breast and has the same appearance as the nodule in the left breast (**H/24**).

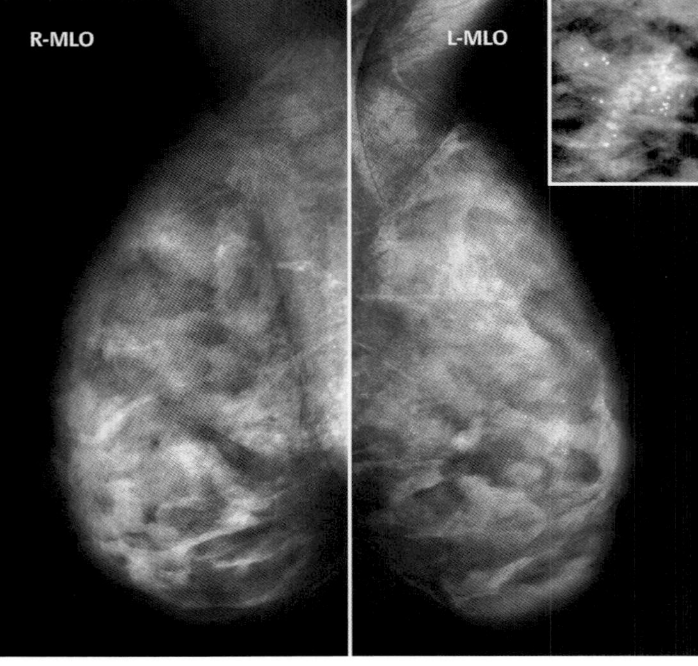


**b** *Bilateral oblique mammograms* show very radiodense breasts (ACR 4) with clustered microcalcifications in the left breast (**d/7** [inset]) (core-needle biopsy was not suspicious). A faint, inhomogeneous density with mixed smooth and scalloped margins is projected over the pectoral muscle in the upper portion of the left breast (**b/11**).

**Question on Fig. 5.126**

*How would you interpret the visible and palpable nodule in the left breast based on the history, core-needle biopsy, and imaging findings?*

(**a**) Papilloma
(**b**) Fibroadenoma
(**c**) Carcinoma

→ **Answer on p. 383**

**Fig. 5.127 A 52-year-old woman underwent previous removal of a left axillary lymph node metastasis (signet ring type) from a mucinous carcinoma (a).** Possible primary tumor: gastric, bronchial, or breast. Mammogram of the left breast shows no suspicious findings (**b, c**). Ultrasound shows ductectasia, which is investigated by fine-needle aspiration (**d**). Cytologic findings are normal (**e**). MRI shows circumscribed enhancement in the *upper inner quadrant* of the left breast (**f**), prompting reinvestigation of the ductectasia by ultrasound-guided core-needle core biopsy, which shows mastitis with no evidence of a primary tumor. The search for a primary tumor includes gastroscopy and thoracic CT, but both are negative. The metastasis is estrogen- and progesterone-receptor-positive (immunohistochemistry 1 week later), raising strong suspicion of breast cancer. But this cannot be verified by physical examination, mammography, or ultrasound. Whole-body PET shows no suspicious hypermetabolic foci anywhere in the body–including the breast and left axillary region–that would suggest gross viable tumor tissue.

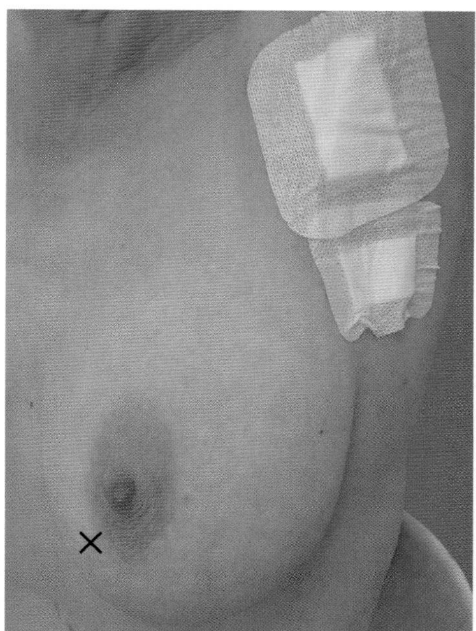

**a** *Appearance* of the left breast following previous removal of an axillary lymph node metastasis. The breast appears clinically normal. X marks the area investigated by fine-needle aspiration and core-needle biopsy.

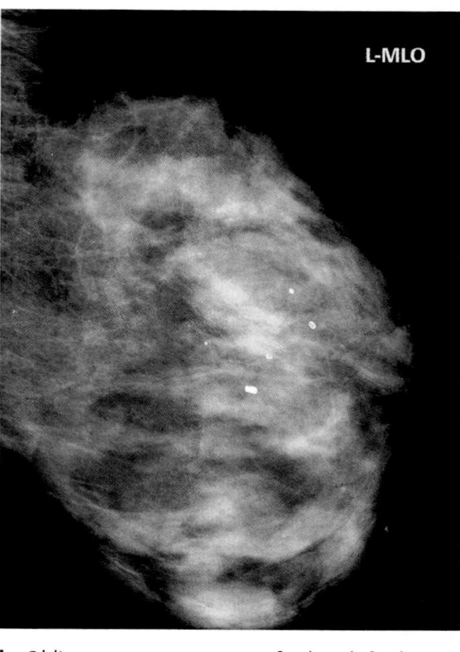


**b** *Oblique mammogram* of the left breast shows a radiodense, inhomogeneous breast with coarse, unsuspicious retroareolar calcifications (ACR 4, BIRADS 2, P**G**MI).

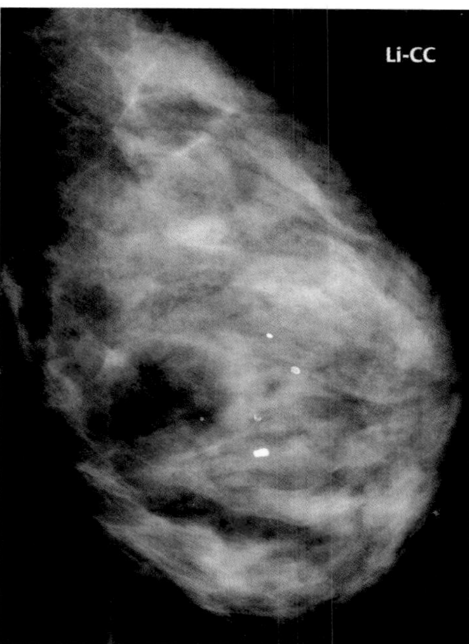


**c** *Craniocaudal mammogram* shows a very radiodense left breast with coarse calcifications (fat necrosis) and no evidence of malignancy (ACR 4, BIRADS 2, **P**GMI).

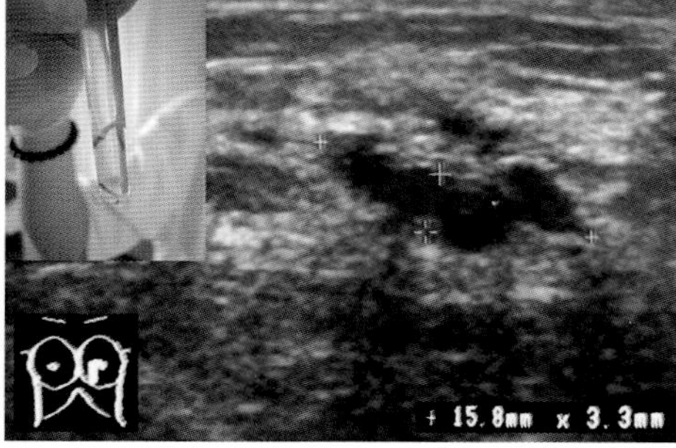


**d** *Sonogram* of the left breast shows a 1.5 cm × 0.3 cm × 0.3 cm periareolar hypoechoic area at the 8-o'clock position consistent with circumscribed ductectasia. *CNB* (see X in panel **a**) yielded four compact tissue cores that *sink in saline tubes* (upper left inset), confirming that they are not composed of fat.

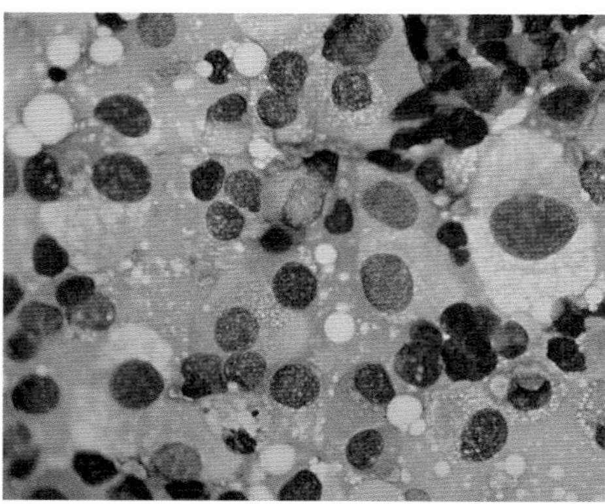

**e** *FNA* of the area marked in **a** yields compact, unsuspicious aggregates of degenerated epithelial cells.

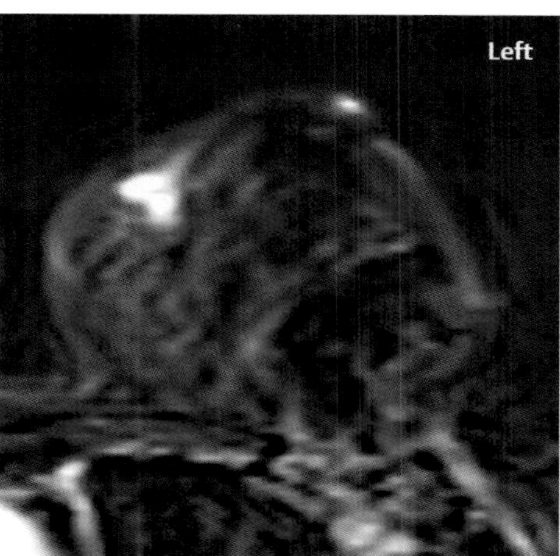


**f** *MR subtraction* image shows an irregular 2 cm area of gadolinium enhancement over the upper inner quadrant of the left breast about 6 cm dorso-medial of mamilla (**S–s/11**). The right breast appeared normal.

**Question 1 on Fig. 5.127**

*Do the sonographic and MRI findings have exactly the same location?*

(**a**) Yes
(**b**) No
(**c**) Uncertain

→ **Answer on p. 384**

**Question 2 on Fig. 5.127**

*What action would you recommend?*

(**a**) Wide excisional biopsy after preoperative localization of the sonographic lesion
(**b**) Excisional biopsy after localization by MRI
(**c**) Withhold breast biopsy because the primary tumor is apparently located elsewhere.

→ **Answer on p. 384**

**Fig. 5.128 A 73-year-old woman presents for mammographic screening.** The patient has nodular breasts and very radiodense mammograms. New clustered microcalcifications appeared between 2000 and 2002 (**a**) and were investigated by digital stereotactic biopsy. *Histology:* sclerosing adenosis. Weeks after the biopsy, the patient noticed increasing firmness in the biopsied breast and presented for several follow-ups thinking that she had an infection. Her doctor drew no conclusions from these visits. She presents again in 2003, this time with a very large breast nodule (**d**). The microcalcifications are unchanged (**b**). Ultrasound shows numerous hypoechoic areas with a combination of scalloped, smooth, diffuse, and ill-defined margins (**c**). Bacteriologic tests are negative.

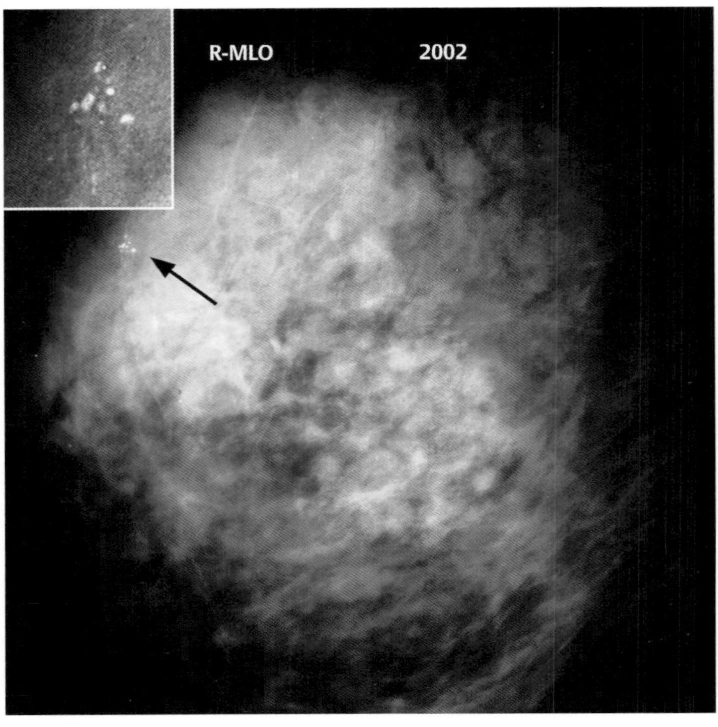


**a** *Oblique mammogram* of the right breast in 2002 shows increased breast density with a new, rosette-like cluster of coarse microcalcifications (inset at upper left). Histology indicated sclerosing adenosis.

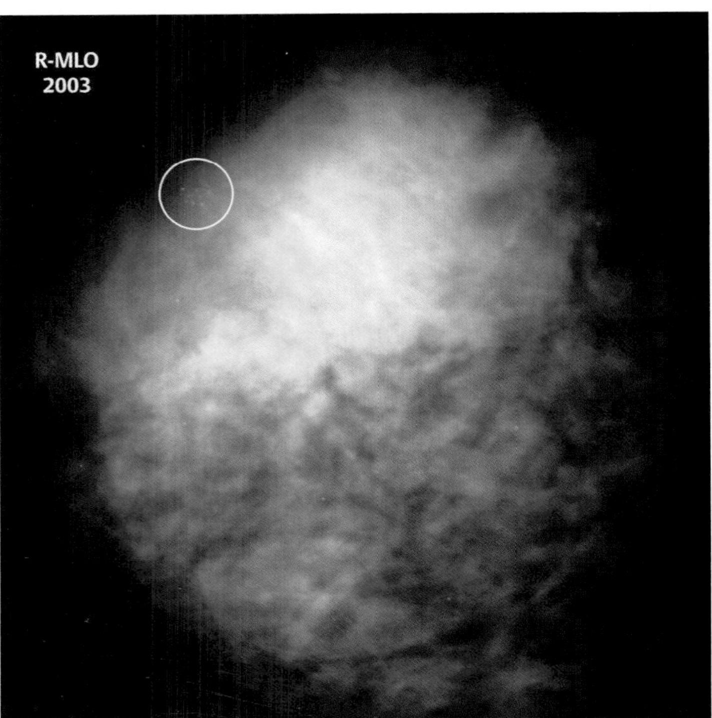


**b** *Oblique mammogram* of the right breast in 2003 shows very high density of the breast parenchyma, especially in the upper quadrants. Calcifications are still visible, are minimally increased, and have a somewhat dustlike appearance (**g/23**, see marker) (no longer clearly visible within the dense tissue).

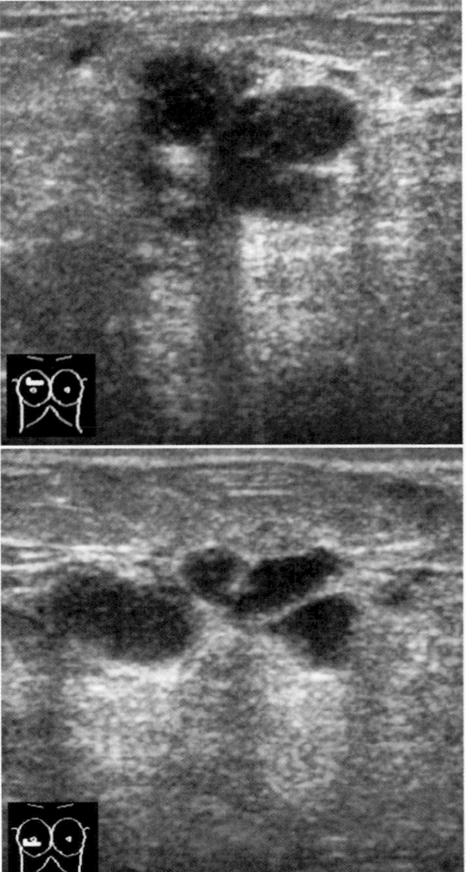

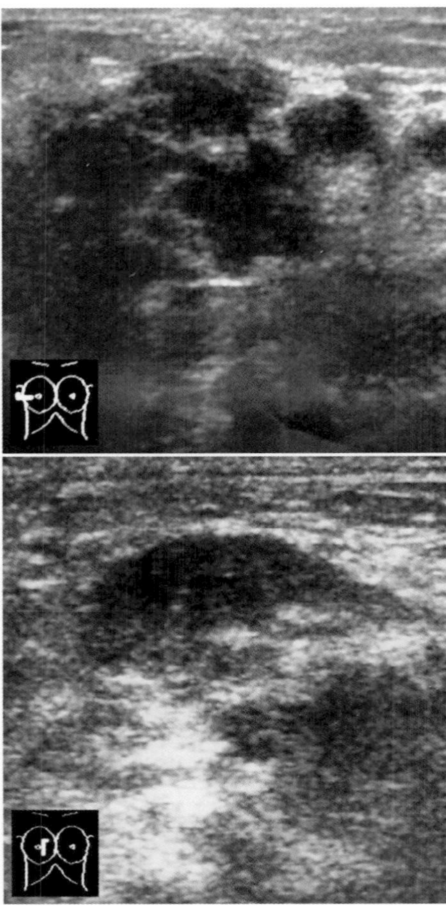

**c** *Sonograms* of various quadrants in the right breast show numerous liquid and solid hypoechoic areas. Fine-needle aspiration is done for bacteriologic testing.

**Fig. 5.128 A 73-year-old woman presents for mammographic screening.** *(continued)*

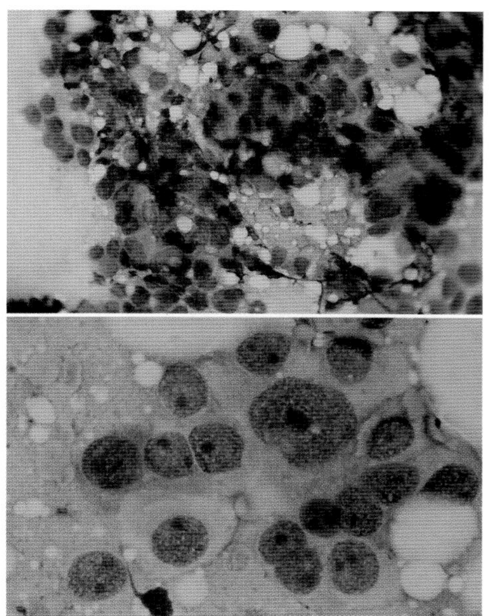

**d** *Cytology* shows a somewhat lobular cluster of cells with enlarged, hyperchromatic (above), very pleomorphic nuclei and fine reticular thinning and disintegration of the nuclear chromatin (below). The findings are typical of this disease.

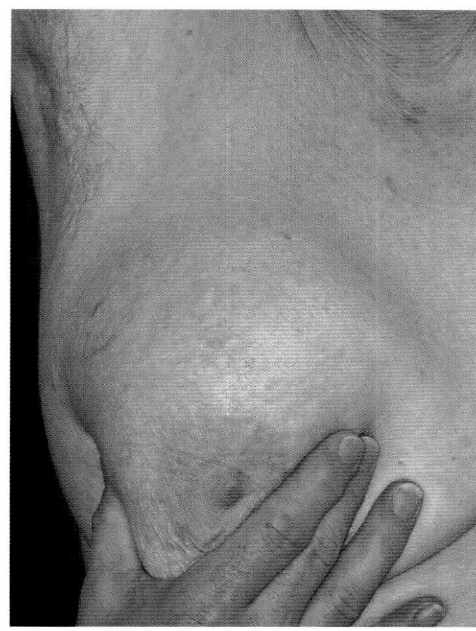

**e** *Clinical appearance* of the right breast. The palpable nodule is pushed upward between the thumb and index finger.

**Question 1 on Fig. 5.128**

*Is there a causal relationship between the clustered microcalcifications and what is happening in the breast?*

(**a**) No
(**b**) Yes
(**c**) Somewhat

→ **Answer on p. 384**

**Question 2 on Fig. 5.128**

*How would you interpret the findings?*

(**a**) Chronic bacterial mastitis with abscess formation
(**b**) Cystosarcoma phylloides
(**c**) Locally advanced carcinoma

→ **Answer on p. 384**

## Possibilities and Limitations of Complementary Investigations

Inspection and palpation, mammography, ultrasound, MRI, and in rare cases PET will usually provide a correct diagnosis when used in conjunction with minimally invasive interventional procedures. The various tests and procedures should be applied selectively and efficiently to yield a cost-effective early diagnosis. No method should be considered a gold standard in itself, and all methods should be aimed at detecting or excluding breast cancer economically at the earliest possible stage with minimal physical and emotional discomfort for patients. Breast ultrasound with high-resolution transducers plays a major role in routine settings, for detecting or excluding breast cancer and for tracking physiological and hormonal changes in the breast parenchyma (see p. 193 ff). Ultrasound has become the most important modality for detecting noncalcifying breast cancers, which are very often missed on mammograms at an early stage, especially in dense breasts and especially in the form of lobular neoplasms. A mammogram-only screening program is definitely a step in the right direction, as it ensures that maximum numbers of women within a certain age group will be screened on a regular basis. But mammographic screening by itself is not effective enough to reduce the number of interval cancers. Single-view mammograms supplemented by inspection, palpation, and breast ultrasound would be the ideal combination for detecting *early* breast cancer and preinvasive lesions in women between 35 and 75 years of age. MRI in younger women with dense breasts and a positive (high risk) family history would also be useful for detecting precancerous lesions that are not detectable by mammography or ultrasound (about 80 % vs. 50 %). Imaging must be done during the proper phase of the cycle (days 7–12) to avoid false-positive findings as well as unnecessary interventional and surgical procedures.

**Figures 5.129–5.138** illustrate the capabilities of complementary diagnostic tests, and several cases illustrate their limitations.

*(continued on p. 275)*

**Fig. 5.129 A 65-year-old woman noticed a movable, tender nodule in the retroareolar area of the left breast 10 days previously (a).** A recurrent serous or bloody discharge from one duct in the right breast has been present for several weeks. Nipple smear cytology is not suspicious. The history includes nonpuerperal mastitis involving the inner portion of the left breast 8 months before.

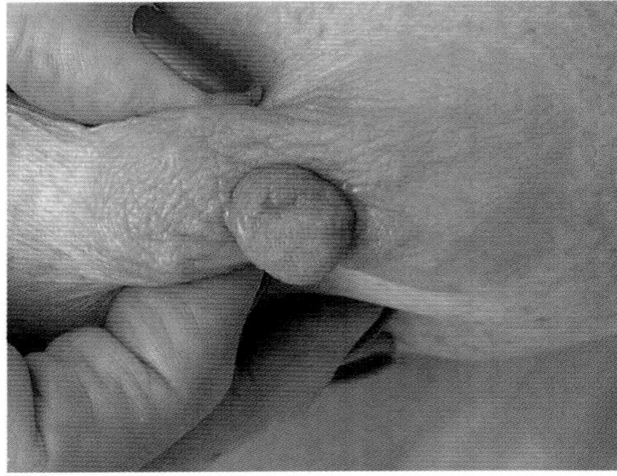

**a** *Physical examination* of the left nipple shows a 1 cm retroareolar nodule. Compression of an ectatic duct at the 11-o'clock position elicits a serous discharge. Otherwise the breast appears normal.

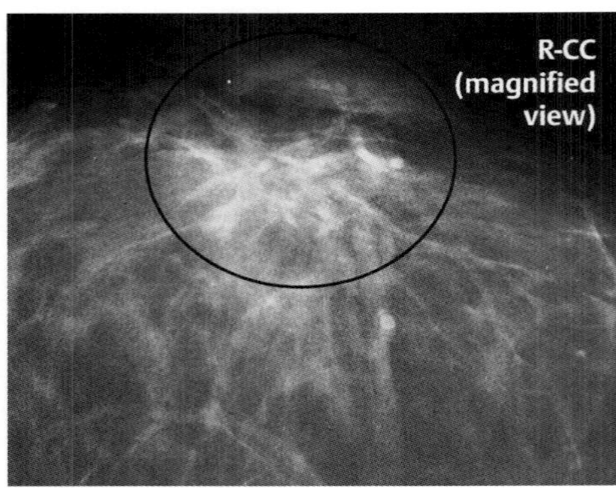


**b** *Craniocaudal mammogram* of the left breast (retroareolar spot view) shows an involuted breast with a transverse, bandlike, retroareolar 3 mm × 11 mm density with indistinct margins and no microcalcifications (ACR 1, BIRADS 3).

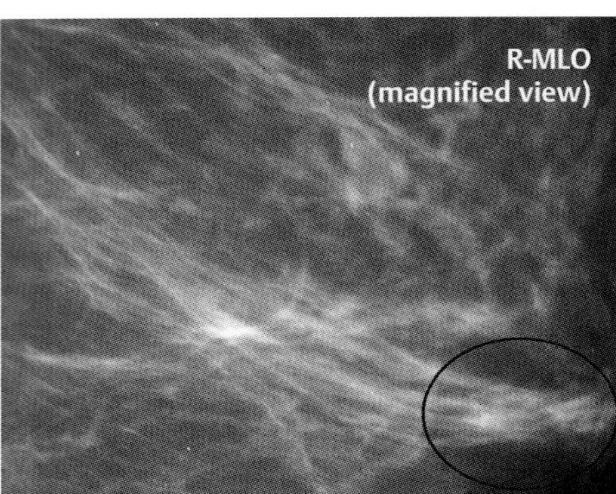


**c** *Oblique mammogram* of the left breast (retroareolar spot view) shows dense, bandlike ducts with a 6 mm-wide inhomogeneous retroareolar density (ACR 1, BIRADS 3).

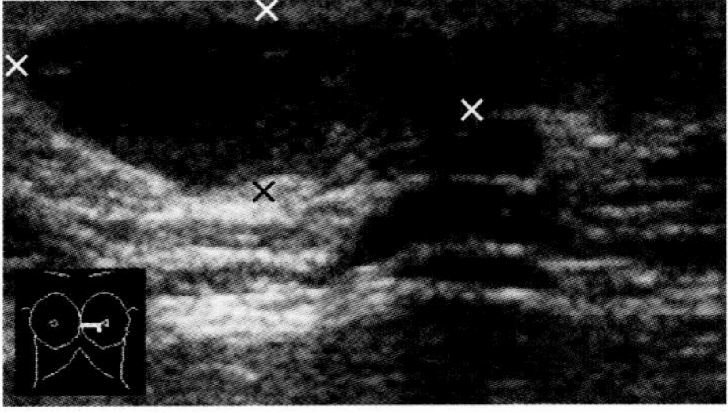

**d** *Sonogram* of the retroareolar left breast shows ductectasia (**a–D/18–19**) with a 4.9 cm × 1.3 cm inhomogeneous, well-circumscribed intraductal density (see marker) (nipple is at upper left).

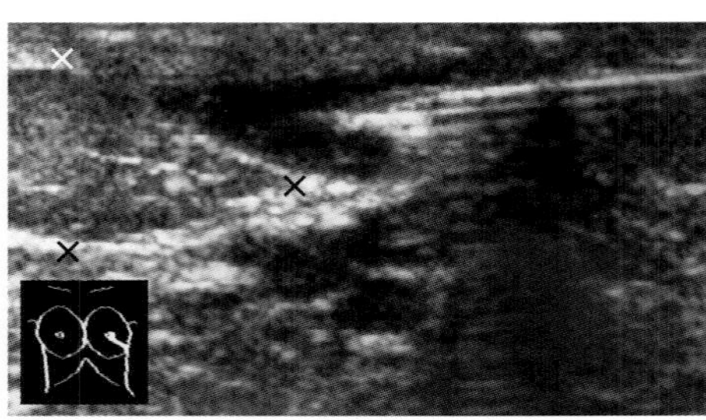

**e** *Ultrasound-guided core-needle biopsy.* Postfire image shows the needle tip within an ectatic duct; to the left of it is the intraductal lesion (see marker).

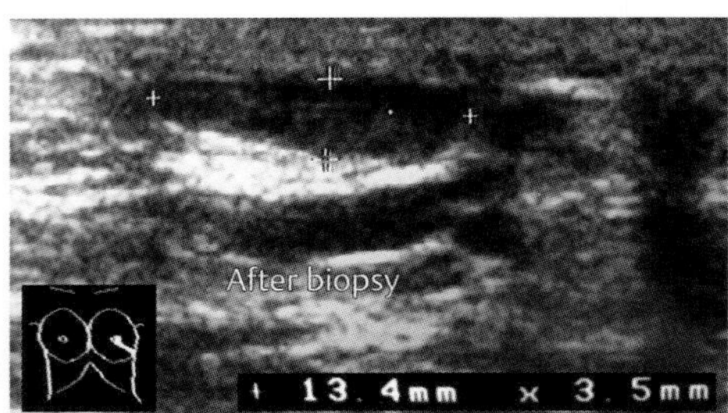


**f** *Retroareolar sonogram* after the evacuation of purulent fluid (**g**). Note persistence of ductectasia with a 1.3 cm × 0.3 cm "residual density". An enlarged duct has been evacuated at **h–J/17**.

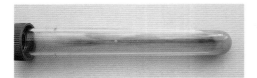

**g** *Core biopsy material.* Reddish-yellow fluid in a plastic tube.

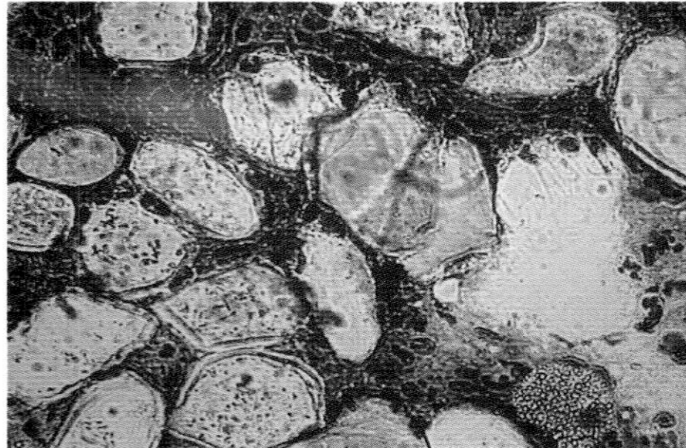

**h** *Cytology* (fluid from the coaxial needle, magnified 20 ×) shows numerous pale cells, relatively plump and misshapen, containing small, mostly eccentric nuclei.

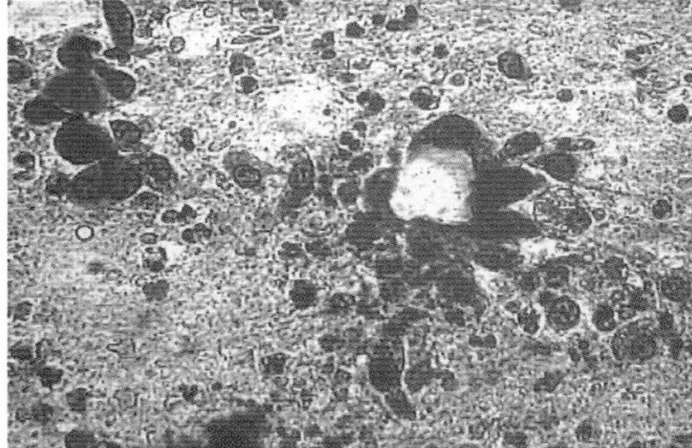

**i** *Cytologic smear* shows a cluster of cells with relatively plump, moderately pleomorphic adenoma nuclei, prominent nucleoli, and basophilic cytoplasm. A cell cluster at **i/11** has engulfed one of the pale cells seen in panel **h**.

**Question 1 on Fig. 5.129**

*How would you interpret the lesion based on the history and the physical and imaging findings?*

(**a**) Benign
(**b**) Malignant
(**c**) Indeterminate

→ **Answer on p. 384**

**Question 2 on Fig. 5.129**

*How would you interpret the retroareolar density?*

(**a**) Ductectasia with plasma cell mastitis
(**b**) Granulating mastitis
(**c**) Ductal carcinoma with an associated inflammatory component

→ **Answer on p. 384**

**Fig. 5.130 A 68-year-old woman presents with a two-day history of a painful infra-areolar swelling in the right breast.** The swollen area measures 2 cm × 3 cm and is associated with circumscribed skin redness present for 24 hours (**a**). There is no skin or nipple retraction. The patient noticed a dark spot in her brassiere, but discharge cannot be elicited at presentation. Percutaneous aspiration of the firm area yields viscous, yellowish debris (**d**).

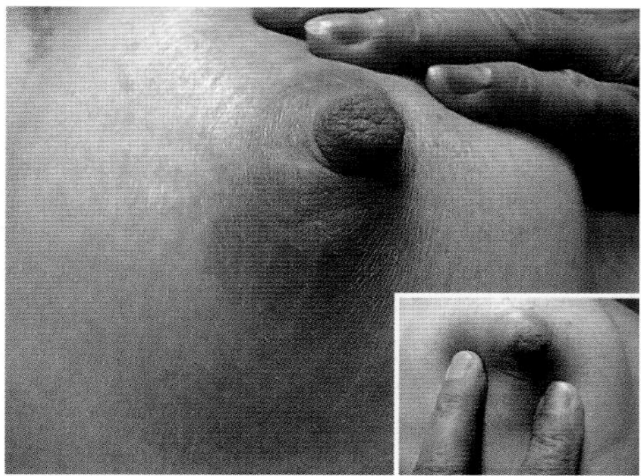

**a** *Clinical inspection* of the right breast shows infra-areolar skin redness at the 6-o'clock position (**k–L/24–25**). A freely movable nodule (inset) is also noted at that location.

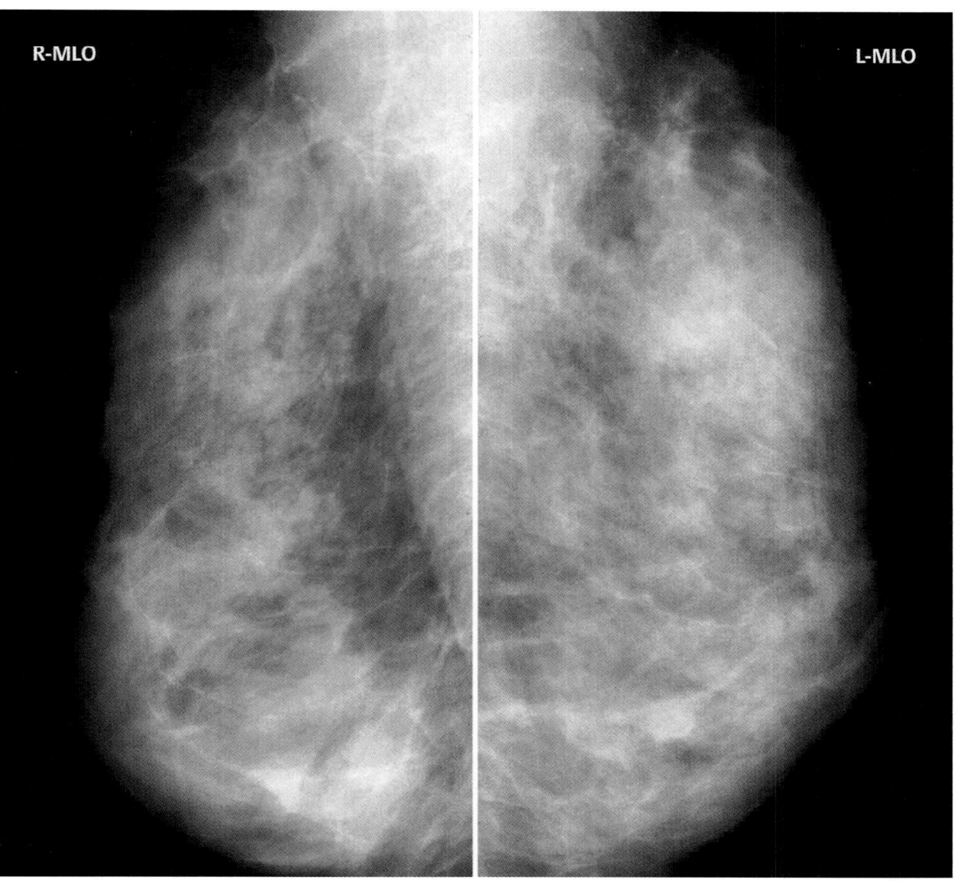


**b** *Bilateral oblique mammograms* show radiodense breasts with a nonspecific density in the upper portion of the left breast (**R–S/21–23**) and lower portion of the right breast (**P–Q/15–16**). No abnormalities are seen in the right retroareolar area (ACR 3, BIRADS 1, P**G**MI).

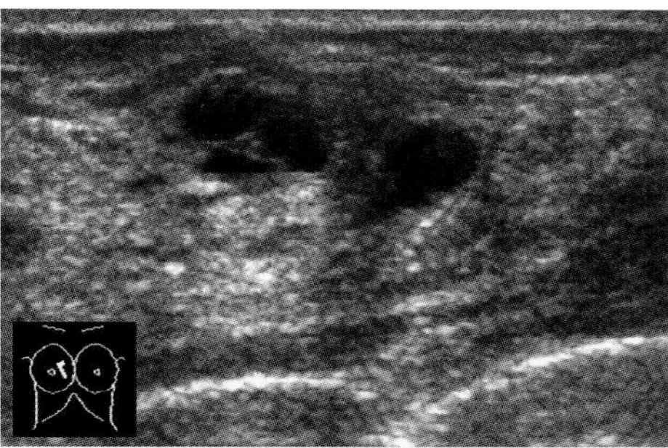

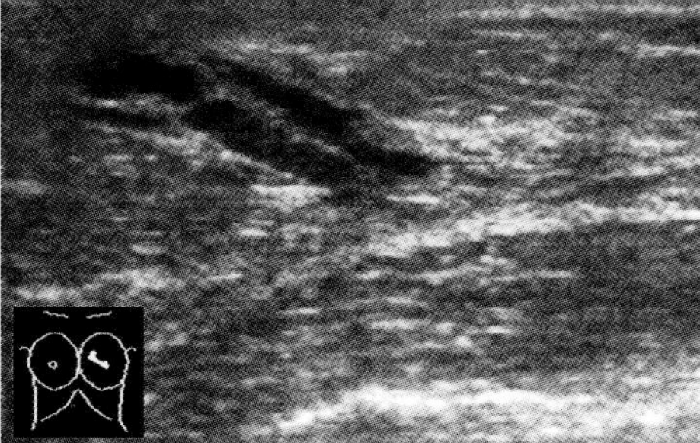

**c** *Sonogram* demonstrates retroareolar ductectasia in the right breast. Scan through the palpable mass shows a relatively well-circumscribed, convex subcutaneous area with dilated, cystlike ductal structures. Scan of the left breast shows ductectasia with smooth duct contours (nipple is at upper left in the image).

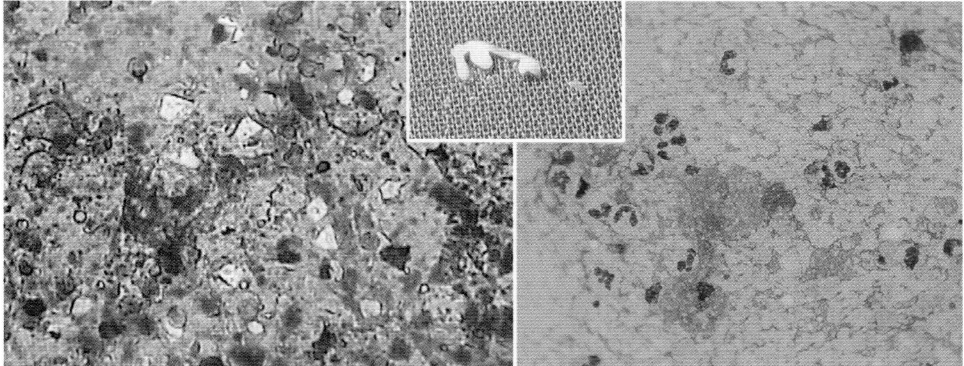

**d** *Fine-needle aspiration* of the right breast. Aspirate expelled onto a glass slide shows fatty debris (top center). Cytology shows pale clumps of cholesterol (left; e.g., **O/10–11**) accompanied by foam cells and inflammatory cells (right).

**Question on Fig. 5.130**

*How would you interpret the nodule?*

(**a**) Ductal carcinoma
(**b**) Ductectasia with retained secretions and associated inflammation
(**c**) Granulating mastitis

→ **Answer on p. 385**

**Fig. 5.131 A 45-year-old woman suddenly noticed a slightly tender infra-areolar firmness in the right breast (a).** The skin in that area is slightly reddened. There is no nipple retraction or discharge.

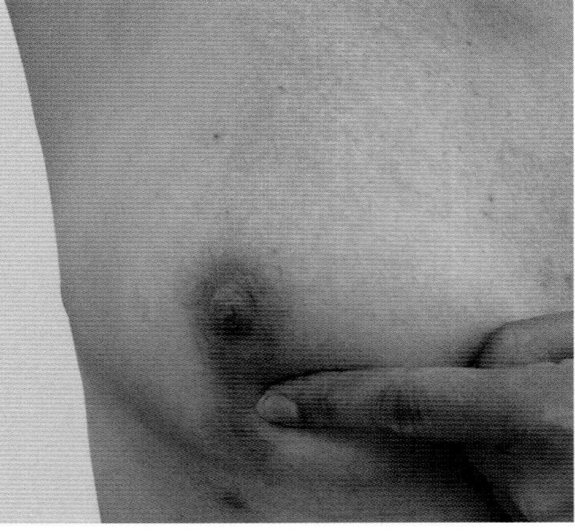

**a** *Physical examination* of the right breast shows slight skin redness below the nipple-areola without skin retraction.

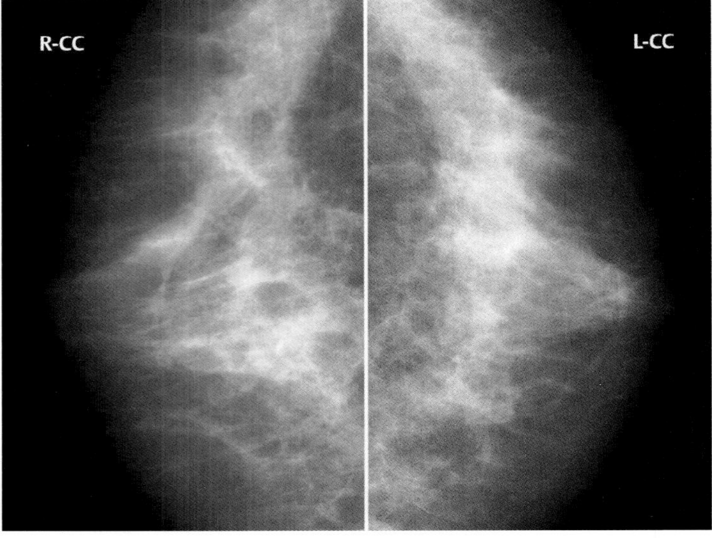


**d** *Bilateral craniocaudal mammograms* show radiodense breasts with inhomogeneities. The deep portion of the breast parenchyma is not fully imaged on either side (ACR 3, BIRADS 2, PG**M**I).

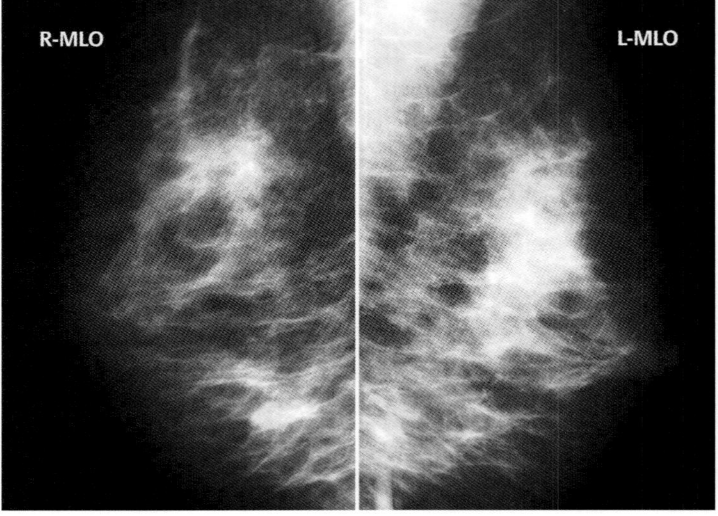


**b** *Bilateral oblique mammograms* show relatively dense breasts with nonspecific densities, including one in the area of the right inframammary fold (**C/15**). The breast parenchyma is not completely imaged on either side; the pectoral muscles cannot be traced to nipple level (ACR 3, BIRADS 2, PG**M**I).

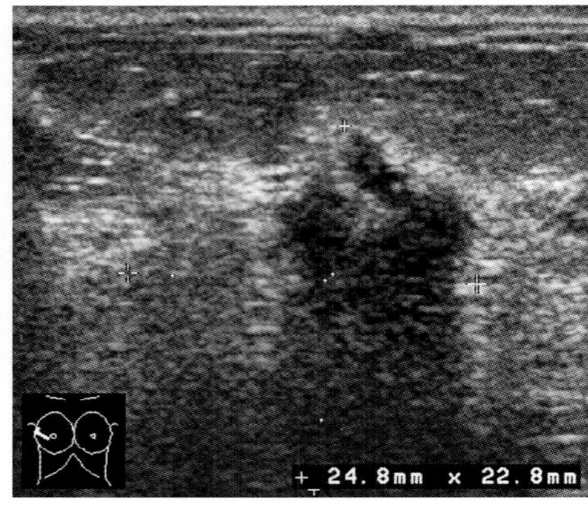


**e** *Sonogram* of the right breast at the site of the palpable mass shows a 2.4 cm × 2.2 cm hypoechoic area with a posterior acoustic shadow, irregular margins, and an echogenic rim (**g–h/14–15**).

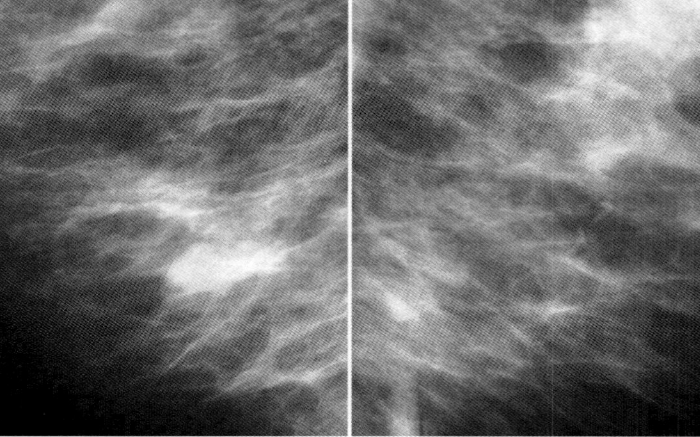

**c** *Bilateral oblique mammograms* (magnified views of the lower quadrants) show nonspecific densities in both breasts, especially on the right side.

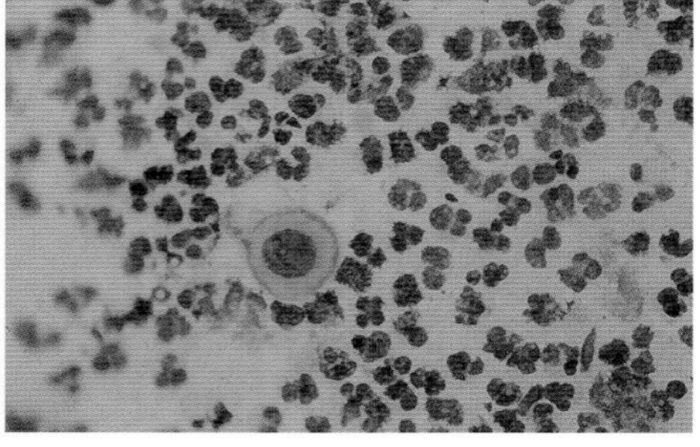

**f** *Aspiration cytology* shows a typical cellular pattern.

**Question on Fig. 5.131**

*How would you interpret these findings?*

(**a**) Invasive lobular carcinoma

(**b**) Acute mastitis

(**c**) Ductectasia with chronic mastitis

→ **Answer on p. 385**

**Fig. 5.132 A 45-year-old woman presents for mammographic screening** with no known trauma history and a positive family history of breast cancer. Mammograms show coarse calcifications in the left breast (**a**). Given her family history, the patient is alarmed by the calcifications and would like a tissue diagnosis.

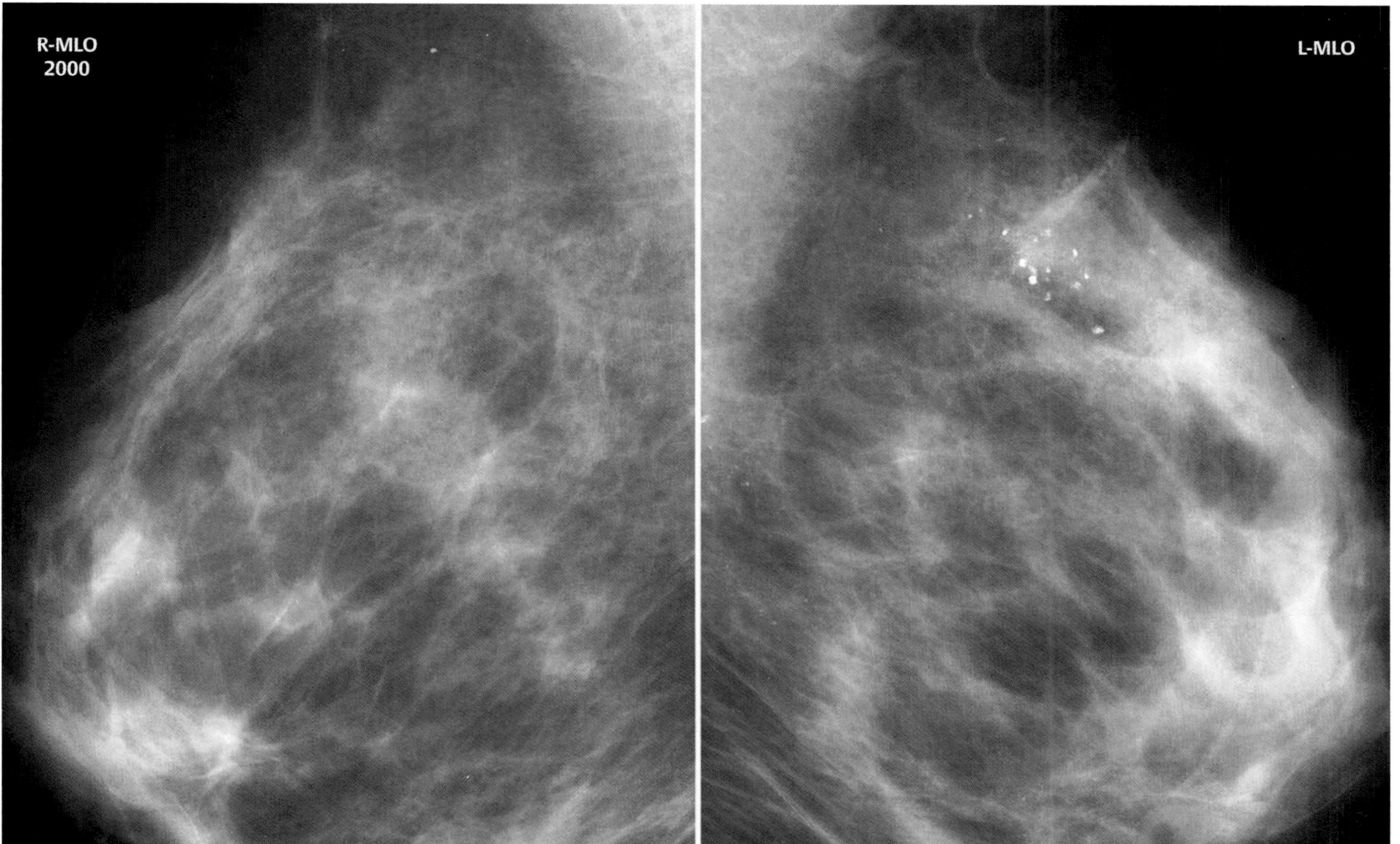


**a** *Bilateral oblique mammograms* in 2000 show radiodense breasts–the left more than the right–with nonspecific inhomogeneities and coarse calcifications in the upper portion of the left breast (**R/22–24**) (ACR 3, BIRADS 2, PG**M**I).

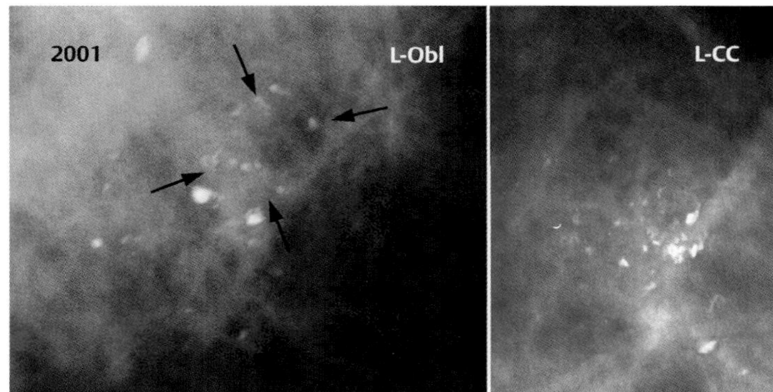


**b** *Oblique mammogram* of the left breast in March, 2001 (magnified view) documents progression of calcifications (ACR 3, BIRADS 3) in the upper part formed like a rosette, similar to blunt duct adenosis (arrows). A *craniocaudal spot view* is shown on the right.

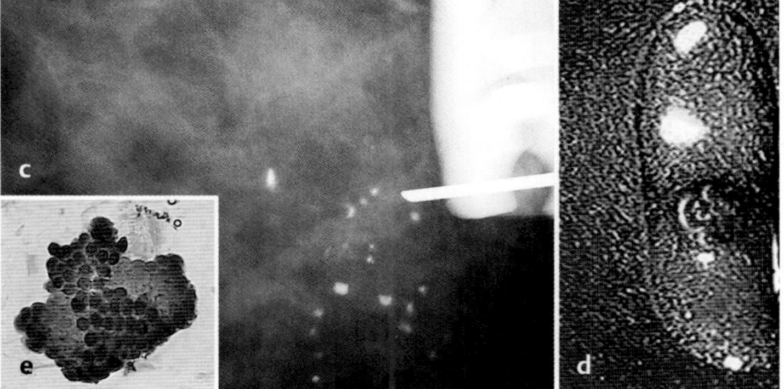


**c** *Digital fine-needle aspiration*. The needle is correctly positioned for aspirating the calcification cluster on a GE Senovision system.
**d** *The aspiration* yields an oily fluid with wormlike paste at the center (**T/10**)).
**e** *Cytology* reveals monomorphic cells in a calcium-rich (blue) liquid.

**Question on Fig. 5.132**

*How would you interpret the calcifying process in the left breast?*

(**a**) Fat necrosis
(**b**) Comedocarcinoma, progressive
(**c**) Granulomatous mastitis

→ **Answer on p. 385**

**Fig. 5.133** **A 60-year-old woman presents with a palpable retroareolar mass in the left breast and no nipple discharge on either side.**

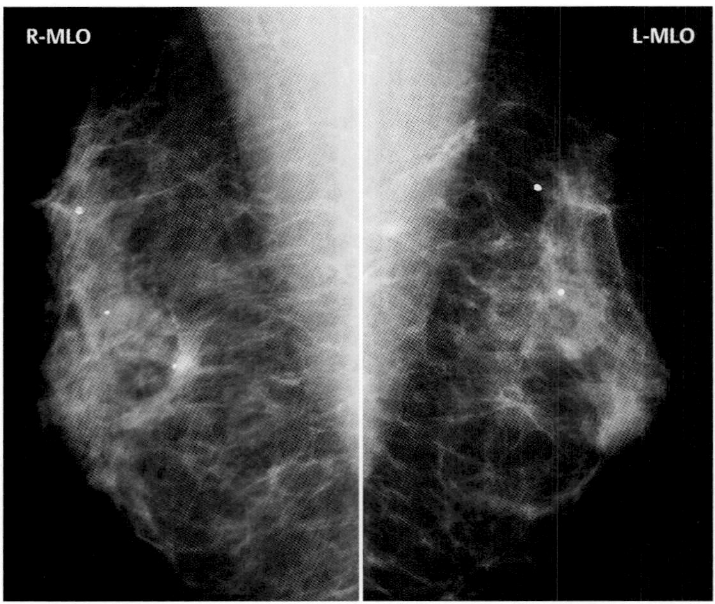


**a** *Bilateral oblique mammograms* show radiolucent breasts with coarse calcifications and a nonspecific density in the right breast (**B/22–23**) (ACR 2, BIRADS 3, **P**GMI).

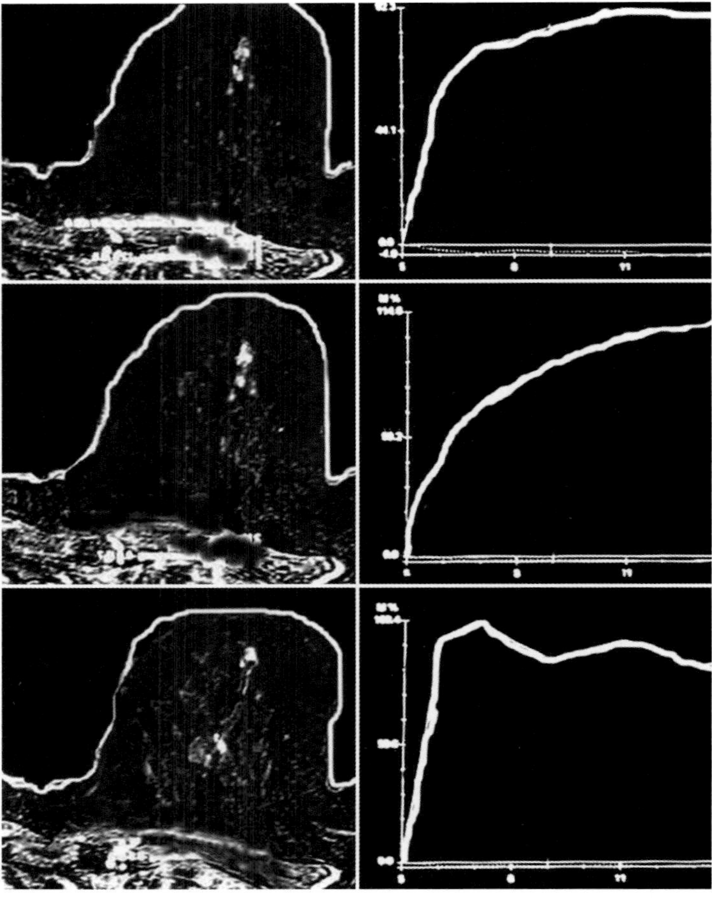

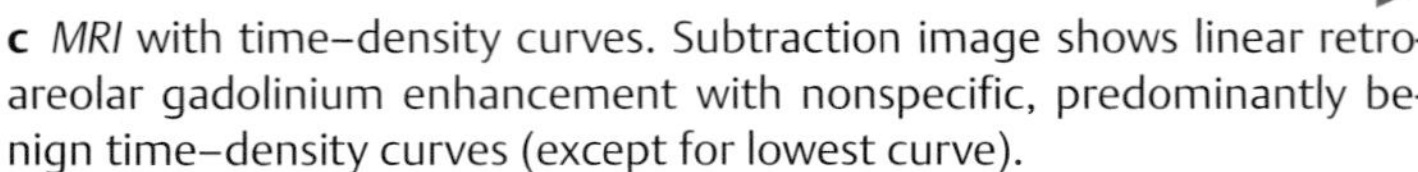

**c** *MRI* with time–density curves. Subtraction image shows linear retroareolar gadolinium enhancement with nonspecific, predominantly benign time–density curves (except for lowest curve).

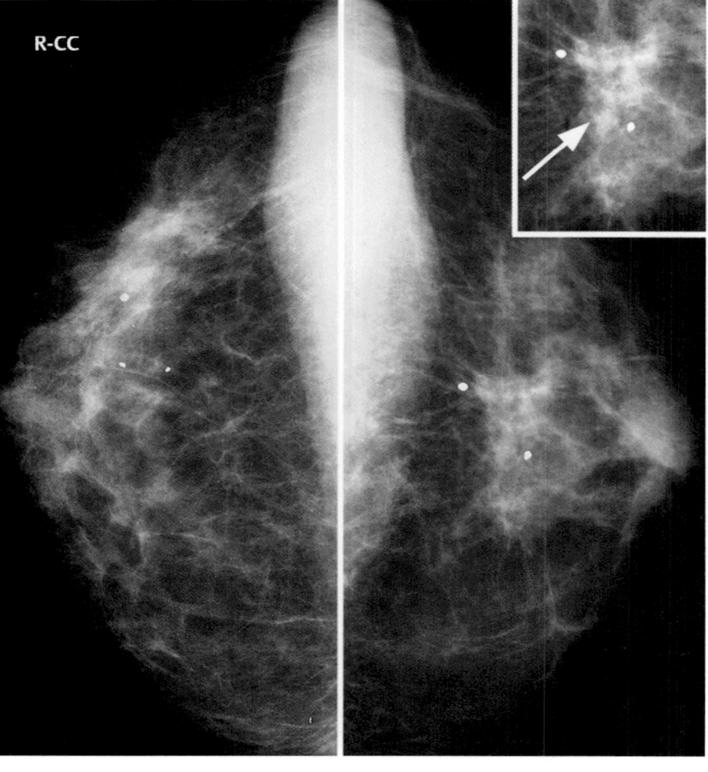


**b** *Bilateral craniocaudal mammograms*. Mammogram of the left breast shows a spiculated, inhomogeneous, retroareolar density (**d/8–9**) with coarse calcifications at its periphery (ACR 2, BIRADS 4, **P**GMI). *Inset:* digital enlargement of the density (arrow).

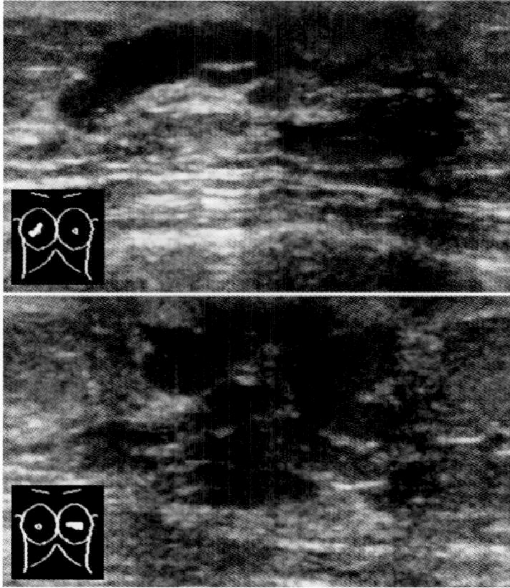

**d** *Sonogram* of the *right* breast (top) shows dilated retroareolar ducts. Scan of the *left* breast (bottom) shows a stellate pattern of ectatic retroareolar ducts.

**Question on Fig. 5.133**

*How would you interpret the retroareolar mass in the left breast?*

(**a**) Invasive ductal neoplasm
(**b**) Papillomatosis
(**c**) Circumscribed focal ductectasia with associated inflammation

→ **Answer on p. 385**

**Fig. 5.134 A 62-year-old woman sustained trauma to the right breast 3 weeks previously** (a large dog jumped up on her and "snagged" her right nipple with its claws). Nipple retraction was present for approximately 2 weeks, unaccompanied by redness or inflammatory signs. Palpation reveals a nonspecific nodular mass in the upper outer quadrant of the right breast. Mammographic and sonographic abnormalities are present.

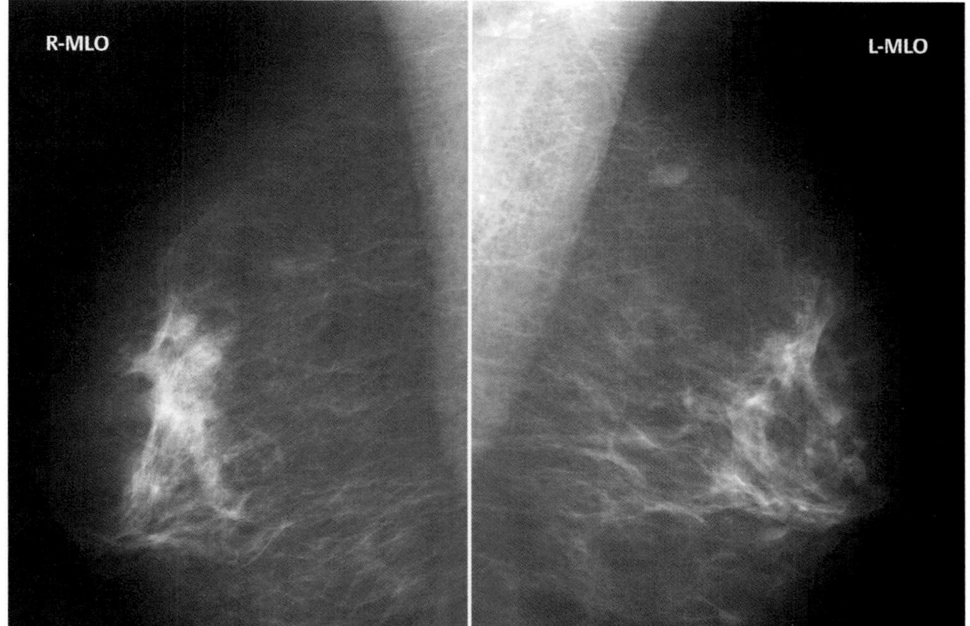


**a** *Bilateral oblique mammograms*. A 2 cm × 4 cm density is visible in the upper portion of the *right* breast (**k–L/20–22**), radiating to the nipple. Image of the *left* breast shows an intramammary lymph node in the axillary recess (**O/24**) (ACR 2, BIRADS 5, **P**GMI).

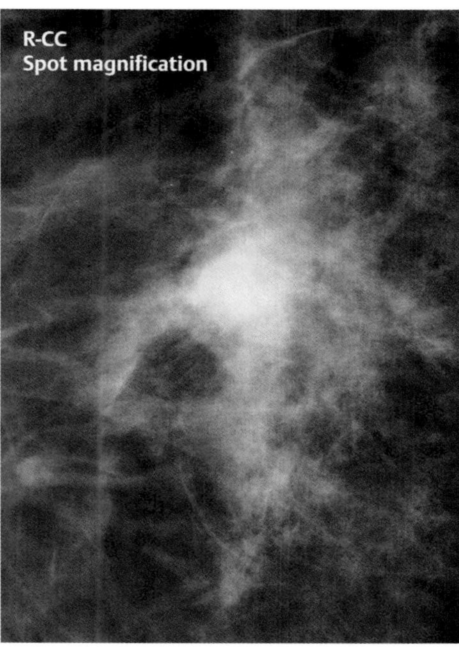


**c** *Craniocaudal magnification mammogram* of the right breast shows a well-circumscribed opacity with inhomogeneous central density and broad extensions radiating toward the periphery and, to a degree, toward the retroareolar area (BIRADS 5).

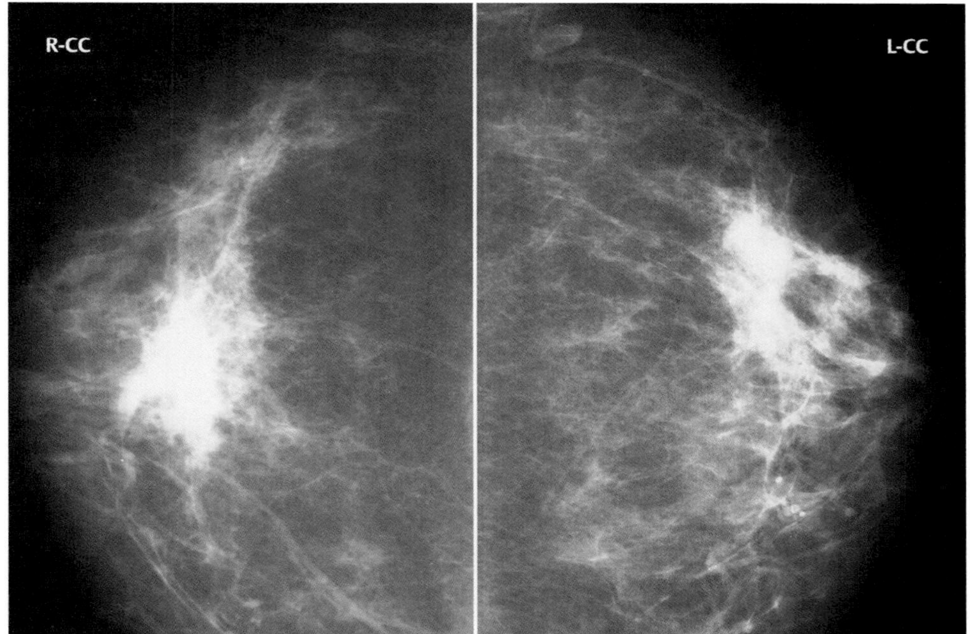


**b** *Bilateral craniocaudal mammograms* show a 1 × 2 cm spiculated retroareolar density in the right breast (**k–l/8–12**). Slightly increased density of the breast parenchyma is also noted on the left side (**o–P/10–11**). The lymph node seen in panel **a** is visible in the axillary recess (**n/14**) (ACR 2, BIRADS 5 right, BIRADS 2 left, **P**GMI).

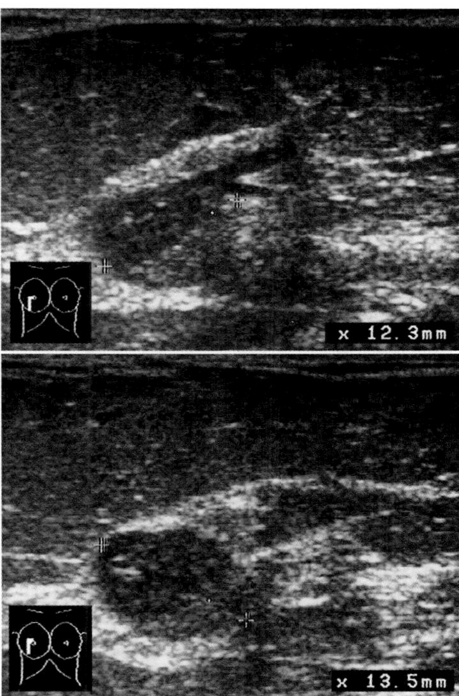


**d** *Sonograms* of the right breast show a well-circumscribed hypoechoic nodule without posterior acoustic enhancement (**R–S/6–7**). The surrounding breast parenchyma is rich in connective tissue and shows no evidence of enlarged TDLUs. Upper image with enlarged lactiferous ducts (**S/12–13**).

▶ **Fig. 5.134e**

**Fig. 5.134 A 62-year-old woman sustained trauma to the right breast 3 weeks previously.** *(continued)*

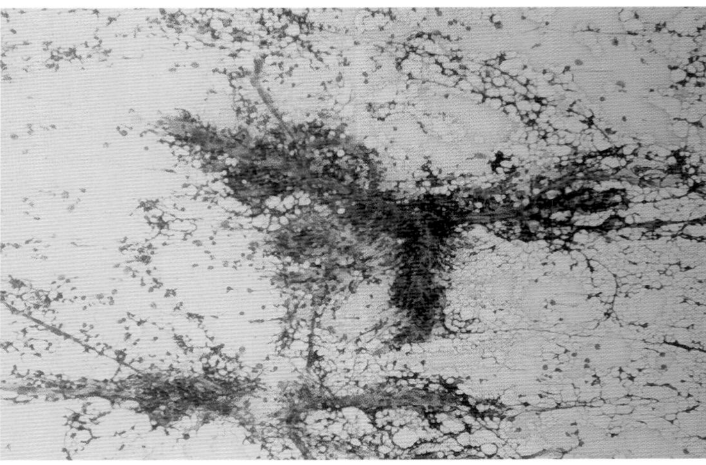

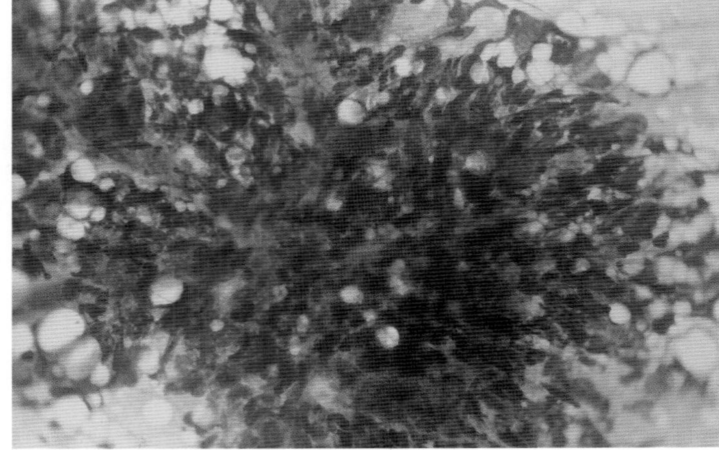

**e** *FNA cytology* shows leukocytes and a granuloma on the left, and the center of the granuloma on the right (see **Fig. 5.135 g**, p. 270).

**Question on Fig. 5.134**

*Which of the following should be included in the differential diagnosis based on the ultrasound findings?*

(**a**) Scirrhous neoplasm (see p. 64)
(**b**) Mucinous carcinoma (see p. 64)
(**c**) Granulomatous mastitis

→ **Answer on p. 385**

**Fig. 5.135 A 34-year-old Albanian woman presents with nonspecific, slightly tender palpable nodules in the lower portion of the right breast.** The nodules were first detected in January, 2002 and were associated with a general feeling of tension in the right breast. Follow-up examination 6 weeks later shows marked deterioration of findings with new, coarse subcutaneous nodules and livid skin discoloration in the lower right breast (**a**). Ultrasound reveals confluent hypoechoic areas with smooth margins (**e**). The left breast appears normal. MRI shows atypical changes in the right breast (**f**). Typical histologic changes are found (**g**).

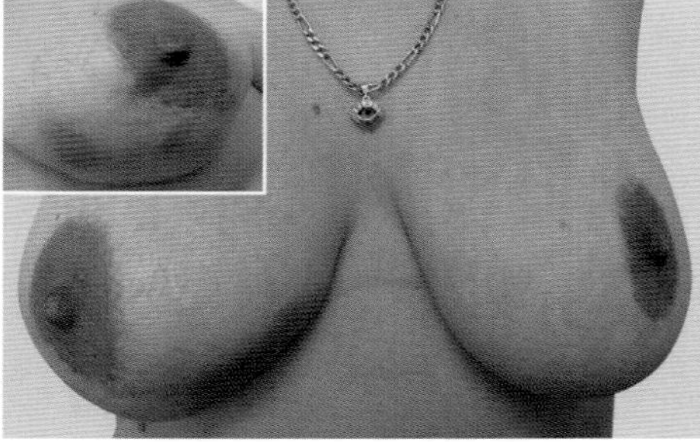

**a** *Clinical inspection*. Both breasts (inset: lower portion of right breast) have a normal configuration with no skin retraction. Reddish-purple skin discoloration is present at the 7 to 9-o'clock positions, extending to the areola. Slight protrusion of the areola is noted between the 8 and 10-o'clock positions (**a/15**).

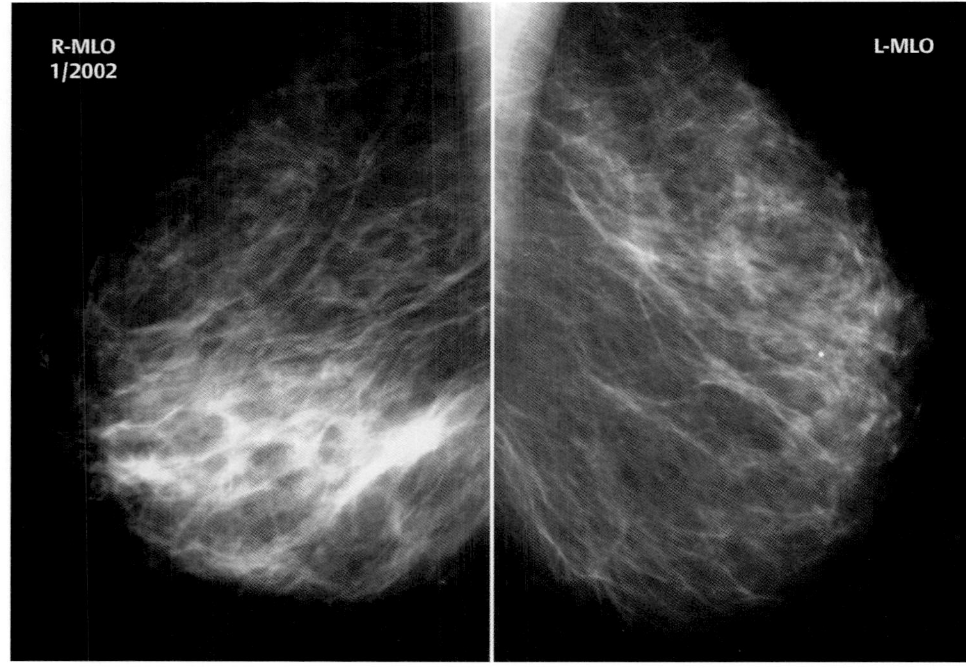


**b** *Bilateral oblique mammograms* in *January*, 2002 (image courtesy of Ulrich Barkow, Stuttgart) show a ground-glass pattern of linear and focal opacities in the lower portion of the right breast. The upper quadrants and left breast appear normal (ACR 2, BIRADS 4, PGMI).

**Fig. 5.135** **A 34-year-old Albanian woman presents with nonspecific, slightly tender palpable nodules.** *(continued)*

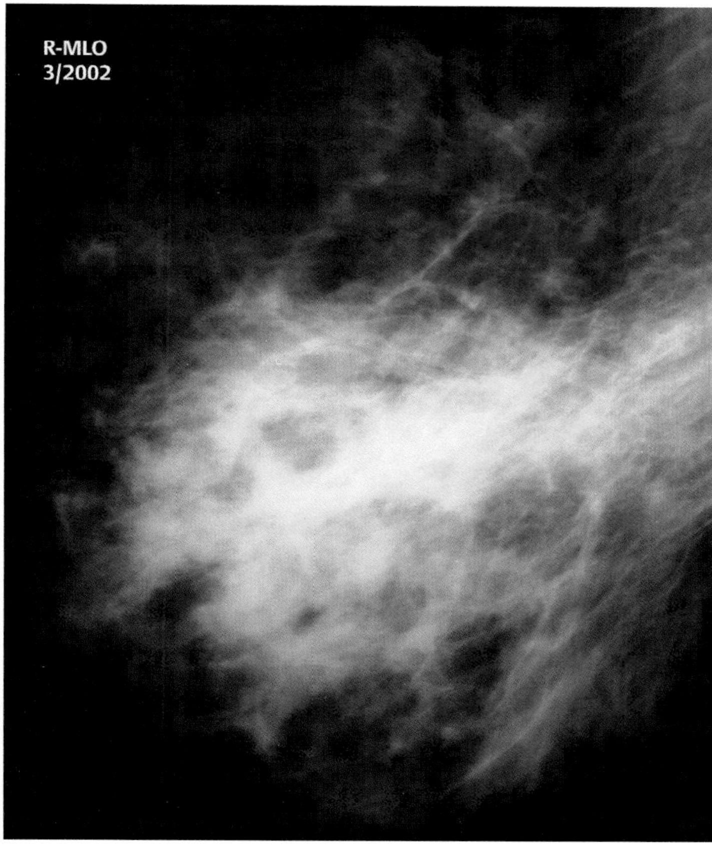


**c** *Oblique mammogram* of the right breast in *March*, 2002. Densities in the lower quadrants have increased dramatically relative to prior images, appearing as confluent patchy opacities that now radiate into the upper quadrants (BIRADS 5).

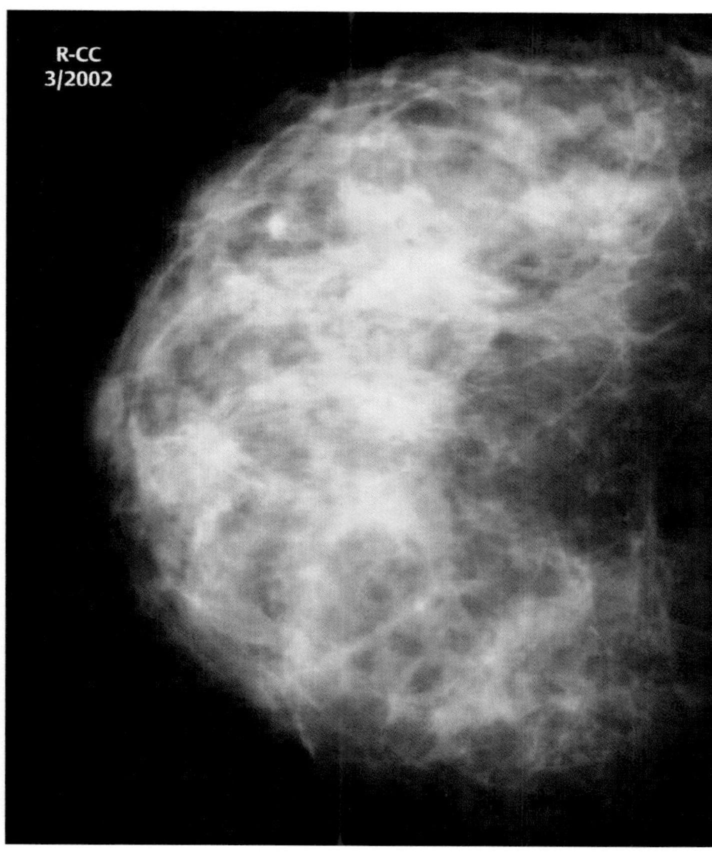


**d** *Craniocaudal mammogram* of the right breast in *March*, 2002 shows confluent, inhomogeneous densities (BIRADS 5, P**G**MI). The left breast is unchanged from January.

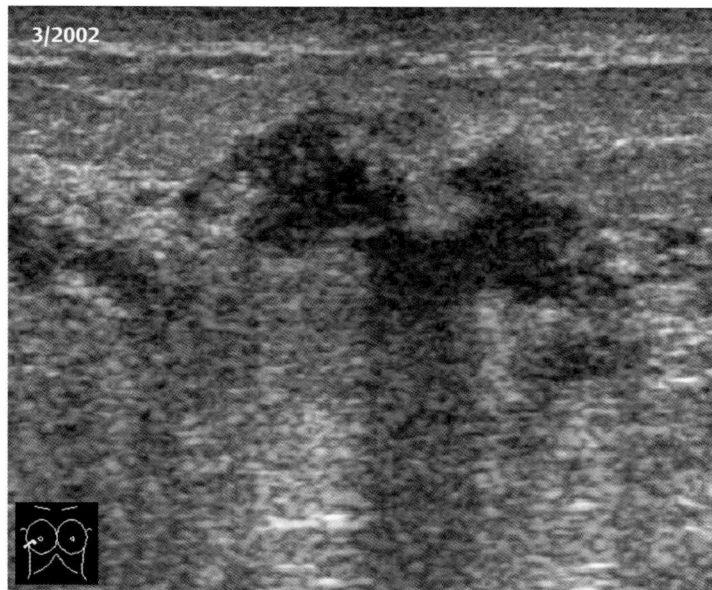


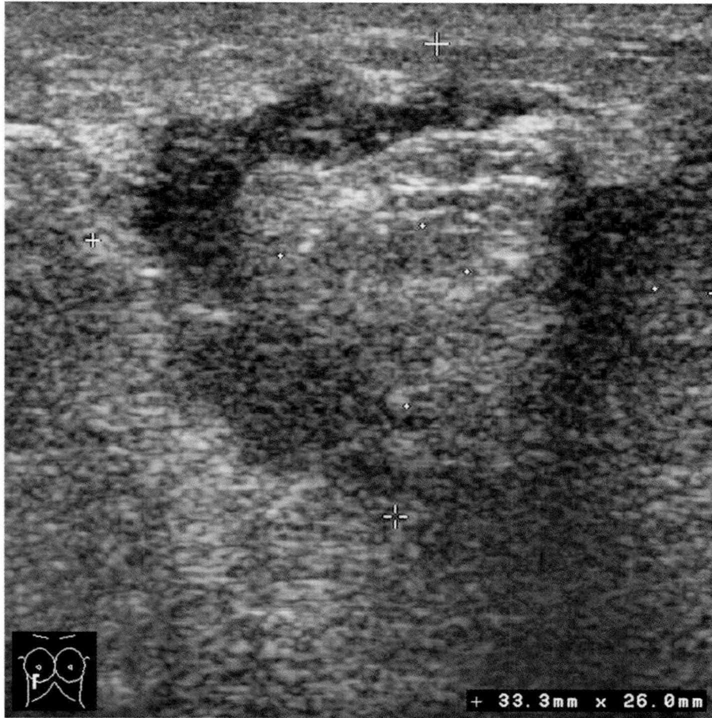


**e** *Sonograms* of the right breast in *March*, 2002, show a hypoechoic, partially liquid area with irregular margins, posterior acoustic enhancement, and possible central necrosis (**L–O/8–11**, and in the right image at **p–T/7–12**).

▶ **Fig. 5.135 f, g**

**Fig. 5.135** **A 34-year-old Albanian woman presents with nonspecific, slightly tender palpable nodules.** *(continued)*

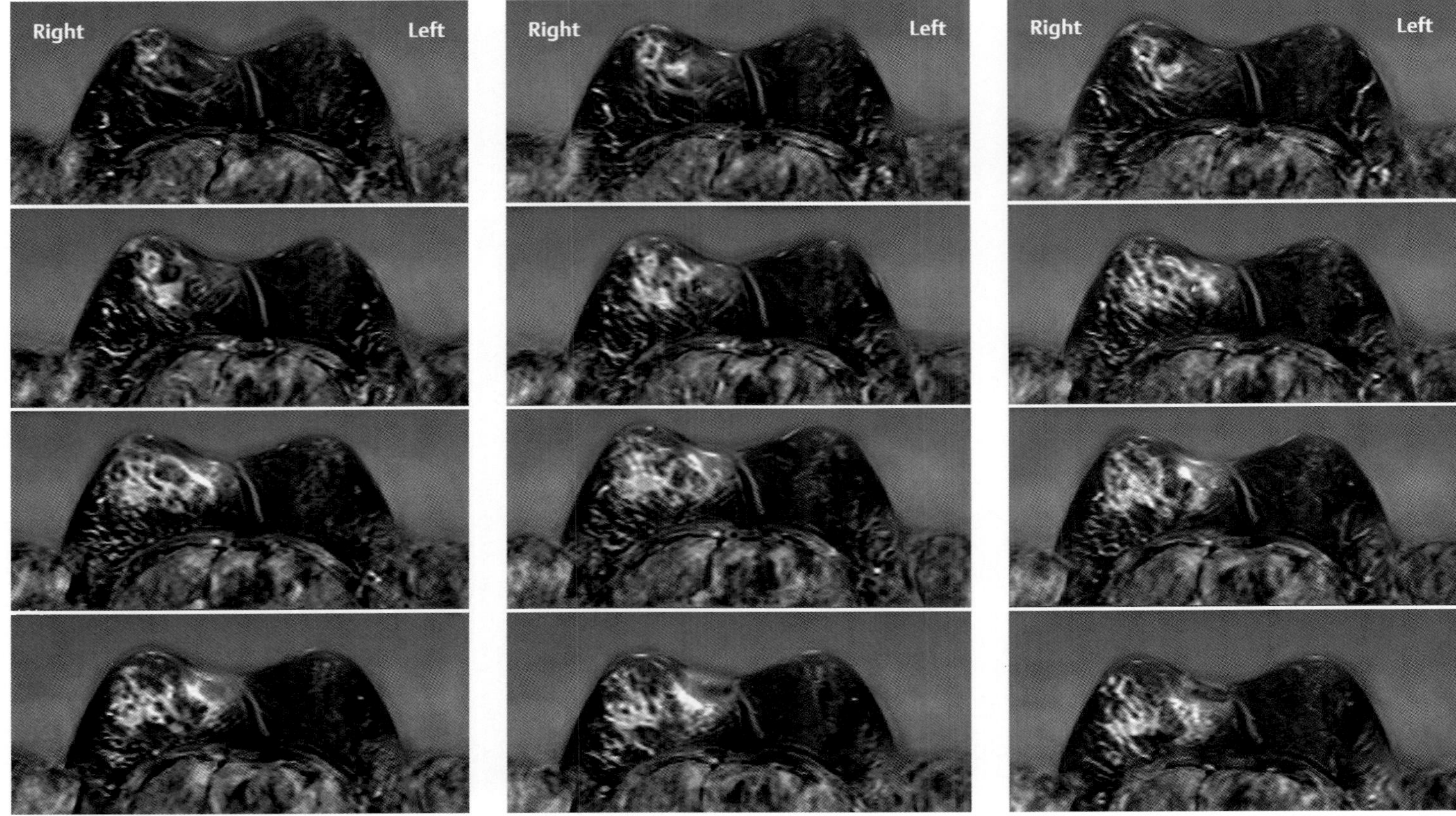


**f** *MRI images* in March, 2002, show a conspicuous, confluent pattern of linear and focal gadolinium enhancement at the same location as the clinical and mammographic findings. The left breast shows no abnormalities.

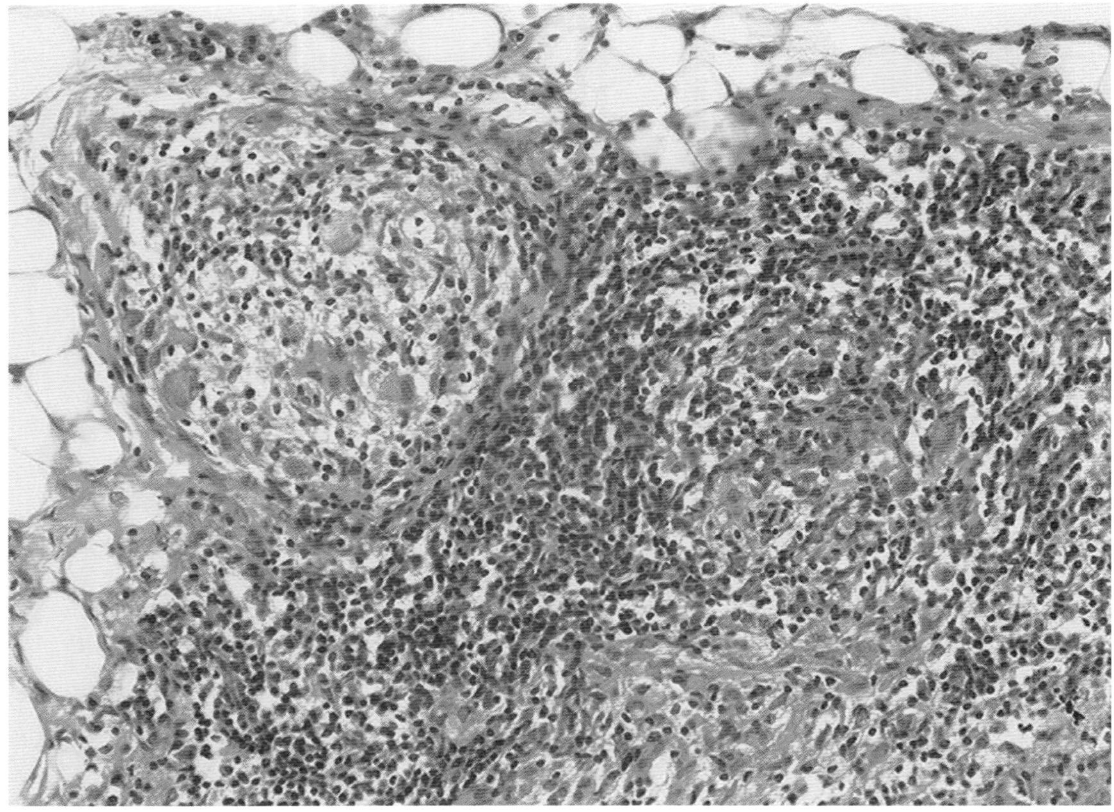

**g** *Histologic section* (16× magnification) shows masses of leukocytes, lymphocytes, and granulomas (e.g., **a–d/ 7–12**) with foreign-body giant cells, some of the Langerhans type.

**Question on Fig. 5.135**

*What is your diagnosis?*

(**a**) Inflammatory breast cancer
(**b**) Angiosarcoma (degenerated hamartoma)
(**c**) Granulomatous mastitis

→ **Answer on p. 386**

**Fig. 5.136 A 50-year-old woman presents with a long history of stabbing pains in the left breast**, most severe in the retroareolar area. No suspicious palpable masses are found in either breast, and there is no skin or nipple retraction. The left areola is larger than the right (**a**). No mammographic abnormalities are found (**b, c**). MRI shows circumscribed retroareolar gadolinium enhancement (**e**), and ultrasound shows a hypoechoic area at that location (**d**). Core-needle biopsy is performed, and the lesion is histologically evaluated (**f**).

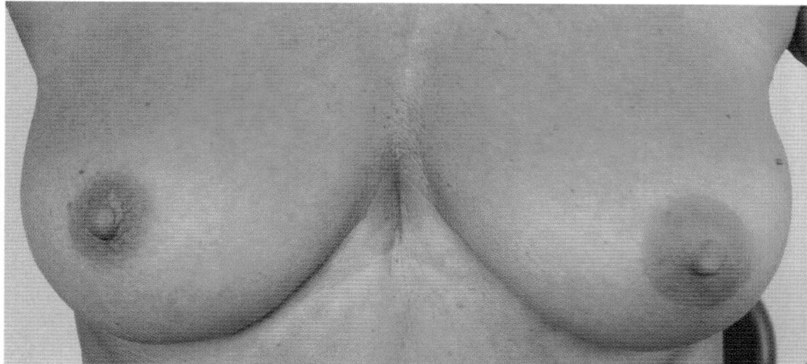

**a** *Clinical inspection* shows asymmetrical areolae with no other visible abnormalities. Inflammatory redness of the skin fold between the breasts is unrelated to the breast process.

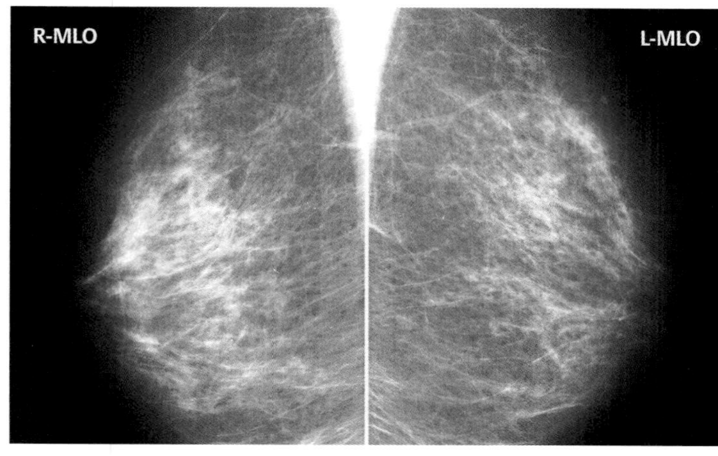


**b** *Bilateral oblique mammograms* document involution of both breasts (ACR 2, P**G**MI).

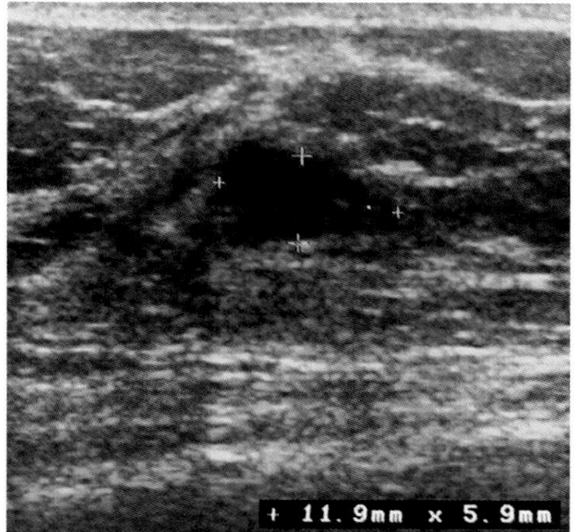


**d** *Sonogram* shows a hypoechoic retroareolar lesion.

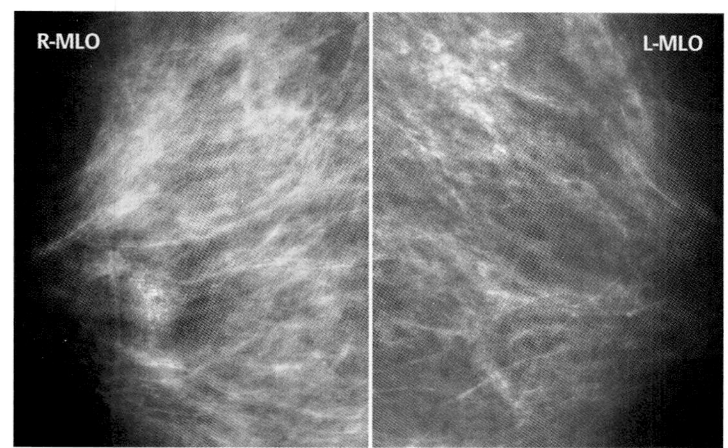


**c** *Bilateral oblique retroareolar magnification mammograms* (3 ×). Possible difference between the two sides?

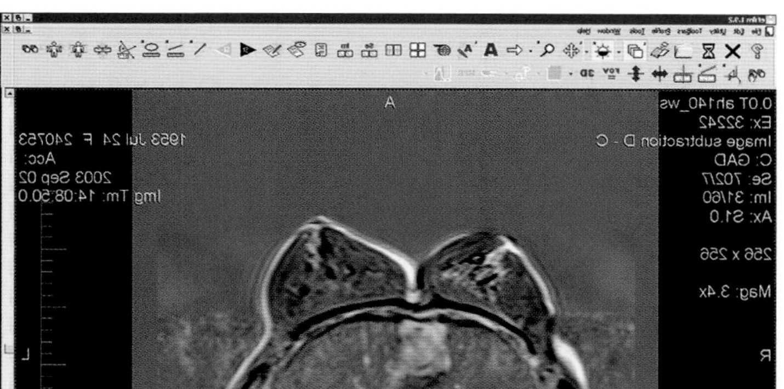

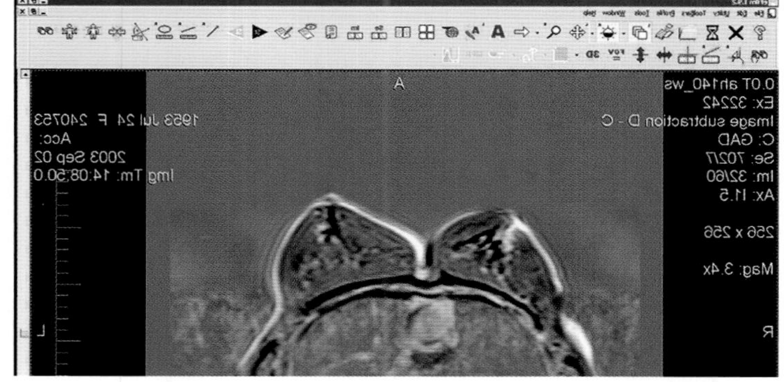

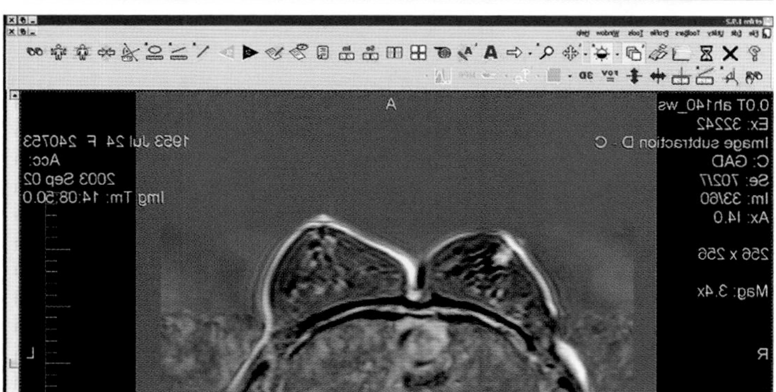

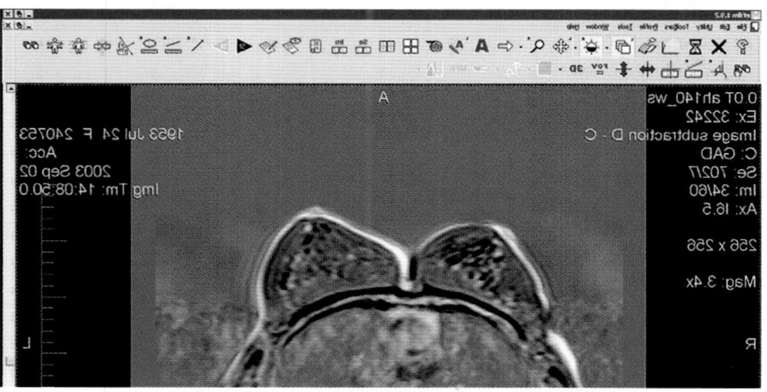

**e** *MR subtraction images* show circumscribed retroareolar gadolinium enhancement.

▶ Fig. 5.136 f

**Fig. 5.136** **A 50-year-old woman presents with a long history of stabbing pains in the left breast.** *(continued)*

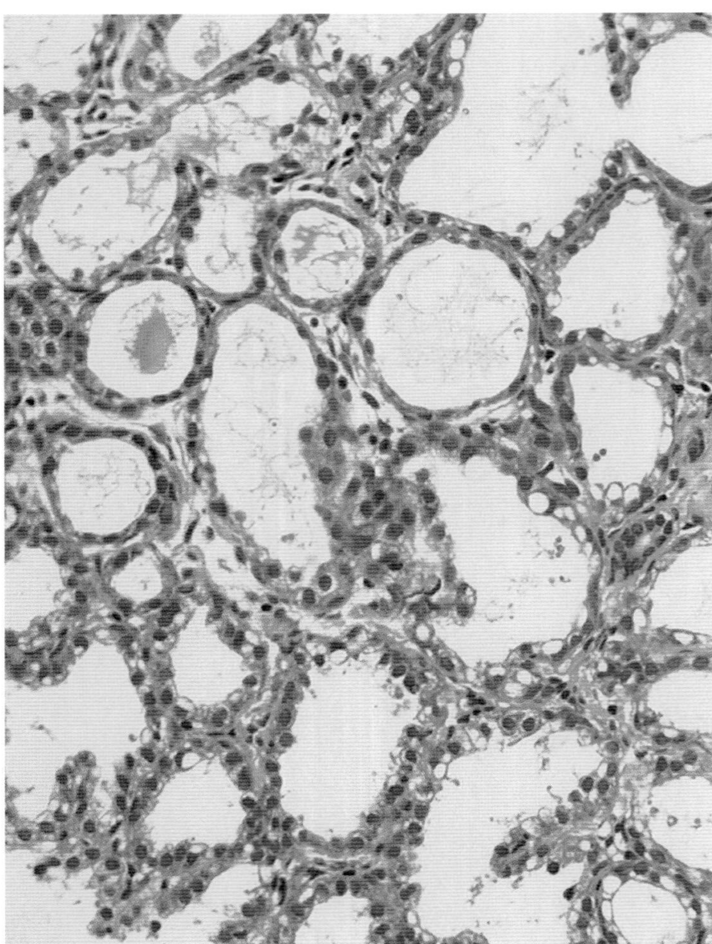

**f** *Histologic section* shows enlarged lobules with uniform cellularity and no atypias. The acini contain secretions.

**Question 1 on Fig. 5.136**

*What does visual inspection reveal in panel a, and what does the finding suggest in view of the patient's complaints?*

(**a**) Inflammatory process
(**b**) Neurologic disorder
(**c**) Tumor-related changes

→ **Answer on p. 388**

**Question 2 on Fig. 5.136**

*Which breast contains the retroareolar focal lesion detected by MRI and ultrasound?*

(**a**) Left breast
(**b**) Right breast
(**c**) Uncertain

→ **Answer on p. 388**

**Question 3 on Fig. 5.136**

*How would you interpret the lesion?*

(**a**) Fibroadenoma
(**b**) Fibrolipoma
(**c**) Lactating adenoma

→ **Answer on p. 388**

**Fig. 5.137** **A 64-year-old woman presents for breast screening.** The patient has no complaints or nodules (**a**). She has suffered from *diabetes mellitus* for years. Mammograms show subtle changes (**b–d**). Ultrasound shows a conspicuous lesion in the upper inner quadrant of the right breast (**e**), corresponding to circumscribed gadolinium enhancement on MRI (**f**). Ultrasound-guided core-needle biopsy is diagnostic (**g**).

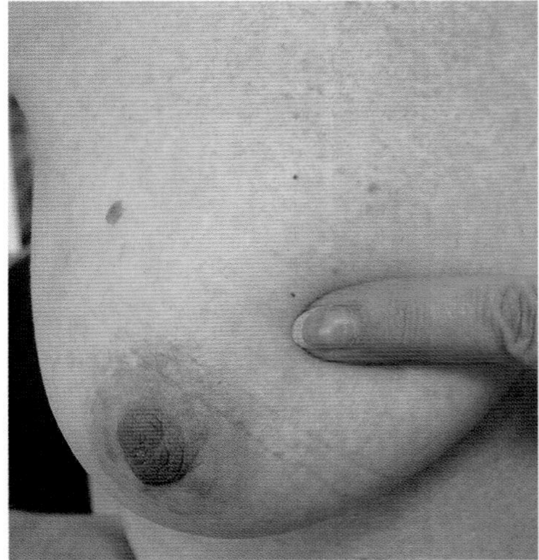

**a** The breast appears *clinically* normal. The finger indicates the site of the mammographic lesion in **d** prior to ultrasound-guided CNB.

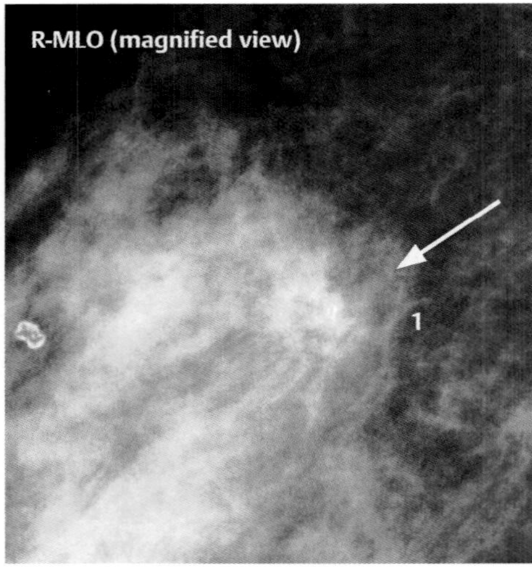


**b** *Oblique mammogram* of the right breast (magnified view of area 1 in **d**) shows a subtle, inhomogeneous density with ill-defined margins and no calcifications.

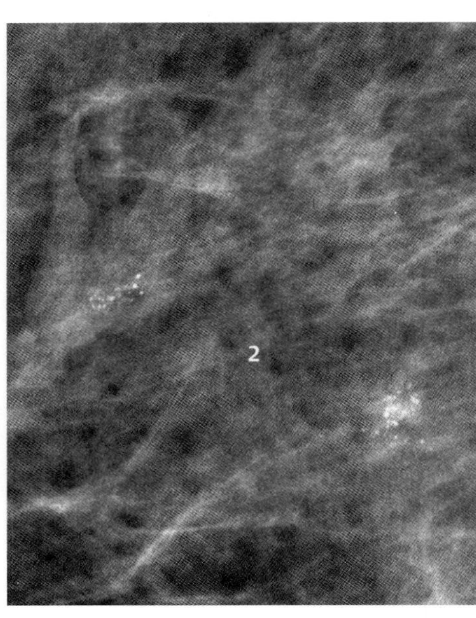


**c** *Oblique mammogram* of the right breast (magnified view of area 2 in **d**) shows two moderately pleomorphic microcalcification clusters (sclerosing adenosis? DCIS?).

**Fig. 5.137** **A 64-year-old woman presents for breast screening.** *(continued)*

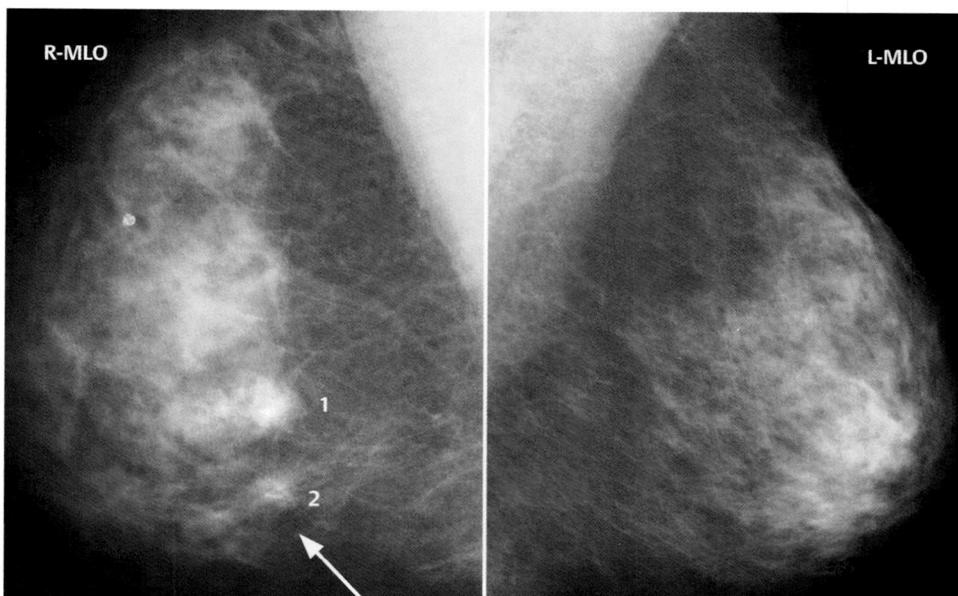


**d** *Bilateral oblique mammograms* provide good visualization of radiodense breasts with periductular fibrosis. Two suspicious foci are visible in the right breast at **l/22** (1) and **l/20** (2) (ACR 3, BIRADS 4 right, BIRADS 3 left, **P**GMI).

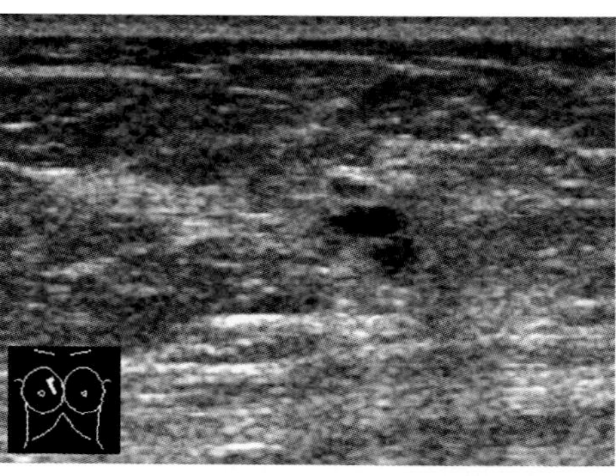

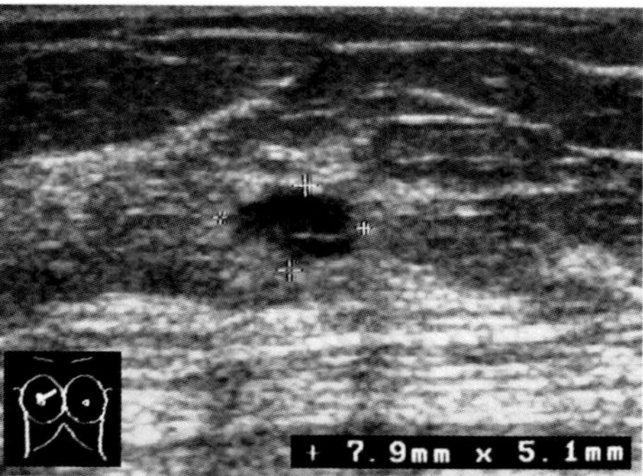


**e** *Sonograms* of the right breast show a 9 mm × 7 mm × 5 mm, partially septated hypoechoic area with irregular margins at 12-o'clock with a 4 mm-wide echogenic rim (**R–S/20–21, r/25**).

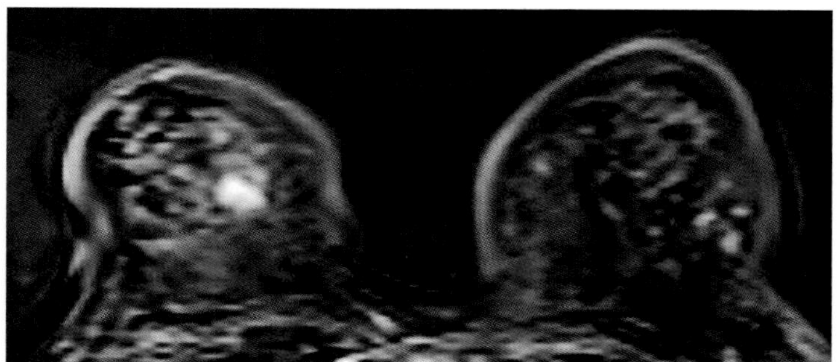

**f** *MR subtraction* images show a 1.5 × 2 cm intensely enhancing lesion with scalloped margins (**L/13**) (slowly rising time–density curve).

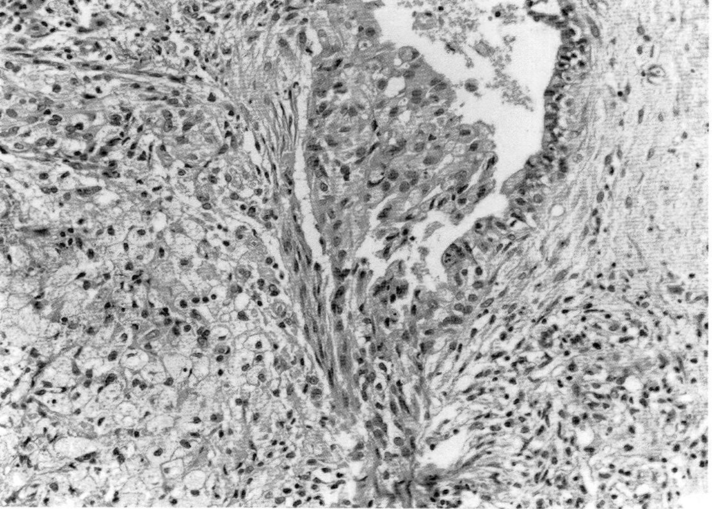

**g** *Histologic section* (lesion 1 from **d**) of an enlarged duct shows nests of foam cells plus lymphocytic infiltration of the duct wall and periductular tissue (image courtesy of Hans-Helmut Dahm, Esslingen).

**Question 1 on Fig. 5.137**

*The lesions detected by MRI and ultrasound correspond to what location in the mammogram?*

(**a**) The upper lesion (no. 1)
(**b**) The lower lesion (no. 2)
(**c**) Neither one

→ **Answer on p. 388**

**Question 2 on Fig. 5.137**

*How would you interpret the upper lesion (no. 1)?*

(**a**) Aggressive fibrosis
(**b**) Lymphocytoid
(**c**) Invasive lobular neoplasm

→ **Answer on p. 388**

**Question 3 on Fig. 5.137**

*How would you explain the discrepancy in lesion size between ultrasound (dark zone) and MRI?*

(**a**) Diffuse tumor infiltration of surrounding tissues
(**b**) Different lesions
(**c**) Inflammatory perifocal reaction

→ **Answer on p. 389**

**Fig. 5.138 A 57-year-old woman had an initial mammogram in 1997 for a cyst in the upper outer quadrant of the left breast.** Two years later the cyst recurs and is aspirated again. This time a pneumocystogram is obtained (**d**) after breast ultrasound (**c**).

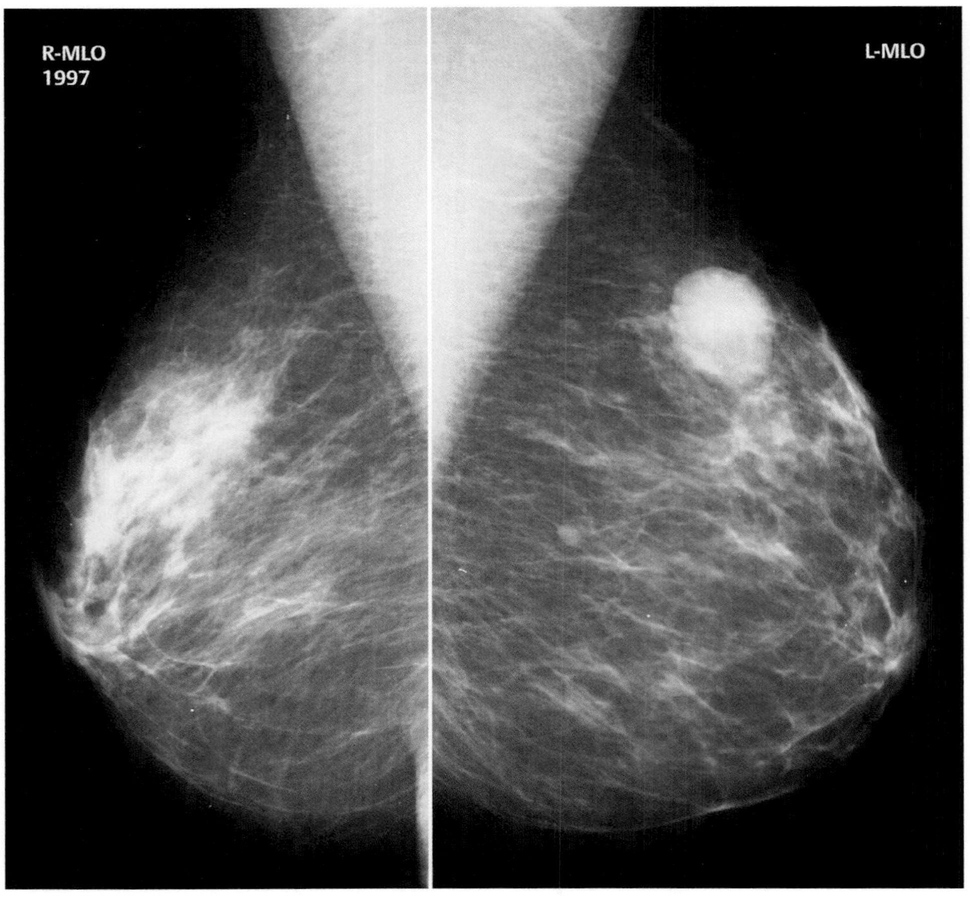


**a** *Bilateral oblique mammograms* in 1997 show an involuted left breast that is slightly less radiodense than the right breast. The upper portion of the left breast contains a 3.0 cm cyst corresponding to a palpable mass at that location (ACR 2 right, ACR 1 left, BIRADS 2, P**G**MI).

**d** *Pneumocystogram* in 1999 (detail from the oblique image) demonstrates the cyst lumen and the irregular basal contours of the cyst wall.

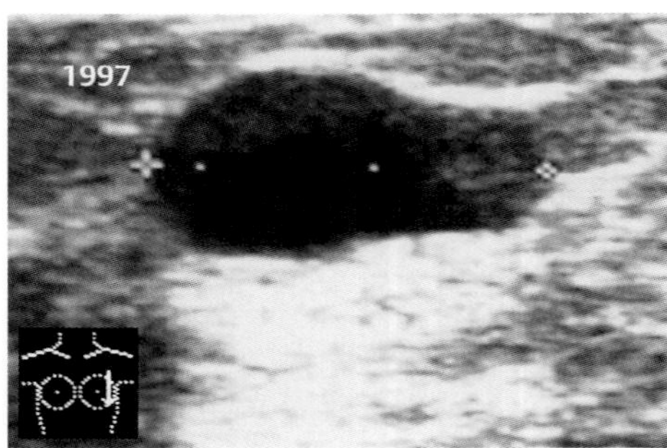


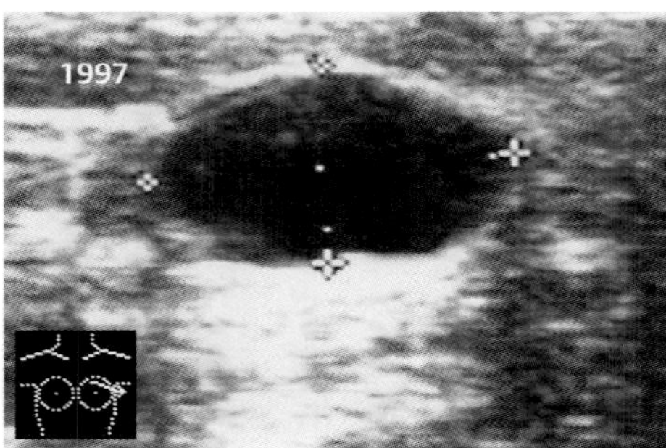


**b** *Sonograms* of the left breast in 1997 show a cyst with a hypoechoic center and strong posterior acoustic enhancement.

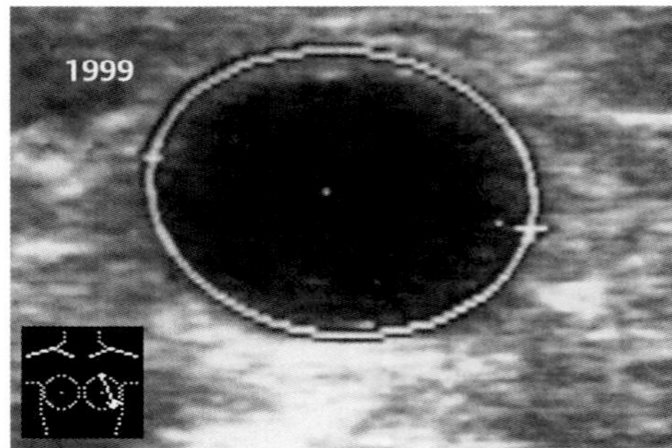


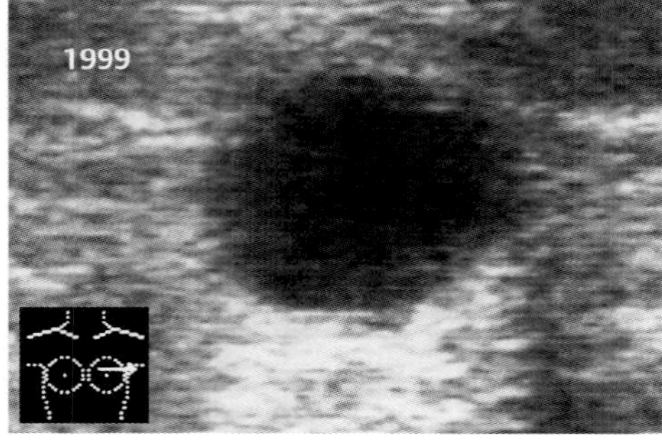


**c** *Sonograms* of the left breast in 1999 show a cyst with the same acoustic characteristics as in 1997.

**Question on Fig. 5.138**

*Did the cyst change between 1997 and 1999?*

(**a**) Yes

(**b**) No

(**c**) Uncertain

→ **Answer on p. 389**

(continued from p. 261)

## Neoplasms in Younger Women

In a review of our own cases, we find that 35% of all invasive neoplasms and 40% of preinvasive lesions were diagnosed in women under 50 years of age (see **Fig. 2.2**, p. 15). The worldwide incidence of breast cancer is rising in women over 35 years of age while it is remaining constant in women under 30 and falling in women 50 years and older. It is reasonable to assume that breast cancer in younger women (25–35 years of age) has a predominantly genetic cause (see p. 13) and that calcifying preinvasive lesions can be detected mammographically as early as 25 years of age in some patients (see **Fig. 5.139**). Breast cancer is practically nonexistent under 18 years of age and is extremely rare from 18 to 25 years of age. Even so, we recently diagnosed breast cancer in an 18-year-old woman with no family history (**Fig. 5.64**, p. 161).

If it is correct that cellular mutations occurring between puberty and first pregnancy can lead to breast cancer (see p. 9), this interval would fall chronologically between approximately 15 and 33 years of age. A mutation occurring in this period could develop into a detectable tumor in 6–16 years, with the result that preinvasive lesions such as DCIS with microcalcifications would be detectable between 25 and 40 years of age. At this age the breast tissue is still relatively radiodense and radiosensitive (Jung 2001), especially between puberty and the first pregnancy (if it occurs). The breast tissue can be more accurately evaluated by ultrasound and MRI than by mammography (only 11% of women under age 35 have a breast density of ACR 1–2). X-rays can also have mutagenic effects in young women.

But if mammography is performed at this age, it should be limited to *one* projection per side. This is adequate for diagnostic purposes and is also prudent from a radiobiologic standpoint. Single-view mammograms can confidently detect or exclude microcalcifications while limiting the radiation dose to about 50% of standard biplane views (see Future Trends, p. 107). With the aid of MRI, single-view mammography, and breast ultrasound, it is possible to detect breast cancer and its precursors at an early stage in women 25–45 years of age who are at risk for the disease. **Figures 5.139–5.143** illustrate the problems that may arise in the imaging and differential diagnosis of breast cancer in women about 40 years of age and younger.

(continued on p. 283)

**Fig. 5.139 Neoplasm in a 27-year-old female judo wrestler.** The patient came for screening due a positive family history of breast cancer (mother and grandmother). Bilateral single-view mammograms (later supplemented by a craniocaudal view of the right breast) show atypical clustered microcalcifications in the prepectoral region of the right breast. Histology reveals moderately well-differentiated DCIS with microcalcifications and a strongly positive estrogen- and progesterone-receptor status. The calcifications are removed by wide excisional biopsy.

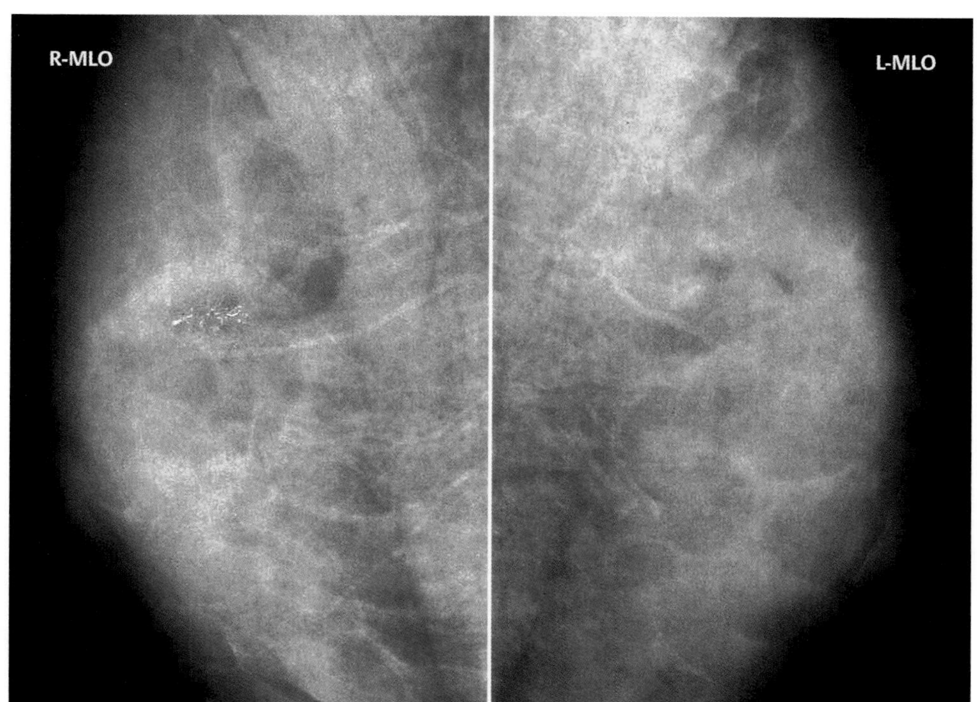


**a** *Bilateral oblique mammograms* show very radiodense breasts (ACR 4, BIRADS 4, **P**GMI) with clustered microcalcifications in the right breast at **L/10**.

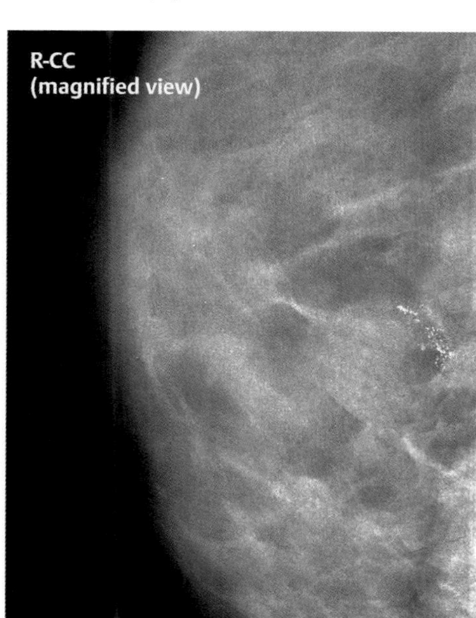


**b** *Craniocaudal mammogram* of the right breast. A cluster of pleomorphic microcalcifications measuring 1 cm × 1 cm × 2 cm is visible at the center of the breast (**T/10**). The breast parenchyma is very radiodense (ACR 4, BIRADS 4, **P**GMI).

▶ Fig. 5.139 c–e

**Fig. 5.139 Neoplasm in a 27-year-old female judo wrestler.** *(continued)*

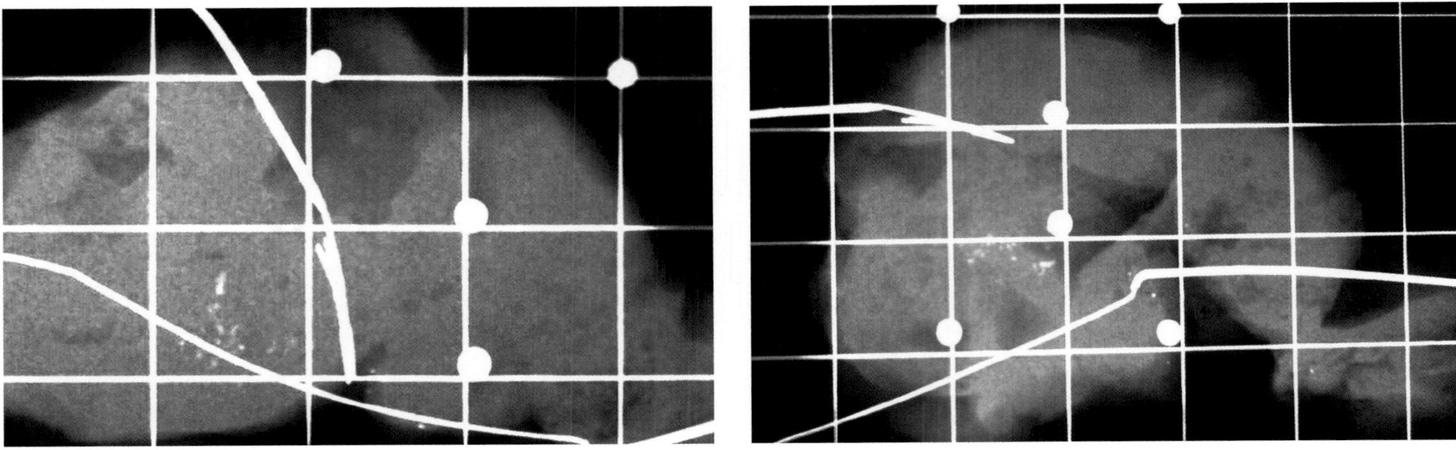

**c, d** *Specimen radiographs* in two mutually perpendicular planes confirm the presence of microcalcifications in the biopsy specimen.

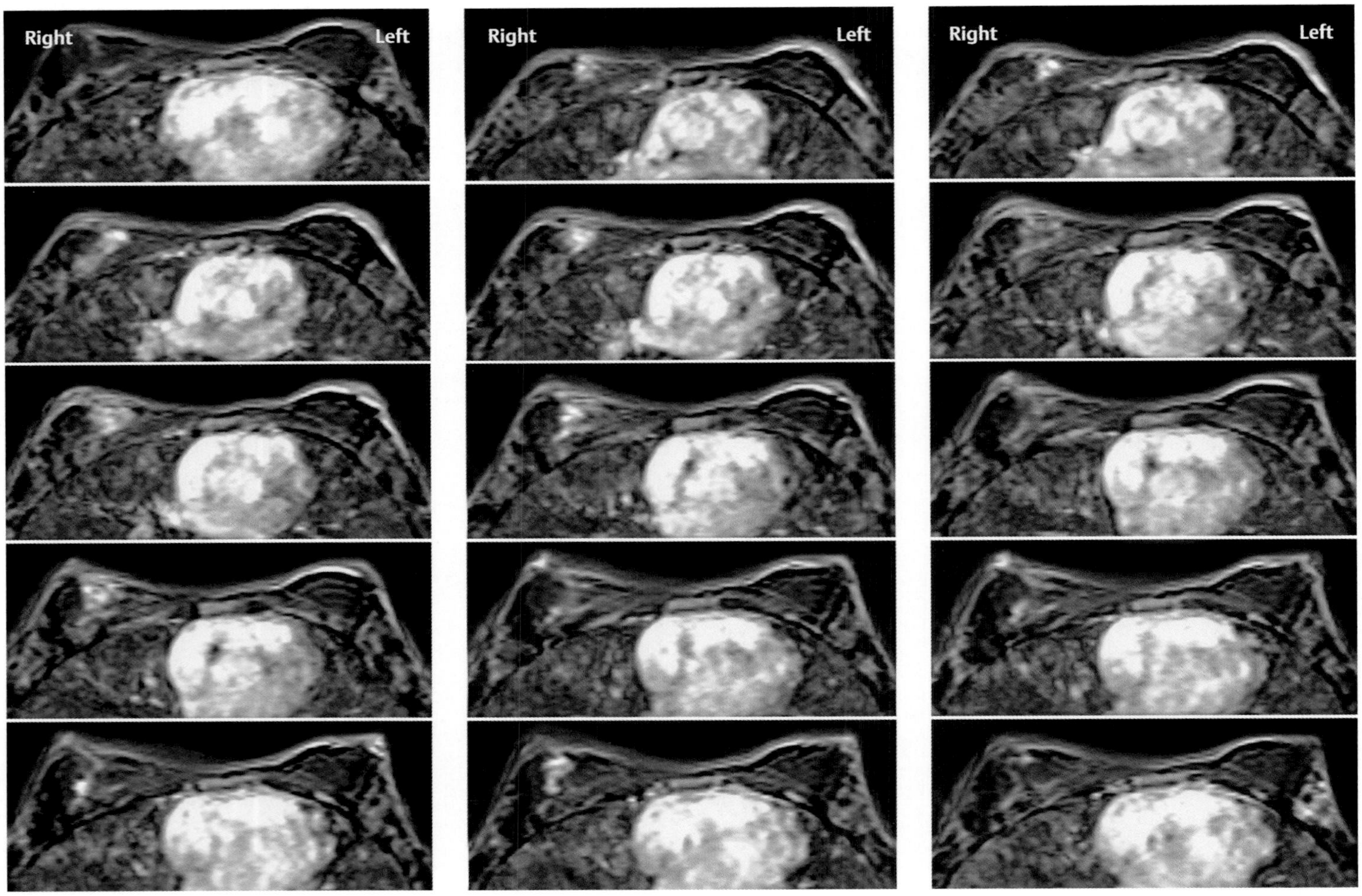

**e** *MR subtraction images* show focal gadolinium enhancement in the area occupied by calcifications in the right breast. The enhancement can be traced to the retroareolar region (e.g., **E/9**), raising suspicion of noncalcifying DCIS outside the calcification area as well. The left breast shows faint, nonspecific gadolinium enhancement at **j/8–9**.

**Question 1 on Fig. 5.139**

*Do the specimen radiographs (c, d) show that the DCIS was removed with clear margins?*

(**a**) No
(**b**) Yes
(**c**) Cannot be determined

→ **Answer on p. 390**

**Question 2 on Fig. 5.139**

*Is nipple involvement likely based on the mammographic findings?*

(**a**) Yes
(**b**) No
(**c**) Cannot be determined

→ **Answer on p. 390**

**Fig. 5.140 A 30-year-old woman presents with a 1.3 cm freely movable nodule in the upper outer quadrant of the left breast (a).** The nodule shows a combination of sharp and ill-defined margins at ultrasound (**c**) and an inhomogeneous, partly cystic internal echo pattern. The nodule is not visible mammographically in the radiodense breast (**b**). Aspiration cytology shows aggregates of different cells (**d**). The nodule shows intense gadolinium enhancement on MRI (**e**). The patient wants very much to conceive, and she becomes pregnant 3 years after removal of the nodule.

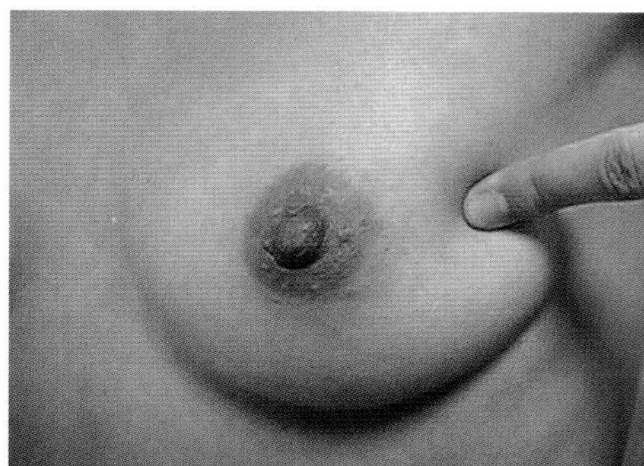

**a** *Clinical inspection* reveals a nodule at the 2-o'clock position in the upper outer quadrant of the left breast. The nodule is not associated with skin or nipple retraction.

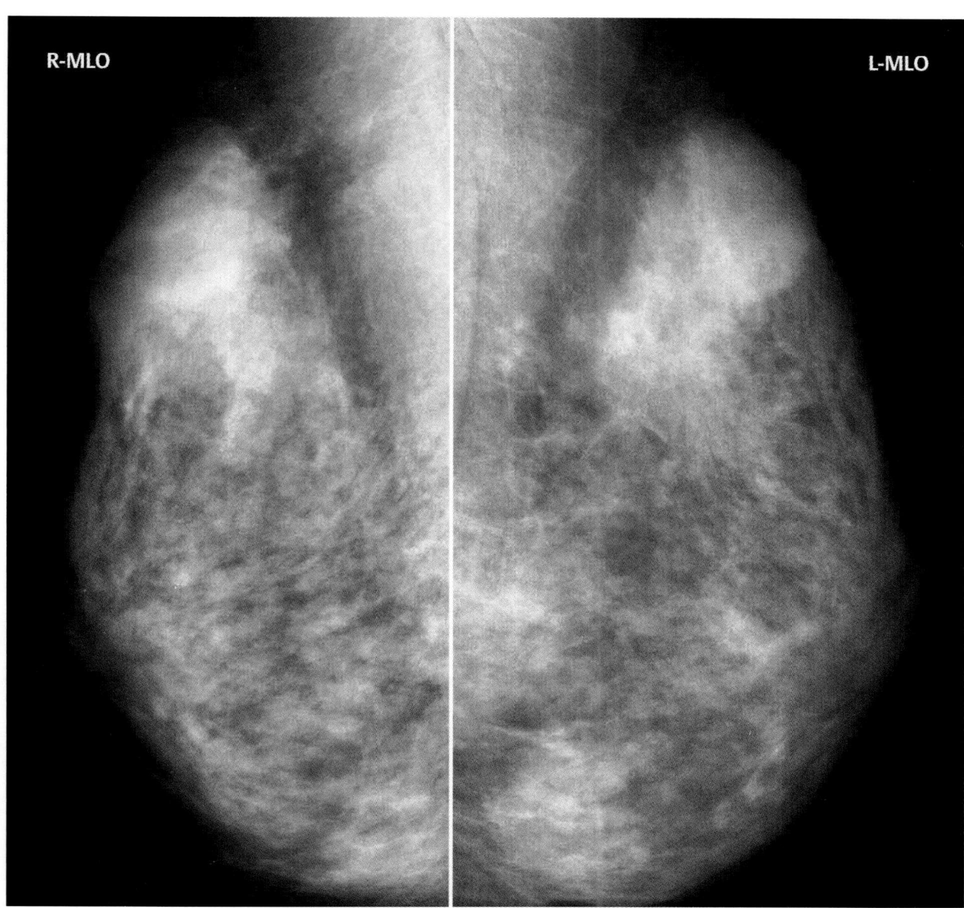


**b** *Bilateral oblique mammograms* show very radiodense breasts with patchy, inhomogeneous opacities superiorly (left **r–s/21–24**) and inferiorly (left **Q–R/14–16**) (ACR 3, BIRADS 2, **P**GMI). Findings are identical in the craniocaudal views.

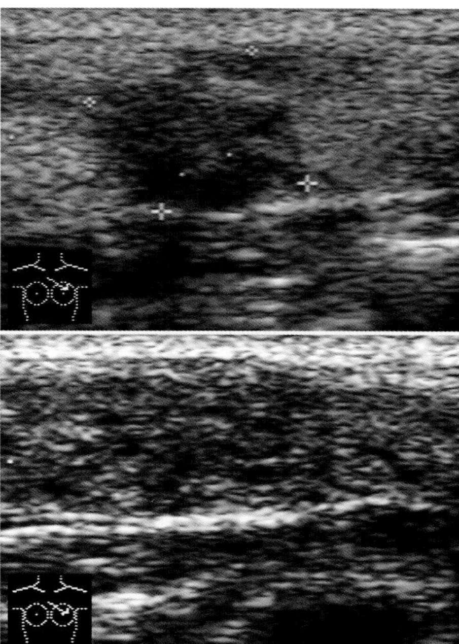

**c** *Sonograms* of the left breast at 2-o'clock (above) show a nodule with smooth anterior margins (**k–l/16–18**) and no posterior acoustic enhancement. The glandular tissue appears normal. An echogenic duct (**k–m/12**) is surrounded by copious stromal tissue (below).

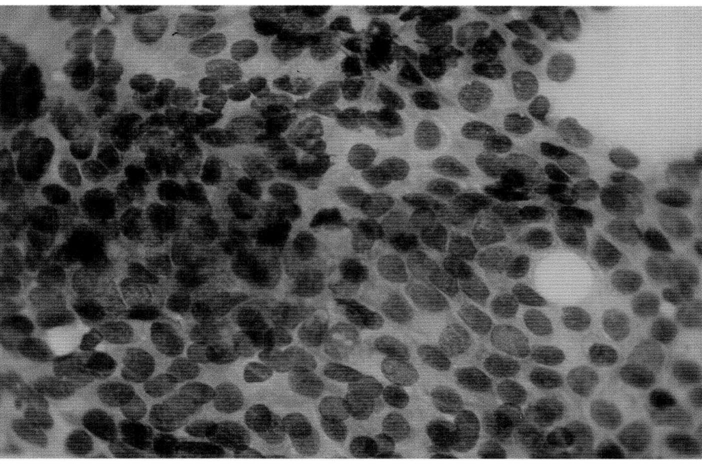

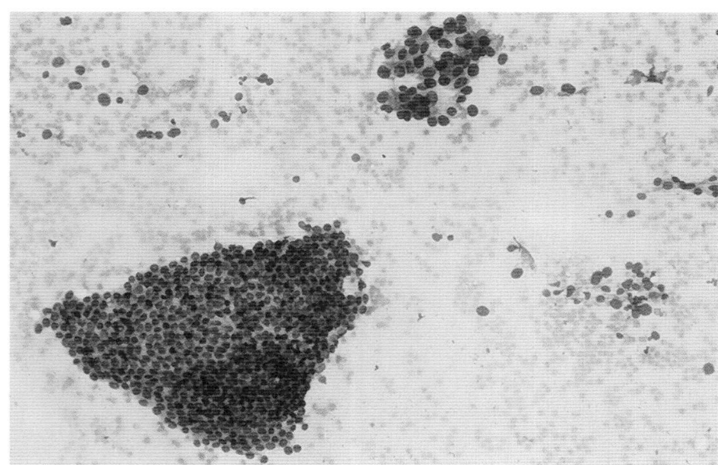

**d** *FNA cytology.* At lower left is a large cell complex with smooth or slightly concave borders and a uniform arrangement of cells. At upper right is a loose cluster of pleomorphic cells, some dissociated.

▶ **Fig. 5.140 e**

**Fig. 5.140 A 30-year-old woman presents with a 1.3 cm freely movable nodule in the upper outer quadrant of the left breast.** *(continued)*

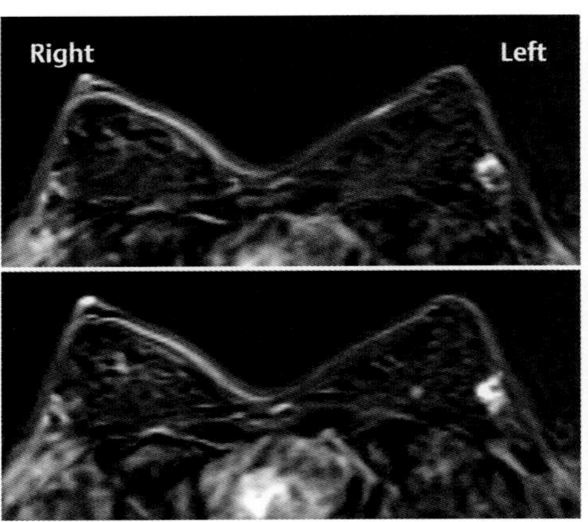


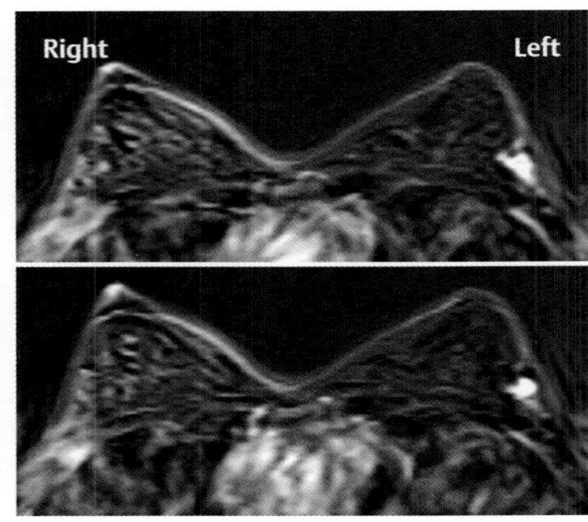


**e** *MR subtraction images* show a smooth nodule in the left axillary recess with fine extensions and intense gadolinium enhancement. The lesion has a benign time–density curve.

**Question 1 on Fig. 5.140**

*How would you interpret the nodule on the left side?*

(**a**) Fibroadenoma
(**b**) Mucinous carcinoma
(**c**) Fibroadenoma with DCIS

→ **Answer on p. 391**

**Question 2 on Fig. 5.140**

*As a rule, should patients be allowed to become pregnant and to nurse following treatment for a tumor or DCIS?*

(**a**) Yes
(**b**) No
(**c**) Only with the healthy breast

→ **Answer on p. 391**

**Fig. 5.141 A 31-year-old woman recently noticed a small, freely movable nodule in the lower inner quadrant of her left breast** at the 8-o'clock position (**a**). Nipple retraction has been present for years but is unrelated to the nodule. She has no family history of breast cancer.

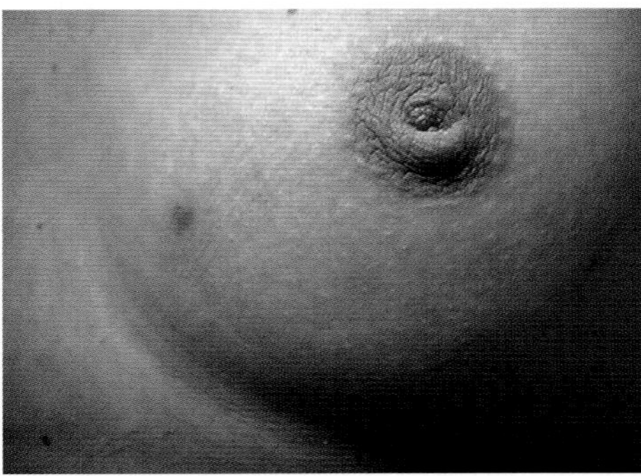

**a** *Clinical inspection* of the left breast (lower inner quadrant) shows skin redness after FNA of the nodule (**B/15**).

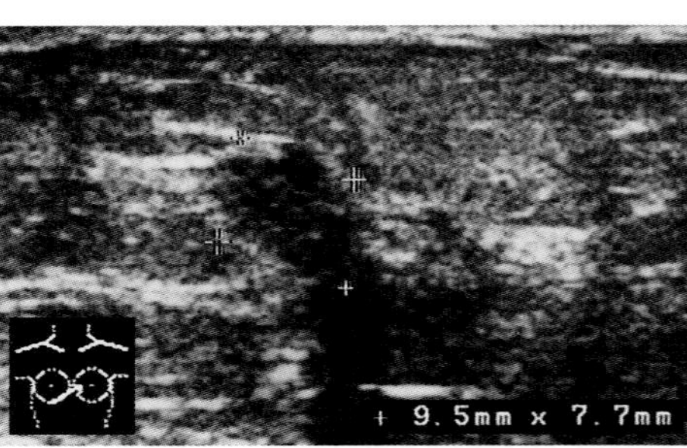


**c** *Sonogram* of the lower inner quadrant of the left breast shows a 10 mm hypoechoic nodule with internal echoes and posterior acoustic shadowing.

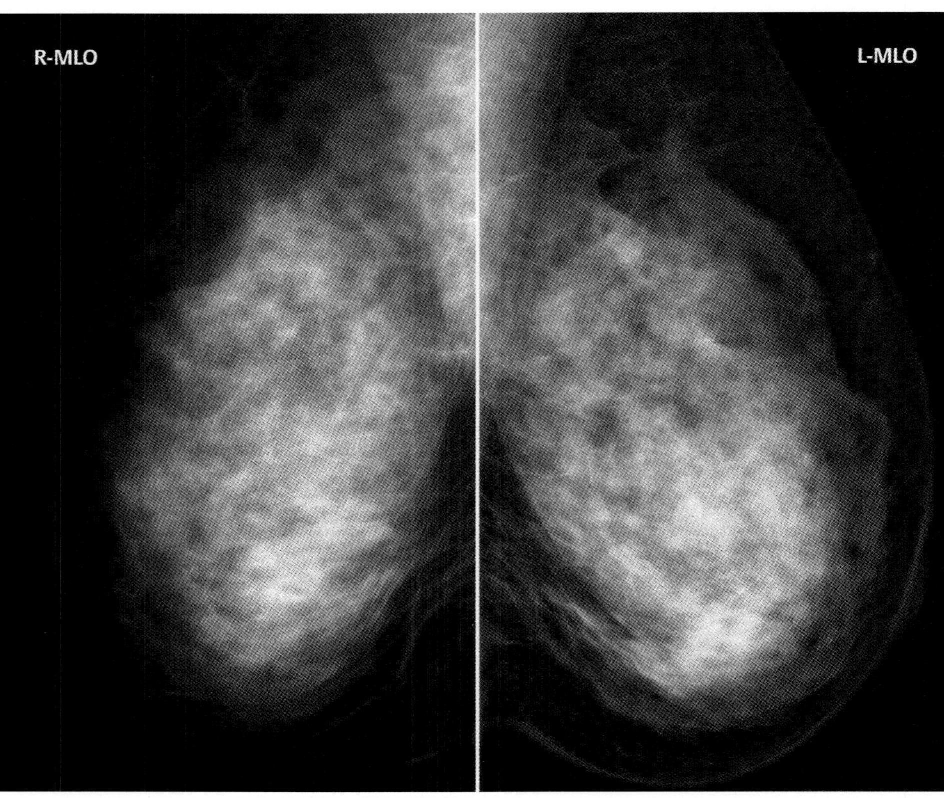


**b** *Bilateral oblique mammograms* show radiodense breasts with confluent opacities (ACR 4, BIRADS 1, **PGMI**). The craniocaudal view shows identical findings with no atypical changes.

**Fig. 5.141** **31-year-old woman with a small, freely movable nodule in the lower inner quadrant of her left breast.** *(continued)*

**d** *FNA cytology* shows a compact cell cluster with large nuclei and an altered nuclear-cytoplasmic ratio, e.g. **k/25, l/25**.

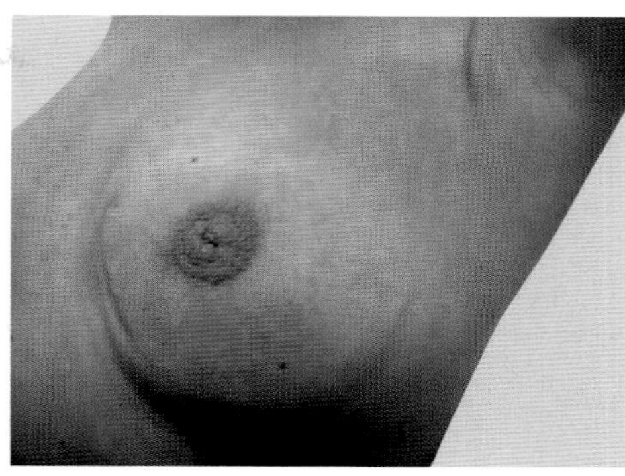

**e** *Physical examination* 2 months after surgical removal of the nodule reveals skin retraction and scarring in the former tumor bed with a small, firm nodule (**n/25**) and infra-areolar skin redness (**O–o/24**). Another scar is visible in the left axilla (**p/27**).

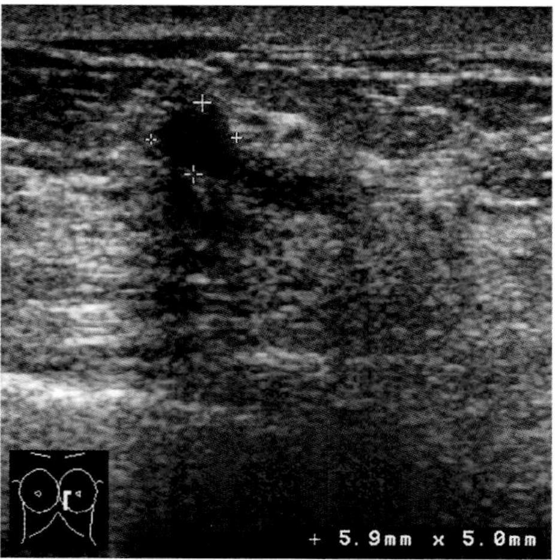


**f** *Sonogram of the left breast* (scar area) shows a smooth-walled lesion 6 mm in diameter with inhomogeneous posterior acoustic shadowing.

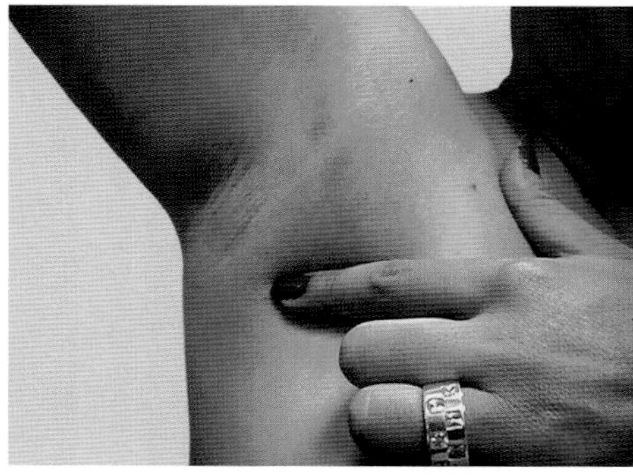

**g** *Clinical appearance* of the right axilla. The patient found a palpable lentil-sized nodule 2 months after surgery on the left breast.

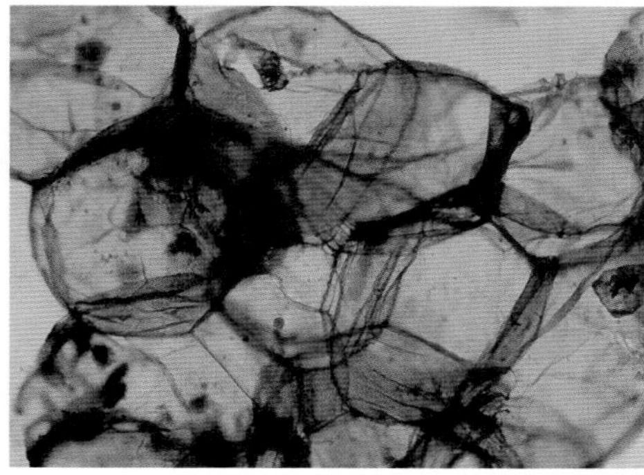

**h** *FNA aspirate* from the right axilla (20 × magnification) contains compact cell clusters that suggest the correct diagnosis.

**Question 1 on Fig. 5.141**

*How would you interpret these findings?*

(**a**) Fibroadenoma
(**b**) Cystosarcoma phylloides
(**c**) Cellular malignancy

→ **Answer on p. 391**

**Question 2 on Fig. 5.141**

*How would you interpret the findings in the left breast 2 months after completion of radiotherapy?*

(**a**) Local recurrence
(**b**) Seroma
(**c**) Oil cyst

→ **Answer on p. 391**

**Question 3 on Fig. 5.141**

*How would you interpret the nodule in the right axilla 2 months after completion of radiotherapy?*

(**a**) Small lymph node
(**b**) Distant metastasis
(**c**) Lipoma

→ **Answer on p. 391**

**Question 4 on Fig. 5.141**

*The patient refused chemotherapy. Is this justified based on the absence of axillary involvement?*

(**a**) Yes
(**b**) No
(**c**) Not relevant

→ **Answer on p. 391**

**Fig. 5.142 A 42-year-old woman presents for breast screening.** She has regular cycles and is currently in the *immediate premenstrual phase.* A subtle, cylindrical mass is noted above the left nipple at the 12-o'clock position. It is not associated with skin or nipple retraction (**a**). No mammographic abnormalities are seen (**b**). Ultrasound and MRI show an atypical change (**c, d**). Ultrasound-guided FNA and CNB are performed at the 12-o'clock position in the left breast.

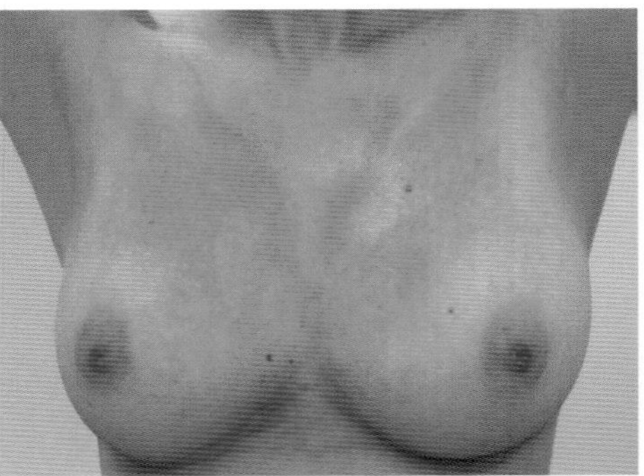

**a** *Clinical inspection* of both breasts with the arms raised shows no skin or nipple retraction.

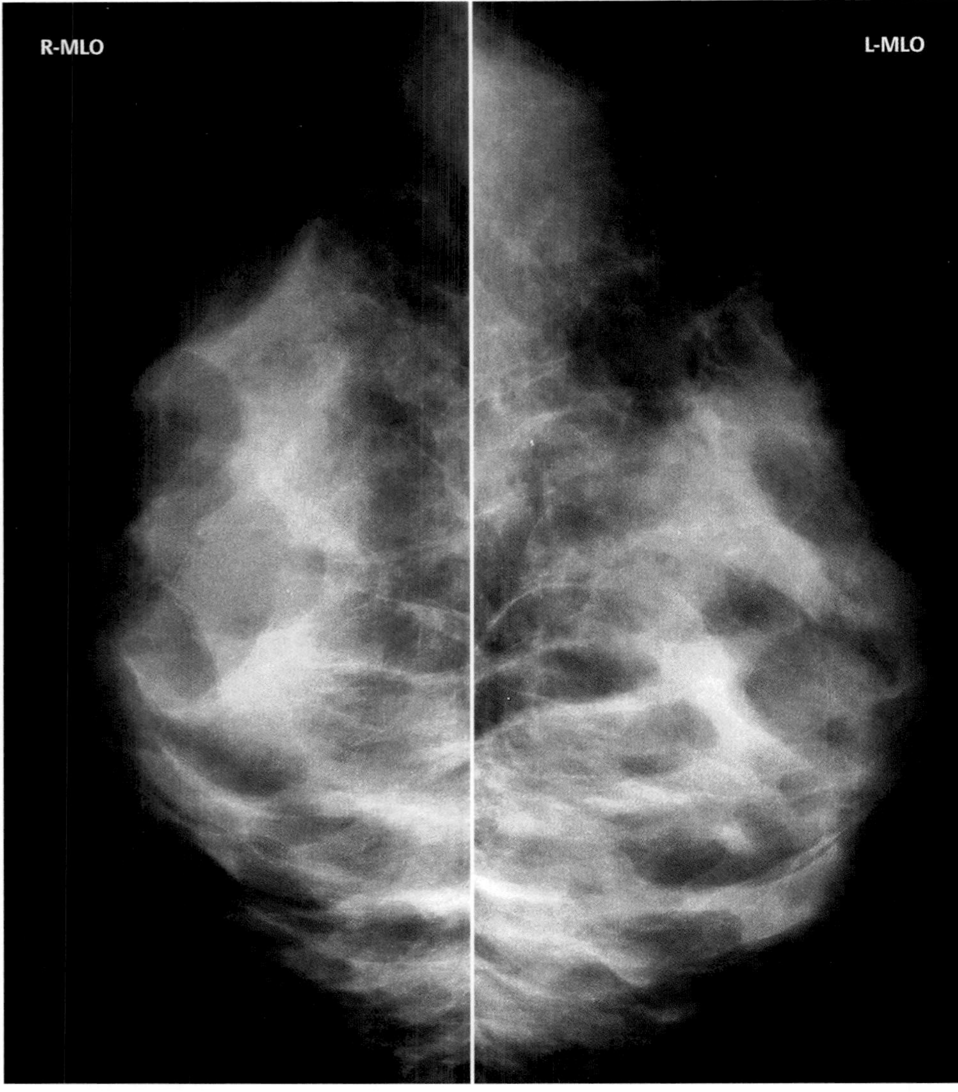


**b** *Bilateral oblique mammograms* show very radiodense breasts. The breasts are completely visualized at the level of the inframammary folds (ACR 3, BIRADS 1, PGMI).

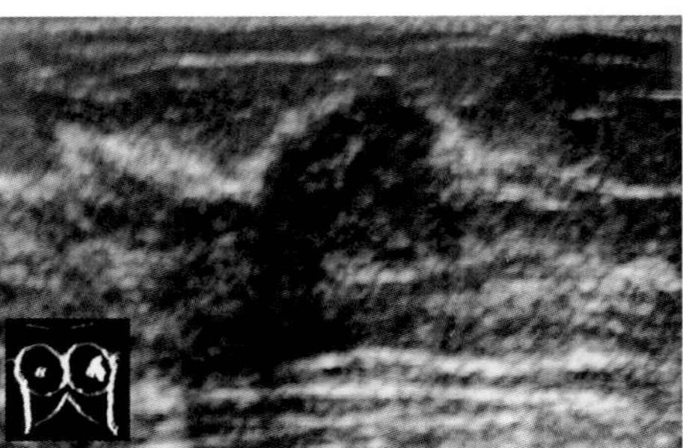

**c** *Sonogram* of the left breast shows a hypoechoic subcutaneous area at the end of two lobes with partial posterior shadowing in stroma-rich parenchyma.

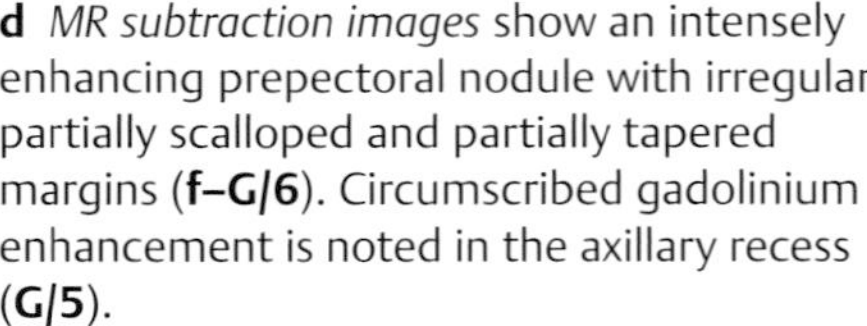

**d** *MR subtraction images* show an intensely enhancing prepectoral nodule with irregular, partially scalloped and partially tapered margins (**f–G/6**). Circumscribed gadolinium enhancement is noted in the axillary recess (**G/5**).

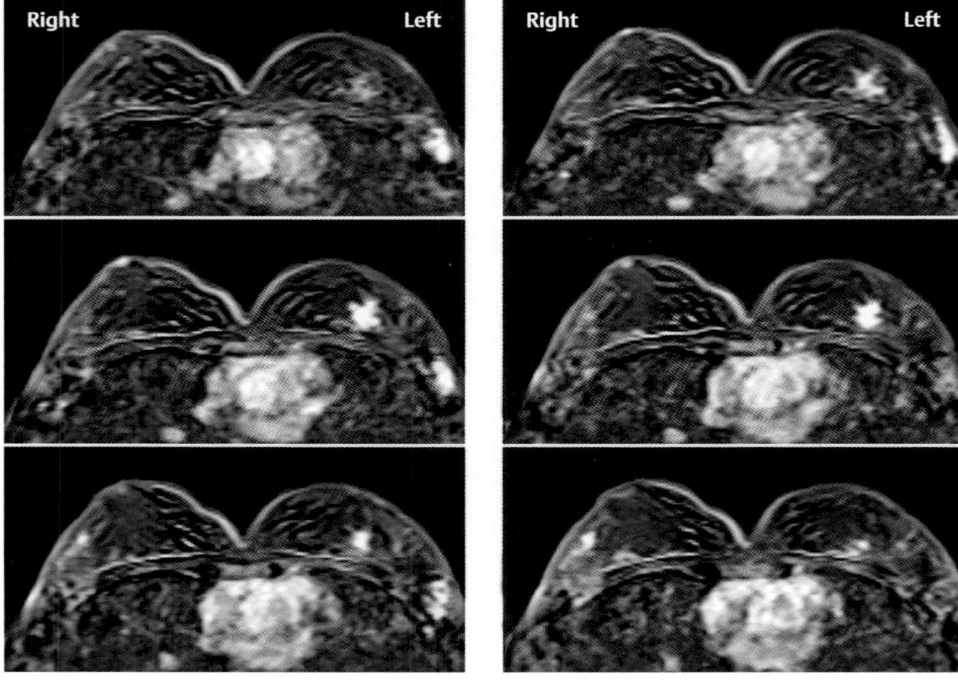

**Fig. 5.142** **A 42-year-old woman presents for breast screening.** *(continued)*

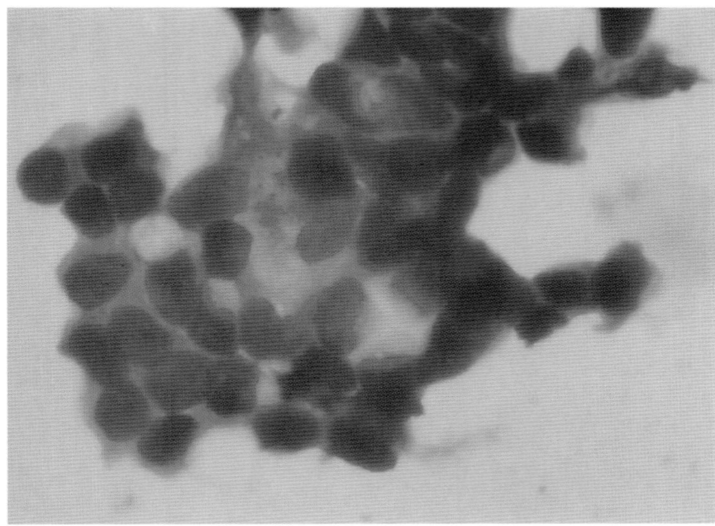

**e** *FNA cytology* shows scant cellular material. A fragment with slightly concave-convex borders contains small, dense, pleomorphic cells.

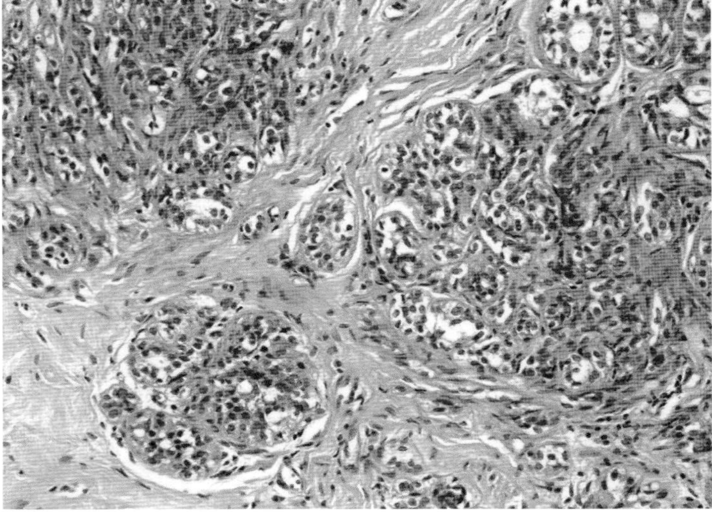

**f** *Histologic section* shows enlarged TDLUs (e.g., **R–t/22–26** and **p–q/21–23**) in stroma-rich surroundings with uniform epithelial cover layers and mild proliferative changes (image courtesy of Hans-Helmut Dahm, Esslingen).

**Question on Fig. 5.142**

*How would you interpret the finding in the left breast?*

(**a**) Sclerosing adenosis
(**b**) Invasive lobular carcinoma
(**c**) Cystosarcoma phylloides

→ **Answer on p. 392**

**Fig. 5.143** **A 39-year-old woman presents with an indeterminate mass in the upper outer quadrant of the left breast.** There is no associated skin or nipple retraction.

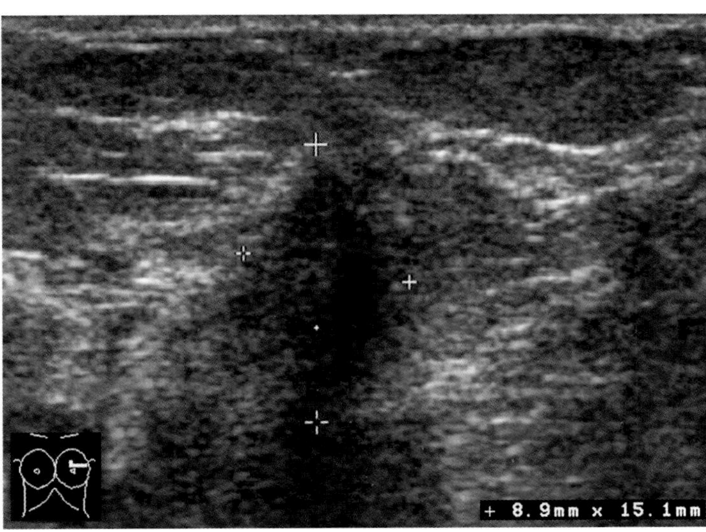


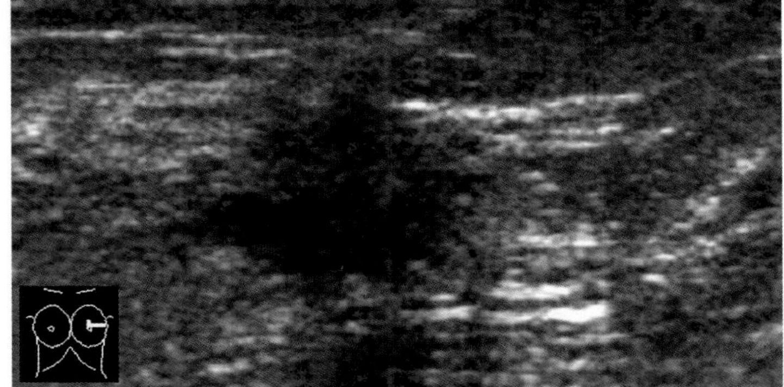

**a** *Sonograms* of the left breast show a hypoechoic 1.5 cm nodule with indistinct margins.

▶ **Fig. 5.143 b–d**

**Fig. 5.143** **A 39-year-old woman presents with an indeterminate mass in the upper outer quadrant of the left breast.** *(continued)*

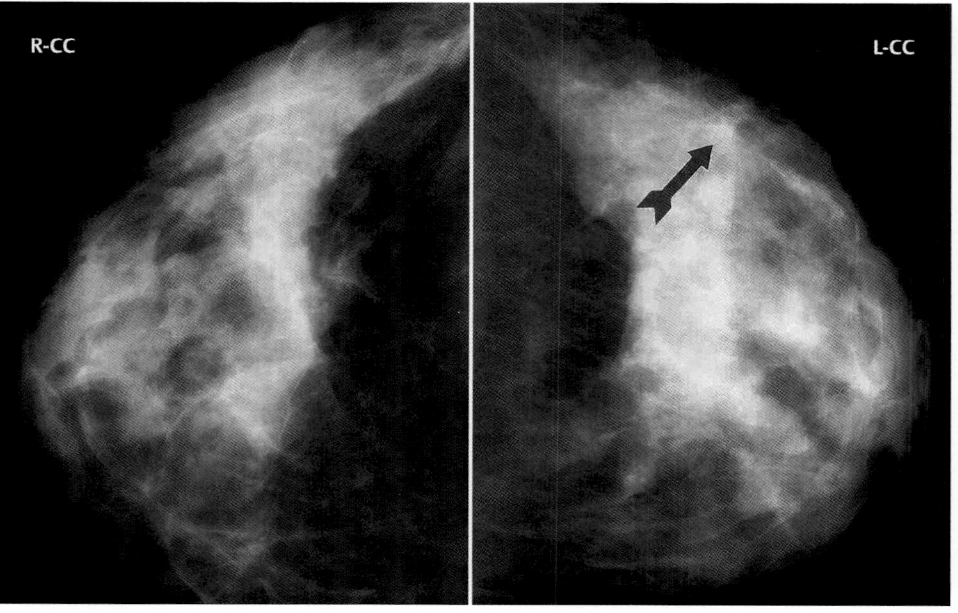


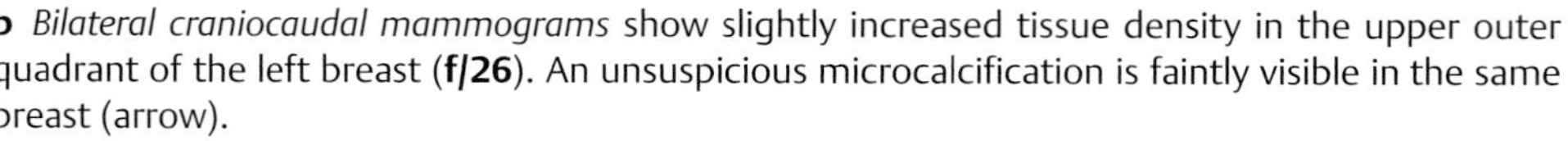

**b** *Bilateral craniocaudal mammograms* show slightly increased tissue density in the upper outer quadrant of the left breast (**f/26**). An unsuspicious microcalcification is faintly visible in the same breast (arrow).

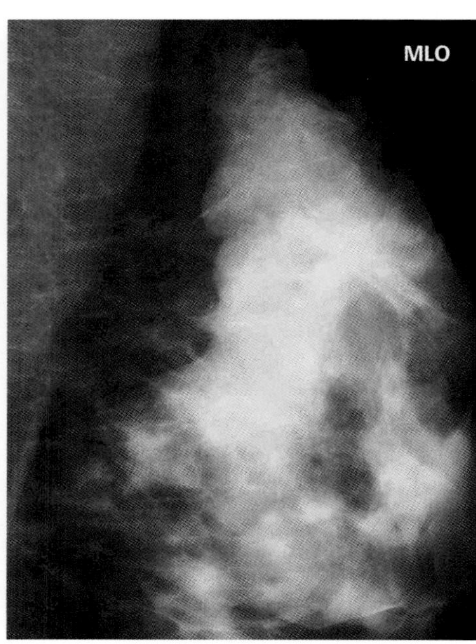


**c** *Oblique mammogram* of the left breast (magnified view). The parenchyma in the upper portion of the breast shows no abnormalities. There is subtle evidence of a stellate density at **i–j/24–25**.

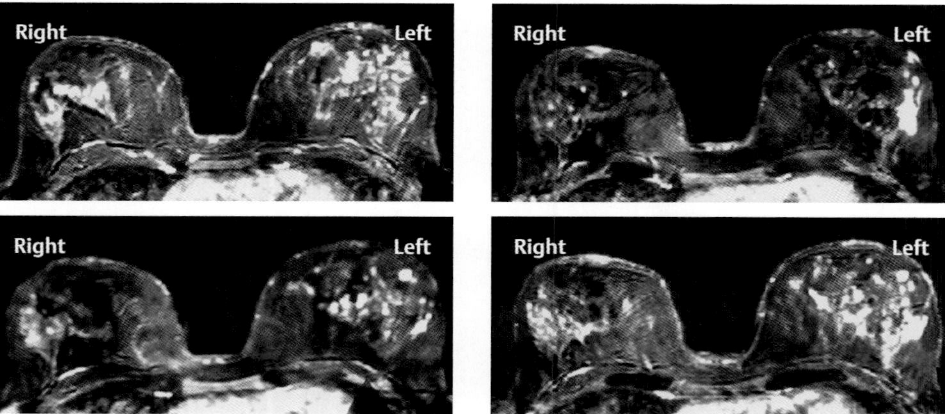


**d** *MR subtraction images* show intense gadolinium enhancements of the left breast nodule (**G/15–16**) and in the surrounding. Increased blood flow is noted throughout the left and the right breast.

**Question 1 on Fig. 5.143**

*How would you interpret these findings?*

(**a**) Fibroadenoma

(**b**) Carcinoma

→ **Answer on p. 392**

**Question 2 on Fig. 5.143**

*In the case of a fibroadenoma and carcinoma: Are other nodules present in the left breast?*

(**a**) Yes

(**b**) No

(**c**) Uncertain

→ **Answer on p. 392**

**Question 3 on Fig. 5.143**

*In the case of a carcinoma: Does it appear that breast-conserving surgery is an option?*

(**a**) Yes

(**b**) No

(**c**) Uncertain

→ **Answer on p. 392**

*(continued from p. 275)*

## Changes during Pregnancy and Lactation—A Special Diagnostic Challenge

A total of 2.8% of all breast cancers occur during pregnancy (Haen et al. 2003). There is no proof that pregnancy adversely affects the course of the disease, and terminating the pregnancy will not improve the cure rates. Pregnancy termination would be indicated only during the first trimester, when chemotherapy would likely produce a teratogenic effect (Haen et al. 2003).

The pregnant breast poses special diagnostic problems due to heavy lobular proliferation and the resultant increase in radiographic breast density (see p. 168). Firmness and nodularity are difficult to interpret in the pregnant breast, and diagnosis tends to be delayed because few pregnant women perform self-examination to detect or exclude breast cancer and are more interested in preparing themselves for the tasks of child care. This explains why pregnant women and young mothers may dismiss or fail to notice even relatively large breast nodules.

Breast changes during pregnancy should be investigated mainly by ultrasound combined with interventional procedures. FNA cytology is not recommended during pregnancy due to the high degree of cellular proliferation, which can mimic atypical changes and cause diagnostic errors. CNB for histologic evaluation is preferred. VB is not essential for the investigation of nodules but may be recommended for lesion removal following diagnostic confirmation by CNB.

Toward the end of pregnancy and especially during lactation, real-time ultrasound can demonstrate milk sloshing in the dilated lactiferous ducts. It is not stationary as in a pipe but is released from the peripheral TDLUs into the duct system mainly in response to the sucking action of the newborn. This phenomenon can be clearly observed with ultrasound during breastfeeding. In pregnant patients with congenital ductectasia, it is relatively common to find calcified secretions as well as prepartum and postpartum mastitis due to the obstruction of milk flow. Usually these conditions do not resolve with the cessation of lactation. "Cheese cysts" may develop from inspissated milk. Lactating adenomas persist even after the end of lactation and may raise problems of clinical and cytologic differential diagnosis due to the atypical appearance of the cells (see **Fig. 5.146f**, p. 287). Every nodule that persists after the cessation of breastfeeding should be investigated by CNB. Lactating adenomas may also occur outside of pregnancy and lactation (see **Fig. 5.136**, p. 271).

It is sometimes difficult to recognize inflammatory carcinoma, which is frequently confused with postpartum mastitis (see **Fig. 5.148**, p. 289). **Figures 5.144–5.148** pertain to pregnancy and lactation, in which the diagnosis relies mainly on clinical findings.

*(continued on p. 291)*

**Fig. 5.144 A 42-year-old woman is still lactating 4 months postpartum.** A week before she suddenly noticed a tense, 4 cm nodule deep to the right nipple measuring 5 cm × 6 cm × 6 cm (**a**). She has no skin or nipple retraction.

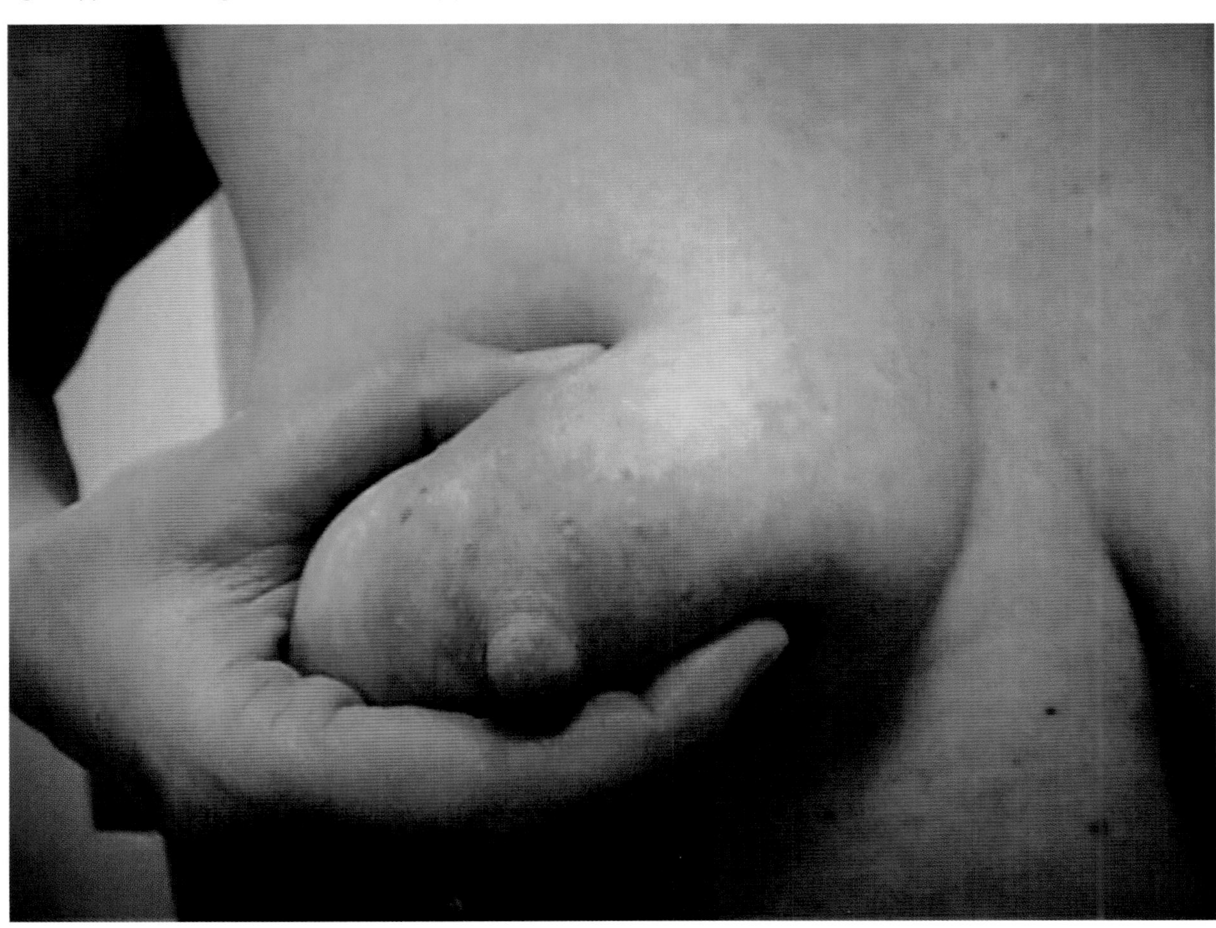

**a** *Clinical examination:* A large, fairly mobile nodule is palpable deep to the right nipple. Pressure on the nodule does not elicit discharge.

▶ **Fig. 5.144 b–e**

**Fig. 5.144** **A 42-year-old woman is still lactating 4 months postpartum.** *(continued)*

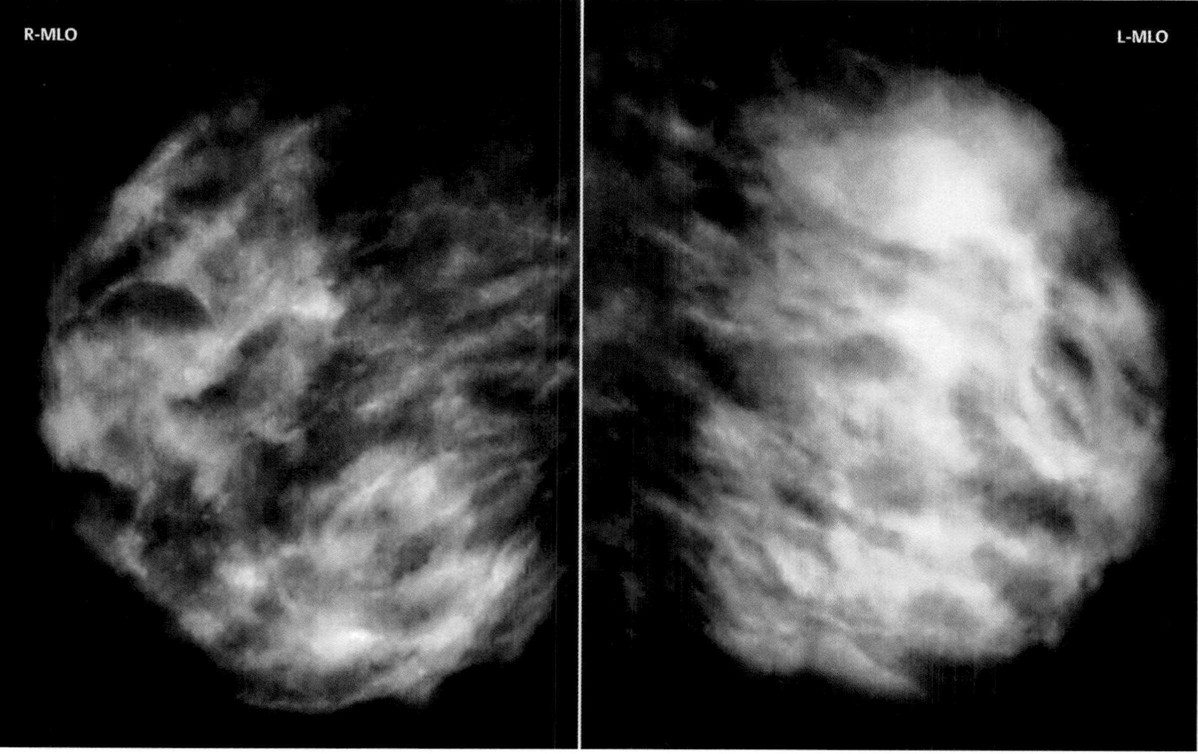


**b** *Bilateral oblique mammograms* show very radiodense breasts, especially on the left side, consistent with lactation (ACR 3, BIRADS 1, **P**GMI).

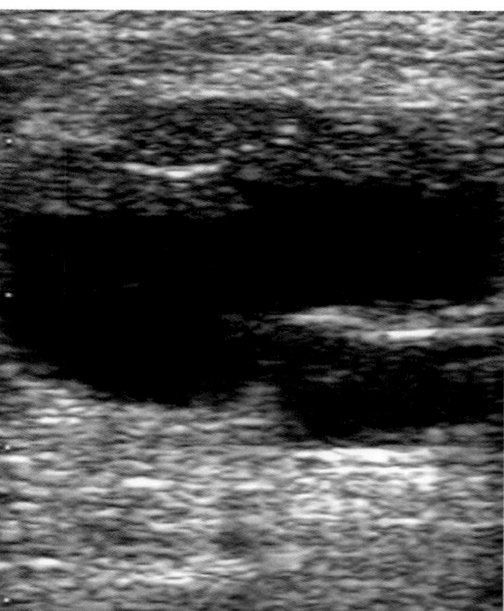

**c** *Retroareolar sonogram* of the right breast shows a large hypoechoic nodule bounded above by a slightly more echogenic layer. The nodule has relatively smooth internal margins.

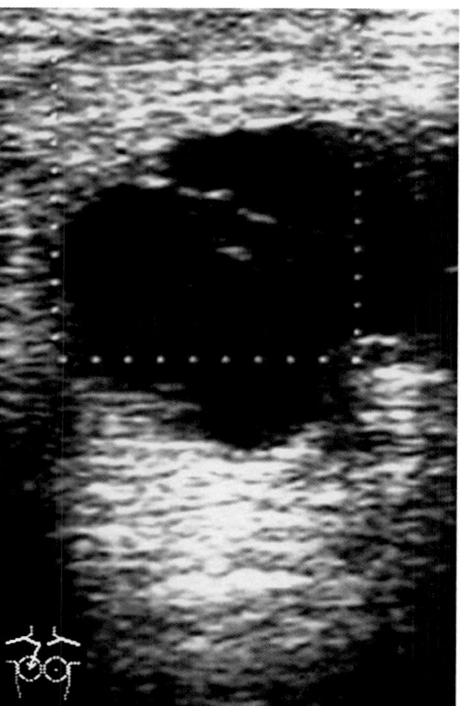

**d** *Sonogram* of the right breast (different plane) shows an echo-free nodule with smooth margins and strong posterior acoustic enhancement.

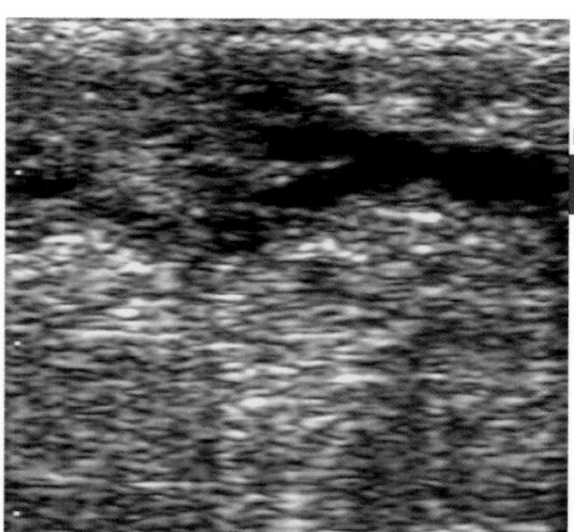


**e** *Retroareolar sonogram* of the left breast shows dilated ducts consistent with lactation (nipple on the right!).

**Question 1 on Fig. 5.144**

*How would you interpret the nodule in the right breast?*

(**a**) Galactocele
(**b**) Simple cyst
(**c**) Medullary carcinoma

→ **Answer on p. 392**

**Question 2 on Fig. 5.144**

*What caused the layer above the hypoechoic nodule at **A–D/15** in **c**?*

(**a**) Cellular proliferation on the galactocele wall
(**b**) “Cheesy” exudate due to stagnated milk flow
(**c**) Artifact due to indentation of the galactocele roof

→ **Answer on p. 392**

**Fig. 5.145** **A 32-year-old woman in her 27th week of pregnancy presents with patchy skin redness and moderate edematous induration of gradual onset affecting the lower half of the left breast (a).** There is no nodularity or regional lymph node enlargement.

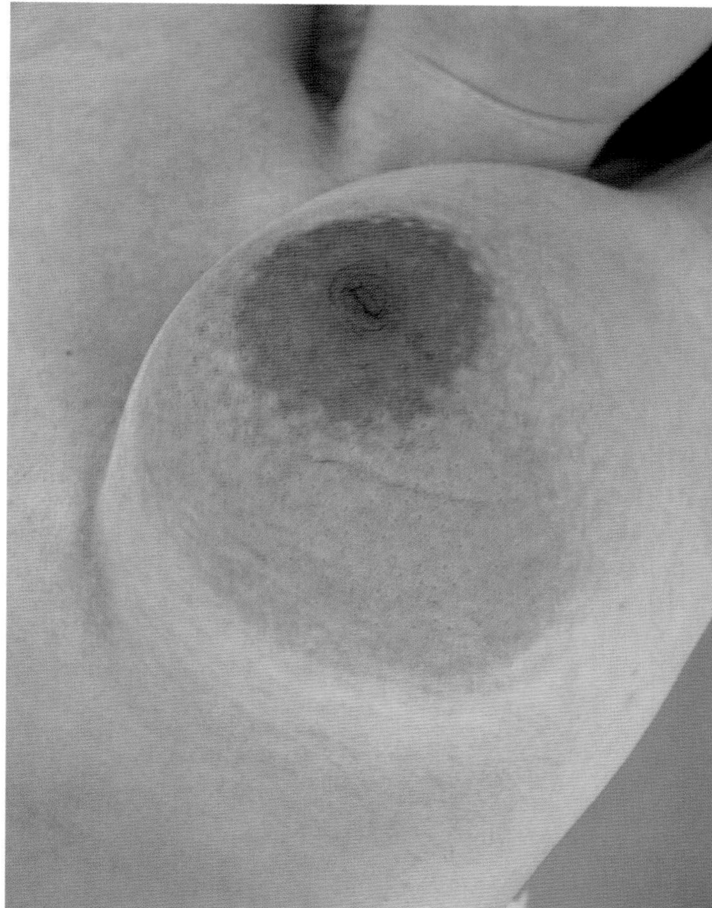

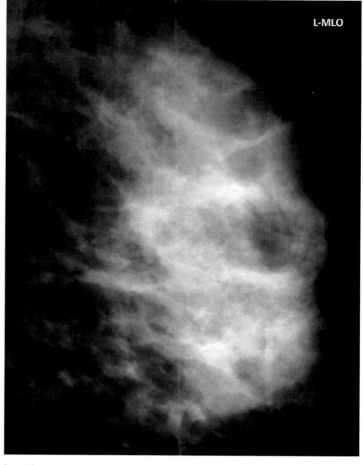

**a** *Clinical inspection*: The left breast viewed from below (with arms crossed behind the neck, above). Inspection reveals a sharply demarcated area of reddish-purple skin discoloration with no nipple irritation and bilateral nipple inversion. There is no orange-peel dimpling of the skin.

L-MLO

**b** *Oblique mammogram* of the left breast shows radiodense breast parenchyma consistent with the 27th week of pregnancy (ACR 3, BIRADS 1, **P**GMI).

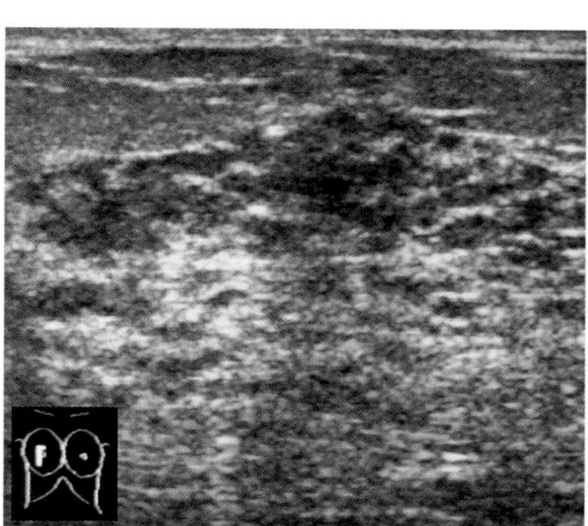

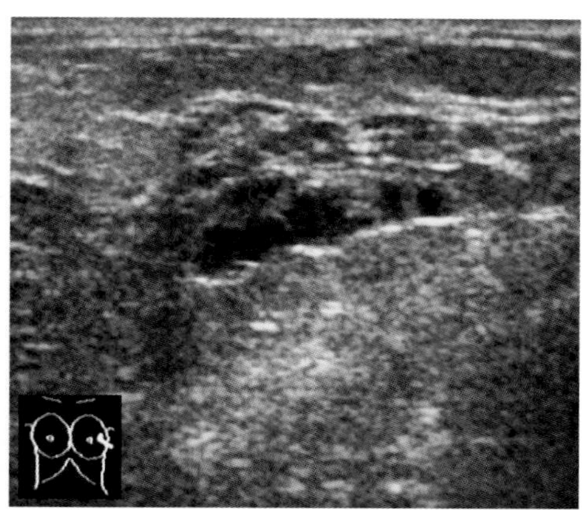

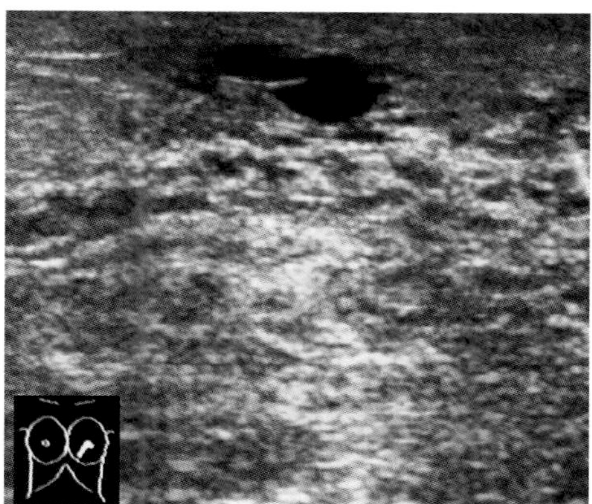

**c** *Sonograms* of the right and left breast show proliferating TDLUs and ductectasia (compare with **Fig. 5.144 e**). There is no evidence of circumscribed disease in the erythematous area and no edematous thickening of the skin.

▶ **Fig. 5.145 d**

**Fig. 5.145 A 32-year-old woman in her 27th week of pregnancy.** *(continued)*

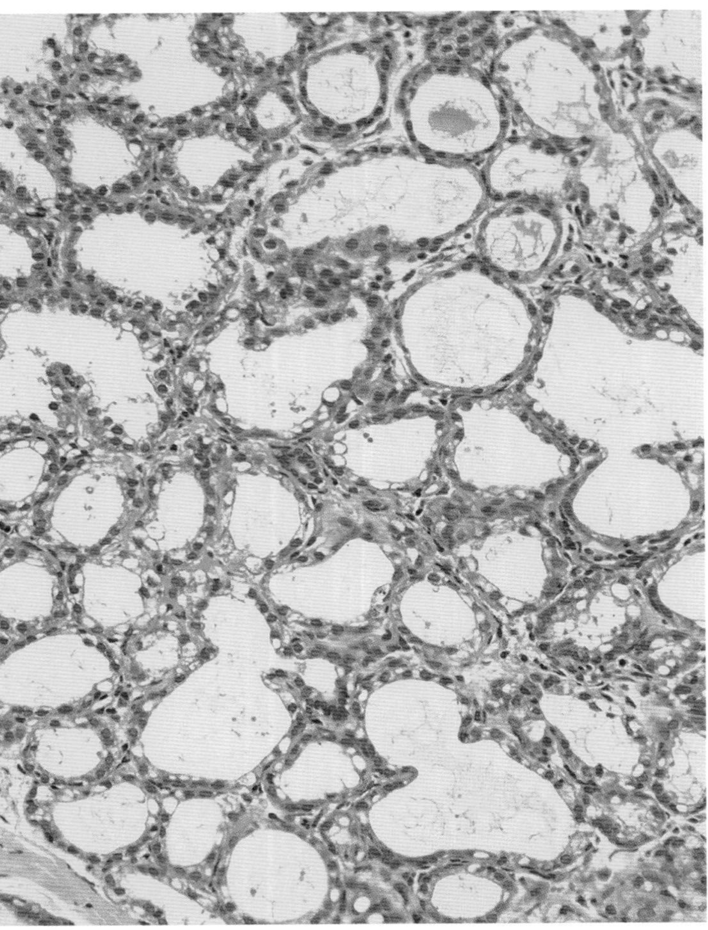

**d** *Histologic section* from a "blind" core-needle core biopsy of infra-areolar glandular tissue during pregnancy. There are interspersed areas in which the lobules show generally increased density and the ducts are greatly increased in number. The acini have large lumina and are lined by secretory epithelium with broad, vacuolated cytoplasm. The ducts contain inspissated secretions. A few lobules are atrophic. The interstitium is loosely infiltrated by lymphocytes. There is no appreciable cellular atypia.

**Question 1 on Fig. 5.145**

*Why was the left breast radiographed in only one plane?*

(**a**) To exclude microcalcifications
(**b**) To decrease radiation exposure
(**c**) To reduce costs
(**d**) All of the above

→ **Answer on p. 393**

**Question 2 on Fig. 5.145**

*What is the cause of the skin redness?*

(**a**) Lactating lobular hyperplasia with an associated inflammatory reaction (lactation nodule)
(**b**) Invasive lobular carcinoma
(**c**) Comedocarcinoma

→ **Answer on p. 393**

**Fig. 5.146 A 32-year-old woman presents with postpartum nodularity in the infra-areolar portion of the right breast.** Two FNAs yield atypical cells (**f**). She has no family history of breast cancer.

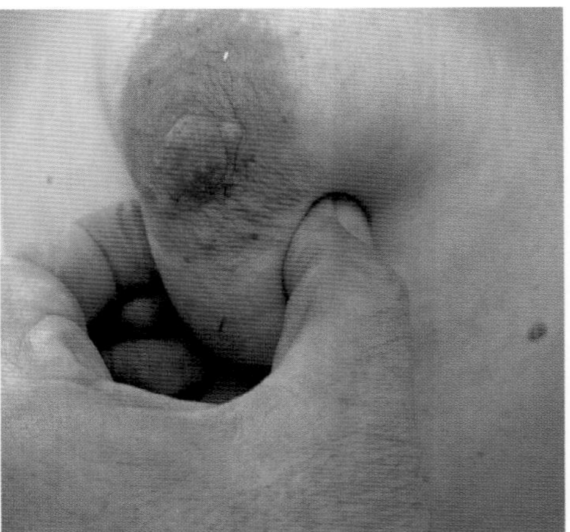

**a** *Physical examination* reveals a freely movable infra-areolar nodule approximately 2 cm in diameter. Pressure on the nodule does not elicit milky discharge.

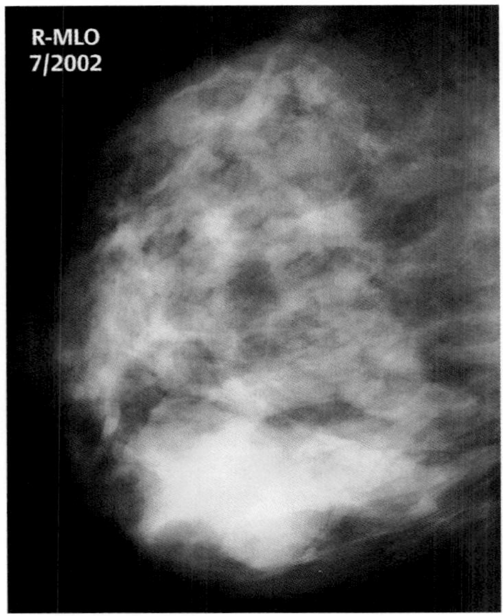


**b** *Oblique mammogram* of the right breast in July, 2002 shows a radiodense breast with a patchy structure and a large, relatively well-circumscribed elliptical opacity measuring 3.5 cm × 2.5 cm that does not contain microcalcifications (**E–G/6–7**) (ACR 2, BIRADS 2, P**G**MI).

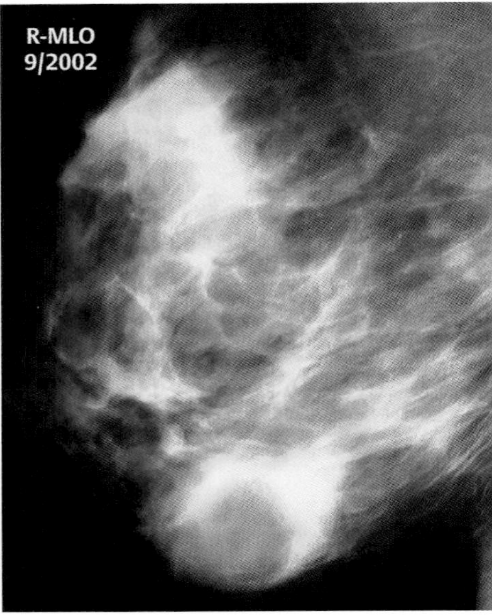


**c** *Oblique mammogram* of the right breast in September, 2002. The nodule has become smaller since the previous mammogram (**h–i/5–7**), and its margins have become more irregular. The glandular tissue is still relatively radiodense. The parenchyma is not completely imaged at the level of the inframammary fold (ACR 2, BIRADS 3, PG**MI**).

**Fig. 5.146** **A 32-year-old woman presents with postpartum nodularity in the infra-areolar portion of the right breast.** *(continued)*

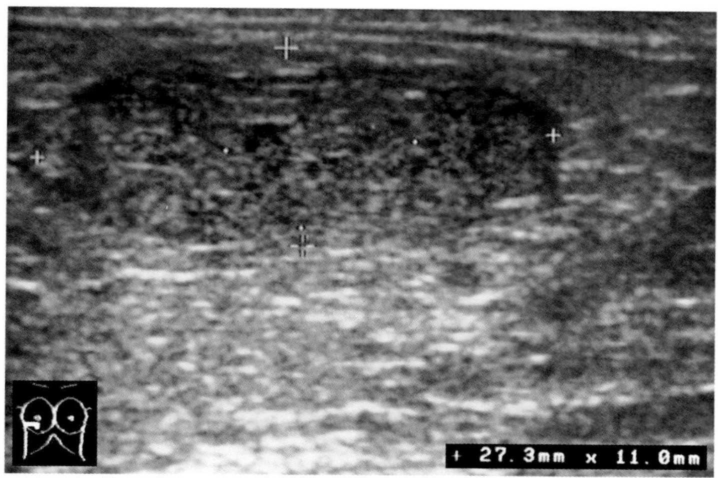


**d** *Sonogram* in July, 2002 shows a 27 mm × 11 mm hyperechoic nodule with smooth margins. The nodule resembles the normal breast parenchyma with proliferating TDLUs (isoechoic).

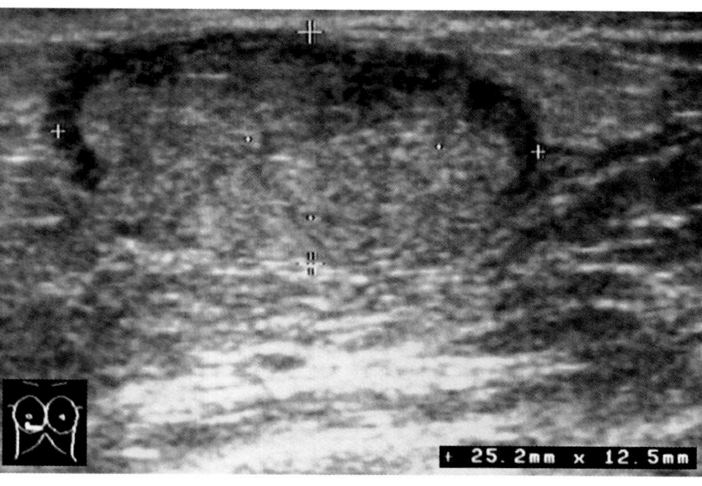


**e** *Sonogram* in September, 2002. Two months later the nodule has become slightly smaller (25 mm × 12 mm). It is lobulated and surrounded by a hypoechoic zone. It appears to be fused to a pseudocapsule at its base.

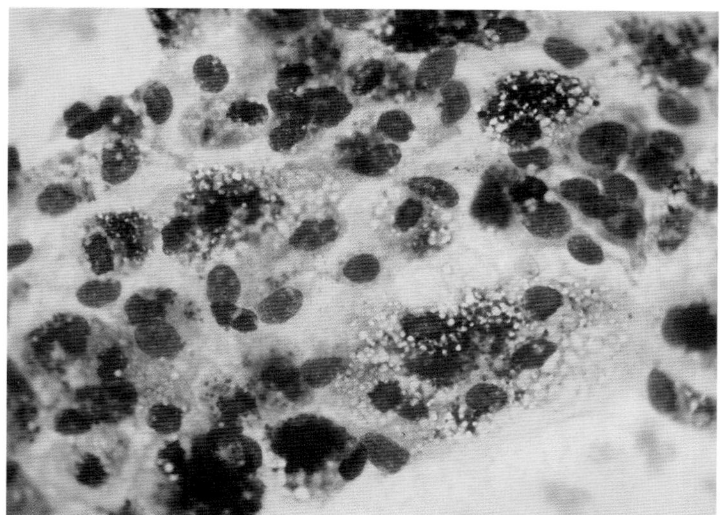

**f** *FNA cytology* of the nodule shows disseminated, elliptical pleomorphic cells interspersed among numerous siderin-laden foam cells. No prominent nucleoli are seen.

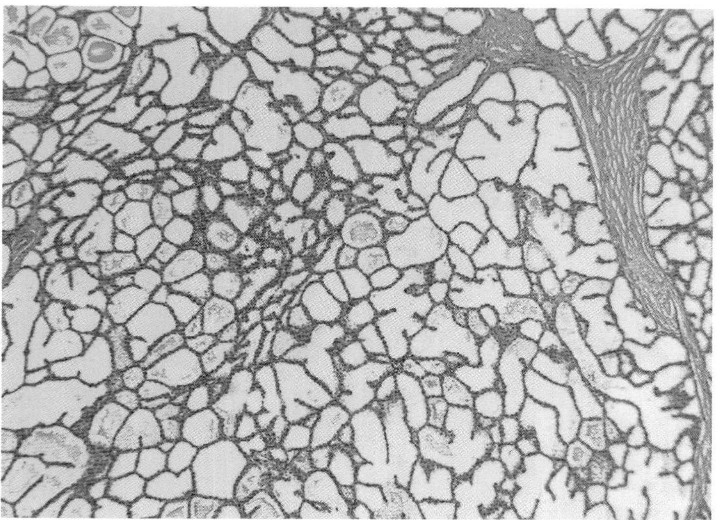

**g** *Histologic section* shows a hypertrophic lobule with greatly enlarged acini lined by lactating epithelium. The nuclei show a partly apical and partly basal distribution and are slightly pleomorphic. Fiber-rich connective tissue is present in a few areas and is loosely infiltrated by lymphoplasmocytes and granulocytes enclosing nests of foam cells (image courtesy of Hans-Helmut Dahm, Esslingen).

**Question on Fig. 5.146**

*How would you interpret the nodule?*

(**a**) Medullary carcinoma

(**b**) Lactating adenoma

(**c**) Intracystic ductal papilloma

→ **Answer on p. 393**

**Fig. 5.147 A 39-year-old woman underwent a previous tumorectomy in the third trimester of pregnancy.** Swelling and edema persisted in the right breast after the cessation of lactation. Ultrasound and MRI now show indeterminate changes. Mammographic findings are also equivocal.

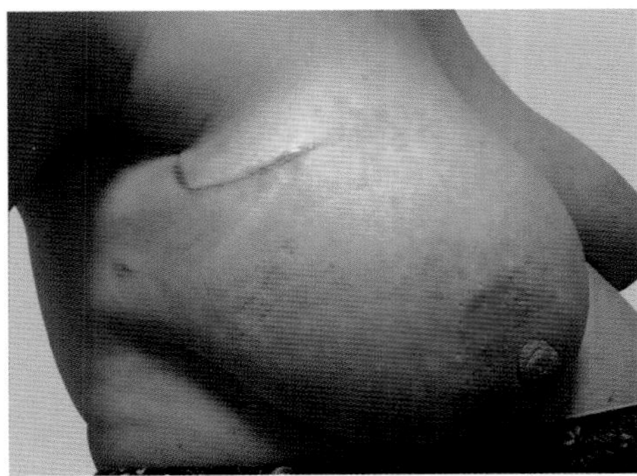

**a** *Clinical inspection* of the right breast shows postpartum swelling and incipient orange-peel dimpling of the skin. A freshly healed lumpectomy scar is visible in the upper outer quadrant.

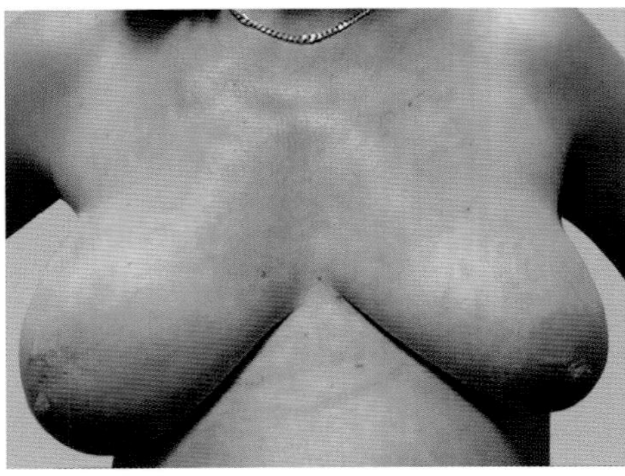

**b** *Bilateral inspection* shows enlargement, swelling, and redness of the right breast with no nipple retraction. Status 2 months after a right-sided tumorectomy.

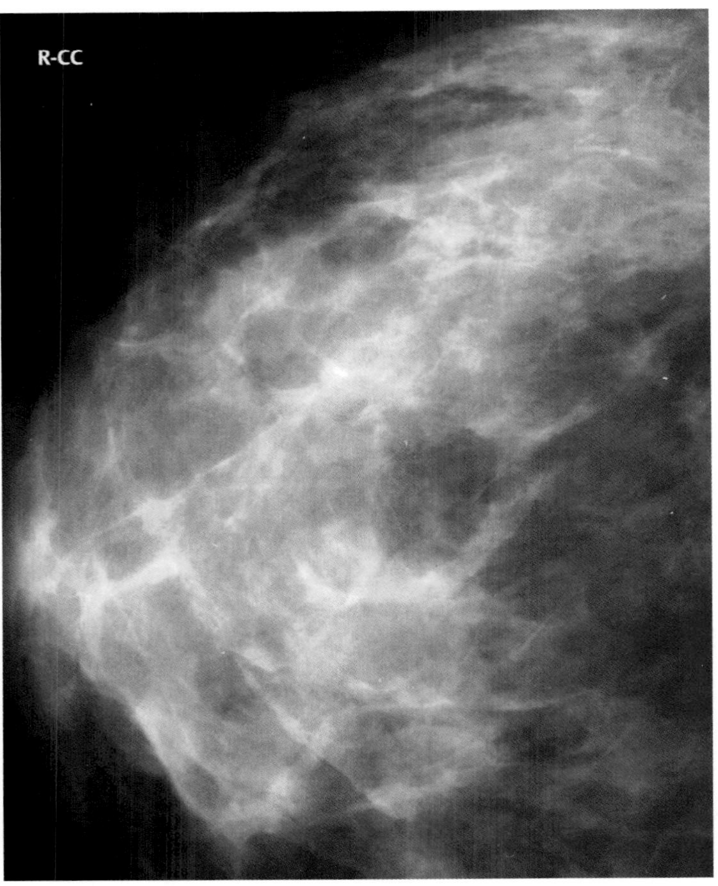


**c** *Craniocaudal mammogram* of the right breast shows radiodense parenchyma with nonspecific opacities (ACR 3, BIRADS?, P**G**MI).

**Question on Fig. 5.147**

*Do the findings indicate a tumor recurrence in the right breast, or are they more indicative of postpartum and postoperative changes with lymphedema?*

(**a**) Tumor recurrence
(**b**) Postoperative changes
(**c**) Uncertain

→ **Answer on p. 393**

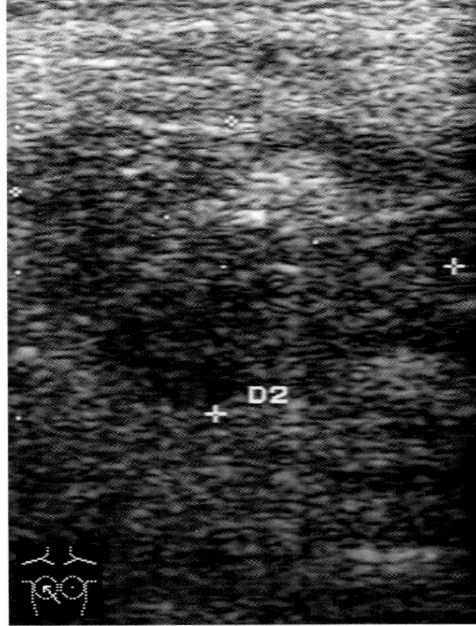


**d** *Sonogram* of the right breast shows postoperative changes with a 3 cm hypoechoic area at the former tumor site (see marker). Diffusely distributed mini-echoes are a result of lymphatic obstruction (so called "salt and pepper"-pattern, see also **Fig. 5.58 d**, p. 368).

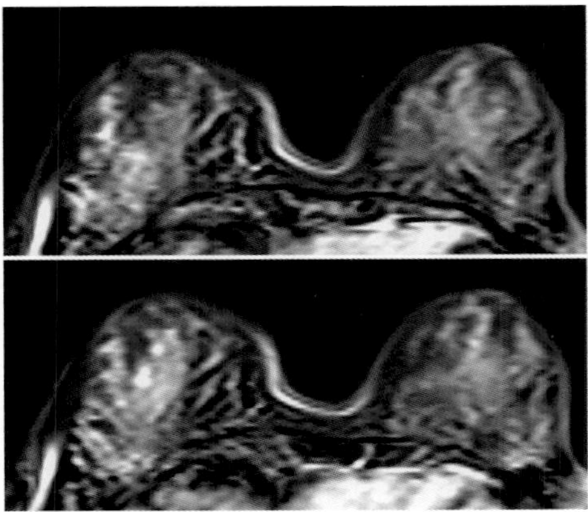

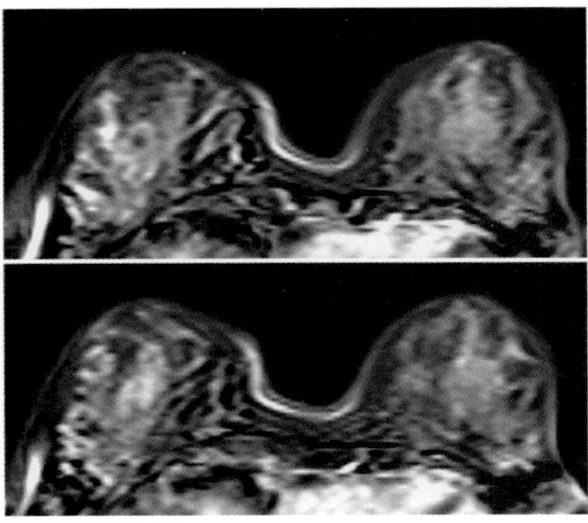

**e** *MR subtraction images* show markedly increased vascularity in both breasts, especially on the right side, with no focal or nodular gadolinium enhancement.

**Fig. 5.148 A 34-year-old woman delivered a child in December, 1998, and nursed until June, 1999.** She first noticed swelling and redness of her left breast in September, 1999. She was assumed to have postpartum mastitis, and the changes responded well to treatment with a prolactin inhibitor. At first the patient was reluctant to have mammograms (radiation concerns), but later she consented so that a malignant process could be excluded (**c**). Ultrasound shows nonspecific hypoechoic areas, especially in the upper portion of the left breast (**e**). MRI shows intense, streaky enhancement in the upper outer quadrant of the left breast (**f**). Puerperal mastitis? Inflammatory neoplasm? Galactostasis?

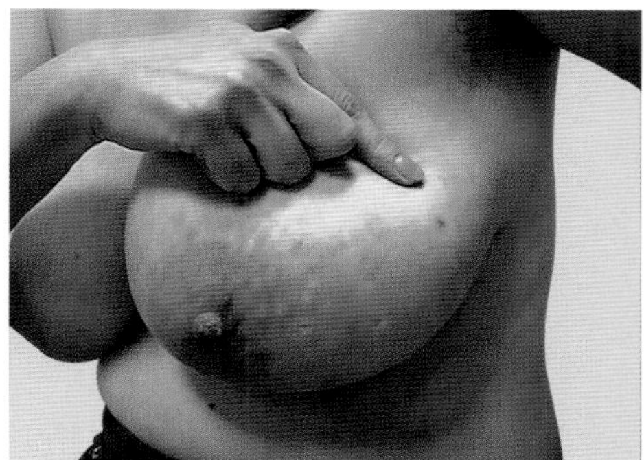

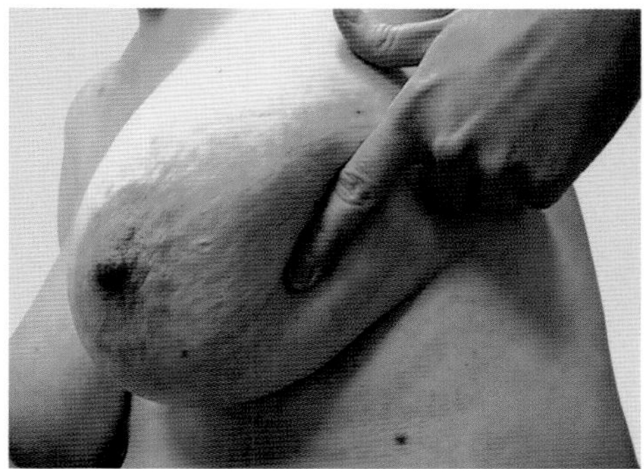

**a, b** *Clinical appearance* of the left breast in October, 1999. Nonspecific masses are present at the 2 and 4-o'clock positions. The left breast is swollen and shows incipient orange-peel dimpling with no skin redness.

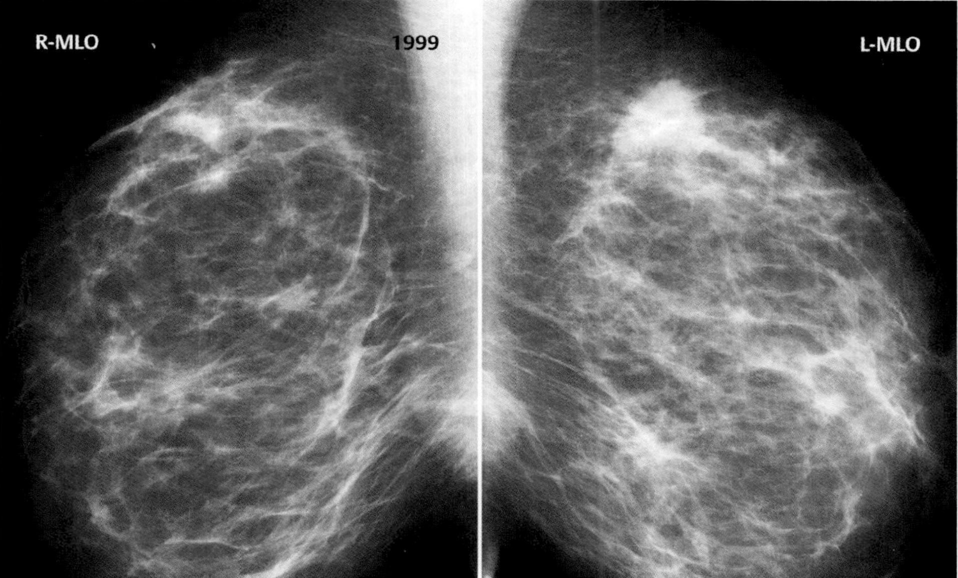


**c** *Bilateral oblique mammograms* in October, 1999 show increased reticular markings in the left breast with two atypical densities in the upper portion (**r/24**) and lower portion of the breast (**R–r/19**) (ACR 2, BIRADS 4, P**G**MI).

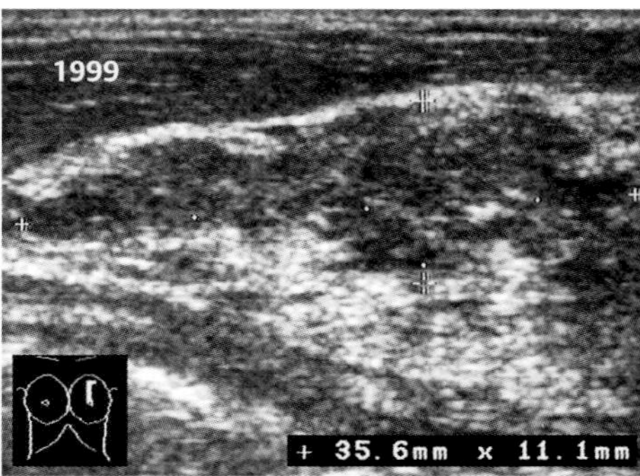


**e** *Sonogram* of the left breast shows a hypoechoic zone with irregular margins.

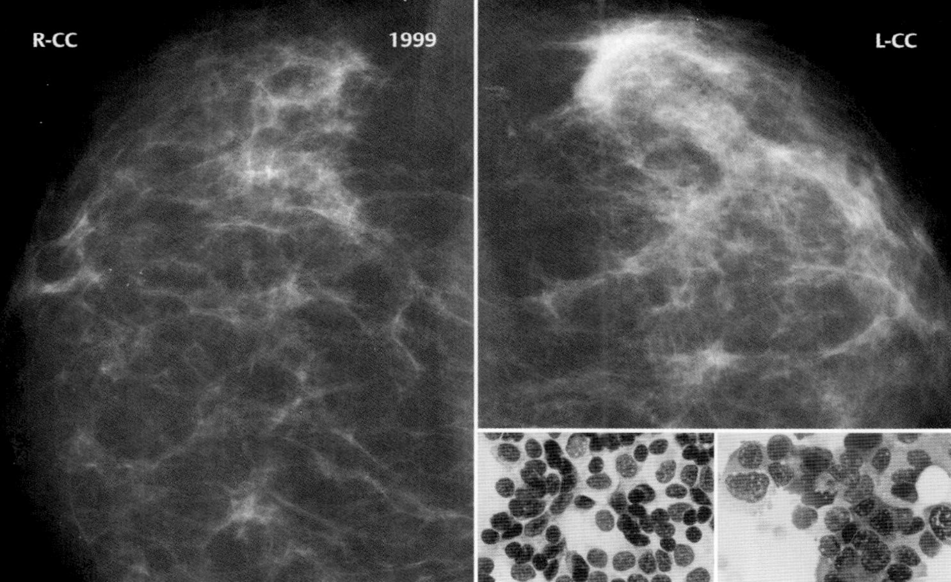


**d** *Bilateral craniocaudal mammograms* show increased reticular markings in the outer quadrants of the left breast. Nonspecific areas of increased parenchymal density are noted in the outer portion of the left breast (**R–S/13–14** cc; **R–S/24** oblique) (ACR 2, BIRADS 3, **P**GMI). Fine-needle aspiration of the upper outer quadrant (lower right corner of image) yielded multiple dissociated cells in which the nuclear-cytoplasmic ratio was shifted in favor of the nuclei.

▶ **Fig. 5.148f**

**Fig. 5.148** **A 34-year-old woman delivered a child in December, 1998, and nursed until June, 1999.** *(continued)*

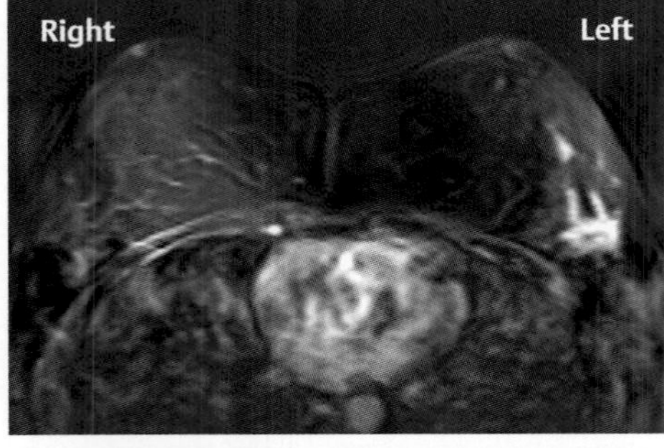


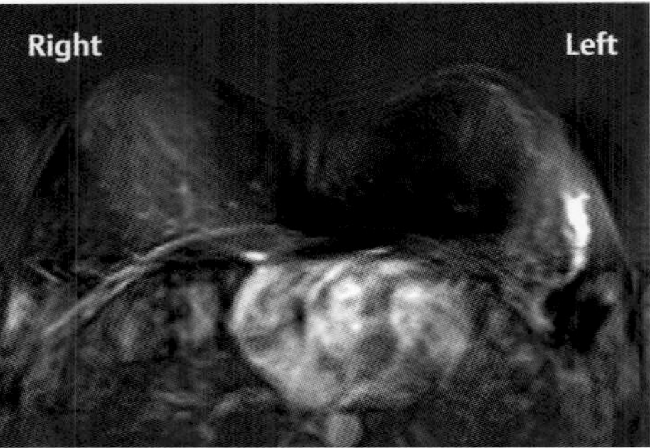


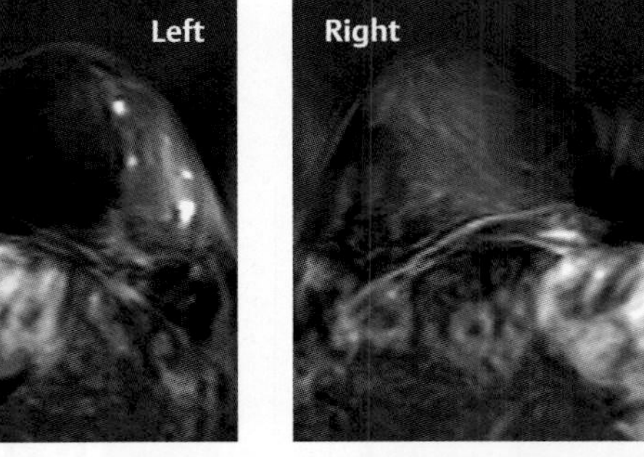


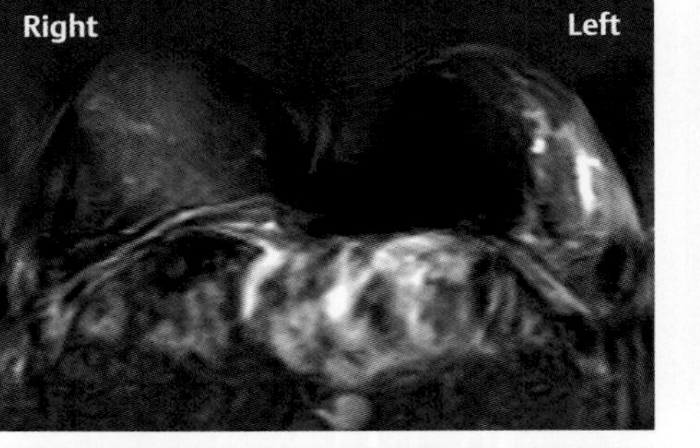


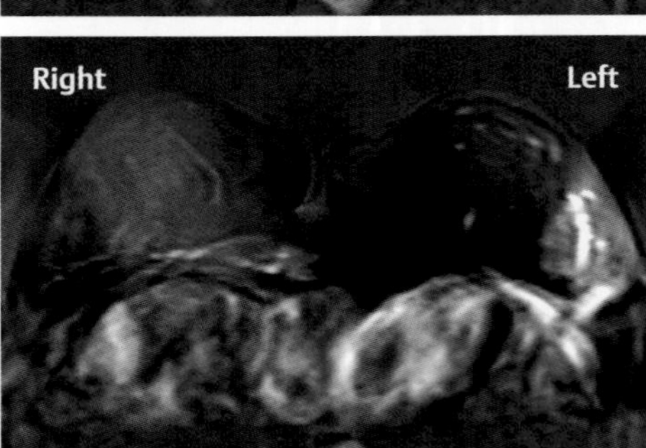


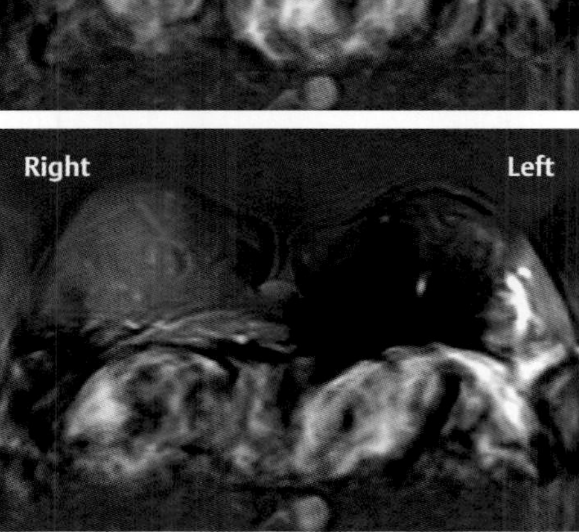


**f** *MR subtraction images* from June 1999 show intense multifocal gadolinium enhancements in the lateral portion of the left breast (p.e. **c/21**) explaining the reticular markings in the mammogramm of the left breast (image sequence from upper left to bottom right).

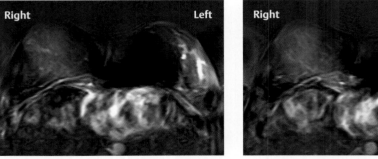

**Question on Fig. 5.148**

*How would you interpret the changes in the left breast?*

(**a**) Galactostasis
(**b**) Postpartum mastitis
(**c**) Inflammatory carcinoma

→ **Answer on p. 394**

(continued from p. 283)

## The Male Breast

### Gynecomastia

The most common disorder of the male breast is gynecomastia, which is caused by a relative predominance of the female sex hormone estrogen and is variable in its extent but usually affects both breasts. The proliferation of connective tissue, ducts, and fat in one or both breasts may cause the glandular tissue to grow from a bean-sized mass to a fully developed mammary gland. Clinical presentation, imaging techniques (**Fig. 5.149**), diagnosis, and interventional procedures are basically the same as in females. The development of gynecomastia is illustrated in **Fig. 5.150**.

(continued on p. 294)

**Fig. 5.149 Imaging and cytologic evaluation of the male breast.** A 23-year-old man presents with a painful retroareolar nodule in the right breast, which has been present for several weeks (**b**). He has a positive family history of breast cancer (mother and maternal grandmother).

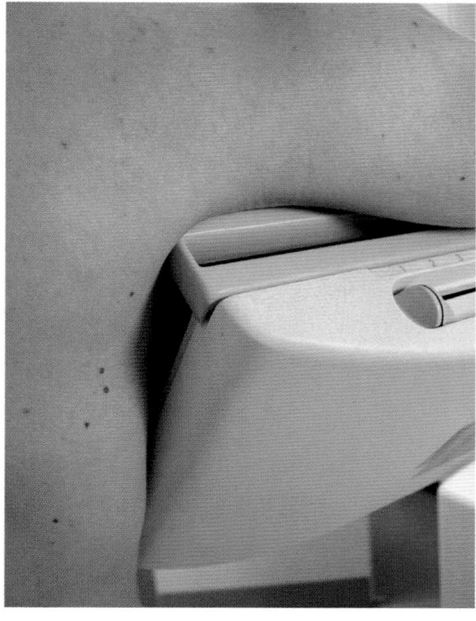

**a** For an *oblique mammogram*, the film holder is positioned at a 45–60° angle behind the posterior axillary fold.

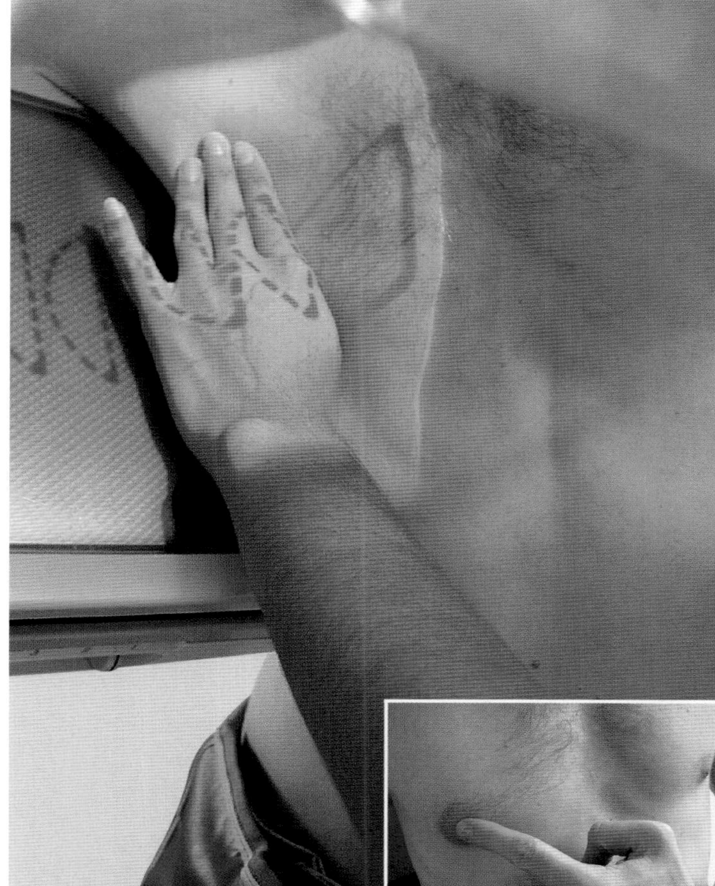

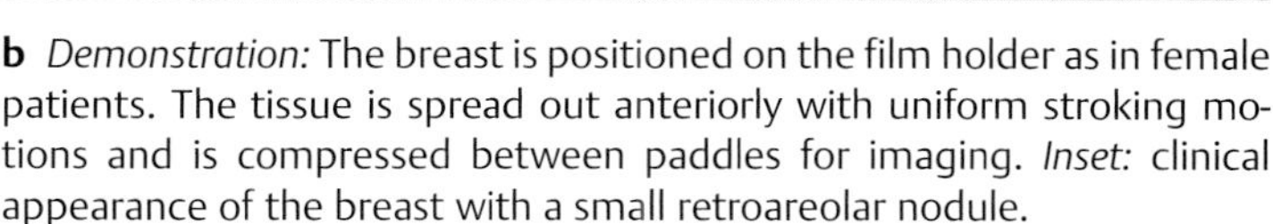

**b** *Demonstration:* The breast is positioned on the film holder as in female patients. The tissue is spread out anteriorly with uniform stroking motions and is compressed between paddles for imaging. *Inset:* clinical appearance of the breast with a small retroareolar nodule.

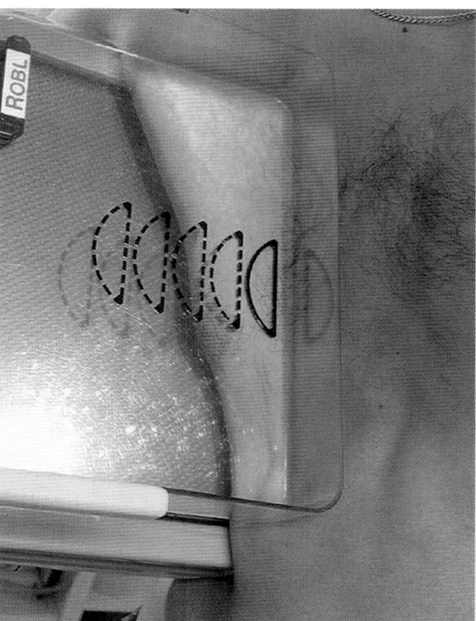


**c** *Demonstration:* The breast is correctly positioned between the compression paddles and film holder, affording a tangential view of the nipple. This projection covers the axillary recess to a level below the humeral head, and the exposure chamber is projected onto the retroareolar region. The craniocaudal view is also exposed as described for female patients.

▶ Fig. 5.149 d–f

**Fig. 5.149 Imaging and cytologic evaluation of the male breast.** *(continued)*

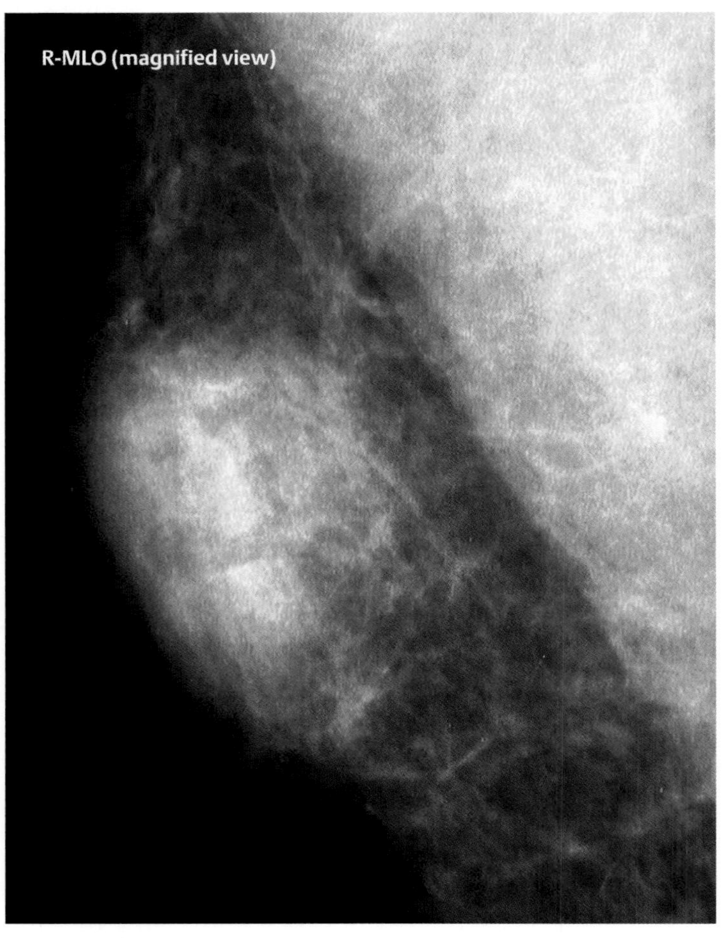


**d** *Oblique mammogram* of the right breast shows an inhomogeneous nodule with ill-defined posterior margins and no calcifications. The pectoral muscle is clearly visualized (ACR 2, BIRADS?, **P**GMI).

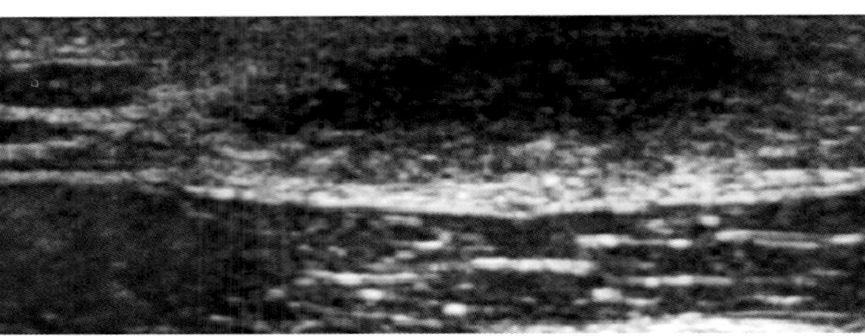

**e** *Ultrasound* shows an elliptical, subcutaneous, hypoechoic nodule with smooth margins, a homogeneous internal echo pattern, and slight posterior acoustic enhancement.

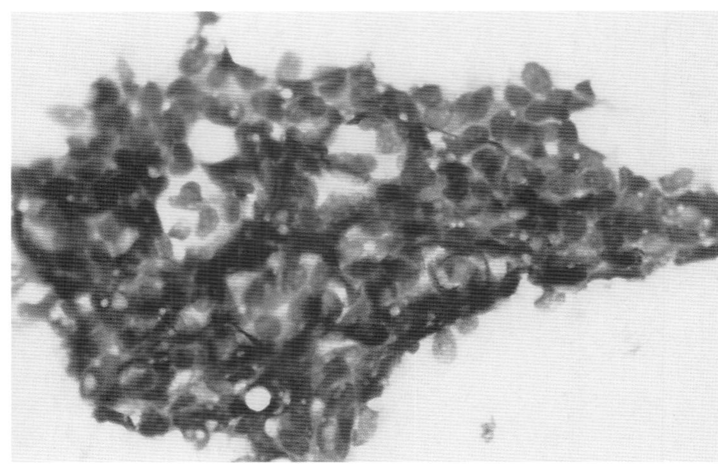

**f** *FNA cytology* shows a compact aggregate of cells with a smooth, concave border and multiple small, crowded glandular cells, most with elliptical nuclei that show some degenerative features.

**Question 1 on Fig. 5.149**

*Is genetic disposition also an important factor in males?*

(**a**) Yes
(**b**) No
(**c**) Unknown

→ **Answer on p. 394**

**Question 2 on Fig. 5.149**

*How would you interpret the retroareolar nodule?*

(**a**) Carcinoma
(**b**) Gynecomastia
(**c**) Ductal papilloma

→ **Answer on p. 395**

**Fig. 5.150** **A 57-year-old man.** For years the patient has taken the diuretic Dehydrosanol-Tri and diclofenac for knee pain and swelling. In 1998 he underwent a left subcutaneous mastectomy for a 2.5 cm nodule (**b**). At that time he also had slight swelling and firmness in the right breast (**a**). A right subcutaneous mastectomy was performed in 2000 for a 3.5 cm tender nodule. Radiographs in 2001 show new retroareolar densities on both sides. Recurrence of gynecomastia? Scars? Carcinoma?

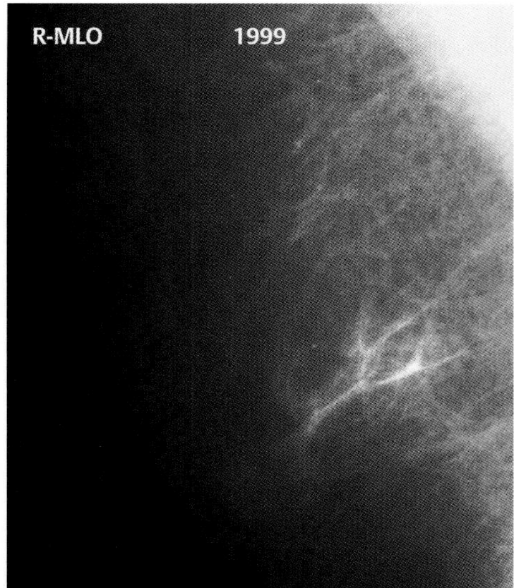


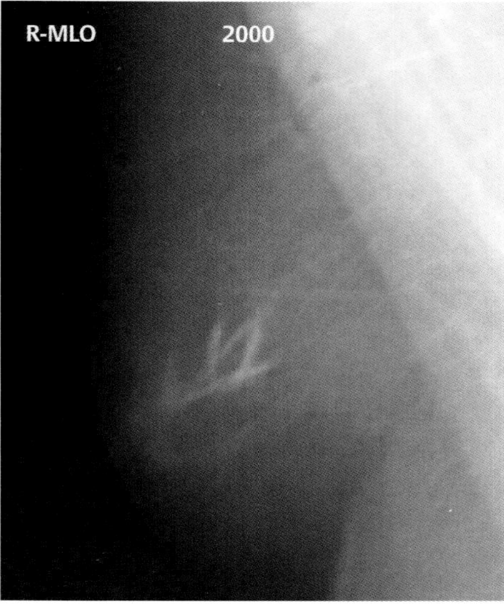


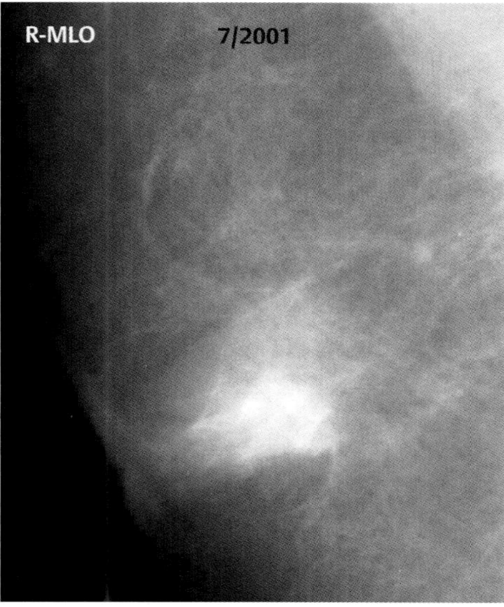


**a** *Oblique mammograms* of the right breast from 1999 to 2001. The image of March, 2000 shows a small focus of retroareolar gynecomastia with marked arborization of the rudimentary glandular tissue (prompting a subcutaneous mastectomy). Reexcision was performed in July 2001.

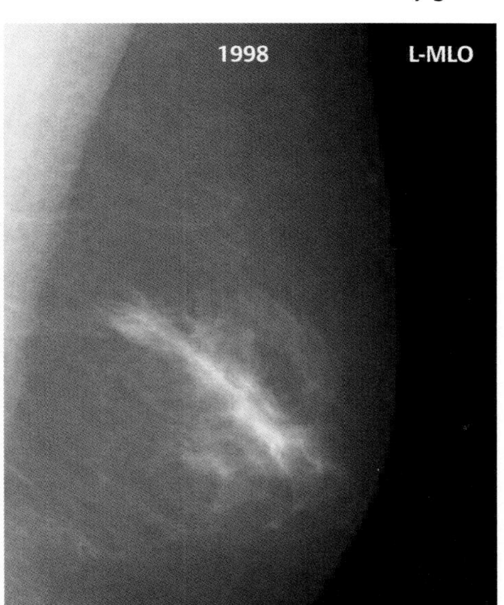


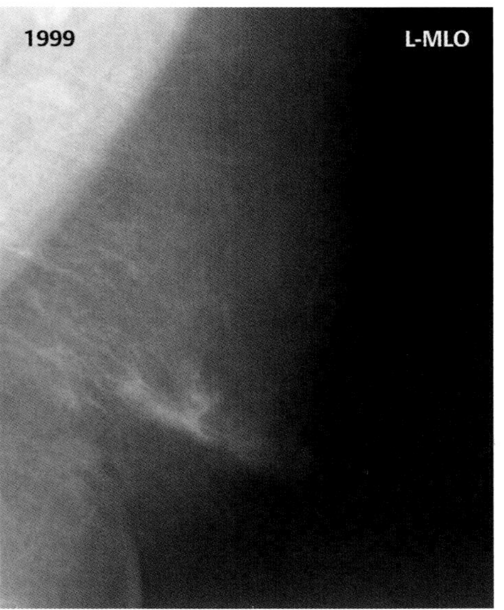


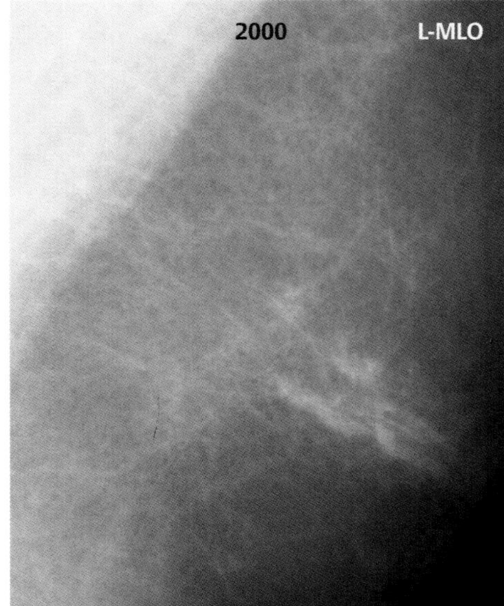


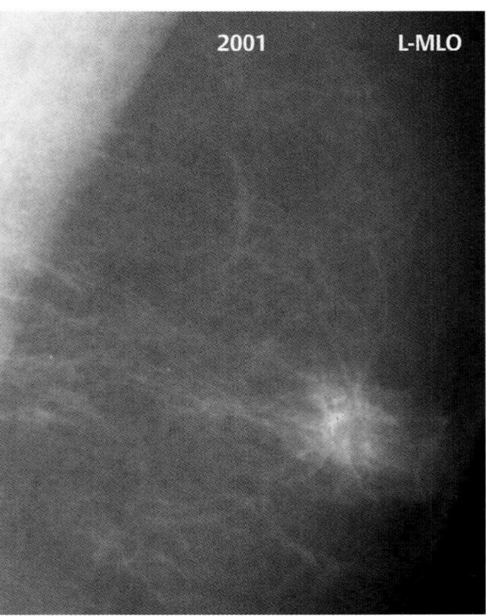


**b** *Oblique mammograms* of the left breast from 1999 to 2001 document the development of gynecomastia.

▶ **Fig. 5.150 c**

**Fig. 5.150** **A 57-year-old man.** *(continued)*

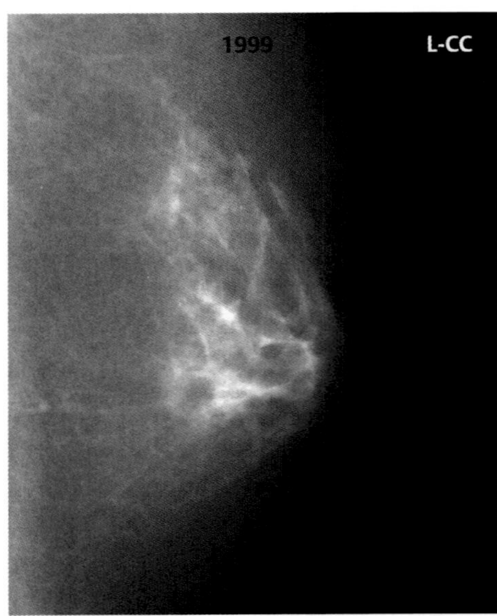


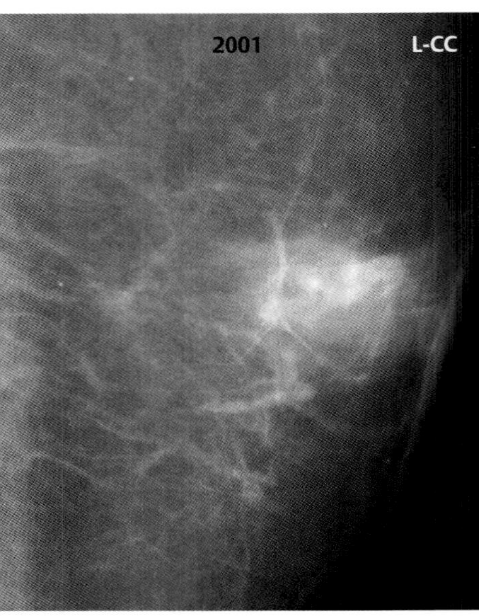


**c** *Craniocaudal mammograms* of the left breast from 1999 to 2001 show pronounced gynecomastia in 1999 (treated by subcutaneous mastectomy in 2000). A new retroareolar density appeared after surgery. (Images courtesy of Martin Jettmar, Geislingen.)

**Question on Fig. 5.150**

*How would you explain the bilateral retroareolar densities in 2001?*

(**a**) Incomplete excision of glandular tissue with recurrence of gynecomastia
(**b**) Scars following subcutaneous mastectomy
(**c**) Malignancy

→ **Answer on p. 396**

*(continued from p. 291)*

Two morphologic stages are distinguished:

- **Florid stage** (first 4 months), characterized by the initial appearance and growth of a painful breast nodule. Histologic examination shows loose, very cellular intralobular stroma with numerous lactiferous ducts and budding ducts devoid of lobules (see **Fig. 5.149i, j**, p. 395). Unsuspicious foci of epithelial proliferation may occur within dilated ducts. Nipple discharge may occur, usually in response to androgenic hormones. Cases of this kind may require evaluation by ductography to exclude an intraductal tumor, especially in patients with bloody discharge. The boundary between the breast parenchyma and surrounding fat is ill-defined.
- **Late stage** (after 1 year). Gynecomastia has been present for some time. Histologic examination shows a firm, fibrous, sometimes hyalinized connective tissue with lactiferous ducts. Lobular structures are usually absent. The histologic findings depend on the duration of gynecomastia and not on its cause.

The following factors may cause gynecomastia:

- Local causes in the mammary gland (heightened response of the breast parenchyma to normal hormone levels in the blood); 80% of newborn males have gynecomastia because of the estrogen-levels of the mother.
- Pituitary hyperstimulation (increased production of somatotropic hormone, gonadotropin, or prolactin by tumors, the pituitary, or hypothalamus).
- Other hormonal factors involving an absolute or relative rise of blood estrogen levels due to adrenal or testicular tumors (Leydig cell tumor, seminoma, chorioepithelioma, teratoma), hepatic cirrhosis, or Klinefelter syndrome.
- Drugs (psychopharmaceuticals, meprobamate, butyrophenone, alpha-methyldopa, rauwolfia alkaloids, ergotamine, digitalis, diphenylhydantoin, spironolactone, thiazides, and other diuretics; marihuana abuse, alcohol, heroin).
- Metabolic disorders and other diseases (e.g., leprous and mumps-related orchitis, pseudohermaphroditism, previous radiotherapy for malignant tumors, neurologic disorders: Friedreich ataxia, dystrophia myotonica, traumatic paraplegia, syringomyelia, sarcoidosis, and tuberculosis; also renal failure and chronic hemodialysis, hypo- and hyperthyroidism, diabetes mellitus).
- Being an HIV carrier under highly active antiretroviral therapy.

Thus, gynecomastia is not a disease entity but a symptom. Adolescent and hormonal forms of gynecomastia usually present with bilateral clinical and mammographic involvement, whereas gynecomastia in men 50–70 years of age is most often unilateral and related to pharmacologic therapy. Carcinoma rarely develops in a setting of gynecomastia, although accurate statistical data have not been reported in the literature.

Hall (1959) distinguished three grades of gynecomastia based on the degree of enlargement:

- **Grade I** is characterized by a large, firm, painless nodule that is freely movable relative to the pectoral muscle. A discrepancy exists between breast volume and the appearance on mammograms, which often show only dense fatty tissue. Mammograms show a retroareolar density with branches radiating toward the periphery, especially in the late stage and in older males, who occasionally have gross calcifications and, less commonly, microcalcifications (see **Fig. 5.152**, left breast).
- **Grade II** is characterized by a firm, movable nodule deep to the nipple. The palpable and radiographic extent of enlargement are identical. Mammograms show an ill-defined, inhomogeneous, triangular retroareolar density. Microcalcifications may occur. A florid stage is usually present. Mixed forms between grade I and grade II may be seen (see **Fig. 5.150 b**).
- **Grade III** denotes uniform breast enlargement, usually bilateral, with no palpable firmness or nodularity. The clinical presentation is the same as in a 17- to 18-year old female. Mammographic extent and density are the same as in a young female breast, making the breast difficult to evaluate by mammography. Ultrasound shows a thin layer of subcutaneous fat.

**Differential diagnosis of gynecomastia:**

- Carcinoma. Radiographic morphology and ultrasound findings are the same as in the female breast. The enlargement is frequently eccentric and unilateral with a bloody or brownish watery discharge. Microcalcifications and skin and nipple retraction are occasionally present (see **Fig. 5.150b**).
- Papilloma. This lesion is associated with discharge, and a nipple smear should be obtained (see **Fig. 5.150a**).
- Fibroadenoma (very rare) and cystocarcoma phylloides
- Fibroma, hemangioma, lymphangioma, myoblastoma, myxoma, myoma
- Metastases from malignant tumors (e.g., malignant melanoma)
- Abscess or inflammatory cyst, chronic and acute mastitis
- Lipoma, pseudogynecomastia
- Atheroma, lipophagic granuloma (e.g., following immunization for typhoid fever)
- Sarcoma

### Male Breast Cancer

Male breast cancer was extremely rare at the turn of the twentieth century. Although this disease is still uncommon today, the numbers are rising, perhaps due to the male use of estrogen as an antiaging product. Approximately 1% of all breast cancers occur in males.

There is a broad consensus in the literature that breast cancer in males has a poorer prognosis than in females. The natural history of the disease is the same in both sexes, although the 10-year survival rate of male breast cancer is only 50%. Usually the diagnosis of breast cancer is entertained too late, and often the disease is diagnosed only after skeletal metastasis has occurred.

**Histologically**, there is no difference between male and female breast cancer. The age distribution is also the same.

The **cause** of male breast cancer is unknown. Its pathogenesis presumably relates to a defect in the production or metabolism of estrogen, because the urinary excretion of this hormone was found to be elevated in three men with a strong positive family history of breast cancer.

**Males from high-risk families should have regular breast screening examinations.**

Brenner et al. (2004) described a man with clinically diagnosed breast cancer who carried a mutation in the *BRCA2* gene and whose tumor was detected by screening mammography. Everson et al. (1976) found infiltrating ductal carcinoma in a total of six men from two different families. Three men in one family who had prophylactic mastectomies were found to have focal intraductal epithelial hyperplasia. In the other family, malignant breast lesions also developed in several women.

Ludwig et al. (2007) reported on a series of 67 men from the Leipzig metropolitan area in Germany. The sex ratio was 1:136 (1 male to 136 female carcinomas) and the average age at diagnosis was 65 years. The authors believe that the etiology may relate to an increased estrogen/testosterone ratio and exposure to various environmental agents. Three-fourths of the neoplasms were hormone-receptor-positive. The overexpression of HER2/neu is as prevalent in males as in females. Ten percent of all male tumors are well-differentiated carcinomas in situ while 75% have a papillary, cribriform, or micropapillary morphology. Ninety percent of invasive carcinomas have a ductal origin. Two percent of male breast cancers exhibit the features of Paget disease. Occasional cases of invasive lobular carcinoma also occur. Medullary, mucinous, and adenoid cystic carcinomas are extremely rare.

Patients present clinically with a firm, relatively fixed, painless, palpable nodule located deep to the nipple. Nipple discharge is occasionally observed. A very small number of male breast cancers exhibit Paget features with typical nipple changes. Skin and nipple retraction are sometimes present (see **Figs. 5.152 a, 5.153 a**).

Male breast cancer has the same radiographic features as in females, and sonographic findings are also identical. CNB can establish the diagnosis without difficulty. If doubt exists, the nodule should be removed by surgical or vacuum biopsy.

The differential diagnosis is the same as for gynecomastia (see above). **Figures 5.151–5.153** illustrate typical changes in the male breast.

**Fig. 5.151 Male breast cancer (comedocarcinoma).** A 64-year-old man had a 5-year history of recurrent bleeding from the right breast. He presents now with a firm, painless, freely movable, bean-sized nodule deep to the nipple.

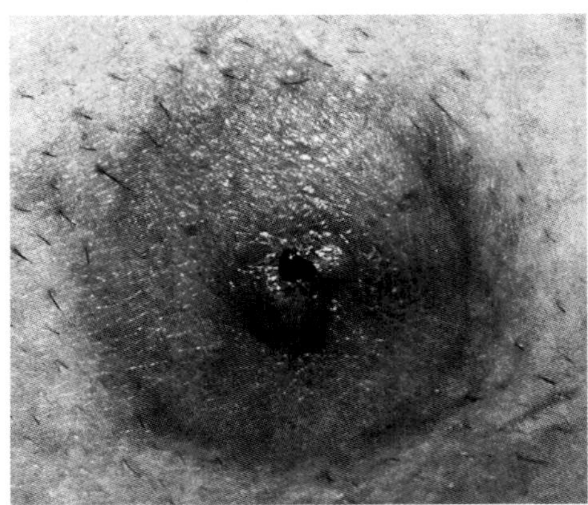

**a** *Clinical inspection* of the right nipple shows bloody discharge from one duct. The nipple is not retracted.

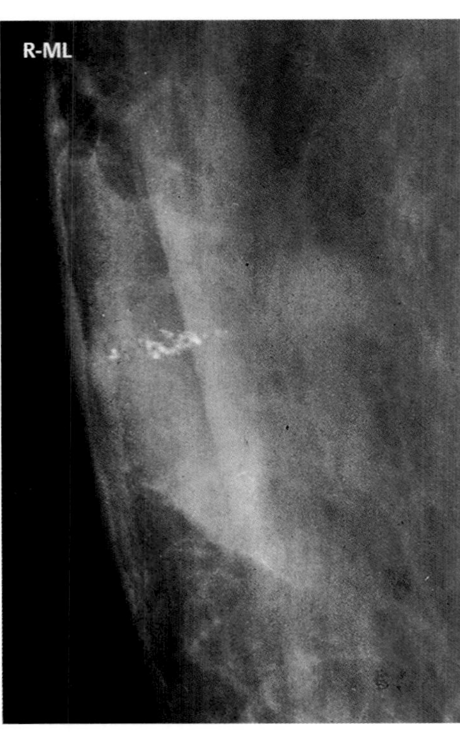


**b** *Mediolateral mammogram* shows a bandlike arrangement of coarse and pleomorphic microcalcifications deep to the nipple. The parenchymal breast tissue is hazy and ill-defined. A tumorlike lesion is not seen (image courtesy of Levente Mitrovics, Ludwigsburg).

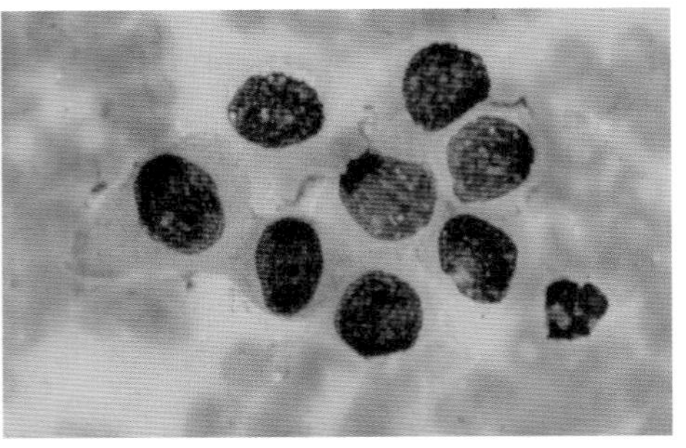

**c** *Cytologic smear* shows relatively large, pleomorphic nuclei consistent with high-grade malignancy. The cells show a finely reticular, disintegrated chromatin pattern.

**Fig. 5.152 Pronounced changes in the right breast of an 82-year-old man (a).** More subtle changes are also present in the left breast (**b**). Ultrasound shows a retroareolar hypoechoic nodule (**c**), while mammograms show bilateral retroareolar densities (**d**).

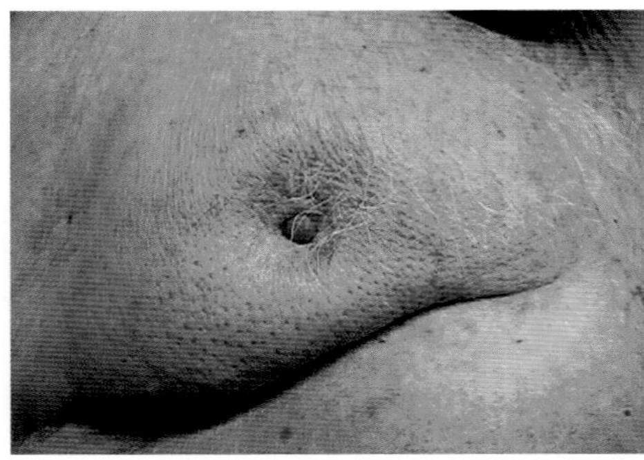

**a** *Clinical inspection* of the right breast with the arm raised: nipple retraction.

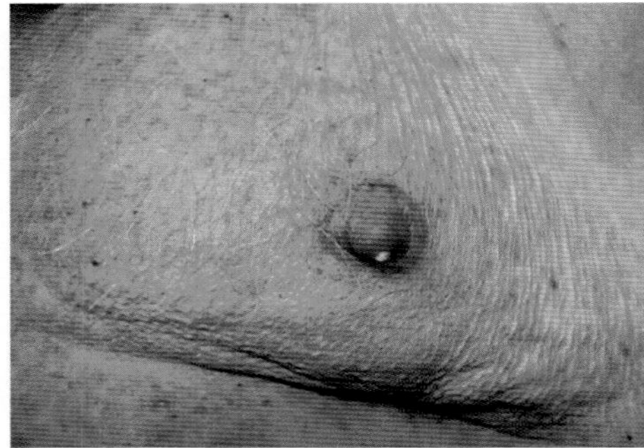

**b** *Clinical inspection* of the left breast shows downward deviation of the nipple with a small fibroma. Areas of skin retraction are visible in the inframammary fold.

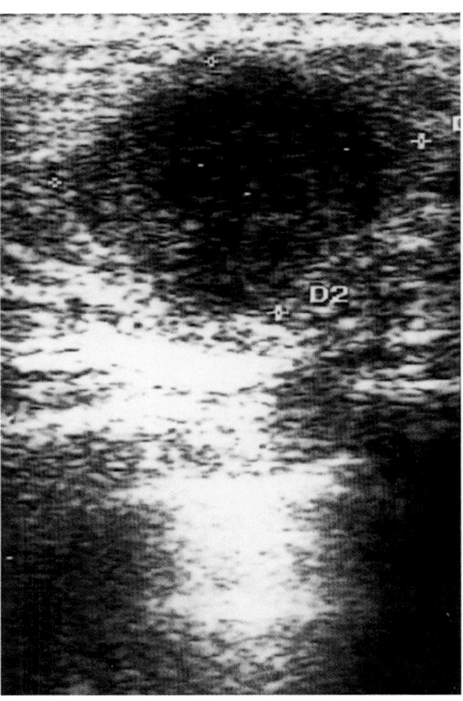


**c** *Sonogram* of the right breast shows a 1.2 cm, relatively well-circumscribed nodule with strong posterior acoustic enhancement.

**Fig. 5.152 Pronounced changes in the right breast of an 82-year-old man.** *(continued)*

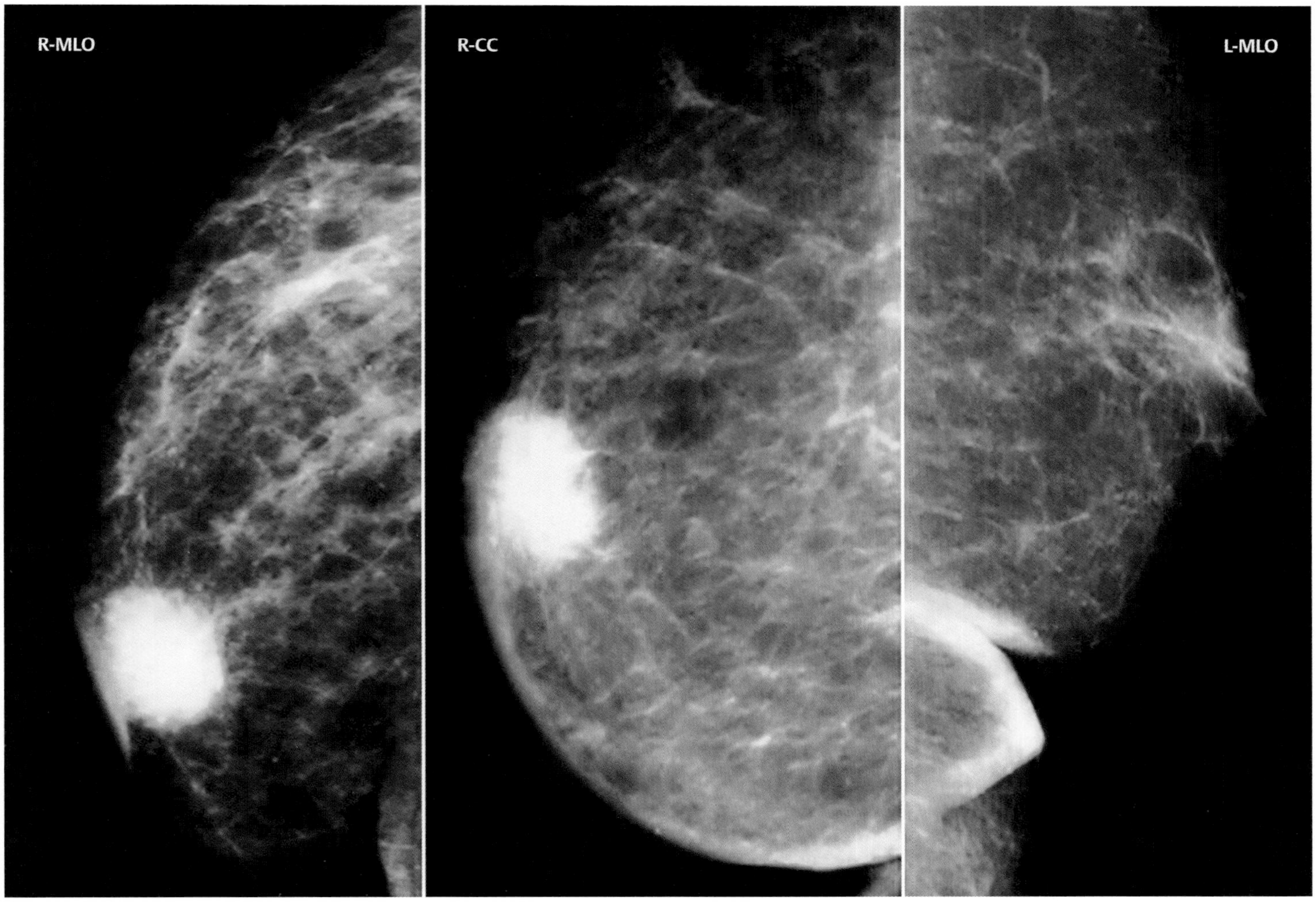

**d** Two *mammographic views* of the right breast and an oblique view of the left breast (image on the right) demonstrate a retroareolar nodule in the right breast and a faint retroareolar density in the left breast consistent with gynecomastia.

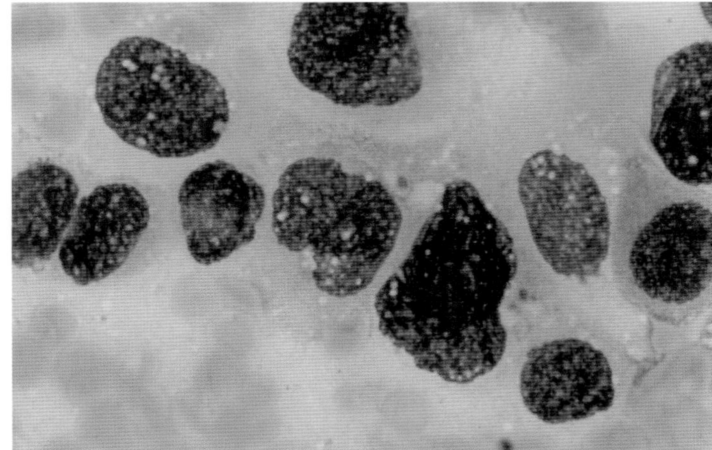

**e** *FNA* (right breast) large polymorphous cells.

**Question on Fig. 5.152**

*How would you interpret the changes in the right breast?*

(**a**) Gynecomastia

(**b**) Cyst

(**c**) Inflammatory carcinoma arising from a very cellular tumor

→ **Answer on p. 396**

**Fig. 5.153 A 67-year-old man presents with a 6-month history of progressive skin retraction on the left breast** relating to a locally advanced carcinoma (**a**). Mammograms show a stellate lesion in the left breast and a nonspecific density in the right breast (**b**). Ultrasound shows a hypoechoic area in the right breast and typical tumorlike findings on the left side (**c, d**). The patient underwent surgery for a high rectal carcinoma in 1993.

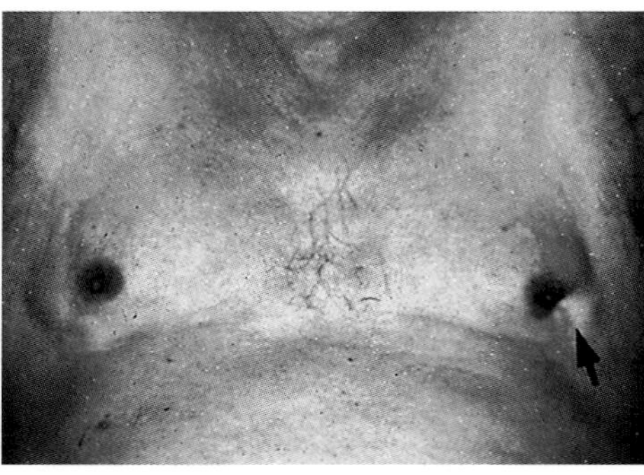

**a** *Clinical inspection* shows marked skin retraction by the left areola at the 4-o'clock position.

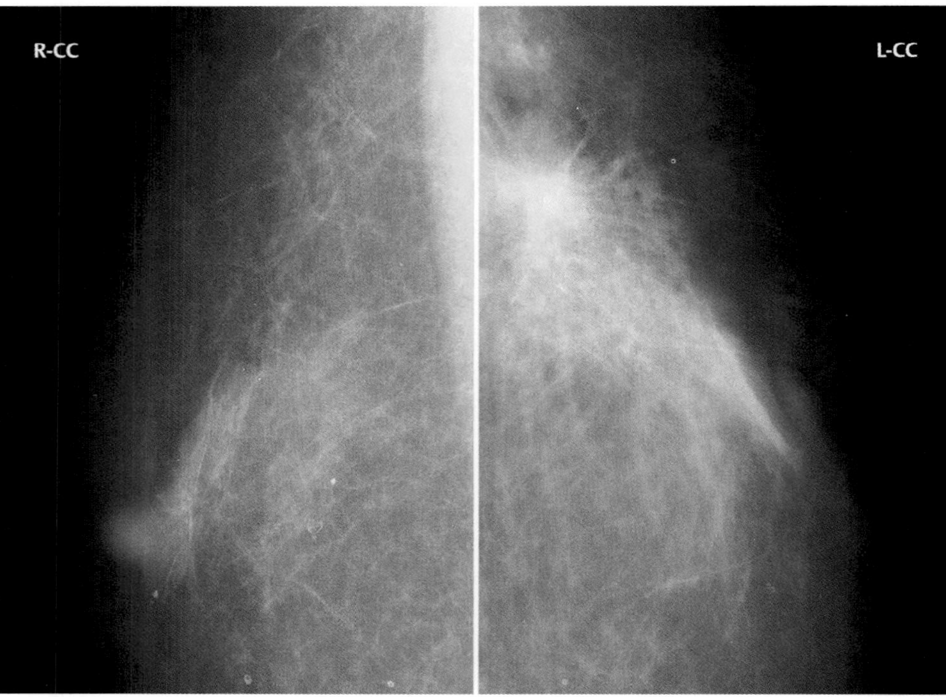


**b** *Bilateral craniocaudal mammograms.* Tumor in the left breast appears as a patchy opacity with spicules radiating to the areola and pectoral muscle (**g–i/20–25**). The right mammogram shows a retroareolar nodule with nonspecific triangular opacities (**E–F/19–21**) (ACR 1, BIRADS 5 on the left, BIRADS? on the right, PG**MI**).

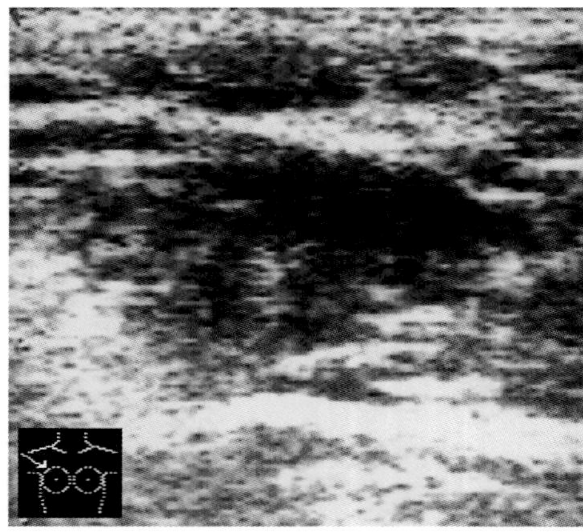

**c** *Sonogram* of the right breast shows a hypoechoic triangular zone (**a–c/17–19**).

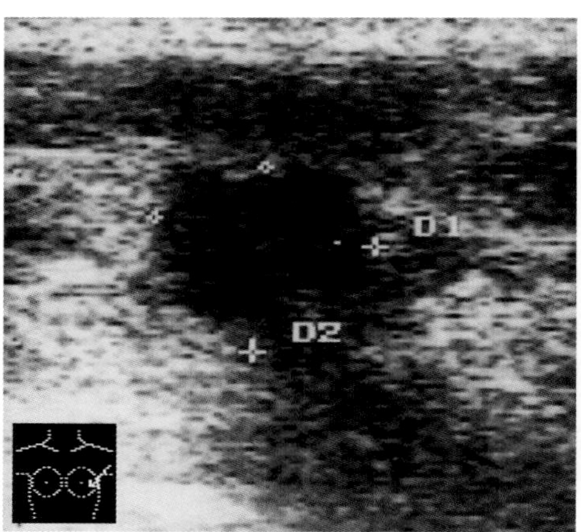


**d** *Sonogram* of the left breast shows a 1.2 cm hypoechoic nodule with relatively smooth margins and a posterior acoustic shadow.

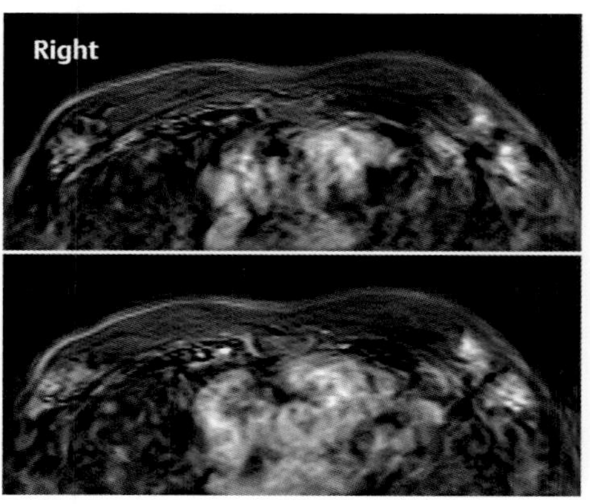


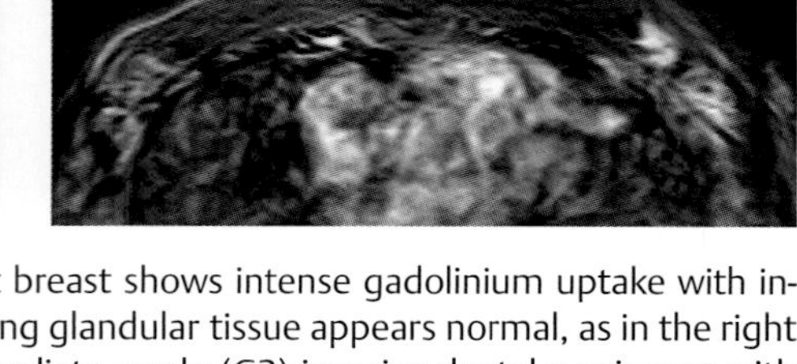

**e** *MR subtraction images.* The tumor in the left breast shows intense gadolinium uptake with involvement of the pectoral fascia. The surrounding glandular tissue appears normal, as in the right breast. *Histology on the left side:* 2.5 cm, intermediate-grade (G2) invasive ductal carcinoma with residua in the remaining gland. There is no evidence of lymph node metastasis.

**Question on Fig. 5.153**

*How would you interpret the retroareolar nodule in the* right *mammogram (**b**)?*

(**a**) Gynecomastia
(**b**) Second carcinoma
(**c**) Nipple-areola in gynecomastia

→ **Answer on p. 397**

# Therapy and Perioperative Management

The histologic result (as detailed in the previous chapter) marks the endpoint of the **diagnostic** work-up. The **treatment** phase for malignant conditions begins in the clinical setting (preferably at a certified breast center) as *perioperative management*.

These services include:

- Preoperative localization of clinically occult lesions
- Sentinel lymph node biopsy
- Specimen radiography with a precise description of the biopsy site
- Postoperative mammography if required.

Perioperative management does not include preoperative liver ultrasound, chest radiographs, or radionuclide bone scans traditionally performed in hospitalized patients. These services can be provided by private radiologists outside the hospital.

Cooperation within the framework inside the hospital should be structured in such a way that the diagnostic unit of a breast center is responsible for preoperative tests (sometimes also including interventional procedures and MRM) and also perioperative management to ensure continuity of the diagnostic chain. In many cases the examining physician has come to know the individual anatomy of the patient better than the surgeon and is more aware of the problems that may arise during wire localization and finding calcifications within the specimen. Preoperative and postoperative conferences (including all disciplines from within and outside the hospital, including breast-care nurses) are very important for discussing all patient-relevant problems that have to take into consideration. The US guidelines play here an important role (Torosian, 2002).

> **!** **The main goal of perioperative management is the complete removal of an occult lesion from the breast (no frozen sections, no reexcision, no MRM or other postoperative tests to diagnose a missed lesion). Whenever possible the lesion should be removed in one step with minimal disfigurement and low morbidity through a limited axillary procedure (sentinel lymph node biopsy).**

Perioperative management significantly improves diagnostic certainty, ensures a more efficient chain of care, and has a major role in determining the eventual outcome. The incidence of local recurrences is the prime indicator of the quality of the healthcare chain. Distant metastases, if they occur, are already present at the time of tumor therapy. Local recurrences, on the other hand, occur only if the tumor was not removed with clear margins, if the sentinel lymph node biopsy (see p. 307) was imprecise, or in patients with subclinical multicentric or multifocal disease, which may lead secondarily to an axillary recurrence (where the axilla was negative at the time of breast surgery). Perioperative management, then, stands or falls with the technical proficiency of the surgeon, radiologist, pathologist, and radiation oncologist and their ability to cooperate with one another. The chain of care described above is only as strong as its weakest link. Every member of the chain should be aware of this.

**Some quantitative criteria for a well-functioning breast center are summarized below** ("IMZE" refers to values at the Interdisciplinary Breast Center of Esslingen, the author's home breast center)

- Ratio of benign to malignant lesions at open biopsy: < 1 : 1 (IMZE 4 : 1)
- Percentage of specimen radiographs (or specimen sonograms) sent to the pathologist after the preoperative localization of nonpalpable lesions: ≥ 90% (IMZE 96%)
- Percentage of ductal carcinomas in situ: ≥ 10%
- Percentage of invasive carcinomas 5 mm or smaller: ≥ 10%
- Percentage of invasive carcinomas 10 mm or smaller: ≥ 20%
- Percentage of invasive carcinomas 20 mm or smaller: ≥ 65%
- Percentage of lymph-node-negative invasive carcinomas: > 75%
- Percentage of women participating in a screening program who state that they were well informed and were involved in the decision-making process beyond informed consent: > 90%
- Percentage of carcinomas detected within 24 months after previous negative mammograms (BIRADS 1–3), i.e., interval cancers/false-negative mammograms: ≤ 50%
- Percentage of interval cancers referred for detailed interdisciplinary analysis: ≥ 95%
- Complete documentation of the parameters necessary for overall quality management in the diagnostic chain: ≥ 90%
- Percentage of detection rates exceeding the observed incidence rate: > 50% (Albert et al. 2008)
- Medium time-span between diagnosis and operation 5–18 days (IMZE 9 days)
- Percentage of BCT (breast-conserving therapy) > 60% (IMZE T1-tumors 87%)
- Percentage of MRM (moderate radical mastectomy) < 10% (IMZE 19%)
- Percentage of SLNB (invasive cancers) > 60% (IMZE 90%)
- Percentage of documentation of pTNM, menopausal status, safety distance, receptor- and Her-2-neu status > 95% (IMZE 100%)
- Percentage of BCT radiation therapy > 95% (Kreienberg et al 2008) (IMZE 98%)

## Preoperative Localization

Clinically occult lesions can be localized with a fine wire marker introduced under **digital stereotactic** or **sonographic** guidance. The localization wire should be placed such that the end of the wire is *in front of* the suspicious area, not behind it (see **Figs. 5.154, 5.155**). This ensures that, dissecting toward the lesion from the areolar rim, the surgeon will encounter the localization wire first before reaching the calcification cluster or nodule. If the wire were placed *behind* the lesion, the surgeon would reach the lesion before encountering the marker, perhaps destroying or significantly damaging the tumor along the way. It is also possible to transfix the lesion with the wire. While this technique gives accurate localization by leaving the nodule or calcification cluster "hanging by a thread," the pathologist may have difficulty processing the altered breast tissue in the case of smaller lesions. These and other details must be decided individually within the team. In any case, the statistical goal is to place the localizing wire no farther than 10 mm from the lesion in no more than 10% of all preoperative localizations (farther in the case of DCIS and ADH than in invasive carcinoma, see p. 45ff.), and its position should be accurately described in both planes.

### Digital Stereotactic Localization

*Digital stereotactic localization* employs basically the same technique as digital stereotactic (ST-) FNA and CNB (see p. 249). It is important to perform the preoperative localization of an occult lesion before the sentinel lymph node procedure because of the *finger radiation dose* (Meades et al. 2009).

After the breast has been imaged in the craniocaudal or lateral projection, a survey view is obtained and the targeted area is placed as close to the center of the image as possible. The mediolateral or lateromedial projection (depending on the location of the calcifications) is better than the craniocaudal approach, for in the event of complications (inflammation, etc.) the patient will not be left with scars or pigmentation changes in the cleavage area.

It would be ideal to approach the lesion from the areola, but this is not possible with the stereotactic units now available.

Sometimes it is necessary to mark the lesion from below, but standard systems for localization in the sitting patient (Senovision, GE, Siemens) do not allow for this approach. Localization can be performed from below in systems where the patient can lie down on the **stereotactic table** (Fischer, Giotto, Lorad). Sometimes when a lesion is suspicious in MRI, it is marked with CT-guided puncture, as the lesions that enhance in MRI will likely also be visible in CT with radiographic contrast medium. This makes a good substitute for MR-guided marking, as the equipment for MRI guidance is very expensive (**Figs. 5.124**, p. 255; **5.157**, p. 304).

When the lesion has been centered in the image, the puncture site is usually numbed with local anesthetic. But because localization requires just one needle insertion, we dispense with local anesthesia and pierce the skin very quickly with the introducer needle. The needle, loaded with the hookwire, is advanced to a position directly in front of the targeted lesion, and two radiographs (craniocaudal and strictly mediolateral) are taken to confirm placement. A good rule is to insert the needle 5–10 mm deeper than indicated on the digital display, because the end of the wire tends to retract slightly during hookwire deployment, needle withdrawal, and the release of breast compression. If the tip of the localization wire is not positioned ideally in front of the lesion, it is better to place it too low than too high. With a lower wire position the surgeon knows that the lesion has been removed when the end of the wire is removed; this is not the case when the wire has been placed too high.

For various reasons, it is not uncommon to get a suboptimal placement of the wire marker. In this case it is better to perform a second localization than to assume that the surgeon will find the lesion anyway. Whenever the placement is not optimal, the radiologist should contact the surgeon and personally explain the situation.

If the location of the lesion is not uniquely defined in the mammogram, craniocaudal and straight lateral projections should be taken prior to localization. It may be helpful to place an adhesive, radiopaque centimeter marker on the skin (see **Fig. 5.119 a, b**, p. 252).

Following definitive placement of the localization wire, craniocaudal and straight lateral projections are taken again to document the relationship of the marker to the targeted lesion. The surgeon should receive a brief written report indicating the most important relevant data and stating whether a specimen radiograph is needed. Most interdepartmental snags occur at the interfaces between preoperative localization, postoperative specimen radiography, and contact with the pathologist.

In former times, breast lesions were localized with a wire marker introduced freehand from the areolar margin. This technique is too imprecise and has become obsolete. Moreover, when a simple metal wire with a hooked end is used (see **Fig. 5.157 f**, p. 305), there is a risk that the wire may migrate a considerable distance toward the chest wall or axilla, making it difficult or impossible for the surgeon to locate and retrieve it during the operation, unless the wire has been anchored by an external clip. The use of X-shaped or curved wires prevents this migration, even when the wire is introduced from the areola (**Fig. 5.156**, p. 303).

Various types of wires and needles can be used for localization and need not be described here. It should be noted, however, that the disadvantage of using a curved wire tip is that it may not fully expand in fibrotic tissue and may occasionally snag the pleura or periosteum when introduced near the pleura (very painful, risk of pneumothorax). Consequently, the author and his colleagues prefer an *X-shaped hookwire*. The advantage is that the opposing prongs prevent wire migration into the breast; the disadvantage is that it can only be removed surgically. Among the many localization wires and needles that are available, each group should select the model that will work best from an interdisciplinary standpoint. For example, the material should not be so thin that the surgeon is likely to sever it while dissecting toward the lesion, and it should not interfere with tissue analysis by the pathologist. Meanwhile, the surgeon should be able to remove the breast lesion with clear margins, and the pathologist should receive an intact specimen that can be accurately evaluated.

Frozen section examination has become obsolete. The guidelines state that more than 70% of all lesions selected for removal should be histological diagnosed prior to surgery (why not 100%?). When quality is lost at the interface between preoperative localization and preoperative specimen radiography (see p. 305) and the correlation with the pathologic management, very often this will adversely affect the overall quality and effectiveness of *early* breast cancer detection.

Preoperative localization is generally done on the day before surgery. There should be no difficulty, however, in performing preoperative localization 2–3 days before surgery (under aseptic conditions, of course). This is important, because it means that localization does not necessarily have to be done in the hospital where the surgery is scheduled in cases where the hospital lacks proper equipment for the procedure. In any event, digital stereotactic biopsy units are very costly and are not always a wise purchase for every hospital, even those that do 50–100 localizations a year.

Whenever possible, localization should be performed through the same needle tract previously used for CNB. This tract marks the approach for the surgeon and should be removed along with the lesion, although inoculation metastases are extremely rare. We have never seen a case of inoculation metastasis in 35 years of practice. While it is known that core biopsy seeds tumor cells along the needle tract, the cells are destroyed by host defenses.

Of course, personal care of the patient during preoperative localization should be as careful and precise as in digital stereotactic (ST-) CNB (see p. 249).

*(continued on p. 305)*

**Fig. 5.154 Preoperative localization. a** Mammogram of a 69-year-old woman with a DCIS in the upper outer quadrant of the left breast. **b** Mammogram of a 64-year-old woman with clustered microcalcifications (ADH) in the upper portion of the left breast. Both lesions were localized with a hookwire placed under digital stereotactic guidance.

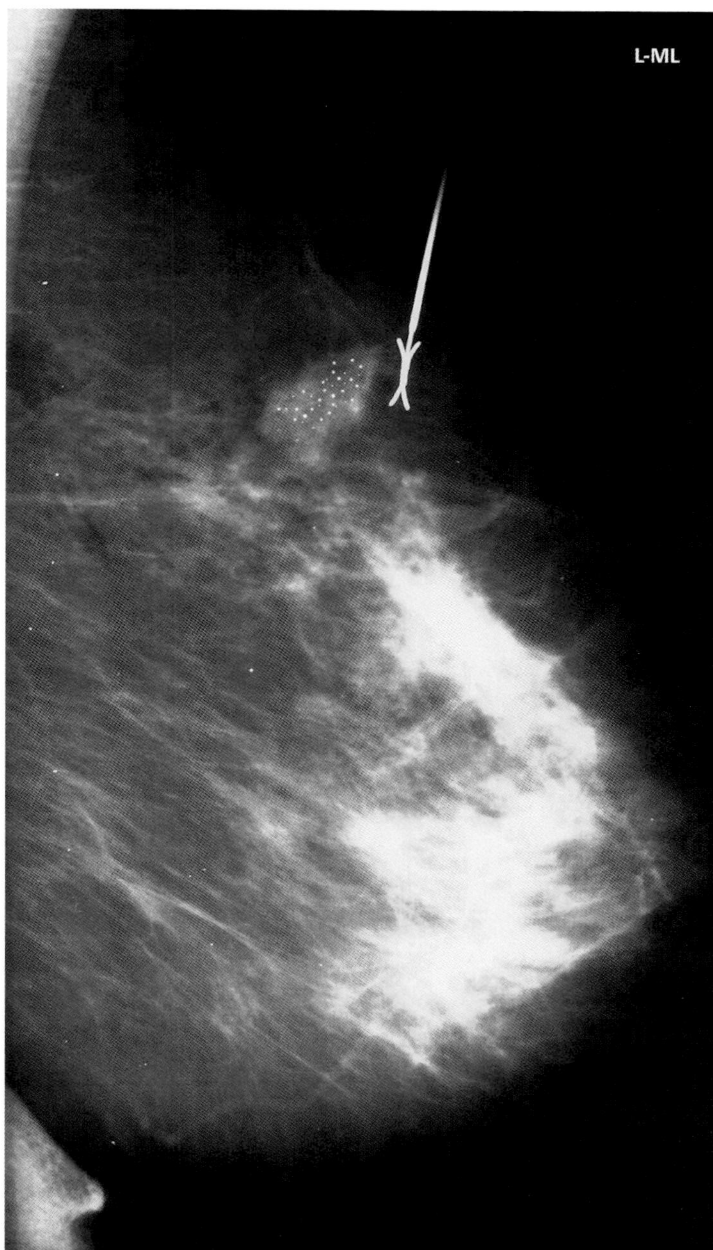


**a** *Mediolateral localization mammogram* of the left breast. Atypical microcalcifications are visible within a suspicious density (**M/21–22**). The tip of the localization wire is anterior to the calcification cluster.

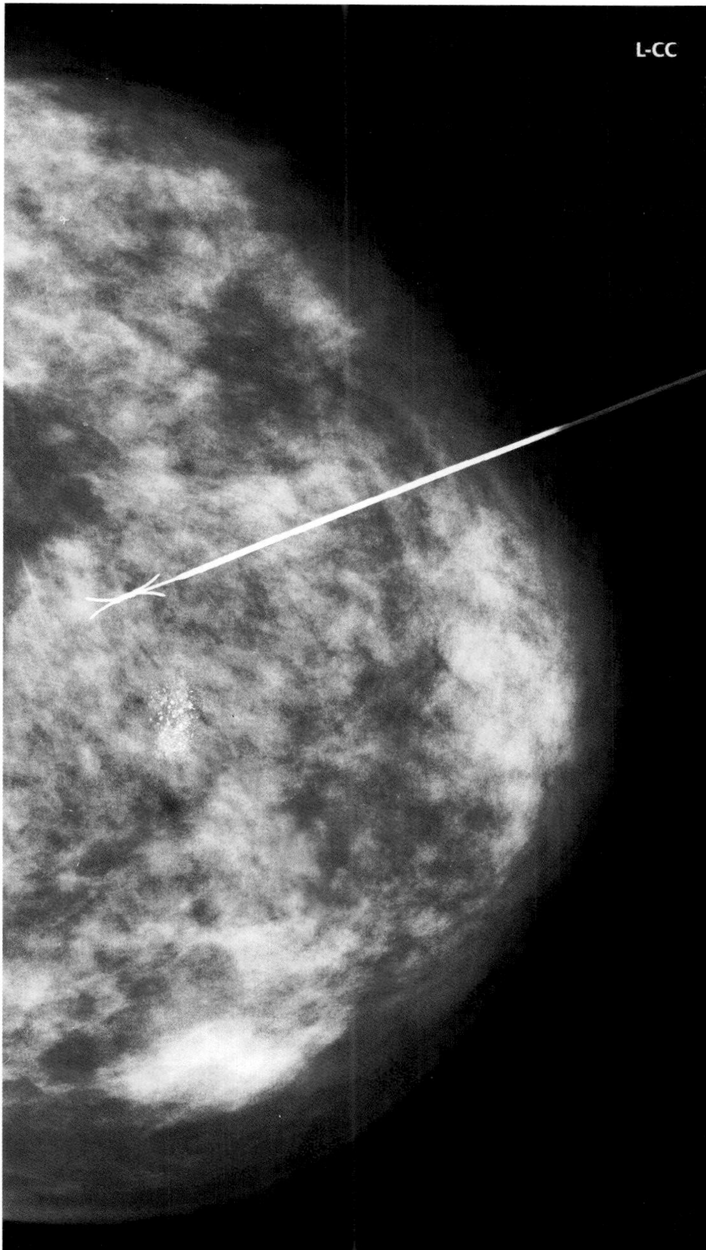


**b** *Craniocaudal localization mammogram* of the left breast (different patient from the one in **a**). The hookwire is 2 cm posterolateral to the calcification cluster (**Q/16–17**).

**Question on Fig. 5.154**

*Which localization is correct for a periareolar approach to the calcifications?*

(**a**) Localization in **a**

(**b**) Localization in **b**

(**c**) Both are equally good

→ **Answer on p. 397**

**Fig. 5.155 Localization problems in a 56-year-old woman** with extensive DCIS in the upper inner quadrant of the left breast. The medial and lateral lesion margins have each been marked with a hookwire. The localization wires may show the surgeon the calcification margins in the craniocaudal view but not in the lateral view.

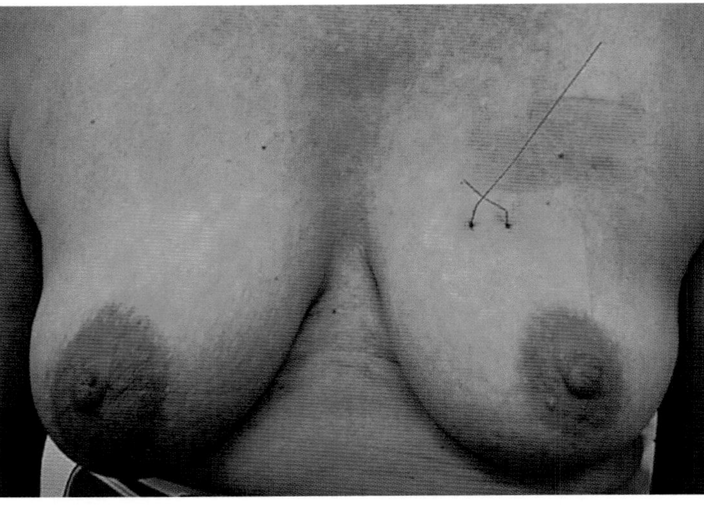

**a** *Clinical appearance* after localization. Two wire markers have been placed in the upper inner quadrant of the left breast.

**Comment:** With DCIS and ADH, the localization wire should be placed 1 cm from the calcification cluster, and an additional 1 cm safety zone should be added for the resection because these lesions are considerably larger than they appear on mammograms (see **Fig. 4.22**, p. 44).

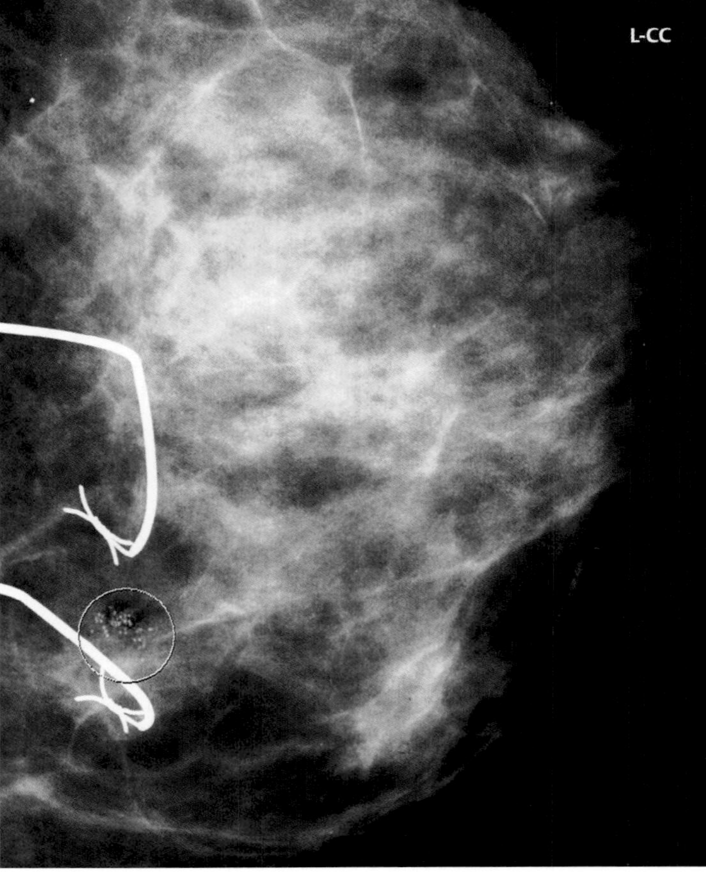


**b** *Craniocaudal mammogram* (localization view) shows the localizing wires correctly positioned at the calcification margins in the vertical plane. If additional wires were placed, they would obstruct the surgeon's view.

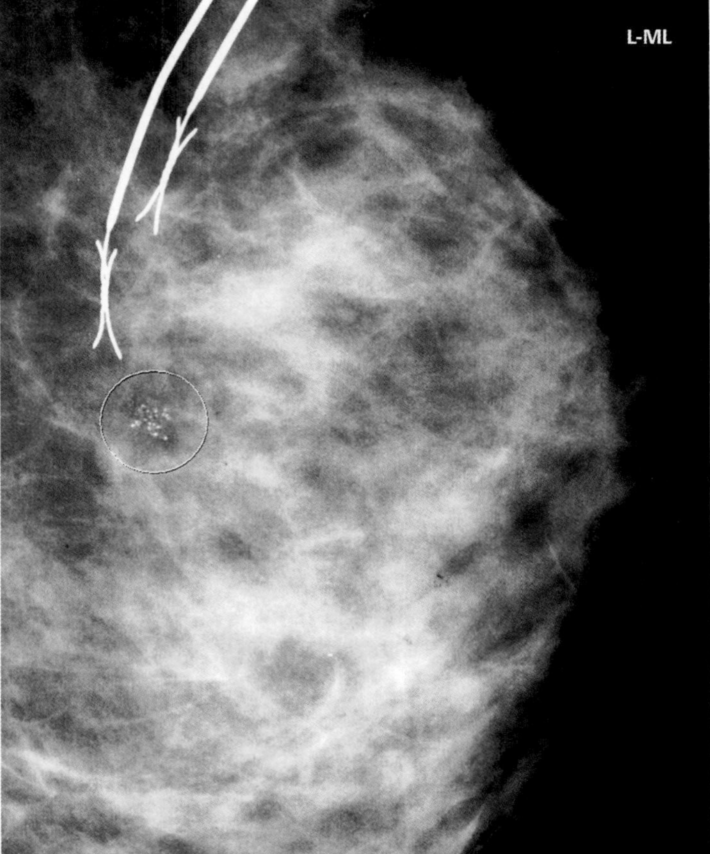


**c** *Mediolateral mammogram* (localization view). Both wires are projected behind and 1 cm above the calcifications, which is unfavorable (see p. 300).

**Fig. 5.156 A 37-year-old woman has a 6 mm palpable nodule in the lower outer quadrant of the right breast.** Mammograms show multiple microcalcification clusters, which are marked with a localizing wire under digital stereotactic guidance. Two surgical specimens contain poorly differentiated (G3) ductal carcinoma in situ (DCIS) with positive margins. The reexcision specimen contains additional DCIS foci with a 2 mm margin of healthy tissue. One specimen contains adenosis with microcalcifications.

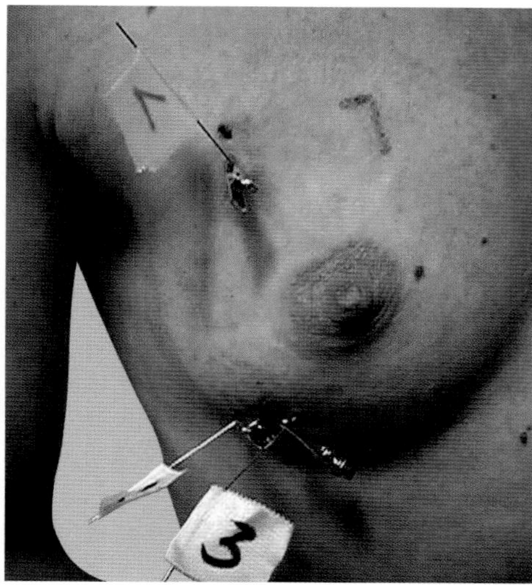

**a** Clinical appearance after wire localization of the three calcification clusters (1 at 11-o'clock position; 2 at 8-o'clock position; 3 at 7-o'clock position).

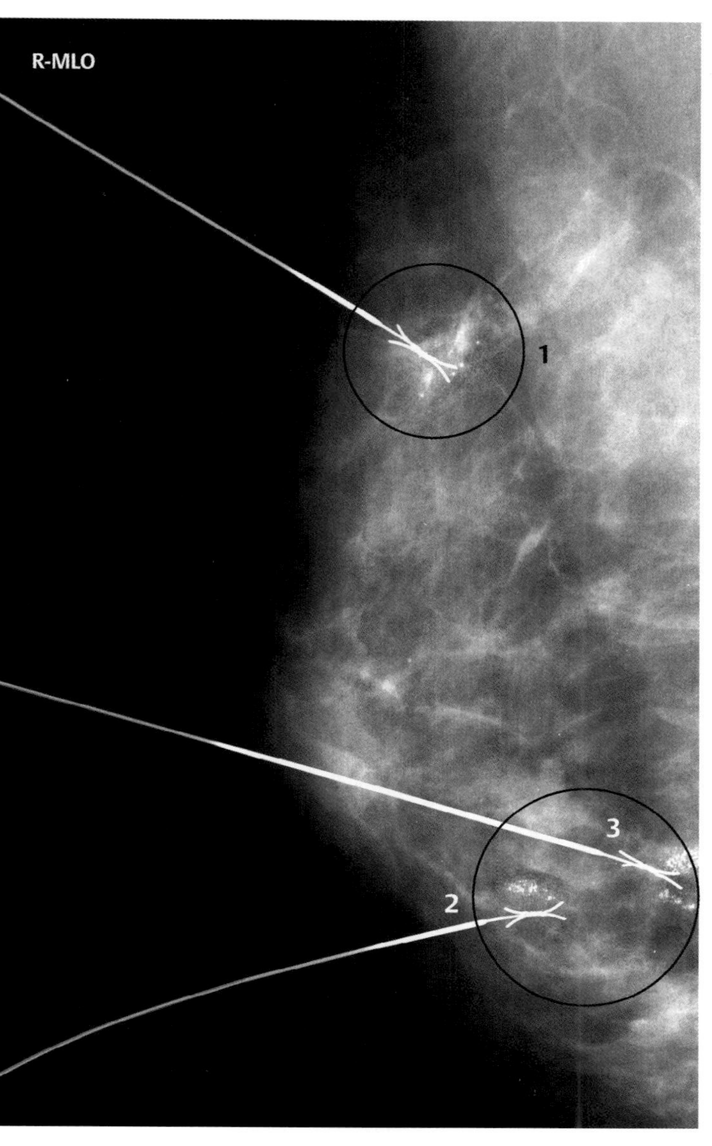


**b** *Oblique mammogram* of the right breast. The calcification clusters have been marked with localizing wires.

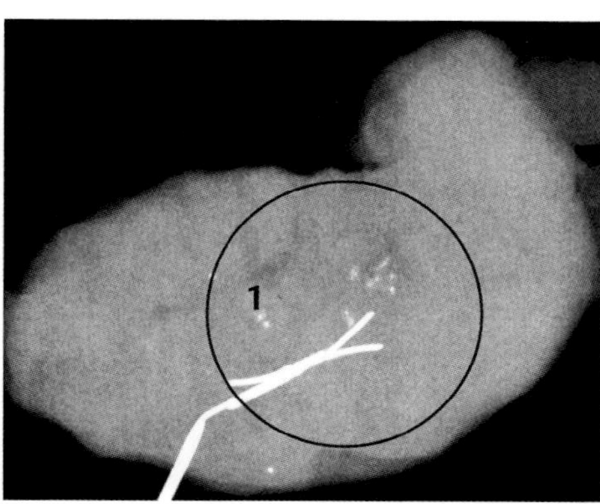


**c** *Specimen radiograph* demonstrates calcification cluster 1 (see **a**).

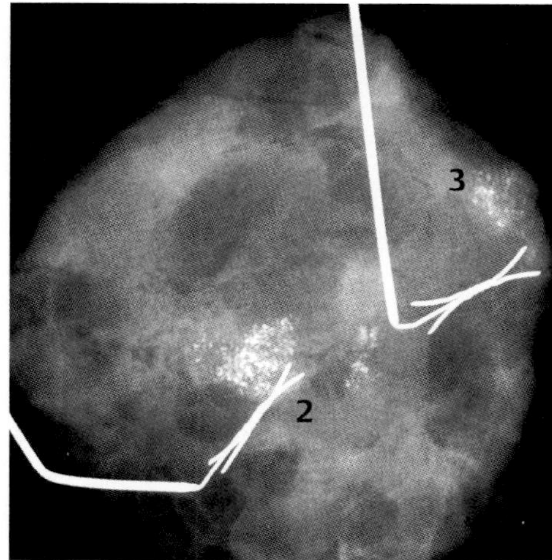


**d** *Specimen radiograph* with calcification clusters 2 and 3 (see **a**). Note that the cluster on the right (3) is at the edge of the specimen. This suggests positive margins and necessitates a reexcision.

**Question 1 on Fig. 5.156**

*Which wire (1–3, see* ***a****) has localized the adenosis?*

(**a**) 1
(**b**) 2
(**c**) 3

→ **Answer on p. 397**

**Question 2 on Fig. 5.156**

*What adjuvant therapy is* unnecessary *in the present case?*

(**a**) Adjuvant hormone therapy
(**b**) Adjuvant polychemotherapy
(**c**) Radiotherapy

→ **Answer on p. 397**

**Question 3 on Fig. 5.156**

*Follow-up mammograms of the treated breast should be taken (according to German guidelines) at what intervals during the first 3 years?*

(**a**) Every 3 months
(**b**) Every 6 months
(**c**) Every 12 months

→ **Answer on p. 397**

**Fig. 5.157 A 56-year-old woman with relatively large, very nodular breasts presents for screening** (inset in **a**). Mammograms show high radiographic breast density (**a, b**). Ultrasound shows an atypical change in the left breast, while MRI shows intense bilateral gadolinium uptake with an enhancing focus in the left breast (**d**). Because MRI-guided localization equipment was not available, localization was directed by computed tomography (**e**), which defines the tumor more clearly than the other modalities. The tumor is excised with clear margins.

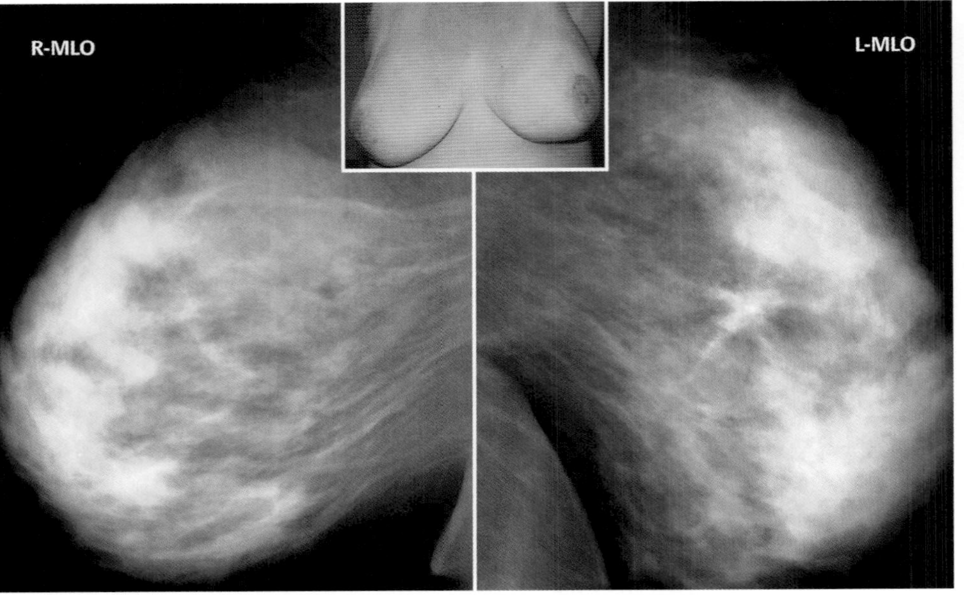


**a** *Bilateral oblique mammograms* show very radiodense breasts with confluent intramammary opacities (ACR 3, BIRADS?, **P**GMI).

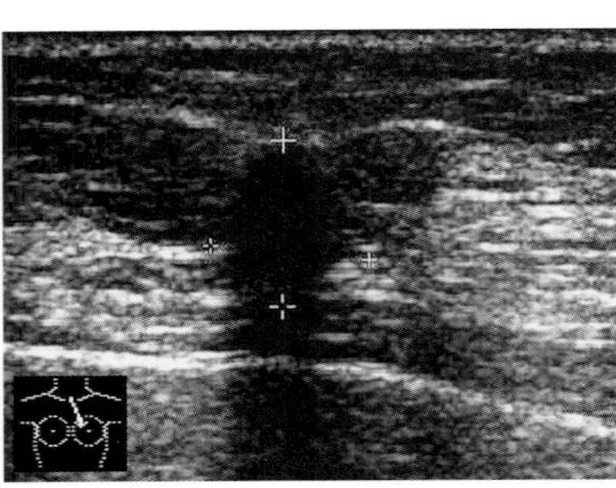

**c** *Sonogram* of the upper inner quadrant of the left breast shows an atypical hypoechoic lesion with internal echoes (**I–i/24–25**).

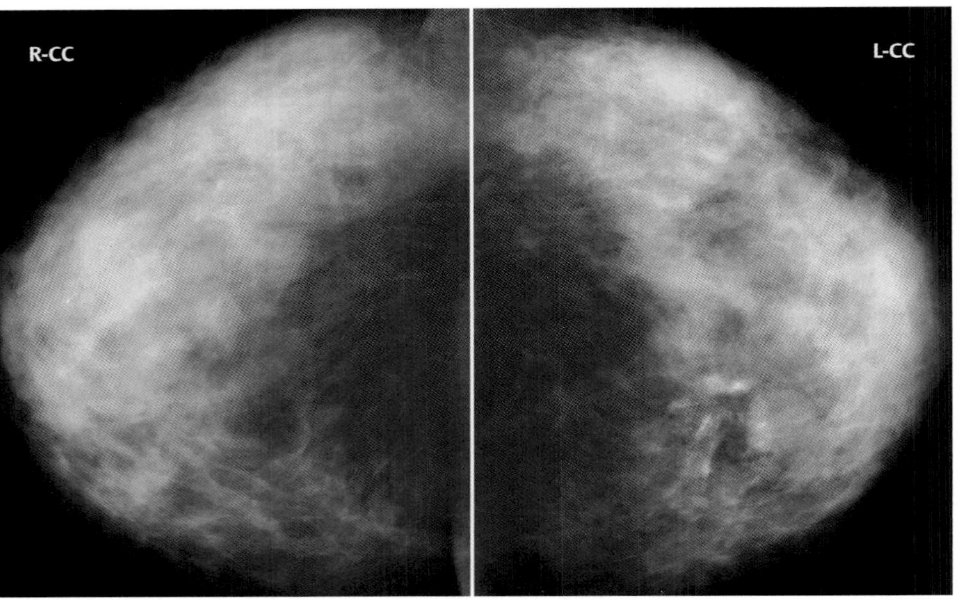


**b** *Bilateral craniocaudal mammograms* show very radiodense, inhomogeneous breasts (ACR 3, BIRADS?, P**G**MI).

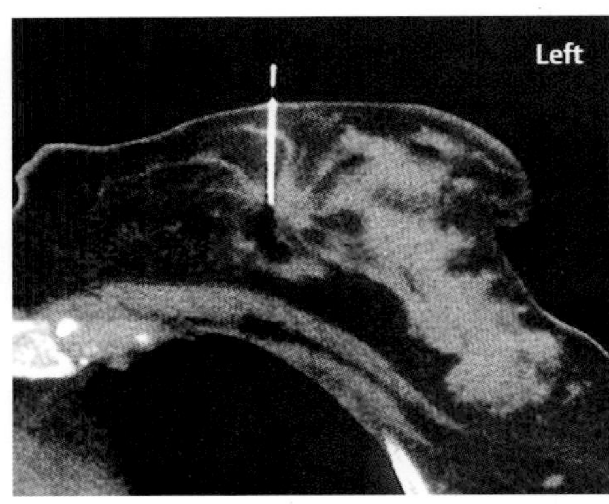


**e** *Spiral CT* shows an approximately 2 cm spiculated lesion in the medial portion of the left breast according to the findings in ultrasound (**c**).

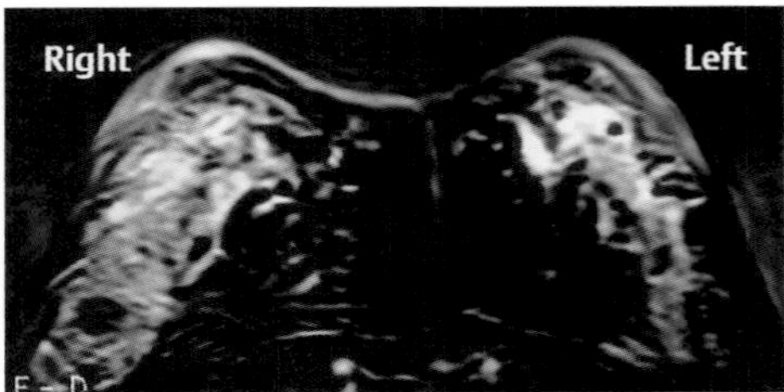


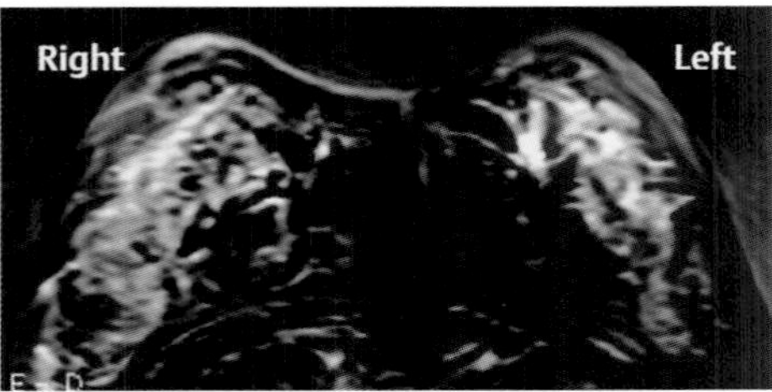


**d** *MR subtraction images* show intense gadolinium uptake in both breasts with focal enhancement in the left breast (**C–c/5**). No enhancement in the area of microcalcifications in the right breast.

**Fig. 5.157 A 56-year-old woman presents for screening.** *(continued)*

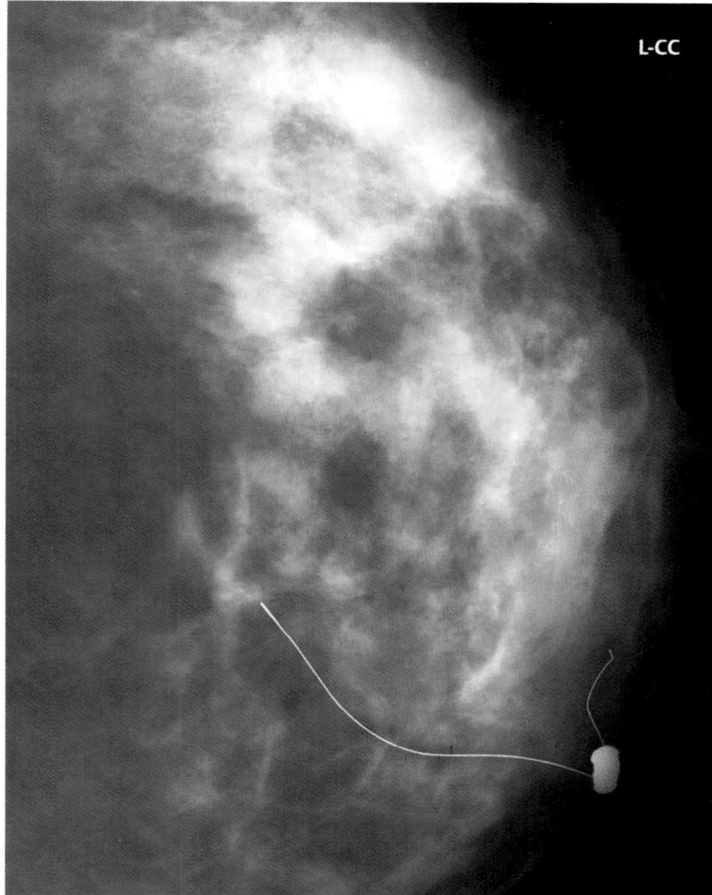


**f** *Craniocaudal mammogram* of the left breast after CT-guided localization. The localization wire has been placed behind the suspicious mammographic lesion. Histology identified the lesion as invasive ductal carcinoma. (Incidentally, the wire marker has a small barb at its tip and would migrate deeper into the breast were it not anchored by an external bead.)

**Question on Fig. 5.157**

*When a tumor is poorly visualized on mammogram:*
*Which modality (**c–e**) is best and most cost-effective for lesion localization?*
(**a**) Ultrasound
(**b**) Magnetic resonance imaging
(**c**) Computed tomography

→ **Answer on p. 398**

#### Ultrasound-Guided Localization

The preoperative localization of sonographically visible lesions should always be performed under ultrasound guidance. This is not only more economical than digital stereotactic guidance but is also more precise, since the lesion can be approached from the areolar margin. This is also the approach that most breast surgeons prefer. In this way the localization wire marks a route to the suspicious lesion and can be removed with the specimen. This also eliminates the need for an additional skin lesion. It is best for the surgeon to perform the localization personally, as this will convey a three-dimensional impression of where the lesion and localizing wire are located.

Even with ultrasound-guided localization, it is good practice to obtain two mammographic projections (craniocaudal and straight lateral) after the procedure, as this will make it easier to evaluate the removal site and also monitor postoperative changes over time.

It is possible to demonstrate the excised tissue in a specimen *sonogram*. Of course, a preoperative specimen radiograph would not be appropriate for ultrasound-localized lesions unless the sonographic lesion were also calcified. In this case the calcifications should be documented in a specimen radiograph (to confirm clear margins). Whenever it is uncertain whether all calcifications or a sonographic lesion have been removed, an immediate postoperative radiograph or sonogram should be obtained with minimal breast compression for confirmation purposes.

The percentage of correctly localized specimens at open biopsy should be > 97% according to guidelines. The ratio of malignant to benign lesions at open biopsy should be > 1 : 1 (i.e., more malignant than benign lesions should be surgically biopsied). The percentage of specimen radiographs for preoperatively localized lesions sent to the pathologist should be > 90%.

The malignant-to-benign ratio in our practice is better than 4 : 1 owing to our policy of confirming diagnoses by preoperative interventional procedures.

## Specimen Radiography of Clinically Occult Lesions

When calcifications are removed from the breast, the surgical specimen should be radiographed during the operation. The ideal solution would be to have a radiography machine in the operating suite. Cabinet radiography systems were once available for specimen radiography (Faxitron), but unfortunately they have largely been abandoned due to high costs. It is necessary, then, to take the

**Fig. 5.158 Microcalcifications and specimen radiography in a 68-year-old woman with confirmed DCIS in the lower inner quadrant of the left breast** (see also **Fig. 4.23**, p. 46). Preoperative localization of the calcifications is performed under digital stereotactic guidance. The margins of the calcification cluster are marked so that the surgeon can see the approximate extent of the resection. With DCIS, it is dangerous to cut too close to the calcification margins. The optimum safety zone is 10 mm. In the case illustrated, breast conservation was not an option because numerous additional uncalcified DCIS foci and a small invasive ductal carcinoma were also found in the breast.

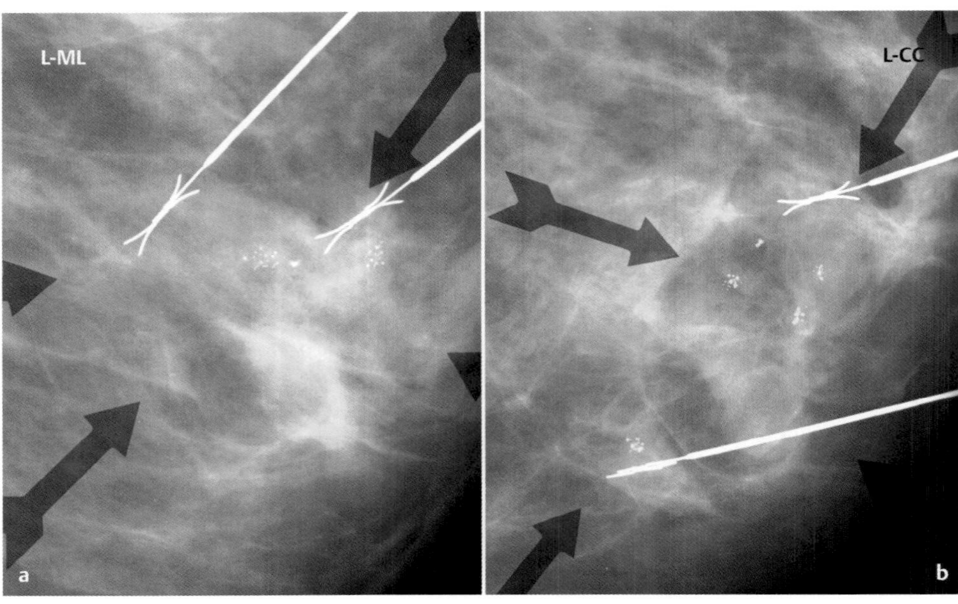


**a** *Mediolateral mammogram* after localization (caudal magnified view). Two hookwires have been placed to mark the approximate margins of the calcification cluster. The dark arrows indicate the area targeted for excision.
**b** *Preoperative craniocaudal mammogram* (magnified view). The calcification margins have been localized in the region of the left inner lower quadrant. The hookwires have been placed approximately 5 mm from the calcifications (dark arrows as explained in **a**).

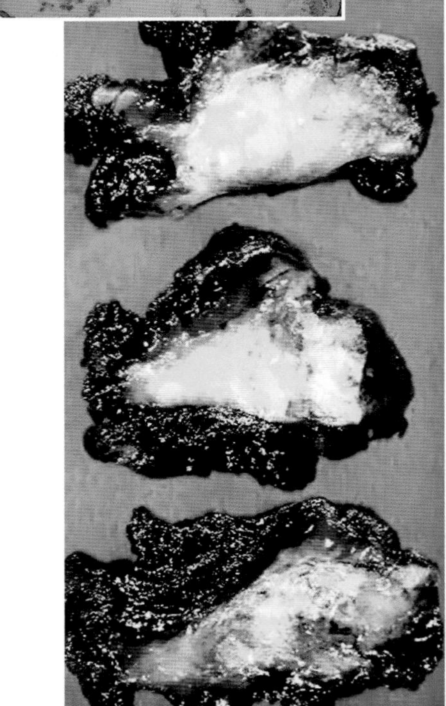

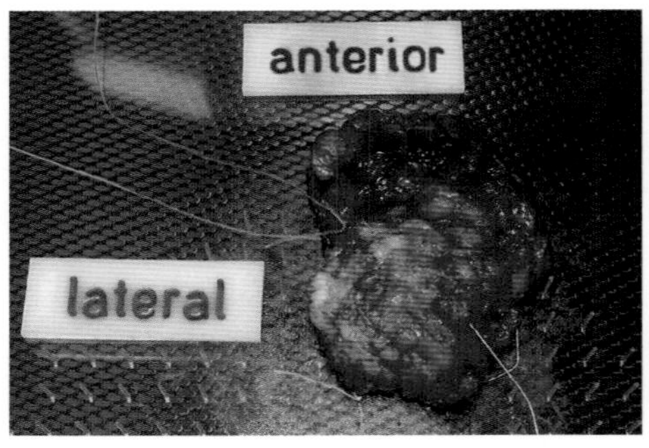


**c** *Surgical specimen* in a Plexiglas breast phantom. The superior wire is short, the lateral wire is long, and the anterior wire is of medium length. The specimen is positioned to match its anatomic orientation within the breast.

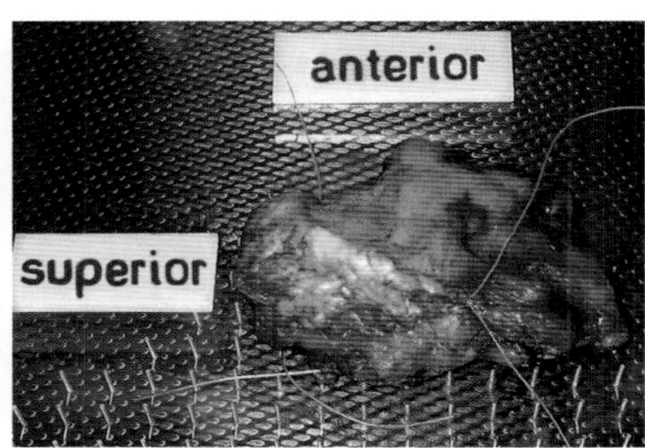


**d** Here the *surgical specimen* has been rotated 90° so that the short wire is pointing upward and the medium-length wire is pointing anteriorly.

**g** *India ink staining of biopsy material.* The *tissue samples* are dipped in India ink. The tissue surface takes up the black stain, making it easier to analyze the fine tissue structure in relation to the specimen surface. The distance from the surface of the nearest tumor focus to the stained surface is the *minimum healthy tissue margin* (upper left of specimen).

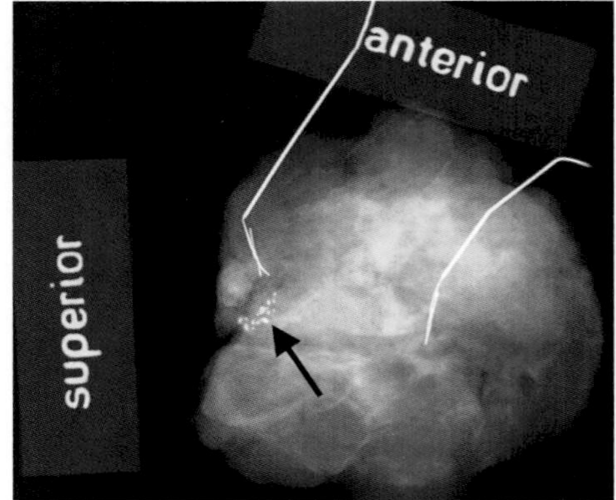


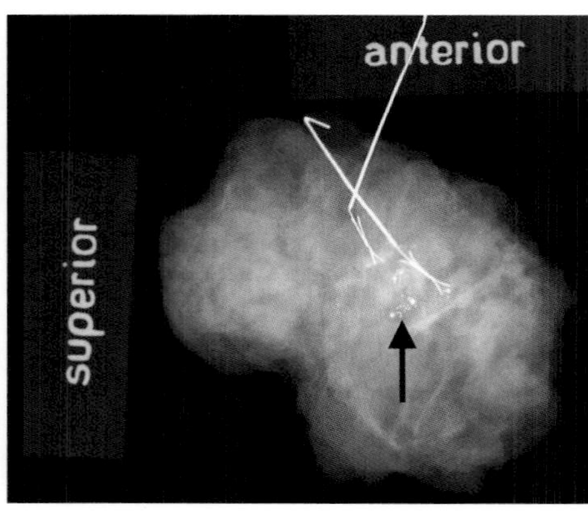


◀

**e** *Specimen radiograph* corresponding to **c**. The calcifications at the lateral edge of the specimen (arrow) show that the DCIS was not removed with clear margins, necessitating a lateral reexcision.

**f** With the *specimen* rotated 90°, the specimen radiograph displays the calcifications at the center of the tissue block (arrow). If this were the only projection taken, it would erroneously suggest that all calcifications had been removed.

excised tissue to radiology. Before the specimen is taken from the operating room, its superior (cranial), anterior and lateral margins must be marked and the specimen should be dipped in India ink (**Fig. 5.158**). Alliteration aids orientation: The **S**uperior localizing wire is **S**hort, the **A**nterior wire is **A**verage (medium) length, and the **L**ateral wire is **L**ong. The specimen is placed in a Plexiglas breast phantom at the same site and orientation as in the native breast, i.e., with the long wire in the virtual craniocaudal plane and the medium-length wire directed anteriorly. The short superior (cranial) wire points upward. The long wire is labeled with a "lateral" x-ray marker and the anterior wire with an "anterior" marker for subsequent radiographic orientation. The same is done in the virtual mediolateral view, labeling the short wire "superior" and the medium-length wire "anterior" (see **Fig. 5.158 c, d**). Each center has a modified system which allows the orientation about the margins of the removed tissue in projection to the entire breast.

The two radiographs in mutually perpendicular planes show precisely where any calcifications encroach upon a specimen margin and where the surgeon may need to excise additional tissue. It is obsolete to x-ray the specimen in only one plane without a breast phantom. A single projection without a phantom cannot uniquely identify the reexcision site based solely on the different lengths of the localization wires. Mutually perpendicular views also provide representative images that are useful for later follow-ups.

If the calcifications appear at the center of the specimen in both projections, no further action is needed. If the calcifications encroach on the specimen margin, the projections indicate the site where reexcision will be needed.

Another option is to mount the specimen on a styrofoam board over a drawing of the breast to indicate its intramammary location. The pectoral side is down, the anterior side is up. Because reexcision cannot be done on the pectoral or anterior sides, the pathologist and surgeon can concentrate on the cranial, medial, and lateral margins of the specimen.

The same method is used to radiograph the reexcision specimen if it contains calcifications and has been localized with wire markers. The technologist (or preferably the physician who performed the localization!) takes the specimen radiograph, original mammogram, and tissue specimen to the pathologist, who can use the radiographs to better appreciate the pathoanatomic relationships of the lesion.

The results of specimen radiography should be documented in writing, preferably in the report on preoperative localization. Frozen section histology is obsolete. Following specimen radiography, the material is embedded in paraffin blocks, paying particular attention to the tumor-free margin. The clear "safety zone" should be at least 10 mm for DCIS and 2 mm for invasive tumors. Safety zones have not been defined for ADH but should be the same as for DCIS. It would be prudent to take a specimen radiograph of the paraffin block or mount the specimen in sequential slices in their proper spatial orientation (as described in the Pathology Appendix to the S3 guidelines). In this way the pathologist can pick out the blocks that actually contain calcifications. The radiologist may mark the calcification site with a single needle to direct the pathologist and also provide a check in case calcifications are not found. Despite its value, however, paraffin block radiography will likely encounter resistance because of significant organizational problems.

Considerable friction may occur at the logistical interfaces between preoperative localization, surgery, specimen radiography, and histologic analysis within a hospital, and individual team members may lose a great deal of time due to unnecessary waiting. All team members should strive to carry out their tasks as quickly as possible.

An efficient routine might run as follows:

- Fifteen minutes before the start the operation, the surgeon informs the radiologist that the marked specimen will be radiographed.
- The radiologist informs his technologist, who prepares the radiography machine and plastic phantom and waits for the specimen (the order of the first two points may be reversed; this can be decided on an individual basis).
- An assistant takes the surgical specimen from the operating suite to radiology. He or she should know where the radiologist is! It is not uncommon for "rookies" to mistakenly take the specimen directly to pathology or some other department.
- The radiologic technologist or physician's assistant mounts and orients the surgical specimen on the breast phantom or styrofoam board as described above and takes a craniocaudal and lateral projection. She takes these images to the physician who performed the localization (if the physician still present, which is not always the case), who calls the operating room and reports the finding (the phone number of the operating room must be indicated on the pathology form if different rooms are used). If calcifications are found at the edge of the specimen, the surgeon can perform a targeted reexcision during the same anesthesia.
- The radiologist or technologist goes to the pathologist and indicates the precise location of the calcifications based on the phantom grid or localizing needle.
- When a definitive histologic diagnosis has been made, all involved parties attend a general postoperative case conference to check the plausibility of the findings, i.e., whether the removed lesion or calcifications are consistent with the changes seen at mammography, MRI, and/or ultrasound. This conference should be scheduled as soon as possible so that any necessary additional radiographs or reexcisions can be performed while the patient is still in the hospital.

## Sentinel Lymph Node Biopsy (SLNB)

*B. Koellner*

The sentinel lymph node procedure can reduce the invasiveness of breast cancer surgery, especially in the axillary region. The goal is to minimize the extent of axillary dissection to prevent postoperative arm edema (**Fig. 5.159**). Basically the sentinel lymph node is identified by scintigraphy, *also* marked with dye, and removed. If the sentinel lymph node is free of cancer, no additional axillary surgery is needed. If the sentinel node is positive, a standard level II axillary dissection with at least 10 lymph nodes is performed.

Localization of the sentinel lymph node is done approximately at the same time as preoperative localization of the breast tumor, and this should be coordinated by the nuclear medicine and radiology staff. We complete preoperative localization before the sentinel node biopsy is done, as this lets the nuclear medicine physician know precisely where the tumor is located and the finger radiation dose is minimized for the physician who performs the preoperative localization (Meades et al 2009).

**Fig. 5.159 Arm edema in a 60-year-old woman** 8 years after a radical axillary dissection on the left side (see also **Fig. 1.2 b**, p. 5). The edema is most pronounced in the forearm. Despite treatment with a compression stocking, the patient had very severe complaints.

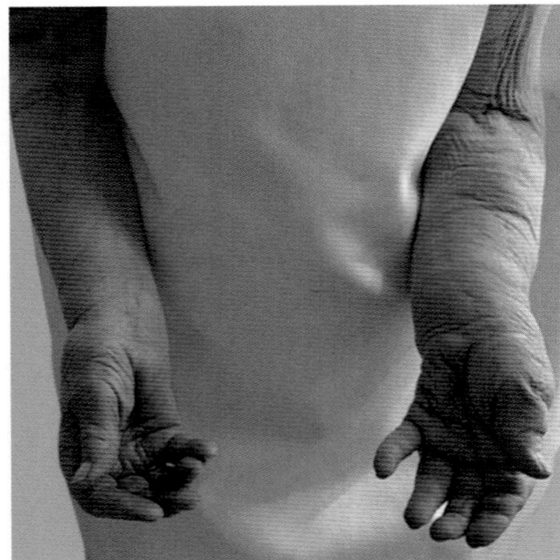

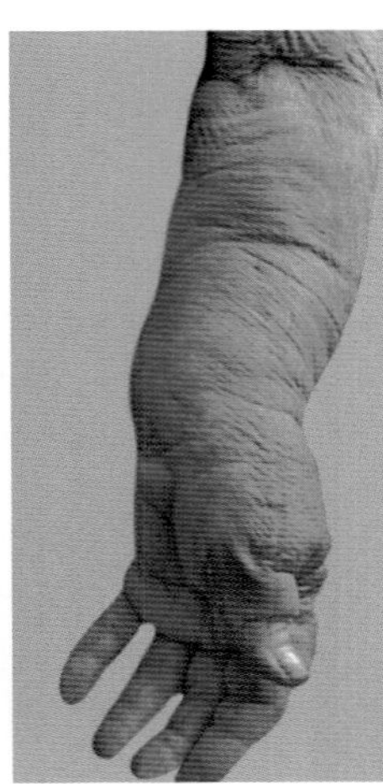

The optimum solution in selected cases would be to inject the radiotracer directly through the introducer needle before placing the peritumoral hookwire, but this requires very close teamwork within the breast center.

### Principle

As early as 1977 efforts were made to detect and localize lymphogenous metastasis of malignant melanoma by injecting patent blue dye at the periphery of the tumor. This procedure had a high false-negative rate, however. It was soon followed by the development of small gamma probes that could be used intraoperatively to detect the accumulation of radiolabeled colloid in lymph nodes (see **Fig. 5.160**).

In cases of invasive breast cancer (or occasional extensive DCIS), surgical treatment consists of removing the tumor with maximum breast conservation and performing an adequate axillary lymph node dissection. The reason for extending the operation into the axilla is to histologically confirm or exclude nodal metastasis and achieve local tumor control, which are important factors in the planning of postoperative care.

The larger the operative field, the more serious the postoperative sequelae may be. One-third of all patients who undergo axillary dissection experience problems such as:

- Impaired venous or lymphatic drainage from the ipsilateral arm, leading to lymphedema (see **Fig. 5.159**)
- Nerve damage resulting in sensorimotor deficits (strength loss, limitation of motion)
- Limitation of motion due to adhesions.

> **!** **The sentinel lymph node is the first lymph node to receive lymphatic drainage from a breast tumor (see Fig. 5.184 j, p. 408) Consequently, it is the most likely site for initial metastasis to occur.**

The combined use of radiolabeled colloid and patent blue dye can provide accurate scintigraphic and visual localization of the sentinel lymph node (SLN). When the identified SLN has been analyzed by modern histologic and histochemical methods, tumor involvement can be confirmed or excluded with 90% confidence. Today, **lymph node staging** can be accomplished with a simple **minimally invasive biopsy**. Data from a number of recent studies in several thousand patients have shed light on the rate of axillary recurrence following SLN biopsy alone (Smidt 2005; Palesty 2006). These data consistently show that fewer than 1% of patients develop clinically apparent axillary lymph node metastasis after SLN biopsy without axillary dissection.

When a negative SLN biopsy is obtained in a patient with breast cancer, staging by axillary dissection may be omitted when certain exclusionary criteria are met, including:

- An early tumor stage: pT1–2 (tumor smaller than 5 cm)
- No definite axillary involvement (by palpation or ultrasound)
- No scars in the breast (previous operations, biopsies) that compromise lymphatic drainage
- Multifocal tumors less than 3 cm apart
- Preoperative confirmation by FNA, CNB, or VB

### Technique of Sentinel Lymph Node Scintigraphy

The basic steps are as follows:

- Informed consent is secured.
- The radiotracer consists of $^{99m}$Tc-labeled nanocolloid (human serum albumin with a particle size < 80 nm) with an activity of approximately 20–30 MBq per injection. The gamma camera requires a LEHR (low-energy high-resolution) collimator with a 256 × 1024 matrix. A gamma probe with a single-hole collimator is used in the operating room and in the nuclear medicine department. This provides an approximately 1–2.5 cm field of view at a tissue depth of 2 cm and can detect separate lymph nodes located 5 cm from the injection site. The probe requires a narrow energy window and good handling ability (Schlag 2001). We use the device made by Neoprobe Corporation (Neo 2000; model 2100), which is equipped with a CdZnTe crystal (**Fig. 5.160**). This probe has a reusable 14 mm detector head with collimator. Sterile transparent sheaths are available for operating room use. Cordless detectors have also become available. Thin lead shields (rolled to 2 mm thickness) are also needed to mask the intense activity at the injection site.
- **Injection:** The tracer is injected interstitially and subdermally at the periphery of the tumor or into the subareolar region of the affected quadrant (occasionally both). Experience has shown that tracer administered by subareolar injection is transported very efficiently via the subareolar lymphatic plexus to the ipsilateral axillary lymph nodes. Deep, intramammary, and mediastinal lymph nodes are rarely visualized by scintigraphy. But a deep peritumoral injection or direct intratumoral injection is more likely to define intramammary and mediastinal lymph nodes via transpectoral lymphatics. Individual circumstances will determine the specific injection technique (**Fig. 5.161**). Skin contamination with $^{99m}$Tc-labeled nanocolloid should be scrupulously avoided. Gentle stroke massaging of the injection site will expedite lymphatic drainage (which is generally stimulated by heat and inhibited by cold).

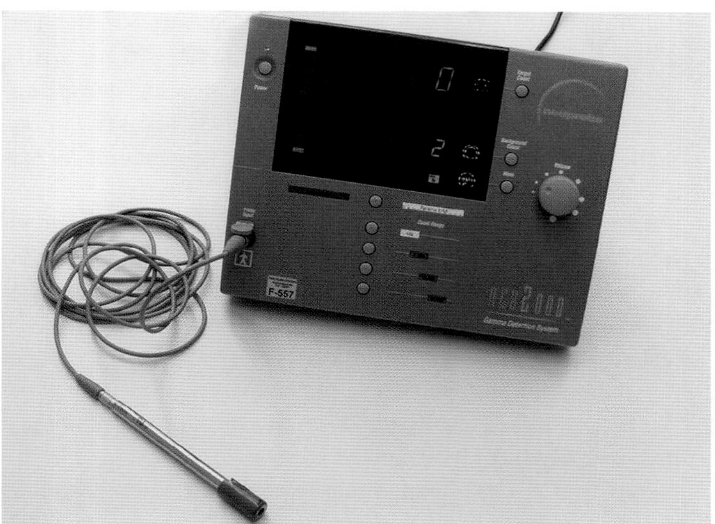

**Fig. 5.160 Gamma probe for sentinel lymph node (SLN) identification,** manufactured by Neoprobe Corp. (Neo 2000, model 2100).

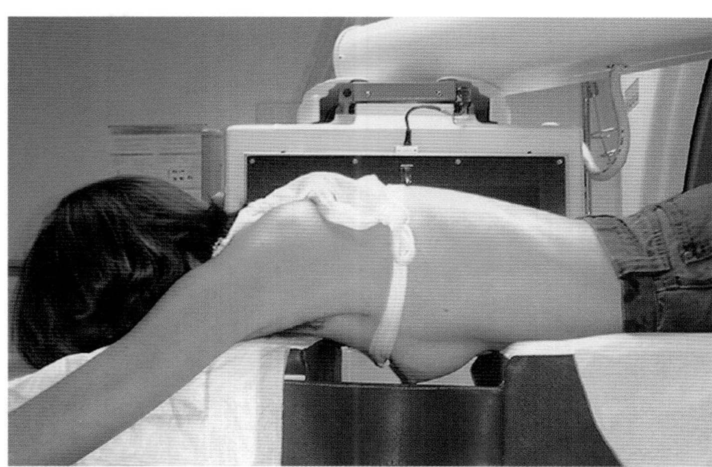

**Fig. 5.162 Sentinel lymph node scintigraphy with a gamma camera.** For lateromedial scanning (see **Fig. 5.164**), the patient lies prone next to the camera detector head.

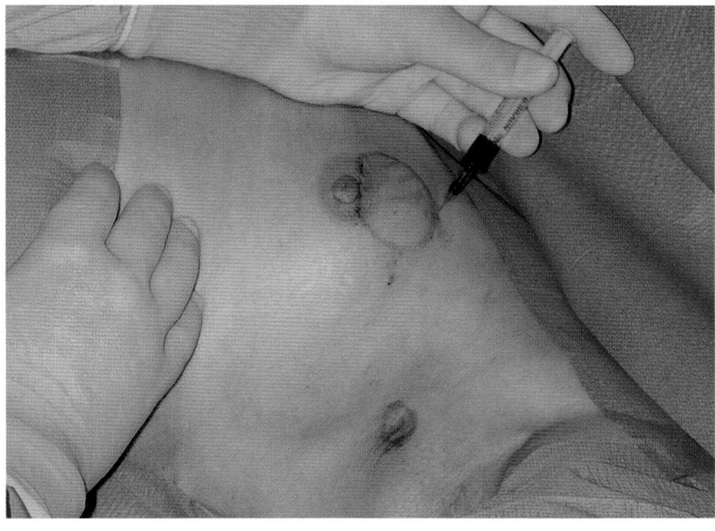

**Fig. 5.161 Supra-areolar injection of patent blue dye.** Injection of the radiotracer in the nuclear medicine department (see skin marking) is followed by the peritumoral injection of patent blue dye. The location of the SLN has been marked on the axillary skin at **c/12**.

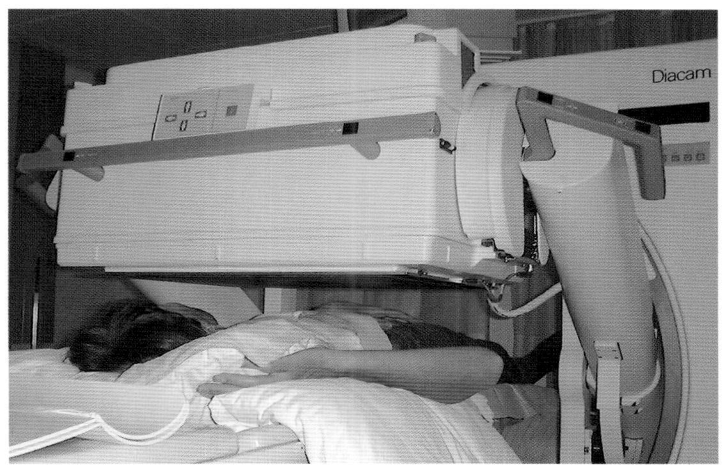


**Fig. 5.163 For anterior scanning of the SLN** (see **Fig. 5.165**), the patient lies supine beneath the detector head.

- **Scanning:** At our institution, the first **gamma camera scans** are taken in the anterior and lateral projections 2–3 hours after radiotracer injection. Scanning may be repeated the next day immediately before the operation.
  - Lateral projection: For the lateral projection, the patient lies prone with the breasts hanging through an aperture in the table to that the breast tissue will not obscure the lymph nodes during the acquisition (**Fig. 5.162**). The arms are extended toward the head of the table. With a point source in the axilla, care should be taken that the axilla is within the camera field of view before image acquisition is begun.
  - Anterior projection: For this projection the patient lies supine with the breast drawn slightly forward and downward with a cloth. The injection site, axilla, sternum, and clavicle should be within the camera field of view (**Fig. 5.163**).

*Tips and Tricks*

- For initial scanning at 2–3 hours postinjection, the first acquisition should be a "fast" (10-second) scan *without* lead shielding of the injection site, followed by a second, 10-minute scan in the same position *with* lead shielding.
- Print out and compare both scans to determine whether a hot spot corresponds to the unshielded injection site or a SLN, especially when the SLN is located close to the injection site (**Figs. 5.164, 5.165**). A slab phantom can be placed behind the patient to outline the body contours (**Fig. 5.167**).
- The injection site should be shielded for immediate preoperative scanning on the following day. The acquisition time for each projection is 10 minutes (**Fig. 5.166**).
- Direct shielding of the injection site with lead prevents flare effects that could obscure faint tracer uptake by the SLN (which accumulates no more than 1% of the administered activity).

**Fig. 5.164 Lateral SLN scan at 3 hours postinjection.** Left image: without lead shielding of the injection site; right image: with lead shielding.

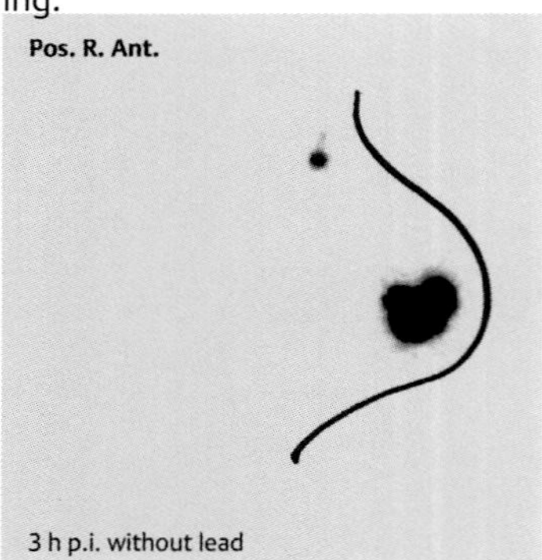


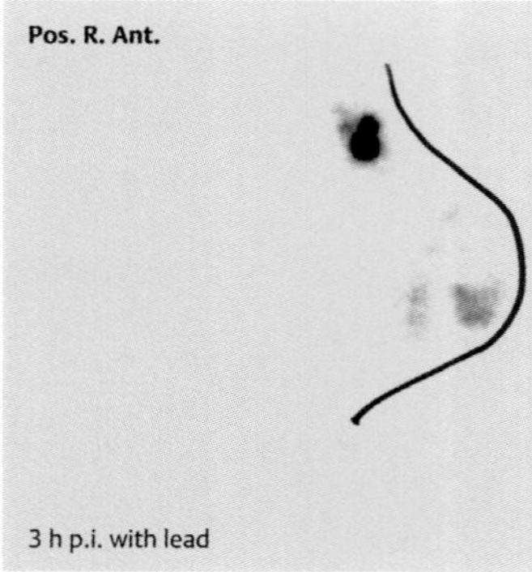


**Fig. 5.165 Anterior SLN scan at 3 hours postinjection.** Left image: without lead shielding of the injection site; right image: with lead shielding.

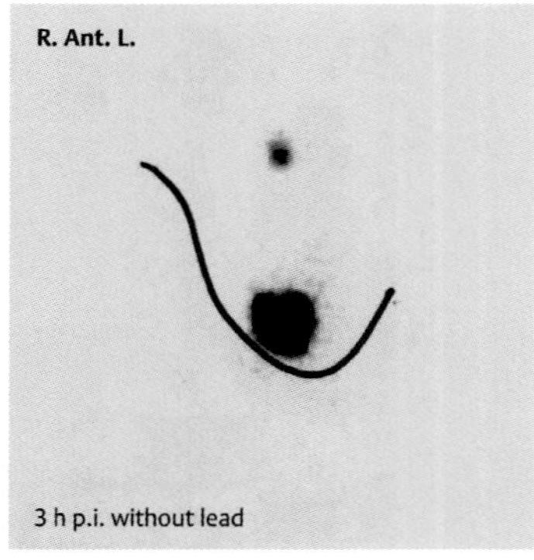


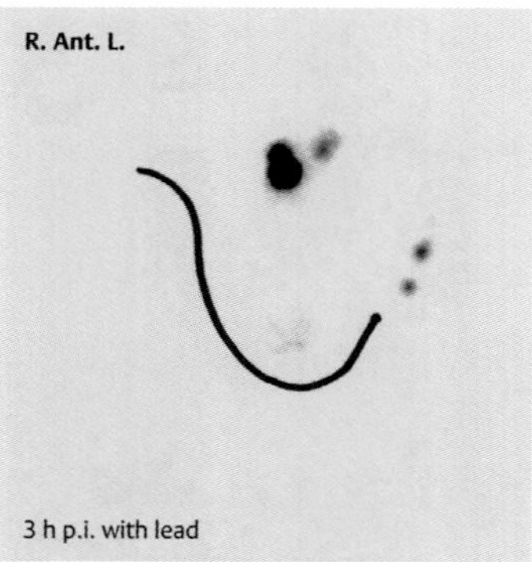


**Fig. 5.166 Immediate preoperative scintiscans** (taken the following day).

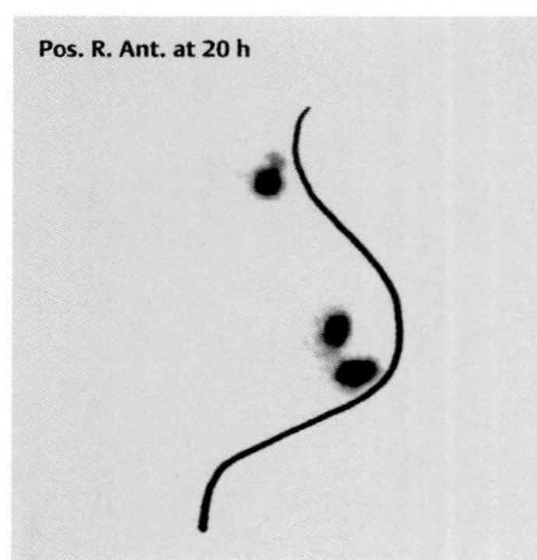


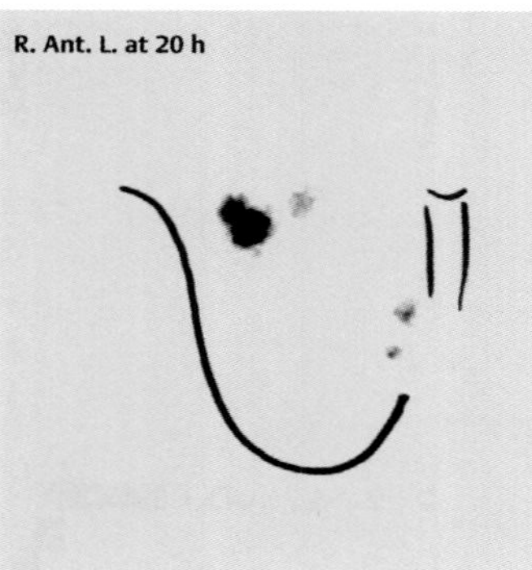


- Aided by a point source, the SLN is identified with the gamma camera and gamma probe no later than 20 hours postinjection, and its location is marked on the skin (see **Fig. 5.161**). The surgeon can mark the SLN in the operating room, or this may be done jointly with the nuclear medicine physician. Mapping a lymphatic pathway may lead to a lymph node that is completely permeated by tumor, and the map should be indicated on the skin. The nuclear medicine report should include the location and number of detected lymph nodes and lymphatics. The tumor is removed first (greatest uptake), followed by the SLN. This order can be reversed to save time, sending the removed sentinel node to pathology while the tumor is being excised.
- For visual identification of the lymphatic pathways (to guide the surgeon), patent blue dye is also injected in the operating room. Dye administered by segmental or subareolar quadrant injection will drain within minutes, producing a visible map of the lymphatics that will aid in planning the incision site (see **Fig. 5.161**). The combination of radiotracer and dye localization allows positive identification of the SLN in more than 98% of cases (our statistics agree with those in the literature). No standards for SLN identification are given in the S3 guidelines.
- All lymph nodes that have been removed should be checked for radioactivity before leaving the operating room. Residual activity is also tested in the operating suite. The activity count and location of the SLNs (level I, level II, and others) and the residual activity in the axilla should be documented. Finally, the number of scintigraphically detected SLNs should be checked against the number of SLNs actually removed. We recommend defining a maximum of three lymph nodes as SLNs.
- Kennedy et al. (2003) found that removing the first three SLNs was 98% accurate in detecting a positive lymph node status. Additional detectable lymph nodes are limited by the count ratio. Lymph nodes that have only one-third activity of the nodes with the greatest uptake in vivo are no longer classified as SLNs and are not removed. Interventional recommendations consistently advise against looking for extra-axillary SLNs because of the potentially greater morbidity (Goldhirsch 2003; Schwartz et al. 2002). Subsequent frozen section histology will determine the need for axillary dissection.

### Sources of Error

The main sources of error are as follows:

- The injection site is too close to the SLN (e.g., tumors near the axilla). In this case no tracer should be injected into the subareolar region of the affected quadrant, and none should be injected cranially to the tumor.
- Tracer contamination of the skin surface. The connection between the needle and syringe must be secure and leakproof. Any activity dripping onto the skin could mimic a SLN during scanning.
- Impaired lymphatic drainage due, for example, to cold (cooling a hematoma after vacuum biopsy or core biopsy), previous surgery or radiotherapy, or lymphatic obstruction by the tumor. This would contraindicate radiolocalization.
- Missing the SLN because the gamma camera field or view does not cover all axillary nodes and lymphatics.
- False-negative SLN biopsy.

Reports in the literature show that when lymph nodes declared negative by frozen section are later examined histologically in paraffin-embedded sections using standard staining methods and immunohistochemical analysis, an incidence of lymph node metastasis up to 5% is found. If lymph node involvement is not detected until after the operation, the patient may be referred for axillary dissection or radiotherapy.

*False-negative findings* may also result from failure to remove affected lymph nodes outside the axilla, such as supraclavicular lymph nodes, deep lymph nodes, and lymph nodes at unusual sites (Gordon et al. 2001).

## Safety Aspects

### *Radiation Dose to Personnel*

The radiation dose to technologists, surgeons, operating room staff, nurses, and cleaning staff is extremely low. The authors of the Consensus Conference state that even pregnant women are not at significant risk. Schlag (2001) offered the following dose estimates: Following the peritumoral injection of 160 MBq of $^{99m}$Tc-labeled nanocolloid, a surgeon standing 0.5 meters from the patient for 20 minutes will receive approximately 0.4 µSv of radiation. The operating room staff and anesthesiologist will receive approximately 0.4 µSv, and the pathologist will receive approximately 0.3 µSv over a period of 10–30 minutes. Thus, the radiation dose to operating room personnel and pathologist is well below the safe dose limit of 1 mSv/year, indicating an absence of significant radiation exposure. (More than 2000 operations a year would have to be performed to reach the dose limit!)

### *Radiation Dose to the Patient*

The whole-body dose for a SLN biopsy is approximately 0.4 mSv, comparable to that in two-view mammography. The injection site receives a dose of approximately 960 mGy, while the injected breast receives 115 mGy (very low) (Schlag 2001).

### *Radioactive Waste in the Operating Room and Pathology*

Radioactive waste and refuse in the operating room and pathology laboratory should be stored in a secure location until the radioactivity decays below the safe limit. Usually this takes 10 half-lives, or approximately 60 hours. Residual waste from pathology should be stored in the nuclear medicine department until its activity has fallen to safe levels.

### *Allergies and Cross-Reactions*

Technetium nanocolloid is generally well tolerated. To date the author and his colleagues have not encountered any allergic reactions to this colloid, although they are possible in theory.

Most reports in the literature have described allergic reactions to the injection of patent blue dye (with a fatal outcome in one case).

**Tip**

**Patent blue dye should not be used in patients who cannot tolerate blue dye in cosmetic products.**

No cross-reactions are known to occur between $^{99m}$Tc-labeled nanocolloid and patent blue dye.

### *Postoperative Complications*

Postoperative complications are less common than after axillary dissection and drainage. As a rule, patients who undergo breast-conserving surgery with SLN biopsy can begin physical exercises earlier due to axillary preservation, and chemotherapy and/or radiotherapy can be initiated at an earlier date.

## Contraindications

Contraindications to the SLN procedure are as follows:

- **Known axillary involvement.** If there is reason to suspect axillary involvement, FNA or CNB may be a useful aid to preoperative decision making. If FNA and CNB are negative, SLN scintigraphy may be performed.
- **Acute hematoma following core biopsy.** This condition is managed by local compression and cooling. SLN scintigraphy would be unsuccessful in the presence of acute hematoma.
- **Multifocal disease.** SLN biopsy is unreliable in cases where tumors are present in multiple quadrants and are located more than 2–3 cm apart.
- **Local tumor spread with lymph node involvement.** In this case SLN biopsy should be done only in an investigational setting after neoadjuvant therapy.
- Previous axillary dissection, previous breast augmentation with incision of the axilla, and previous lymph node biopsy are relative contraindications to SLN biopsy (Gordon et al. 2001).

**Previous reduction mammoplasty** is a relative contraindication. It is essential to have unobstructed lymphatic drainage between the tumor and lymph node. Reduction mammoplasty is not a contraindication in patients with a tumor in the upper outer quadrant.

## Results

Minimally invasive surgery with SLN scintigraphy provides **accurate tumor staging** because the pathologist receives only the lymph nodes that are most likely to be involved by tumor. Occasionally this may be the case with lymph nodes detected a short distance away from the presumed location.

The **lower postoperative morbidity** of SLN biopsy compared with axillary dissection and its greater diagnostic accuracy are important arguments for the SLN procedure. Suga et al. (2004) described lymphography with the interstitial administration of an oily radiographic contrast medium (lipoidol) as a possible alternative to nuclear medicine imaging of the SLN. These authors injected 2 mL of undiluted lipoidol at peritumoral and retroareolar sites, massaged the injection sites, and obtained multislice spiral CT scans of the breast and axilla 5 minutes later. The results were compared with SLN identification with patent blue dye. Negative lymph nodes and especially positive lymph nodes (which are not opacified by the injected medium) can be clearly identified and distinguished from one another by CT mapping with 3D reconstructions. Scintigraphy cannot identify metastatically involved lymph nodes.

Sentinel lymph node biopsy in skilled hands is a good **alternative to routine axillary dissection** (see **Fig. 5.168**). The St. Galen Consensus Conference in 2003 characterized the procedure as an acceptable method for the determination of nodal status. Controlled studies show that the SLN can be identified in up to 98% of cases and reflects axillary lymph node status in 95–97% of cases. To date we have had a SLN detection rate >98% at the IMZE breast center in more than 600 examinations.

Axillary lymph node metastasis is a rare occurrence following a negative SLN biopsy. We believe that surgeons who practice the procedure should participate in studies. We also feel that special attention should be given to the supra- and infraclavicular fossae during follow-up care (see **Fig. 5.184**, p. 335 and 407 f).

**Fig. 5.167 Sentinel lymph node scintigraphy.** A cobalt-57 slab phantom was placed behind the patient during scanning to outline the body contours. When the injection site is covered with lead, three lymph nodes in the right axilla show intense tracer uptake while two successive lymph nodes show faint uptake. The upper images are anterior projections; the lower images are right lateral projections.

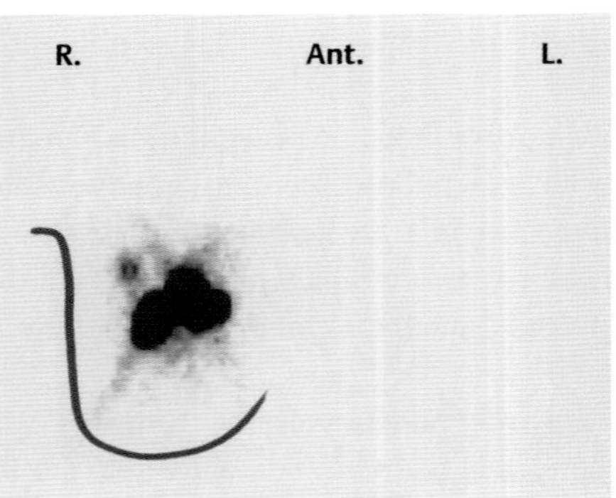


Without lead, 2.5 h p.i.

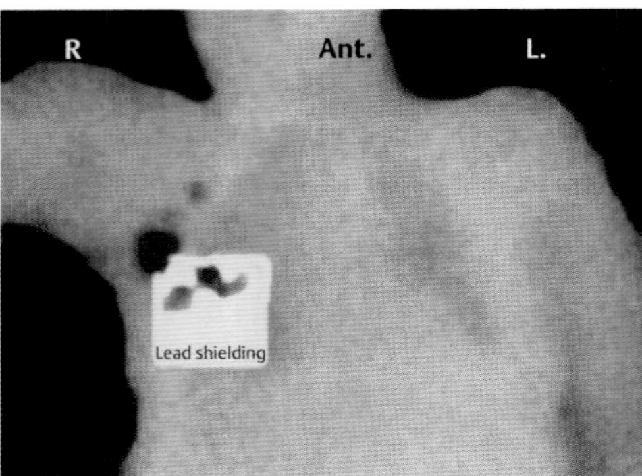


With lead, 2.5 h p.i.

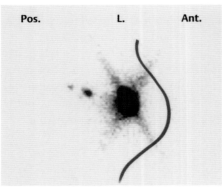

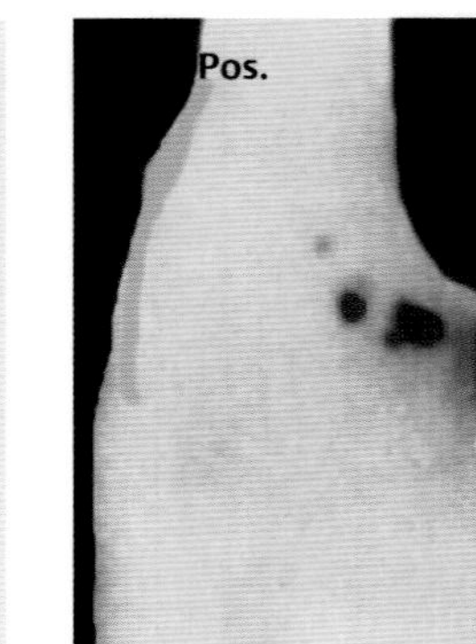


Without lead, 2.5 h p.i.

With lead, 2.5 h p.i.

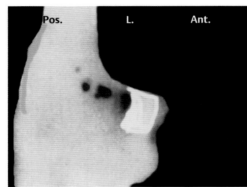

**Question 1 on Fig. 5.167**

*Do the scintiscans indicate a malignant process?*

(**a**) No
(**b**) Yes
(**c**) Indirectly

→ **Answer on p. 398**

**Question 2 on Fig. 5.167**

*If a positive sentinel lymph node is found, a left axillary dissection should be performed to what level?*

(**a**) Level I
(**b**) Level II
(**c**) Level III

→ **Answer on p. 398**

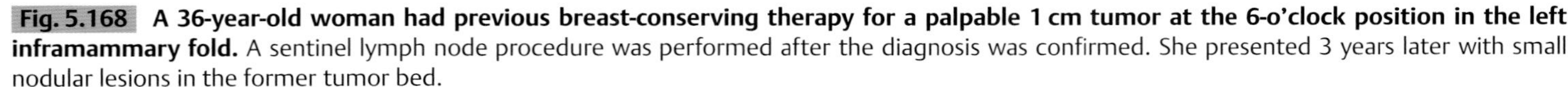

**Fig. 5.168 A 36-year-old woman had previous breast-conserving therapy for a palpable 1 cm tumor at the 6-o'clock position in the left inframammary fold.** A sentinel lymph node procedure was performed after the diagnosis was confirmed. She presented 3 years later with small nodular lesions in the former tumor bed.

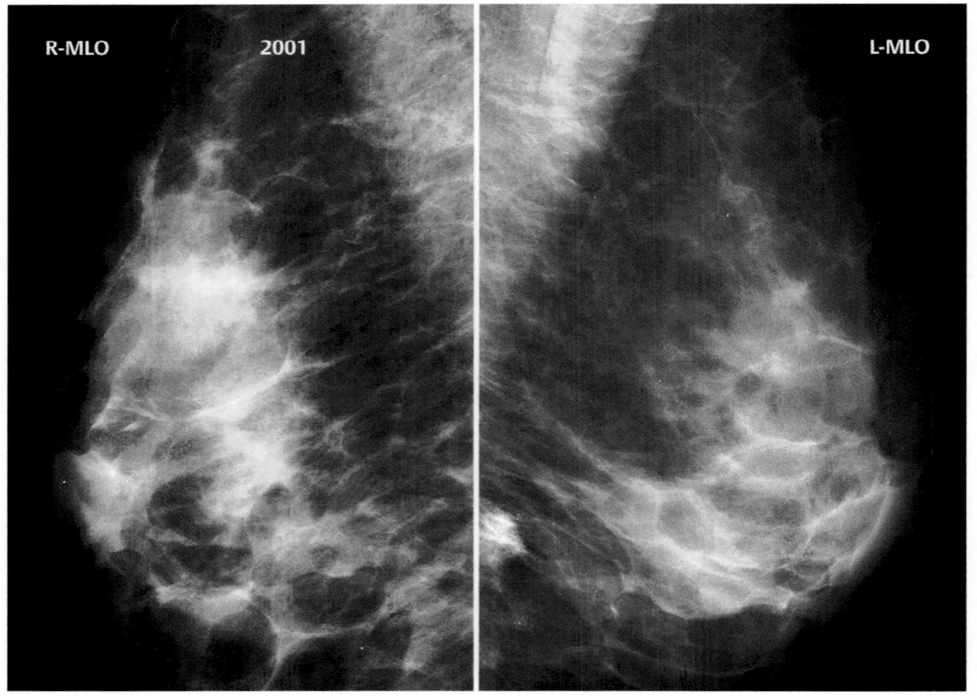


**a** *Bilateral oblique mammograms* in 2001 show moderately radiodense breasts with a well-circumscribed 1 cm nodule above the inframammary fold on the left side (**d/5–6**). Due to incomplete imaging of the inframammary fold, the posterior portion of the nodule is not fully visualized (ACR 2, BIRADS 4, PG**MI**).

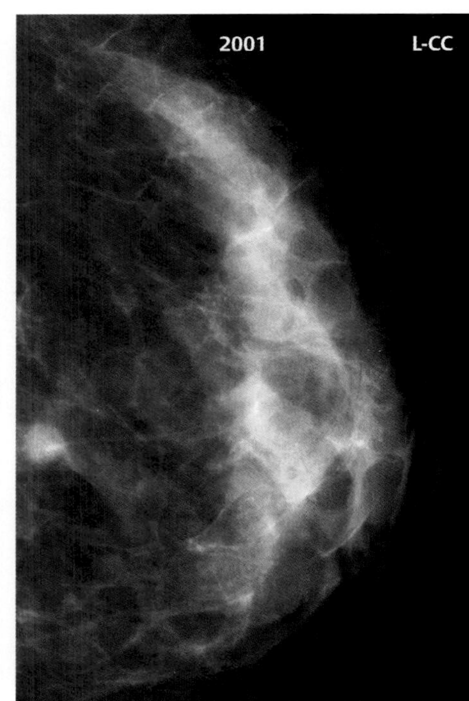


**b** *Craniocaudal mammogram* of the left breast in 2001 clearly demonstrates a 1 cm nodule with slightly irregular margins (**H/7**) (ACR 2, BIRADS 4, **P**GMI). Histology indicated a very cellular neoplasm.

**Fig. 5.168** **36-year-old woman, previous breast-conserving therapy for a palpable 1 cm tumor at the 6-o'clock position in the left inframammary fold.** *(continued)*

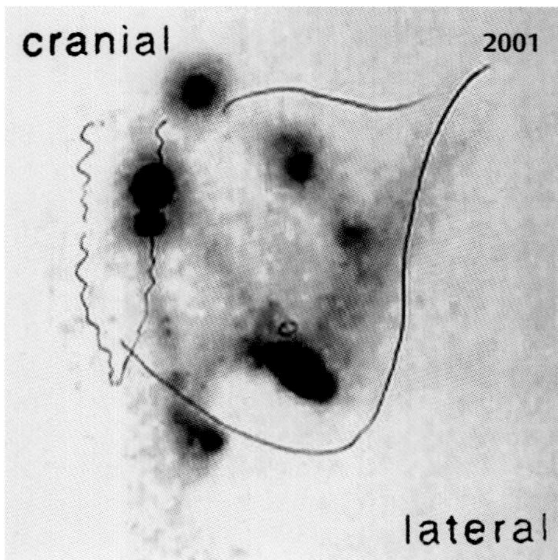


**c** *Sentinel lymph node* procedure on the left side in 2001. With a tumor in the inframammary fold, the scan shows uptake by retrosternal and clavicular lymph nodes without involvement of the left axilla.

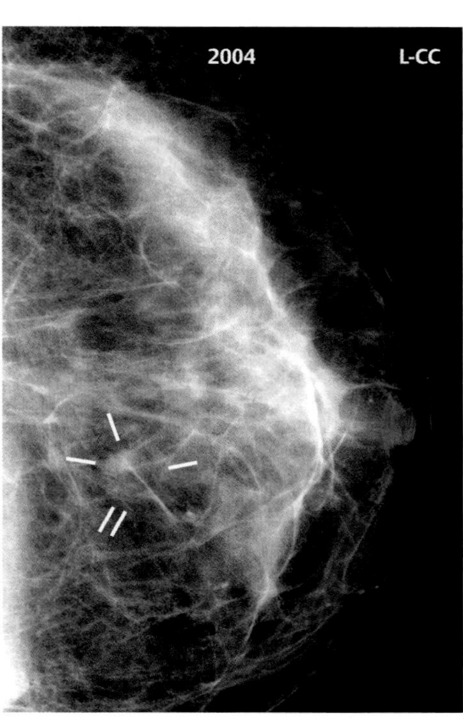


**d** *Craniocaudal mammogram* of the left breast in 2004 shows scar tissue 3 years after tumor removal and postoperative radiotherapy. A small nodular density is visible (see marker) near the primary tumor from 2001.

**Question on Fig. 5.168**

*What would be the most appropriate treatment if a malignant process is found?*

(**a**) Removal of the clavicular lymph nodes and radiotherapy over an additional sternal field

(**b**) Removal of the clavicular lymph nodes plus removal of the retrosternal lymph nodes via sternotomy

(**c**) Radiation to the axillary, clavicular, and retrosternal lymph nodes without axillary dissection

→ **Answer on p. 398**

If other lymph nodes located in close proximity to the SLN seem suspicious at operation due to their size or appearance, they should be removed along with the sentinel node and examined. If they are found to contain metastases, the SLN biopsy should not be classified as false-negative.

When the gamma camera and probe are used for preoperative localization and the gamma probe and patent blue dye are used intraoperatively, the rate of false-negative findings is less than 5%.

On the basis of the Consensus Conference held in Philadelphia in April, 2001 (Gordon et al. 2001) and later consensus conferences held until 2005 (Kühn 2005), which were attended by international experts in surgery, pathology, radiology, radiation oncology, nuclear medicine, and medical oncology and reflected the experience of several thousand SLN procedures, it was determined that the introduction of SLN biopsies at hospitals involves a **learning phase**. As soon as SLN biopsies show a 98% rate of agreement with concomitant axillary dissections performed in approximately 20–30 patients, it may be concluded that the learning phase is complete and SLN biopsy can be done as an alternative to axillary dissection.

> **!** **The SLN procedure can spare many women the significant morbidity of conventional axillary dissection, but success requires close cooperation among all involved disciplines—nuclear medicine, radiology, gynecology, surgery, and pathology.**

## Treatment-Related Reactions, Complications, and Errors

Even when the guidelines are taken into account and optimum interdepartmental links are established within a breast center, there are still typical treatment-related reactions and complications with which the breast diagnostician must be familiar. Examples are shown in this section. The illustrative cases are not limited to breast cancer operations, as any surgical procedure on the breast may cause changes that are sometimes difficult to interpret and require differentiation from a malignant process. Significant treatment errors should not happen in a certified breast center, but they do occur. The doctor–patient relationship is a central concern. The majority of lawsuits result from poor demeanor, arrogance on the part of the attending physician or staff, or disparaging comments made by treating physicians in reference to colleagues. Errors should never be swept under the carpet but must be discussed within the team in a manner that addresses and corrects their cause. Finger-pointing is useless and should be avoided. The smaller the circle of problem solvers, the more efficiently can solutions be devised (case conferences!).

Physicians who perform mammography must be familiar with treatment-related changes to avoid misinterpretations. Scars in particular are often mistaken for a local recurrence of breast cancer. MRI can differentiate scars from recurrent tumors, and intensely enhancing lesions can be investigated by digital stereotactic or ultrasound-guided CNB or preferably VB, which yields more material.

Whenever possible, treatment-related reactions and complications should be corrected promptly before any long-term morbidity can develop (arm edema, scarring, breast disfigurement, etc.).

The most common treatment errors are as follows:

- Removing a palpable or sonographically visible lesion without mammography and preoperative histologic confirmation (interventional procedures). Potential results: positive tumor margins, need for reexcision, second tumor in the clinically healthy breast (omission of preoperative MRI), and additional lesions in the treated breast (see **Fig. 5.144**, p. 283).
- Imprecise localization, causing residual tumor to be left in the breast (see **Fig. 5.176**, p. 324).
- Missed tumors due to disregard of mammographic or ultrasound findings and failure to localize atypical calcifications (see **Fig. 5.169**, p. 314 f).
- Metastatic surgery for curative intent without knowledge of the whole-body status (PET; see **Fig. 5.184**, p. 335).

**Figures 5.169–5.179** illustrate common but preventable complications and errors.

**Fig. 5.169 Treatment of breast carcinoma, postoperative changes, and localization problems** in a 42-year-old woman with three lesions (**1**) at the 12-o'clock position in the upper portion of the left breast, clustered microcalcifications (exclusion of DCIS) (**2**), and a 1.4 cm suspicious lesion (histology: mucinous carcinoma without axillary lymph node involvement) (**3**). The right breast contains a sonographic lesion 7 mm in diameter (**a**). The patient presents postoperatively with three scars in both breasts (**d**). Because histology of lesion (**1**) in **a** showed no microcalcifications, a new oblique view of the left breast is taken and both breasts are examined sonographically. Ultrasound still shows the lesion in the right breast, now accompanied by a scar located at the 3-o'clock position (**d**). The lesion was not marked preoperatively by image-guided localization, but was removed under "palpable guidance." The mucinous carcinoma in the left breast had originally been removed with clear margins. The nodule in the right breast could also be removed after sonographic localization. The SLN procedure was positive, detecting two sentinel nodes (**e**).

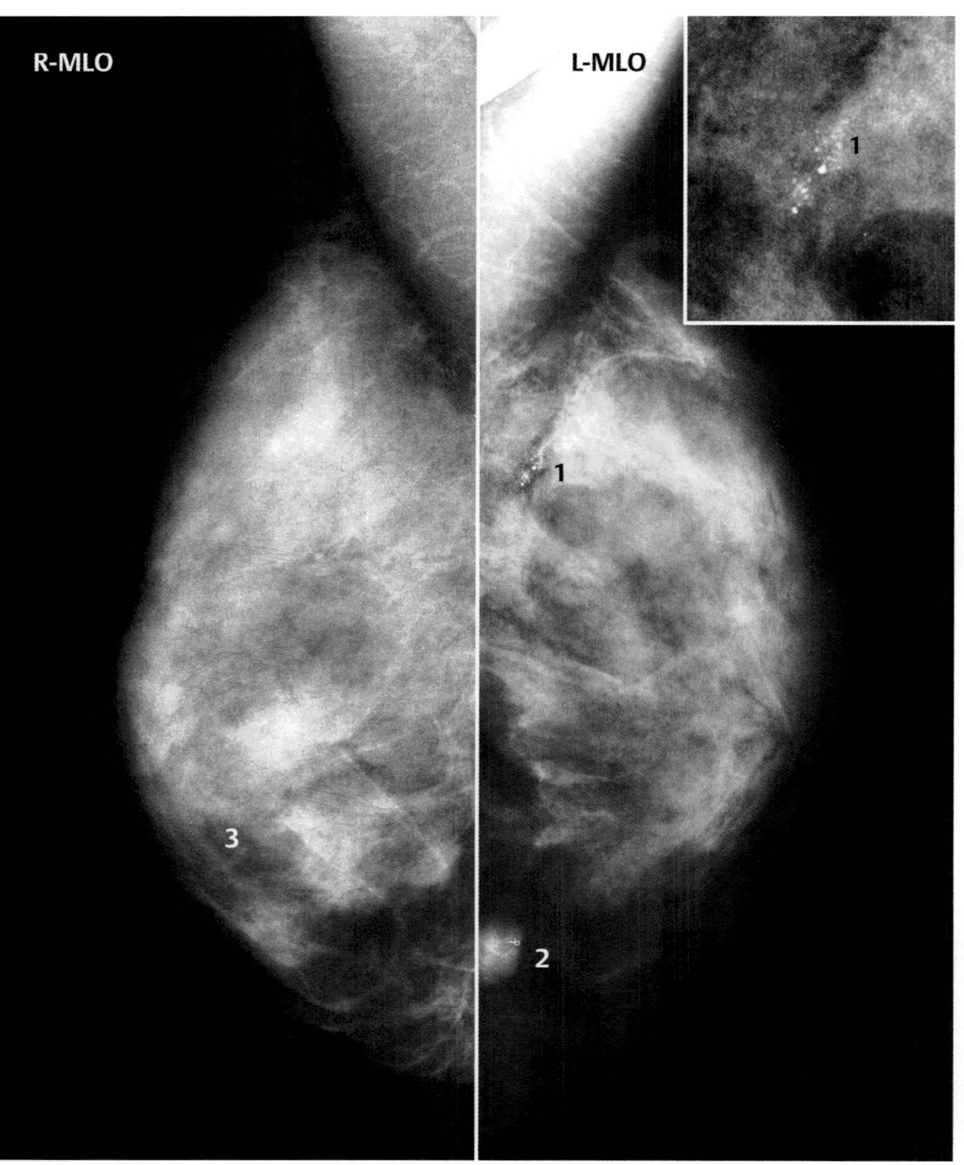


**a** *Bilateral oblique mammograms* (preoperative) show very radiodense breasts. A nodule with mixed smooth and scalloped margins is visible in the left inframammary fold (**2**), and clustered microcalcifications are visible in the upper portion of the breast at the 12-o'clock position (**1**).

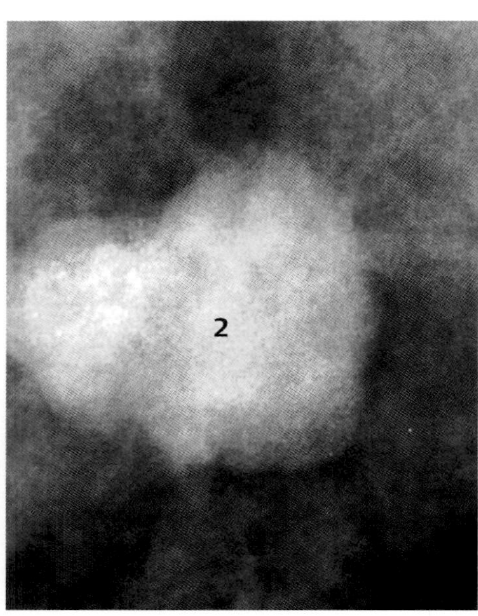


**b** *Oblique mammogram* of the left breast (magnified view) shows clustered microcalcifications next to fine punctate microcalcifications covering an area of 1 cm × 1 cm.

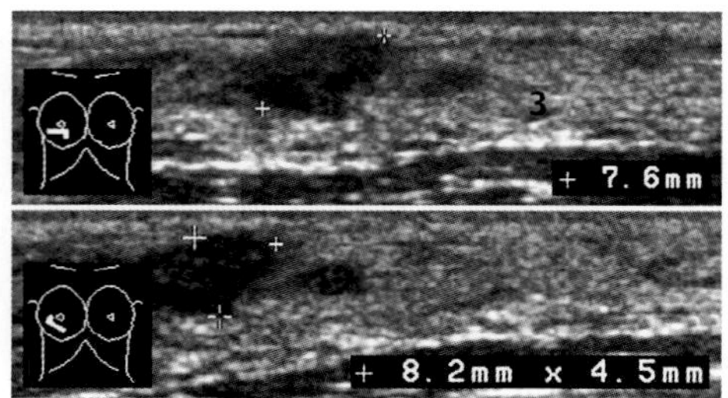


**c** *Sonograms* of the right breast show a 7 mm nodule with mixed smooth and ill-defined margins and no posterior acoustic enhancement (**3**).

**Fig. 5.169 Treatment of breast carcinoma, postoperative changes, and localization problems.** *(continued)*

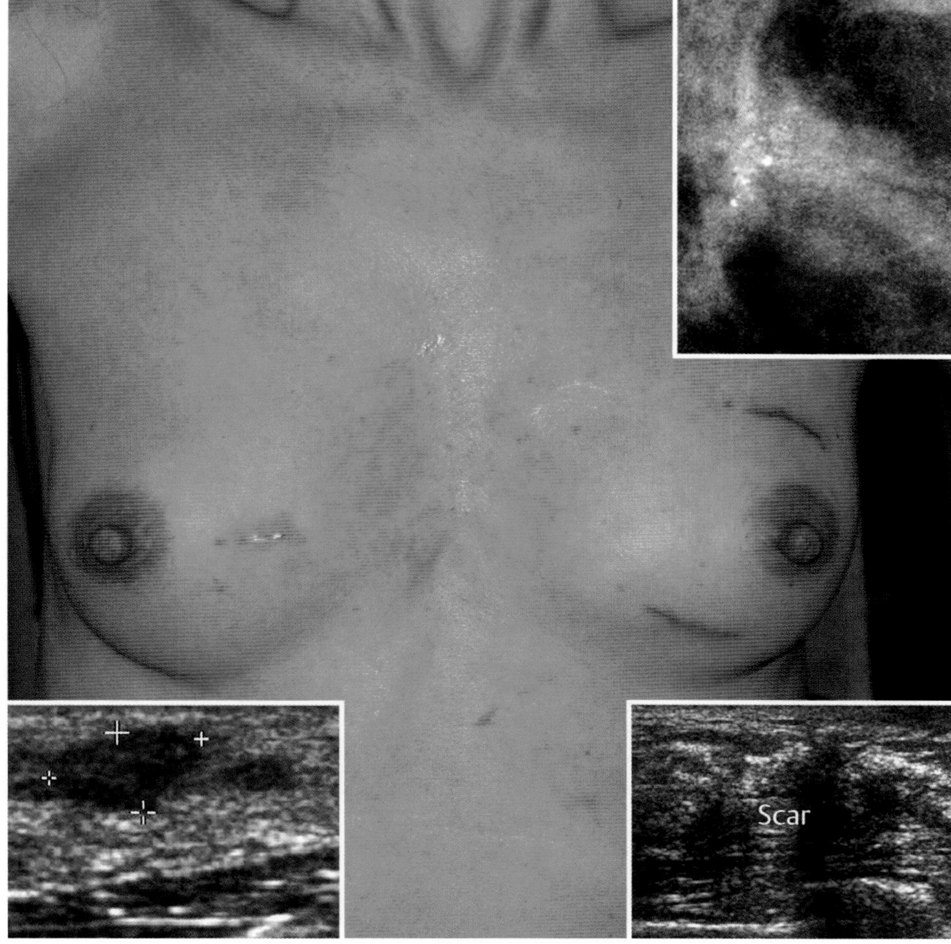


**d** *Clinical appearance* 4 weeks after surgery. Two scars are visible on the left breast and one on the right breast at the 3-o'clock position. Postoperative skin depression is noted at the site of the excised mucinous carcinoma in the *left* inframammary fold. The insets show the corresponding mammographic and sonographic changes at this time.

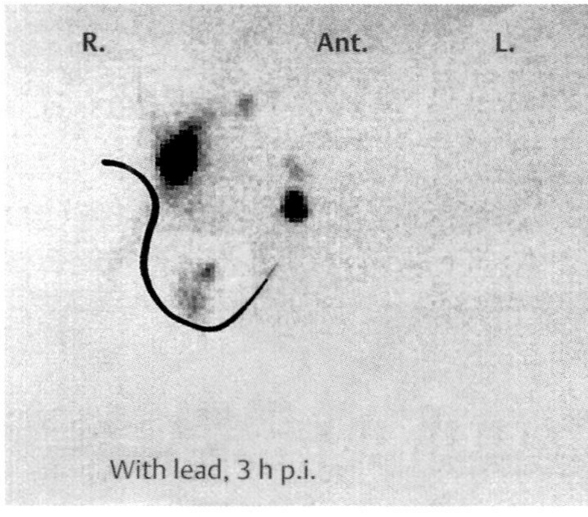


**e** *SLN examination* of the right breast, from which a well-differentiated (G1) tubular carcinoma 7 cm in diameter was finally removed.

**Question 1 on Fig. 5.169**

*Approximately what percentage of the microcalcifications in the upper portion of the left breast (**b**) were removed?*

(**a**) Up to 100%
(**b**) Up to 50%
(**c**) 0%

→ **Answer on p. 399**

**Question 2 on Fig. 5.169**

*Is the suspicious sonographic lesion in the right breast (histology: well-differentiated tubular carcinoma) located within the scarred area at the 3-o'clock position (compare panel **c**)?*

(**a**) Yes
(**b**) No
(**c**) Uncertain

→ **Answer on p. 399**

**Question 3 on Fig. 5.169**

*Two sentinel lymph nodes are visible in the scintiscan of the right breast. Which should be removed?*

(**a**) The axillary lymph node
(**b**) The axillary and sternal lymph nodes
(**c**) None

→ **Answer on p. 399**

**Fig. 5.170 Microcalcifications were removed from the left breast of a 74-year-old woman in 2000, with benign histology.** Mammograms in 2002 show ringlike lucencies in the left breast (**a, b**). Ultrasound shows fibrocystic changes in the right breast and an irregular hypoechoic lesion in the left breast (**e**).

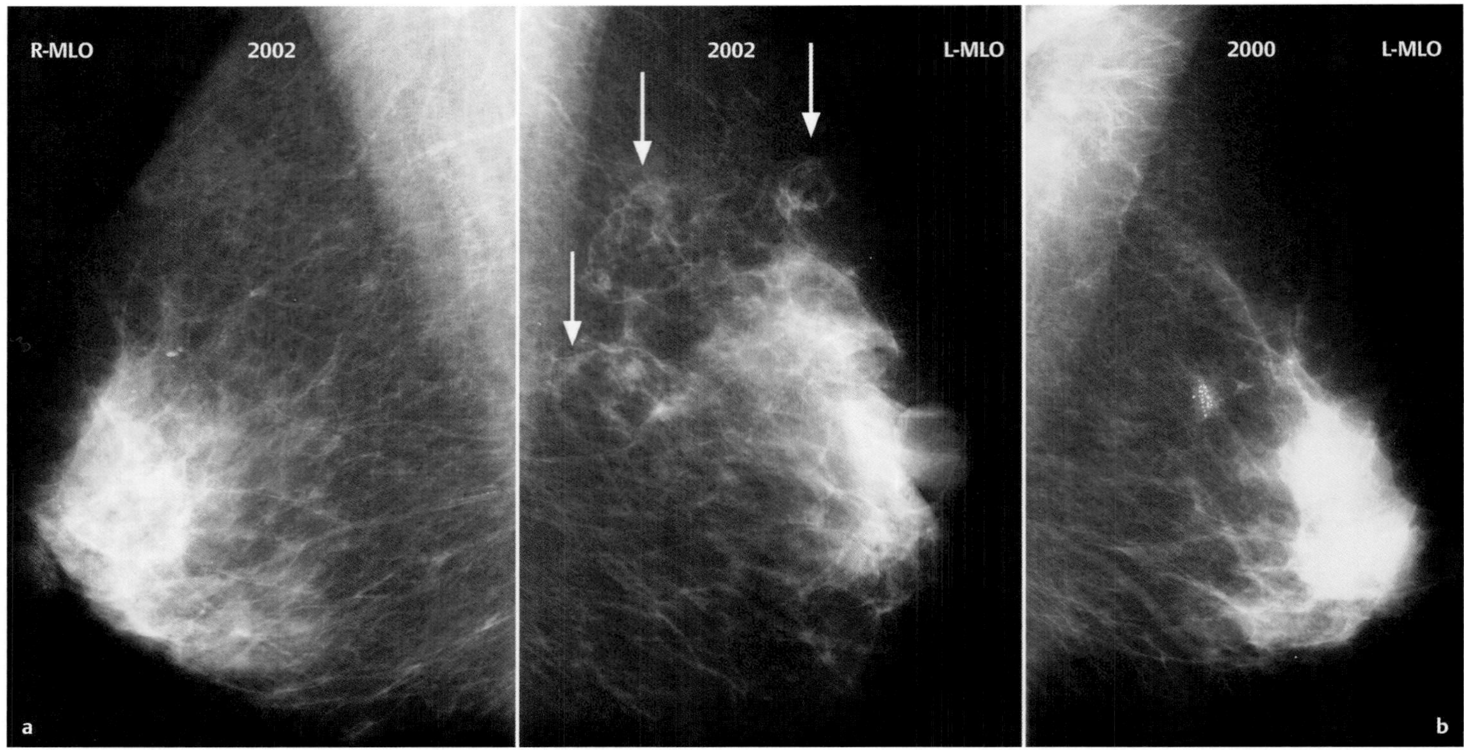


**a** *Bilateral oblique mammograms* in 2002 show scalloped lucencies in the upper outer quadrant of the left breast (arrows) with dense honeycomb-like borders. The right breast appears normal (ACR 3, BIRADS?, **P**GMI).

**b** *Preoperative oblique mammogram* of the left breast in 2000 shows a normal-appearing radiodense breast prior to calcification (**I/21**) removal (ACR 3, BIRADS 4, P**G**MI).

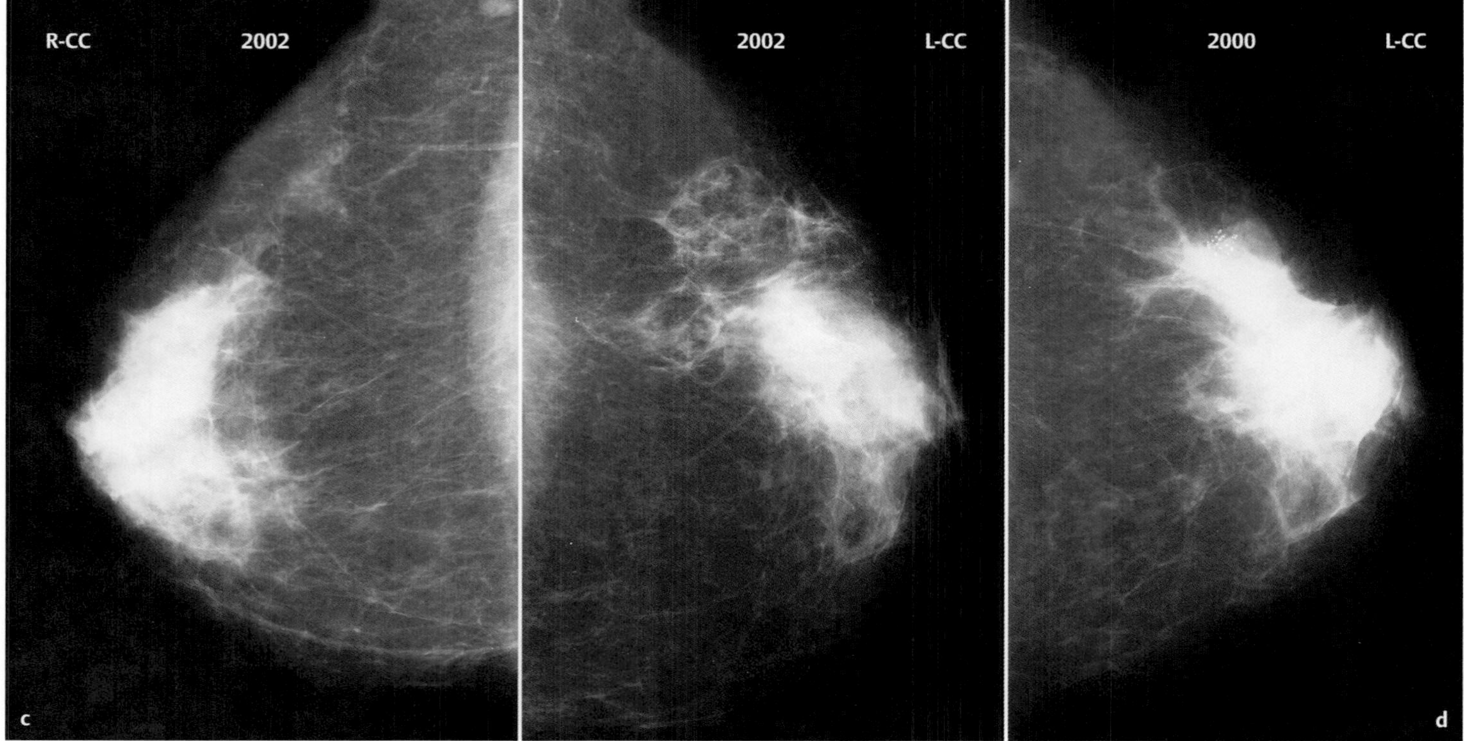


**c** *Bilateral craniocaudal mammograms* in 2002 show honeycomb lucencies in the upper left breast (**e–f/9–11**). The right breast appears normal. A small lymph node is visible in the right axillary recess (**d/14**) (ACR 2, BIRADS 1, **P**GMI).

**d** *Preoperative craniocaudal mammogram* in 2000 shows a radiodense left breast with indistinct borders and scattered, microcalcifications (**I/10**). Status before removal of the microcalcifications (ACR 3, BIRADS 4, P**G**MI).

**Fig. 5.170** **Microcalcifications were removed from the left breast of a 74-year-old woman in 2000, with benign histology.** *(continued)*

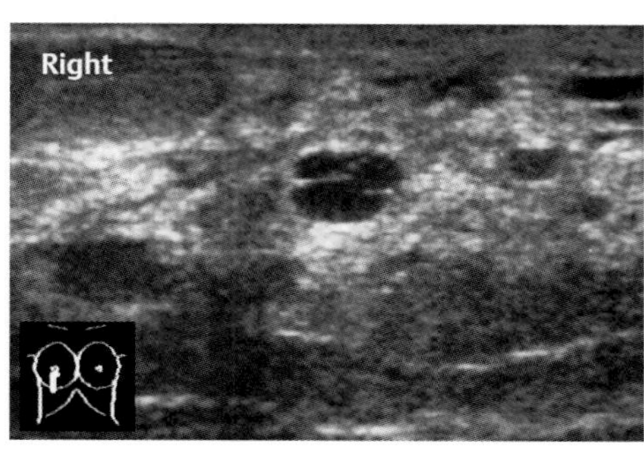


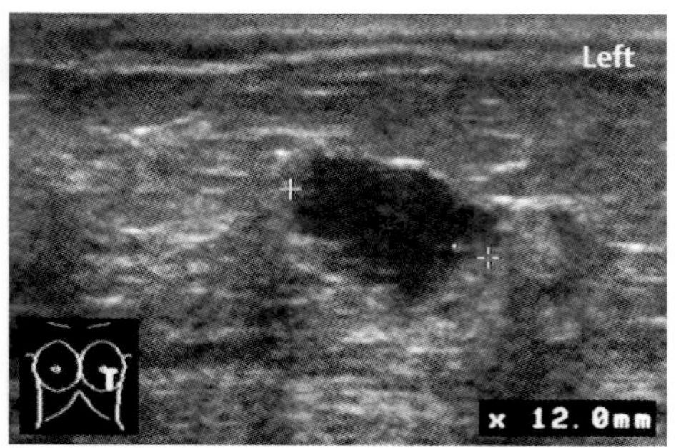


**e** *Sonograms* of both breasts. Microcysts are visible in the right breast (**l/26**). The left breast contains irregular hypoechoic lesions with slight posterior acoustic enhancement (**o–p/5–6**).

**Question on Fig. 5.170**

*How would you interpret the changes in the left breast?*

(**a**) Carcinomatous lymphangitis
(**b**) Mastitis
(**c**) Postoperative oil cysts

→ **Answer on p. 400**

**Fig. 5.171** **Problems after reduction mammoplasty in a 61-year-old woman.** This patient underwent a reduction mammoplasty 2 years previously. She presents now with relatively severe point tenderness in the scarred area of each breast, more pronounced on the right side (**a**). Preoperative mammograms (**b**). Postoperative mammograms (**c**) show basally confluent densities in the painful areas of both breasts.

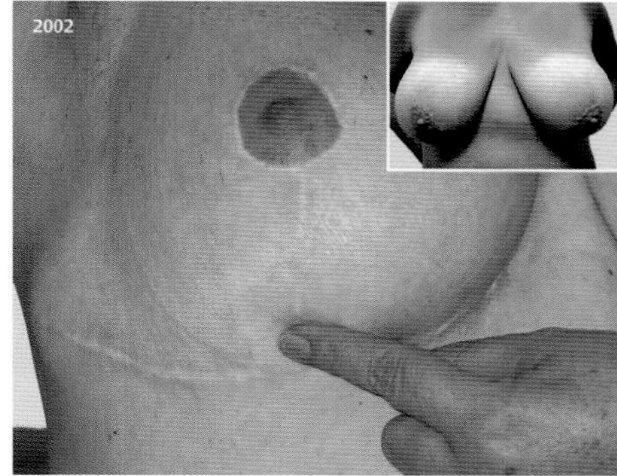


**a** *Postoperative physical examination* of the right breast elicits severe point tenderness in the area of the inframammary scar. Palpation detects possible nonspecific areas of increased firmness but no palpable nodule. The breast parenchyma is tense on both sides. Similar complaints are present in the left breast (inset at upper right: appearance before reduction mammoplasty).

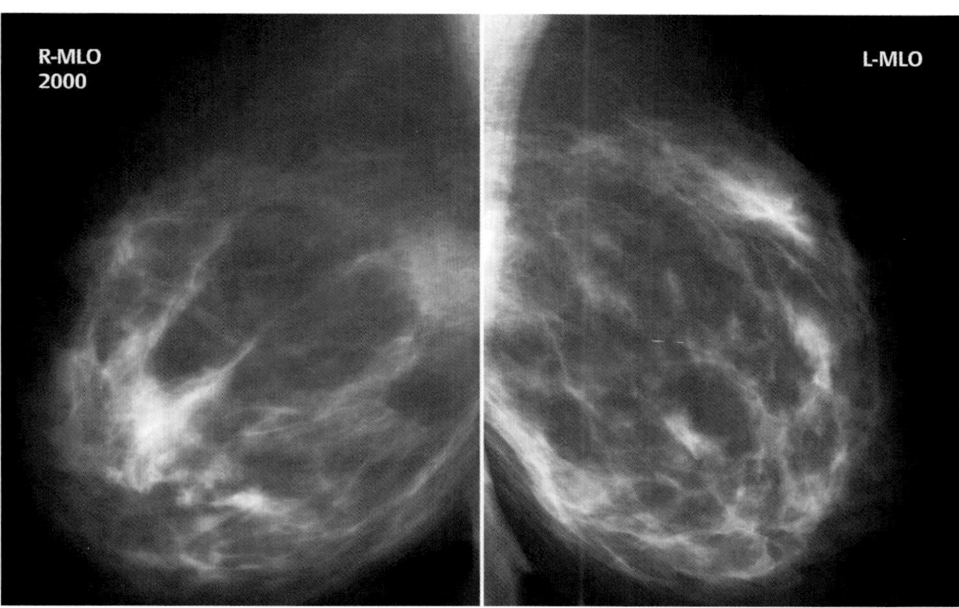


**b** *Bilateral oblique mammograms* before reduction mammoplasty show very large breasts with focal opacities, more pronounced on the right side (**O–o/13–15**) (ACR 2, BIRADS 1, P**G**MI).

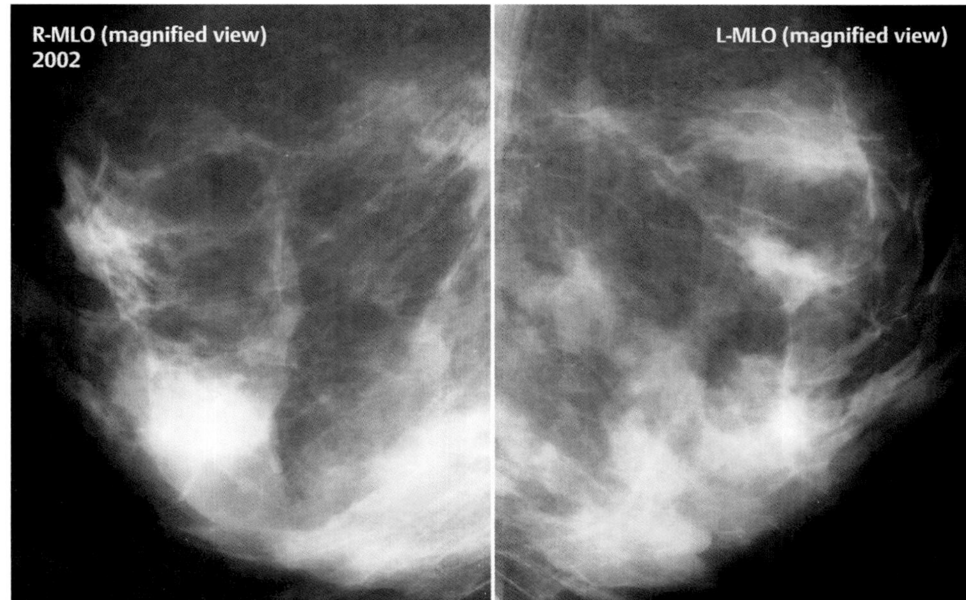


**c** *Bilateral oblique mammograms* after reduction mammoplasty (magnified views of the lower portions of both breasts) show inhomogeneous, cloudy opacities (**n–T/3–6**) that are most pronounced in the inframammary fold of the right breast (see panel **a**) (ACR 4, BIRADS 2, PG**MI**).

▶ **Fig. 5.171 d, e**

**Fig. 5.171 Problems after reduction mammoplasty in a 61-year-old woman.** *(continued)*

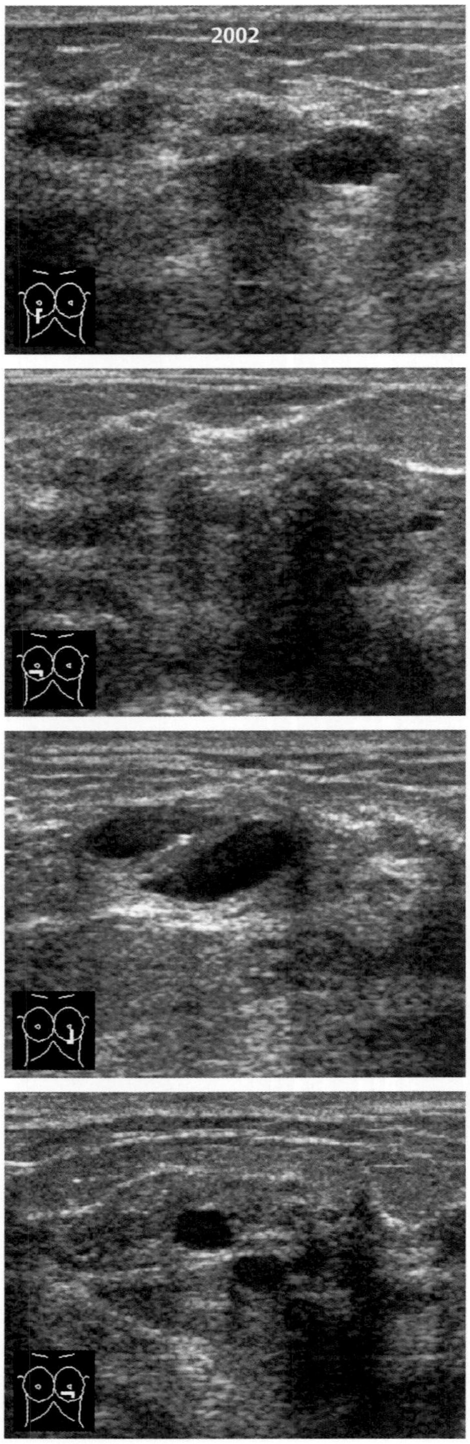

**d** *Infra-areolar sonograms* of the right and left breasts (2002) show numerous hypoechoic, inhomogeneous areas, mostly with smooth margins and some with liquid contents.

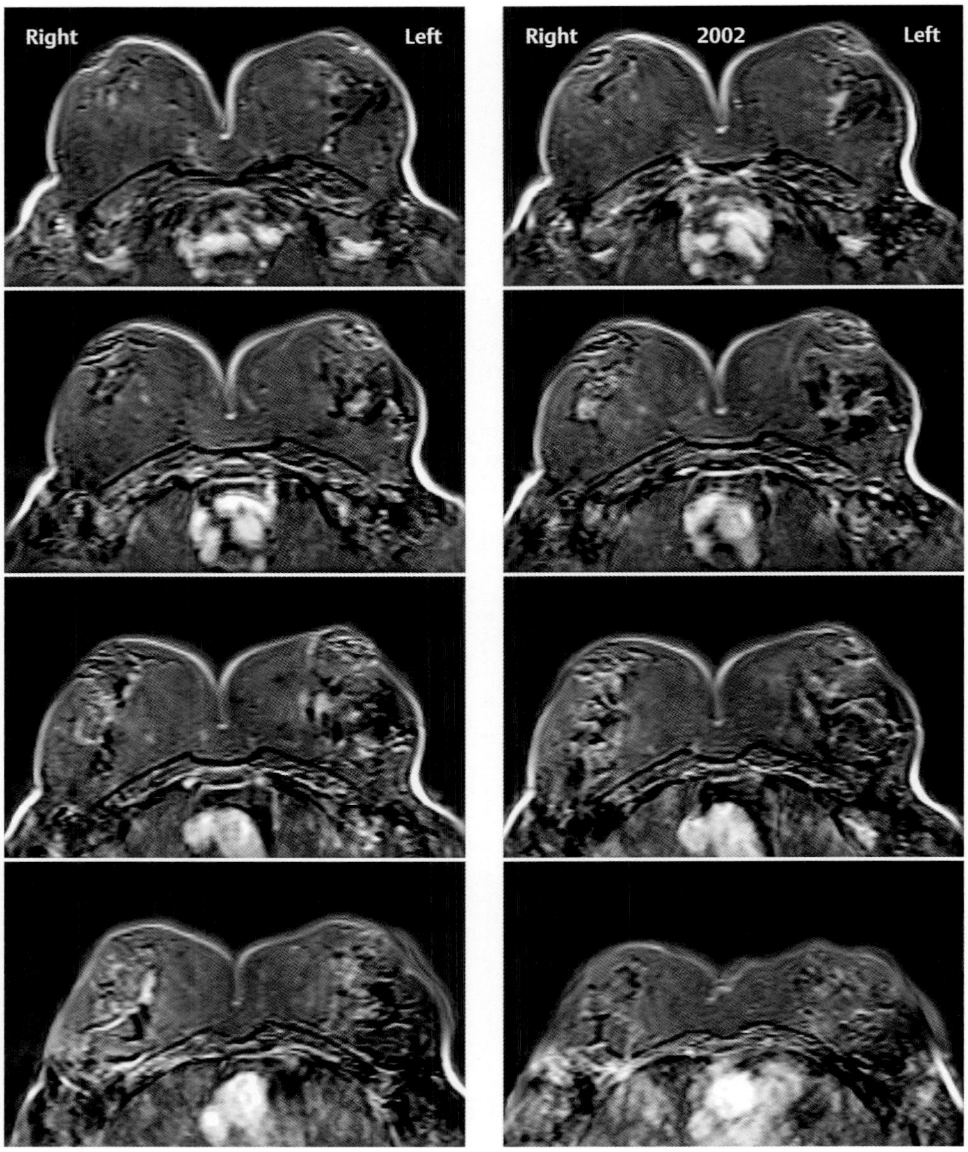

**e** MR subtraction images (2002) show streaky areas of discrete inhomogeneous gadolinium enhancement in the lower quadrants accompanied by cystlike lesions beside artefacts (**f–g/13–14, 17–18, 22** left breast; **E/18, H/22** right breast).

**Question on Fig. 5.171**

*How would you interpret the infra-areolar changes?*

(**a**) Fat necrosis with oil cysts

(**b**) Scar tissue with inflammatory changes

(**c**) Epidermal cysts after reduction mammoplasty

→ **Answer on p. 400**

**Fig. 5.172 A 60-year-old woman underwent a tumorectomy in the right breast (a)**. She presented 5 days after excision of an 8 × 5 × 3 cm tissue block containing a firm tumor up to 3.3 cm in size extending to the posterior edge of the specimen. At histology the tumor was found to be 1.3 cm from the anterior and medial specimen margins. *Histologic diagnosis:* invasive ductal carcinoma of variable differentiation (G 1/2) with a very small posterior clear margin. The patient refused reexcision and axillary dissection. New imaging studies are ordered to exclude residual tumor tissue in the breast (**b, c**).

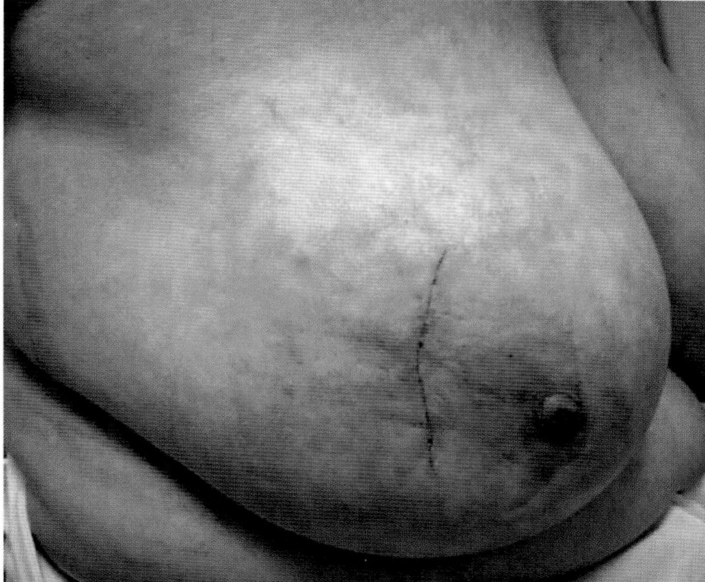

**a** *Clinical appearance* of the right breast 5 days after tumorectomy and closure with intracutaneous sutures.

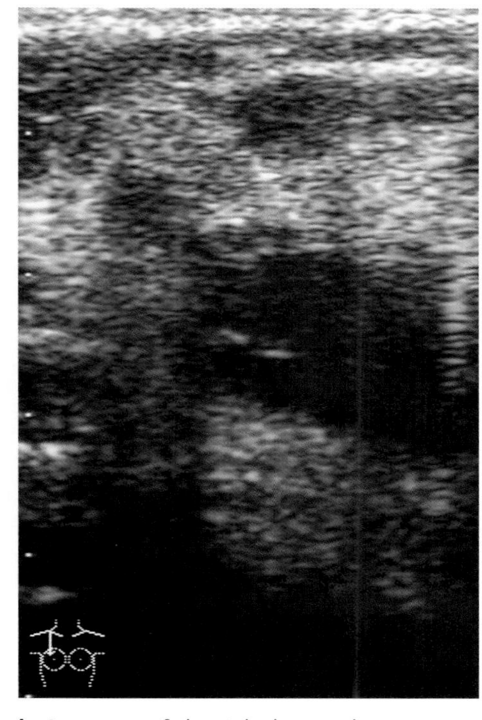

**b** *Sonogram* of the right breast shows a post-operative seroma with smooth borders and a echogenic rim caused by hematoma.

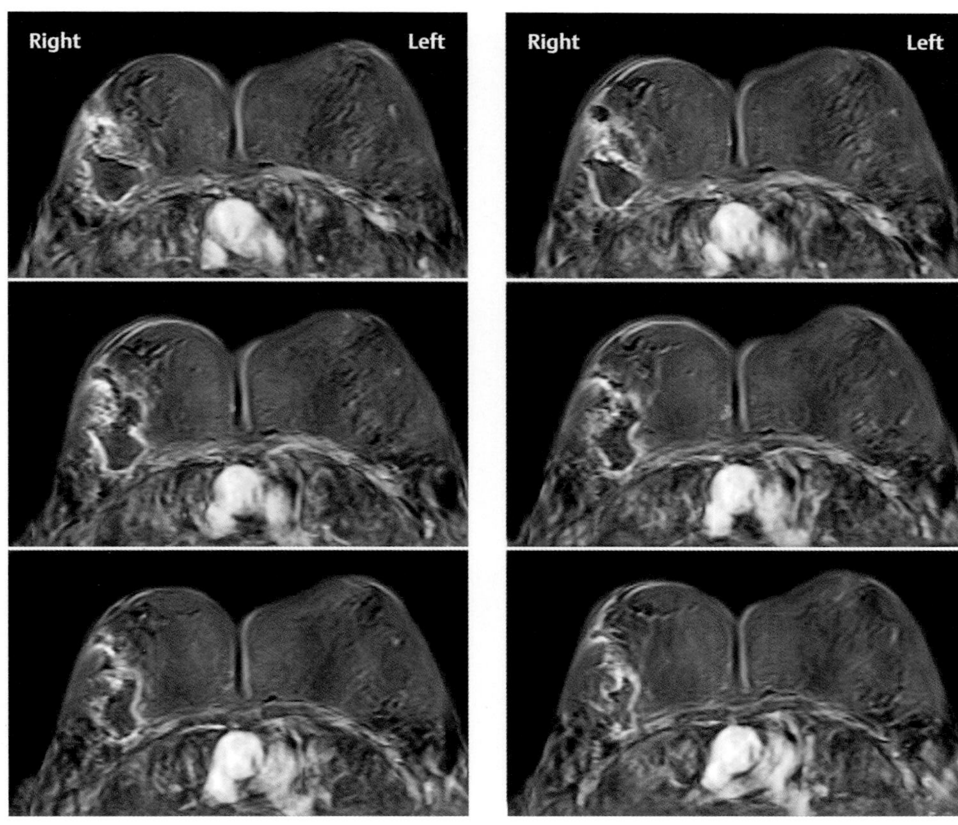


**c** *Series of MR subtraction images* show intense gadolinium enhancement at the periphery of the surgical cavity in the right breast, especially anteriorly (**k/12, 8–9, 4–5** etc.).

**Question on Fig. 5.172**

*How would you interpret the enhancing areas around the surgical cavity?*

(**a**) Residual tumors after an incomplete tumorectomy
(**b**) Granulation tissue 5 days post-operatively
(**c**) Both are possible

→ **Answer on p. 400**

**Fig. 5.173 A 51-year-old woman underwent left breast-conserving surgery in 1998** followed by radiotherapy. One year later she presents with slowly progressive swelling of the left breast and orange-peel dimpling of the skin (**a**). Mammograms show increased density of the left breast with no circumscribed tumor nodules (**b**).Ultrasound shows enlarged lymphatics (**c**). MRI shows no abnormalities (**d**). The patient is asymptomatic with no local warmth of the left breast and no lymph node enlargement.

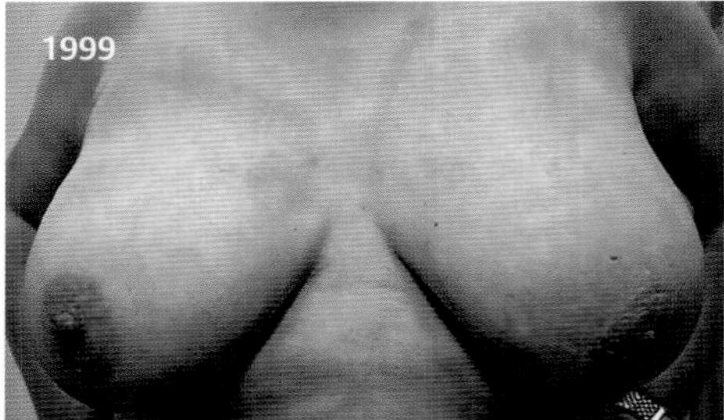


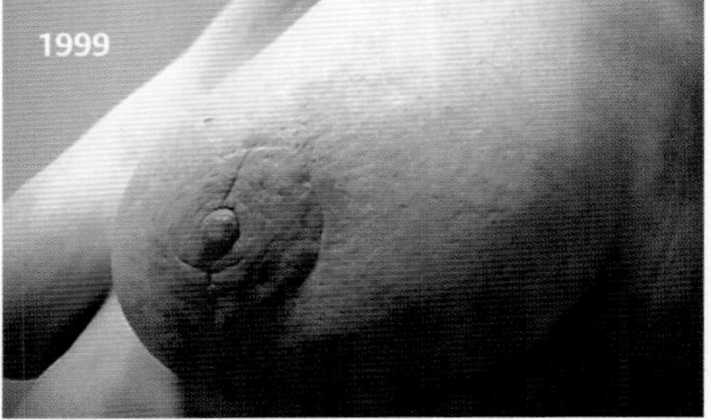


**a** *Bilateral clinical appearance*. The left breast is enlarged and shows orange-peel skin dimpling. Increased venous markings are noted on the nonoperated right breast. A periareolar scar is visible between the 1 and 5-o'clock positions on the left breast (below). A slight skin depression is visible at the former tumor site. Orange-peel skin dimpling is most pronounced in the areola (**B–c/19–21**).

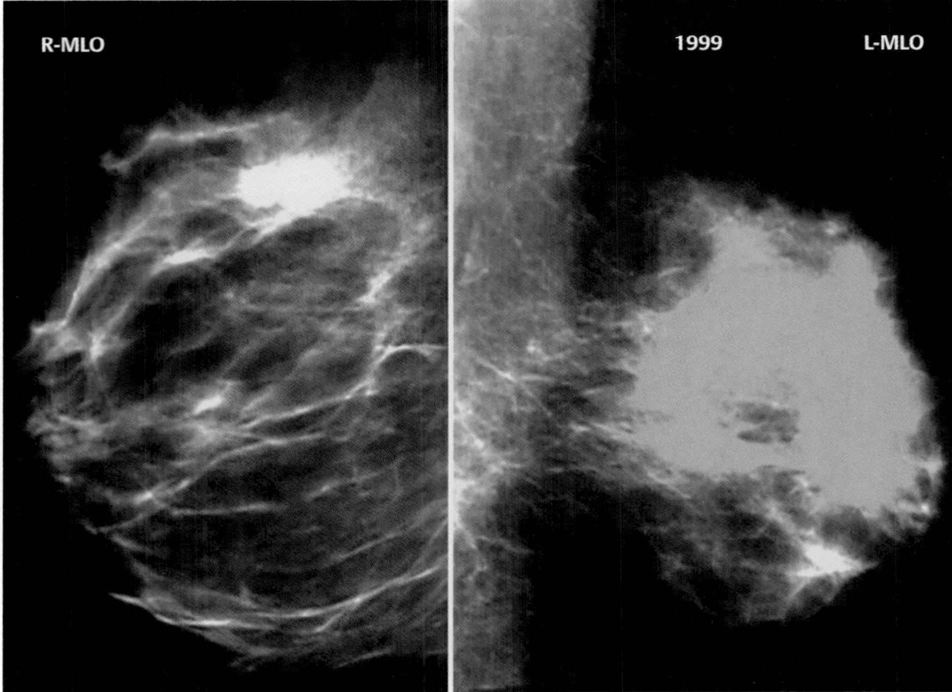


**b** *Bilateral oblique mammograms* show greatly increased density of the left breast (**h–J/18–23**) (ACR 3) with no microcalcifications. The right breast appears normal aside from a circumscribed upper density (**F–f/23–24**), which is not visible in the second projection (ACR 2, BIRADS 2, PGMI).

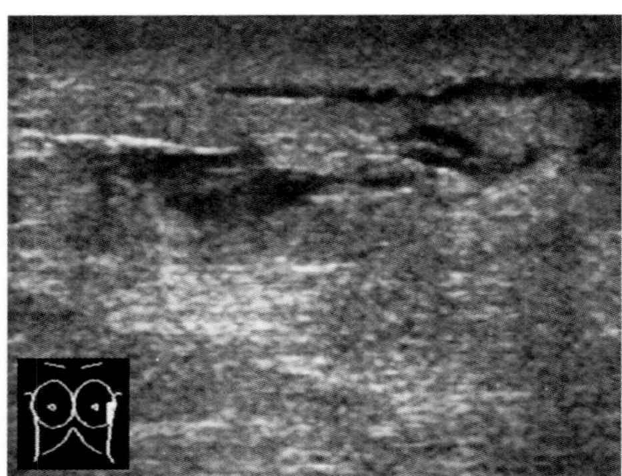

**c** *Sonogram* of the left breast shows enlarged subcutaneous lymphatics in the axillary recess with skin thickening (**a–D/14**) and pooling of lymphatic fluid (**a–D/12–13**).

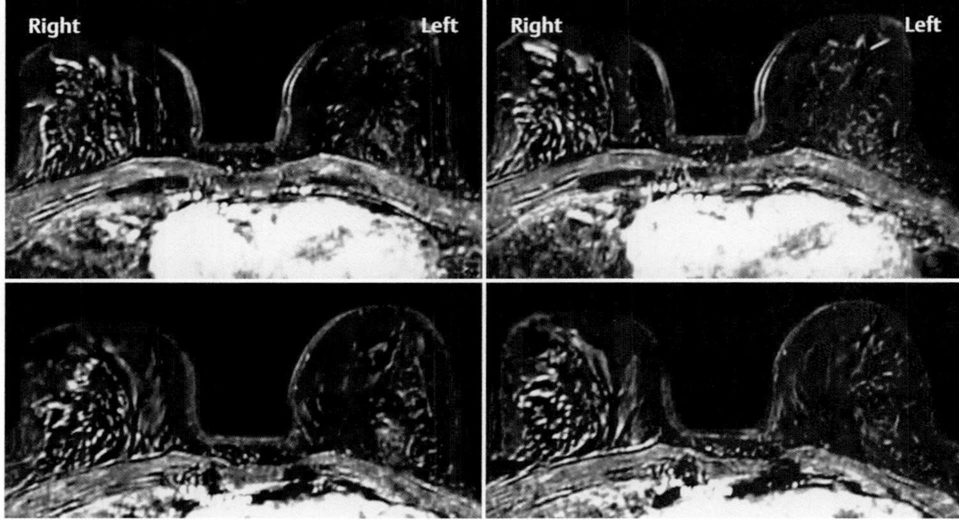


**d** *MR subtraction images* in 1999 show a uniform, harmonious distribution of gadolinium enhancement with no evidence of a local proliferative process.

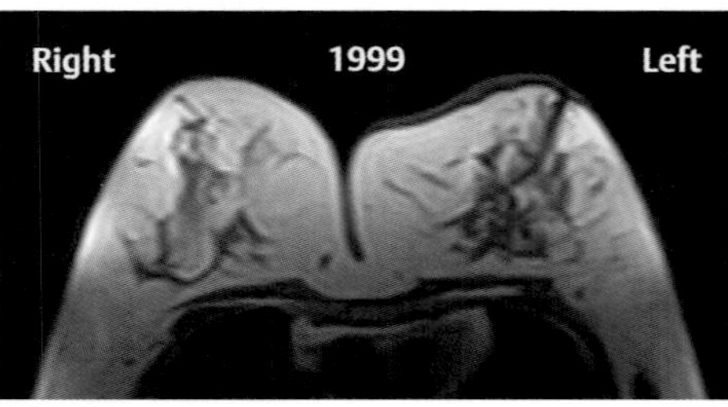


**e** *MRM* without contrast medium shows increased density of the left breast with no increase in subcutaneous markings but with medial skin thickening (**b–c/6**) (compare with features of inflammatory carcinoma, **Fig. 4.34** f, p. 65, and p. 72).

**Question on Fig. 5.173**

*How would you interpret the swelling of the left breast 1 year postoperatively?*

(**a**) Carcinomatous lymphangitis

(**b**) Lymphedema following breast-conserving therapy

(**c**) Nonpuerperal mastitis

→ **Answer on p. 400**

**Fig. 5.174** **A 62-year-old woman underwent bilateral reduction mammoplasty 10 years ago and presents with no clinical abnormalities.** Prior mammograms are unavailable.

R-MLO

L-MLO

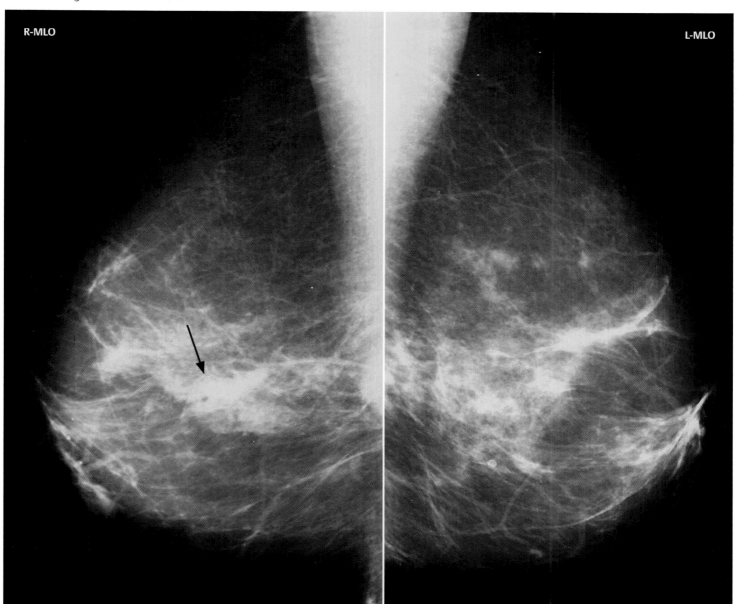

**a** *Bilateral oblique mammograms* show focal scars in both breasts (**M–n/17** right breast, **p–s/18–19** left breast) 10 years after reduction mammoplasty.

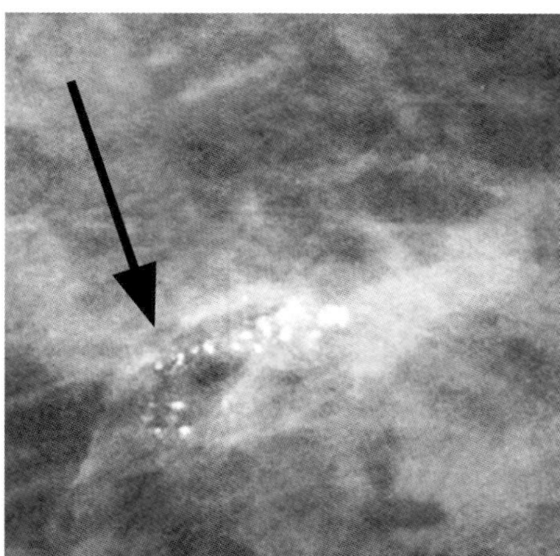

**b** *Magnification mammogram* shows a cluster of relatively pleomorphic microcalcifications in the right breast (arrow) (ACR 2, BIRADS 4b, **P**GMI).

▶ **Fig. 5.174c, d**

**Fig. 5.174 62-year-old woman underwent bilateral reduction mammoplasty 10 years ago, no clinical abnormalities.** *(continued)*

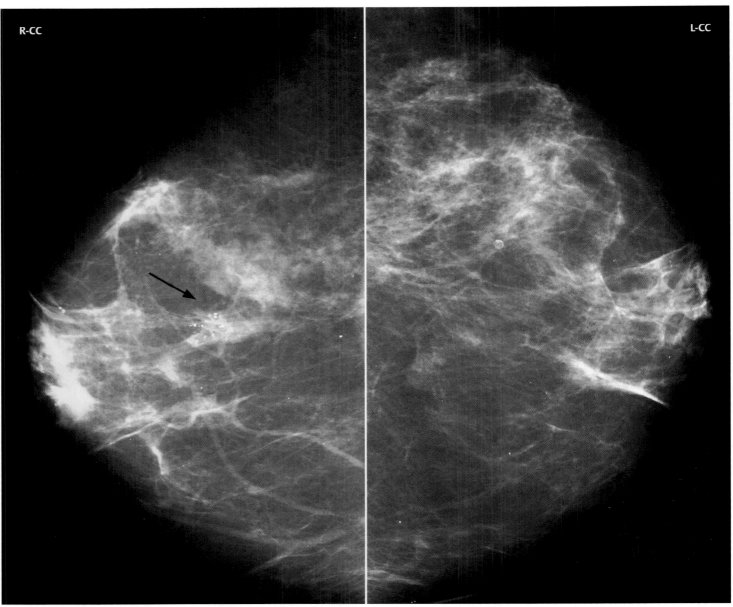

**c** *Bilateral craniocaudal mammograms* show cicatricial changes in the left breast (e.g., at **h–j/17** and **f–h/21–24**) and a Y-shaped cluster of pleomorphic calcifications in the right breast (ACR 2, BIRADS 4b, PG**M**I).

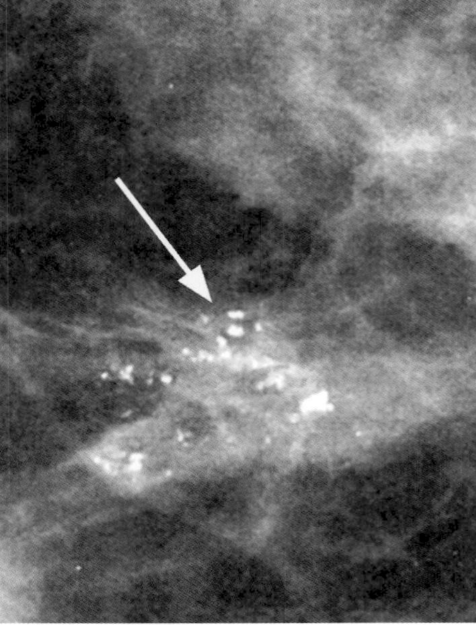

**d** *Magnification mammogram* of the central area in **c** shows coarse calcifications within stroma-rich glandular tissue.

**Question on Fig. 5.174**

*What is the cause of the calcifications?*

(**a**) Fat necrosis
(**b**) DCIS
(**c**) Cannot be determined

→ **Answer on p. 401**

**Fig. 5.175 Postoperative nipple discharge in a 54-year-old woman** who underwent previous right breast-conserving excision of a 2.4 cm tumor in the axillary recess. Seroma collections in the former tumor bed were removed several times by percutaneous needle aspiration. Later the patient developed a milky, blood-tinged nipple discharge. The discharge ceased for a time after radiotherapy but recurred several months later. Ultrasound still demonstrates a large seroma in the upper outer quadrant of the right breast (**c**), which is treated by percutaneous aspiration. Instillation of contrast medium into the residual cavity yields the mammograms shown in **a** and **b**.

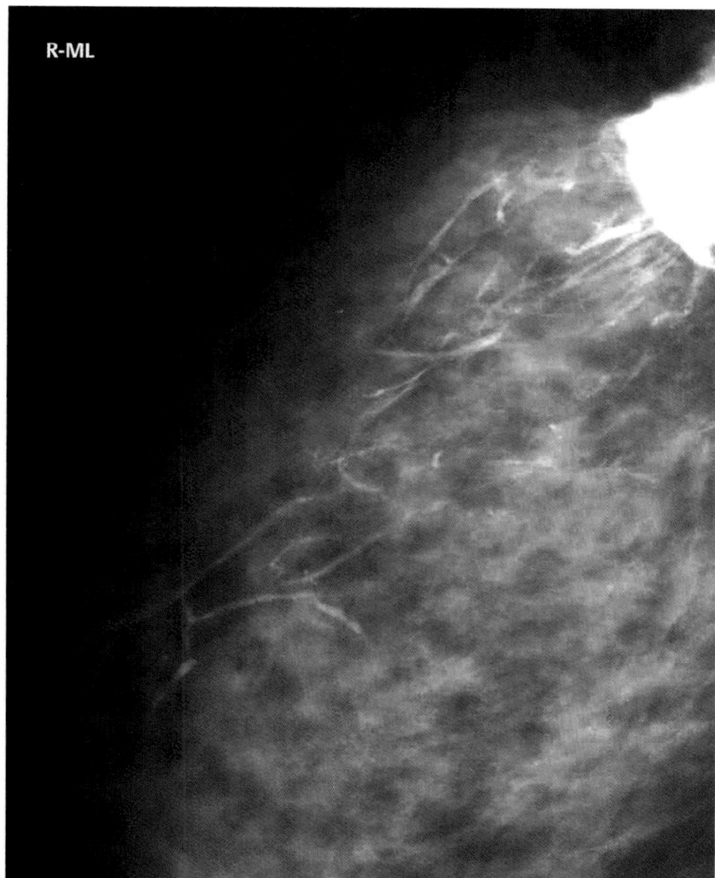


**a** Oblique mammogram (magnified view) shows lactiferous ducts with irregular borders in the upper outer quadrant of the right breast (**a–E/16–23**).

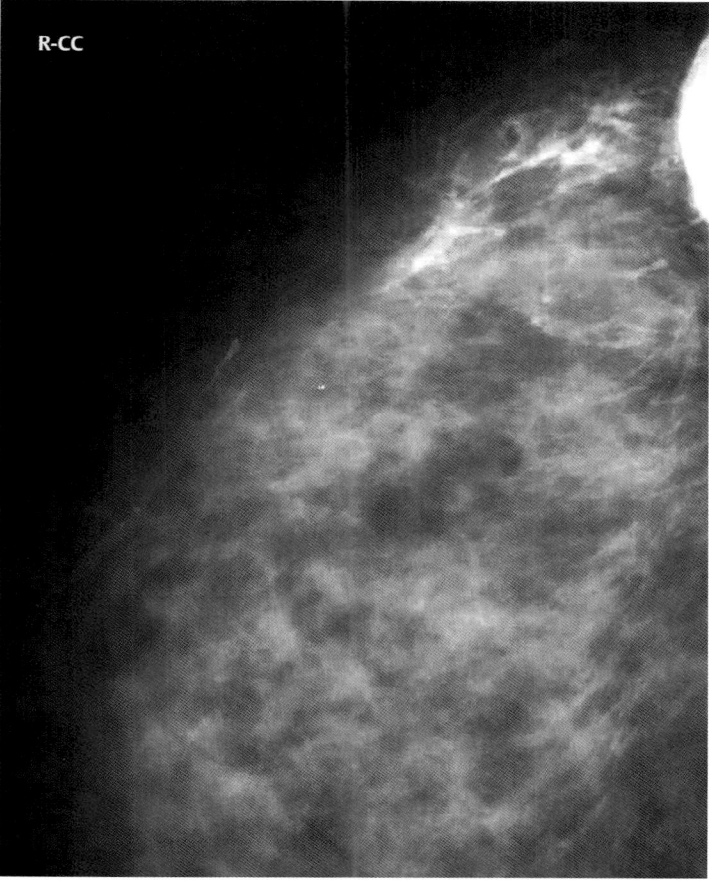


**b** Craniocaudal mammogram of the right breast (magnified view of the lateral quadrants) shows poorly opacified ducts with irregular borders (**h–J/21–24**).

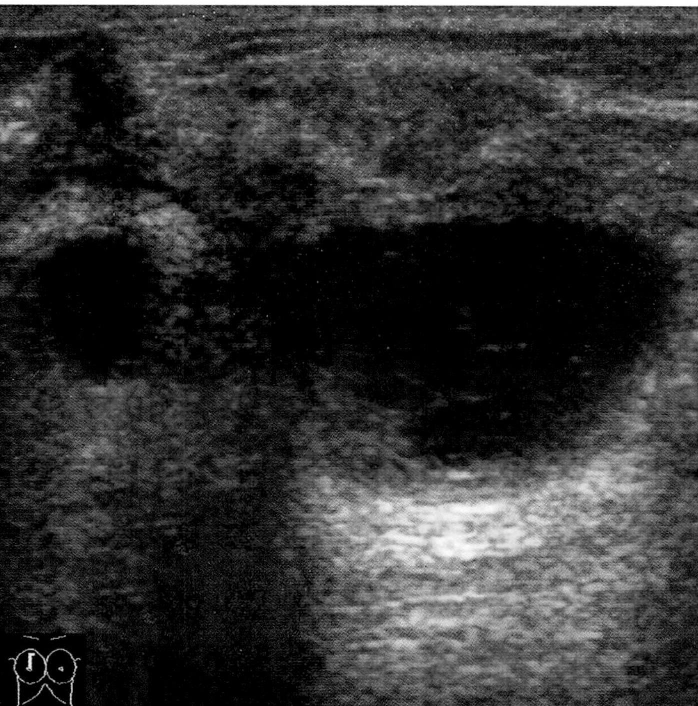

**Question on Fig. 5.175**

*What is the cause of the recurrent nipple discharge?*

(**a**) Communication between the irradiated seroma cavity and duct system

(**b**) Ductectasia with papillomatosis

(**c**) Ductal neoplasm

→ **Answer on p. 401**

**c** Sonogram 4 months after the completion of radiotherapy shows two seromas of different sizes with ill-defined borders (**L–M/7–9**). A small, subcutaneous, hypoechoic area (**k/11**) is visible in the area of skin necrosis. Inflammatory?

**Fig. 5.176 Atypical operative technique in a 43-year-old woman** with a presumed fibroadenoma in the upper outer quadrant of the left breast based on sonographic findings. A lumpectomy was performed, and histology revealed *invasive carcinoma* with both ductal and lobular elements and an extensive intraductal component (EIC, see p. 75). The tumor had not been removed with clear margins. Preoperative mammograms were not obtained, and preoperative sonograms were unavailable. The patient, with cutaneous sutures still in place (**a**), presents now for determination of further action. Mammograms show extensive atypical calcifications in the axillary recess (**c**). MRI shows residual axillary tumor (**d**), which is confirmed histologically. SLN scintigraphy shows tracer uptake in axillary, clavicular, and sternal lymph nodes (**e**).

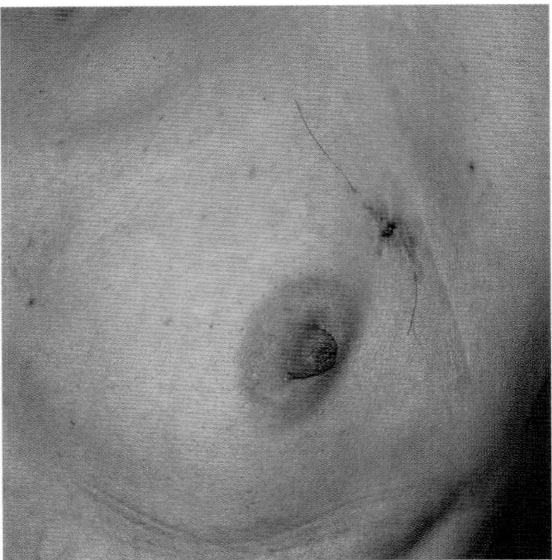

**a** *Clinical appearance* of the left breast following local excision of a presumed fibroadenoma (palpable nodule). A cutaneous suture is still in place, and there is lateral deviation of the nipple.

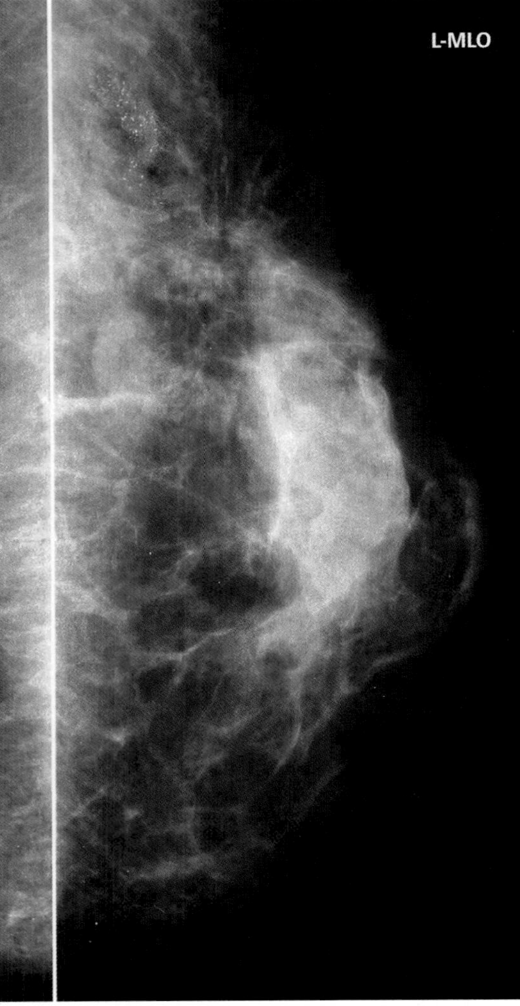


**b** *Bilateral craniocaudal mammograms* show a lateral tissue defect in the left breast (**h–I/22**). Microcalcifications are visible at the axillary periphery of the breast (**H/23–24**).

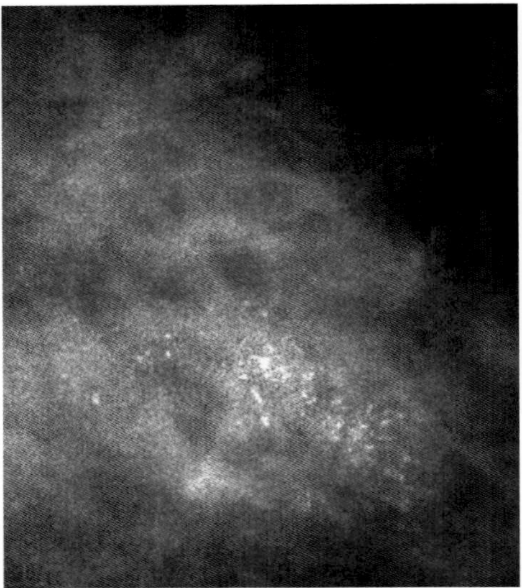

**c** *Magnification mammogram* of the left axillary recess shows atypical pleomorphic calcifications.

**Question on Fig. 5.176**

*What aspect of the second operation (reexcision) in this case did* not *conform to recommended guidelines?*

(**a**) The omission of preoperative mammography and localization of the calcifications
(**b**) The sentinel lymph node procedure
(**c**) Preoperative MRM

→ **Answer on p. 402**

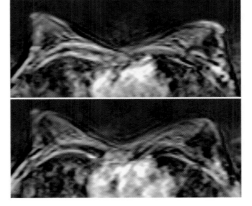

**d** *MR subtraction images* show nonspecific gadolinium enhancement on the axillary side of the surgical cavity (**G/5+8**) (identical to the calcifications).

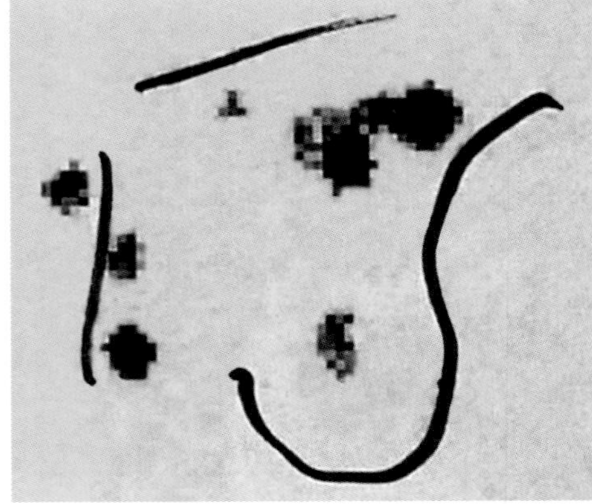

**e** Sentinel lymph node scintigraphy shows axillary, infraclavicular, and retrosternal uptake.

**Fig. 5.177 Kaposi sarcoma versus inflammatory carcinoma in a 72-year-old woman** who underwent left breast-conserving surgery and completed her *course of radiotherapy 20 days previously*. She presents now with intense redness of the irradiated breast, swelling of the areola, yellowish-white crusts on the nipple, itching, and burning pain.

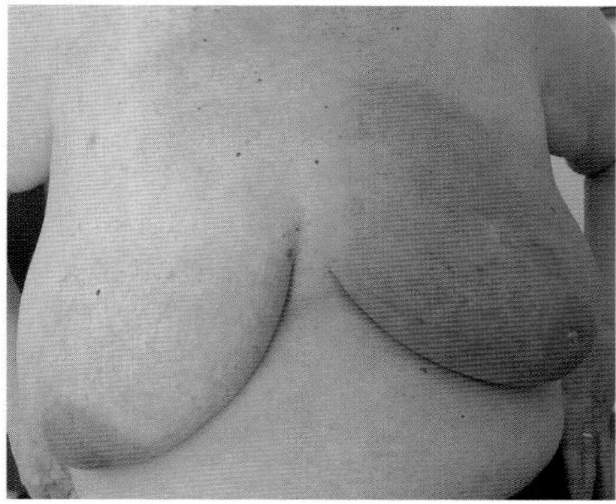

**a** *Clinical inspection* shows intense redness of the left breast with swelling of the areola (**m/23**). A scar is visible a handwidth above the left nipple. The right breast appears normal.

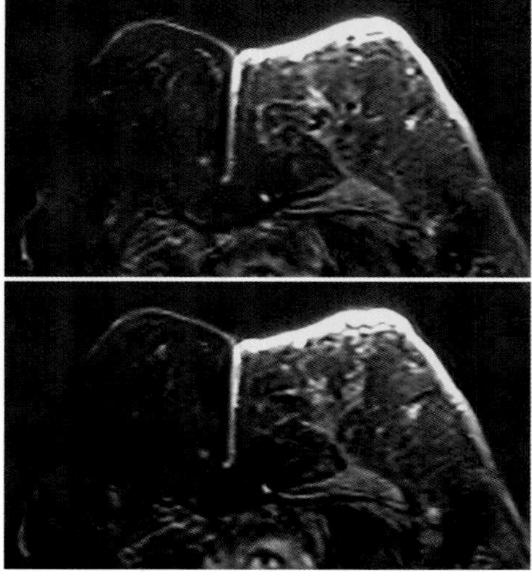

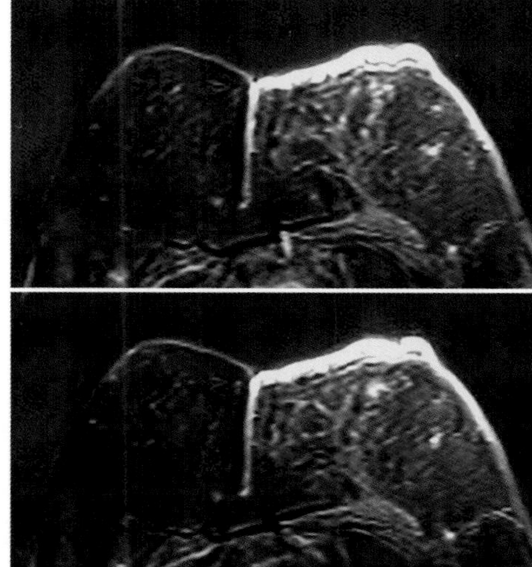

**b** *MR subtraction images* show no focal areas of intramammary gadolinium enhancement. The thickened skin of the left breast does show gadolinium uptake (**o–p/22+26**).

**Question on Fig. 5.177**

*How would you interpret these findings?*

(**a**) Radiodermatitis following radiation to the breast

(**b**) Kaposi sarcoma (angiosarcoma)

(**c**) Inflammatory carcinoma

→ **Answer on p. 402**

**Fig. 5.178 Treatment regimen for locally advanced breast cancer in a 57-year-old woman** with a recurrent milky nipple discharge on the left side. Progressive swelling of the left breast has been present for the past week. Histology shows poorly differentiated ductal carcinoma with axillary lymph node involvement (up to 2 cm in diameter). She has a strongly positive estrogen receptor status, positive progesterone receptor status, and strongly positive HER-2/neu status. The case is followed from 1998 to 2003. *Question:* What is the best treatment?

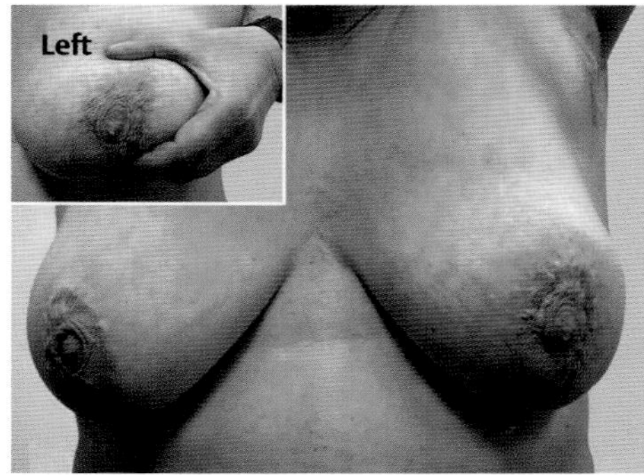


**a** *Clinical appearance* in October, 1998. The left breast is slightly enlarged. There is incipient orange-peel dimpling of the periareolar skin with deep pores. The left nipple is not retracted, while slight nipple retraction is noted on the right side. Inset at upper left: 8 cm mass in the left breast. (Further clinical progression is shown in panels **i–k**, p. 404.)

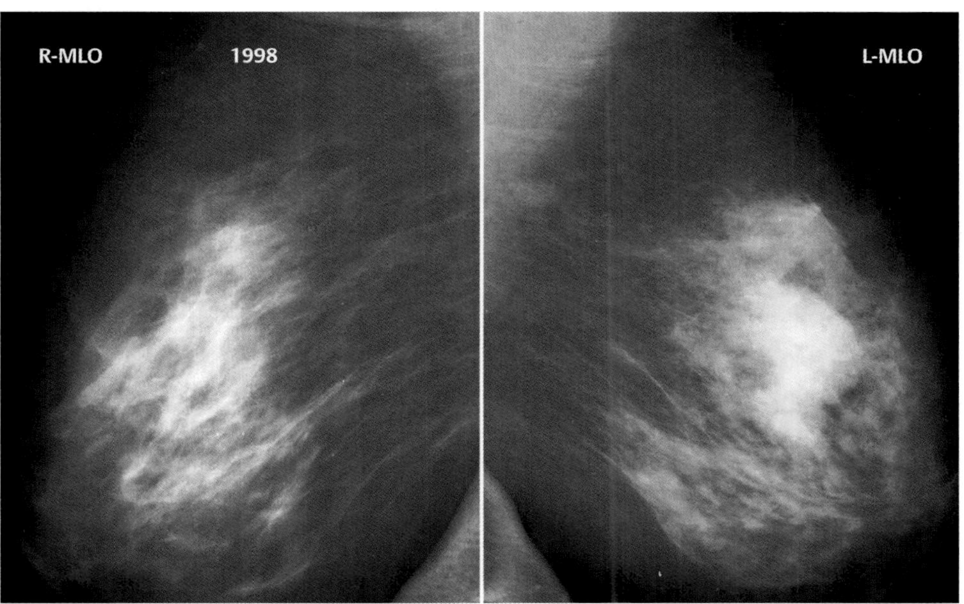


**b** *Bilateral oblique mammograms* show very radiodense breasts with an inhomogeneous, ill-defined opacity in the left breast extending from the nipple to the upper border of the breast parenchyma (**S–T/6–9**). No microcalcifications are visible (ACR 3, BIRADS 4, PGMI). (Further mammographic progression is shown in panel **g**, p. 403.)

▶ **Fig. 5.178 c–f**

**Fig. 5.178 Treatment regimen for locally advanced breast cancer in a 57-year-old woman.** *(continued)*

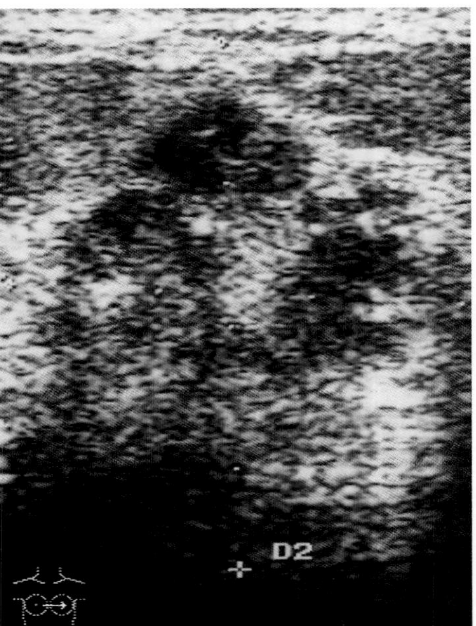


**c** *Sonogram* through the central portion of the left breast shows numerous confluent, hypoechoic nodules with an echogenic rim and posterior acoustic shadowing. This pattern is suspicious for malignancy. High-level echoes in surrounding tissues are consistent with lymphatic obstruction.

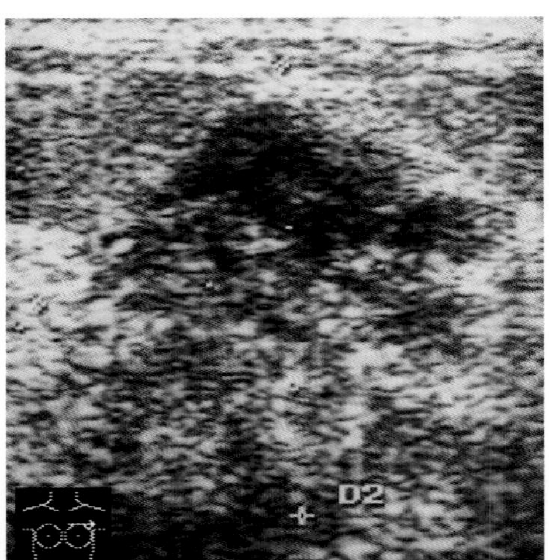


**d** *Sonogram* of the left axilla shows a 30 mm × 27 mm hypoechoic nodule with inhomogeneous internal echoes. High-level echoes in the surrounding tissue suggest *lymphatic obstruction.*

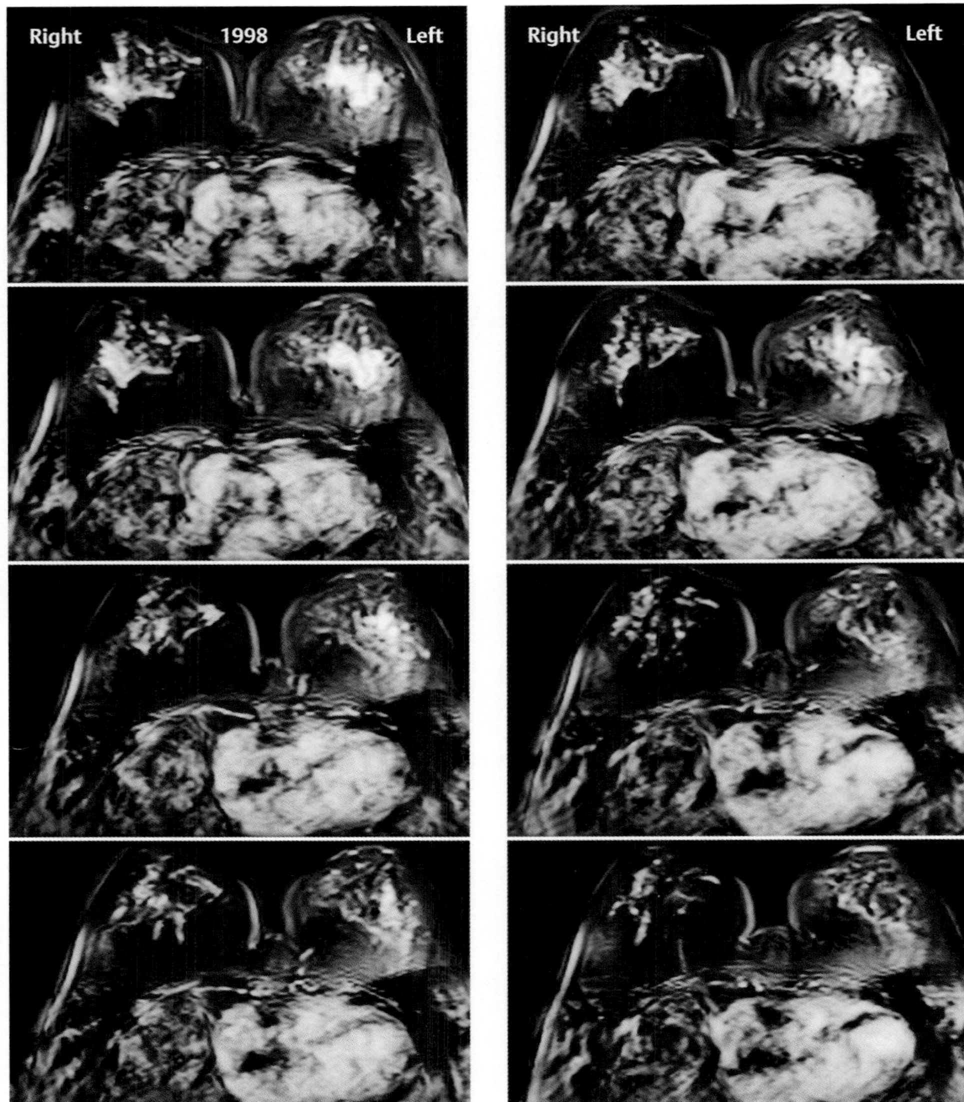


**f** *MR subtraction images* show a mixed diffuse and confluent-nodular pattern of intense tumorlike gadolinium uptake in the left breast (**f–G/22–23**). A tumorlike pattern of gadolinium enhancement is also noted in the retroareolar right breast (**e/23**) and axillary recess (**d–E/21 + 25**) (biopsy was not performed on this side, however). The findings suggest a locally advanced tumor stage with axillary lymph node involvement in the left breast and no detectable distant metastases (compare with PET in **e**). (MRM is consistent with a tumor also in the right breast; see further progression in panel **h**, p. 404.)

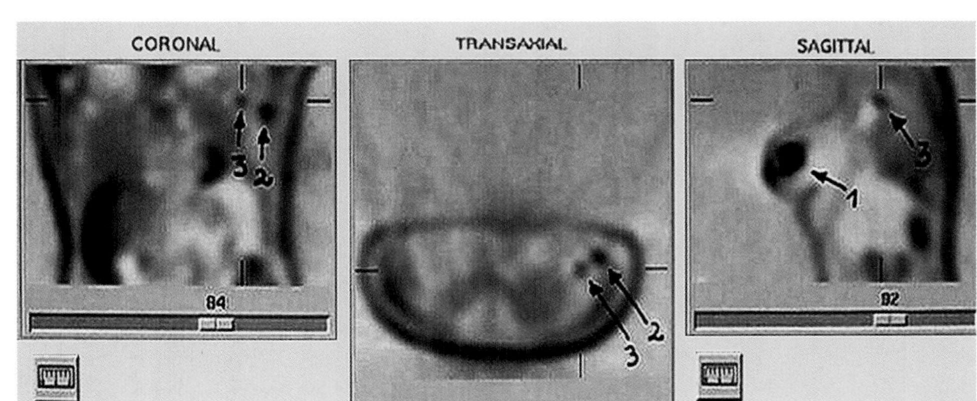


**e** *Positron emission tomography (PET)* shows marked glucose hypermetabolism in the tumor-bearing region of the left breast (**1**). Multiple lymph nodes are detected in the axilla (**2, 3**). There is no evidence of tumor in the right breast or distant metastases (image courtesy of Bernhard Hörr, Plochingen).

**Question on Fig. 5.178**

*What primary treatment regimen would you recommend?*

(**a**) Left mastectomy with adjuvant hormonal therapy and chemotherapy
(**b**) Radiotherapy with adjuvant hormonal therapy and chemotherapy
(**c**) Chemotherapy (neoadjuvant/primary) followed by surgical excision, radiotherapy, and adjuvant hormonal therapy

→ **Answer on p. 403**

**Fig. 5.179 Mastitis, generalized lymphadenopathy, or inflammatory carcinoma?** A 55-year-old woman presents with redness and swelling of her left breast that has been increasing for several weeks (**a, b**). An enlarged lymph node is palpable in the left supraclavicular fossa at the junction of the subclavian and internal jugular veins (**c**). Computed tomography additionally shows enlarged lymph nodes in the left axilla and at the jugulosubclavian venous junction in each supraclavicular fossa (**f, g**). Mammography shows relatively dense glandular tissue in both breasts with no striking asymmetry. The left breast is slightly more radiodense than the right, consistent with CT findings (**e**). The lymph node in the left supraclavicular fossa is investigated by FNA, which yields debris and scattered suspicious-looking cells. *A punch* biopsy taken from the skin of the left breast shows edema with no evidence of inflammatory carcinoma.

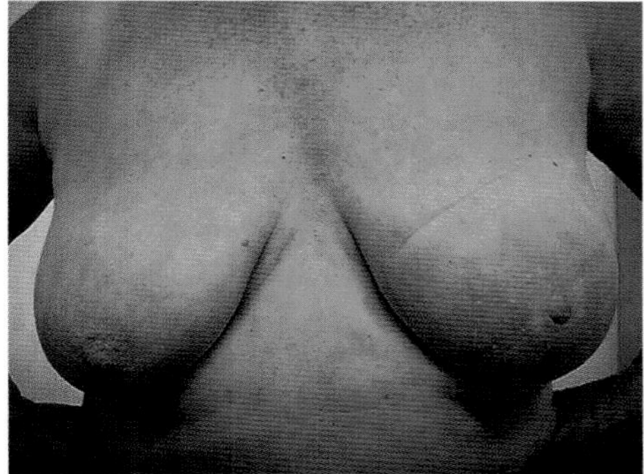

**a** *Clinical appearance* of both breasts. The left breast is slightly enlarged, reddened, and shows incipient orange-peel dimpling of the skin.

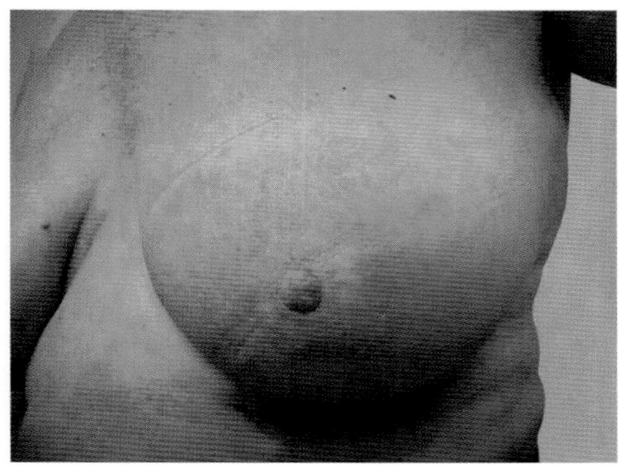

**b** *Close-up view* of the left breast shows swelling, redness, and orange-peel skin.

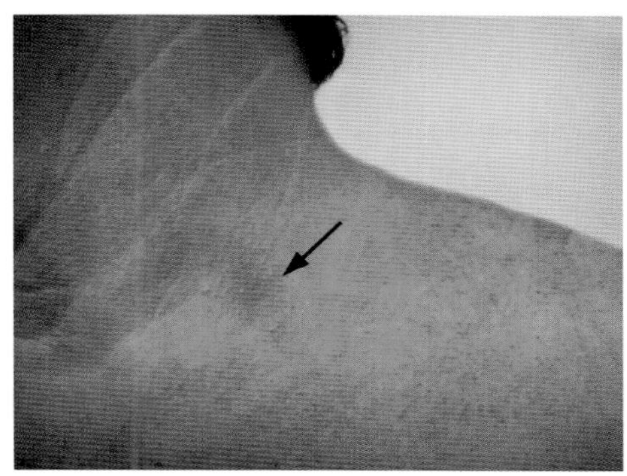

**c** *Clinical appearance* of the left supraclavicular fossa. A lymph node is palpable at the junction of the left subclavian and internal jugular veins (arrow, compare with **g**) and is investigated by fine-needle aspiration.

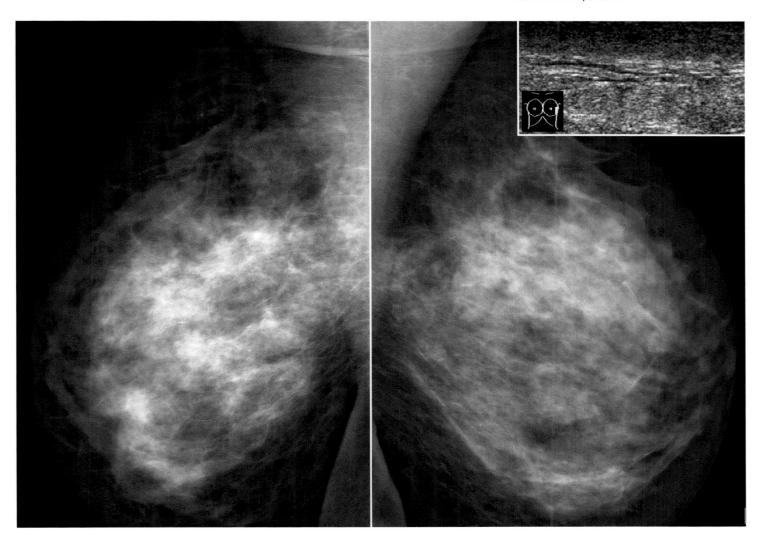

**d** *Bilateral oblique mammograms* show radiodense breasts with no suspicious circumscribed lesions (ACR 3, BIRADS 2, P**G**MI). *Inset: Ultrasound* shows dilated subcutaneous lymphatics in the axillary recess.

▶ **Fig. 5.179 e–g**

**Fig. 5.179 Mastitis, generalized lymphadenopathy, or inflammatory carcinoma?** *(continued)*

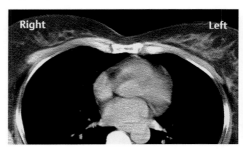

**e** *Computed tomography* of the chest (magnified view of both breasts). The left breast parenchyma is more radiodense than the right (**c/26–27**).

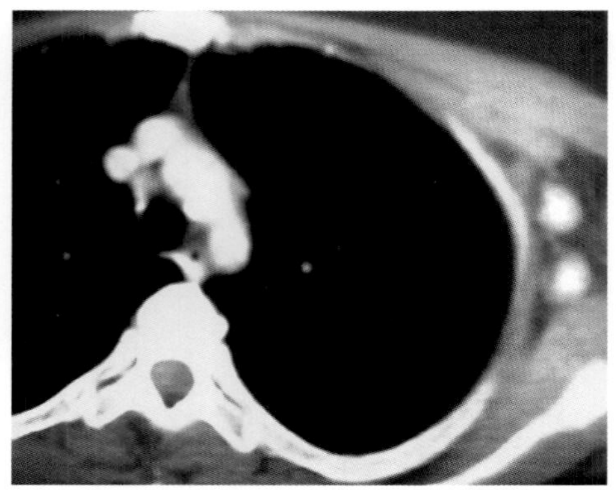

**f** *Computed tomography* (magnified view of the left axilla) demonstrates two enlarged axillary lymph nodes (**G/24–25**).

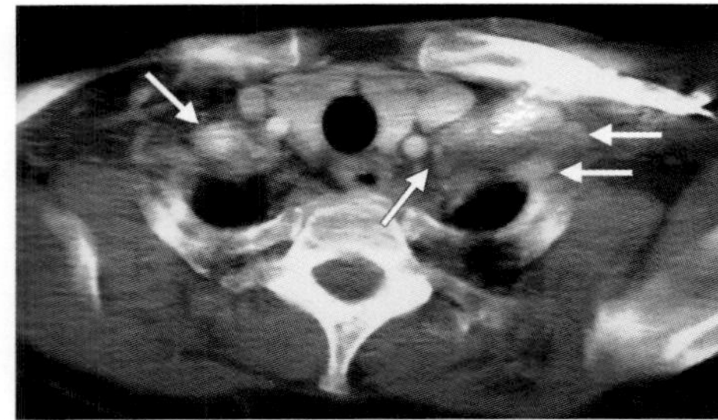

**g** *Computed tomography* (junction of right and left subclavian and internal jugular veins, thyroid gland) shows enlarged lymph nodes on both sides (arrows). The lymph node on the left side is investigated by fine-needle aspiration.

**Question 1 on Fig. 5.179**

*What is your diagnosis?*

(**a**) Inflammatory carcinoma with lymph node metastases in the axilla and supraclavicular fossa
(**b**) Nonpuerperal mastitis with inflammatory lymphadenopathy
(**c**) Generalized lymphadenopathy with lymphedema in the left breast

→ **Answer on p. 405**

**Question 2 on Fig. 5.179**

*Does the skin biopsy (punch biopsy) exclude inflammatory carcinoma?*

(**a**) Yes
(**b**) No
(**c**) Uncertain

→ **Answer on p. 405**

# Postoperative Changes and Follow-Up

Follow-up examinations are scheduled so that local recurrences, lymph node involvement, and distant metastases can be detected and treated without delay. From a psychological standpoint, follow-up enables doctors to reassure patients that their treatment has been effective and their cancer has not returned. Experience has shown that it is better to see the glass as "half full" rather than "half empty," even when the doctor has made a mistake and must correct it.

*The treated breast should be followed at 6-month intervals for 2–3 years* (depending on the stage and aggressiveness of the treated tumor), then once a year thereafter like the healthy breast. Today, follow-up examinations consist only of mammograms of the operated and clinically healthy breasts. In women treated for invasive cancer (not DCIS!), it is consistent with guidelines but not essential to schedule mammograms at 6-month intervals for 3 years. A more reasonable approach is to examine both breasts at 6 months and then at yearly intervals thereafter, because with current treatments (excision with clear margins, postoperative irradiation, systemic therapy) it is unlikely that a recurrence will develop during the first 2 years. Moreover, patients tend to become anxious and apprehensive for up to 2 weeks before their scheduled follow-up visit.

Follow-up visits should include mammograms, sonograms, and if necessary magnetic resonance images. MRI should be scheduled between two mammogram appointments if possible to provide a tighter and more effective control net. Typical findings include postoperative changes due to scar formation, organized hematomas, seroma formation, foreign body reactions, infra- and supraclavicular lymph node metastases, and many more. The examiner must be familiar with these changes to avoid misinterpretations and unnecessary repeat biopsies. Examples are shown in **Figs. 5.180–5.185**.

*(continued on p. 337)*

**Fig. 5.180** **A 63-year-old woman underwent right breast-conserving surgery** for comedocarcinoma (T1b N0 M0, G3) first diagnosed in June, 1998. She received a standard course of radiotherapy to the breast from July to August, 1998, in addition to tamoxifen. Recovery was complicated by wound healing problems requiring multiple revisions and a latissimus dorsi musculocutaneous flap. She presents now with new, rapidly enlarging, slightly itchy reddish-purple skin eruptions on the operated breast without any pain (**a, b**).

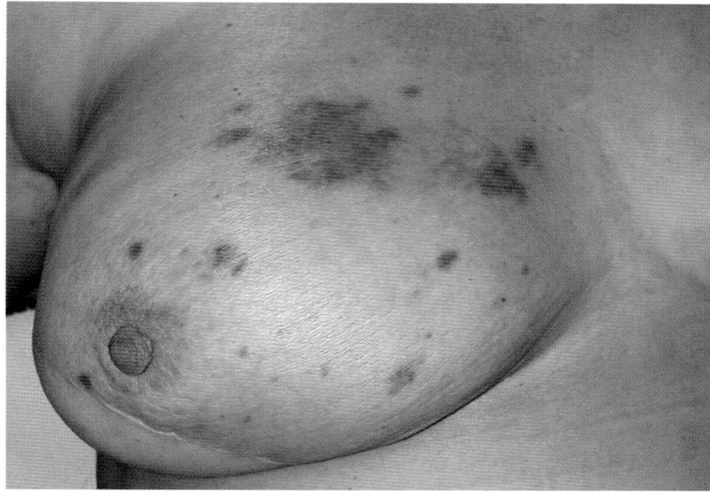

**a** *Clinical appearance* of the right breast. A long infra-areolar scar is present. Reddish-purple macular skin changes are visible about the areola accompanied by a large, patchy skin eruption with irregular margins closer to the chest wall.

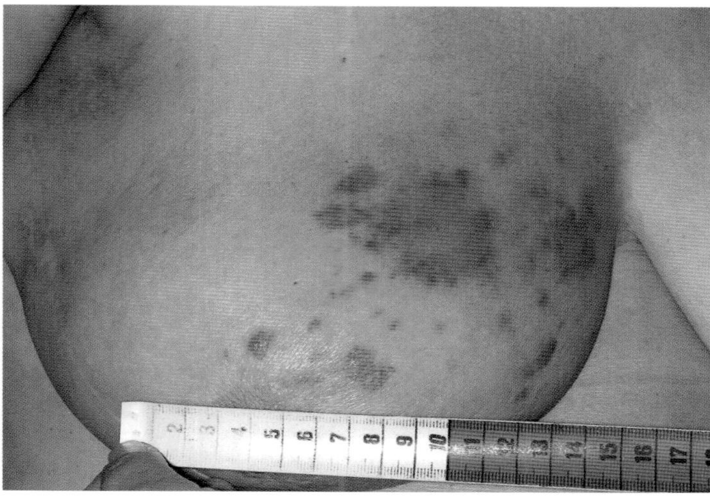

**b** *Clinical appearance* of the right breast 2 months later. The skin lesions have increased in size (images courtesy of Holger Jost, Esslingen).

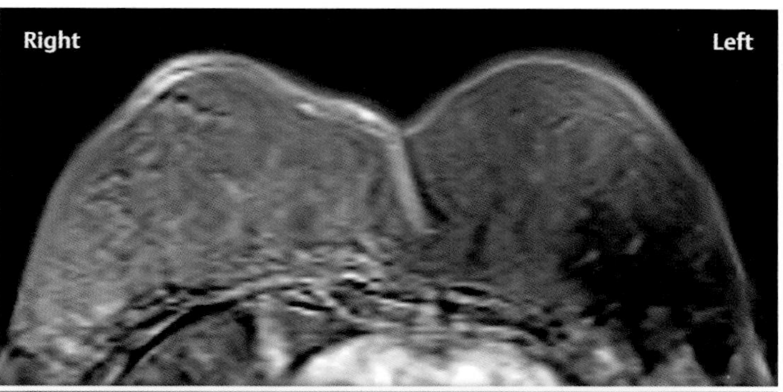


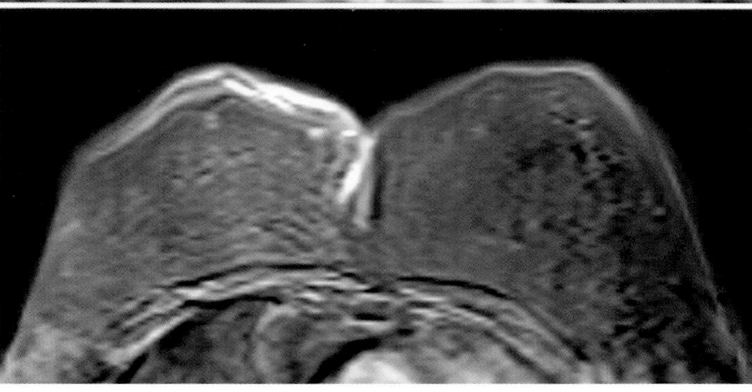

**c** *MRI* shows no intramammary lesions but does show intense gadolinium enhancement of the irradiated skin.

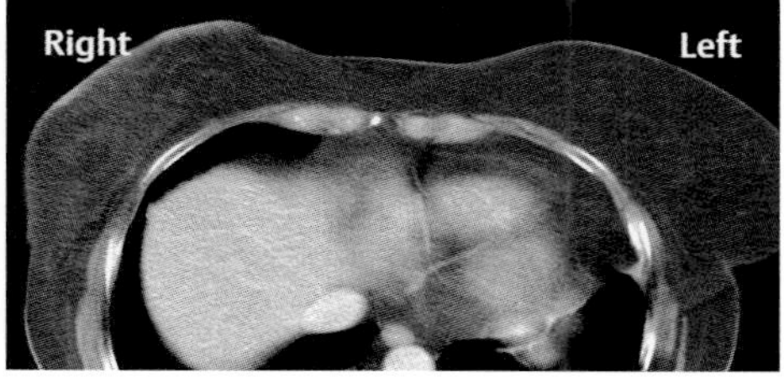


**d** *Computed tomography* shows a circumscribed increase in skin density with no intramammary abnormalities. The left breast appears normal.

**Question on Fig. 5.180**

*How would you interpret the skin changes?*

(**a**) Atypical vascular lesion (angiosarcoma) following radiotherapy (Kaposi sarcoma)

(**b**) Shingles

(**c**) Trophic skin changes due to protracted wound healing problems

→ **Answer on p. 405**

**Fig. 5.181 Follow-up visit.** Scar, local recurrence, or postirradiation changes in a 47-year-old woman who underwent right breast-conserving surgery and radiotherapy in July, 1994. Two reexcisions were performed for recurrent tumors (November, 1994, and January, 1996). She presents now with skin flattening and retraction at the original tumor site.

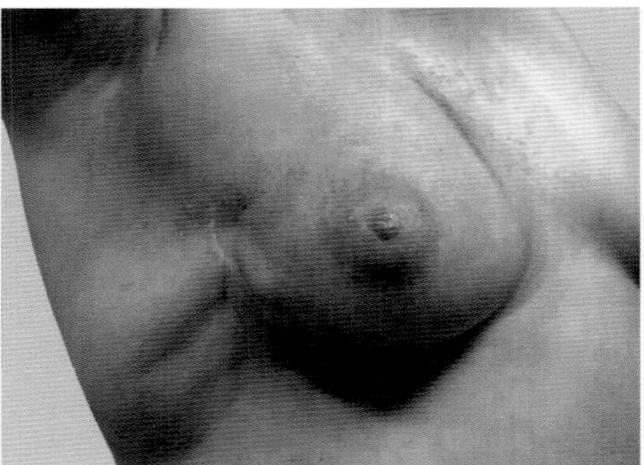

**a** *Clinical inspection* of the right breast shows postoperative scarring and skin retraction on the lateral side of the breast near the chest wall.

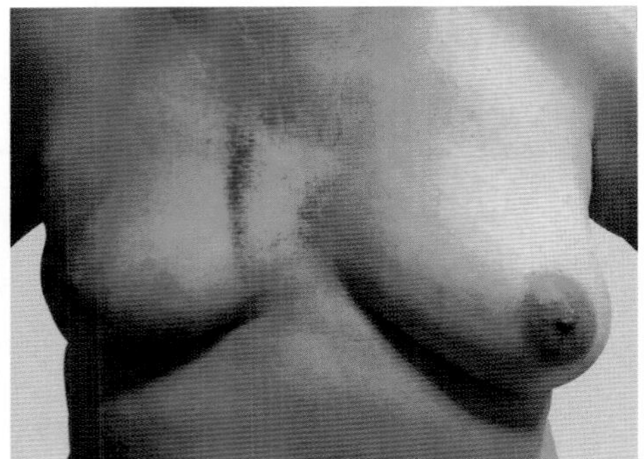

**b** *Clinical inspection* of both breasts shows that the right breast is markedly smaller than the left. Linear telangiectasia appears as a vertical mark to the right of the sternum (**e/24–25**).

R-MLO

L-MLO

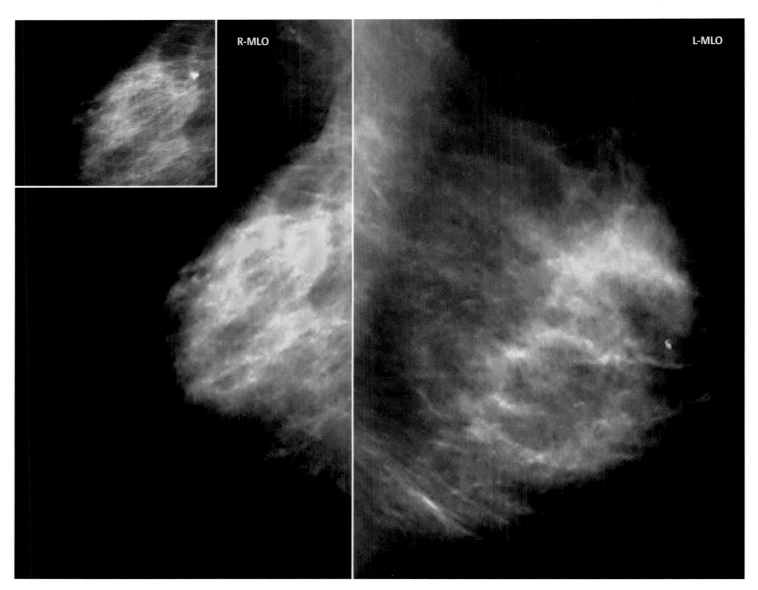

**c** *Bilateral oblique mammograms* in 1996 show a very radiodense right breast with inhomogeneities following multiple reexcisions (**D–E/12–14**). The survey view and the spot view of the upper quadrants (inset) both show nonspecific densities (**B–c/16–18**) (ACR 3, BIRADS?, PG**MI** right, **P**GMI left).

**Fig. 5.181 Follow-up visit.** *(continued)*

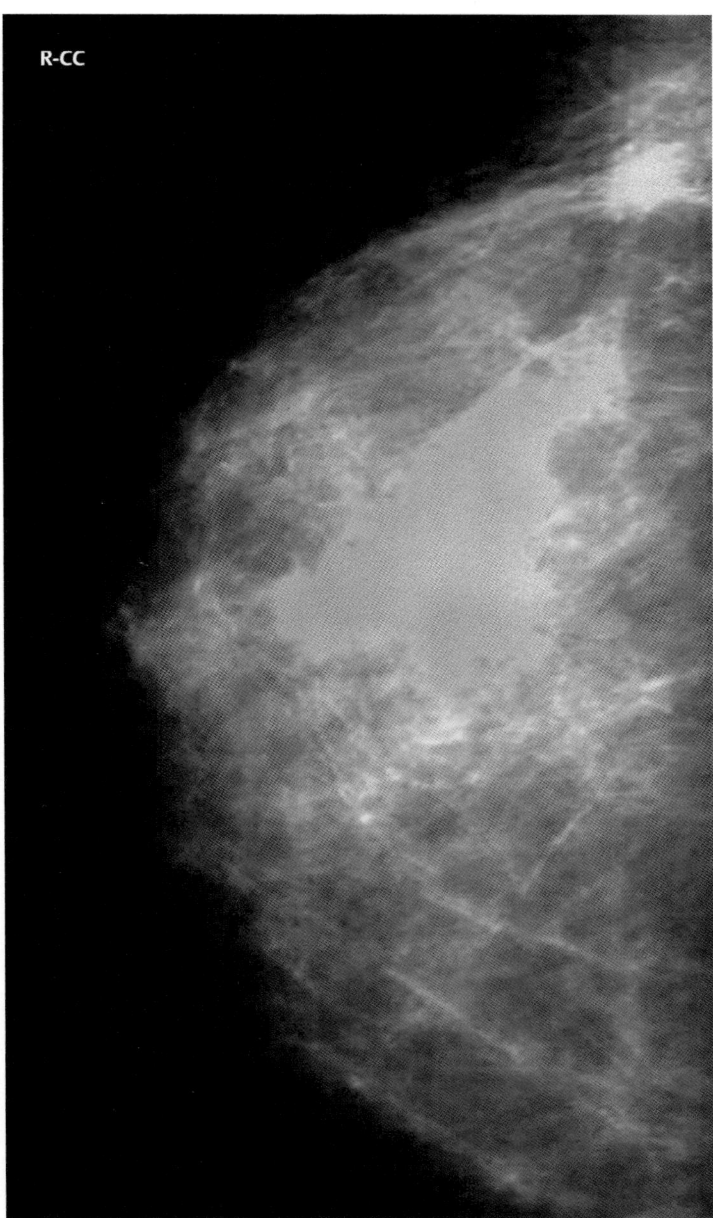


**d** *Craniocaudal mammogram* of the right breast in 1996 shows radiodense glandular tissue with focal retraction and spiculated tissue on the lateral side (**O/25–26**).

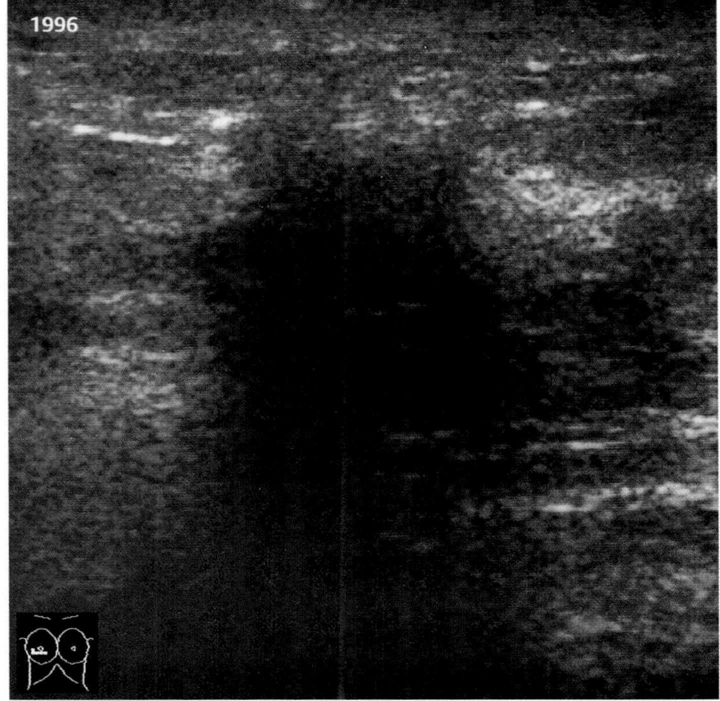


**e** *Sonogram* of the upper outer quadrant of the right breast in 1996 shows a broad scar with a posterior acoustic shadow. Color duplex scan did not show increased vascularity in surrounding tissues.

**Question 1 on Fig. 5.181**

*How would you interpret the skin changes over the inner quadrants?*

(**a**) Congenital telangiectasia
(**b**) Acute mastitis
(**c**) Radiation-induced changes with fibrosis

→ **Answer on p. 405**

**Question 2 on Fig. 5.181**

*Are inspection, palpation, mammography, and ultrasound sufficient for a follow-up examination of the right breast?*

(**a**) Yes
(**b**) No

→ **Answer on p. 405**

**Fig. 5.182 Scar, local recurrence, or summation artifact?** A 56-year-old woman found a nodule in her right breast 1 year earlier (2000). Her left breast seemed normal, but when she presented for examination a malignant tumor was also detected in the left breast (**a**) (both poorly differentiated ductal carcinomas; right T1c N0 M0 G3, left T1c Nx M0 G3); The diagnosis was confirmed by CNB. PET showed no evidence of distant metastasis. Prior to *neoadjuvant chemotherapy*, the tumor was removed from the right breast, followed by removal of the left tumor. Radiotherapy to both breasts was followed by a good cosmetic result. Mammographic follow-up now detects a spiculated density at the former tumor site in the right breast (**e**) associated with circumscribed skin retraction (**d**).

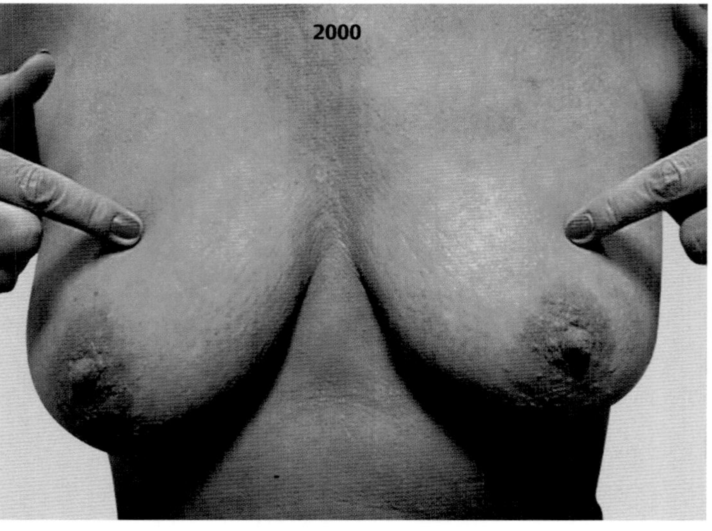


**a** *Clinical aspect*: Nodules are palpable in the left and right breasts.

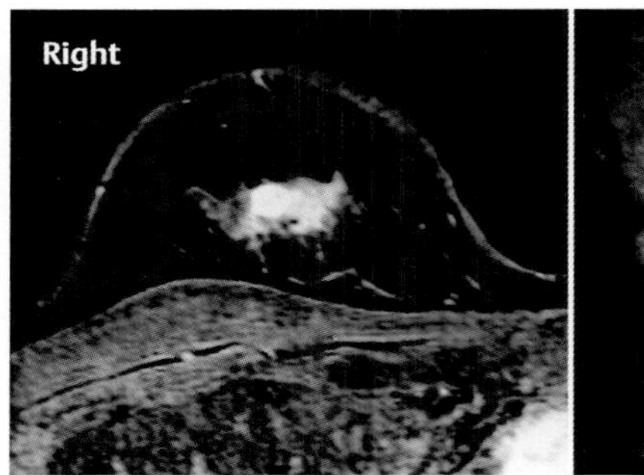


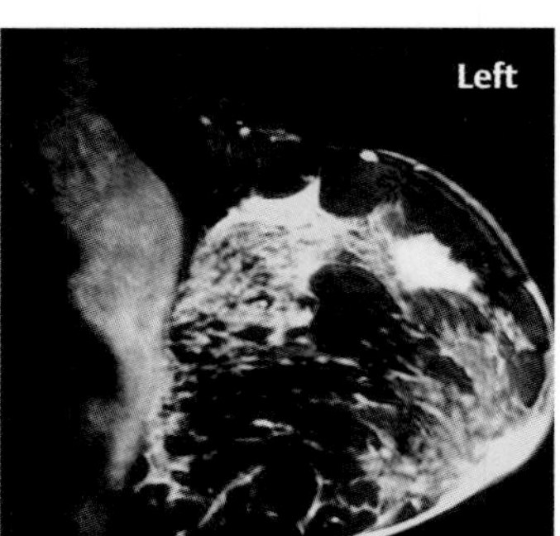


**c** *MRM subtraction* images show gadolinium-enhancing tumors in both breasts (right coronal, left sagittal). Conformance to the shape of a mammary lobe is most clearly appreciated in the sagittal image.

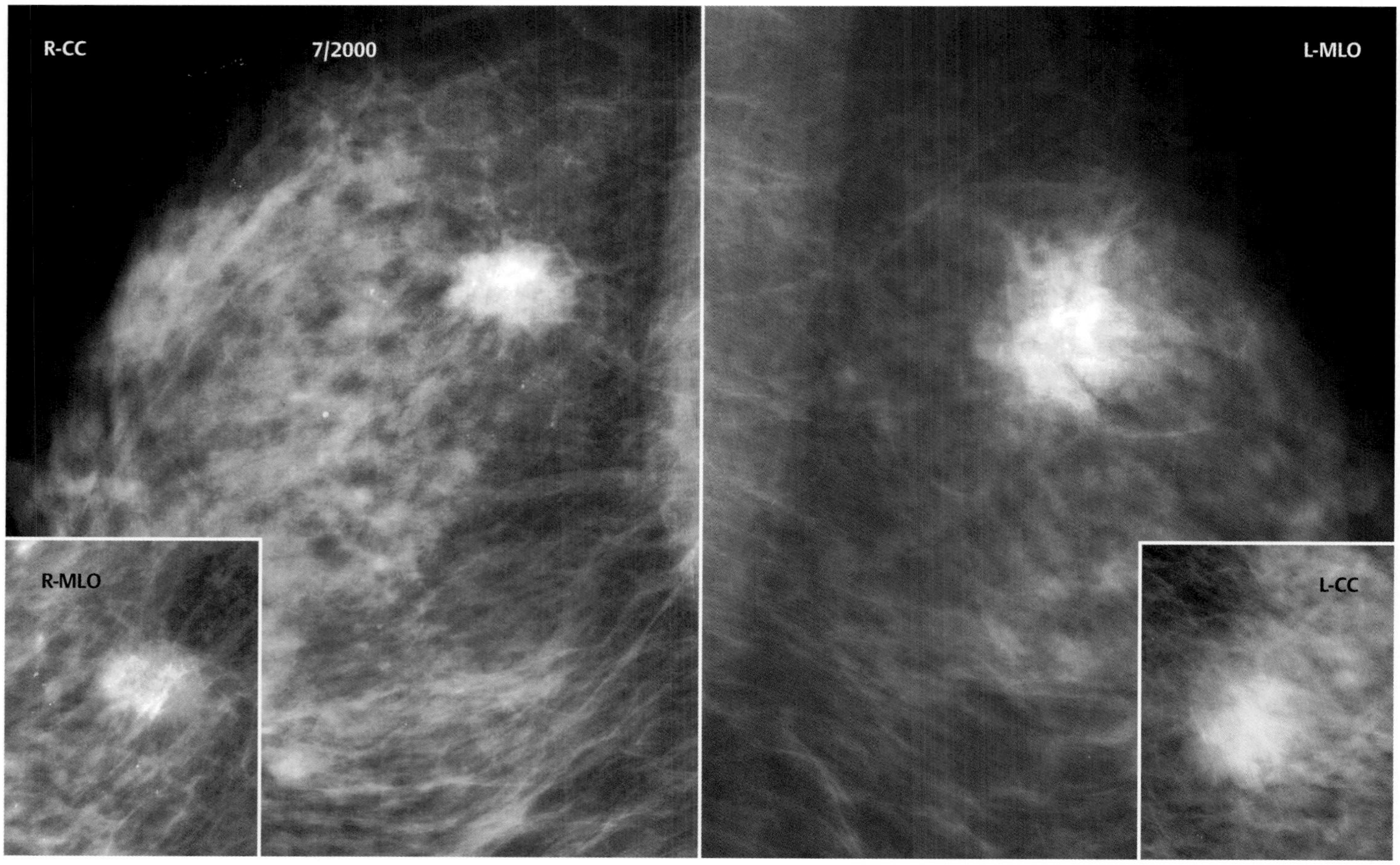

**b** *Craniocaudal mammogram* of the right breast and oblique mammogram of the left breast in July, 2000. *Left breast:* 2 cm tumor in radiodense glandular tissue with mixed scalloped and spiculated margins and associated bulging of the skin. *Right breast:* 1 cm spiculated nodule in the lateral portion of the breast associated with heavy periductal fibrosis. The pectoral muscle is only partly imaged (ACR 2, BIRADS 5 both sides, **P**GMI both sides). *Insets:* corresponding magnified views in the second plane.

**Fig. 5.182 Scar, local recurrence, or summation artifact?** *(continued)*

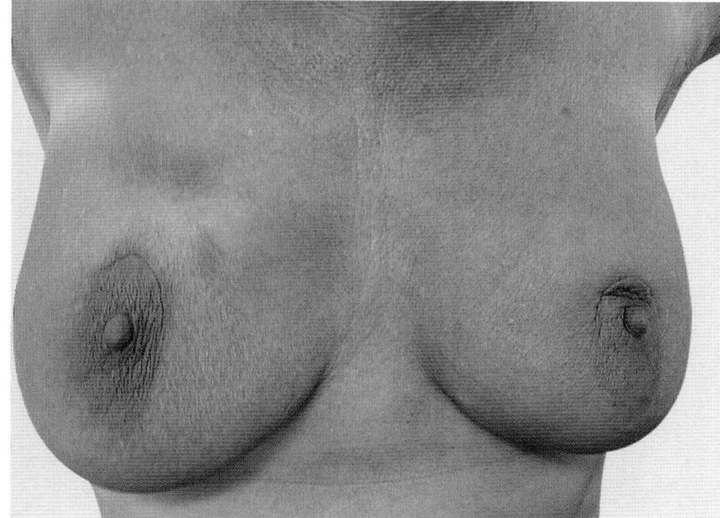

**d** *Posttreatment appearance* in February, 2001. Circumscribed skin retraction is noted at the former tumor site in the right breast (**k–L/25**) with apparent buckling of the medial skin (**l/24**). The left breast shows retraction of the areola at the 12-o'clock position (**n/23**). Bilateral hyperpigmentation of the skin is noted after the completion of radiotherapy.

**Question on Fig. 5.182**

*How would you interpret the mammographic density at* ***O–o/14–15*** *in the right breast?*

(**a**) Tumor excision scar

(**b**) Local recurrence

(**c**) Summation artifact

→ **Answer on p. 406**

R-MLO 2/2002 L-MLO

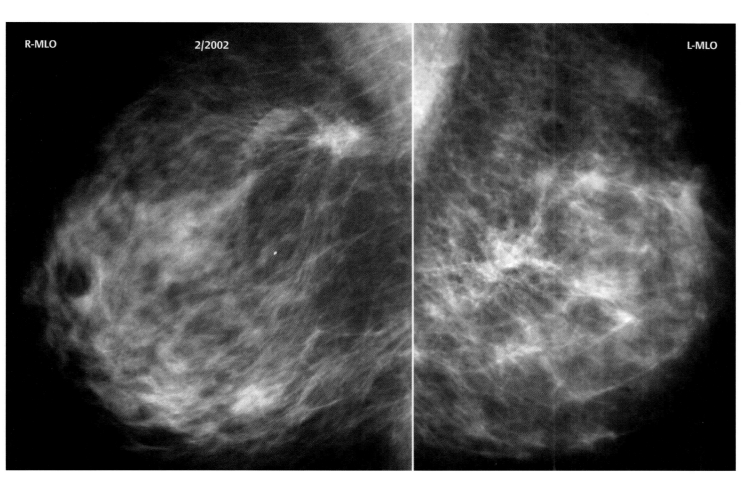

**e** *Bilateral oblique mammograms* in February, 2002 show a spiculated density at the former tumor site in the right breast (**O/13–14**). Despite radiotherapy, the remaining glandular tissue is more radiolucent than in **b** in response to hormonal and chemotherapy. Fibrosis is visible at the former tumor site in the left breast (**Q–S/9–12**).

**Fig. 5.183 Inspection and mammography in the follow-up of a 57-year-old woman who underwent left breast-conserving surgery.** Lymphedema is still present. The left breast appears normal at ultrasound. MRI shows no suspicious changes in either breast. The goal is to evaluate the right breast.

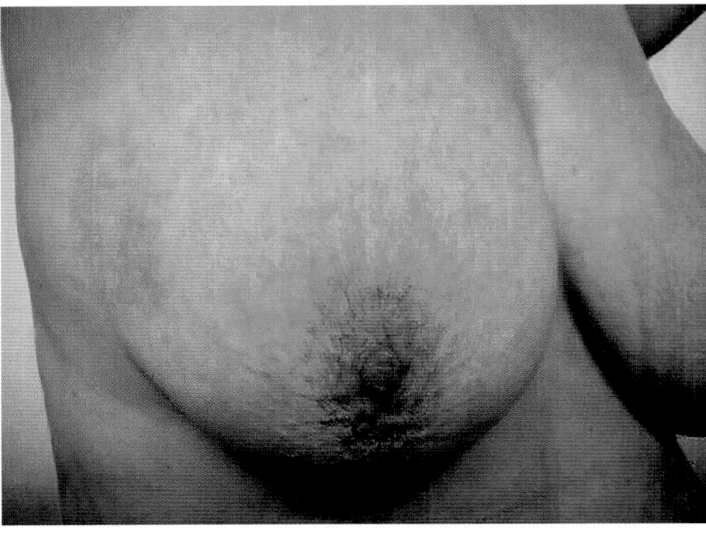

**a** *Clinical appearance* of the right breast following previous breast-conserving therapy of the left breast.

**Question on Fig. 5.183**

*Are the findings suspicious for a tumor?*

(**a**) No

(**b**) Yes, based on clinical findings and mammograms

(**c**) Yes, based on mammograms. No based on clinical findings

→ **Answer on p. 406**

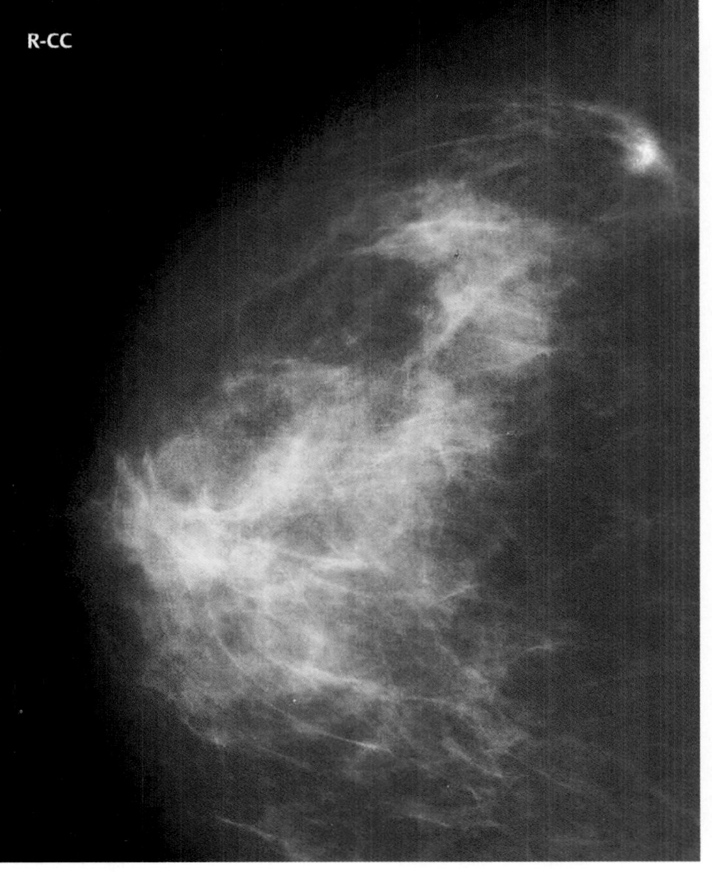


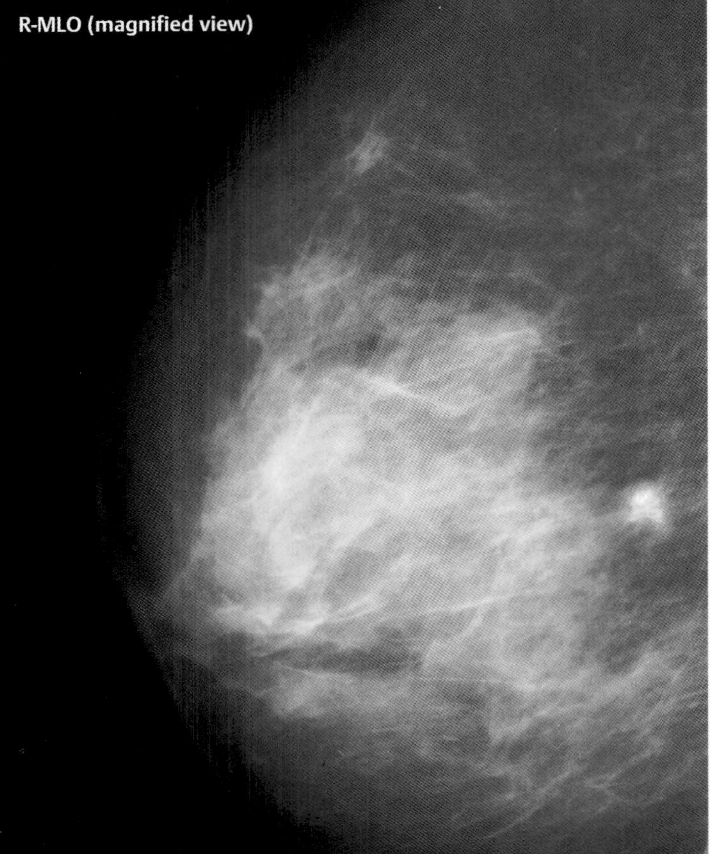


**b** *Craniocaudal* (left) and *mediolateral* (right) *mammograms* of the right breast show radiodense breast parenchyma with small focal densities (ACR 2, BIRADS?, PGMI).

**Fig. 5.184 Inspection and palpation in tumor follow-up.** Three of the four patients shown below have elevated tumor markers with no mammographic or sonographic abnormalities. Each patient can be correctly diagnosed by inspection and palpation. Only one of these women has a benign condition.

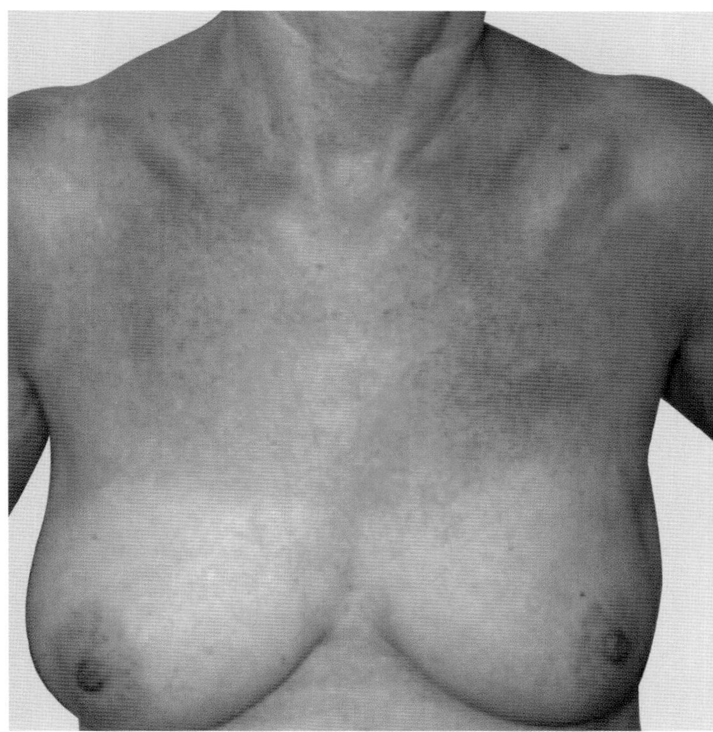

**a Patient A.** A 42-year-old woman who underwent previous left breast-conserving surgery.

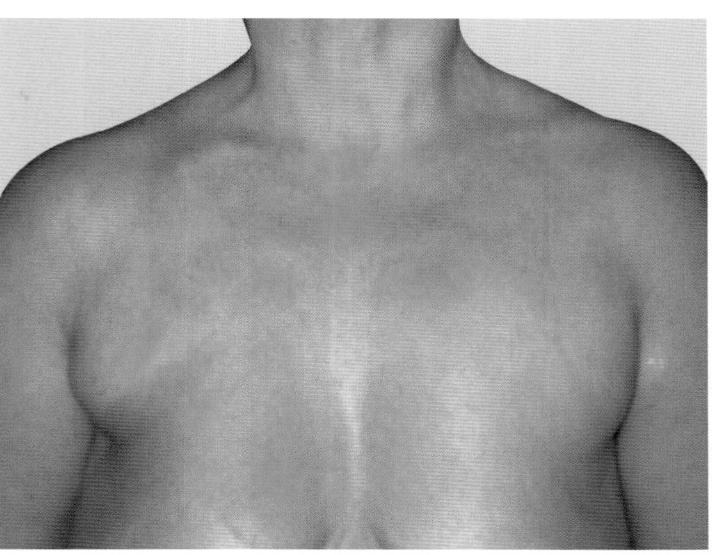

**b Patient B.** A 56-year-old woman who underwent previous right breast-conserving surgery.

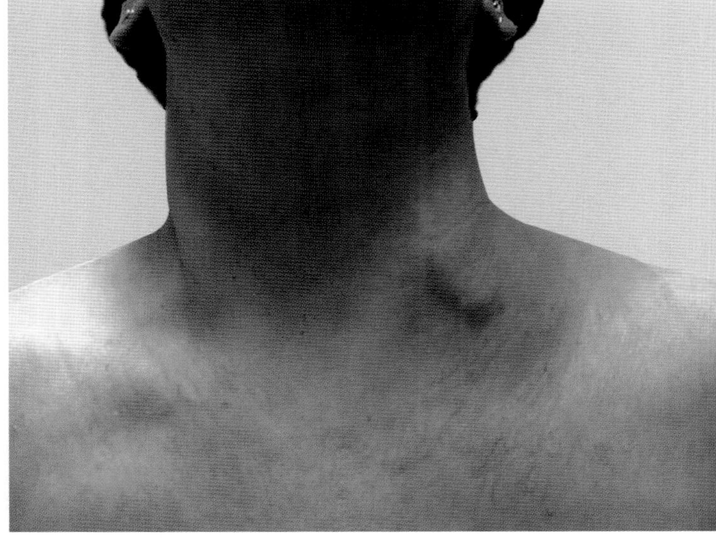

**c Patient C.** A 47-year-old woman who has abnormal CT findings in the left breast.

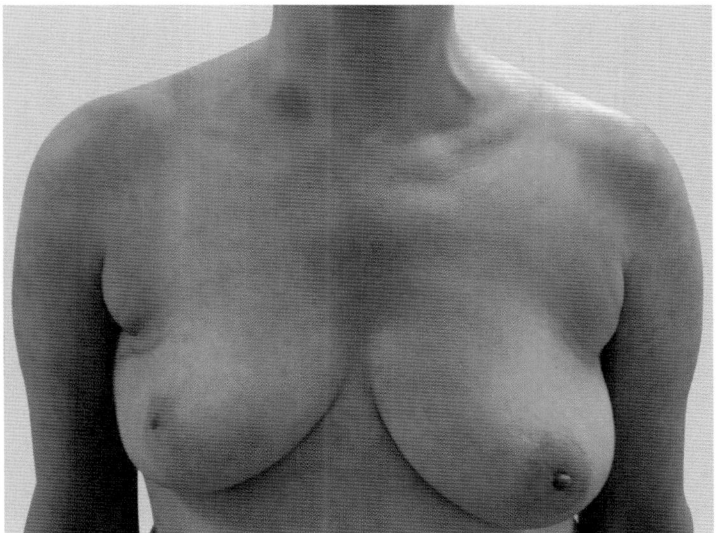

**d Patient D.** A 47-year-old woman who had a previous hysterectomy for endometrial cancer and also underwent right breast-conserving surgery.

**Question on Fig. 5.184**

*All four women have a visible abnormality in the neck and shoulder region. Only one patient has a subcutaneous lipoma. Which one?*

→ **Answer on p. 407**

**Fig. 5.185 Differentiation between scar and local recurrence by FNA and MRI in a 65-year-old woman.** Two years previously the patient underwent excision of a locally advanced tumor in the left breast. A large postoperative seroma formed at the surgical site and in the axilla (**a**). Follow-up mammograms 2 years later demonstrate a stellate scar (**b**). Ultrasound shows a hypoechoic area in the area of the former seroma (**c**). MRI shows intense, suspicious gadolinium enhancement in the region of the scar (**d**). Fine-needle aspiration yields unsuspicious cellular material and debris. Further course of action?

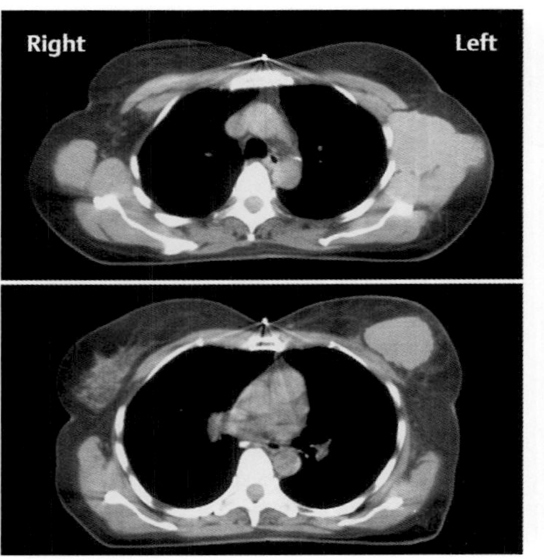


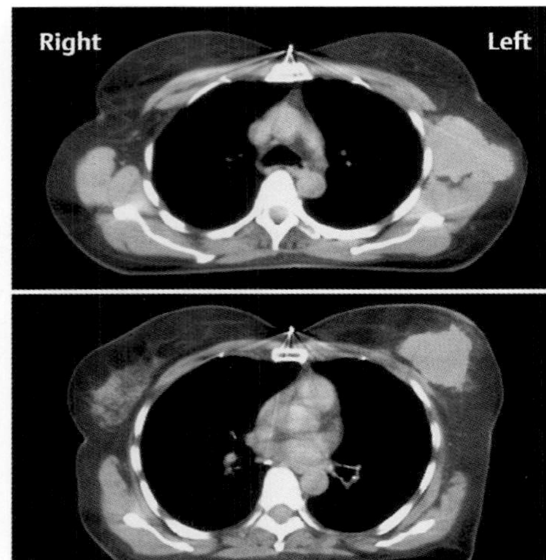


**a** *Postoperative computed tomography* for planning radiotherapy. Scans show an extensive seroma at the operative site (**C–c/22, f–G/22**) and in the left axilla (**c/24, f–G/24**).

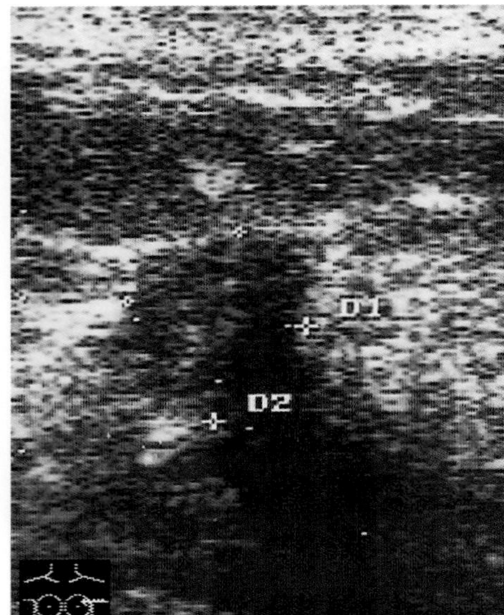


**c** *Sonogram* of the left breast *2 years later* in the former tumor bed (site of previous seroma) shows a hypoechoic area with smooth margins and a posterior acoustic shadow.

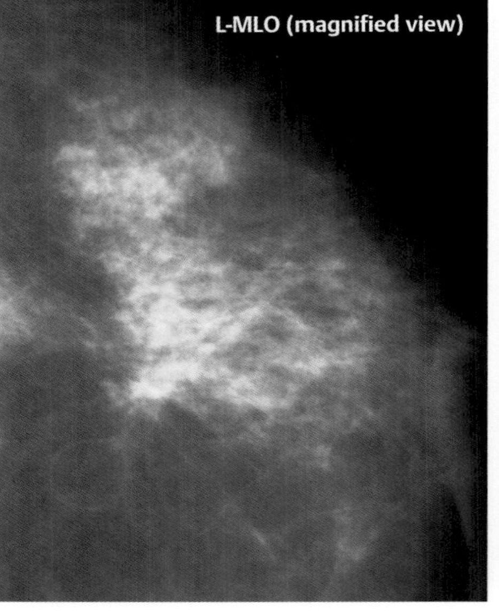


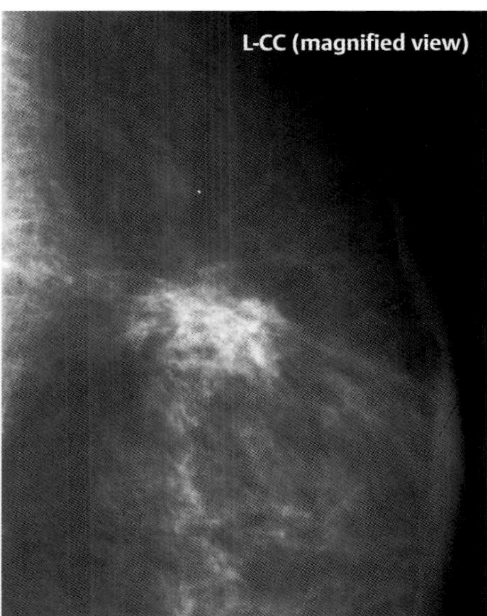


**b** *Oblique* and *craniocaudal* (left) *mammograms* of the left breast *2 years later* show a stellate density at the former tumor site consistent with a scar.

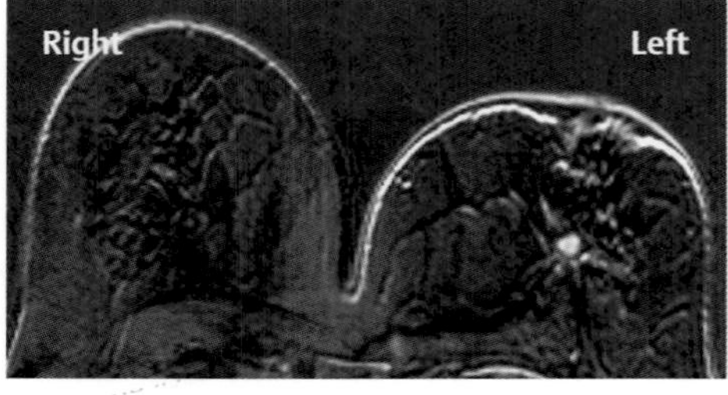


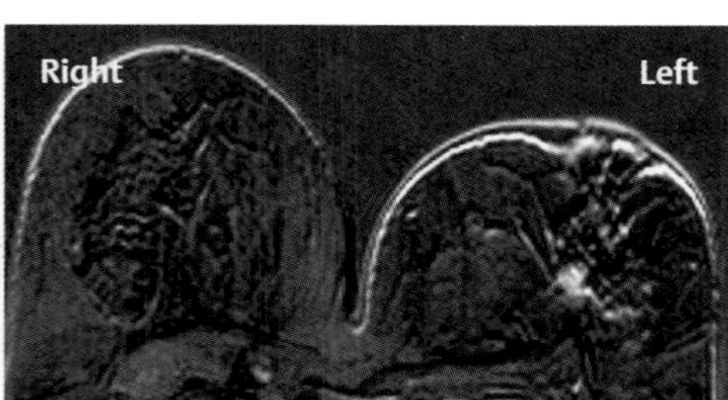


**d** *MR subtraction images* show intense, suspicious gadolinium enhancement of the scarred area (**c+G/5**).

**Question on Fig. 5.185**

*What action would you recommend with unsuspicious cytology and positive MRI?*

(**a**) Follow-up in 6 months
(**b**) Operative treatment
(**c**) Immediate CNB or vacuum biopsy under sonographic, digital stereotactic or MRI guidance

→ **Answer on p. 409**

(continued from p. 328)

Clinical as well as mammographic, sonographic, and MRI findings in the postoperative breast may raise problems of differential diagnosis that often lead to a false-positive interpretation. Scars are the principal source of confusion as they may cause skin and nipple retraction, architectural distortion on mammograms, hypoechoic tumorlike zones on sonograms, and often an intense gadolinium enhancement on MRI when imaged 3–6 months postoperatively (with or without radiotherapy) due to granulation tissue formation and inflammatory tissue reactions.

The use of MRI alone greatly limits our ability to make an accurate benign–malignant differentiation because of the irregular patterns of gadolinium enhancement that occur in both benign and malignant lesions. At present, MRI is approximately 100% sensitive for detecting invasive cancer in the nonoperated breast, while reports on its specificity range widely from 37% to 97% in the recent literature (Kuhl and Braun 2008).

Postoperative changes are most easily interpreted in cases where a thorough preoperative diagnosis has been made. Granulation tissue and scars tend to become smaller over time, while recurrent tumors tend to enlarge. In patients who have had radiation to the breast, cells display radiogenic changes that may be mistaken for a recurrence when evaluated by FNA (see **Fig. 5.168e**, p. 399; **Fig. 5.188**, p. 342 f).

Scars may cause ductal enlargement or stenosis (on ductograms) and calcifications. Fat necrosis with calcifications may pose problems of differential diagnosis at the periphery of excisions when viewed 6–12 months postoperatively (see **Fig. 5.106**, p. 229 f). This condition may be confusing even when it occurs earlier than it would take for malignant calcifications to form in a local recurrence. Care should be taken that all malignant calcifications have been removed with a healthy tissue margin. Thus, two-view postoperative mammograms should always be obtained after the removal of DCIS, either immediately before the patient is discharged or 2–3 months after the operation. Additional follow-ups are then scheduled at 6-month intervals for the next 2 years and at 1-year intervals thereafter. Single-view mammograms are usually adequate for this purpose, using the projection that most clearly defines the operative area. Ultrasound should be added in radiodense breasts.

A special challenge is posed by aesthetic breast reconstructions, especially with silicone implants (see p. 212). In the examination of older silicone implants, the patient should be informed that compression mammography may damage the implant. This is an extremely rare occurrence—but disclosure is better than becoming entangled in a lawsuit.

In the mammographic examination of breast implants (except for subpectoral cosmetic augmentation), the examiner should use as little breast compression as possible. Two and sometimes three projections should be obtained in all cases.

Almost all breast implants undergo fibrous encapsulation, resulting in the formation of wavy surface ridges. Frequently the implant is ruptured, but this does not mean that free silicone has entered the breast parenchyma. The tough fibrous capsule that forms around the implant is sufficient to contain the silicone.

Yearly MRI and ultrasound follow-ups are recommended for women with breast implants, MRI being the more sensitive modality for detecting implant damage. Addition of ultrasound (which shows a typical "snowstorm" pattern of implant rupture caused by intramammary silicone) can establish the diagnosis with reasonable certainty (Harris et al. 2004), but it depends on the reason for insertion of implants. It is appropriate after BCT in young women. For cosmetic reasons follow-ups every 2–3 years are sufficient if there are no problems (pain, lump, change of form, and so on).

Because the routine use of **sentinel lymph node biopsy** (see p. 307) has resulted in less-aggressive treatment of the axilla, there may be a greater theoretical risk of lymph node metastases occurring at higher levels, even with a negative SLN biopsy, than with the older, more radical axillary clearance procedures. This should not have major practical consequences, however, because lymph nodes that drain directly to level III can also be identified by SLN detection and can therefore be removed if necessary. Among 600 SLNBs the authors found no residual or follow-up metastasis in the axilla or above.

There are extranodal lymphatic pathways that may bypass the sentinel lymph node. For this reason, special attention should be given to the supraclavicular fossa and especially the infraclavicular fossa in follow-up examinations. Lymph node metastases are frequently missed at these sites due to the subtlety of metastases that form beneath the pectoral muscle or within the fossae (see **Fig. 5.184 b**, p. 335). On the other hand, subcutaneous lipomas are easy to detect and their benignancy can be established easily and economically by FNA (see **Fig. 5.184 a**, p. 335).

**Tip**

**PET scanning should be used for the staging of locally advanced tumors that have received neoadjuvant therapy and have metastasized to the axilla. PET can detect or exclude distant metastases and direct the planning of treatment.**

There is no reason why women already treated for breast cancer should not be readmitted to a screening program on a long-term basis, as it is also important to maintain surveillance of the healthy breast.

MRI is of major importance in the follow-up of women who have undergone breast-conserving therapy. It should be performed every 12–18 months in all breasts with a density of ACR 3 or higher, preferably scheduling it between mammography and ultrasound or perhaps in conjunction with these two modalities.

**Chest radiographs, hepatic ultrasound, skeletal examinations, radionuclide bone scans**, and the regular determination of **tumor marker levels** are unnecessary in follow-up settings. This is because these tests are costly, have a low diagnostic yield, are time-consuming, and are distressful for many patients—especially when false-positive findings are obtained. But in cases where metastasis is detected or presumed based on clinical manifestations, it is appropriate to determine tumor marker levels (CEA, CA 18–5, CA 19–9, CA 27–29, etc.) to evaluate therapeutic response. Of course, imaging studies (radiography, MRI, CT, PET, etc.) are also appropriate for this indication. An essential goal of follow-up is the early detection of local recurrence and of second tumors in the clinically healthy breast. Early detection alone has far-reaching implications and can prevent the development of disseminated disease. Should metastasis occur, the survival-time is limited and has not increased for the past 40 years. But the quality of life has improved during this time.

In 1995, a central office for breast cancer follow-up was established in Germany within the framework of a field study called

"Quality Assurance in Breast Cancer Follow-Up." Conducted by the Comprehensive Cancer Center (OSP) in Stuttgart (Germany) under the direction of Professor Else Heidemann, in cooperation with the Institute for Medical Information Processing at the University of Tübingen (Germany) (Professor H.-K. Selbmann), the goal of the project was to compare **symptom-oriented follow-up** with **conventional follow-up** in terms of survival time and disease-free survival while also developing a quality management system for breast cancer follow-up in the Stuttgart region (Heidemann and Rössle 2004). The basic structures for quality management include a reminder system for doctors and patients, the documentation of follow-up data after testing for completeness and plausibility, and the reporting of data back to primary caregivers for evaluating the quality of results. An interim evaluation showed that mammographic follow-ups, which are essential for the detection of cancer recurrence, were performed far too infrequently. This emphasized the importance of reminding both doctors and patients of upcoming mammogram appointments.* The study also found a number of discrepancies between patients' statements in quality-of-life questionnaires and the findings of physicians who took the patients' histories, especially with regard to shortness of breath, pain, and weakness/fatigue. These discrepancies were reported to the attending physician in a separate note. Newsletters were sent to patients at irregular intervals informing them of various topics relating to breast cancer follow-up. In addition, FAQs were compiled, answered, and distributed to all participating patients in a newsletter. Many physicians in private practice were enrolled in the project. There were also colleagues who declined to participate despite the willingness of their patients. The reason given was lack of adequate compensation for follow-up services; eliminating this problem would certainly induce more physicians to participate in the project. Surveys by the authors have shown that women would be happy to participate in the project and would derive an added sense of security from the additional care.

Symptom-oriented follow-up has advantages over standard "technique-oriented" follow-up with respect to total survival. It is true that most patients would prefer a more technically oriented follow-up with greater emphasis on imaging (MRI, CT, etc.), which is costly but inefficient. They rely more on sophisticated studies in the hope of alleviating their fears. While this attitude is understandable, it overlooks the fact that equivocal findings may give rise to new concerns, or that elevated tumor markers may raise suspicion of metastases, which are usually excluded by further cost-intensive tests.

In a cost analysis in the United States comparing a *minimalistic* follow-up regimen with a more *intensive* (imaging-based) follow-up program over a 5-year period, it was found that the average cost of the intensive program, at 5735 USD, was more than five times that of the simpler regimen, which averaged 1025 USD. This would result in an annual cost saving of 821 million USD with no demonstrable negative impact on patient survival (Stemmler et al. 2006).

There is no difference in the probability of survival between conventional follow-up and symptom-oriented follow-up. The following factors were found to be statistically significant in terms of survival probability:

- Disease stage (UICC)
- Age (50 years or younger, > 50 years)
- Type of surgical procedure
- Receptor status (positive, negative)

Other factors such as *tumor grade* or the presence of *multiple primary tumors* were not found to be statistically relevant. These and other studies have shown that regularly scheduled imaging procedures should be replaced by a follow-up protocol that puts greater emphasis on the investigation and treatment of patients' complaints.

It would be desirable to have this kind of quality management available not just in Stuttgart but throughout Germany and the rest of the world. A trend toward symptom-oriented care has become evident in English-speaking countries in recent years (Harris et al. 2004). One future solution might be the creation of an internet container (e.g., the IWC company) with ODS-Easy software that could be accessed by large numbers of specialists and radiologists in private practice.

## Local Recurrence

Local recurrence is detected mammographically in one-fourth to one-half of women who have undergone breast-conserving therapy (Harris et al. 2004). The main clinical manifestations of local recurrence are skin retraction, local firmness, and the appearance of mammographic densities, microcalcifications, and architectural distortion (**Figs. 5.186, 5.187**). *Ultrasound* cannot distinguish between local recurrence and scar tissue. *Magnetic resonance imaging* typically shows new areas of gadolinium enhancement. This finding is particularly significant when a baseline has been established, and so pre- and postoperative magnetic resonance images should be available. A local recurrence may affect the breast following breast-conserving therapy and may involve the chest wall following mastectomy.

An intramammary local recurrence is occasionally difficult to distinguish from fat necrosis. According to published reports, calcifications form earlier in fat necrosis than in tumors. Closely related to local recurrences in the breast are changes due to intramammary metastases from tumors in other organs (very rare!) and breast changes due to the obstruction of lymphatic drainage. Possible causes of lymphatic obstruction are axillary lymph node metastases, nonmalignant lesions in the axilla, and axillary and retrosternal scarring. Intramammary metastases typically present as well-circumscribed round nodules that have a multicentric distribution in the breast. Their cause is easily established by FNA. Cutaneous metastases (fortunately rare today) do not present problems of differential diagnosis. It can be more difficult to diagnose disseminated disease. The possibility of distant metastasis should be considered in all cases where a slow-growing breast cancer has been missed, and PET should be performed if distant metastasis would have therapeutic implications (see p. 227).

* At our center in Esslingen (IMZE), we have solved this problem with single-view mammography (see p. 105). Patients receive single-view mammograms only if they are on time for their follow-up visits. Otherwise we obtain two views per breast. The efficacy of this system for "rewarding punctuality" has been impressive.

**Fig. 5.186** **Right breast of a 70-year-old woman** who underwent repeated operations and core biopsies from 1977, each yielding a diagnosis of fibroadenoma or scar. Years ago she had a cystosarcoma phylloides tumor removed from the right breast. Her breast became progressively smaller over the course of treatment. In 2001 her gynecologist noted firmness in the right breast and diagnosed fibrosis, prompting surgical excision. Core biopsy was performed in January, 2004 again yielding a diagnosis of scar tissue.

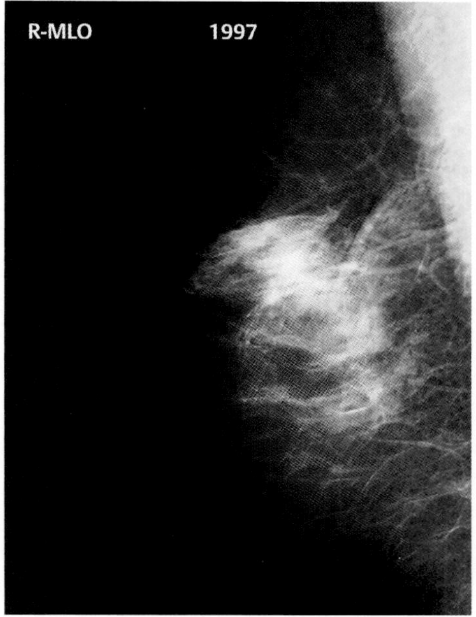


**a** *Oblique mammogram* in 1997 shows a nonspecific density in the upper portion of the radiodense right breast. A local excision was performed, and the lesion was identified histologically as fibrosis.

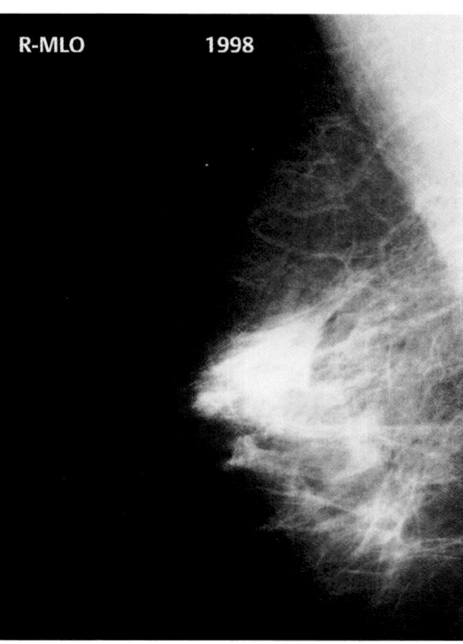


**b** *Oblique mammogram* of the right breast in 1998 shows nonspecific increased retroareolar density.

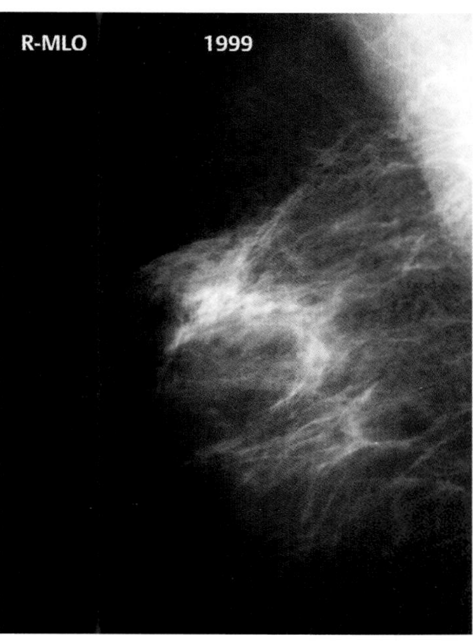


**c** *Oblique mammogram* of the right breast in 1999. Previous surgical biopsy yielded a diagnosis of fibrosis and scar tissue.

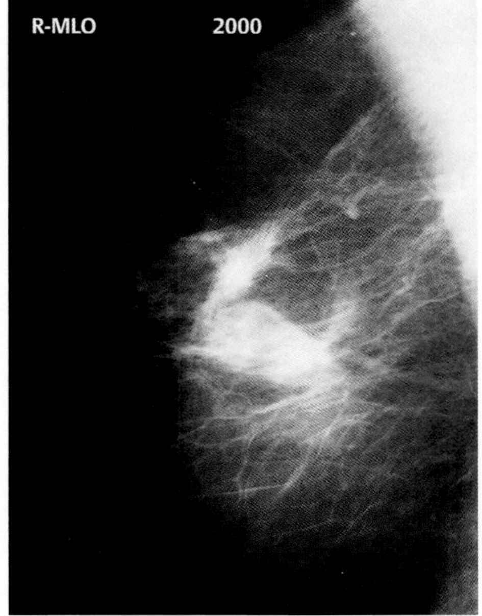


**d** *Oblique mammogram* of the right breast in 2000 shows increasing retroareolar density in the indurated glandular tissue. CNB indicated fibrosis.

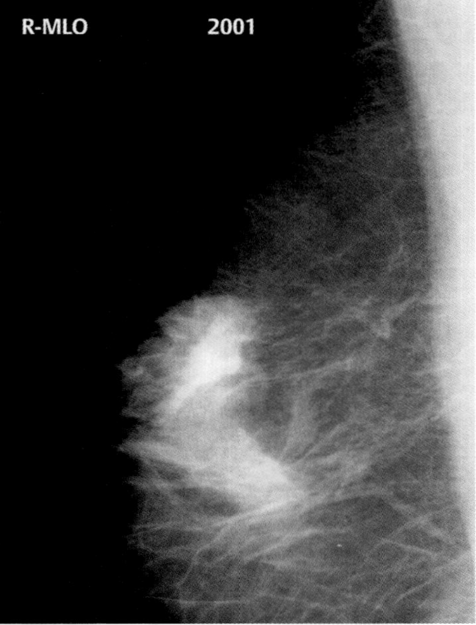


**e** *Oblique mammogram* of the right breast in 2001. The gynecologist mistrusts the core needle biopsy result and performs an open biopsy, which again yields scar tissue and fibrosis.

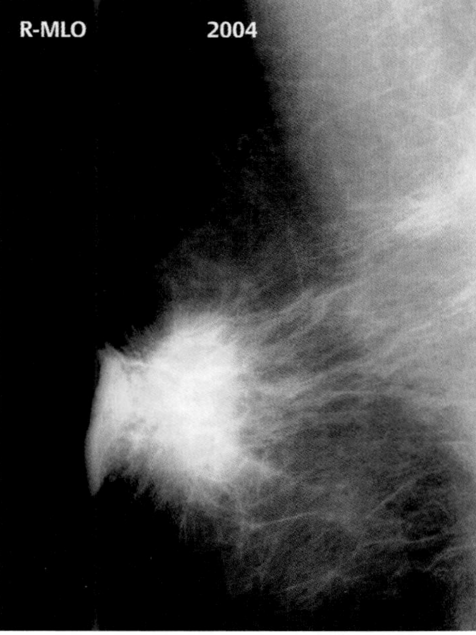


**f** *Oblique mammogram* of the right breast in February, 2004. Another CNB is performed for increasing breast firmness, and histology indicates a scar.

**Question on Fig. 5.186**

*How would you interpret the findings?*

(**a**) Chronic aggressive fibrosis

(**b**) Breast carcinoma that was missed in numerous biopsies (by the surgeon and pathologist)

(**c**) Recurrence of cystosarcoma phylloides

→ **Answer on p. 409**

## Intramammary, Regional, and Generalized Metastasis

The treatment protocol for distant metastasis is different from that for local disease.

Imaging procedures are not used to screen for distant metastases during follow-up. The former practice of obtaining yearly thoracic and skeletal radionuclide scans and hepatic ultrasound scans is now considered obsolete. These tests have no real therapeutic implications, for while they permitted the earlier initiation of treatment for metastases, they had no real benefit in terms of survival time or quality of life. Today, treatment with aromatase inhibitors and Zoladex may benefit patients, but this remains to be seen—for once distant metastasis has occurred, a cure is no longer possible. The later the patient learns that her cancer has metastasized, the better her quality of life. This does not mean that we should lie to a patient with confirmed metastasis and offer a benign diagnosis as the cause of her complaints. On the contrary: even patients with confirmed metastasis will benefit from being actively involved in their plan of treatment. Sehouli et al. (2004) reported on an initial nationwide patient survey in Germany that addressed the question of how patients with metastatic breast cancer perceive their treatment. They were surprised to learn that the internet is a major source of information for women with metastatic breast cancer. Surveys like this one, which was presented at the 26th German Cancer Congress in Berlin, are designed to advance the following goals:

- Assess the need for information and disclosure
- Identify deficits in clinical management
- Discern reasons for patient compliance and noncompliance
- Generate working hypotheses and discussion material for possible solutions
- Establish a foundation for prospective studies

The average age of the women who responded to the survey was 49.5 years. Based on the information supplied by the women interviewed, the initial consultation in which the diagnosis was reported lasted an average of 15 minutes (0–300 minutes). To see whether their doctor recommended the appropriate treatment, 74.9% of the women used the internet, 56.7% sought a second opinion, and 25.4% asked their family doctor. Some 95% of the responders wanted to consult an independent expert source, but 73% were unaware of such an institution. Most of the participants—86.3% and 82%—believed that their treating physician was the best information source for learning more about adjuvant and palliative treatment options, respectively.

The US National Cancer Institute presents a very helpful index of *questions and answers* (www.cancertopics/treatment/breast) about metastatic breast cancer and the principles of treatment (surgery, radiation, chemotherapy/hormone therapy/complementary and alternative treatment, and so on). The website of the European Federation of Neurological Societies (EFNS) from Soffietti et al. (2006) (www.efnsguidelinesondiagnosisandtreatmentofbrain-metastasis) can be recommended, in particular for questions of diagnosis and treatment of cerebral metastasis.

Patients tended to feel well informed when their treatment was discussed within the framework of an overall treatment plan (54.9%). Half of the patients (50.6%) asked their doctors for information on enrolling in clinical studies. Almost all the patients wanted detailed information on the side-effects of their chemotherapy. Approximately 50% of the women wanted complete and understandable doctor–patient conferences that were tailored to the patient's individual wants and needs. The patients recommended the following changes:

- Even orthodox physicians should offer alternative therapies (55%).
- Physicians should take more time for explanations (50.2%).
- Doctors should cooperate better among themselves (39.2%).

These and other patient recommendations are summarized in **Table 5.14**.

Patients receive much of their information from medical brochures, TV broadcasts, support groups, etc. (**Table 5.15**). This suggests possible areas of improvement in every practice, and every physician involved in the treatment of cancer patients should implement modifications and innovations based on personal experience.

Incidentally, when it comes to the treatment of metastases it is important to determine whether the lesions are actually metastatic to the breast or whether they originate in some other organ. In rare cases, for example, an atypical pattern of metastasis may suggest that a first or second tumor is metastatic thyroid cancer, which would be treatable with radio-iodine unless prior iodine administration (e.g., in radiographic contrast medium) has eliminated this option.

**Table 5.14 Interim analysis of a survey question answered by 503 women:** "If you could make three changes in your treatment for breast cancer, what would they be?" (multiple answers possible; total answers *n* = 1499) (Sehouli et al. 2004).

| Answers | Frequency (%) |
|---|---|
| The total length of treatment should be shorter. | 12.0 |
| There should be better cooperation among doctors. | 39.2 |
| Doctors should take more time for explanations. | 50.2 |
| The treatment should not cause hair loss. | 19.4 |
| Better treatment for pain. | 7.4 |
| Better treatment for fatigue. | 26.8 |
| More medications to control vomiting. | 11.4 |
| Better treatment for headaches. | 2.4 |
| Nursing care should be improved. | 7.6 |
| Treatment results should be reported to patients more often. | 25.0 |
| The treatment should be more effective. | 24.6 |
| Doctors should offer alternative treatments. | 55.0 |

**Fig. 5.187 Examination of a 61-year-old woman 6 years after right mastectomy (a).** A nonspecific mass is noted in the area of the thoracic scar. FNA of the mass yields atypical cells from a papillary tumor. Ultrasound shows an elliptical, hypoechoic area on the chest wall with posterior acoustic enhancement (**b**). Subsequent excision of the palpable mass yielded a histologic diagnosis of *lipoma*.

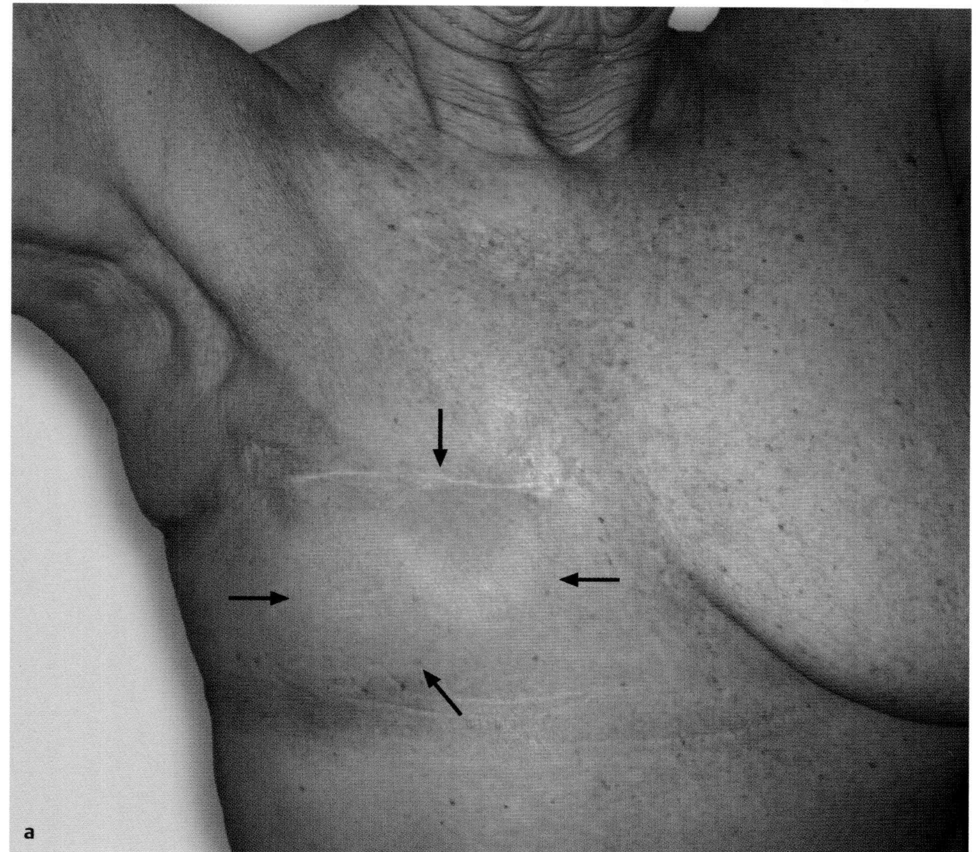

**a** Aspect of thoracic wall with bulging beneath the scar (arrows).

**Question 1 on Fig. 5.187**

*Is there is plausible connection between the sonographic/cytologic findings and the histologic findings?*

(**a**) Yes

(**b**) No

→ **Answer on p. 409**

**Question 2 on Fig. 5.187**

*What anatomical structure is involved?*

(**a**) Rib

(**b**) Soft tissues

(**c**) Pleura

→ **Answer on p. 409**

**Table 5.15 Effectiveness of various information sources from the patients' perspective** ("What sources of information have you found most helpful in learning about treatment options?" multiple answers possible) (Sehouli et al. 2004).

| Answers | Frequency (%) |
|---|---|
| **Adjuvant therapy** | |
| Treating physician | 86.3 |
| Patient brochures | 30.4 |
| TV broadcasts | 5.0 |
| Support groups | 21.1 |
| Internet | 55.3 |
| Family doctor | 18.3 |
| **Palliative care** | |
| Treating physician | 82.0 |
| Patient brochures | 25.6 |
| TV broadcasts | 6.0 |
| Support groups | 22.6 |
| Internet | 57.1 |
| Family doctor | 14.3 |

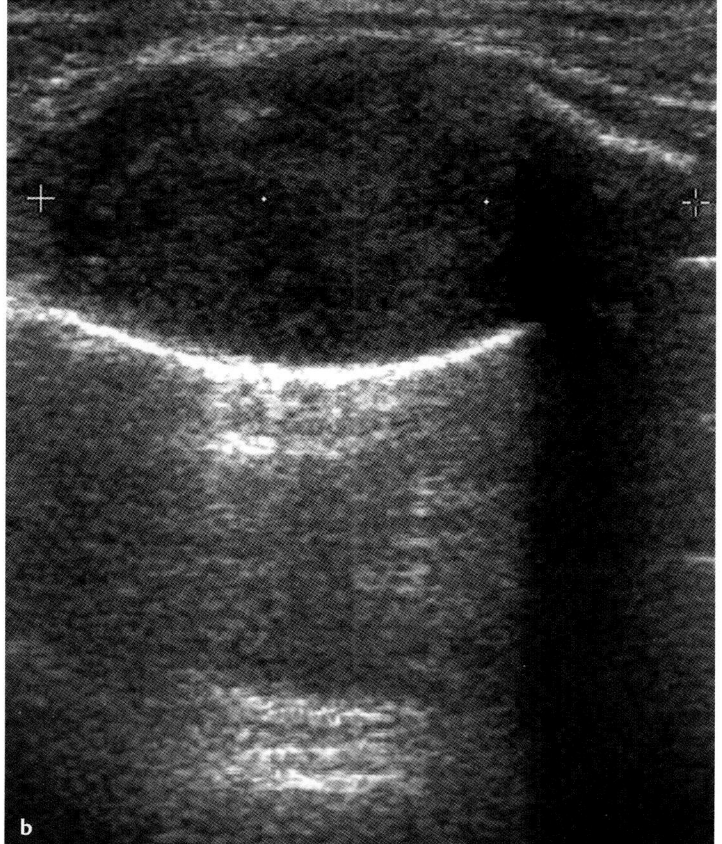

**b** Ultrasound of the bulged area.

**Fig. 5.188 Second opinion. A 63-year-old woman who noted a nonspecific palpable mass in her left breast in September, 2006.** Mammography showed no abnormalities (**a, b**). A colleague recommended ultrasound. In December, 2006, physical examination (**f**, left), ultrasound (**d**), and MRI (**e–g**) revealed an *extensive invasive lobular carcinoma*. The tumor was hormone-receptor-negative and showed high expression of HER2/neu. This prompted a cycle of primary (neoadjuvant) chemotherapy, which led to very rapid tumor regression (**h–l**). An excisional biopsy from the original tumor in July, 2007 confirmed that complete remission had occurred. In January, 2008, fat necrosis and an oil cyst were found at the excision site (**k**), and mammograms showed cicatricial changes in that area (**i**). Trastuzumab (Herceptin) since August of 2007 for the overexpression of HER2. In early 2008 regression of all tumors including a left axillary metastasis (histologically confirmed before chemotherapy) (**d, g**). **How do possible distant metastases respond to this treatment regimen?**

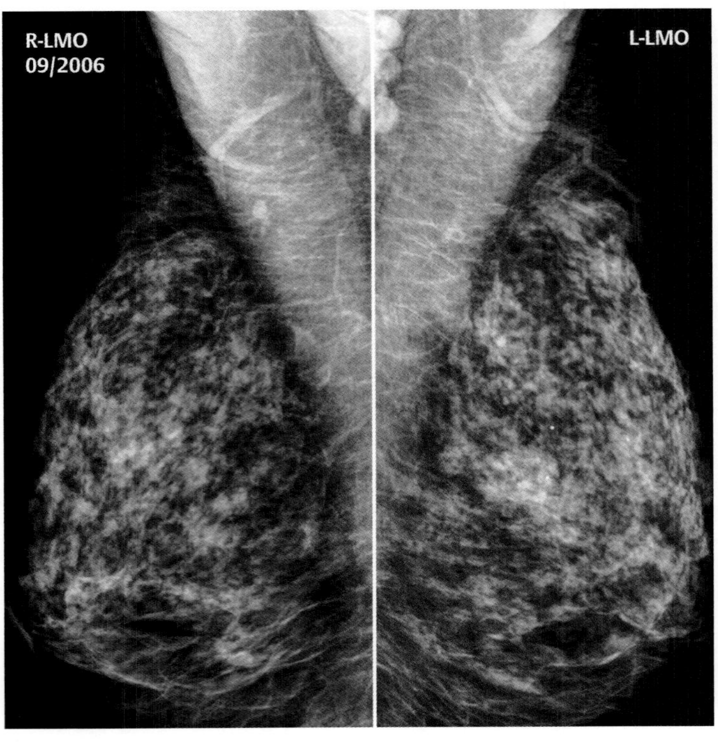


**a** *Bilateral oblique mammograms* in September, 2006 are normal. Notable findings are increased periductular markings and a prominent left axillary lymph node.

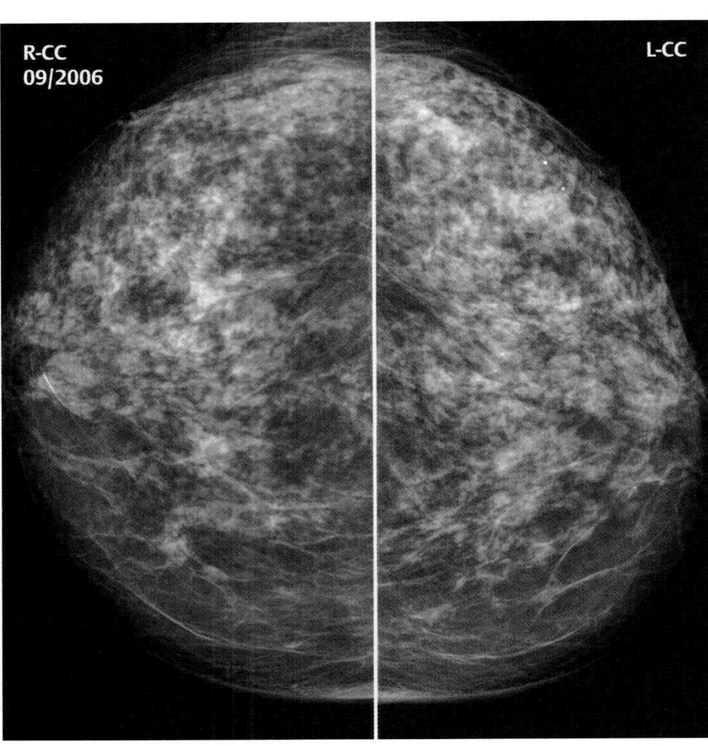


**b** *Bilateral craniocaudal mammograms* in September, 2006 show no evidence of a malignant process (ACR 3, BIRADS 1, P**G**MI).

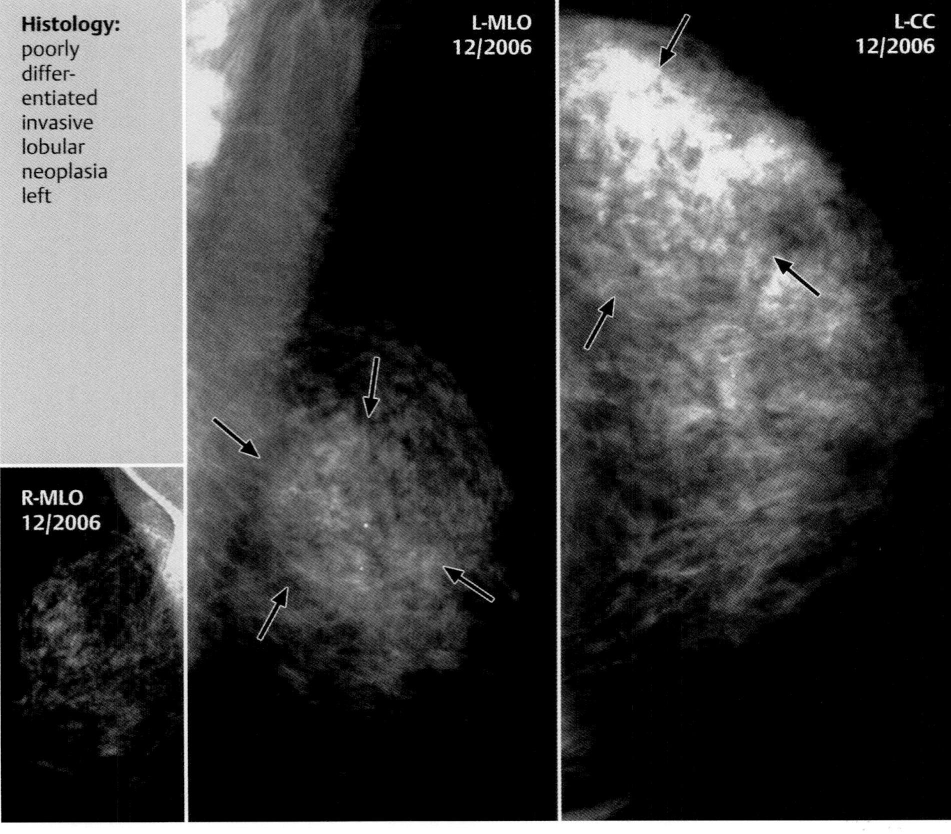


**c** *Biplane mammograms* of the left breast and an *oblique mammogram* of the right breast in December, 2006 show nonspecific increased parenchymal density in the outer quadrants of the left breast between the 1 and 4-o'clock positions relative to the previous examination (ACR 3, PG**M**I, BIRADS 4). The left axillary lymph node is markedly enlarged. No abnormalities are seen in the right breast.

**Fig. 5.188 Second opinion. 63-year-old woman who noted a nonspecific palpable mass in her left breast.** *(continued)*

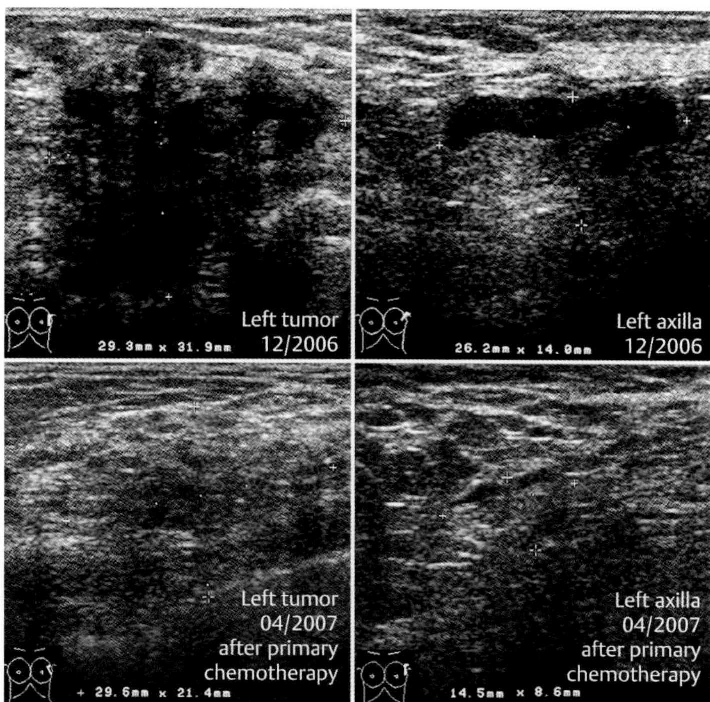


**d** *Ultrasound* in December, 2006 (upper two images), and follow-up scans after primary chemotherapy in April, 2007 (below). Ultrasound in 2006 shows an extensive tumor with hypoechoic, inhomogeneous elements and irregular margins measuring 3 cm × 3 cm × 4 cm. A greatly enlarged lymph node with a broad rim is visible in the left axilla due to the locally advanced neoplasia. Images 4 months later document complete tumor regression (lower left) and complete normalization of the left axillary lymph node (lower right).

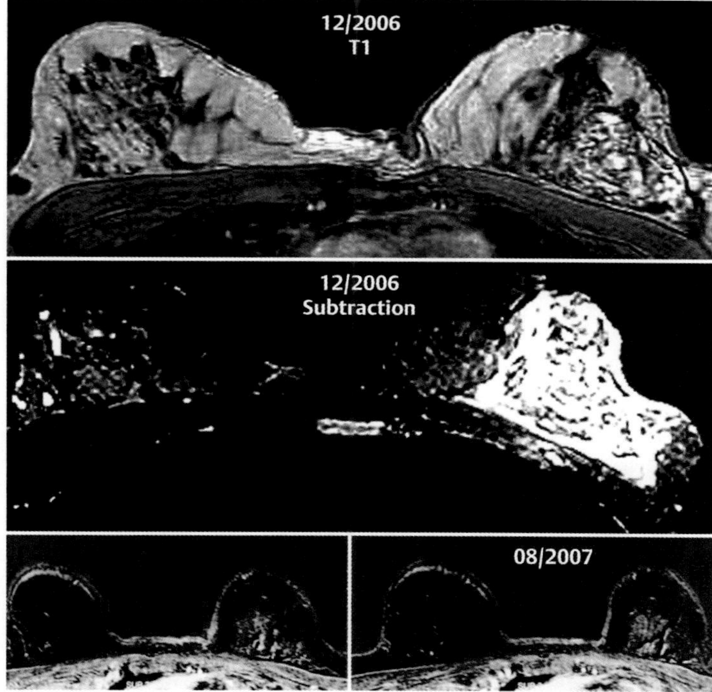


**e** *MRI* in December, 2006 (upper two images) and August, 2007 (lower image). In the T1-weighted *subtraction image* inhomogeneous zone surrounded by a thin capsule in the lateral portion of the breast. The tumor has not produced a mass effect or retraction signs in surrounding tissues.
The *subtraction image* after contrast administration shows marked reticular gadolinium enhancement that clearly reveals the diffuse pattern of tumor growth (see also panel **f**).

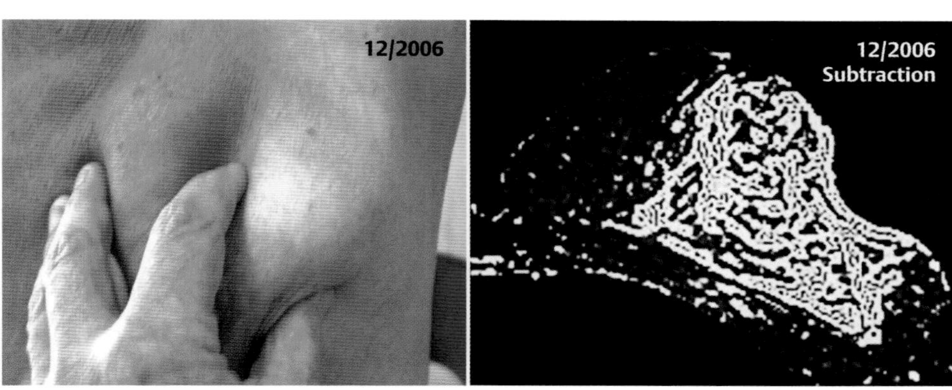


**f** *Physical examination and MRI* in December, 2006. The extensive lobular tumor shows slight changes at mammography and very pronounced changes on MRI. Tumor growth is oriented along normal glandular structures, and MRI shows a typical absence of mass effect and retraction. This explains the frequently normal mammographic findings associated with this type of lesion, with palpable findings suggestive of tumor infiltration.

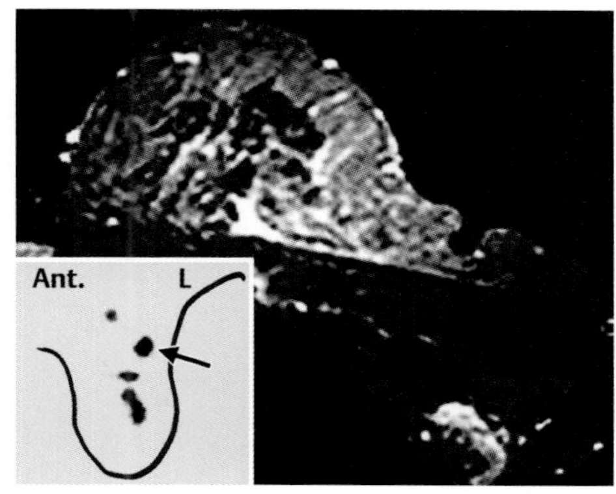


**g** *MRI* of the left breast and axilla and corresponding sentinel lymph node (inset lower left). A lymph node in the left axilla shows intense peripheral gadolinium enhancement. Core-needle biopsy of this node gave histologic proof of *metastatic involvement*. The enlarged, metastatic lymph node (**S/9**) is labeled in the sentinel image (arrow). It regressed completely in response to primary chemotherapy, and a tumor was not found on subsequent axillary dissection.

▶ **Fig. 5.188 h–l**

**Fig. 5.188 Second opinion. 63-year-old woman who noted a nonspecific palpable mass in her left breast.** *(continued)*

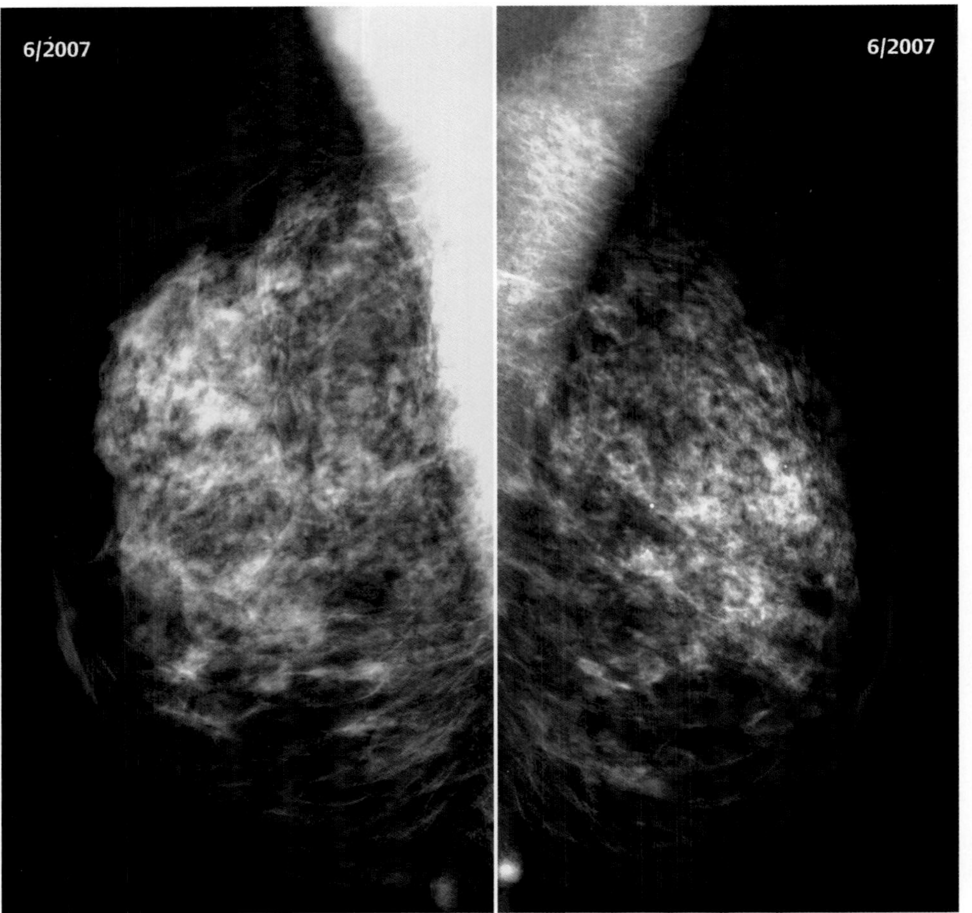


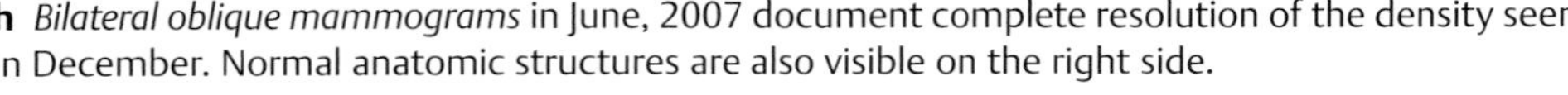

**h** *Bilateral oblique mammograms* in June, 2007 document complete resolution of the density seen in December. Normal anatomic structures are also visible on the right side.

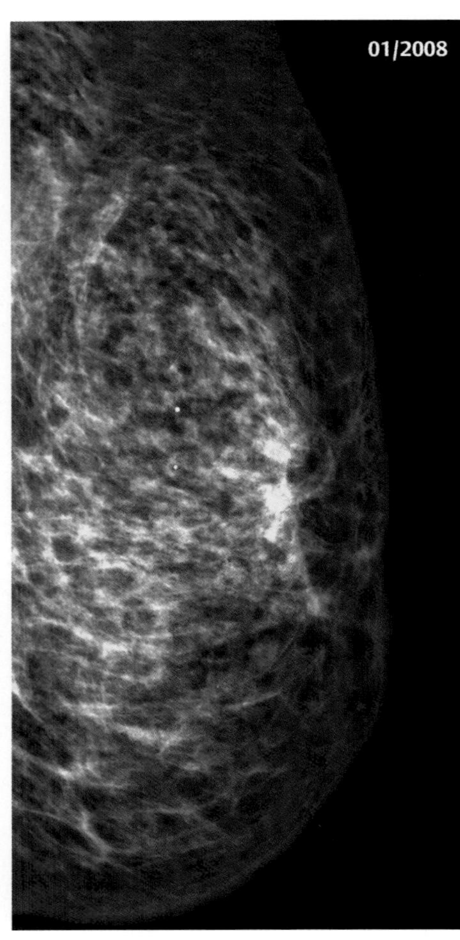


**i** *Oblique mammogram* of the left breast in January, 2008 shows a nonspecific supra-areolar density (**i/21–22**) consistent with *fat necrosis* relative to the previous examination.

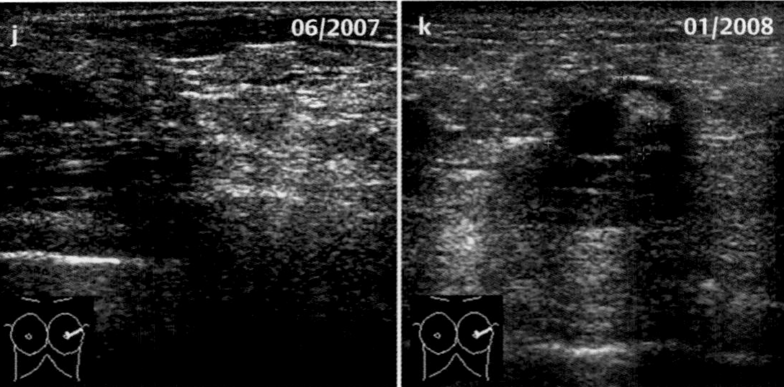


**j** *Ultrasound* in June, 2007 documents complete tumor regression. The rest of the breast parenchyma is rich in connective tissue (**b–C/10–12**). **k** *Ultrasound* in January, 2008 (see mammogram **i**). Excisional biopsy is followed by fat necrosis (**E/11–12**) and an oil cyst (**d/11–12**). There is no evidence of new tumor growth.

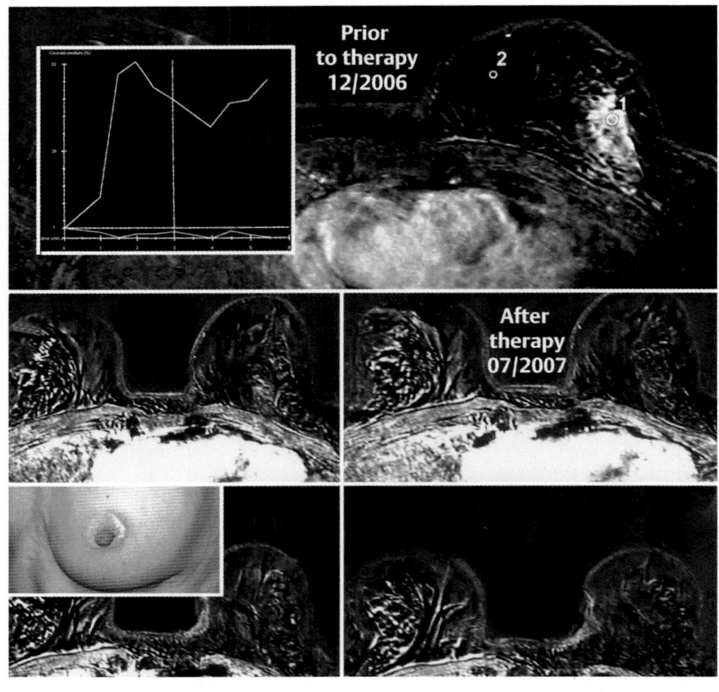


**l** *MR images* before (December 2006, upper image) and after primary chemotherapy (July 2007, lower 4 images) document complete tumor regression. The time–density curve (upper inset) is typical of a neoplasm. *Lower inset:* View of the left breast after chemotherapy and radiation shows hyperpigmentation of the breast and a depigmented scar in the areola. Otherwise the breast appears normal and is free of palpable abnormalities.

**Question on Fig. 5.188**

*What is the effect of the therapy in this case (neoadjuvant chemotherapy and tratozumab) on distant metastases?*

(**a**) Acts equally well on the primary tumor and on *all* metastases.

(**b**) Acts well on primary tumor and peripheral metastases (lung, liver, bone) but has little effect on cerebral metastases.

(**c**) Acts very well on cerebral metastases but poorly on other metastases.

→ **Answer on p. 409**

# Answers

*Page numbers in parentheses indicate the location of the figure in the main text.*

### Answer for Fig. 4.14 (p. 37)

**Answer (b) is correct. Extensive DCIS in the right breast** was found throughout the breast at operation, necessitating a simple mastectomy. Concomitant examination of the lower axillary lymph nodes showed nonspecific lymphadenitis. Surgery is indicated whenever malignancy is suspected; short- and long-term follow-ups only delay the diagnosis. Of course, the breast parenchyma was already infiltrated by tumor in 2001 but this was not detected.

*FNA* of the palpable mass yielded atypical cells, while retroareolar CNB revealed ADH. This fact, plus the diffuse mammographic changes, suggests an extensive atypical proliferative process in which inflammation is a nonspecific feature accompanying ductectasia with nipple retraction (several-year history).

**Lesson:** The clinical changes in this case (except for diffuse breast enlargement) were only the tip of the iceberg—the presenting features of a typical noncalcifying DCIS, which could have been diagnosed as early as 2001 by a careful analysis of the mammogram.

### Answer for Fig. 4.20 (p. 41)

**Answer (c) is correct. The process is difficult to classify based on calcification pattern and has a somewhat malignant appearance.** The calcium particles are pleomorphic, but they consistently conform to the anatomic structures of the breast parenchyma. Vacuum biopsy revealed *adenosis with extensive calcifications* and showed no evidence of carcinoma.

The calcifications gradually regressed over time as the degree of lobular proliferation declined with ageing. Comedo calcifications in ductectasia would be more homogeneous and would show a more linear pattern conforming to the ducts (see **Fig. 5.49a–d, h**, p. 140 f).

**Lesson:** Calcifications in the breast are not static but change with the functional activity of the TDLUs. Malignant calcifications may increase or disappear (see **Fig. 4.21**). Benign calcifications will often regress over time. A benign–malignant differentiation should be accomplished during the initial work-up, at least by CNB or vacuum biopsy (see p. 230).

**Fig. 4.20**

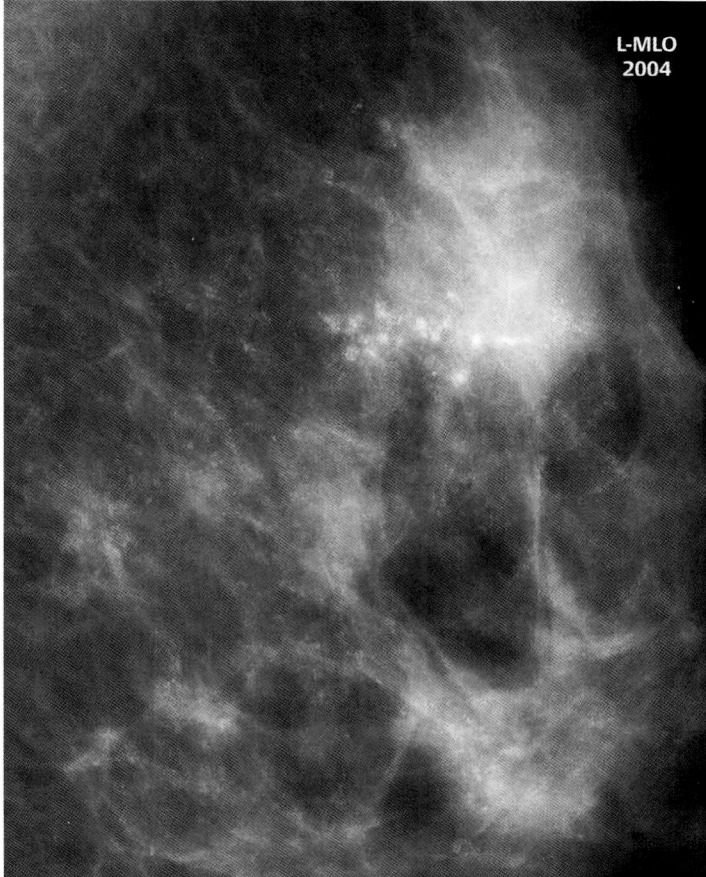


**c** *Oblique mammogram* of the left breast in September, 2004. The calcifications have regressed relative to June, 2000 (see **b**), i.e., they have become smaller and more pleomorphic.

**d** *Oblique digital magnification mammogram* of the left breast. The calcifications in the magnified view now have a more hazy, dust like appearance than in image **b**.

### Answer for Fig. 4.22 (p. 44 f)

**Answer (b) is correct. DCIS (G2).** The Van Nuys index was 6 points. Estrogen and progesterone receptors were positive. Despite their relatively uniform appearance (BIRADS 4a), the calcifications were investigated by digital stereotactic CNB.

The *mammographically* visible calcifications covered an area of only 1 cm. After multiple reexcisions the DCIS was removed with clear margins and was ultimately found to have a total extent of 4.4 cm. This is typical for ADH and DCIS, where visible calcifications are just the tip of the iceberg. The histological findings are usually far more extensive.

Given the size of the precancerous lesion, a normal-appearing sentinel lymph node was removed.

*Ultrasound* findings were normal. Therefore *invasive carcinoma* also seems unlikely. However, this does not guarantee that carcinoma is absent.

The location of the calcifications made it unlikely that they were related to the known *fibroadenoma* that had been present for years. The calcifications were located at the 11-o'clock position, whereas the fibroadenoma was at the 2-o'clock position. The calcifications had recently appeared, while the fibroadenoma had a long history (although this does not necessarily exclude fibroadenoma calcifications).

*Blunt duct adenosis* is characterized by a typical rosette calcification pattern (see **Fig. 5.132 b**, p. 265), which was not present in this case.

### Answer for Fig. 4.23, Question 1 (p. 47)

**Answer (b) is correct. The mammograms of the left breast show an asymmetry** at **f–J/5–13** (oblique), **p–S/18–21** (cc) and suspect microcalcifications at **l–i/4–6** (oblique) and **r–s/18–19** (cc) (BIRADS 4). The density visible in the oblique view of the right breast becomes diffuse in the craniocaudal view. *Ultrasound* shows no abnormalities.

### Answer for Fig. 4.23, Question 2 (p. 47)

**Answer (b) is correct. The calcifications are malignant.** The calcifications in the left breast are new, as they were not visible in the previous examination. They are inhomogeneous, multifocal, and have a mixed pleomorphic and stippled morphology (see **Fig. 5.158 a, b**, p. 306). The calcifications were removed, but without clear margins. Ultimately, the discovery of additional noncalcifying *DCIS* foci throughout the breast necessitated a mastectomy (see localization procedure in **Fig. 5.158**, p. 306). This is an impressive example of how extensive the noncalcifying portion of DCIS may be—the few calcifying areas in the mammogramm are the tip of the iceberg.

The small hypoechoic foci seen at ultrasound are not cysts in this case (no posterior acoustic enhancement). *Ultrasound-guided CNB* yielded elements of a cribriform-type *moderately differentiated DCIS* as well as *ADH* with microcalcifications.

### Answer for Fig. 4.23, Question 3 (p. 47)

**Answer (b) is correct. The left breast has an inhomogeneous architecture.** It is noteworthy that the left breast, when compared with the right, has a discrete inhomogeneous and patchy structure in all areas, especially the upper inner quadrant, caused by the multifocal growth of the tumor.

### Answer for Fig. 4.24 (p. 48 ff)

**Answer (a) is correct. The right breast appears mammographically normal**, even in high-quality images. *Ultrasound* examination of the right breast revealed a 1.8 cm × 1.3 cm tumor in the sternal recess, where the patient had noticed a firmness (**i**). It is also visible on the *MR* subtraction image (**j**), although the rest of the right breast appears normal.

Ultrasound-guided *CNB* in both breasts yielded elements of a *moderately differentiated invasive ductal carcinoma (G2)*. The tumor location is shown in panel **k** of the figure. Following the biopsy, a circumscribed hematoma is visible above the tumor (CNB was very painful due to the proximity of the pectoral fascia.)

**Lesson:** Breast ultrasound should include the clavicular, sternal, abdominal, and axillary recesses, because tumors growing in those areas will generally go undetected on mammograms (see **Fig. 5.54 a, b**, p. 146, and **Fig. 5.61 a**, p. 157 f).

The patient underwent *right breast-conserving surgery*. She requested the same treatment for the left breast, and again the tumor was removed with clear margins. The right breast did not receive postoperative radiation as requested by the patient.

Concomitant examination of the lower axillary lymph nodes showed nonspecific lymphadenitis. *Surgery* is indicated whenever malignancy is suspected; short- and long-term follow-ups only delay the diagnosis. Of course, the breast parenchyma was already infiltrated by tumor in 2001 but this was not detected. In 2008, the patient revealed bone metastases.

**Fig. 4.24**

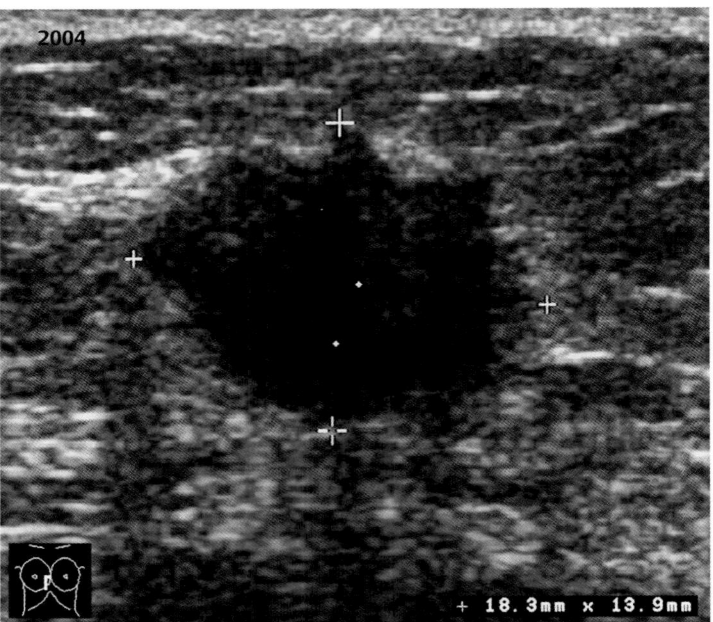


**i** *Presternal sonogram* of the right breast in 2004 shows in the sternal recess (see marker) a 1.8 cm × 1.3 cm hypoechoic nodule with ill-defined margins, typical of a malignant tumor.

**Fig. 4.24** *(continued)*

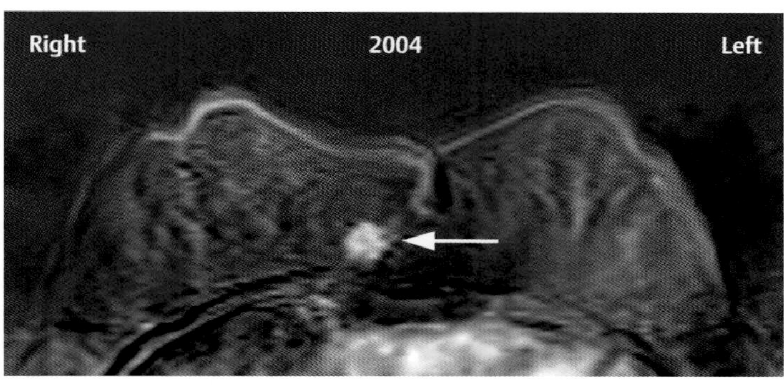


**j** *MR subtraction* image in June, 2004, shows intense gadolinium enhancement of the presternal mass (arrow).

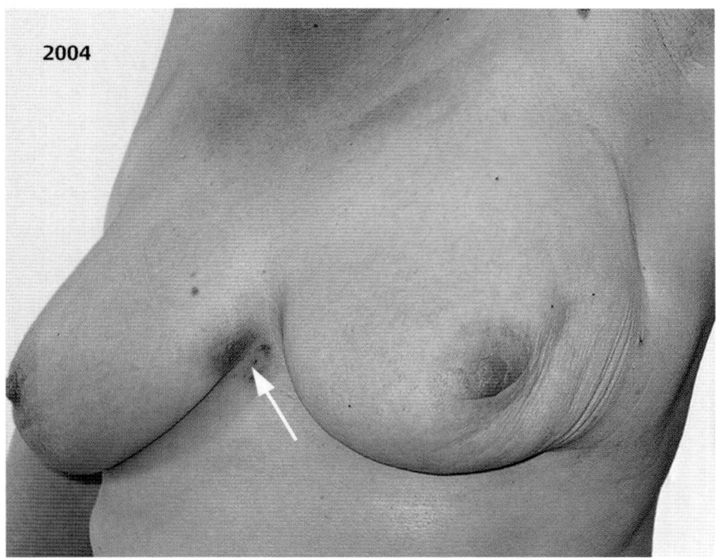


**k** *Clinical view*: Postoperative skin retraction of the left breast is noted after surgery in 1998. A presternal hematoma (arrow) appeared after fine-needle biopsy of the tumor at that site in 2004.

### Answer for Fig. 4.25 (p. 52)

**Answer (d) is correct. Malignant calcifications were not removed with clear margins.** Calcifications are located close to the excised margins in the upper portion of the specimen radiograph at **c–d/ 26–27**. This means that calcifications and tumor tissue may have been left in the breast.

The three pathologists submitted the following diagnoses:

- Multifocal *microcystic adenosis* with associated calcifications and areas of mild ductal epithelial hyperplasia. Core biopsy also yielded focal lobular epithelial hyperplasia with no atypias.
- Mild, *atypical ductal hyperplasia* of the breast. The hyperplasia is moderately estrogen-receptor-positive and moderately progesterone-receptor-positive.
- Very *well-differentiated intraductal carcinoma*. Long-term Tamoxifen therapy would be sufficient if the breast is closely followed by mammography and ultrasound and no additional microcalcifications are found at excisional biopsy (reference pathologist).

During the next two years, more atypical calcifications appeared at the previous surgical site. The calcifications were now classified as *adenosis* by a different pathologist (who did not know the previous diagnosis). The patient, distressed by this point, again sought the opinion of the author, who advised her to trust the latest diagnosis and take a wait-and-see approach.

### Answer for Fig. 4.26, Question 1 (p. 53)

**The lesion is located in the right retroareolar area at k–l/22 (oblique) and 13 (cc).**

### Answer for Fig. 4.26, Question 2 (p. 53)

**Answer (c) is correct. Intracystic papilloma with focal ADH.** The nodule was surgically removed. Histologic examination also confirmed microcalcifications (not visible on mammograms). *Ultrasound* indicates a central cystic degenerative papilloma. Cytology did not indicate ADH. There was no evidence of invasive carcinoma.

A *fibroadenoma* would not cause nipple discharge. The discharge would be inconsistent with *medullary carcinoma*.

**Lesson:** ADH may be hidden in a papilloma, fibroadenoma, or other benign tumor and is difficult to detect cytologically in this setting.

### Answer for Fig. 4.27, Question 1 (p. 54)

**Answer (d) is correct. A pathologic process is located in the right breast** at **a–C/21–23** (oblique view) and **A–D/11–15** (craniocaudal view) in the mammograms of 1996. The atypical cells (tumor cells from the duct system) are an indication for contrast ductography of the right breast and for MRI. Both studies were performed 3 months later.

Meanwhile (1997), the densities in the right breast increased significantly (**i, j**). *Ultrasound* shows small, ill-defined focal hypoechoic areas in the upper outer quadrant of the right breast, some with associated shadowing (**g, h**). *Ductography* of the right breast shows a moderately ectatic duct system with cutoffs that are suspicious for an intraductal process (**l, m**). The duct system in the upper outer quadrant of the right breast shows intense gadolinium enhancement on *MRI* (**k**). The changes were already present in 1996 but were not identified as abnormal until 3 months later, when the patient demanded an explanation for her galactorrhea, prompting an assessment by ductography and MRI.

### Answer for Fig. 4.27, Question 2 (p. 54)

**Answer (b) is correct. Noncalcifying intraductal carcinoma (DCIS).** *Histology* showed extensive DCIS. Local excision in the upper outer quadrant did not yield clear margins, and it was necessary to proceed with mastectomy. The lymph nodes were clear. The tumor was estrogen-receptor-negative and markedly progesterone-receptor-positive.

In-situ carcinoma (DCIS) does not always calcify, especially when it is rapidly progressive as in this case. Within 3 months, the entire upper outer quadrant was infiltrated from the axillary recess.

Fig. 4.27

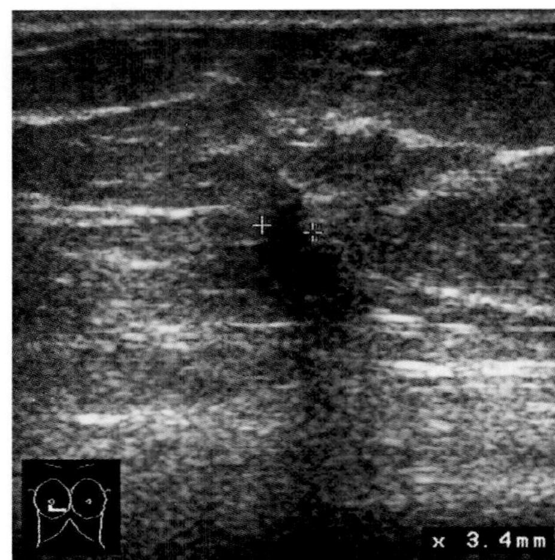


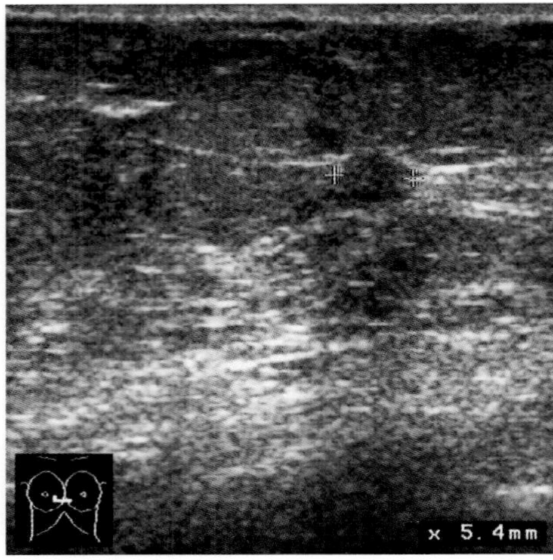


**g, h** *Sonogram* of the right breast in January, 1997 shows small hypoechoic areas with posterior acoustic shadowing (11 MHz).

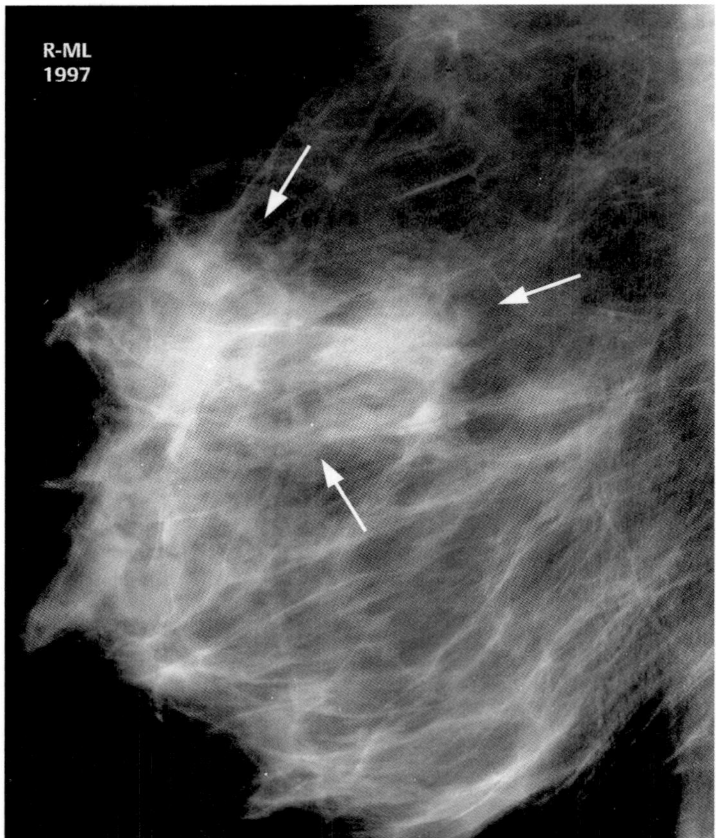


**i** *Mediolateral mammogram* in January, 1997 shows increased parenchymal density in the upper portion of the right breast (corresponding to coordinates **a–c/21–23** in the 1996 mammogram, **a, b**).

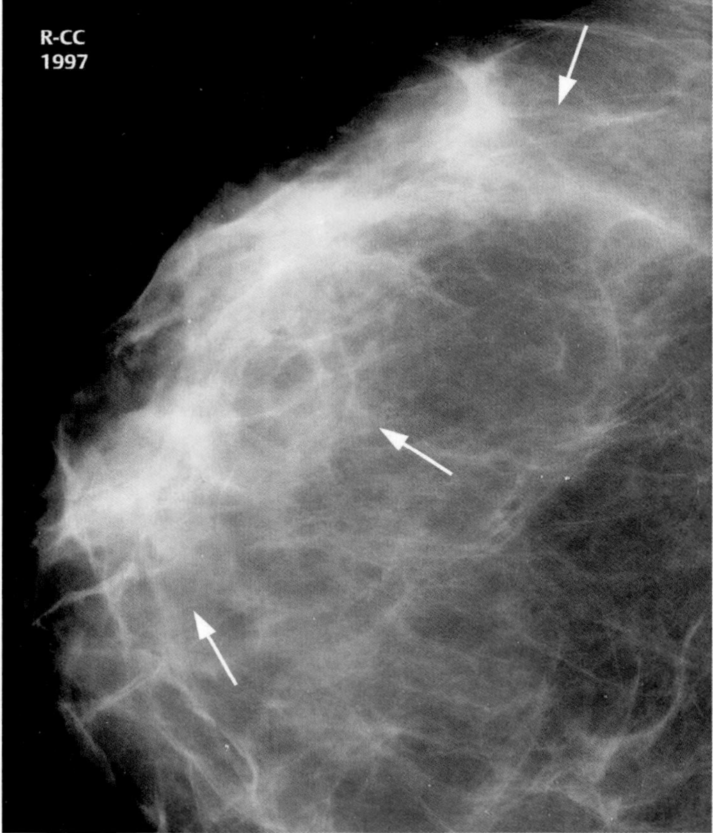


**j** *Craniocaudal mammogram* in January, 1997 shows nonspecific increased density of the parenchyma in the lateral portion of the right breast (arrows) with significant progression relative to the prior examination (corresponds to coordinates **A–D/11–15** in the 1996 mammogram, **c, d**).

Fig. 4.27 *(continued)*

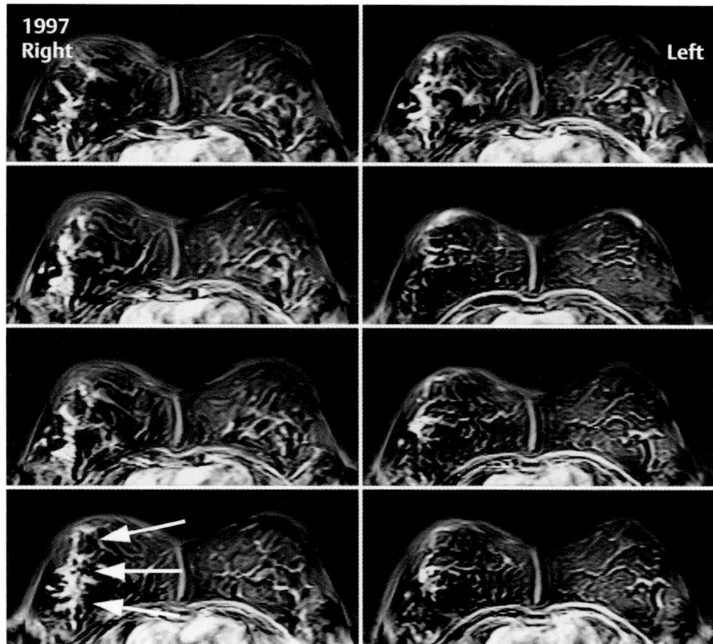


**k** *MR subtraction image* in January, 1997 shows intense gadolinium enhancement with prominent ducts (before ductography) in the upper outer quadrant of the right breast (arrows). The left breast appears normal.

ADH and DCIS are usually more extensive than mammograms and contrast ductography would suggest.

The rapid tumor growth is remarkable since the tumor was graded histologically as G1.

Unilateral *involution* of the left breast (unusual) is not supported by the atypical cytology on the right side. The same applies to right-sided *mastitis in ductectasia.*

There was no need to investigate the *left breast* by ductography.

## Answer for Fig. 4.28 (p. 55)

**Answer (b) is correct. DCIS not removed with adequate margins.** The specimen radiograph does contain the main calcification cluster, but the mammogram shows linear calcifications conforming segmental to the duct system and extending into the retroareolar region. The initial resection should have extended into that region, therefore. Even multiple reexcisions could not remove the calcifications with clear margins, and it was necessary to proceed with mastectomy.

Fig. 4.27

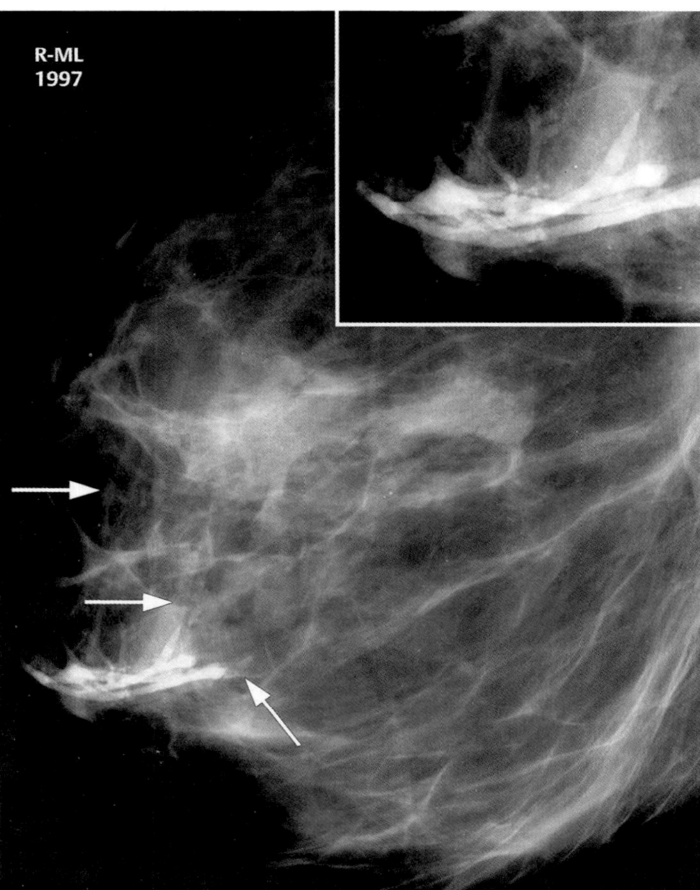


**l** *Mediolateral ductogram* of the right breast in February, 1997 shows opacification of the retroareolar ducts with peripheral duct cutoffs (arrows) (see magnified view at upper right).

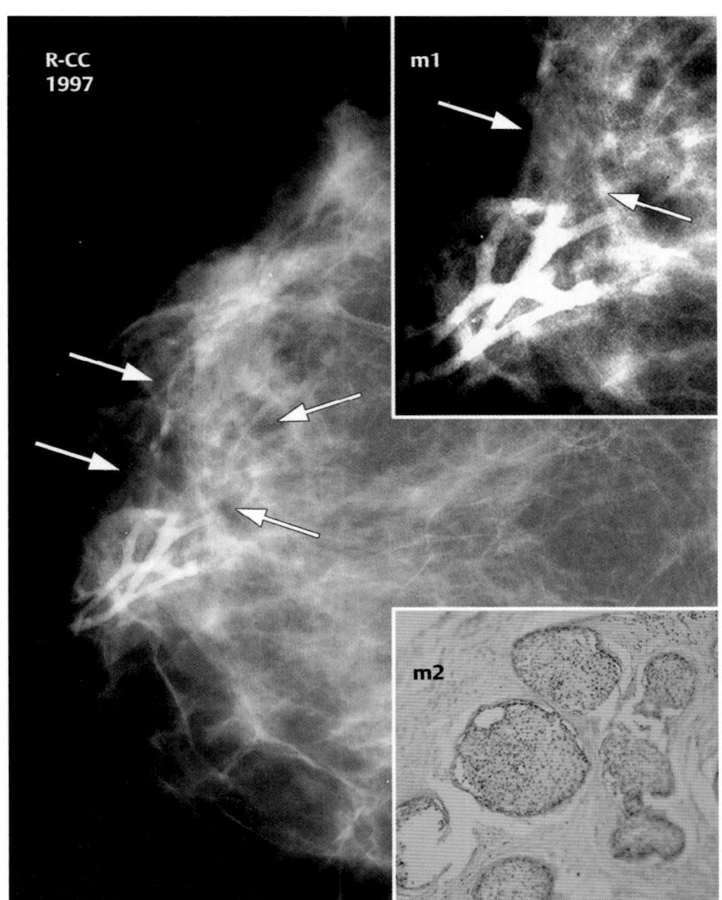


**m** *Craniocaudal ductogram* of the right breast in February, 1997 shows broadened retroareolar ducts and peripheral duct cutoffs (arrows). **m2** The "extinction" of ducts in the contrast ductogram corresponds histologically to infiltration of the ducts by DCIS tumor tissue.

### Answer for Fig. 4.29 (p. 57)

**Answer (b) is correct. Poorly differentiated invasive ductal cancer (G3)** 0.4 cm in diameter and an extensive intraductal component (EIC) with an overall diameter of 1 cm in a glassy, inhomogeneous lump (**i**). No metastases were found in 17 axillary lymph nodes.

The smaller lateral lesion (**F/24** in **b**) is a *fibroadenoma.*

Fibrocystic changes and intraductal papilloma were also found in the mastectomy specimen following complete excision of the invasive carcinoma.

Even initial *MRI* in 1997 (**f**) shows an extensive intraductal component (EIC) and may also show the ductal hyperplasia described by the pathologist. Because the *DCIS* 1997 was a G1 lesion, the MRI finding does not necessarily represent a recurrent tumor. Fat necrosis may also calcify and have similar MRI features, but the second tumor is located 2–3 cm posteromedial to the first tumor and thus slightly outside the primary operative area (see panels **e** and **k**).

*Papilloma* would be a possibility. Whenever microcalcifications appear after DCIS has been diagnosed, they should be histologically investigated (by FNB or vacuum biopsy). Short-term follow-ups are not appropriate and would only delay necessary curative treatment.

### Answer for Fig. 4.30 (p. 59)

**Answer (c) is correct. Medullary carcinoma does not cause calcifications.** It has round or scalloped margins and does not cast an acoustic shadow at ultrasound. Because of its high cellularity, it shows posterior acoustic enhancement similar to a cyst.

*Histology of the calcifications:* small focal *lobular carcinoma in situ* with microcalcifications. There is no histologic evidence of invasive carcinoma.

> **!** **LCIS can occasionally be detected by the presence of microcalcifications, but this is much less frequent than with DCIS (though not all areas of DCIS calcify). LCIS therefore does not occur exclusively in proximity to benign changes.**

### Answer for Fig. 5.1 (p. 79)

**Answer (b) is correct. Hyperkeratotic areas and keratoma formation.** If *Paget disease* were present, the changes would be related to the retroareolar duct system and would be accompanied by redness and possible bleeding from the nipple and/or areola. Thus, these changes and the cytologic pattern are not at all typical of Paget disease or of *shingles*, as shingles is always accompanied by pain (see **Fig. 5.77**).

*Seborrheic warts* are a common finding in older women. The central crusting of the nipple is harmless. It is a symptom of ductectasia and is caused by inspissated discharge from the very often enlarged retroareolar ducts.

### Answer for Fig. 5.2 (p. 79 f)

**Answer (b) is correct. Extensive fat necrosis.** The laser treatments apparently caused this, which increased significantly over the 12-month period.

*FNA* yields lipophagic cells but no epithelial cells suspicious for neoplasia. *Histology* shows organized and calcified areas of fat necrosis with no evidence of malignancy. The *MRI* changes are caused by the hemangioma. There is no evidence of circumscribed nodularity. The *sonographic changes* stem from the calcifications and not from a malignant process.

### Answer for Fig. 5.3 (p. 81)

**Answer (b) is correct. Folliculitis.** It is unclear to what extent the changes are related to neurodermatitis. Bacteriology excluded a fungal infection (actinomycosis) and tuberculosis. The abscess does not communicate with the duct system, so it is not a result of *ductectasia with plasma cell mastitis.* The lesion was removed by local excision and the further course was uneventful. The changes in this case are not consistent with *Paget disease.*

### Answer for Fig. 5.4 (p. 81)

**Answer (a) is correct. Psoriasis lesion**, several of which can be found at other sites on the patient's body (especially the elbow).

*Neurodermatitis* does not have the typical glistening, cornified layer on the epidermis. *Shingles* occurs predominantly on the back rather than in the breast region (see **Fig. 5.7**). Mammograms and sonograms are normal.

### Answer for Fig. 5.5 (p. 82)

**Answer (c) is correct. Circumscribed scleroderma** is a benign process that is treated with Contractubex Compositum ointment. If the lesion continues to progress and additional lesions appear, high-dose penicillin therapy may be considered.

The absence of lesions elsewhere on the body does not support a diagnosis of *neurodermatitis. Carcinomatous lymphangitis* is excluded by the overall clinical appearance and the normal mammograms and sonograms.

### Answer for Fig. 5.6 (p. 82ff)

**Answer (a) is correct. Inflammatory breast cancer** (BIRADS 4b) on the left side, despite the absence of orange-peel skin dimpling.

It is curious that the changes in the left breast were initially associated with a circulatory disturbance. The history is also remarkable, and the patient may have exaggerated certain details, although this type of report is not unusual for a normal clinical setting (even at certified centers). This observation also highlights the potential dangers of interventional procedures. In this case, 7 months passed from initial clinical changes to definitive diagnosis. The inflammatory carcinoma was eventually diagnosed by *ultrasound-guided CNB,* because the lesions were clearly visible at ultrasound and were

Fig. 5.6

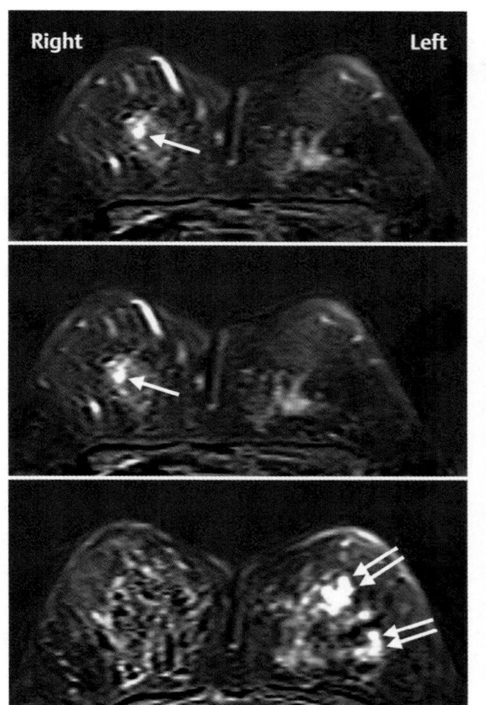


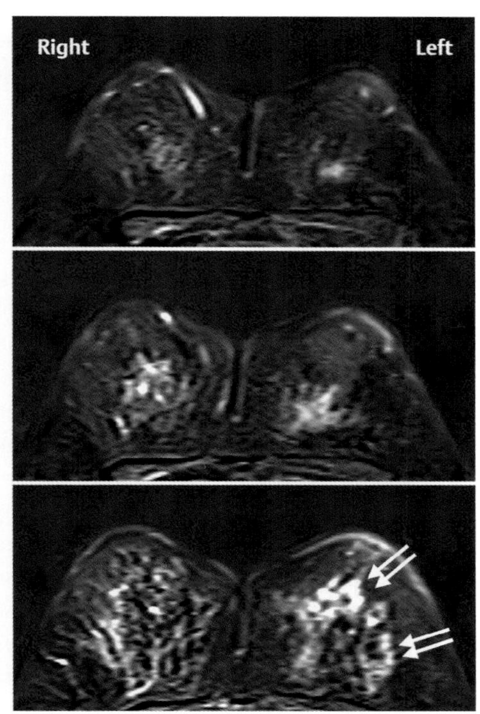


**g** *MR subtraction image* shows diffuse foci of gadolinium enhancement in the left breast (see double arrows). The right breast shows intense parenchymal blood flow with local proliferation at the upper border of the breast (see arrows).

easily biopsied. *Vacuum biopsy*, incidentally, is generally better for diagnosing because it can sample a greater amount of material (see p. 230).

Treatment consisted of primary (neoadjuvant) chemotherapy. Mastectomy or local radiotherapy may be appropriate, depending on chemotherapy response.

MRI of the left breast shows diffuse gadolinium enhancement indicating involvement of the entire breast (**g**). The lesion in the right breast also enhances. Because mammograms and sonograms are both suspicious for a tumor, *preoperative CNB* of the right breast was ordered but subsequently forgotten. Follow-ups showed no evidence of a second tumor as of 2008. *Thrombosis of the left subclavian vein* would not have caused circulatory impairment but would have caused swelling of the left breast and arm. *Obstruction of lymphatic drainage* appears unlikely because of the small, suspicious hypoechoic areas detected at ultrasound. The MR findings are not consistent with lymphatic obstruction or venous thrombosis.

## Answer for Fig. 5.7 (p. 85)

**Answer (b) is correct. Shingles** with small, segmental skin eruptions conforming to the distribution of the spinal nerve. A typical shingles rash is preceded by pain that radiates in bands to the chest and upper abdomen. The changes in the right breast are due to radiation-induced fibrosis with cutaneous erythema due to obstructed lymphatic drainage. The shingles is unrelated to the changes in the breast.

*Cutaneous metastases* are excluded by the segmental arrangement of the lesions, the absence of nodularity about the skin lesions, and the absence of cutaneous or distant metastases elsewhere in the body.

*Postirradiation changes* would be homogeneous rather than focal. Changes on the back, which occur rarely, would conform to the radiotherapy portal and would appear as diffuse redness with increasing hyperpigmentation.

Fig. 5.7

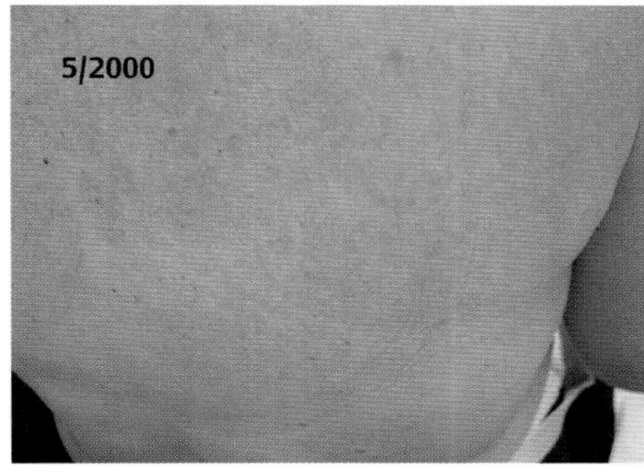


**f** *Clinical appearance* of the back 2 years later.

## Answer for Fig. 5.8 (p. 86)

**Answer (c) is correct. First-degree frostbite**. The patient cooled the breast by the direct application of ice packs to the skin for several days. This resulted in frostbite, which regressed spontaneously over the next 3 months. The skin appeared completely normal one year later (**c**).

*Carcinomatous lymphangitis* does not develop within a few weeks. Inflammatory infiltrates following the percutaneous aspiration of an abscess would be possible. Cultures did not reveal a causative organism, so multiple skin abscesses are unlikely.

Fig. 5.8

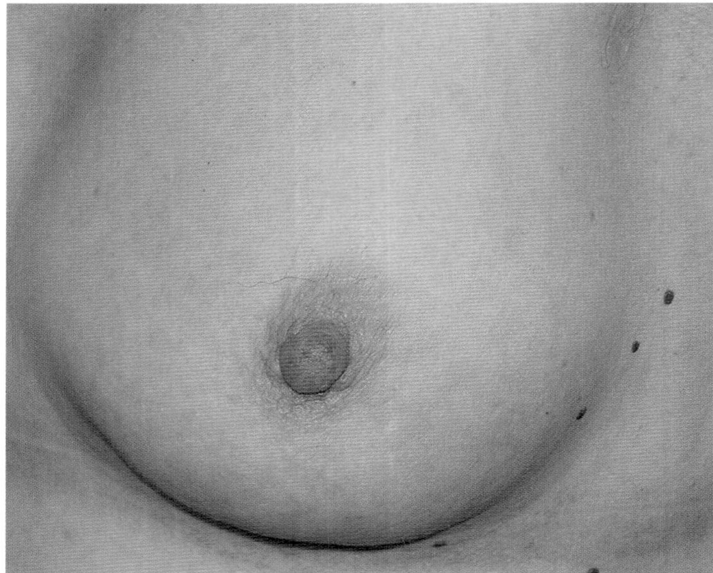

**c** *Clinical appearance* of the left breast. The skin changes regressed over a 1-year period.

### Answer for Fig. 5.9 (p. 87)

**Answer (b) is correct. REM syndrome**. Mucous deposits may be minimal in the early stage of this disease.

We know from experience that REM syndrome responds well to Resochin (initial dose of 250 mg/day until response, then 125 mg/day). If the complaints are purely cosmetic, one should be more hesitant in selecting patients for this unconventional therapy (Professor Gerd Lischka, Universitäts-Hautklinik Tübingen, Germany).

The differential diagnosis would include *a well-differentiated lymphoma*, but there is insufficient clinical and histologic evidence to support this diagnosis. The second differential would be *lupus erythematosus*, but comprehensive laboratory tests excluded that disease.

Bilateral shingles is excluded by the location and homogeneity of the erythema (see **Fig. 5.7 c**).

### Answer for Fig. 5.10 (p. 87)

**Answer (a) is correct. Horner syndrome** on the right eye (miosis, ptosis, enophthalmos) as well as generalized dissemination of *bilateral breast cancer.*

The skin on both breasts shows carcinomatous lymphangitis (**i**, p. 354). The breast is mottled by areas of extreme firmness and is no longer radiolucent on *mammograms* (**f**). *Ultrasound* reveals multiple tumorlike lesions (**h**).

Previous ultrasound 4 years ago showed several small, atypical hypoechoic foci (**g**), which were classified as nonmalignant and were not investigated further. Repeated pathologic analysis of the breast tissue after *reduction mammoplasty* did not yield any new findings other than the previous diagnosis of Prechtel grade II fibrocystic change with proliferative foci.

*Histology: bilateral moderately differentiated invasive lobular carcinoma* with small foci of lobule-like infiltrates composed of atypical epithelial cells.

Answers (**b**) and (**c**) are synonyms for Horner syndrome, which includes the following clinical features:

- Miosis (not responsive to cocaine drops)
- Ipsilateral disturbance of lacrimation
- Ipsilateral anhidrosis
- Hypotonia of the ipsilateral globe
- Ipsilateral heterochromia iridis and (rarely) facial hemiatrophy

**Lesson:** This case illustrates the difficulties posed by dense breast parenchyma combined with postreduction-mammoplasty scarring and equivocal sonograms. The tumors grew practically under the

Fig. 5.10

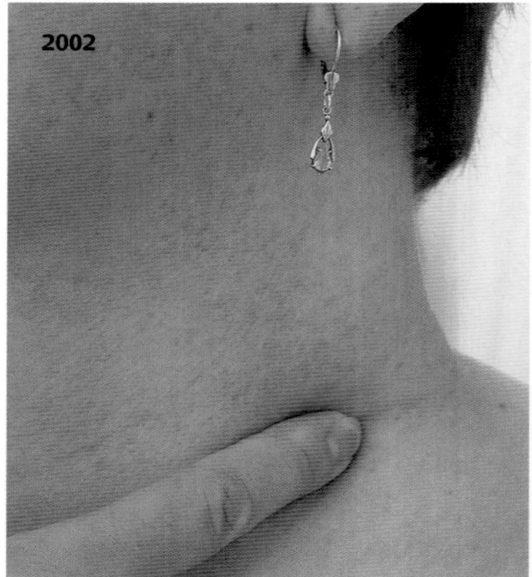


**b** *Clinical inspection* reveals nodularity on the left side of the neck.

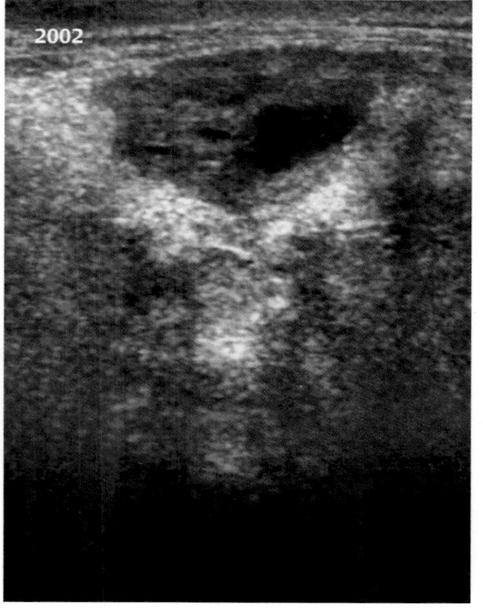


**c** Sonogram of the nodular area shows enlarged lymph nodes. The central hypoechoic area is a necrotic metastasis.

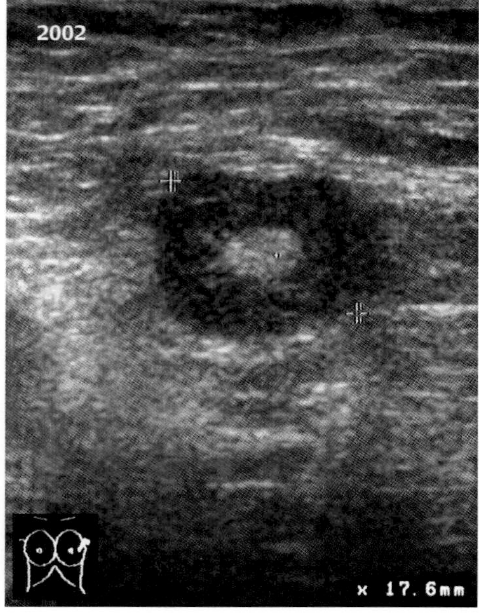


**d** *Sonogram* of the left axilla shows enlarged lymph nodes with a narrow, fatty sinus consistent with lymph node metastasis.

**Fig. 5.10** *(continued)*

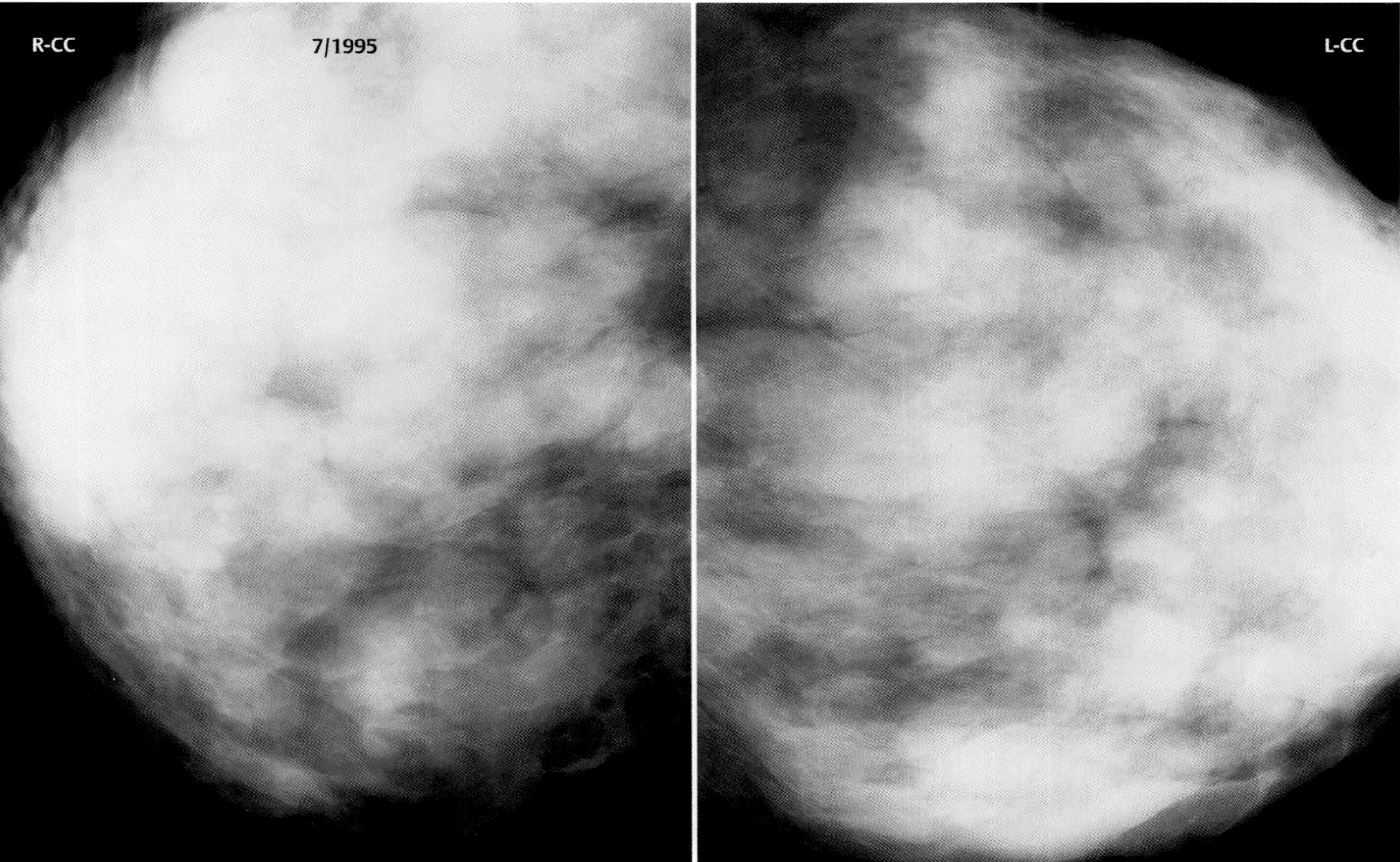


**e** *Bilateral craniocaudal mammograms* in July, 1995, prior to reduction mammoplasty. Eight images were taken on each side due to the large size of the breasts at that time (PGMI). The breasts are too radiodense for meaningful evaluation (ACR 4). CAD revealed several calcific foci, especially on the left side, that were histologically benign (not shown).

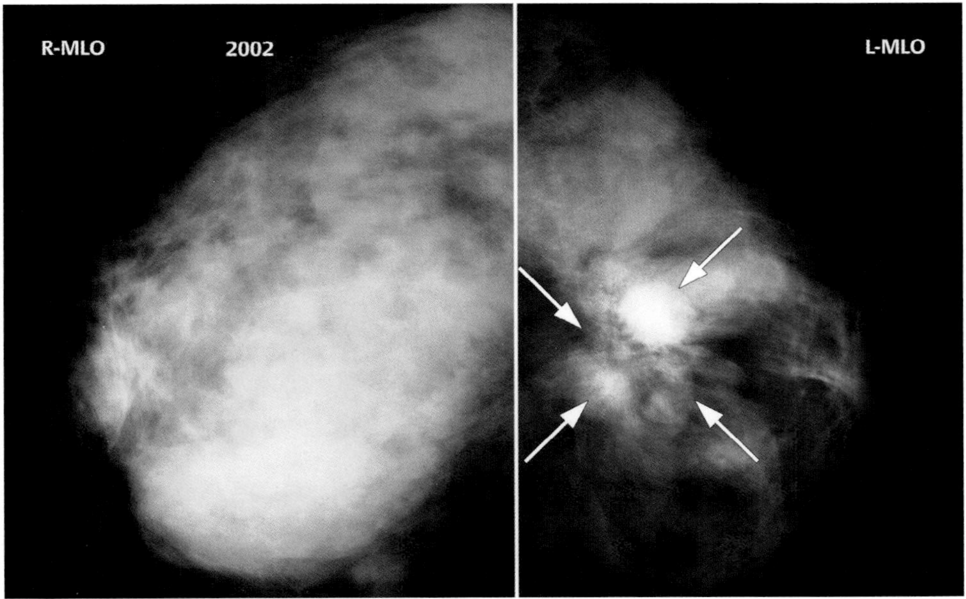


**f** Oblique mammogram in 2002, seven years after bilateral reduction mammoplasty, shows increased density relative to the earlier examination in 1995. The right breast shows homogeneously dense breast parenchyma with confluent, coarse patchy densities. The left breast shows a central, stellate, tumorlike density (arrows).

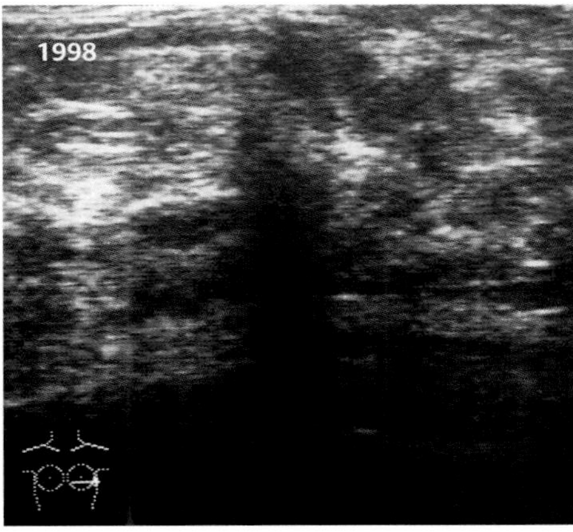


**g** Sonogram of the lower portion of the left breast in April, 1998 shows hypoechoic areas, some with associated acoustic shadowing. Multiple cysts and scars are seen following bilateral reduction mammoplasty.

▶ **Fig. 5.10 h, i**

Fig. 5.10 *(continued)*

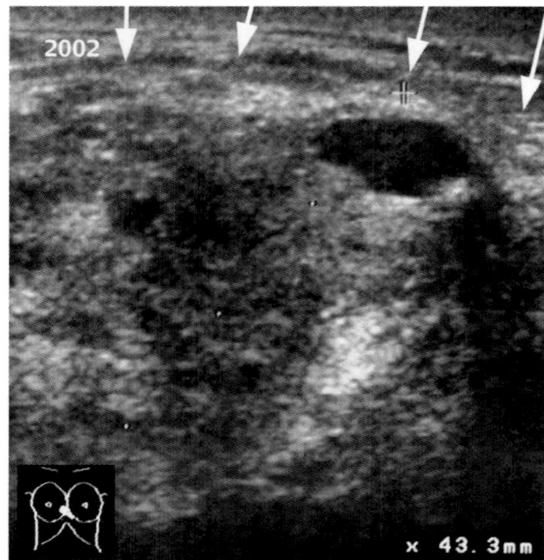


**h** Sonogram in September, 2002 shows one of numerous well-circumscribed nodules with hypoechoic contents and darker necrotic areas. These findings indicate very cellular foci of bilateral, multifocal lobular carcinoma.

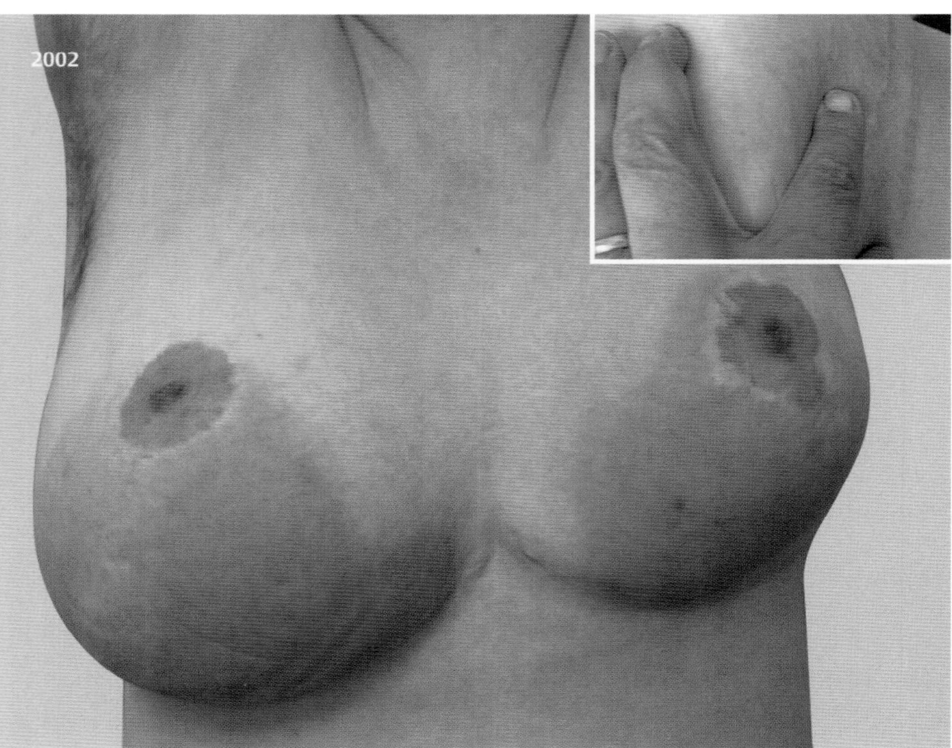


**i** Clinical inspection of both breasts after bilateral reduction mammoplasty shows pronounced reddish-brown discoloration of the lower quadrants. The left breast is smaller than the right. Gross nodularity is present in both breasts (inset at upper right). A mammogram could not be taken or evaluated in 2002 because of the very hard nodular tissue (ACR 4).

nose of the radiologist who took the yearly mammograms! The ocular changes and breast redness appeared approximately 6 weeks before a diagnosis was made. It is remarkable that *cranial CT* and a *thyroid scan* were ordered to investigate the Horner symptom complex even after the abnormal mammographic findings were known. Clinical examination of the cervical lymph nodes, including palpation and a simple FNA, would have advanced the diagnosis much more than the costly and complex imaging studies.

## Answer for Fig. 5.11 (p. 88)

**Answer (c) is correct. Neoplasm in the retroareolar region** of the *right* breast. Localization: oblique **B–b/12–14**; cc **a–B/2–4**).

*Ultrasound* reveals a retroareolar hyperechoic area (**d**), and *MRI* shows intense retroareolar enhancement in the area of the tumor (**e**). *FNA* of the retroareolar area yields tumorlike cells (Pap V) (**f**). The patient underwent mastectomy and was still free of disease 12 years later.

**Lesson:** This case illustrates that *nipple deviation* is not a normal finding, even if it has been present for several years. It should continue to be questioned and diagnostically pursued. This case was complicated by the fact that the left breast also showed slight lateral nipple deviation due to previous surgery.

Fig. 5.11

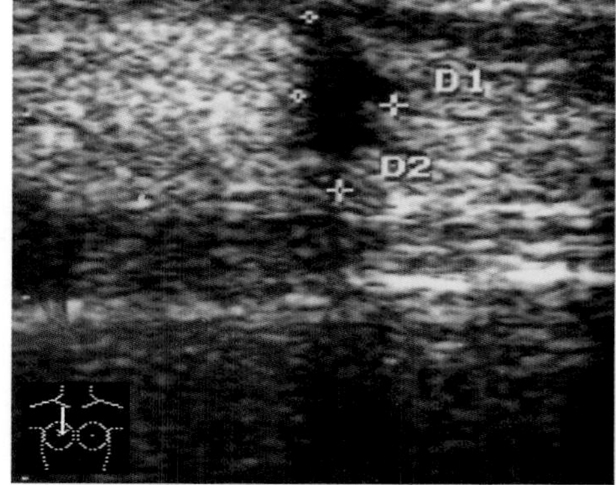


**d** *Sonogram* of the right retroareolar region shows a 1 cm × 1.5 cm hypoechoic area with slight acoustic shadowing (see marker).

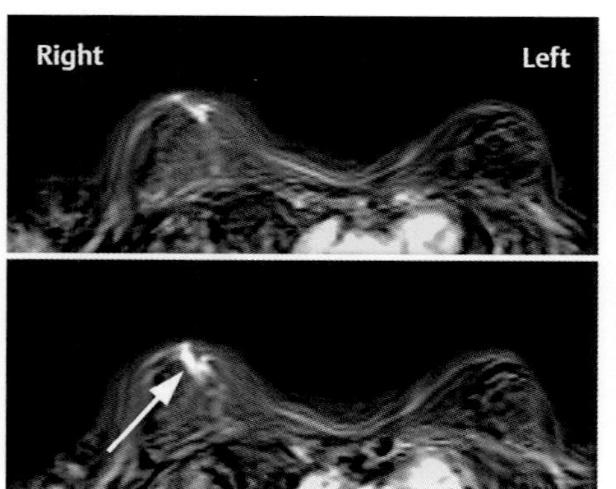


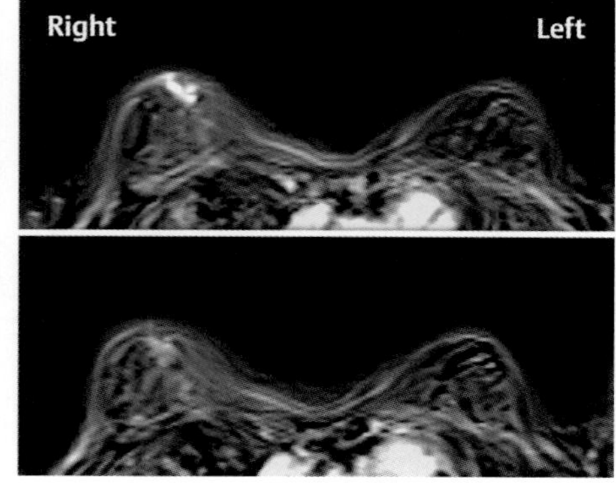


**e** *MR subtraction image* after gadolinium administration shows intense retroareolar enhancement in the right breast (arrow).

**Fig. 5.11** *(continued)*

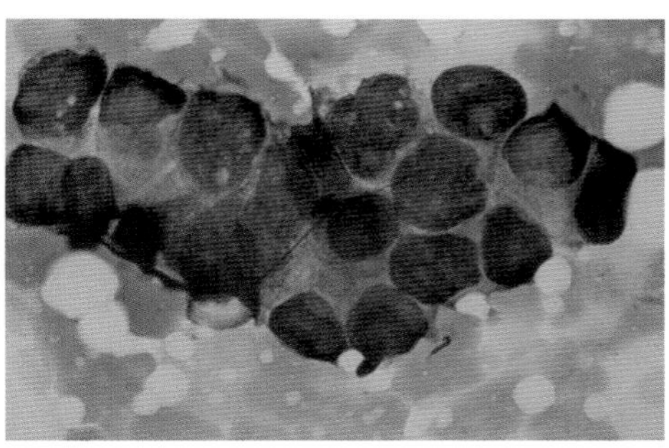

**f** *FNA cytology* (from **d**) yields myriad tumorlike epithelial cells. *Histology* reveals *poorly differentiated, invasive lobular breast carcinoma*. The tumor was excised with clear margins (PT1a, RO).

**Answer for Fig. 5.12** (p. 89)

**Answer (b) is correct. Mucocele**. There is a retroareolar invasive ductal carcinoma (G2) that has not invaded the areola, causing only a mucocele of the nipple (**a**). Histology showed absence of nipple involvement. *Mammography* showed very prominent periductal markings and a thickened right nipple (**b**). The mucocele appears to fill the nipple on *ultrasound* (**d**). The coaxial needle used for *CNB* retrieved copious amounts of mucus (**e**).

*Paget disease* is not consistent with the smooth plaque surface and its smooth margins relative to the nipple (see **Fig. 5.52 c**, p. 364). The normal cytology also excludes Paget disease as well as an *abscess due to ductectasia* (see **Fig. 5.3 b**, p. 81, **Fig. 5.129**, p. 262).

**Lesson:** Not all carcinomas lead to *Paget disease*, even when retroareolar proliferation has occurred. The patient had been aware of the areolar changes for months, as the mucocele had abolished the natural contractile response of the areola to stimulation (**a**).

**Answer for Fig. 5.26** (p. 111)

(**a**) PGMI (craniocaudal skin folds **n–O,23–24**)
(**b**) ACR 2
(**c**) BIRADS 4b left (**p/23** cc, **Q/8** oblique), BIRADS 1 right
*Histology: Invasive ductal carcinoma (G3)* of the left breast.

**Answer for Fig. 5.27** (p. 112)

(**a**) PGMI
(**b**) ACR 3
(**c**) BIRADS 4b left (**E–e/20–21** cc, **F–f/10** oblique), BIRADS 1 right
(**d**) Yes, ultrasound
*Histology: Invasive ductal carcinoma (G1)* of the left breast. **The tumor can be detected only by careful comparison of the mammograms of both breasts!**

**Answer for Fig. 5.28** (p. 113)

(**a**) PGMI (lateral portion of breast incompletely imaged)
(**b**) ACR 3
(**c**) BIRADS 4a left, densities in the left breast (**n–o, 23–26** cc, **o–p/6–9** oblique), BIRADS 1 right
(**d**) Yes, ultrasound and CNB
*Histology: Adenosis* in the left breast.

**Answer for Fig. 5.29** (p. 114)

(**a**) PGMI
(**b**) ACR 2
(**c**) BIRADS 4b left (**e–F/21–22** cc, **F/12** oblique), 2 right (**B/7**)
(**d**) Yes, ultrasound and CNB
*Histology: Invasive ductal carcinoma (G2)* of the left breast. The right breast contains a small cyst, visible only in the oblique view (**B–b/6–7**).

**Answer for Fig. 5.30** (p. 115 f)

(**a**) PGMI (the breasts are incompletely imaged at the level of the inframammary fold in the oblique projections)
(**b**) ACR 2
(**c**) BIRADS 4b left (tissue appears asymmetrical in the lower inner quadrant of the left breast (**n–O/16–17** cc, **n/3–4** oblique). The tumor was missed on initial examination, and the patient returned a year later with an *interval carcinoma* (see panel **c**, p. 116).

**Answer for Fig. 5.31** (p. 117)

(**a**) PGMI (pectoral muscle is incompletely imaged in the oblique and cc projections on both sides)
(**b**) ACR 3
(**c**) BIRADS 4b left (**n–O/23–25** cc, **n–O/8–11** oblique), BIRADS 1 right
(**d**) Yes, ultrasound and CNB.
*Histology: Invasive ductal breast carcinoma (G2)* of the left breast.

No signs of retraction are visible in the area around the tumor (see p. 64).

**Answer for Fig. 5.32** (p. 118)

(**a**) PGMI (the pectoral muscle is incompletely imaged on the right side due to previous treatment; a skin fold is visible on the right side)
(**b**) ACR cc 3, oblique 2
(**c**) BIRADS 4b left in 2003 (circumscribed density at upper left **D–E/23–24** cc, **i/24** oblique), BIRADS 1 right
(**d**) Yes, ultrasound and CNB
*Histology: Sclerosing adenosis*. The density was only faintly visualized on follow-up films taken one year later in 2004 (panel **c**).

**Answer for Fig. 5.33** (p. 119)

(**a**) PGMI
(**b**) ACR 3
(**c**) BIRADS 4b right (a faint stellate density appears near the chest wall at **N/19** cc, **m–N/9** oblique), 1 left
(**d**) Magnification mammography
*Histology: Invasive ductal carcinoma (G2)* of the right breast.

**Answer for Fig. 5.34** (p. 120 f)

(**a**) PGMI craniocaudal; PGMI oblique (the portion containing the tumor near the chest wall in the upper outer quadrant of the right breast is cut off)
(**b**) ACR 3
(**c**) BIRADS 4b right (**c–D/20–21** cc; **O–o/15** oblique). The prepectoral portion of the tumor is cut off; 4b left (visible in both views of the left breast: **F–f/20–22** cc, **P–Q/7–10** oblique).
(**d**) Yes, ultrasound plus CNB
*Histology:* Bilateral *invasive lobular carcinoma (G2).*

**Answer for Fig. 5.35** (p. 122)

(**a**) PGMI (2006)
(**b**) ACR3
(**c**) BIRADS 2
(**d**) No
Right prepectoral nodule (fibroadenoma) with smooth margins and uniform density (**e1**). The nodule is clearly visible at ultrasound (**e1**) and was previously visible in the 2004 examination. By contrast, the retroareolar carcinoma is not visible on mammograms and appears sonographically as a faint, hypoechoic, benign-appearing nodule (**e**). The clinical presentation of skin retraction (arrows, **d**) is suggestive of carcinoma. On *MRI*, the fibroadenoma and retroareolar mass shows equal degrees of gadolinium enhancement (**f**), but both lesions show the same slow-rise type of time–density curve, which is typical of a benign process.

*Core biopsy histology:* intermediate-grade (G2) invasive lobular carcinoma (Department of Pathology, Esslingen).

**Fig. 5.35**

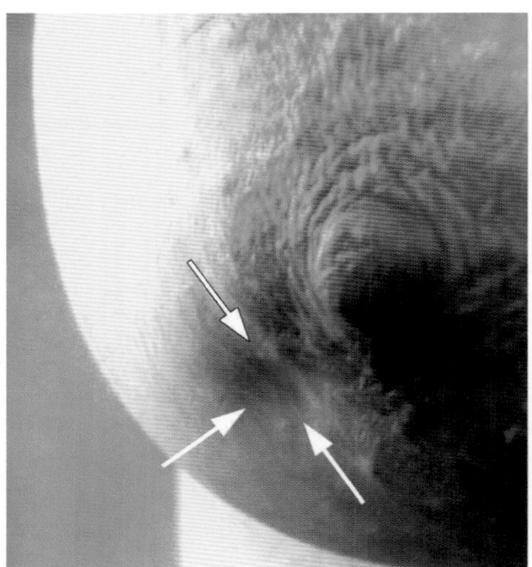

**d** *Clinical appearance of the right breast* (lateral nipple region): circumscribed retraction (arrows) of the areola and skin (suspicious).

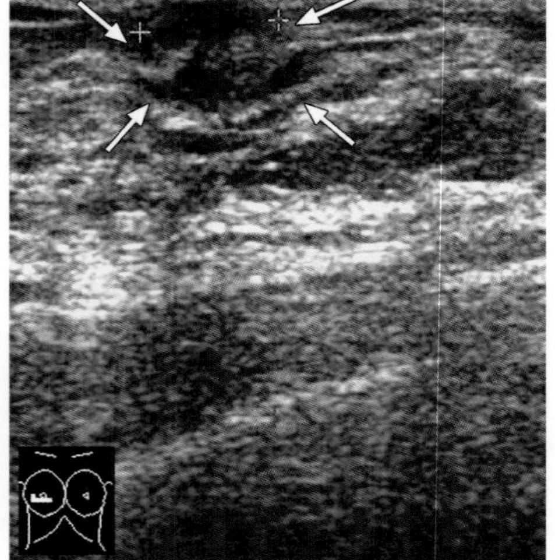

**e** Retroareolar *sonogram* at the skin retraction site (tumor) shows a well-circumscribed hypoechoic nodule (arrows) with irregular internal echoes and no acoustic enhancement (marker).

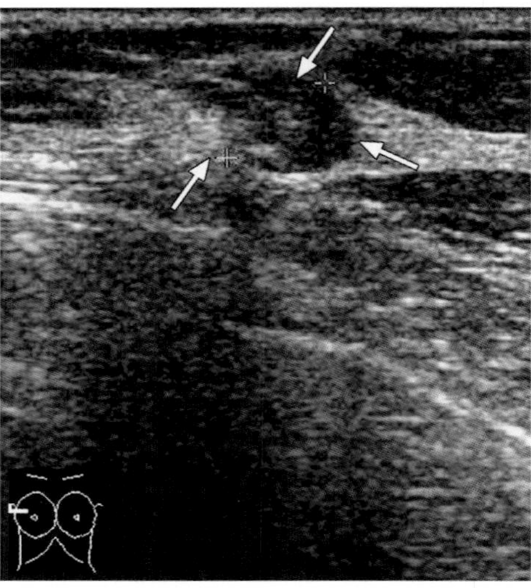

**e1** *Sonogram* of the upper quadrant at 12-o'clock (fibroadenoma) shows a smooth nodule (arrows) with irregular internal echoes and faint posterior enhancement.

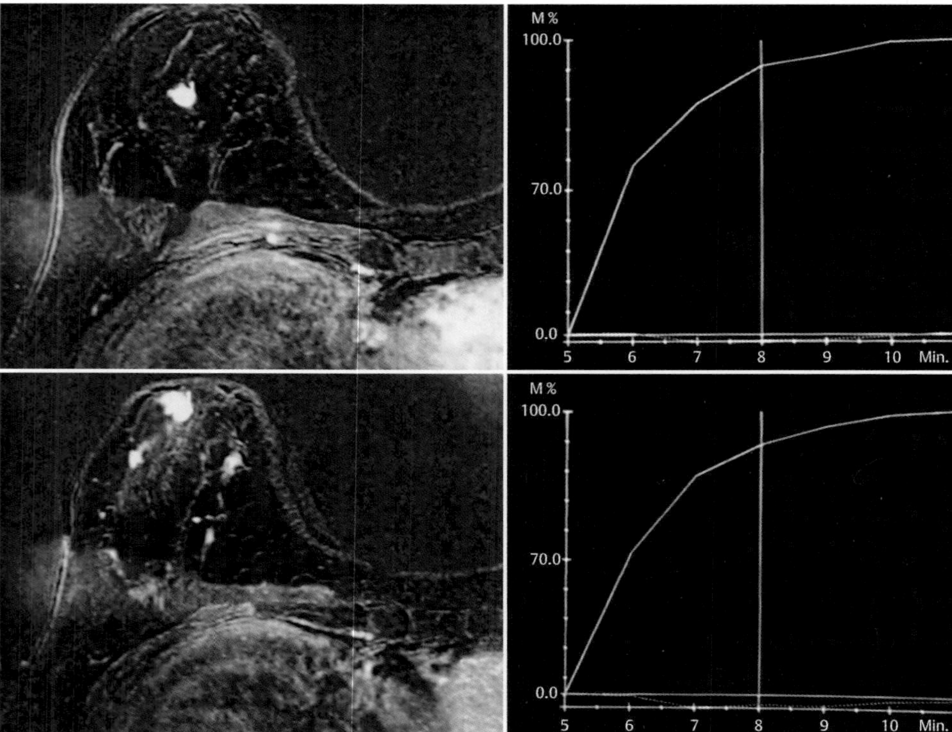


**f** *MRI* shows two nodules with time–density curves typical of benign nodules. The retroareolar lesion (lower image) is a carcinoma with irregular margins (skin retraction!). The central lesion (image above) is a fibroadenoma.

*Physical examination was the key to early cancer detection. The patient herself, incidentally, failed to notice the skin retraction.*

**Answer for Fig. 5.36** (p. 123)

(**a**) PGMI (pectoral muscle incompletely visible)
(**b**) ACR 3
(**c**) BIRADS 1
(**d**) Recall: no

*Cell-rich DCIS with an invasive component in the right breast, fibroadenoma in the left breast.* The DCIS was not detected by mammography, including magnification views (**c, d**). The tumor is located in the upper inner quadrant of the right breast. It has smooth margins and shows very intense gadolinium enhancement on MRI (**e**). A similar nodule in the left breast exhibits the time–density curve of a fibroadenoma. Color duplex vividly demonstrates the vascularity at the ▶

**Fig. 5.36**

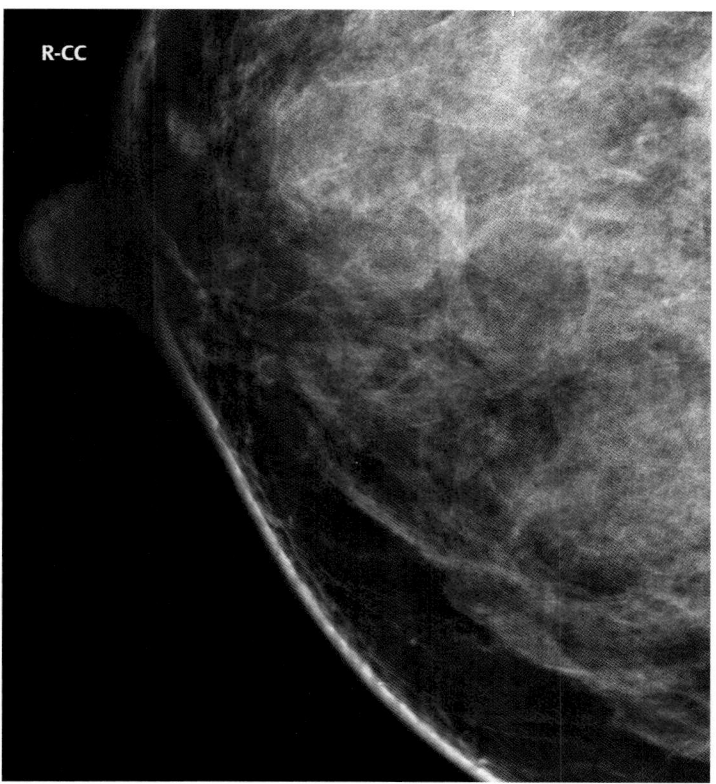


**c** *Mammography:* craniocaudal *spot film* of the upper inner quadrant of the right breast with a fine focus.

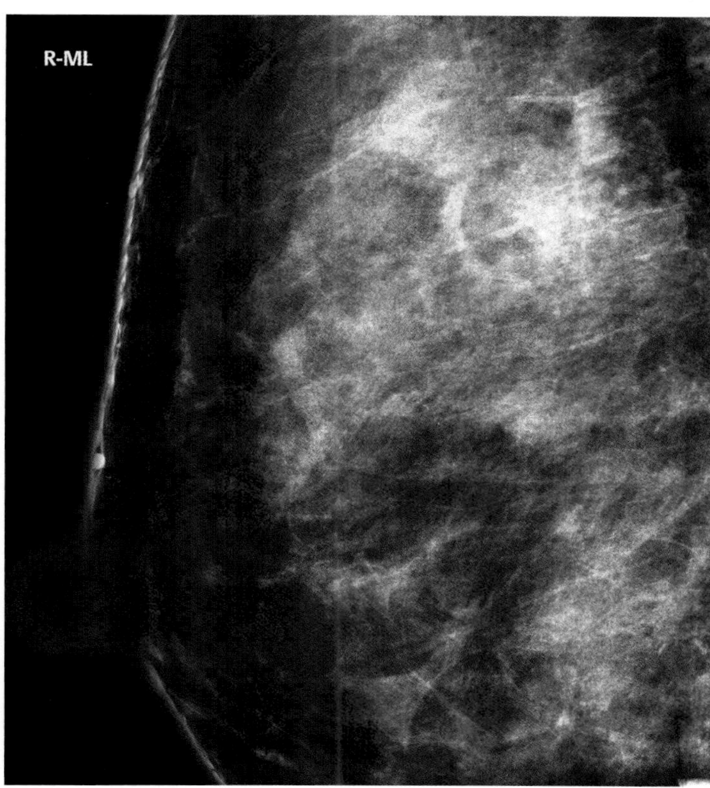


**d** *Mammography:* mediolateral *spot film* of the upper inner quadrant with a fine focus.

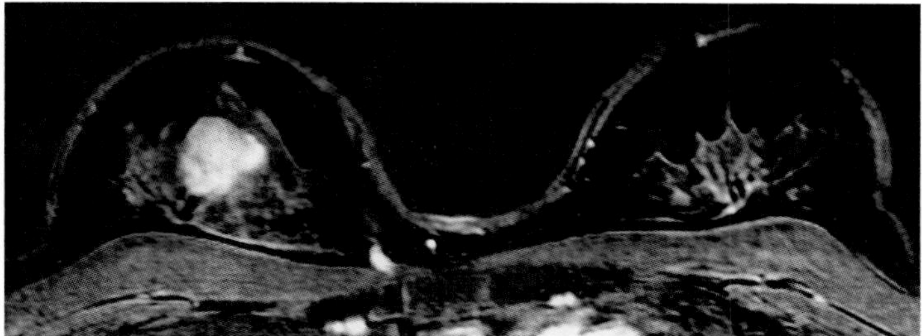

**e** *MRI:* Subtraction images show an intensely enhancing nodule with smooth margins in the upper inner quadrant of the right breast (cancer).

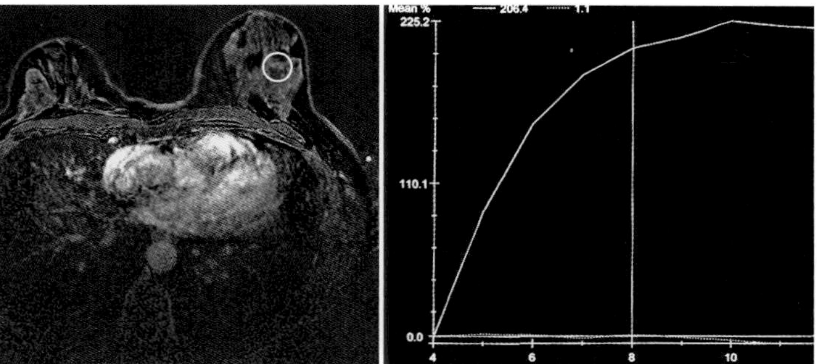


**f** *MRI* of a small nodule in the upper outer quadrant of the left breast with a benign time–density curve.

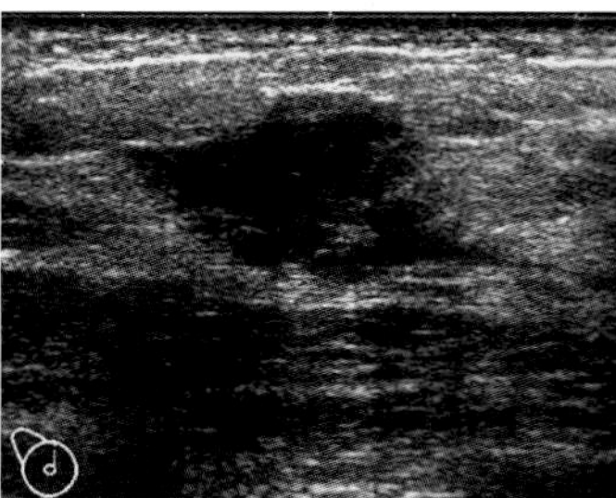

**g** *Sonogram* of *cancer* in the right breast shows an almost 2 cm hypoechoic nodule with a combination of smooth margins and ill-defined medial margins and irregular internal echoes.

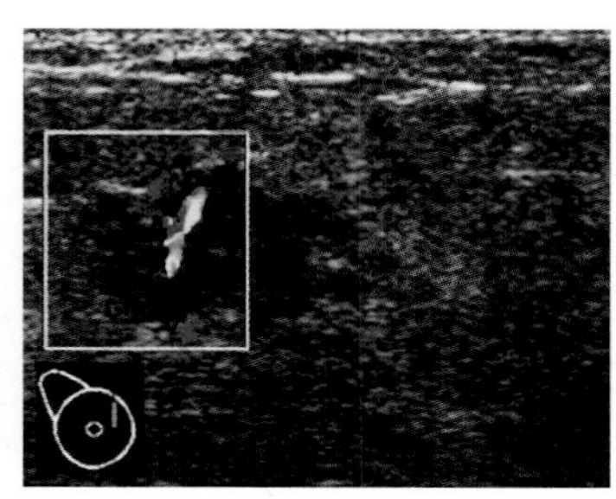

**g1** *Color duplex* shows increased vascularity even in the tumor interior.

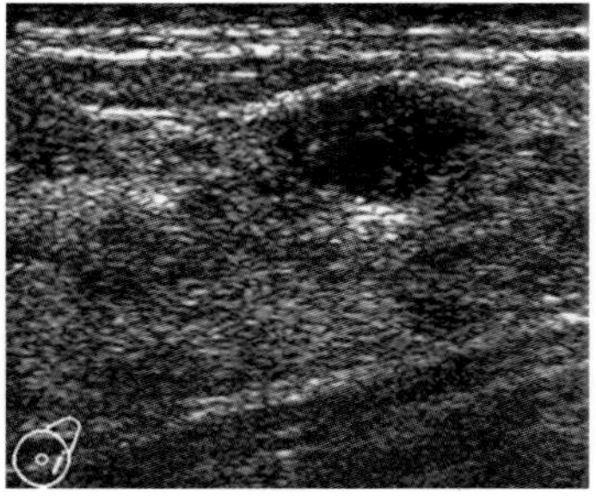

**h** *Sonogram* of the left *fibroadenoma* shows smooth margins and scattered internal echoes.

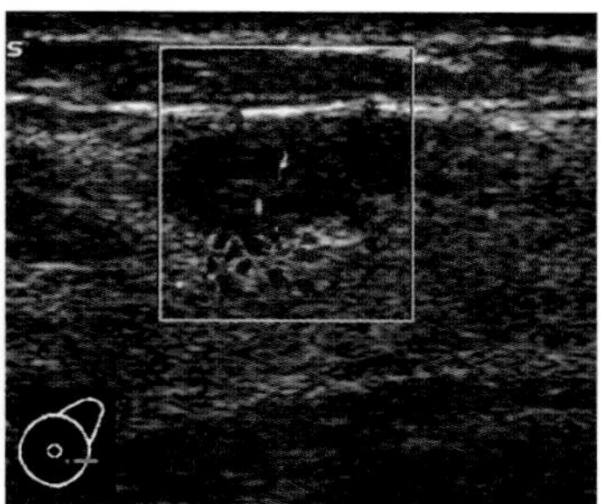

**h1** *Color duplex* of the fibroadenoma mainly shows increased peripheral vascularity accompanied by isolated central vessels (images courtesy of Gebhard Wittlinger, Schorndorf).

center and periphery of the malignant tumor (**g 1**). The lesion is clearly visible at ultrasound, showing smooth inner margins and internal echoes. The fibroadenoma in the left breast is also clearly demonstrated by ultrasound and shows increased peripheral vascularity (**a, h 1**).

### Answer for Fig. 5.37 (p. 124)

(**a**) **P**GM**I** 2004 (PGM**I** in 2002 and 2003—pectoral muscle incompletely imaged, skin fold at **d/25–27**)
(**b**) ACR 3
(**c**) BIRADS 1 in 2002, BIRADS 4 in 2003 (at **D/7–8**), BIRADS 5 in 2004 on left side (**i/7–8**), BIRADS 1 in 2004 on right side.
(**d**) No in 2002. Yes, ultrasound and CNB in 2003 and 2004.
*Histology: Invasive ductal carcinoma (G2).* **The tumor was missed in 2003.**

### Answer for Fig. 5.38 (p. 125)

(**a**) PGM**I** (the pectoral muscle and inframammary fold are not imaged in the oblique view)
(**b**) ACR 2
(**c**) BIRADS 4b left (**q–R/8–9** cc, **q–R/21–22** oblique), 4a right (**N/24–25** oblique, **N/11** cc)
(**d**) Yes, ultrasound and CNB both sides.
*Histology:*
Left breast: *Invasive ductal carcinoma (G2).*
Right breast: *Adenosis* in the upper outer quadrant.

### Answer for Fig. 5.39 (p. 126)

(**a**) P**G**MI—lateral parts of breast parenchyma not imaged
(**b**) ACR3
(**c**) BIRADS 1
*Recall:* yes: ultrasound, because of the inhomogeneous densities and because of the right nipple discharge noted at mammography. No tumor visible on mammograms!

A *1.2 cm invasive ductal carcinoma* is present in the upper inner quadrant of the right breast. The dilated duct provides a landmark for identifying the affected duct and lobe within the breast parenchyma (**c**). Because of the presence of Paget-like cells in the smear, a punch-biopsy of the nipple was also done (histology: *Paget disease*).

*Ultrasound* shows a well-circumscribed hypoechoic tumor at the 1-o'clock position in the upper inner quadrant (**d**). The tumor is also clearly defined by *MRI* and shows an abnormal time–density curve (**e**). Another focus is found in the prepectoral region (arrow in **e**). Because this prepectoral lesion cannot be localized by ultrasound or mammography, it is not biopsied. Despite an atypical time–density curve, it is treated like a fibroadenoma and left within the breast. The patient underwent a standard quadrantectomy with the removal of the nipple because of Paget disease (tumor area with arrow) (**f**) (Thorsten Kühn, IMZE Esslingen).

**This example and the examples below (Figs. 5.39–5.54) illustrate the principle that mammography alone cannot ensure the early detection of breast cancer. The current gold standard should be physical examination plus mammography plus ultrasound.**

**Fig. 5.39**

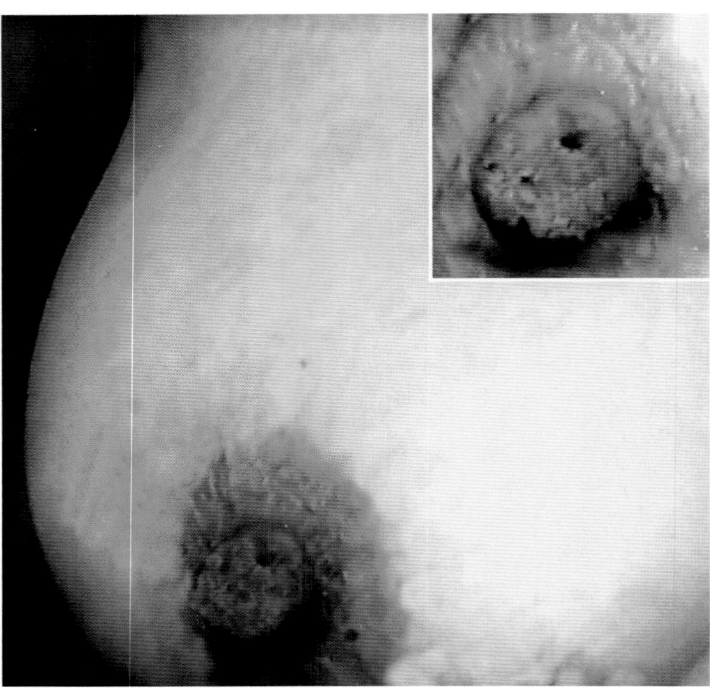

**c** *Clinical appearance* of the right breast and nipple (inset). Serous nipple discharge from a dilated duct is visible at the 1-o'clock position. The tumor is located in the associated mammary lobe. No clinical sign of the histologically proven Paget disease.

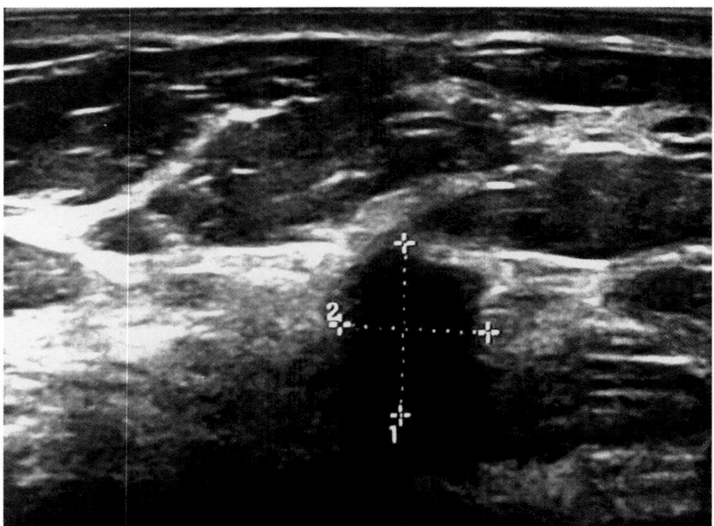


**d** Sonogram of the right breast at the 1-o'clock position shows a relatively well-circumscribed, hypoechoic nodule measuring 1.0 cm × 1.2 cm. There is no other evidence of focal lesions in this breast.

> ***Tip***
>
> Even when detected in a screening examination, atypical nipple discharge requires further investigation.
> The pathology underlying discharge from an isolated duct is always located in the associated segment of the breast. Thus, discharge from the upper inner quadrant of the nipple originates in the upper inner quadrant of the breast, discharge from the lower outer quadrant of the nipple arises in the lower outer quadrant of the breast, and so on.

**Fig. 5.39** *(continued)*

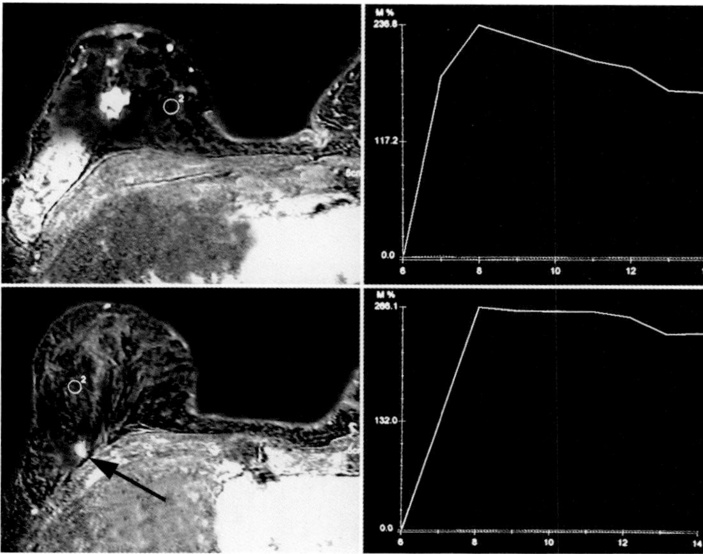

**e** *Subtraction MRI* shows a central nodule at the 1-o'clock position with intense irregular gadolinium enhancement and a malignant-type time–density curve. On the lateral chest wall is a second, 8 mm nodule in the peripheral portion of the same lobule (arrow), also showing a somewhat malignant-type time–density curve. Note the small gadolinium depot between the central tumor and the nipple.
*Ultrasound-guided CNB* of the central nodule was done. (The prepectoral lesion was not biopsied because it was not visible by ultrasound or mammography and an MRI biopsy apparatus was not available at the time.)
*Histology*: *invasive ductal papillary carcinoma* (G2) without nodal metastases. Morbus Paget of the nipple with tumor infiltration of retroareolar ducts.

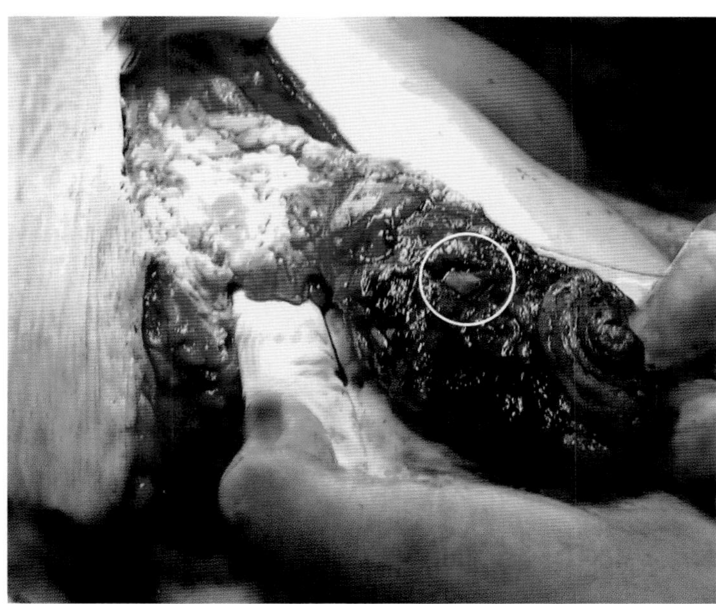

**f** *Intraoperative view.* After blue staining of the affected lobe, a quadrantectomy was performed with resection of the nipple and the lobe to the chest wall (the prepectoral lesion was not found). The further course was uneventful, and the patient was still disease-free at 3 years (images courtesy of Thorsten Kühn, IMZE Esslingen, Germany).

## Answer for Fig. 5.42 (p. 132 f)

**Answer (c) is correct. Artifacts.** The calcifications are mammographic artifacts caused by powder on the skin (clotrimazole 2%, Tannolad lotion).

Powder in the inframammary fold and also in skin warts can produce tumorlike artifacts.

Skin wart and pseudomicrocalcifications are documented in **d** and **c** in a magnification view.

**Fig. 5.42**

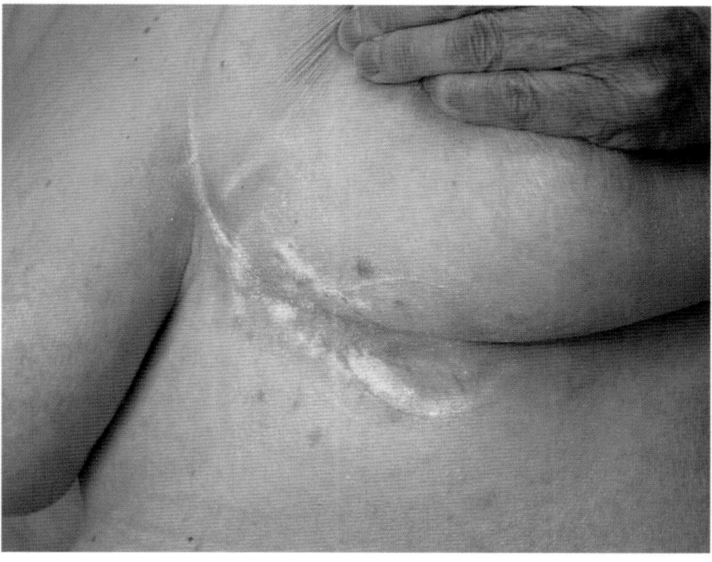

**c** *Clinical inspection*: Apparent "microcalcifications" in the left breast are caused by powder placed in the inframammary fold for a skin rash.

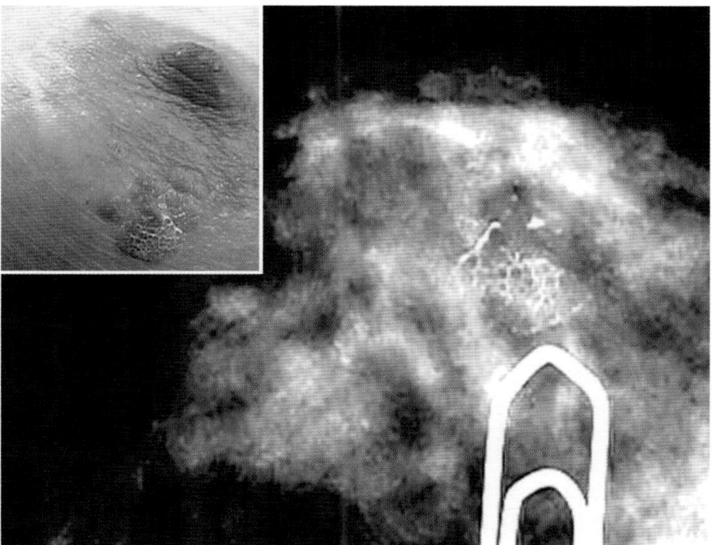

**d** *Mammography* (magnified craniocaudal view) shows an atypical reticular "calcification pattern" caused by cream residues in a hyperkeratotic skin wart (upper left image). **Consider a cutaneous source whenever this pattern is found in a mammogram!** Because the wart is very flat, it lacks the typical halo often seen with skin tumors.

**Answer for Fig. 5.43** (p. 134)

(**a**) No. Asymmetry is caused by a tissue defect. (The technical assistant must notice the scar!)
(**c**) Routine follow-up in 2 years.
Recall is unnecessary when the breast is assessed by visual inspection. The nipple and retroareolar space are absent due to previous severe mastitis. The opacity in the right breast (**B–c/8–10** cc, **B–c/18–20** oblique in panel **b**) represents normal breast parenchyma.

**Fig. 5.43**

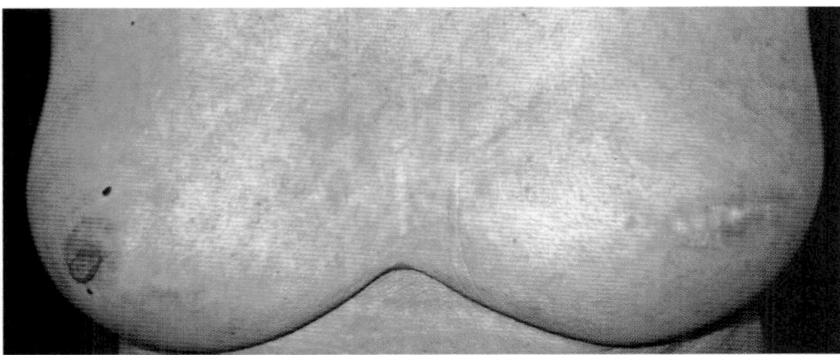

**c** *Clinical appearance* 10 years after resection of the left nipple.

**Answer for Fig. 5.44** (p. 135)

**Answer (b) is correct. Recall.** A 1 cm × 1 cm × 2 cm, inhomogeneous, crescent-shaped opacity is visible in the left axillary recess (at **o/25** in panel **a**). It could be DCIS, especially if the lesion is visible at the prepectoral level in the craniocaudal view. The opacity is actually caused by a *tick bite*, which is visible as a slightly red ring-shaped area on the skin.

*Ultrasound* examination of this region (**d**) shows a subcutaneous, comet-tail-shaped hypoechoic area, a dilated lymph vessel (lymphangitis).

**Fig. 5.44**

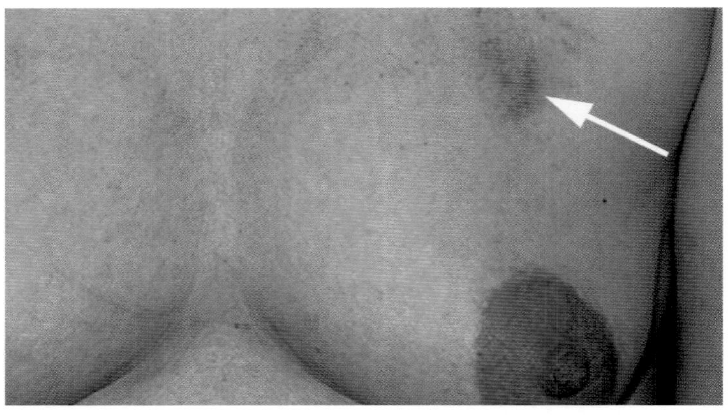

**c** *Clinical inspection* of the breast shows that a slightly red area caused by an insect bite is visible at the 12–1-o'clock position projected into the upper outer quadrant of the left breast.

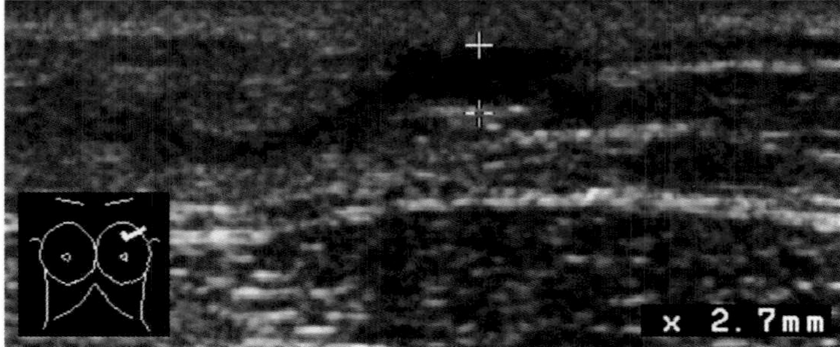


**d** *Sonogram* of the left breast shows a subcutaneous 7 cm × 3-mm hypoechoic area with a ductlike acoustic irregularity extending medially from it.

**Answer for Fig. 5.45** (p. 136)

**Answer (c) is correct. Skin lesion.** The lesion is unrelated to the lymph nodes. On *inspection* of the breast (**b**), a *skin wart* is found on the chest wall that was projected into the axilla in the oblique view. There is no lymphadenopathy. In the same manner, a skin lesion on the breast could also be projected over the breast parenchyma.

**Fig. 5.45**

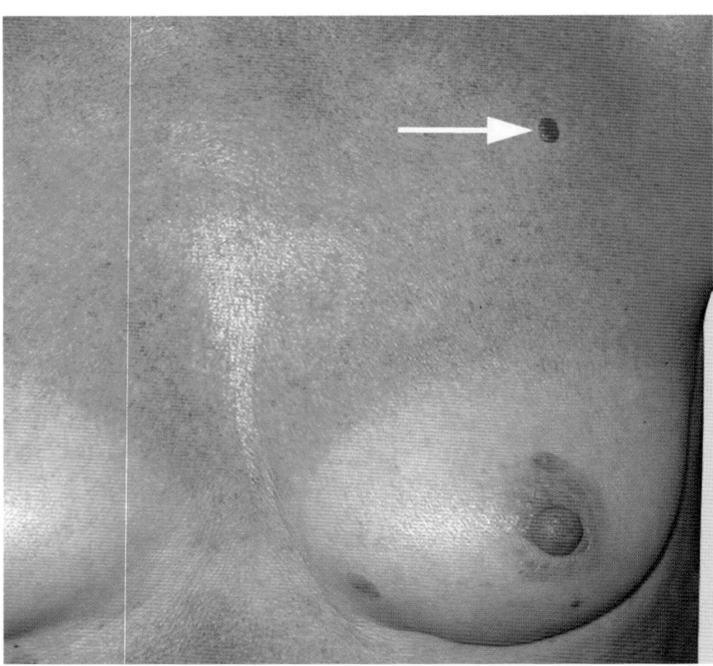

**b** *Clinical inspection* of the left breast reveals a small, prepectoral skin lesion at the 12-o'clock position.

## Answer for Fig. 5.46 (p. 137)

**Answer (a) is correct. Routine follow-up** because of harmless comedo-calcification. Aside from this the mammograms appear normal. **But:** *Ultrasound* shows a 1.2 cm × 0.8 cm × 0.8 cm hypoechoic area in the lower inner quadrant of the right breast (**c**) suspicious for a malignant neoplasm. Ultrasound-guided *CNB* was performed, and rapid staining of material from the coaxial needle already revealed tumorlike cells (**d**).

*Histology:* moderately differentiated invasive *ductal* carcinoma.

**Note:** Knowing the ultrasound findings, we can just discern a faint round opacity among the calcifications on the mammograms (panel **a** [inset], **k/24**).

**Fig. 5.46**

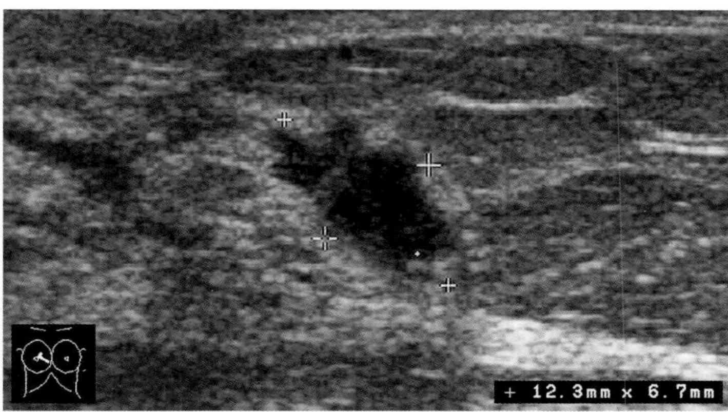


**c** *Sonogram* of the lower inner quadrant of the right breast shows a suspicious 1.2 cm × 0.7 cm hypoechoic area with scalloped margins.

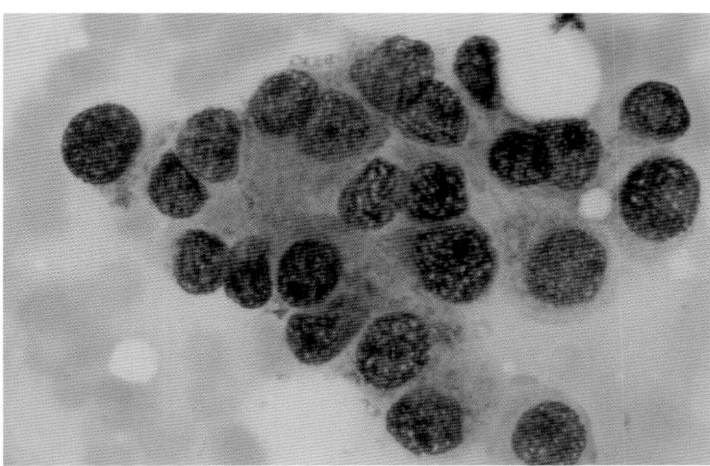

**d** *FNA cytology* shows multiple rows of compact, syncytium-like aggregates of cells arranged in rosette-like clusters. The cells have pleomorphic nuclei, coarse chromatin, and enlarged nucleoli (rather suspicious for *lobular* carcinoma).

## Answer for Fig. 5.47 (p. 138)

**Answer (b) is correct. BIRADS 4a.** A nonspecific density with ill-defined margins is present in the axillary recess on the left side (**E–e/24–25**).

The patient noticed a mass at the 2-o'clock position in her left breast (**c**). *Ultrasound* shows a 1.3 mm × 1.2 mm × 9.0 mm nodule with slightly ill-defined margins at that location (**d**). *FNA* shows the cytologic features of fibroadenoma (**e**). *Excisional biopsy* and *histology* revealed *multifocal breast carcinoma*, necessitating a mastectomy.

When the clinical, sonographic, and histologic findings are compared with the mammographic changes, the latter seem relatively subtle and could easily be missed by an untrained eye. Furthermore, the lateral quadrant of the breast is cut off in the craniocaudal projection (panel **b**), which means that the tumor-affected area is not imaged. This case illustrates the limitations of FNA. The ultrasound findings were also interpreted as *fibroadenoma*, although critical inspection shows slightly ill-defined margins, which should have been an indication for CNB in this patient.

**Fig. 5.47**

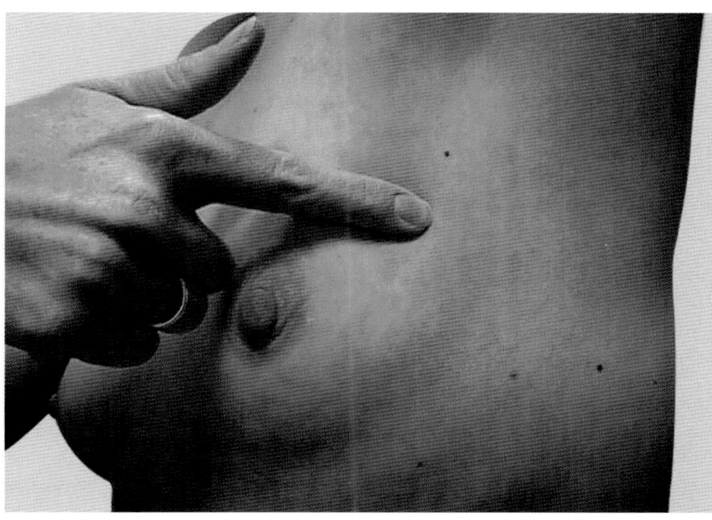

**c** *Physical examination* of the left breast reveals a nonspecific firmness between the breast parenchyma and axillary recess.

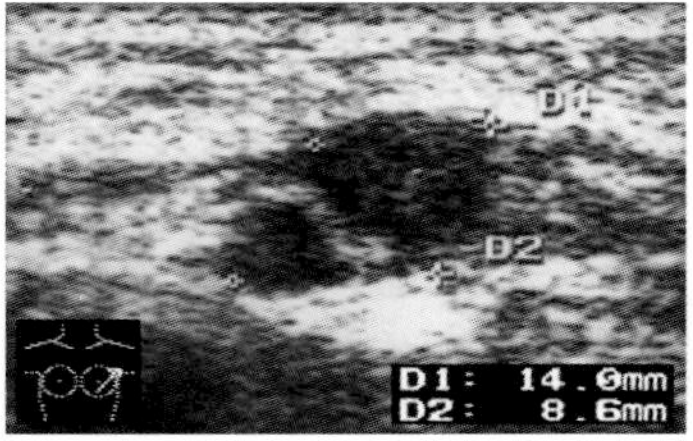


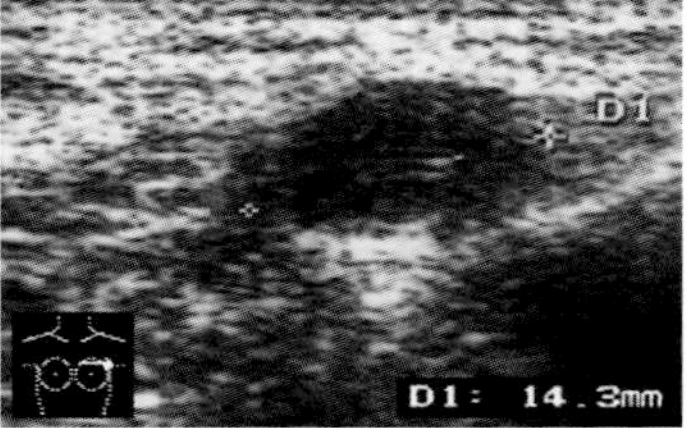


**d** *Sonogram* of the upper outer quadrant of the left breast shows a 1.4 cm × 1.4 cm × 0.9 cm nodule with ill-defined margins, internal echoes, and questionable necrosis located directly on the pectoral muscle. Cytology yielded an erroneous diagnosis of fibroadenoma.

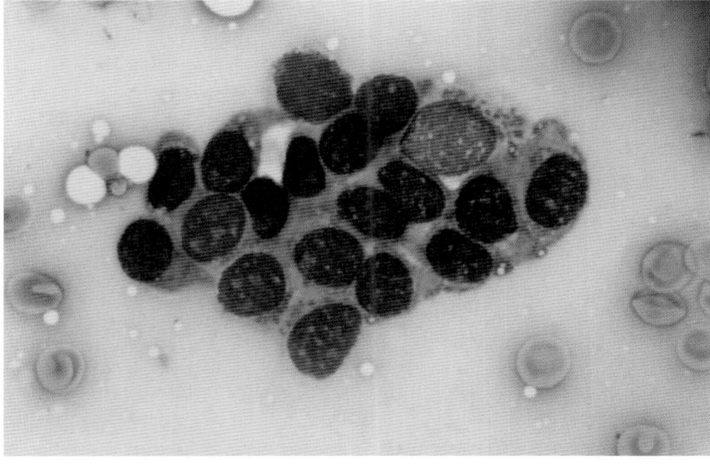

**e** *FNA cytology* shows compact cell clusters with bipolar basket cells (e.g., **q–R/7–8**) and a uniform cell pattern that is suspicious for fibroadenoma. (*Histology* revealed *well-differentiated ductal carcinoma*.) What were supposed to be basket cells were actually elliptical, compressed cancer cells. The nuclear-cytoplasmic ratio is strongly shifted in favor of the nuclei.

### Answer for Fig. 5.48 (p. 139 f)

**Answer (a) is correct. The invasive focus is in the left breast.** The G1 DCIS is located in the upper outer quadrant of the right breast (oblique **l/25**, cc **m/13**). As usual, it is detected by the presence of microcalcifications (**c**). It grows slowly and has time to calcify (see **Fig. 4.34 d**, pp. 65, 67). The invasive G3 carcinoma in the left breast grows rapidly without calcifying (or else the calcifications have already regressed; see **Fig. 4.21**). The intense gadolinium enhancement on *MRI* supports the diagnosis of an *invasive tumor* in the left breast, while the absence of enhancement about the calcifications in the right breast is suggestive of *G1-DCIS*. Because of its rich blood supply, the invasive G3 tumor was easy to detect and localize by *CT* after bolus contrast injection, although the enhancement of the nodule was neutralized by the metal on the localization images (**g**).

**Further course to 2008:** no local recurrence and good cosmetic results (**h**). A *stellate scar* is visible in the area around the excision site on the left side (**i**).

**Note:** The carcinoma in the left breast was detected incidentally by MRI, which had been ordered to investigate the calcifications in the right breast. Ultrasound showed nothing suspicious on either side. In every case that requires surgical intervention, preoperative MRI should be performed to exclude second and multicentric tumors and establish a baseline for postoperative follow-ups.

**Fig. 5.48**

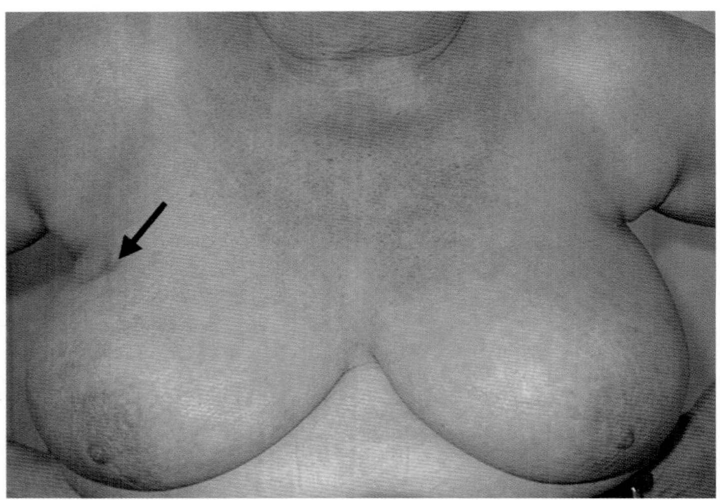

**h** *Clinical inspection* 6 years after bilateral treatment shows a very good cosmetic result. A scar is visible on the right breast (arrow).

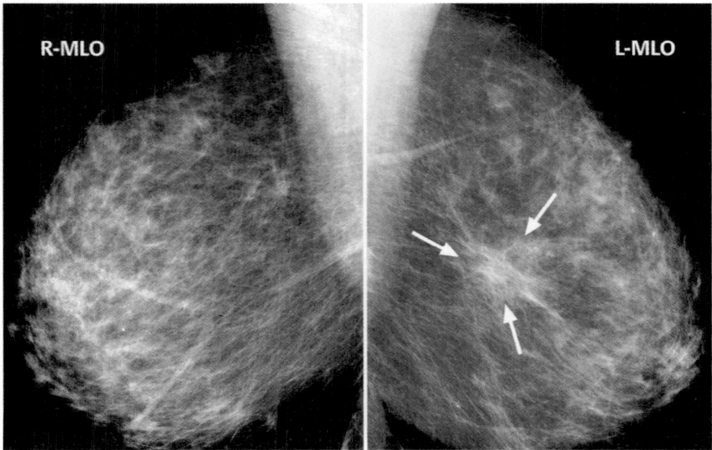


**i** *Bilateral oblique mammograms* 6 years after treatment show a stellate scar at the former tumor site in the left breast (arrows). The right breast appears normal.

### Answer for Fig. 5.49 (p. 140 f)

**Answer (c) is correct. Morphological confirmation by FNA/CNB.** Even cysts that appear harmless at ultrasound should at least be morphologically confirmed by FNA. *Ultrasound-guided CNB* was performed on both lesions (**f**). The nodule near the chest wall was an *apocrine carcinoma* (**g**), and the nodule near the nipple was a small *cyst*. Although the apocrine carcinoma appears mammographically and sonographically benign, suspicious scalloped margins are visible in the specimen radiograph (**h**). The sonogram is not typical of a simple cyst. Posterior acoustic enhancement is absent; the linear shadows from tangential wall segments create the impression of acoustic enhancement.

**Fig. 5.49**

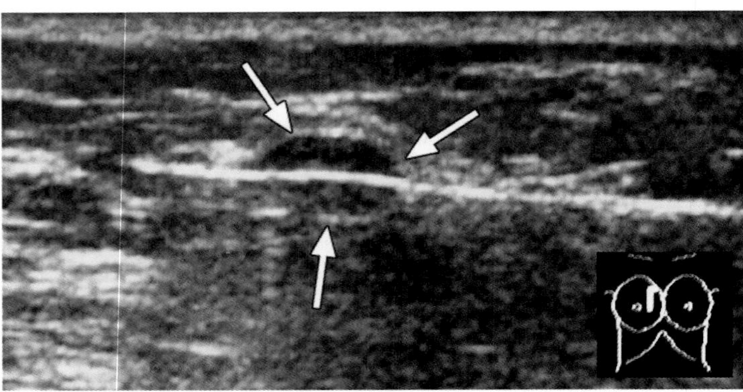

**f** *Ultrasound-guided CNB* of the nodule near the chest wall. The biopsy needle is at the center of the nodule (arrows).

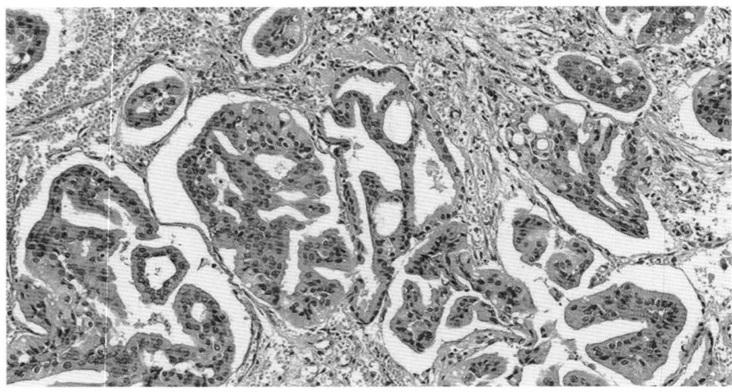

**g** *Histology* shows an *apocrine neoplasm* with proliferating atypical apocrine cell aggregates in enlarged ductules (image courtesy of Hans-Helmut Dahm, Esslingen).

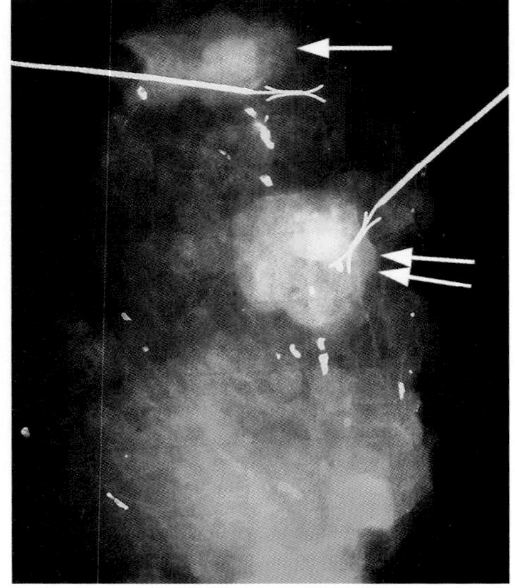

**h** *Specimen radiograph*. Both lesions have been localized. The upper lesion is a *cyst* (arrow). The lower lesion is an *apocrine carcinoma* with scalloped margins (double arrow) surrounded by unsuspicious calcifications (plasma cell mastitis).

**Fig. 5.50**

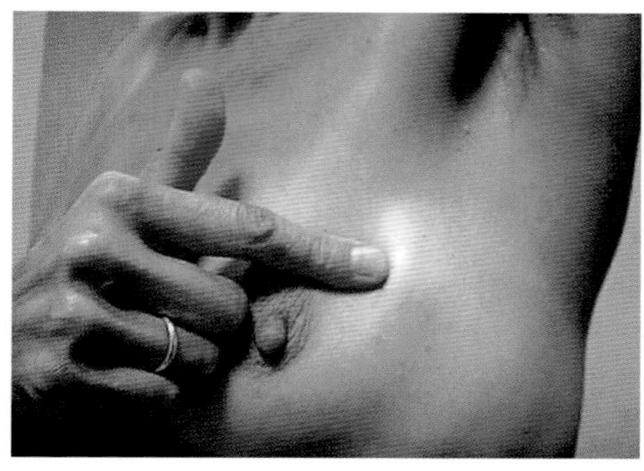

**d** *Physical examination*: A lentil-sized nodule is palpable in the left breast at the 2-o'clock position.

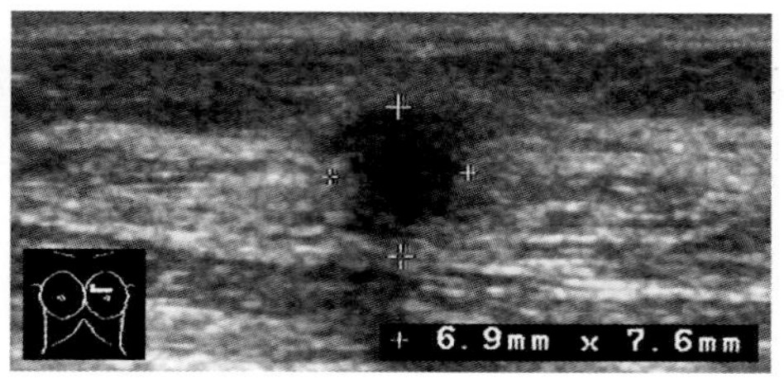


**e** *Sonogram* of the left breast shows a suspicious 7 mm hypoechoic nodule with indistinct margins (S-BIRADS 4).

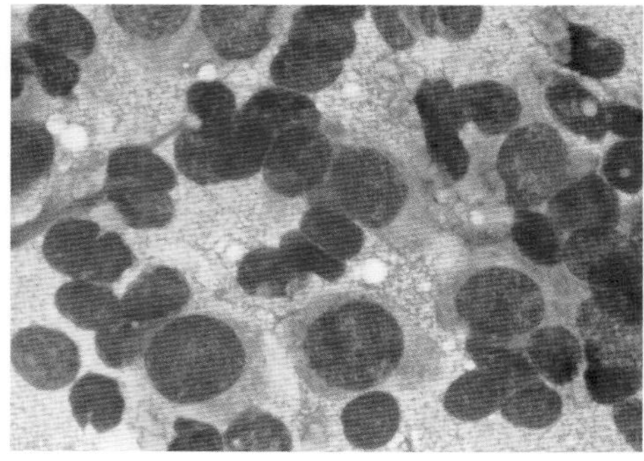

**f** *FNA cytology* reveals separate (dissociated), moderately pleomorphic tumor cells (Pap V).

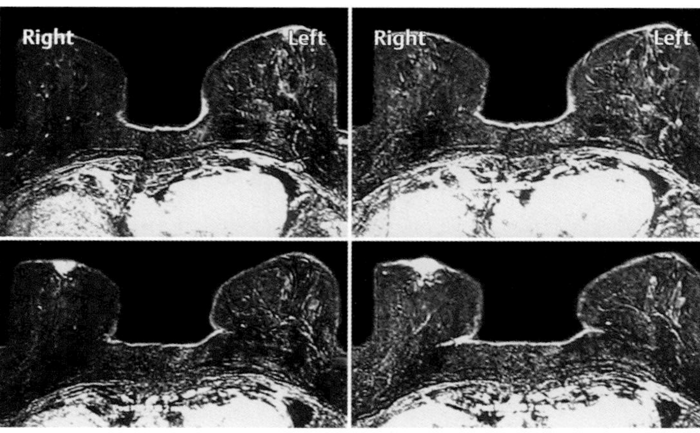


**g** *MR subtraction* image. No enhancement is visible in both breasts.

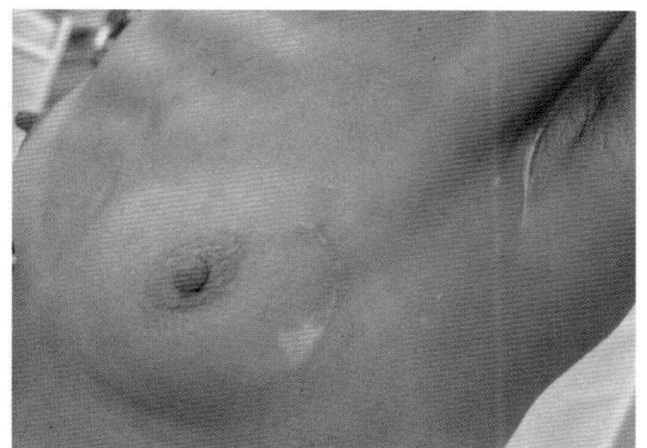

**h** *Clinical inspection* 3 years after surgery shows depigmentation of the scar in vitiligo.

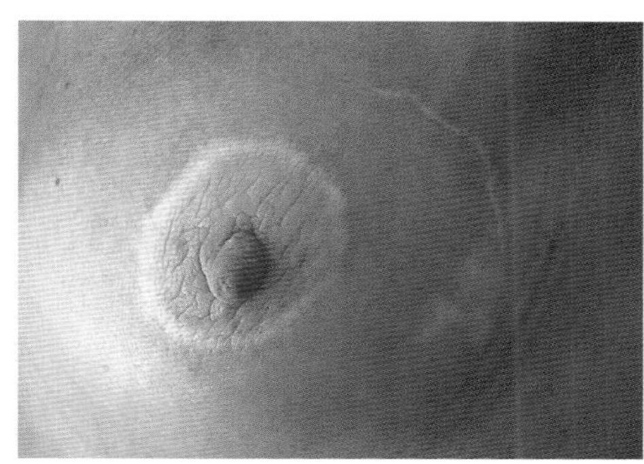

**i** *Clinical inspection* 4 years after surgery shows depigmentation of the scar and areola in vitiligo.

### Answer for Fig. 5.50, Question 1 (p. 141 f)

**Answer (c) is correct. Vitiligo.** The patient has a vitiligo with foci located near the right axilla, in the presternal area, and above the left areola. These changes do not require histologic investigation.

### Answer for Fig. 5.50, Question 2 (p. 141 f)

**Answer (c) is correct. Because of the radiographic density.** Ultrasound scanning is necessary due to the radiographic density of the breast (ACR3) and especially because of small focal densities (**r–S/13**) seen in the upper outer quadrant of the left breast.

At *clinical investigation* a freely movable lentil-sized nodule is palpable in that quadrant (**d**), and *ultrasound* shows a 7 mm focus with ill-defined margins at that location (**e**). Ultrasound-guided *FNA* of the lesion yields suspicious epithelial cells (**f**). Remarkably, *MRI* does *not* show gadolinium enhancement in the left breast (**g**).

**Course to 2008:** no local recurrence and no second tumor in the right breast. The patient developed additional foci of vitiligo about the areola and surgical scar (typical of this disease) (**i**). Depigmentation of the left nipple is a result of radiotherapy.

**Note:** Patients with vitiligo should be informed of this complication (further depigmentation of scars and radiotherapy fields) prior to surgery. The slight deviation of the left nipple toward the lower outer quadrant is unrelated to the tumor in this case.

### Answer for Fig. 5.51, Question 1 (p. 142 f)

**Answer (c) is correct. There is no difference between the two examinations in both breasts.** It cannot be determined which pairs of images are from 2002. Generally there is no difference in the mammographic findings, aside from a few nonspecific densities at various sites. In fact images **a** and **b** are from 2001, images **c** and **d** are from 2002. The semicircular opacity in the right inframammary fold (**m–N/13–14**) is a summation effect, also visible in the previous view.

Fig. 5.51

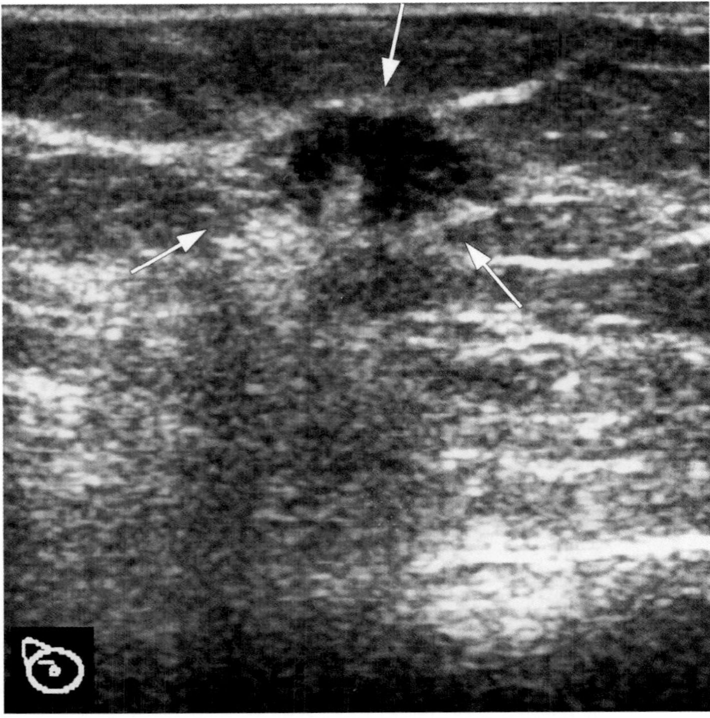

**e** *Sonogram* of the upper outer quadrant of the right breast in 2002 shows a 10 mm × 6 mm × 6 mm cystlike lesion at the 11-o'clock position in the axillary recess. *Histology*: *invasive ductal neoplasm*.

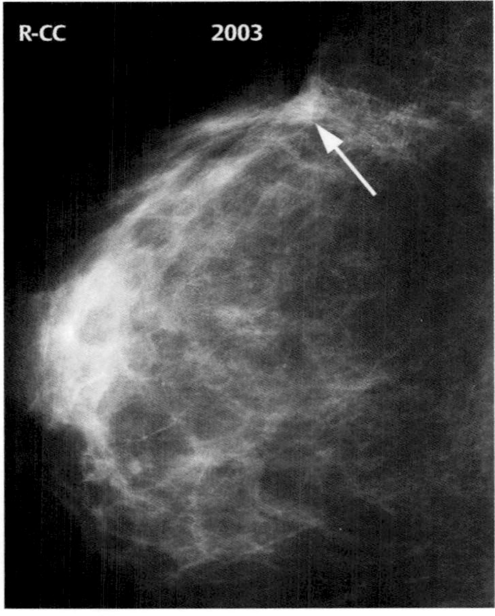


**f** *Craniocaudal mammogram* of the right breast in 2003 shows stellate densities at the excision site consistent with scarring (arrow).

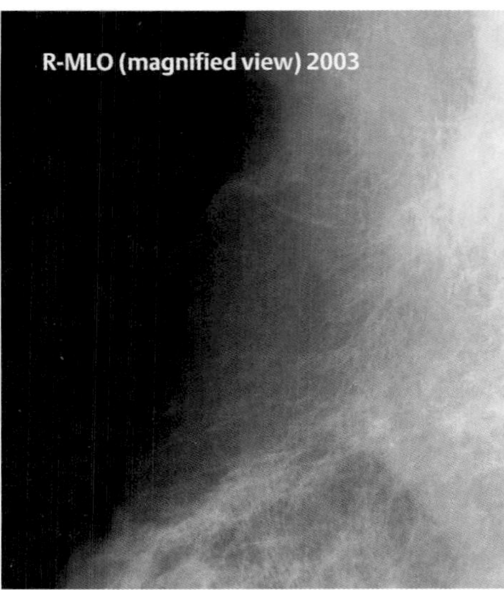


**g** *Mediolateral oblique spot film* of the upper outer quadrant of the right breast shows cicatricial changes at the excision site with no evidence of local recurrence (images courtesy of Bernd Hörr, Plochingen).

### Answer for Fig. 5.51, Question 2 (p. 142 f)

**Answer (c) is correct. Further examination is necessary due to the radiographic density** (ACR 2) of the breast and a subtle, nonspecific opacity in the upper outer quadrant of the right breast (**c**, oblique: **L–I/16–17; d**, cc: **L–M/7–8**). *Sonography* (7.5 MHz) of the right axillary recess shows two foci that extended into the anterior axillary fold (**e**).*CNB* reveals *multifocal invasive ductal carcinoma (G2)*. The scar is seen on right mammogram from 2003 in **f** and **g**.

**Note:** In breasts with a density of ACR 2 or higher, single-view mammography plus ultrasound is recommended instead of two-view mammograms, even in patients with no palpable or mammographic abnormalities (see p. 105). Knowing the ultrasound findings, we can recognize a small focal density that enlarged slightly from 2001 to 2002. In an ACR 2 breast 5 mm large *non calcifying* cancers could be overlooked.

### Answer for Fig. 5.52 (p. 144)

**Answer (c) is correct.** Ultrasound was added due to the radiographic breast density (relative, due to the patient's age).

*Ultrasound* examination was definitely indicated but showed no abnormalities. In this case *visual inspection* of the breast suggests the correct diagnosis. The patient has a *Paget carcinoma* of the right breast. *Mammograms* were also taken but were unremarkable.

Fig. 5.52

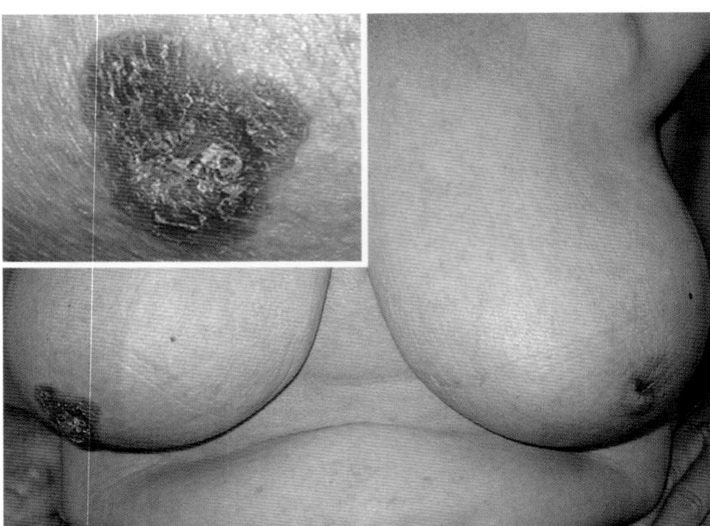

**c** *Clinical inspection* of the right breast reveals advanced *Paget disease* of the nipple and areola. *Histology: DCIS* with involvement of the nipple, no retroareolar tumor invasion. Unsuspicious nipple inversion is noted on the left side.

**Answer for Fig. 5.53** (p. 145)

**Answer (c) is correct. Recall** is indicated due to the suspicious lesion in the left breast. There is a small, suspicious focus in the left breast at **R/25** (BIRADS 4). Despite the high radiographic density, the small lesion is visible in the oblique projection when the two views are compared closely. It was not imaged in the craniocaudal view (perhaps a good case for tomosynthesis!). When the mammographic findings are known, the lesion can be located with *ultrasound* (**b**). The nodule is visible in the *specimen radiograph* and is visualized in its entirety (**c**).

Even if the lesion were not detected, recall would still be necessary based solely on the high mammographic density of the breast. Answer (**b**), then, would not be incorrect.

**Fig. 5.53**

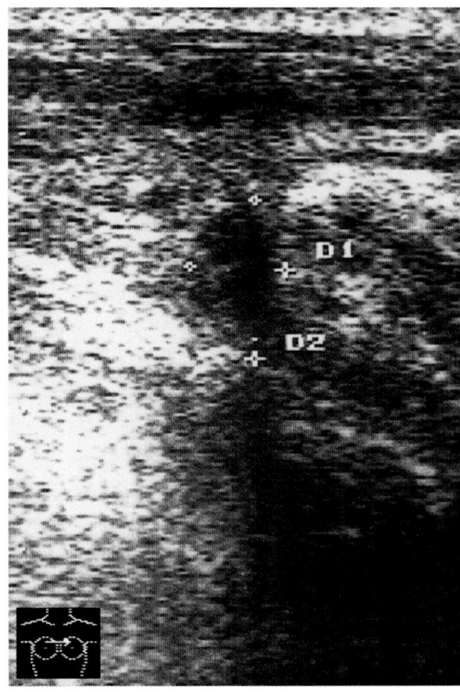


**b** *Sonogram* (5 MHz) of the upper inner quadrant of the left breast shows a 6.5 mm × 11.5 mm nodule with relatively smooth margins and posterior acoustic shadowing.

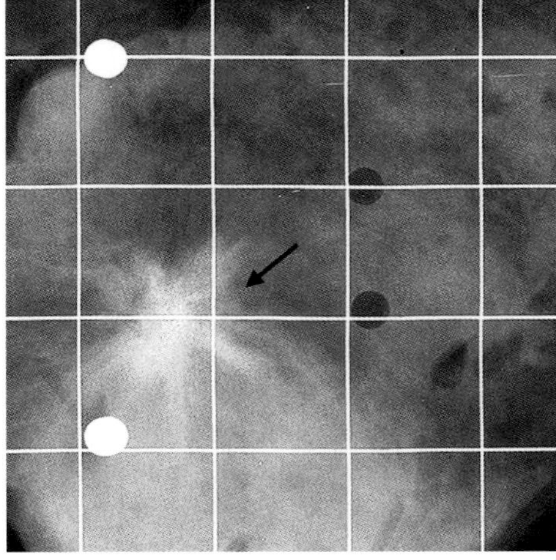

**c** *Specimen radiograph* shows the entire tumor (arrow) with an approximately 1 cm margin width, also visible in the other plane (not shown).

**Answer for Fig. 5.54, Question 1** (p. 146 f)

**Answer (b) is correct. The tumor is located outside the image planes** (see survey image **d** at upper left). When performing *MRI*, the technologist and physician should make sure that the suspicious area is actually imaged. In this case it is not possible to evaluate the tumor and its immediate surroundings, although the images do exclude multicentricity in the left breast and/or a second tumor > 5 mm in the right breast.

**Answer for Fig. 5.54, Question 2** (p. 146 f)

**Answer (b) is correct. The tumor originated in the clavicular recess** (see **Fig. 5.61a**, p. 157) of the left breast. It is surrounded by normal breast parenchyma, some of which has already been infiltrated by carcinoma. The pectoral fascia and muscle are not involved. The effect visible in the sonogram (**c**, upper) is caused by pressure from the ultrasound probe on the tumor. The *spot film* in **b** shows absence of pectoral muscle involvement, and the pathologist did not describe invasion of the pectoral fascia or muscle. The history refutes the notion that the tumor is not visible on *MRI* because it contains too much stroma. The tumor is a very cellular neoplasm that contains only scant stroma.

**Note:** Tumors located outside the breast parenchyma in the axillary, clavicular, medial, or inferior recess are not detectable in screening examinations (see **Fig. 4.24 e**, p. 50 and **i–k**, p. 346). Usually they are detected clinically, more or less fortuitously, when the patient finds a palpable nodule. This underscores the importance of *self-examination*. *Ultrasound* is also important and should include scans of the various recesses. The *spot film* in **b** (p. 146) was taken *after* the palpable mass had been found.

**Answer for Fig. 5.55** (p. 148 f)

**Tumors are present in both breasts.** The right breast has two lesions located at **n–O/18–19**, and the tumor in the left breast is located at **S/20** (see also enlarged lymphnode [metastasis!] in the left axilla **p–Q/27**). In retrospect, the tumor in the right breast should have been detected mammographically in 2001, and the tumor in the left breast should have been visible with ultrasound (given a normal tumor doubling time of 212 days). Unfortunately, the *ultrasound* examination in 2001 was forgotten.

## Answer for Fig. 5.56, Question 1 (p. 150)

**Answer (b) is correct. Benign papillomatous nevus cell nevus** (*histologically* identified).

The nevus was an incidental finding. The patient presented for screening mammography with a pathologic process.

## Answer for Fig. 5.56, Question 2 (p. 150)

The tumor (invasive neoplasm) is located in the left breast at **F/22.** The calcifications are located at **h/20–21** (DCIS? adenosis?).

**Histology:** *1.4 cm moderately differentiated invasive ductal carcinoma.* The tumor was excised with clear margins. The remaining parenchyma contained extensive adenosis with microcalcifications. The left sentinel lymph node contained a small metastatic focus > 0.2 mm in diameter (G2). Axillary exploration showed reactive hyperplasia of 12 lymph nodes with no additional metastases. This is striking when we consider that tumor diagnosis was delayed by 5 years (!). The rounded broad density in the right breast in panel **a** at **C–D/18–21** was fibrosis, with no change over the years.

**Fig. 5.56**

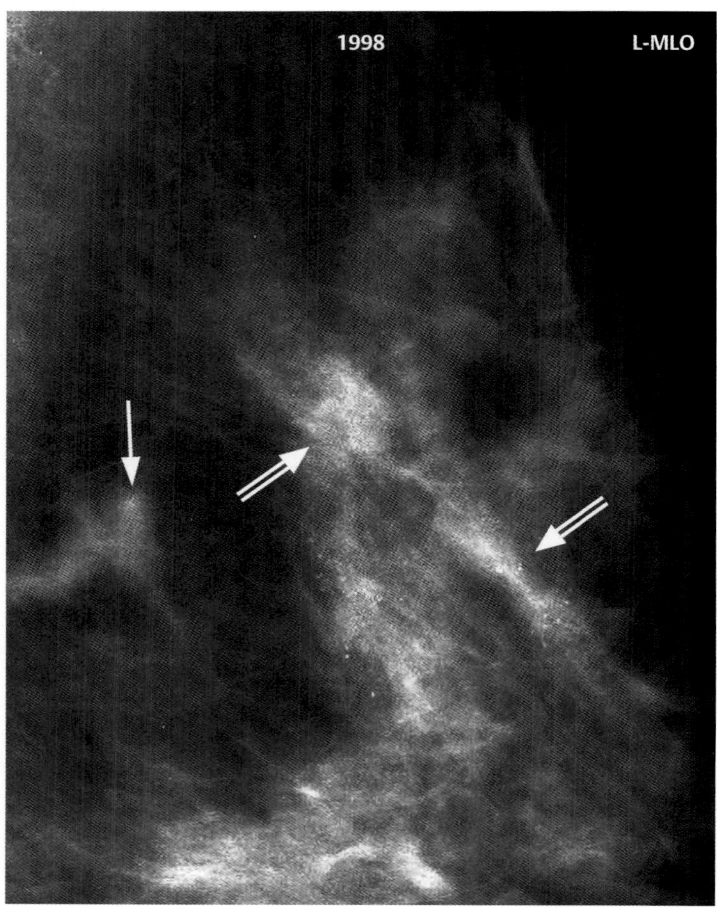


**c** *Oblique mammogram* of the left breast in **1998** (magnified view of upper breast) shows a nonspecific density at the site where the tumor was later detected (arrow). Atypical microcalcifications extend down to the nipple above (double arrows).

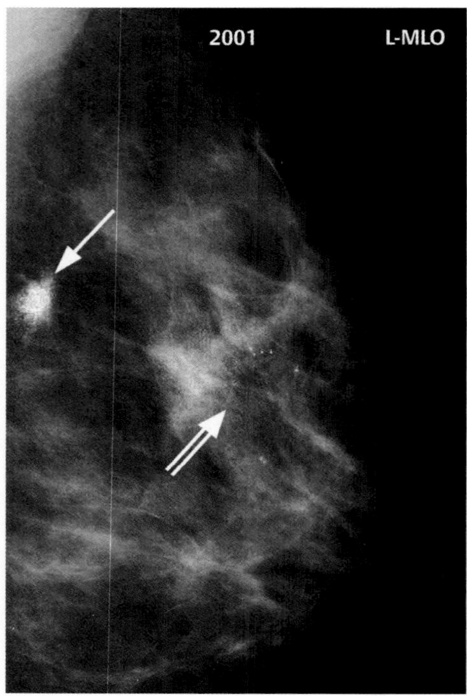


**d** *Oblique mammogram* of the left breast in **2001** (magnified view) shows a tumor mass of irregular density (arrow) associated with increased microcalcifications (double arrow).

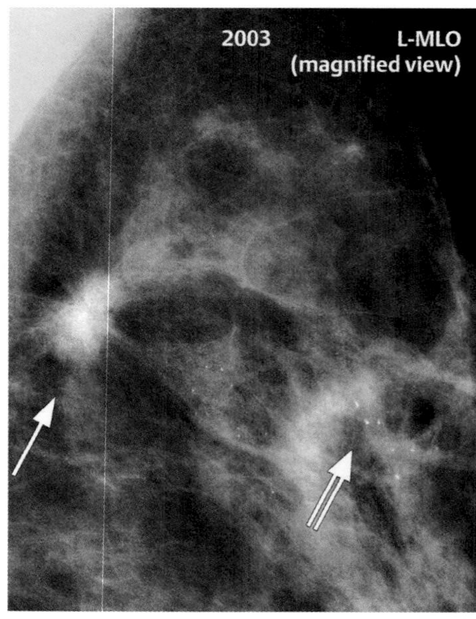


**e** *Oblique mammogram* of the left breast in **2003** shows a prepectoral 1.5 cm stellate tumor (now palpable) (arrow). The calcifications between the tumor and nipple have increased (double arrow). The tumor could not be seen in the craniocaudal view until 2003 due to positioning errors but still should have been detected in 2001.

**Fig. 5.57**

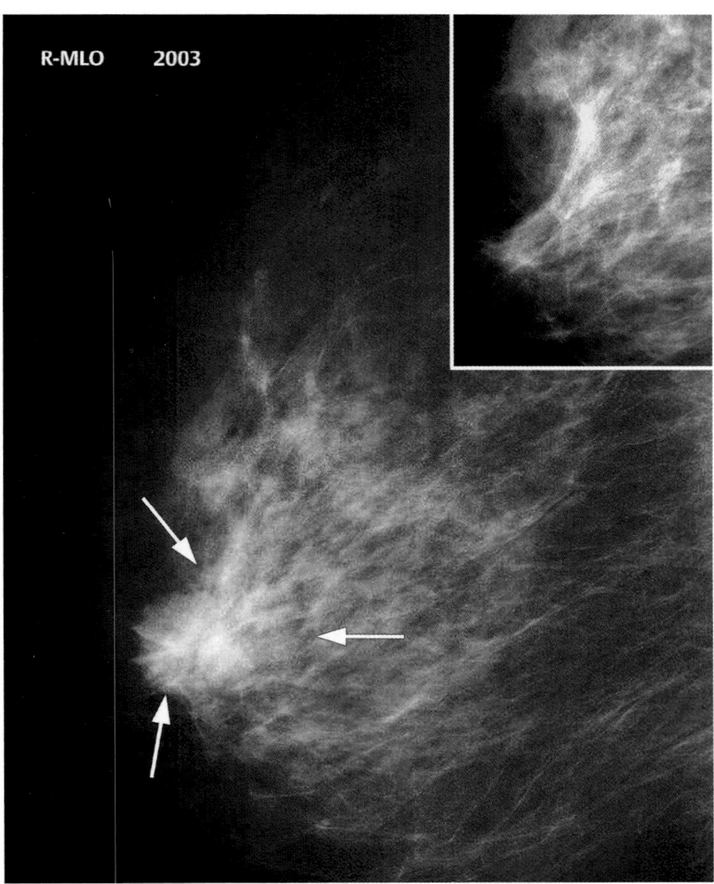


**b** *Oblique mammogram* of the right breast in June, **2003** shows a lobulated retroareolar tumor with spiculations radiating toward the nipple (arrows). (Magnified view at upper right compares the right retroareolar area in **2001** with the new tumor mass.)

**c** *Sonogram* (7.5 MHz) of the right breast in 2003 shows a 1.6 cm × 1.7 cm tumor with mixed scalloped and spiculated margins. The discrepancy between actual tumor size (2.5 cm) and sonographic size (1.5 cm) results from the echogenic halo (bright zone) surrounding the tumor (arrows).

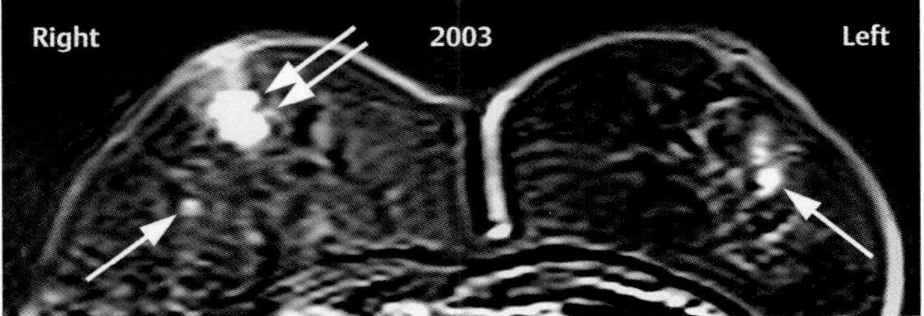


**d** *MR subtraction image* shows scalloped gadolinium enhancement radiating into the retroareolar region (double arrow). A small satellite lesion is visible behind the main tumor (arrow), and a small enhancing focus is visible in the left breast (arrow) (the left breast did not undergo treatment, only follow-up; no tumor at that site as of 2009).

## Answer for Fig. 5.57 (p. 151)

The tumor is located at **k/18**. The ductal markings are noticeably more dense in the parenchyma behind the tumor than they are in the left breast.

Two years later, a 2.5 cm spiculated tumor developed in the right breast (**b, c**). It shows intense gadolinium enhancement on MRI (**d**) and typical nipple retraction (**e**). Extensive infiltration of the ducts was already present 2 years earlier (right breast at **K–N/18–23**, denser than in the left breast), although a circumscribed tumor nodule was not visible on mammograms. Ultrasound (ACR 2) was not performed in 2001 because the breast appeared sufficiently radiolucent. The nodule and infiltrated ducts may already have been visible sonographically at that time (given a normal doubling time of 212 days) and may have shown ductal enhancement on postgadolinium MRI (see **Figs. 4.27 k**, p. 349, and **Fig. 4.29 f**, p. 56). The left breast shows no abnormalities after 5 years (2008) despite nonspecific gadolinium enhancement in MRI.

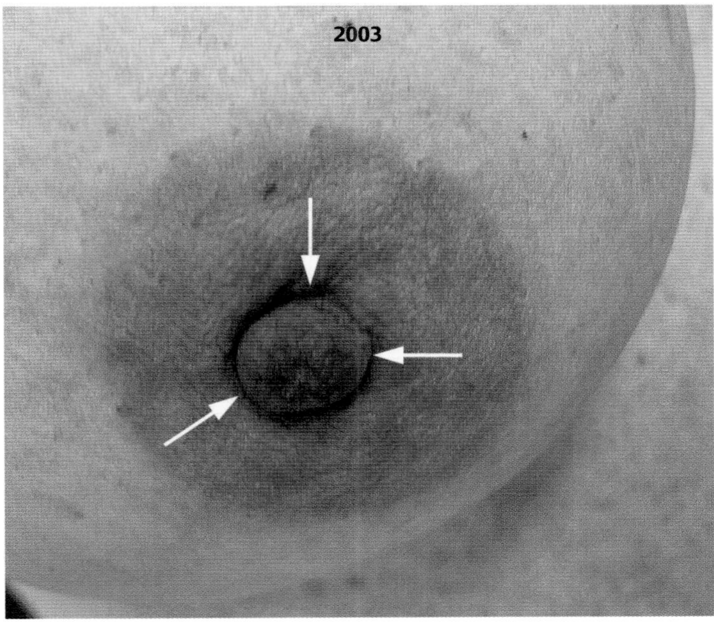


**e** *Clinical inspection* of the right breast shows malignant-type nipple retraction with a crescent-shaped depression at the nipple–areola junction (arrows).

**Answer for Fig. 5.58** (p. 152)

The tumor is located in the left breast at **H–h/22–23** (calcifications) and **i/19–21** (nodule).

**Note:** The invasive retroareolar tumor and the peripheral intraductal component (**h/24**) were already present one year earlier (**a**) but were not detected by *mammography* or *ultrasound. MRI* was withheld at that time because there was no urgent indication to justify the cost.

**Lesson:** Little things can have a big impact: The delay in diagnosis, while only one year, had significant health consequences for this elderly woman. The radical axillary dissection (without sentinel node biopsy) caused the arm edema that continues to be her principal complaint (**h**). The costs for lymph drainage therapy in this patient have greatly exceeded what it would have cost to do an MRI in 1997.

**Fig. 5.58**

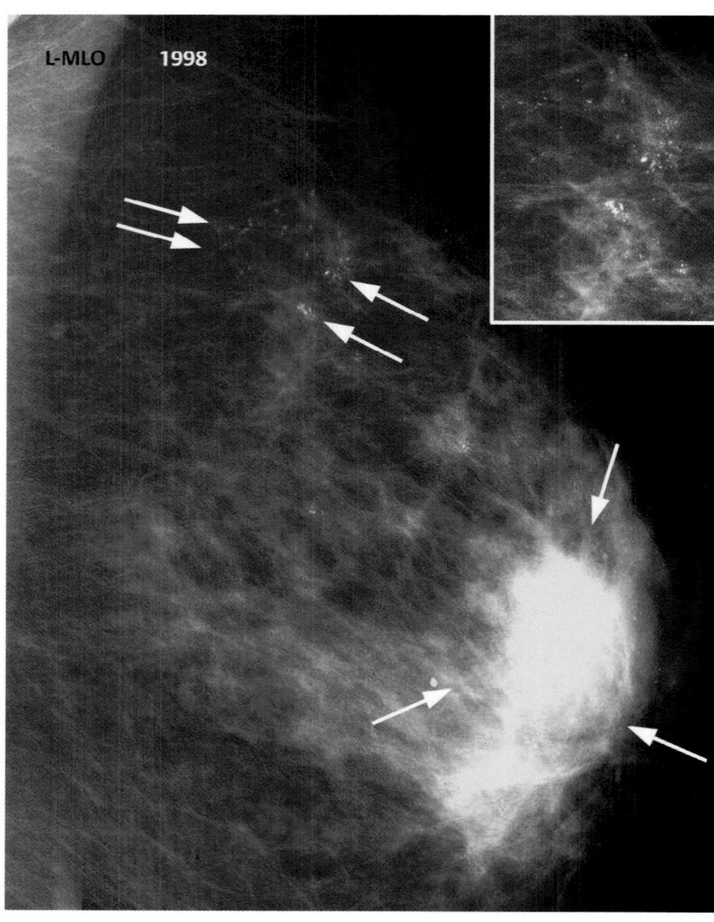


**b** *Oblique mammogram* of the left breast in October, **1998** shows a large retroareolar tumor and microcalcifications in the upper quadrants (double arrows) that show marked progression relative to 1997 (see magnified view at upper right and compare with upper right inset in **a**, p. 152) (arrows).
*Histology: multifocal, poorly differentiated invasive ductal carcinoma* with mucinous elements and an extensive intraductal component (EIC), appearing mammographically at **H/24**. The largest tumor nodule is retroareolar. The mastectomy specimen contained remnants of invasive ductal carcinoma and also DCIS. Twenty-five axillary lymph nodes were removed and all were negative.

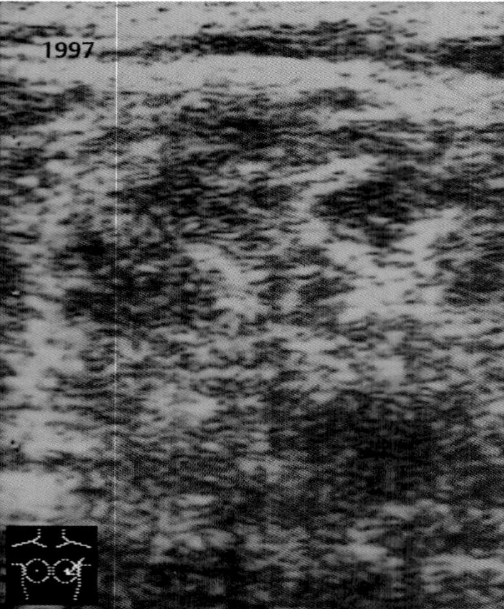


**c** *Sonogram* (5 MHz) of the left breast in November, 1997 shows a nonspecific mottled echo pattern. MRI was recommended (but not performed!). By current standards of practice (2008), this region would be investigated by FNA, CNB, or vacuum biopsy (s. interventional procedures, p. 230).

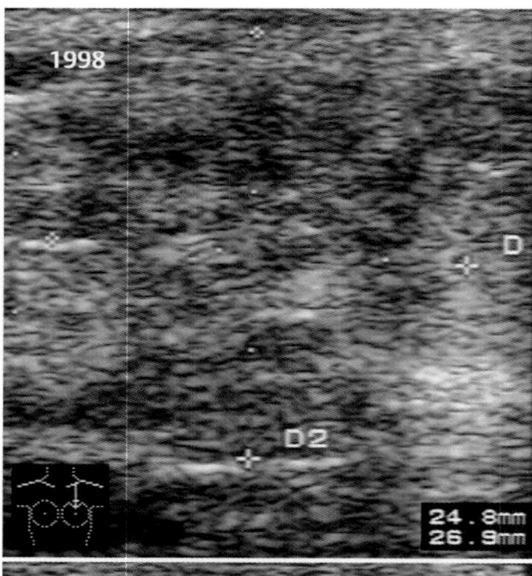


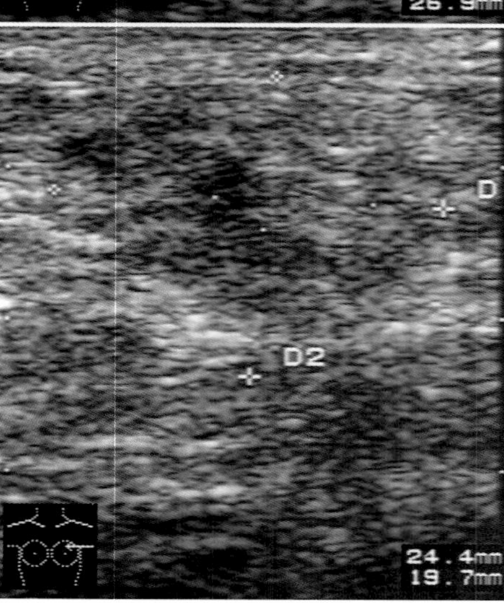


**d** *Sonogram* (7.5 MHz) of the left breast in October, 1998 shows a 2.6 cm × 2.4 cm × 1.9 cm hypoechoic area (see marker) with scalloped margins and a posterior acoustic shadow. Bright internal echoes in a "salt and pepper" pattern are visible in and around the tumor (lymphedema) (see **Fig. 5.147 d**, p. 288). The lymphedema is most pronounced in the periareolar region of the left breast in **f**.

Fig. 5.58 *(continued)*

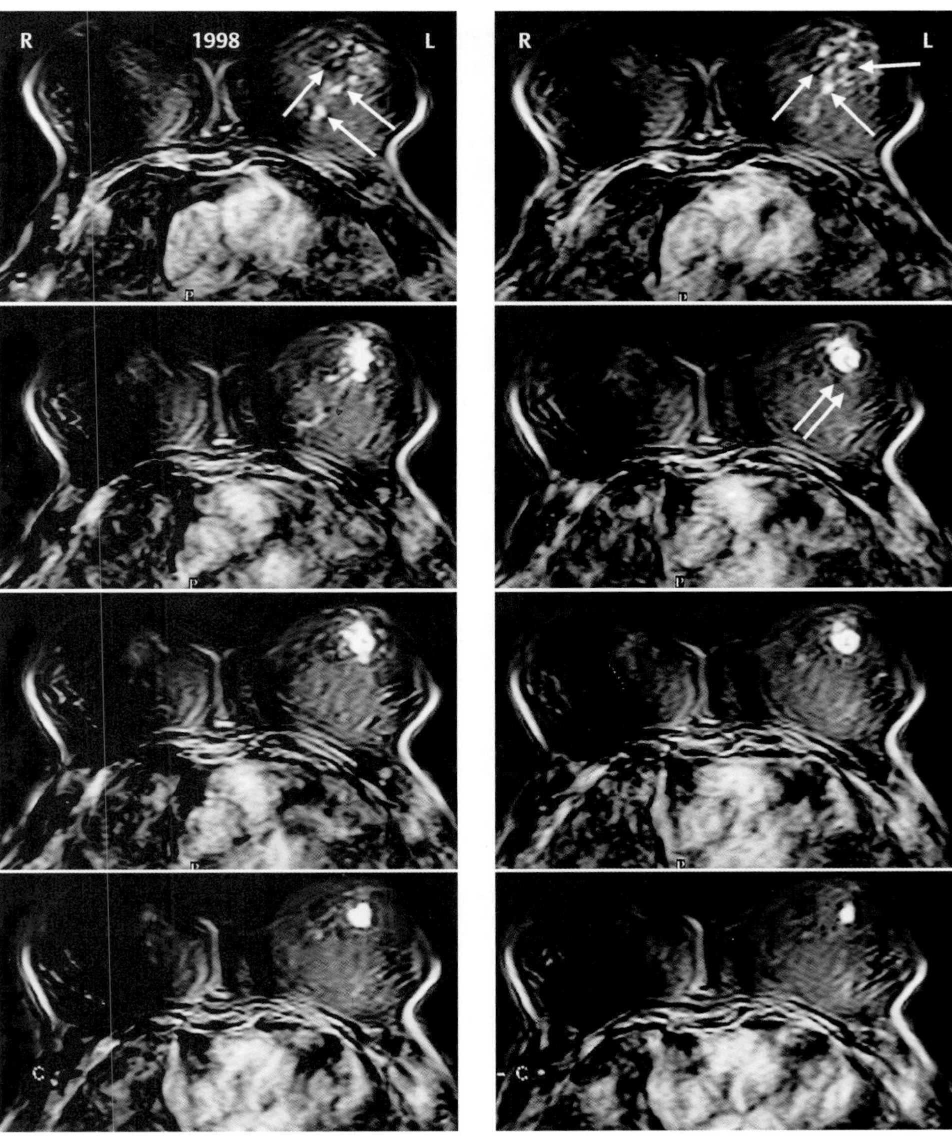


**e** *MR subtraction* images in 1998. The intraductal component (EIC) is clearly visible in the upper images (arrows). It extends into the retroareolar region and is in contact with the large retroareolar mass, which measures 3 cm × 4 cm × 4 cm (double arrow).

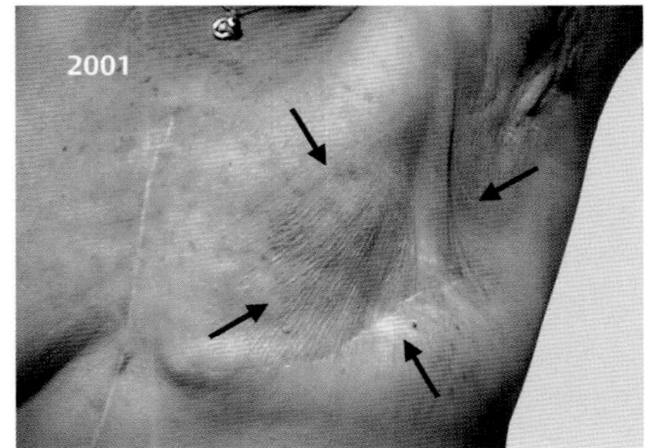


**g** *Clinical appearance* in 2001 of the left chest wall and axilla after modified mastectomy and axillary dissection. *Excerpt from the 1998 medical report:* "The patient has had a normal postoperative course. There is still slight limitation of shoulder motion, for which physical therapy is recommended. The patient was discharged in good condition." The cosmetic results at 3 years are poor. Cutaneous atrophy is noted (arrows). The sternal scar is from a bypass operation.

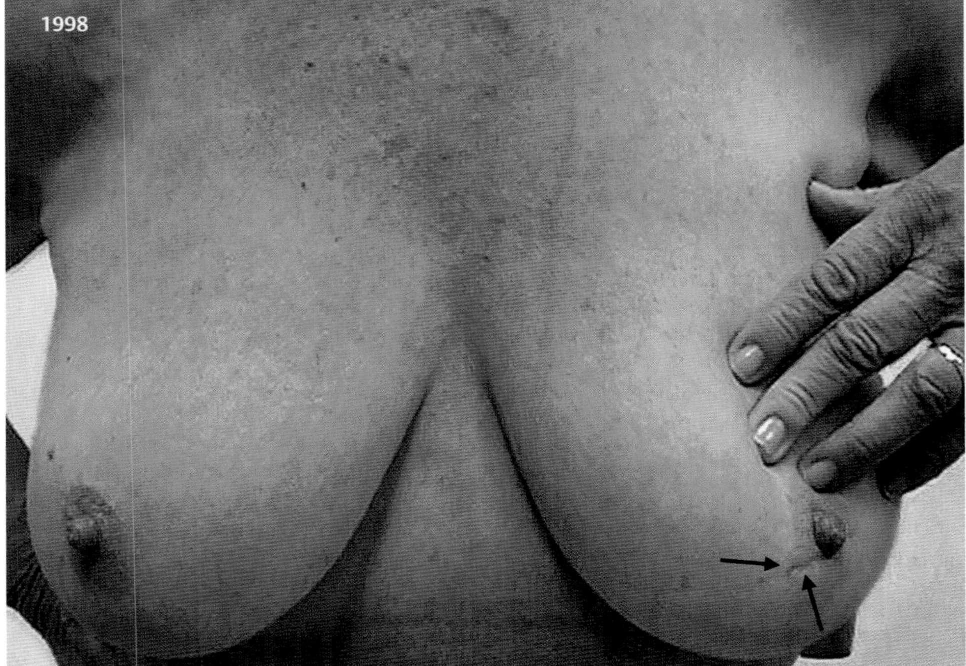


**f** *Physical examination* in **1998** shows diffuse firmness in the upper portion of the left breast with no nipple retraction or circumscribed nodularity. There is edematous swelling of the left areola (arrows).

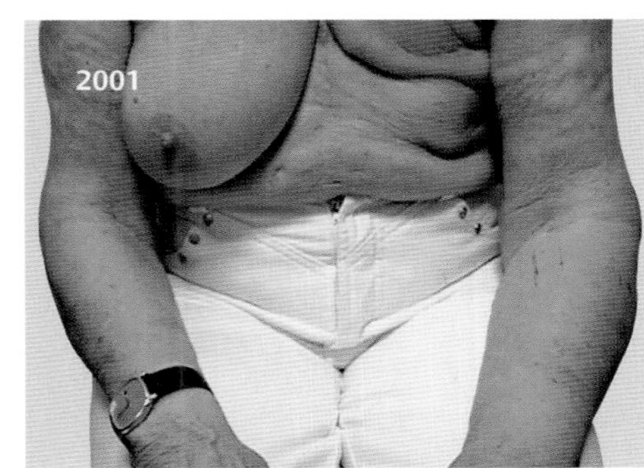


**h** *Clinical appearance* in 2001, 3 years after mastectomy and axillary lymphadenectomy (removing 28 uninvolved axillary nodes). Extensive arm edema is present on the left side. If sentinel node biopsy (see p. 307) had been performed, the patient could have been spared this complication.

## Answer for Fig. 5.59 (p. 153)

The tumor is located in the right breast at **L/22**. It was not detectable on conventional mammograms in 1993.

*Physical examination, mammography*, and *ultrasound* did not detect a tumor when the patient was examined previously in 1991. Two years later the patient was suddenly found to have diffuse firmness of the right breast with extensive malignant calcifications (**d**). The tumor grew at an explosive rate. The diagrams from the *physical examination* (**f–i**) confirm that "something was wrong" in both breasts between 1989 to 1993, especially in the left breast.

**Lesson:** It is very rare for tumors to grow this swiftly (volume doubling time (see p. 20) approximately 50 days; weakened host defenses?). Tumors of this kind are almost never detected at an early stage, especially without benefit of digital mammography (**e**). Diagnosis is even more difficult when clinical changes in the healthy breast distract attention from the affected breast. The patient died 2 years later with disseminated disease.

**Fig. 5.59**

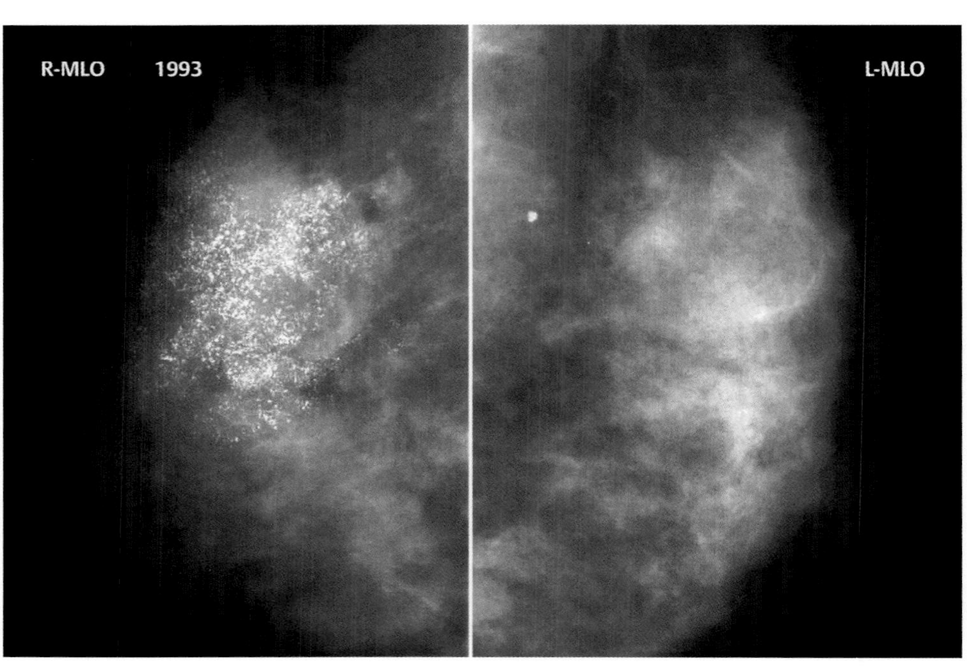


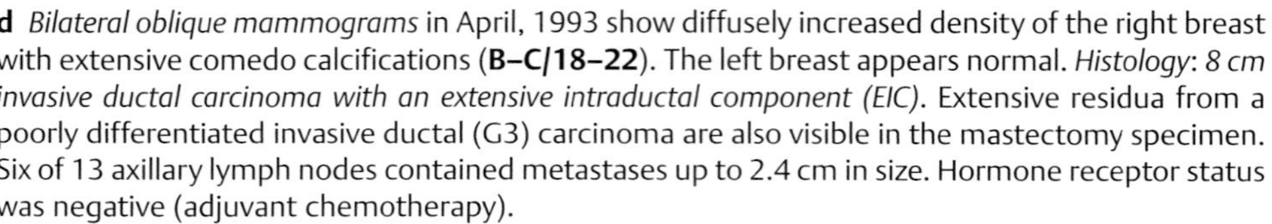

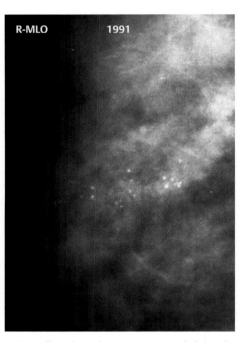

**d** *Bilateral oblique mammograms* in April, 1993 show diffusely increased density of the right breast with extensive comedo calcifications (**B–C/18–22**). The left breast appears normal. *Histology: 8 cm invasive ductal carcinoma with an extensive intraductal component (EIC).* Extensive residua from a poorly differentiated invasive ductal (G3) carcinoma are also visible in the mastectomy specimen. Six of 13 axillary lymph nodes contained metastases up to 2.4 cm in size. Hormone receptor status was negative (adjuvant chemotherapy).

**e** *Digitally enlarged mammogram* of the right breast in 1991. *Secondary digitization* of the images with window leveling revealed initial calcifications in the supra-areolar region (**L/22** in **a**, p. 153) (the ability to manipulate contrast and density is a major advantage of digital mammography over conventional mammography).

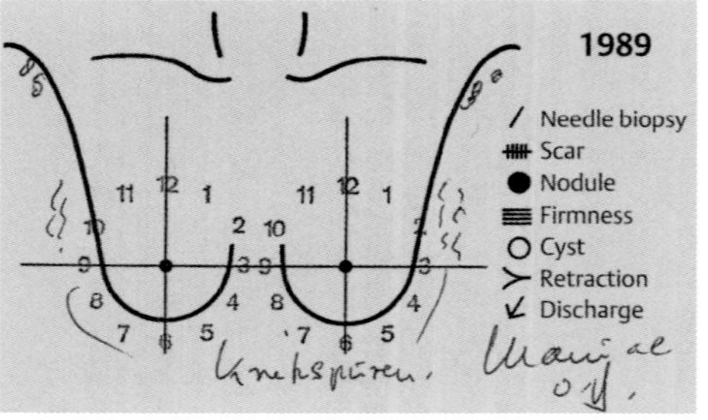


**f** *Breast diagram* from an examination in September, 1989 records enlarged axillary lymph nodes and bilateral scratch marks on the lateral chest wall (chronic pruritus?).

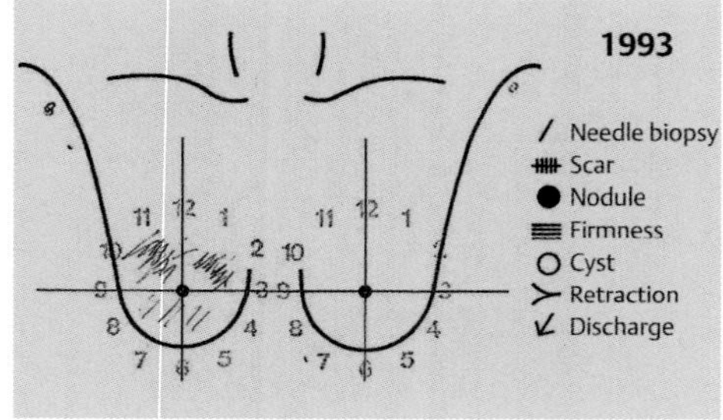


**h** *Breast diagram* from April, 1993 records bilateral enlargement of axillary lymph nodes and diffuse firmness in the right breast.

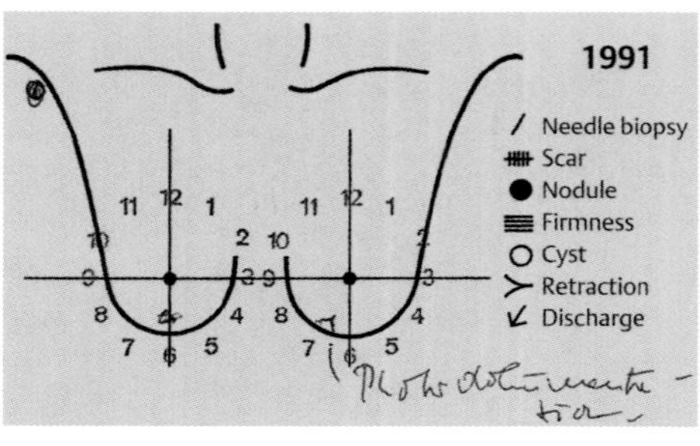


**g** *Breast diagram* from July, 1991 documents slight skin retraction on the lower inner quadrant of the left breast (**c**, p. 153) and a small nodule in the lower portion of the right breast at the 6-o'clock position. The axillary lymph nodes are enlarged.

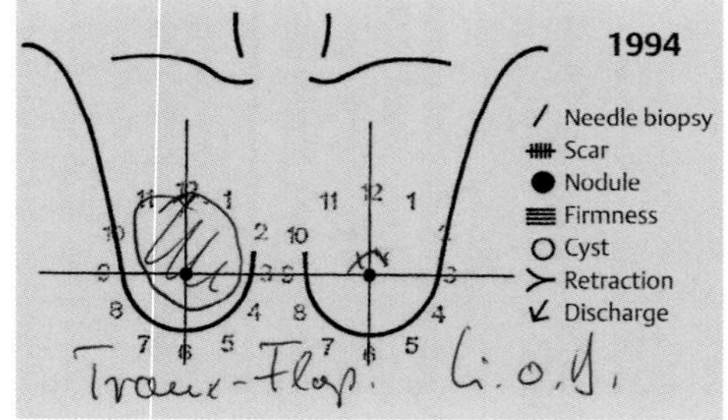


**i** *Breast diagram* from April, 1994 following TRAM flap reconstruction of the right breast and mirror-image biopsy of the left breast documents normal scarring and histology. The left breast is normal.

**Answer for Fig. 5.84, Question 1** (p. 194 ff)

**Patient A: Chronic lymphocytic leukemia. Patient B: metastases. Patient C: Normal axillary lymph node. Patient D: Sarcoidosis.**

**Patient A:** *Chronic lymphocytic leukemia.* The lymph nodes in both axillae were still small when the patient was previously examined in 2001. A small nodule that was barely visible in the right breast in 2001 has enlarged; it is one of the lymph nodes involved by leukemia (see also **H/26–27**). The diagnosis was already known 2 years earlier and cannot be based purely on the mammographically suspicious lymph node. The lymph node definitely has an abnormal echo structure (**n**), and this would have required further investigation if the disease had not already been known. After chemotherapy, the lymphnode changes regress completely (**o**).

**Patient B:** Axillary lymph node *metastases from breast cancer.* Nodal metastases have developed from a neoplasm in the right breast. Despite retroareolar surgery two years earlier, FNB now confirms a locally advanced tumor in that area (small hematoma above the right areola). Thus, the tumor was either missed or left alone at surgery. The patient had 24 positive axillary lymph nodes. Nipple retraction on the right side is caused by the neoplasm and not by previous surgery (see **Fig. 5.57e**, p. 367) (same patient as **Fig. 5.57**, p. 151).

**Patient C:** *Normal axillary lymph node.* Ultrasound shows the typical appearance of normal lymph nodes, but only histologic examination can exclude or confirm micrometastases in cases of malignancy.

**Patient D:** *Sarcoidosis.* The lymph nodes are greatly enlarged and appear to show fatty infiltration.

*Histology: mostly fatty tissue.* The specimen includes a 0.5 cm lymph node fragment in which the lymphatic tissue is permeated by confluent epithelioid cell granulomas. The latter contain numerous multinucleated *Langerhans giant cells.* There is no evidence of caseating necrosis (tuberculosis), atypical cells, or malignancy. The findings are consistent with sarcoidosis. The right axillary lymph nodes show pathologic changes, while the left axilla is clinically and sonographically normal

**Answer for Fig. 5.84, Question 2** (p. 194 ff)

**Answer (b) is correct. Lipoma.** Based on its sonographic and cytologic (not shown) features, the nodule in the elbow is not sarcoidosis but a harmless lipoma that has been present for years. It has the same sonographic appearance as the fatty infiltration of axillary lymph nodes, however.

**Answer for Fig. 5.85** (p. 197)

**Answer (a) is correct. The arm edema is caused by obstruction of venous (and lymphatic?) drainage.** *Ultrasound* clearly demonstrates the dilated venous vessels in the right axilla and shows progressive hourglass-shaped narrowing (**c, K/13–14**). Findings of this kind should be investigated by contrast venography and/or Doppler ultrasound to assess the need for stent implantation. Obstruction of venous drainage is further supported by increased venous markings located in the right shoulder region (**a**) and projected over the pectoral muscle in the right oblique mammogram (**b, P–p/23–26**).

**Fig. 5.84 Lymph node regression under chemotherapy.** Images **n** and **o** illustrate the principle that lymph nodes may regain their normal shape and size after the resolution of systemic diseases like patient A.

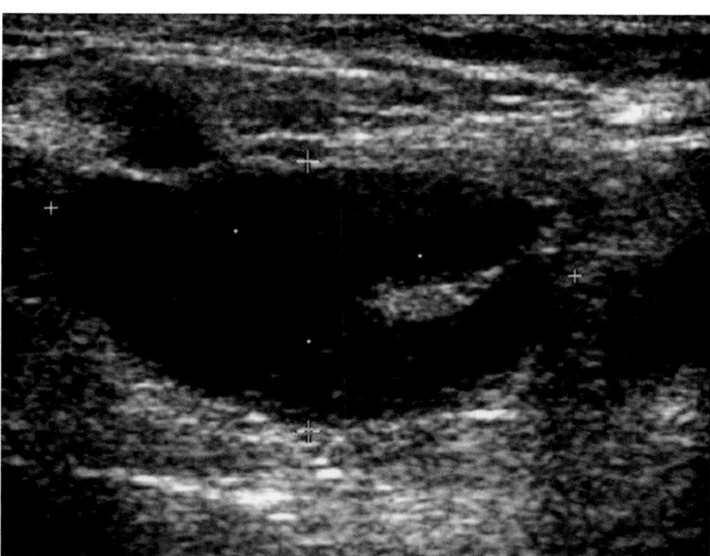

**n** *Sonogram* of the right axilla *before treatment* for *chronic lymphocytic leukemia* shows a greatly enlarged lymph node with a compressed fatty hilum.

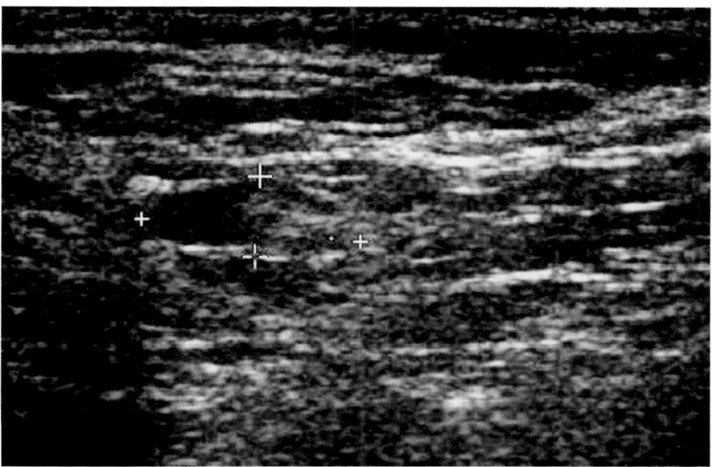

**o** *Sonogram* of the right axilla *after chemotherapy* shows regression of all lymphadenopathy. The lymph nodes have regained a normal size and structure (see marker).

**Lesson:** Breast-conserving treatment is usually followed by a search for axillary lymph node metastases. *Vascular status* is usually disregarded but may have significant consequences in affected women, although collateral vessels can compensate for venous stenosis. Stent insertion was withheld in this case because *Doppler ultrasound* did not detect a functionally active stenosis.

**Answer for Fig. 5.86** (p. 198)

**Answer (b) is correct. Neurinoma.** This patient has an apparent vascular aneurysm. Cytologic and ultrasound findings and the reported pulsations are consistent with an aneurysm and do not support *medullary carcinoma* or a *lymph node.* A neuroma was found at operation, however.

## Answer for Fig. 5.87 (p. 199)

**Answer (a) is correct. Lymph node metastasis.** Two distinct zones are visible in the lymph node at ultrasound: a hypoechoic (darker) zone that is consistent with tumor tissue and a hyperechoic zone (panel **b K–l/16**) representing the former fatty lymph node hilum. *CNB* histology showed that the lymph node was permeated by clusters of tumor cells.

*Lipomatosis* of the lymph node would cause it to become more isoechoic to surrounding fat (see **Fig. 5.84 m**, p. 196). Although a *fibroadenoma* would not be unusual in this area (arising in heterotopic breast parenchyma), it is excluded by ultrasound and cytologic findings.

**Lesson:** Lymph drains from the periphery of the node (cortical follicle) to the hilum and on to the next lymph nodes. Thus, *lymph node metastases occur chiefly in the periphery and should be sought there.* Cystic lymph node changes may be found in association with malignant lymphoma, lymphangioma, HIV-associated angiomatosis, and Kaposi sarcoma (see **Fig. 5.180**, p. 329) (Hollerweger et al. 2008).

## Answer for Fig. 5.88 (p. 200)

**Answer (c) is correct. Invasive ductal carcinoma with EIC.** *CNB* at three different sites yielded DCIS. During *surgery*, portions of an invasive tumor with an EIC were found along with multiple axillary lymph node metastases. The enlarged axillary nodes seen in the *mammogram* (**e/25–26**) do not support a diagnosis of DCIS alone but suggest an invasive tumor with an EIC and lymph node involvement.

**Lesson:** Ultrasound is the simplest and most economical way to evaluate the lymphatic pathways and detect pathologic changes that can be further investigated by FNA and, in special situations, by CNB.

## Answer for Fig. 5.90, Question 1 (p. 204)

**Answer (c) is correct. The radiographic density** of the breasts (especially behind the right nipple) requires *physical examination* (**d**) and *ultrasound* (**f**). Also *MRI* (**g**), and *FNB* (**e**) were performed in this patient.

**Fig. 5.90**

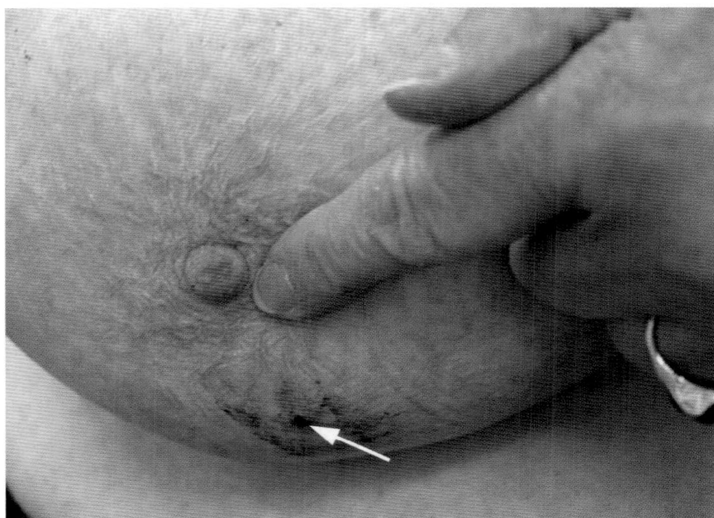

**d** *Physical examination* shows firmness on the right medial side of the areola (at the 3-o'clock position). The skin-perforation of CNB is marked with an arrow.

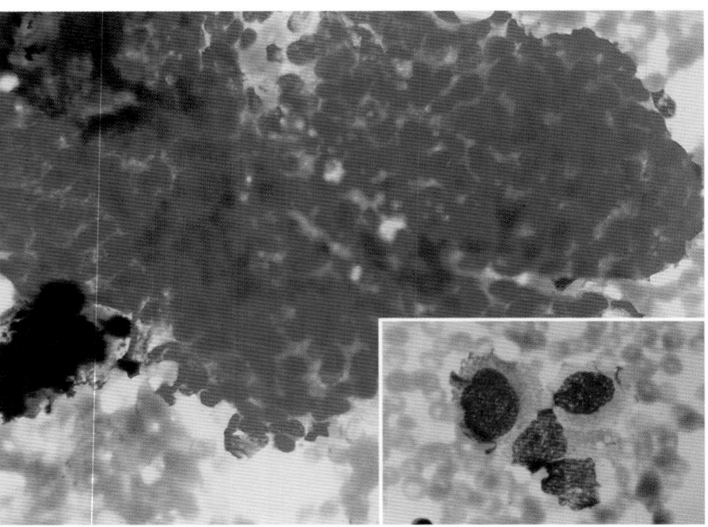

**e** *CC-cytology* (a CNB with simultaneous cytologic examination from a contact-smear (see p. 231) shows a cluster of numerous lobular cells with nuclear crowding (magnification 100×). *Inset* shows a group of four tumor cells with an altered nuclear-cytoplasmic ratio and enlarged, malignant hyperchromatic nuclei with a jagged nuclear membrane and loose premitotic chromatin composed of small fibrils (magnification 1000 ×).

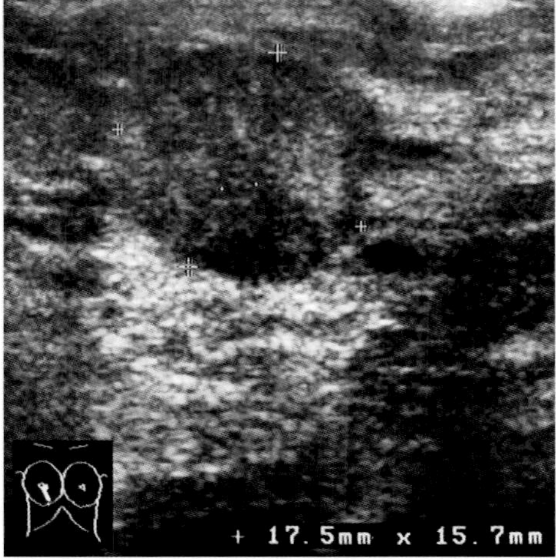


**f** *Sonogram* shows a hyperechoic nodule with smooth margins and posterior acoustic enhancement (see marker).

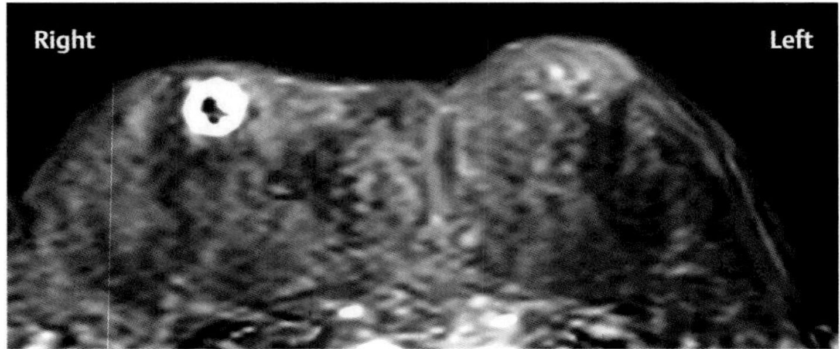


**g** *MRI* shows a smooth, intensely enhancing ringlinke nodule with central necrosis (**G–g/6**) (see **Fig. 4.34 b**, p. 64, and **Fig. 4.41 b**, p. 70).

### Answer for Fig. 5.90, Question 2 (p. 204)

**Answer (a) is correct. Invasive lobular carcinoma** of the right breast (G2), which was managed by *breast-conserving therapy* with removal of the nipple.

A *papilloma* or *fibroadenoma* seldom make an unsharp shadow in mammography.

**Note:** The skilled diagnostician did, of course, detect the nodule by mammography (**B/20–21** oblique, **a–B,10–12** cc).

**Lesson:** In *every* breast with a radiographic density of ACR 3 or higher (see p. 98), ultrasound must be performed to exclude a neoplasm.

*This would be necessary in about 60% of all cases, as indicated by the ACR distribution that has been documented by the author and his colleagues:* ***ACR 1 = 5%, ACR 2 = 35%, ACR 3 = 53%, ACR 4 = 7%****. At least sixty percent of all women* should *be screened by ultrasound in addition to mammography. This would detect 12% of carcinomas rather than 8% (Berg et al. 2008). The addition of breast ultrasound has a false-positive rate of approximately 5% (Buchberger 2005).*

### Answer for Fig. 5.91, Question 1 (p. 205 ff)

**Patient A: Answer (a) is correct. The nodule is located in the lower inner quadrant of the left breast** (at approximately **N/17** oblique, **s/17–18** cc).

The nodule cannot be accurately assessed on *mammograms*, and *ultrasound* should always be added in breasts with a lump. The palpable nodule could have been investigated at once by *ultrasound-guided FNA*. As it was, the lesion was reexamined 3 months later and *MRI* was performed—an unnecessary and costly detour that risked delaying the diagnosis. A palpable nodule does not require further imaging evaluation. *FNA* cytology or *CNB* can readily determine whether the lesion is malignant or benign.

### Answer for Fig. 5.91, Question 2 (p. 205 ff)

**Patient B: Answer (c) is correct.** The nodule is located in the left breast at the coordinates **e/21** (oblique) and **e/9** (cc). The *MR image* was deliberately reversed right-to-left and the sonogram is shown without markers. In all honesty, would you not have been inclined to tell the patient that she was healthy on the basis of only her mammograms?

**Lesson**: Especially in the case of younger patients with high risk for developing breast cancer, mammographic screening alone is insufficient for the confident exclusion of a tumor.

### Answer for Fig. 5.91, Question 3 (p. 205 ff)

**Patient A:** In reality *fibroadenoma* time–density curve seems to be *invasive carcinoma.*

**Patient B:** In reality *invasive carcinoma* time–density curve seems to be *fibroadenoma.*

**Patient C:** In reality *DCIS* time–density curve seems to be *mastopthy.*

**Note:** Time–density curves on MRI are on one hand important, on the other hand weak and not the only diagnostic parameter for the differential diagnosis of atypical clinical, mammographic, and sonographic findings. Relying only on the curves would result in frequent misdiagnoses. Blind trust is not enough.

The fact that *DCIS* (case C) was detected as a palpable nodule with skin retraction is not unusual. A preinvasive lesion is indistinguishable from an *invasive* tumor by its cytologic and ultrasound features. On mammogram as well, ill-defined margins (**I**) are not necessarily a sign of invasiveness. The DCIS occurred without calcifications. *Fibroadenomas* do not cause skin retraction.

## Answer for Fig. 5.92 (p. 208 f)

**Answer (c) is correct. Lobular neoplasm** (G3) and 8 of 24 lymph nodes are involved. The tumor was removed with clear margins only at reexcision. Its total diameter was 2.1 cm. The *sonogram* is definitely abnormal, as is the cell cluster retrieved by *FNA*. The *mammogram* is not completely normal. The visible density on the left side appears benign, which is not consistent with histologic findings (**e**).

The *axillary lymph nodes* are an important mammographic indicator of malignancy. The two lower lymph nodes (panel **c N/25**) have definitely become larger and more dense relative to the previous examination. They were metastatically involved.

The continual size increase and cytologic findings do not support a diagnosis of *fibroma*, while the ultrasound findings of ill-defined margins and a slightly echogenic rim would not be consistent with *fibroadenoma*. As of 2008 the patient was still free of disease.

**Lesson:** It is noteworthy that *MRI* did not show gadolinium enhancement despite the G3 tumor classification, and extensive axillary involvement. Thus, a normal MRI does not prove that a sonographically suspicious lesion is benign.

## Answer for Fig. 5.93 (p. 210)

**Answer (b) is correct. The MRI changes are a result of keloids** (**e**). Because the radiologist read the MR images without actually seeing the patient, he was unaware of the keloids. Also, the tumor that he described at the 9-o'clock position in the right breast could not be verified, and so the proposed operation was canceled.

The *mammographic* density (**b, c**) and *sonographic* changes (**d**) were also caused by keloids and scars.

**Lesson:** Every MRM examination should include inspection and palpation of the breast and should be correlated with mammographic and ultrasound findings. If this had been done here, the keloids would have accounted at once for the MRI findings.

Surgery on the right breast in 2000 to remove tissue at the 9-o'clock position in the upper outer quadrant would not have prevented the second tumor that developed 4 years later in the same breast in the inner upper quadrant (**g, h**).

**Fig. 5.93**

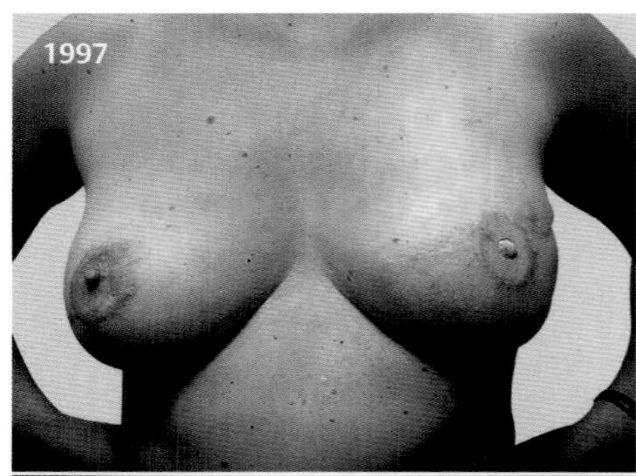


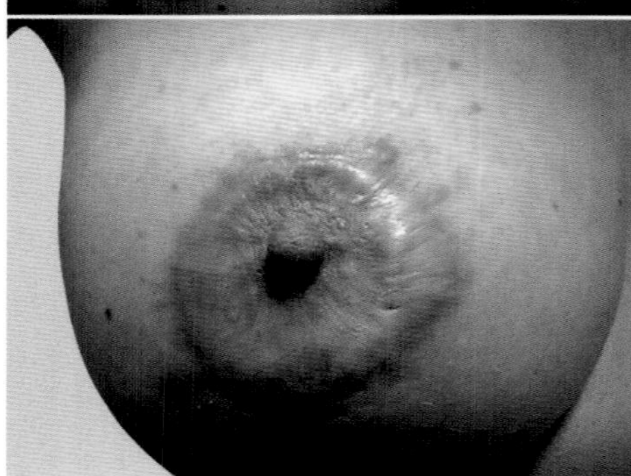

**e** *Clinical appearance. Keloids* are present on both breasts. Mastectomy was done on the left side with silicone implant reconstruction, and massive keloids are visible on the right breast.

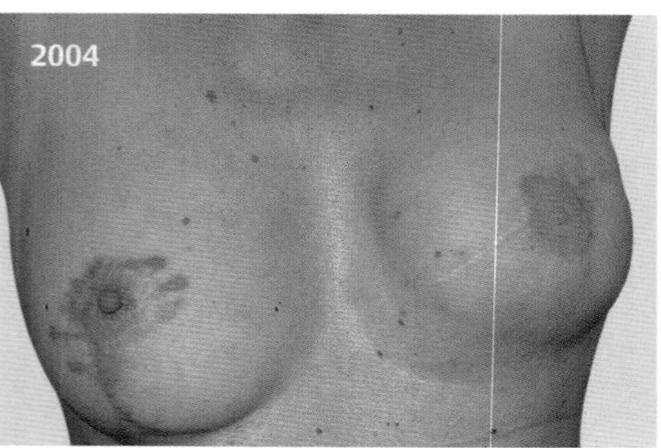


**f** *Clinical appearance 8 years later.* Keloid formation after various forms of treatment (laser) in 2004. Improvement is noted on both sides, but changes are still pronounced on the right side. There are no palpable abnormalities.

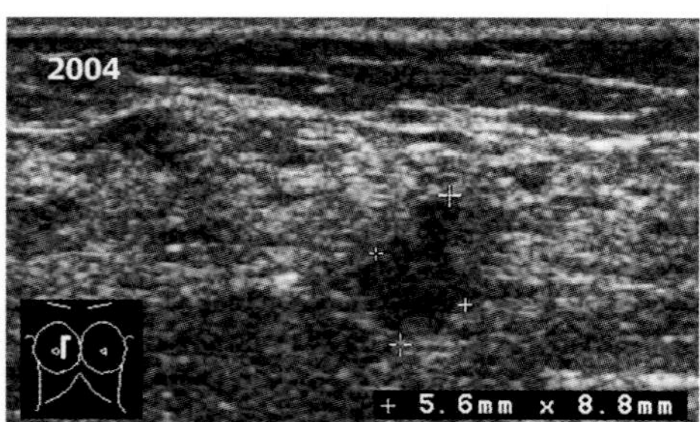


**h** *Sonogram* in *2004* of the medial right breast shows a nonspecific hypoechoic area that is suspicious by its progression.

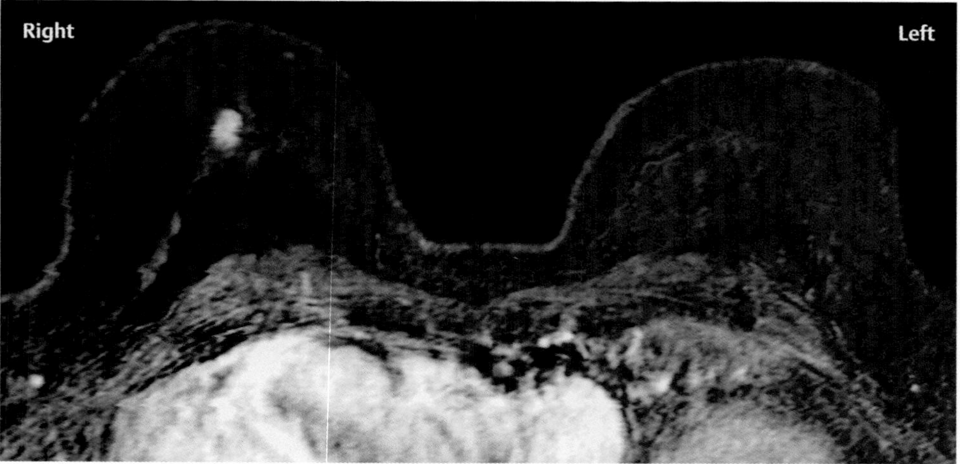


**g** *MRM in 2004* shows atypical focal gadolinium enhancement in the right retroareolar region (*histology:* invasive ductal carcinoma).

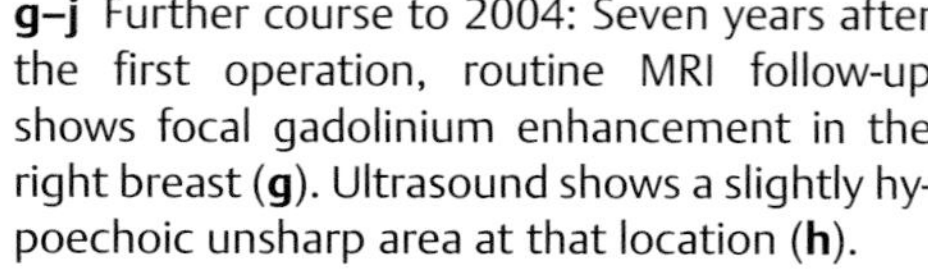

**g–j** Further course to 2004: Seven years after the first operation, routine MRI follow-up shows focal gadolinium enhancement in the right breast (**g**). Ultrasound shows a slightly hypoechoic unsharp area at that location (**h**).

Fig. 5.93 *(continued)*

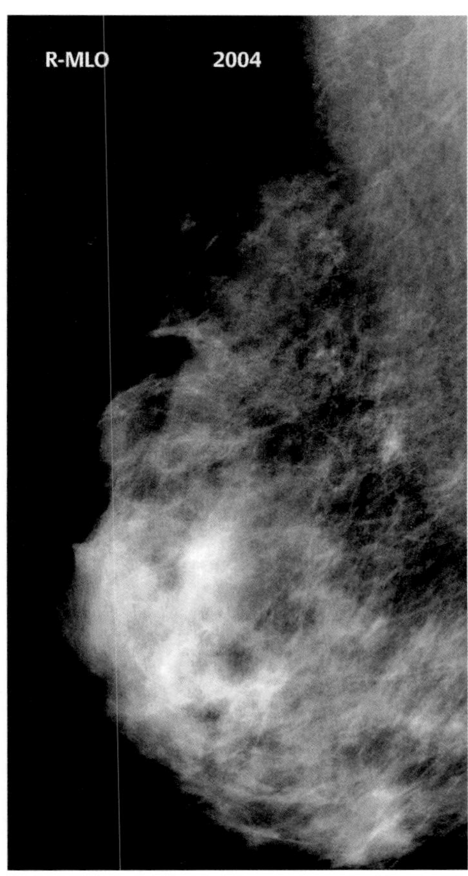


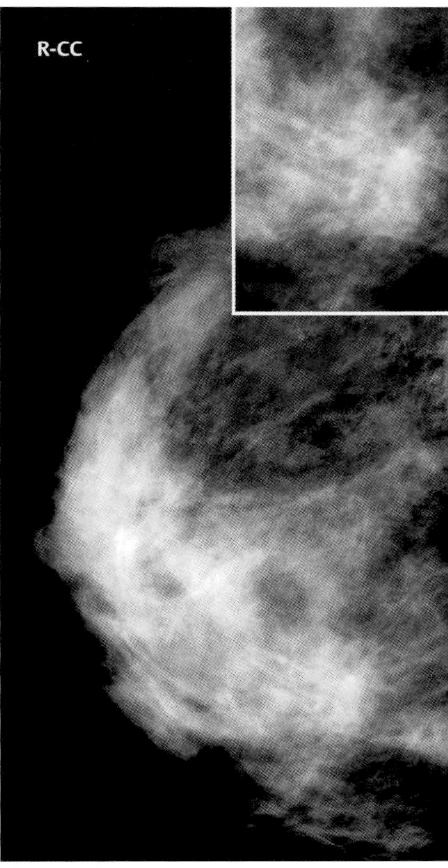


**i** *Oblique mammogram* (digital) 2004 of the right breast after reduction mammoplasty shows pronounced keloid formation and nonspecific opacities in the retroareolar region. No significant changes are noted relative to the previous examination with *analog* mammography (**b**, p. 210).

**j** *Craniocaudal mammogram* (digital) 2004 of the right breast shows retroareolar scarring along with nonspecific opacities. With some imagination, we can perceive a small, focal, slightly spiculated medial density (**P–p/17–19**) (see inset) that was not present in the prior examination with *analog* mammography (**c**, p. 210). This site coincides with the focus seen at ultrasound (**h**).

*Histology: 1 cm × 0.6 cm × 0.6 cm invasive ductal carcinoma*. Further course is unknown.

**Answer for Fig. 5.94** (p. 211)

**Answer (b) is correct. The patient has mastitis.** Several *CNBs* were taken from this area and showed interstitial lymphocytic infiltration. The *subacute mastitis* was most likely caused or exacerbated by an inflammatory duct stricture (**g**). The inflammation led to increased blood flow in the right breast, clearly visible on *MRI*. Remarkably, severe clinical complaints were not reported in that region of the breast. The redness cleared completely in 2 weeks without treatment (**f**). *Ultrasound* still shows proliferating TDLUs (**g**), but some improvement is noted relative to the previous examination in May of 2004 (**h**). The microcalcifications were investigated in November, 2004, and DCIS was identified. The DCIS was unrelated to the inflammation.

Fig. 5.94

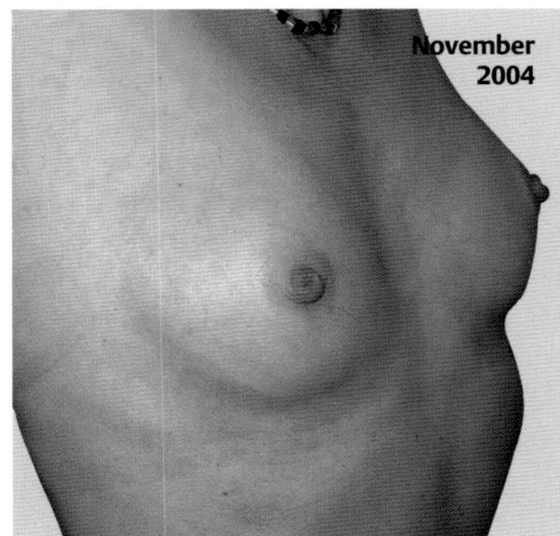


**f** *Clinical inspection* of the right breast in November, 2004. The breast has a normal external appearance.

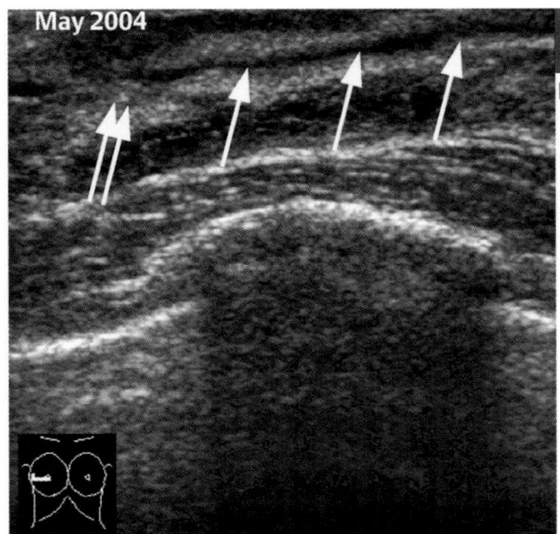


**g** *Sonogram* of the upper outer quadrant of the right breast in May, 2004 shows broadened and confluent linear TDLUs (**n–p/13**) and an enlarged duct (arrows) with a possible stenosis (double arrow) that could be responsible for the spread of inflammation into the axillary recess.

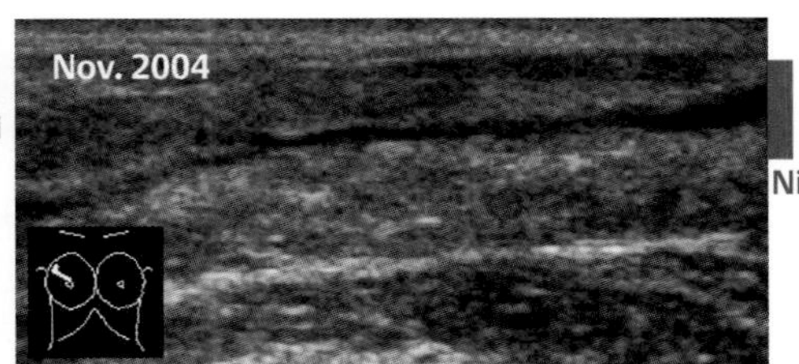


**h** *Sonogram* of the right breast in November, 2004 shows slight regression of lobular proliferation. The duct is still enlarged (**q–T/13–14**) and now shows no sign of stenosis. The DCIS diagnosed at this time (**b**, p. 211) was not visible at ultrasound.

## Answer for Fig. 5.95, Question 1 (p. 214)

**Answer (c) is correct. TRAM flap reconstruction.** The horizontal scar on the upper abdomen (in **a** at **b–C/23**) and the circumscribed density in the inner part of the breast (vascular pedicle) (**h–5**) are from a TRAM flap reconstruction. It is impossible to distinguish mammographically between a latissimus dorsi flap, a TRAM flap, and an autologous fat graft.

**Lesson:** Twenty percent of breast reconstructions are composed of muscle, the rest of fat.

## Answer for Fig. 5.95, Question 2 (p. 214)

**Answer (a) is correct. The local recurrence is in the left breast.** *Mammograms* show a 1 cm, inhomogeneous, ill-defined opacity at that site surrounded by muscle and fat at **H/25–26** (oblique) and at **h/5–6** (cc) inside the muscle/vascular pedicle, which in this case runs transversely through the breast (and forms a central diamond-shaped density in **b** at **H–i/21–24**). The *local recurrence* is visible in both projections.

Only scars from the reduction mammoplasty are visible in the right breast.

**Lesson:** The vascular pedicle in breast reconstructions should not be mistaken for a recurrence (although in this case the local recurrence is projected over it in **c** at **h/6**).

## Answer for Fig. 5.95, Question 3 (p. 214)

**Answer (a) is correct. Yes, the recurrence is located in the upper inner quadrant** (**a**) and causes a visible skin bulge above the scar on the left side near the chest wall (**C/25**). The patient noticed the lump several months earlier.

**Lesson:** Clinical examination with inspection and palpation is important in the follow-up of aesthetic breast reconstructions. MRI may be a useful screening tool after aesthetic breast reconstructions in cases where the healthy breast is radiodense or when it is necessary to differentiate between a scar and local recurrence, but not in this case.

## Answer for Fig. 5.96 (p. 215)

**Answer (b) is correct. Free silicone injections** formerly done by plastic surgeons, mostly in Africa and Indonesia, to tighten the breast. With a *ruptured silicone* implant, the silicone would be less uniformly distributed and portions of the implant would be visible. In this case only globules of silicone gel are visible.

Most of the silicone has gravitated inferolaterally and clumped together, which explains the circumscribed firmness in the lower portion of the right breast.

*Hydatid cysts* of this sort would be unusual. They would appear less dense, and the individual cysts would not be so well-defined.

**Lesson:** Free intramammary silicone injections prevent both the early and late detection of malignant tumors by physical examination, mammography, and ultrasound. It is theoretically possible that MRI could detect the gadolinium enhancement of tumor tissue, but it is unclear how the scar and granulation tissue activated by the silicone globules would respond.

## Answer for Fig. 5.97, Question 1 (p. 216 f)

**Answer (c) is correct. Multifocal tubulolobular carcinoma** that required multiple reexcisions, culminating in mastectomy. The mastectomy specimen did not contain residual tumor. Numerous LCIS lesions and retrograde malignant transformation (see **Figs. 4.11, 4.12**, p. 31) of individual ducts are present in addition to the invasive tumor (pT1c G2 pN0 [0/12] M0).

*Treatment:* EC regimen of adjuvant polychemotherapy and Tamoxifen (20 mg/day) for 5 years. The tumor consists of many small foci distributed diffusely in the breast. Numerous cancer precursors are present but there is no lymph node involvement. This supports the diagnosis of a relatively nonaggressive tubular carcinoma that escaped mammographic and sonographic detection for years. It was ultimately the patient's internist who referred her for the inpatient investigation of palpable abnormalities.

A *medullary carcinoma* would not have gone undetected for 4 years without metastasizing. A *comedo-type DCIS* would have formed calcifications.

## Answer for Fig. 5.97, Question 2 (p. 216 f)

**Answer (c) is correct. TRAM-flap reconstruction.** *MRI* subtraction image shows intense vascularity of the *healthy right breast* extending from the pectoral muscle into the nipple. The *operated left breast* consists mainly of fat tissue with peak gadolinium uptake occurring at the inferior prepectoral pull-through site of the TRAM flap (**s/25–26**). This tissue does not extend to the nipple, which would contraindicate breast-conserving surgery (also contraindicated by the multifocality). Only a TRAM flap procedure would account for these MRM findings. A latissimus dorsi flap would have its vascular pedicle near the axilla.

The *left breast* shows typical *mammographic* lucency and uniformity after fat/muscle implantation compared with the healthy side (**f**). *Ultrasound* of the left breast shows only fatty tissue (**g**), while ultrasound of the healthy *right breast* shows fibrotic breast parenchyma (**h**) without proliferating TDLUs. The cosmetic result is excellent (**i**).

**Lesson:** Mammography is unreliable in a radiodense breast may cause a delay in diagnosis, in this case from 1997 to 2001. This is not the fault of mammography but of the diagnostician, who failed to employ additional procedures and relied entirely on mammograms. Fortunately for the patient, the tumor was a relatively slow-growing and indolent *tubulolobular carcinoma*, which did not metastasize despite the long-delayed diagnosis. The faulty diagnostic workup in this case contrasted with the excellent work of the plastic surgeon. The patient is still free of disease 8 years postoperatively (2009).

Fig. 5.97

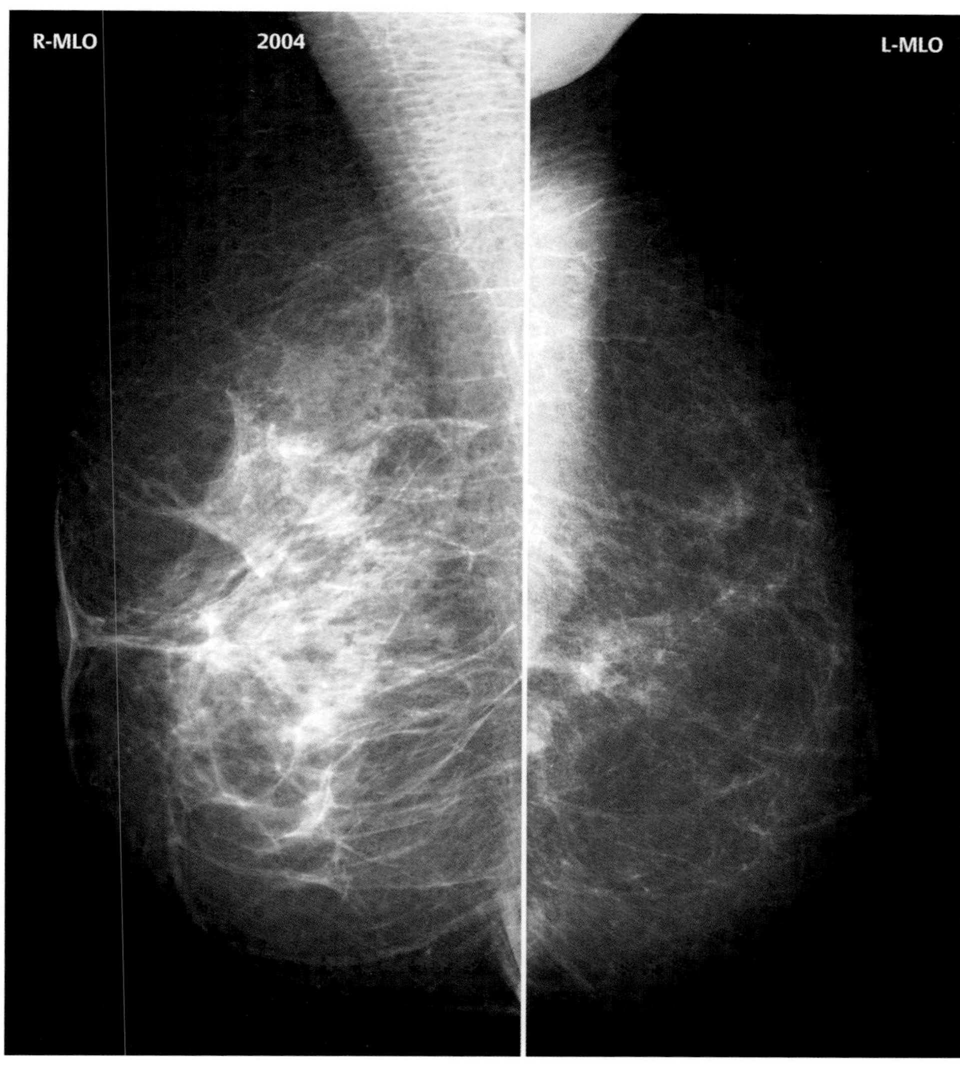


**f** *Bilateral oblique mammograms* in 2004 show a normal-appearing right breast with architectural distortion following excisional biopsy (ACR 3). The left breast shows increased lucency (ACR 1) due to fatty tissue of the TRAM flap–rectus muscle with nonspecific focal densities (**n–O/18**), especially about the vascular pedicle of the flap (see **e**, p. 217).

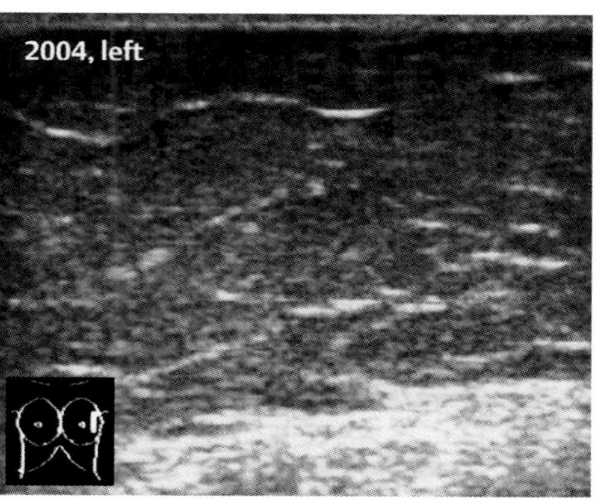


**g** *Sonogram* of the left breast in 2004 shows a uniform echo pattern typical of fatty tissue.

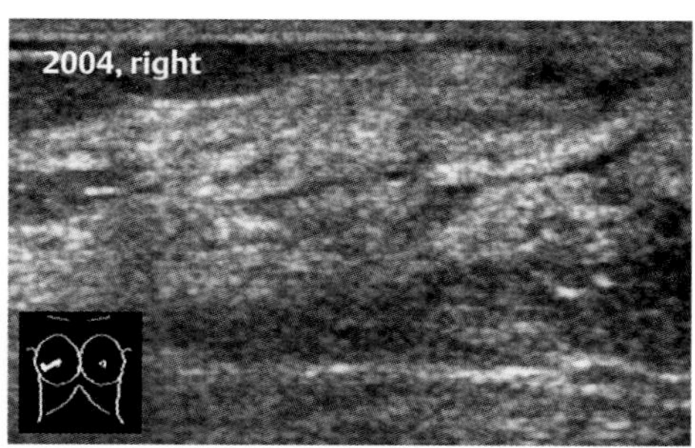


**h** *Sonogram* of the right breast in 2004. The parenchyma in the lower outer quadrant is rich in *inter*lobular stroma and contains a slightly enlarged duct (**s–T/19–20**).

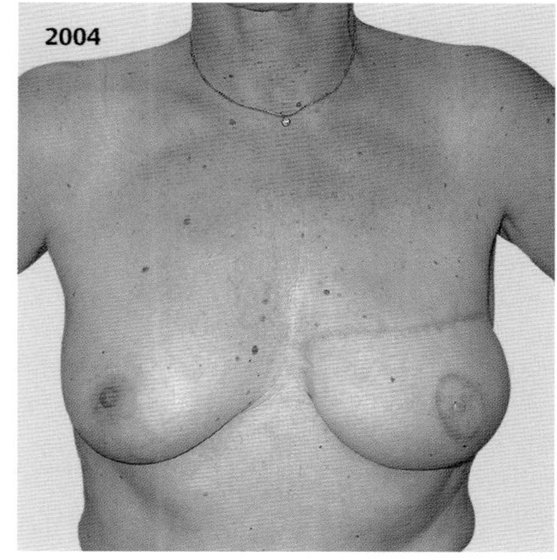


**i** *Clinical inspection* in 2004 shows a very good cosmetic result after a TRAM flap reconstruction of the left breast. A horizontal mastectomy scar and a reconstructed, nonpigmented nipple are visible on the left side.

**Answer for Fig. 5.98, Question 1** (p. 218)

**Answer (c) is correct. Soybean oil implants (Trilucent)**, which are very radiolucent (density factor of oil = 0.8; density factor of water = 1.0; density factor of silicone = 2.0). Because soybean oil is so lucent, the surrounding breast tissue is easier to evaluate and microcalcifications can be detected better than with saline or even silicone.

Trilucent soybean oil implants (www.trilucent.com) have been pulled from the market due to questionable side-effects (implant rupture can apparently incite local inflammatory reactions in the breast).

**Answer for Fig. 5.98, Question 2** (p. 218)

**Answer (c) is correct. Adaptation to breast shape.** Implants must be pliable enough to create smooth transitions in the breast contours (**a**). For this reason, all implants develop folds and wrinkles (which are clearly visible in these images) that may be mistaken for ruptures (see **Fig. 5.101**). A *deflated* implant has a similar appearance, whereas a *ruptured* implant would show signs of capsular disruption.

**Lesson:** Folds are a normal finding in breast implants. They are accentuated by fibrous encapsulation and may also accompany capsular ruptures, although the contents of a ruptured capsule will extravasate into the surrounding tissue, leaving behind a partially filled lumen. Normally, however, implants guarantee a good cosmetic result.

### Answer for Fig. 5.99 (p. 218 f)

**Answer (c) is correct.**

**The deformation is caused by bilateral implant rupture with severe fibrosis of the capsula.** The implant in the right breast is completely collapsed and floating within the outer capsule. When the pectoral muscle contracts, the posterior wall of the capsule that is fused to the pectoral muscle is pulled upward. Because the silicone implant is ruptured and offers no resistance, the breast appears deformed. Both implants were removed and replaced with a good cosmetic result (Michael Greulich, Stuttgart).

The *sonograms* are explained by silicone within the outer capsule, interrupted by portions of the inner capsule of the implant (see *MRI* **c**).

**Lesson:** The curved lines represent the collapsed implant shell. This *linguini sign* is the hallmark of an intra- or extracapsular implant rupture.

### Answer for Fig. 5.100 (p. 220 f)

**Answer (b) is correct. The inner capsule enclosing the silicone has ruptured and the silicone has drained into the outer water-filled capsule.** The echo pattern visible on sonogram is caused by the deflated inner capsule and the silicone in the water-filled interspace.

A simple gel bleed would be present if the inner and outer capsules were intact and the water-filled chamber contained silicone oil. A complete rupture of the inner and outer shells (the host capsule) would cause silicone extravasation around the implant, which has not occurred here. An incomplete rupture of the inner silicone capsule was confirmed at operation.

The slight skin irregularities visible in the infra-areolar region of both breasts are caused by moderate fibrous encapsulation. They are unrelated to the intracapsular rupture and do not signify a local recurrence.

### Answer for Fig. 5.101, Question 1 (p. 221)

**Answer (a) is correct. Trophic skin change.** The vascular layer of the subcutaneous fat has become thin and fibrotic due to the mastectomy and radiotherapy. Pressure from the implant has also compromised blood flow, resulting in trophic skin changes. Cool skin (unlike mastitis!) and livid discoloration are typical findings. A capsular tear is not visible on the images (compare with the subcutaneous fat layer at left).

### Answer for Fig. 5.101, Question 2 (p. 221)

**Answer (b) is correct. Ultrasound shows a "snowstorm" pattern (N–P/9–11)** posterolaterally at the level of a small implant leak (differential diagnosis: gel bleeding). This leak has no practical implications. It is noteworthy that the patient complained of acute pain radiating to the axillary recess. The pain (presumably from the leak) disappeared after one year. The nodule visible in **a** (at the 8-o'clock position) could be a small silicone granuloma.

### Answer for Fig. 5.102, Question 1 (p. 222 f)

**Answer (a) is correct. Single-lumen implant.**

### Answer for Fig. 5.102, Question 2 (p. 222 f)

**Answer (a) is correct. Gel bleed.**

**Lesson:** Gel bleed is manifested by a silicone collection within the intact host capsule (see **e3**)

### Answer for Fig. 5.103, Question 1 (p. 225)

**Answer (a) is correct. Cosmetic breast augmentation** with silicone implants. She had large, ptotic breasts at a younger age and underwent a reduction mammoplasty with reimplantation of the nipples, evidenced now by the scarring on the areola (**a–c**). Parenchyma is visible in each breast on *mammograms* and *MRI* (**d, e**).

**Lesson:** Following the massive proliferation of TDLUs during pregnancy (see p. 170), some women experience a marked regression of glandular tissue without subsequent regeneration of fat and connective tissue. This may cause initially well-formed breasts to become disfigured.

### Answer for Fig. 5.103, Question 2 (p. 225)

**Answer (b) is correct. The nodule results from an old implant leak,** a "confined" perforation of the outer capsule with a calcified foreign-body granuloma.

*Gel bleed* appears sonographically as a snowstorm pattern of opacities around the implant. The leak is clearly visible on ultrasound. The small pleomorphic calcifications next to the coarse calcification have a morphology and arrangement that are suspicious for DCIS, so *CNB* was performed without malignancy.

**Lesson:** Ultrasound can clearly demonstrate implant leaks with associated reactive granulation tissue formation. Ultrasound and MRM can provide an adequate evaluation of breast implants, including their posterior wall. Calcifications, on the other hand, require mammography (preferably digital) for an adequate evaluation.

### Answer for Fig. 5.104 (p. 226)

**Answer (a) is correct. Inflammatory exudate.** Previous needle aspiration under ultrasound guidance yielded serous fluid that did not contain suspicious cells.

The cause of the exudation is unclear. It may be posttraumatic. The breast implant is not displaced. Cytologic findings are normal, and MRI does not show abnormal gadolinium enhancement (Image **b2**, p. 226 courtesy of Stefan Krämer, Esslingen).

Because the fluid production didn't stop, the implant was exchanged and the outer shell removed and histologically analyzed (**c**).

Fig. 5.104

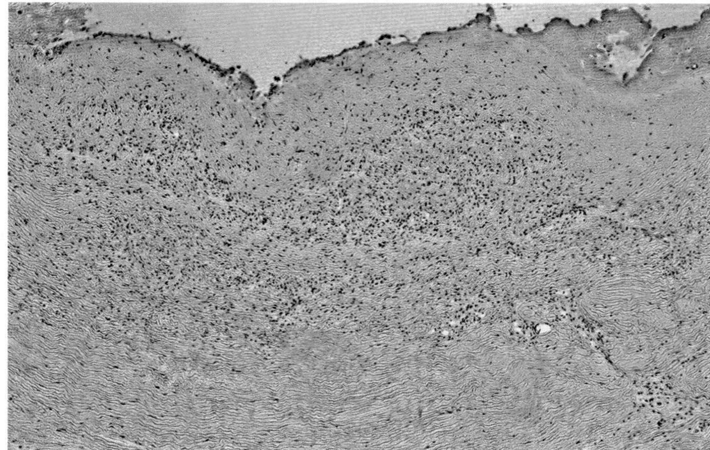

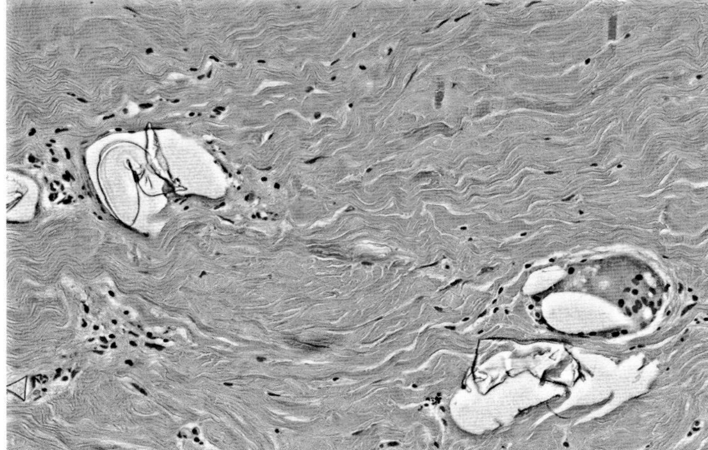

**c** *Histology:* Sparse round cell infiltrates are present in the external capsule as evidence of chronic inflammation (above). Capsule particles closer to the implant contain foreign-body (silicone) inclusions (below) (p. e. **N–O/15–17**) (images courtesy of Jörn Sträter, Esslingen).

### Answer for Fig. 5.105 (p. 227 f)

**Answer (c) is correct. No evidence of recurrence was found in the left breast and axilla.** The scarred area (**c, r–S/9**) (**f, C/13**) below the skin retraction was investigated by percutaneous biopsy, which showed no sign of local recurrence. Similarly, nothing suspicious was found in the left axilla. This case was investigated further by *PET scanning* (**j**). *PET* revealed a lymph node metastasis at the junction of the left subclavian and internal jugular veins and a hypermetabolic focus within the abdomen. Presumably this lesion is not a metastatic process arising from the breast but a separate intra-abdominal tumor with an associated nodal metastasis at the left jugulosubclavian venous junction (the patient is known to have atrophic gastritis). Gastrointestinal studies showed no evidence of disease. The patient was in considerable distress, but as of 2007 there was still no evidence of a pathologic process in either in the breasts or in the abdomen. The tumor markers fell spontaneously to normal levels.

The value of PET in the search for metastases is also illustrated by the case of a *different 60-year-old woman* found to have rising tumor marker levels after the successful treatment of a breast neoplasm. Her mammograms and sonograms were normal, but PET showed hypermetabolic foci about the left hilum (**k**) that were suspicious for metastases. The chest radiograph showed nothing suspicious in that area, but CT confirmed the finding.

**Lesson:** The routine determination of tumor marker levels is problematic in patients who are feeling well. This test often causes needless concern with its high false-positive rate (up to 70% of patients with rising tumor markers and no previously known metastasis). That was not the case here. A suspicious structure was found in the upper gastrointestinal tract in the presence of known atrophic gastritis, and a possible lymph node metastasis was found at the junction of the left subclavian and internal jugular veins. PET eliminated the need for many other tests but did not reassure the patient. She has felt sick (and perhaps is sick) since she was informed of the PET findings.

Fig. 5.105

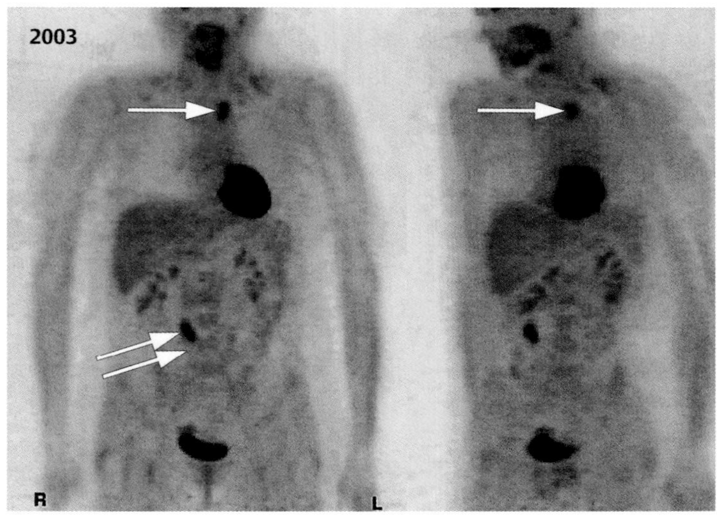


**j** *PET scans* (AP and 45° oblique views) taken in June, 2003 show no tumorlike lesions in the left breast or axilla. Lymph node uptake is visible at the *junction of the left subclavian and internal jugular veins* (arrow) and is *projected over the upper gastrointestinal tract* (double arrow). The findings are suspicious for an abdominal tumor that has metastasized to the jugulosubclavian venous junction and is unrelated to the breast process.

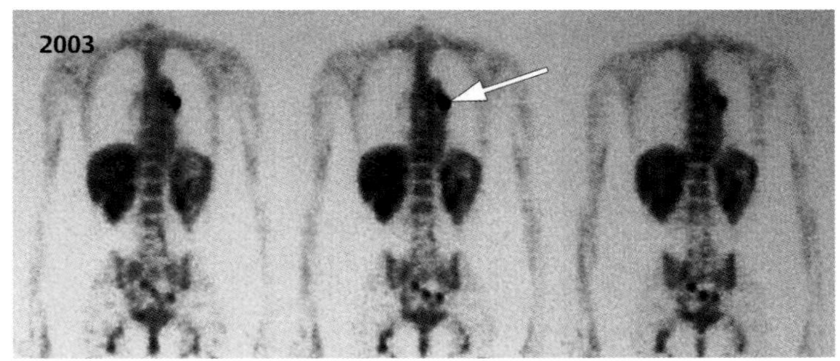


**k** *PET scans* in a different 60-year-old patient treated for a breast tumor show small, hypermetabolic hilar lymph nodes on the left side (arrow). Two years later the patient died as a result of lymph-node and hepatic metastases (images **j** and **k** courtesy of Bernhard Hörr, Plochingen).

### Answer for Fig. 5.106 (p. 229 f)

**Answer (a) is correct. Fat necrosis has developed in the operated breast.** The only hypermetabolic area on the *PET* scan corresponds to a benign, clinically visible change. It is gratifying to diagnose harmless fat necrosis based on a high-tech workup, but it is also very costly. When the *MRI* and *PET* diagnosticians could not commit themselves to a benign diagnosis, *FNA* followed by *CNB* gave quick confirmation of fat necrosis.

**Lesson:** PET/CT is a very useful tool, but rigorous selection criteria should be applied to its use and the results should have therapeutic implications. PET/CT was not indicated in the present case, but the patient herself (a doctor) requested it.

### Answer for Fig. 5.109 (p. 240 f)

**Answer (c) is correct. 2 cm.** Because the notch in the biopsy needle is 2 cm long, *fibroadenomas* and *papillomas* of that size can be removed. This can be done in 10–15 passes when an 8-gauge needle is used. Even larger nodules (up to 3 cm) can sometimes be removed because the needle is maneuverable and nodular remnants can be successfully located and removed. After 20 samples have been taken, however, hematomas make the breast tissue difficult to visualize with *ultrasound*, and residual nodules often cannot be identified. Success can be determined at once or by reexamining the patient at 6–12 months.

**Note:** It is *not* absolutely necessary to remove all portions of a fibroadenoma, for example. Remnants will be reabsorbed by the body or walled off by a capsule and will not cause clinical problems. For instance, if two-thirds of a nodule is histologically benign, it is reasonable to assume that the rest of the nodule does not contain atypical cells. The lesion can be completely removed in a second sitting if desired. *Primary operative treatment* would be indicated for multiple fibroadenomas or nodules more than 2 cm in diameter.

> *The vacuum biopsy of nodules in the nipple region should be performed with special care. The vacuum may draw the nipple into the retroareolar space, injuring or even completely resecting it.*

### Answer for Fig. 5.111 (p. 242)

**Answer (b) is correct. The adhesive patches (EMLA) are for topical anesthesia.** The patches, impregnated with lidocaine and prilocaine, should be applied to the affected nipple at least 60 minutes prior to ductography. They reduce the pain associated with catheterization of the ducts. Local anesthesia of the nipple is usually unnecessary when ultrathin needles are used (**c, d**). Because the EMLA patches take a relatively long time to act, a local anesthetic can also be injected in a circular pattern *around* the areola if necessary to produce local anesthesia of the nipple within seconds.

**Lesson:** Conventional ductography is not widely performed and has become a kind of interventional procedure at some centers. Ductography is not painful when performed with an ultrathin catheter by an experienced examiner. Pain can be prevented if desired by applying skin patches or directly injecting a local anesthetic solution around the areola (not the nipple!). In this example and many other cases, nipple discharge will resolve spontaneously within a few weeks unless it is caused by a papilloma or malignancy.

> *The nipple should be sealed with liquid collodion to prevent leakage of contrast material during mammographic compression.*

### Answer for Fig. 5.112 (p. 243 f)

**Answer (a) is correct. Intraductal debris is never adherent to the duct wall. The inner surface of the duct is smooth.** Debris can be pushed away from the wall on all sides with the ultrasound probe (although this criterion is very vague). This cannot be done with *papillomas*, which are tethered by a basal vascular pedicle (see **Fig. 5.110 b**, p. 241). This is why the duct is mostly dilated or seldom stenotic while the duct wall has an irregular contour. *Intraductal debris* may have smooth or scalloped margins, similar to a papilloma, and it may calcify like a papilloma (see chronic plasma cell mastitis, for example).

**Lesson:** Ductography and ultrasound cannot positively distinguish between papilloma and intraductal debris. Digital magnification can be helpful in some situations, and ultrasound-guided FNA or CNB is naturally recommended in doubtful cases.

### Answer for Fig. 5.114 (p. 245)

**Answer (b) is correct. The discharge is caused by a fibrocystic nodule with cysts and papillomas.** The fibrocystic nodule is clearly visualized at ultrasound.

**Fig. 5.114**

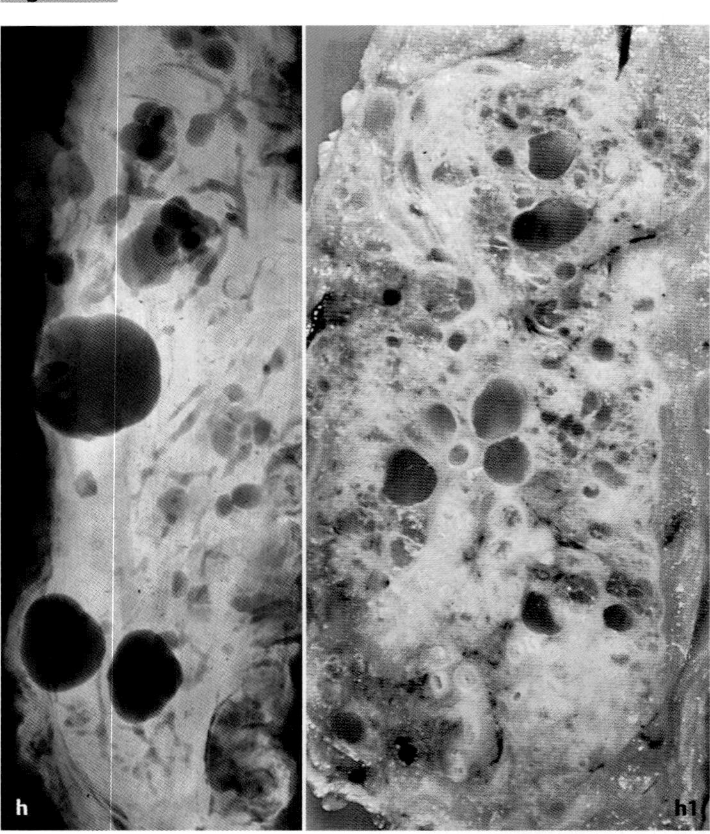


**h** *Specimen radiograph* of a fibrocystic nodule (different patient, 10 × magnification) shows features of microcystic lobular degeneration. Ducts and cysts are filled with air (dark areas). The nodule is histologically benign. A similar nodule appears in **b, c**, and **d** (p. 245).
**h1** *Macroanatomy:* fibrocystic nodules with numerous lobules and ducts showing cystic dilatation.

The *ductogram* shows only the main duct with a cyst, which is visible at **b/17** on the *sonogram* (**d**). The other hypoechoic foci are probably cysts with *intracystic papillomas.*

*CNB* showed fibrocystic changes with unsuspicious foci of intracystic epithelial proliferation. The smear from the nipple was consistent with *papillomatosis.* The patient was advised to have the nodule removed by ultrasound-guided vacuum biopsy, which confirmed the diagnosis. Panel **h** shows a fibrocystic nodule with proliferative foci in small cysts. Additional fibrocystic nodules and occasional discharge were found in the right breast until 2008, but there was no evidence of a malignant process and no additional papillomas were found.

**Lesson:** Mammography, ductography, cytology, ultrasound, and MRI are often excellent complementary modalities for investigating lesions associated with nipple discharge.

### Answer for Fig. 5.115 (p. 246)

**Answer (c) at r/13 is correct. Ultrasound shows two ductal papillomas (l/13** in panel **a**) in continuity with the ectatic ducts (see **d** and **e**). The lesions were successfully removed by SO-VB and since then the patient has been free of complaints. *Operative removal* would have been far more costly and invasive and would have caused greater disfigurement of the relatively small breast than vacuum biopsy. The papilloma was not visible on mammograms (see panel **a**). Papillomas typically appear on ductograms as smooth, round or oval filling defects within the usually dilated ducts (when nipple discharge is present). They can be magnified and analyzed more closely using digital technology. In many cases they can also be imaged sonographically and easily removed by vacuum biopsy (see panels **f–i**).

**Lesson:** In every case of protracted galactorrhea with dilated ducts in an otherwise normal ductogram, the peripheral duct segments should be examined with ultrasound to exclude papillomas. This is particularly important if the ductectasia can be traced into the periphery as in the present case. Ductectasia tends to develop between papilloma and nipple when the papilloma is located at the end of the duct. But if it is located in the midportion of the duct, the entire duct will become ectatic from nipple to periphery (**Fig. 5.112**, p. 243). (The reason for this is unknown but most likely involves a functional disturbance of the duct.) Unilateral circumscribed ductectasia is always suspicious for a papilloma. Peripheral papillomas reportedly undergo malignant transformation more frequently than lesions located near the nipple (Bässler 1978).

Digital imaging technology is extremely helpful in the analysis of intraductal papillary changes (see panels **f–i**).

**Fig. 5.115**

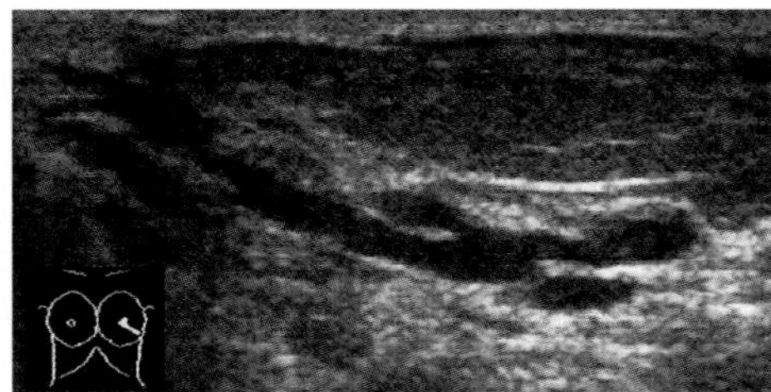

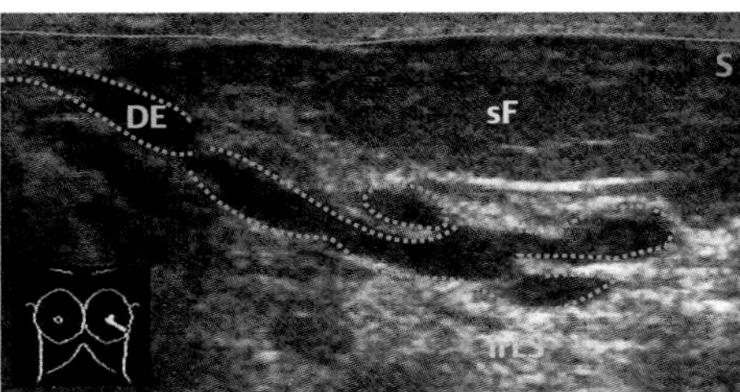


S = skin
sF = subcutaneous fat
IrLS = interlobular stroma
DE = ductectasia

**c** *Sonogram* of the retroareolar area of the left breast shows pronounced ductectasia with no evidence of a papilloma (see **b**, p. 246).

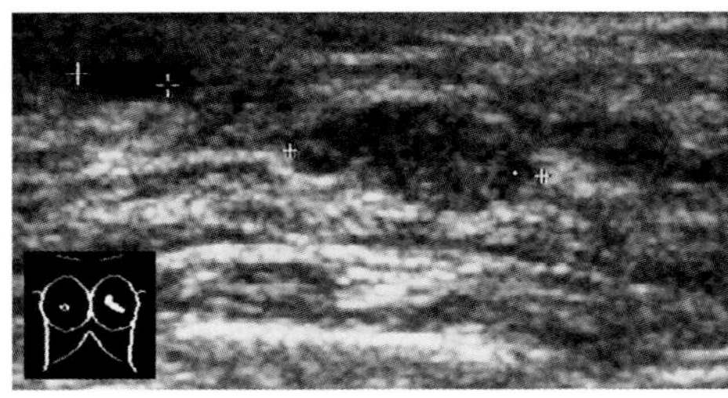

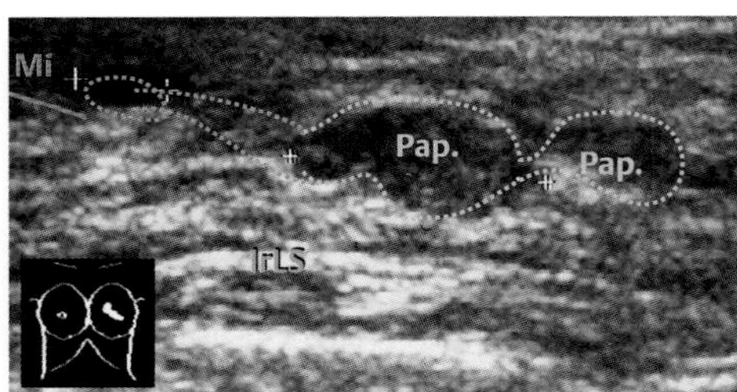


Mi = milk duct
Pap. = papilloma
IrLS = interlobular stroma

**d** *Sonogram* of the supra-areolar area of the left breast (continued from **c**) shows an ectatic duct segment at upper left. Solid intraductal structures (papillomas) are visible to the right of the duct.

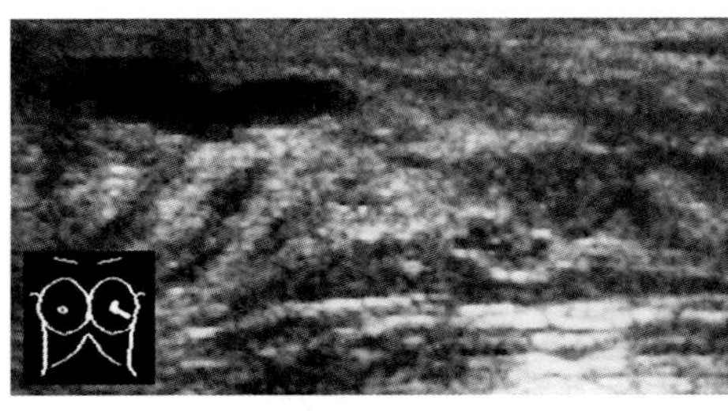

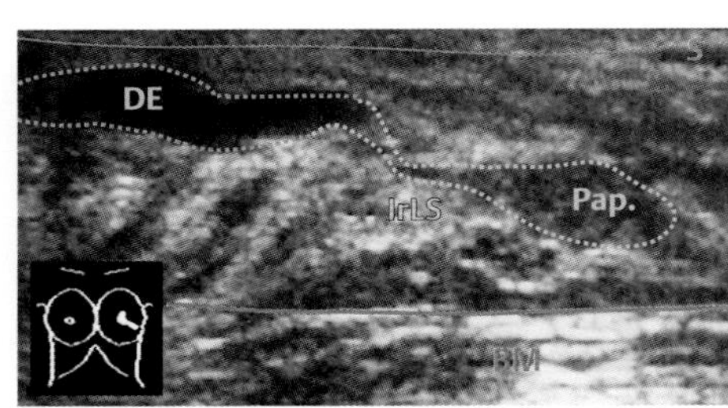


S = skin
DE = ductectasia
Pap. = papilloma
IrLS = interlobular stroma
BM = pectoral muscle

**e** *Sonogram* of the infra-areolar area of the left breast shows an ectatic duct with an intraductal papilloma in continuity with the duct.

▶ Fig. 5.115 f–i

**Fig. 5.115** *(continued)*

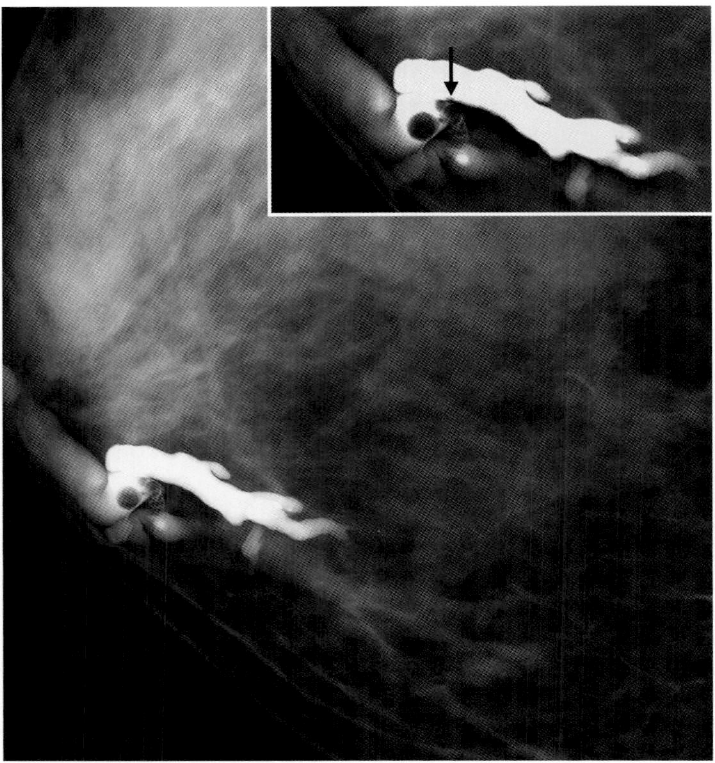

**f** Ductogram of a different patient shows ductectasia and a small papilloma.
**g** Inset: second papilloma in a digital magnification view (arrow). The outlines of the duct are smooth.

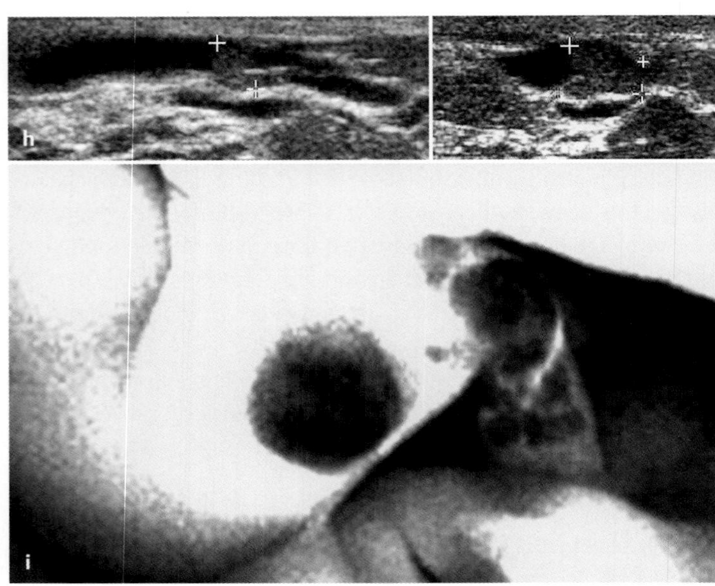

**h** Sonogram shows a dilated duct (dark) and localized papilloma (see marker).
**i Ductography:** magnified view of the ectatic duct with a papilloma at the center of the image and additional papillomas at the periphery (compare **g**). The sonographic correlate appears in **h**.

*With circumscribed ectasia of the retroareolar ducts and abnormal nipple discharge, the breast should always be scanned with ultrasound to look for a ductographically occult papilloma. Ductectasia is mostly caused by papilloma.*

### Answer for Fig. 5.116 (p. 247)

**Answer (a) is correct. Intraductal papilloma.** The lesion is a relatively long, pedunculated intraductal papilloma arising from portions of the duct near the chest wall (a pedunculated papilloma grows "with the flow" rather than against it). The lesion appears noninvasive because it is outlined by contrast medium and is not in contact with the duct wall. It is possible, of course, that a malignancy exists at the base of the pedunculated lesion (**p/21** in **b**), but this would be extremely rare, especially with papillomas near the nipple. There was no evidence of malignancy in the present case.

The cells found in connection with the bloody galactorrhea are typical of *papilloma. Ductectasia* with intraductal debris can produce a similar pattern, but the cells would usually be foam cells with fatty debris, not portions of papilloma.

The *MR* image is also typical of papilloma, although a similar image would result from ductectasia with intraductal debris and accompanying *plasma cell mastitis* as well as from *DCIS.*

### Answer for Fig. 5.117, Question 1 (p. 247 f)

**Answer (a) is correct. Intracystic papillomas.** The gadolinium enhancement on *MRI* would not be consistent with mural debris, which rarely occurs in this intracystic form. The bloody cyst contents are inconsistent with massive ductectasia with fatty wall debris. *Papillary cystic carcinoma* would not occur in small, focal wall deposits. Ultimately, of course, we cannot exclude the possibility that one of the papillomas is undergoing malignant transformation (see **Fig. 5.138 g**, p. 390). *Histology* in this case identified the lesions as benign intracystic papillomas. Until 2009 no evidence of another papilloma or carcinoma.

### Answer for Fig. 5.117, Question 2 (p. 247 f)

**Answer (b) is correct. Blood clot.** The cyst contains a blood clot resulting from vacuum biopsy. Subsequent *FNA* yielded bloody contents while *CNB* identified the nodule as an organizing blood clot, which could not be completely aspirated.

### Answer for Fig. 5.118 (p. 250)

**Answer (a) is correct. Biopsy from the lateral side** provides adequate room for maneuvering the needle. Using a longer coaxial sheath would not be advantageous, as it would not leave enough room for the biopsy needle. Biopsy from the anterior (nipple) side would not improve the situation due to the short distance between the skin and microcalcifications. In any case, the anterior approach would not be an option with standard biopsy equipment.

**Lesson:** Generally the needle should be introduced along the longest available path from skin to microcalcifications so that the outer sheath can be anchored as deeply as possible within the breast.

**Answer for Fig. 5.119** (p. 253 f)

**Answer (c) is correct. The procedure of choice depends on clinical response, locality, and histology.** A large hematoma developed after *vacuum biopsy* (**f**). Compare **j** from different patient. *Ultrasound* showed an organizing hemorrhage (**g**) that was liquefied with Hirudoid compresses until it could be aspirated with a large needle, leaving only a small residue behind (**i**). The hematoma resolved completely by 6 months and nipple discharge did not recur (**f**, upper right).

**Lesson:** The question whether vacuum biopsy is adequate treatment depends on whether the papilloma has been removed and discharge has resolved. If this is the case, no further treatment is needed. If bloody nipple discharge persists, vacuum biopsy can be repeated or the lesion can be operatively removed. *Operative treatment* is definitely indicated if histology shows atypical cells consistent with ADH or DCIS.

**Fig. 5.119** An example of intracystic hemorrhage.

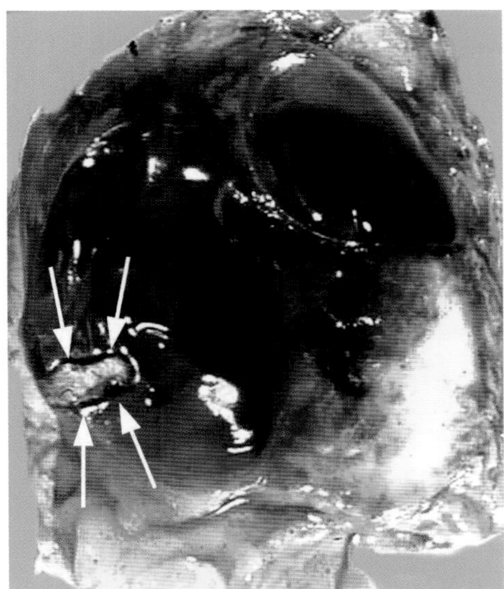

**j** *Gross specimen* contains a small intracystic papilloma (arrow) with heavy bleeding into the adjacent cyst wall (image courtesy of Klaus Prechtel, Starnberg).

Not all papillomas can be removed by vacuum biopsy. Subcutaneous lesions are often inaccessible and require surgery. On the other hand, even papillomas located directly behind the areola can be effectively removed by vacuum biopsy, usually aided by ultrasound guidance.

If they cannot be removed by vacuum biopsy, the duct should be removed radially to the nipple, processed, and histologically examined along with the periductal tissue (Urban 1963).

> *Be careful, incidentally, when performing vacuum biopsy in proximity to large vessels (often visualized because of typical calcifications!). In some circumstances the vacuum may draw vascular segments into the biopsy chamber, causing extensive vascular damage (hematoma) and, very rarely, an arteriovenous (AV) fistula (Hahn et al. 2008).*

**Answer for Fig. 5.125, Question 1** (p. 257)

**Answer (a) is correct. Clinical and mammographic findings are identical when viewed in the oblique projection (b, c).**

**Answer for Fig. 5.125, Question 2** (p. 257)

**Answer (a) is correct. The nodule is very cellular.** *Cytology* reveals large clusters or cells with concave borders. The nodule has smooth, lobulated margins (see p. 69) and is not associated with skin retraction. *MRI, mammography*, and *ultrasound* all display a nodule with smooth, lobulated margins. Ultrasound also shows posterior acoustic enhancement suggestive of very cellular or fluid contents.

**Answer for Fig. 5.125, Question 3** (p. 257)

**Answer (c) is correct. Cytology indicates fibroadenoma with some cell atypias.** The cells are of various sizes and have prominent nucleoli but still maintain a clustered arrangement.

Malignancy cannot be positively excluded based on cytologic findings. The diagnosis of benign fibroadenoma was made after *CNB*. Both nodules were then removed by VB.

**Lesson:** Many patients are greatly distressed by false-positive or equivocal cytologic findings. The results of CNB are more reliable.

> *Most false-positive cytological diagnoses result from fibroadenomas.*

**Answer for Fig. 5.126** (p. 258)

**Answer (c) is correct. The nodule is a carcinoma (lobular).** *Mammographic* findings are consistent with *fibroadenoma. CNB* also suggests fibroadenoma with some atypias (histology 1, see below), perhaps because tissue was sampled from another lesion. The *sonograms* show a malignant process. A smooth margin is visible in the upper sonogram, but central inhomogeneities are also present. The lower image shows ill-defined margins and hypoechoic central structures, which are not typical of fibroadenoma.

*Biopsy* was recommended after the pathologist described nuclear pleomorphism, but the patient did not comply. When follow-up was done several months later, the nodule had increased in size and a repeat *CNB* (histology 2) revealed *lobular carcinoma*.

*Histology 1*: The specimen consists mostly of very *fibrous connective tissue* with areas of hyalinization and a loose arrangement of lobules and excretory ducts. Some of the lobules are thickened. Increased cellularity and *slight nuclear pleomorphism* are noted. Isolated small-caliber ducts contain layered basophilic calculi. Atypical cells are not seen.

*Histology 2*: Areas of *invasive lobular breast carcinoma* are seen. The patient (a physician herself) disputed the definitive diagnosis and opted to undergo a bilateral mastectomy based on the *MRI* findings (which also showed a nodule in the right breast). But besides the palpable nodule in the left breast, no other malignant foci were found in either breast, and the lymph nodes were found to be clear. The *SLN* procedure (**e**) shows a parasternal lymph node, which is not unusual for a tumor located in the inner quadrants or at the upper quadrant boundary.

**Note:** Even long-standing breast nodules may undergo malignant change. Even when imaging findings appear to be benign, subtle changes seen with just one modality (in this case ultrasound) should be critically evaluated. In our case, ultrasound-guided vacuum biopsy could have helped to establish the diagnosis more quickly. VB was recommended to the patient following CNB, but she refused it due to the generally benign histology of the biopsy specimens.

Fig. 5.126

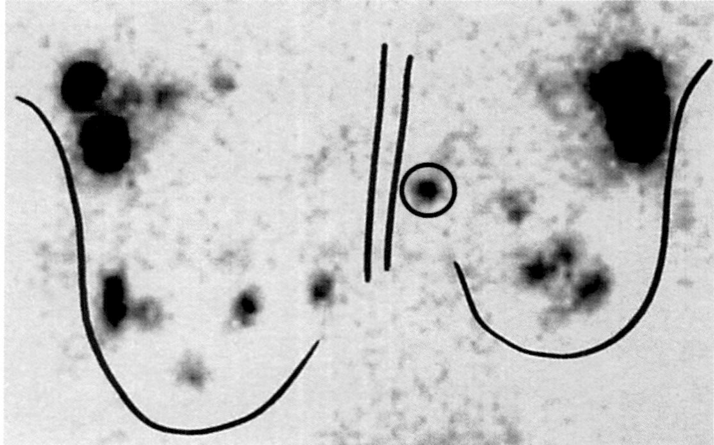

**e** *Sentinel lymph nodes.* The parasternal sentinel node (marker) shows increased uptake following radiotracer injection in the upper portion of the left breast. The SNL procedure was done also on the *right* side based on apparent MRI evidence of a second tumor (see panel **d**), but its presence was not confirmed (MRI false-positive in the right breast).

### Answer for Fig. 5.127, Question 1 (p. 259)

**Answer (b) is correct. The foci are not identical.** This was the diagnostic error. The area of gadolinium enhancement is located closer to the sternum than the ductectasia seen at ultrasound. The diagnostician was misled by the ductectasia and missed the diagnosis. A report from the University Women's Hospital in Tübingen describes the tumor location as 4 cm medial to the nipple, while primary FNA and CNB were performed 1 cm from the areola. The apparent nuclear pleomorphism seen at FNA is a result of inflammatory degenerative changes (note the loose nuclear chromatin pattern).

### Answer for Fig. 5.127, Question 2 (p. 259)

**Answer (b) is correct. The area of gadolinium enhancement was marked on MRI with a localization coil, followed by mammographically guided wire localization of the coil.**

*Histology* showed a 1.6 cm *moderately differentiated invasive lobular carcinoma* associated with pronounced *carcinomatous lymphangitis.* The lesion was excised with clear margins (tumor stage: pT1c G2 pN1 Biii-17/28). Seventeen of 28 lymph nodes were involved.

It was unnecessary to search for an unknown primary tumor (CUP syndrome, see p. 202) outside the breast because the *PET* findings were normal and the metastasis was estrogen- and progesterone-receptor-positive. It is noteworthy, however, that PET imaging in this case was false-negative in the breast and also in the axilla, where an axillary lymphadenectomy had not yet been performed.

**Note:** It is unusual for a moderately differentiated (G2) lobular carcinoma to develop such pronounced carcinomatous lymphangitis and spread from the inner quadrant to involve almost the entire axilla without producing clinical changes in the breast. Essentially this could occur only with a lobular cancer. It is also sobering to note that PET was unrewarding despite the intense tumor enhancement observed on MRI.

### Answer for Fig. 5.128, Question 1 (p. 260 f)

**Answer (a) is correct. No, there is no relationship between calcifications and findings in the breast.** The *sclerosing adenosis* changed very little during the previous 18 months. The calcifications remained the same, while the surrounding breast parenchyma became more dense.

### Answer for Fig. 5.128, Question 2 (p. 260 f)

**Answer (c) is correct. Locally advanced carcinoma (lobular).** The adenosis is unrelated to the breast tumor, which is a 19 cm × 12 cm × 6.5 cm *moderately differentiated (G2) lobular invasive carcinoma.* The *mastectomy* excision margins are clear. Surprisingly, no metastases were found in any of the 14 axillary lymph nodes that were examined. Tumor classification: T3 N0–0/14–Mx G2).

The increasing size and firmness, which the patient dismissed as a postbiopsy infection, could theoretically have been caused by *chronic mastitis,* but the breast never showed warmth or redness and bacteriologic tests were negative. *Cystosarcoma phylloides* may grow to a huge size, and expansile growth is not associated with nipple-areolar retraction.

The locally advanced *lobular carcinoma* developed literally under the nose of the attending physicians. It was most likely present in November of 2000; it was definitely present by 2002 but was not detected mammographically or sonographically in the dense breast. The diagnostician was completely focused on the microcalcifications and biopsied them without noticing the tumor growing alongside them.

**Lesson:** Lobular carcinoma is frequently missed on mammograms and is occasionally missed by ultrasound and cytology as well. It may grow to an exceptionally large size, often causing the patient to insist upon surgery. The absence of axillary lymph node involvement is surprising and can be explained only by the rapid tumor growth, which is not unusual with lobular carcinomas. (see **Fig. 5.188**, p. 342).

### Answer for Fig. 5.129, Question 1 (p. 262)

**Answer (a) is correct.** The lesion is most likely benign.

### Answer for Fig. 5.129, Question 2 (p. 262)

**Answer (a) is correct. Ductectasia with plasma cell mastitis.** The ductectasia is responsible for the recurrent inflammation.

*Cytology* yields granulocytes, protein precipitates, histiocytic lipophagic giant cells (foam cells, **h**), and epithelial and plasma cells showing inflammatory changes (**i**). Cytology supports a diagnosis of *chronic suppurative mastitis.* The residual intraductal opacity after *CNB* (**f**) is consistent *with inflammatory granulation tissue. Ultrasound* suggests that the opacity may also be a *papilloma* or *intraductal carcinoma,* but these lesions are associated with a discolored or bloody discharge and are almost never accompanied by suppurative mastitis.

The *mammographic* changes are nonspecific and may reflect a *papilloma, ductal carcinoma (Paget type),* or *ductectasia.*

The retroareolar nodule and other clinical features are also nonspecific. The purulent, bloody discharge may signify *plasma cell mastitis with ductectasia* or an *intraductal papilloma*.

*Surgical exploration* of the retroareolar region is unnecessary. A persistent discharge is best managed by ultrasound-guided retroareolar vacuum biopsy with removal of the ectatic ducts. Twelve months later the patient was asymptomatic without further treatment and remained so through 2009.

### Answer for Fig. 5.130 (p. 263)

**Answer (b) is correct. The nodule is caused by ductectasia with retained secretions,** as indicated by the fatty debris (**d**). *FNA* cytology of ductectasia most commonly yields fat crystals with cholesterol clumps and foam cells with a large cytoplasmic rim and eccentric nuclei. Individual inflammatory cells are also found. Ductectasia is clearly visualized by *ultrasound*, and the nodular mass is a result of concomitant periductal inflammation. This condition is relatively mild, and skin redness was present for only a short time.

A *carcinoma* is not associated with this kind of debris. Even *chronic granulating mastitis* does not produce fatty debris and has a much more protracted course. Four weeks later, no abnormalities were found in the breast by ultrasound or palpation (other than bilateral ductectasia). There was no need for an operative or interventional procedure (e.g., vacuum biopsy).

### Answer for Fig. 5.131 (p. 264)

**Answer (b) is correct. Acute mastitis,** which has clinical, mammographic, and sonographic features that resemble a *lobular invasive malignancy*. The *cytologic smear* indicates *acute mastitis* with inflammatory cells (leukocytes, lymphocytes, histiocytes). The changes resolved spontaneously within 2 weeks. The cytologic findings definitely exclude *lobular carcinoma*. The *mammographic* changes are fairly nonspecific. An echogenic halo at *ultrasound* may be caused by an inflammatory process (marginal edema?) as well as a malignancy.

### Answer for Fig. 5.132 (p. 265)

**Answer (a) is correct. Fat necrosis.** This diagnosis is supported by the coarse liponecrotic calcifications (**b**), which increased significantly months after *aspiration biopsy (FNA)*. The calcifications do not look malignant; calcium flecks of this kind are unusual even with an aggressive comedocarcinoma. The rosette-like arrangement resembles blunt duct adenosis (see **f**). *Fat necrosis* is also indicated by the oily fluid and vermiform and pasty debris at the center of the oil drop that was obtained at *FNA*. The cells also appear benign (**e**).

A progressive *comedocarcinoma* would not only involve the area of calcifications but would also spread into the periphery. This process is completely localized, however, and the calcifications are regressing (**f**). Even in the absence of a known trauma history, it is still likely that the patient has posttraumatic fat necrosis with oil cysts.

*Chronic granulomatous mastitis* is not associated with coarse calcifications of this kind and is not accompanied by liponecrosis or oil cysts. It is unnecessary to remove the calcifications by vacuum biopsy or even open surgery.

**Fig. 5.132**

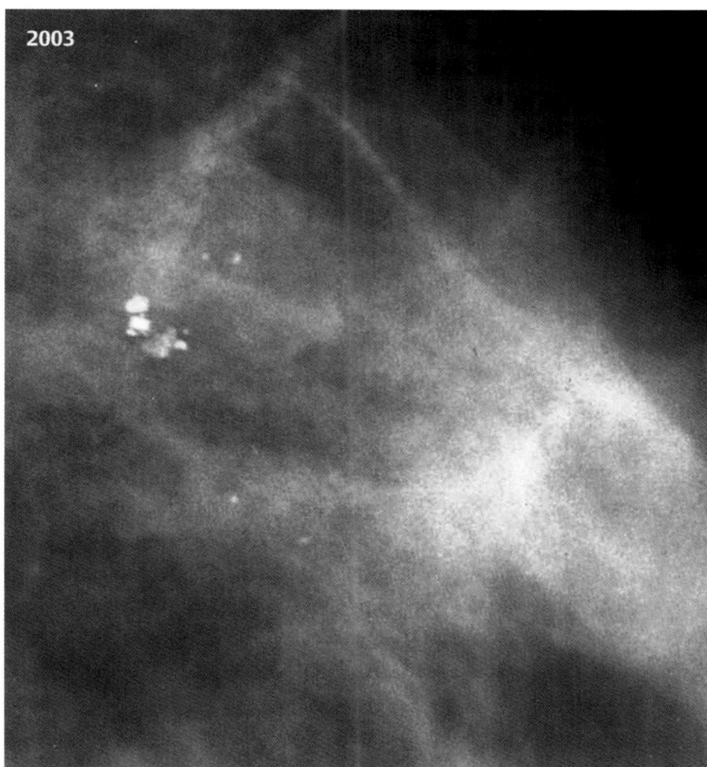


**f** *Oblique mammogram* of the left breast in 2003 (magnified view) documents spontaneous regression of the calcifications, showing only a few residual, unsuspicious particles.

### Answer for Fig. 5.133 (p. 266)

**Answer (c) is correct. Circumscribed focal ductectasia with accompanying inflammation.** The mass is produced by confluent areas of ductectasia. *Ultrasound* does not show intraductal proliferation. The *MRI* findings are referable to *concomitant inflammation*. The flocculent calcifications around the mass are suggestive of recurrent mastitis. The *mammographic* findings are suspicious for a malignant process. It is noteworthy that the change is visible only as a summation effect in the craniocaudal view and is not visible in the oblique view.

There is no need for operative treatment. It would be appropriate to consider removing the ductectasia by vacuum biopsy, but this procedure was withheld in the present case.

### Answer for Fig. 5.134 (p. 267 f)

**Answer (c) is correct. Granulomatous mastitis.** The *mammographic* findings appear suspicious and suggest a stellate scirrhous cancer, but the multifocal lesions seen at ultrasound consistently have smooth margins and a hypoechoic center (indicating a very cellular or mucinous process). *Ultrasound* shows extension of these structures into the periphery with some intraductal extension (**d**). The absence of acoustic enhancement behind the nodule does not support the diagnosis of a mucinous process in this case. *Cytology* shows a typical, predominantly fibrous granuloma with surrounding inflammatory cells.

*CNB* indicates granulomatous mastitis, which was treated with cortisone. The patient declined surgery and vacuum biopsy.

**Lesson:** The cause of *granulomatous mastitis* is unknown. Trauma to the breast may contribute to the development of this disorder. Extension of the granulomatous mastitis along the duct system (probably initiated by claw trauma to the nipple) caused nipple retraction, which is somewhat unusual in granulomatous mastitis.

The discrepancy between the mammographic (stellate) and sonographic (lobulated) lesion appearance and the mild clinical changes (except for nipple retraction in this case) is noteworthy in *granulomatous mastitis*.

### Answer for Fig. 5.135 (p. 268 ff)

**Answer (c) is correct. Granulomatous mastitis.** This is rapidly progressive case (see **Fig. 5.134**, p. 267). The initial impression was *angiosarcoma*. The histologic diagnosis was established by *CNB*. *Bacteriologic tests* were negative and showed no evidence of tuberculosis, actinomycosis, etc. The CRP level of 10 mg/100 mL was significantly above normal (5 mg/100 mL). The findings are consistent with an acute inflammatory process. *Angiosarcoma* would be a possible diagnosis, as it is not unusual for this lesion to spread throughout the breast within 2 months. But the diffuse spread in the breast is more consistent with *inflammatory breast cancer* (predominant involvement of the lower breast quadrants and the absence of orange-peel skin do not support this diagnosis) or an *inflammation*.

The further course was dramatic. In response to cortisone and amoxicillin, an extensive system of fistulous tracts developed with confluent subcutaneous fluid collections (**h**). Some of the fistulae broke through the skin (**i**), and cortisone was discontinued. A final trial of amoxicillin for several months was proposed, to be followed by subcutaneous mastectomy if the therapy was ineffective. After the patient spent 5 months in her homeland Albania, her symptoms regressed (without therapy) and she had normal mammographic, MRI, and sonographic findings (**j, k**).

The fistulous openings healed, leaving only a bluish-purple skin discoloration. No new inflammation occurred as of **2008**, and the patient was free of complaints.

*Granulomatous mastitis* is histologically similar to *tuberculosis* and *sarcoidosis*. *Tuberculosis* and *actinomycosis* were excluded in this case by bacteriologic testing. The cause of granulomatous mastitis is unknown. Cortisone administration actually worsened the patient's condition. It is uncertain whether amoxicillin therapy ultimately contributed to her recovery. It seems likely that the changes would have resolved spontaneously after the patient returned to her homeland.

**Fig. 5.135**

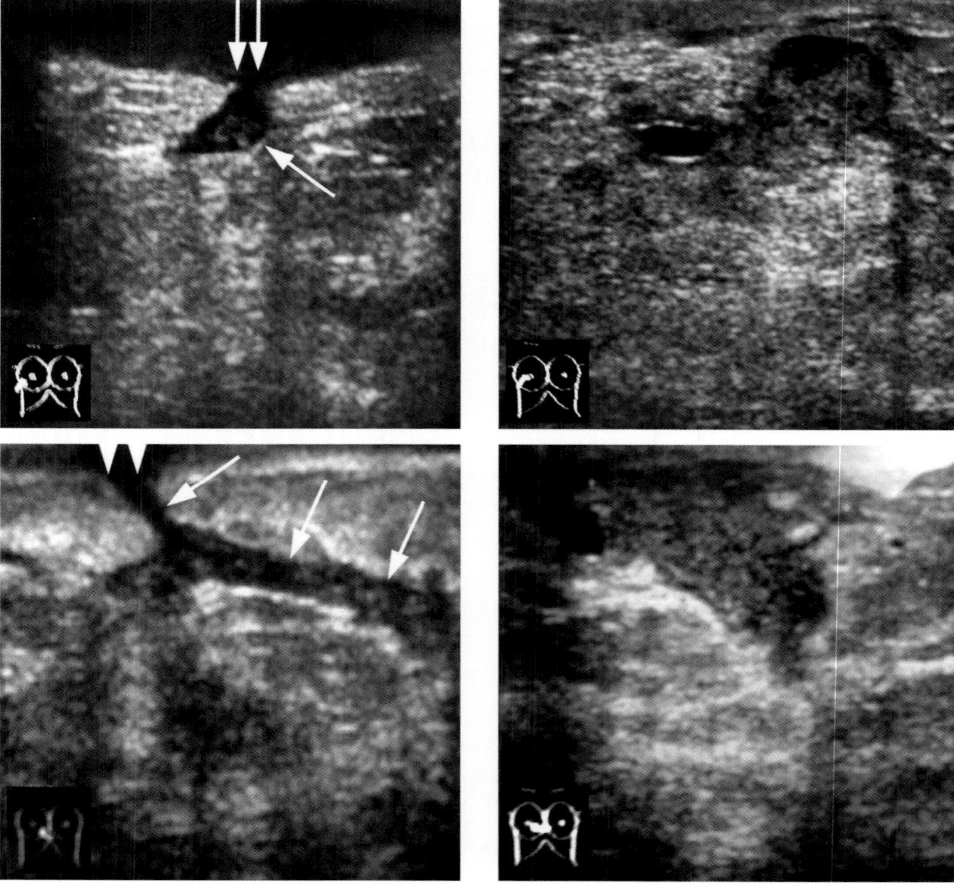

**h** *Progression of ultrasound findings.* The patient developed extensive intramammary fistulous tracts containing a watery serous fluid that drained spontaneously through cutaneous fistulae. The tracts are bordered by well-circumscribed hypoechoic areas with posterior acoustic enhancement.

**Fig. 5.135** *(continued)*

9/2002
2/2003
11/2003
5/2004

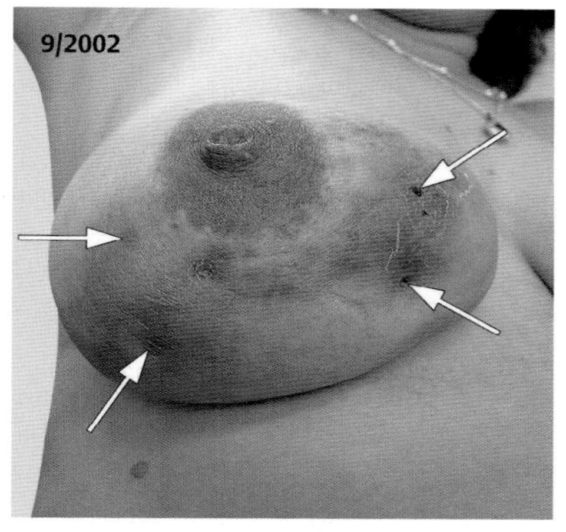

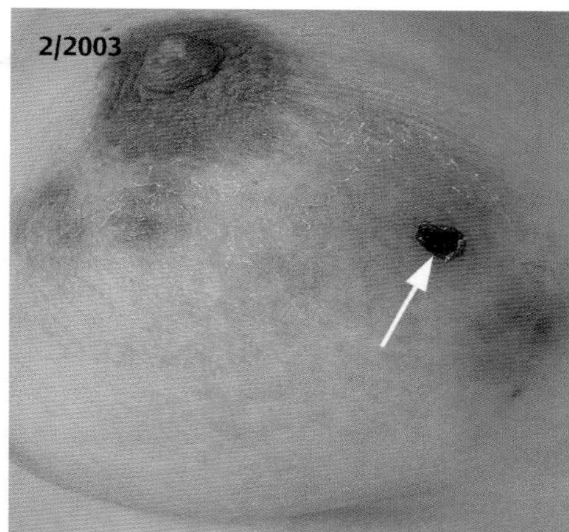

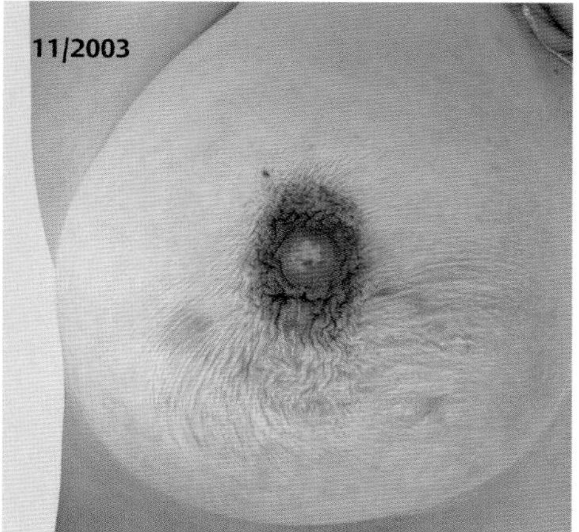

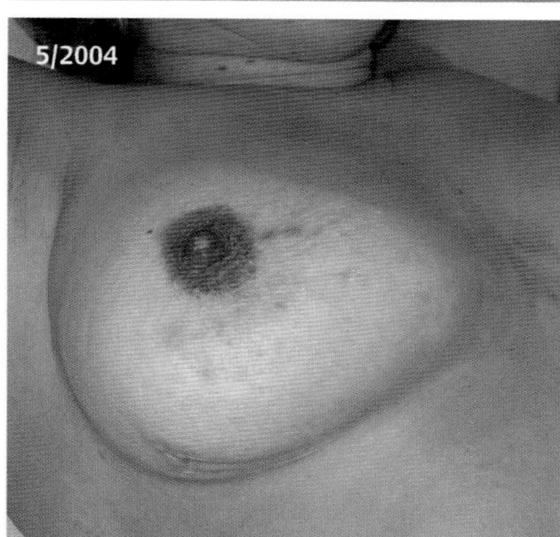

**i** *Clinical appearance* of the right breast over time shows increasing reddish-purple discoloration of the lower breast quadrants, fistula formation, and the complete regression of changes by November, 2003.

▶ **Fig. 5.135k**

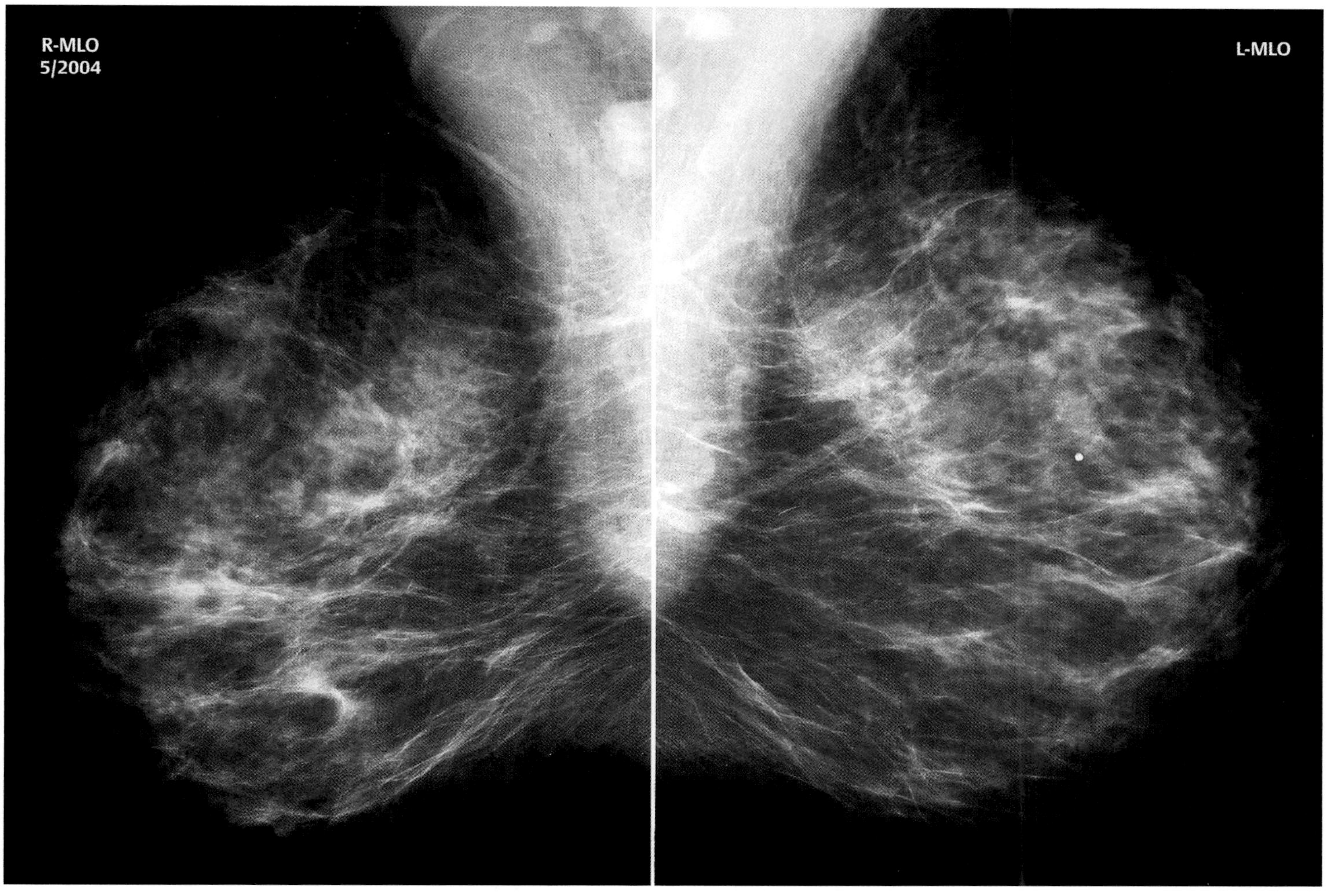

R-MLO
5/2004
L-MLO

**j** *Bilateral oblique mammograms* in May, 2004 show no abnormalities (ACR 2, BIRADS 1, **P**GMI). A lymph node on the right side is still slightly enlarged (**O/13**).

**Fig. 5.135** *(continued)*

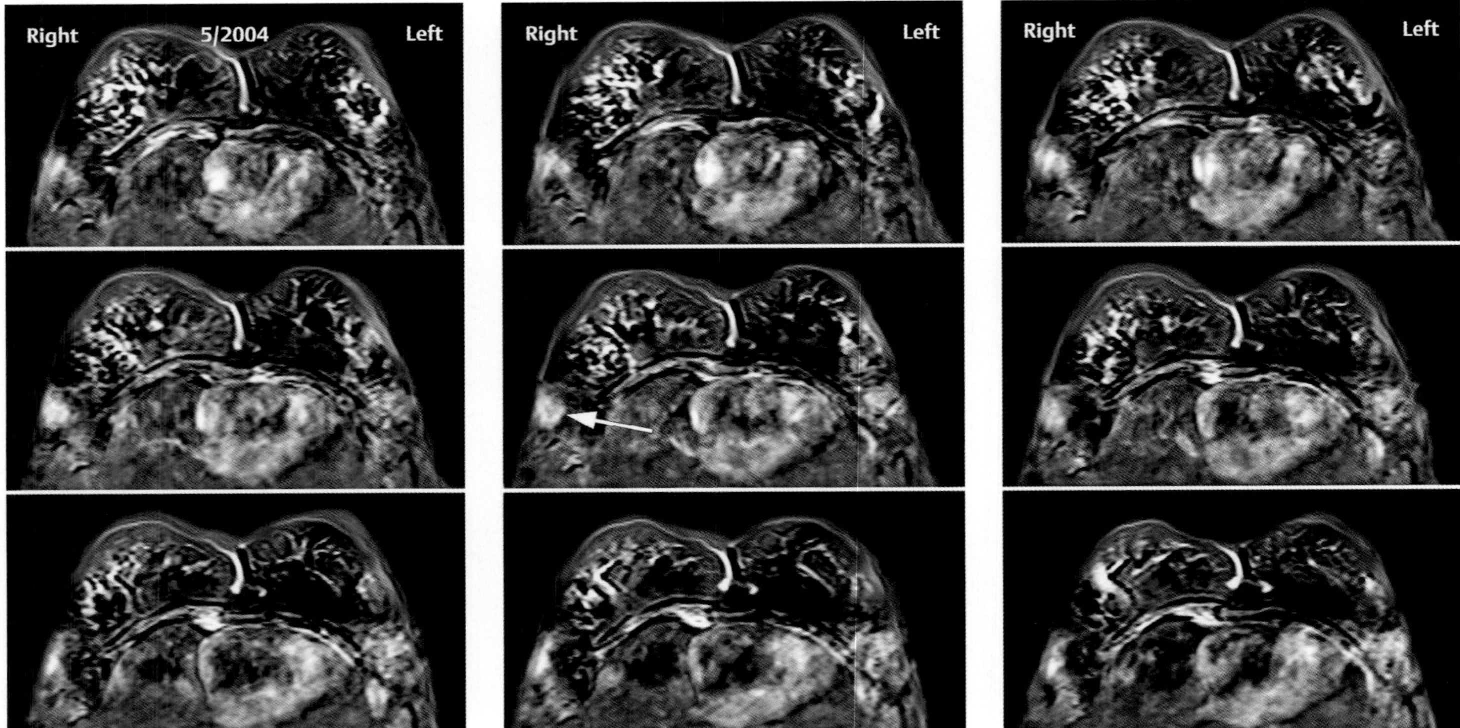


**k** *MR images* in November, 2003, still show slightly increased gadolinium uptake in the right breast, especially in the axillary recess (arrow) (corresponding to the enlarged intramammary lymph node visible in **j**). Otherwise the changes have almost completely resolved compared with the initial images (**f**, p. 270).

### Answer for Fig. 5.136, Question 1 (p. 271 f)

**Answer (b) is correct. A neurologic disorder** is the most likely cause of the lancinating retroareolar pains and atonic left areola, which is smooth and looks larger than the right areola. The exact cause of the pain is unclear (vertebrogenic? neurogenic?). The persistent complaints focused the patient's awareness on the left breast, leading her to believe that there was a lesion there.

### Answer for Fig. 5.136, Question 2 (p. 271 f)

**Answer (b) is correct. The lesion is in the right breast.** Because the patient consistently described severe pain in the left breast, the physician interpreting the MR images also focused on that side. He failed to notice that he was viewing the MR images with the right and left sides reversed. The lesion is actually located in the right breast. The patient noticed this error herself when she was given the images to take home, scrutinized them, and found that it was not the left breast but the right breast that showed contrast enhancement. *Ultrasound* scans were then obtained (**d**), and the findings prompted investigation by ultrasound-guided *CNB*.

### Answer for Fig. 5.136, Question 3 (p. 271 f)

**Answer (c) is correct. Lactating adenoma.** The lesion is a relatively rare lactating adenoma, which was not palpable and caused no complaints. The benign lesion was not surgically removed. The right-sided lesion made the patient less hyperaware of her left breast, but the cause of that pain was still a mystery.

**Lesson:** Haste is the worst enemy of an accurate diagnosis. Reversed images and a nervous patient may lead to diagnostic errors. The loss of areolar muscle contraction in one breast should raise suspicion of a vertebrogenic or neurogenic cause.

### Answer for Fig. 5.137, Question 1 (p. 272 f)

**Answer (a) is correct. The MRI and ultrasound findings correspond to the upper lesion (no. 1).** Microcalcifications (like those in the lower portion of the breast at 2) are not visible on *ultrasound*. A DCIS lesion may exhibit *MRI* changes (see p. 37). The apparent discrepancy between the clinical and mammographic location is caused by the oblique projection. When the lesions are localized in relation to the nipple, their locations coincide.

### Answer for Fig. 5.137, Question 2 (p. 272 f)

**Answer (b) is correct. Lymphocytoid mastitis.** This type of mastitis most commonly affects premenopausal women with more than a 20-year *history of diabetes*. It may be caused by an immune reaction to exogenous insulin or by an autoimmune process (possibly combined with Hashimoto thyroiditis or rheumatoid arthritis) (Völker et al. 2008). This disease may form masses up to 6 cm in diameter, usually without microcalcifications. Rare cases may occur in nondiabetics. Mammograms show focal or asymmetrical mammary fibrosis, as in the present case.

*Lobular carcinoma* may display similar MRI and ultrasound features but does not have septations and does not show such marked density variations within the nodule. Even so, lobular carcinoma was the presumptive diagnosis prior to *CNB*.

*Aggressive fibrosis* may show gadolinium enhancement on MRI, but it would not appear *sonographically* as a hypoechoic structure with smooth margins and posterior acoustic enhancement.

### Answer for Fig. 5.137, Question 3 (p. 272 f)

**Answer (c) is correct. Accompanying inflammation is the cause.** *MRI* shows the acute inflammatory process (hypoechoic at ultrasound) plus the chronic inflammatory process (echogenic rim at ultrasound), so the lesion only appears larger on MRI when the echogenic rim is not included in the sonographic measurement. *Acute and chronic granulating processes* are easily mistaken for malignancies because they often lack the posterior acoustic enhancement that is typically associated with fluids.

Four days later the lesion was no longer detectable by ultrasound (probably due to intralesional hemorrhage). Six-month follow-up showed no abnormalities at ultrasound or MRI. The calcifications (2, **c**) were investigated by *CNB* one year later because they had increased in number and size. Histology revealed *sclerosing adenosis.*

**Lesson:** The other side of the coin: without modern technology for early breast cancer detection, the patient would have been spared considerable distress. The local mastitis would have been scarcely detectable on mammograms, and the patient had no complaints.

### Answer for Fig. 5.138 (p. 274)

**Answer (a) is correct. Yes, the cyst margins showed some degree of change.** They were very smooth in 1997, but *pneumocystography* in 1999 showed irregular basal contours (**d**) and *ultrasound* showed ill-defined margins (**c**). Though subtle, these findings are still meaningful with respect to the further course. The patient did not return for follow-up mammograms until 4 years later (2003), having noticed that the palpable cyst had enlarged and there was retraction of the overlying skin. She also noticed a palpable nodule in her left axilla. *Mammography* (**e**) and *ultrasound* (**f**) show unequivocal signs of a malignant process.

**Lesson:** As a rule, cysts do not undergo malignant change. But this case proves that malignant transformation may occur in rare instances or that cysts may be invaded by an extrinsic tumor (see **g**). In retrospect, changes can be recognized in the cyst wall, even if they are very subtle. This is still no reason to schedule regular follow-up examinations for cysts. Breast cysts are almost a normal finding in women over age 35, and their malignant transformation is very rare.

**Fig. 5.138**

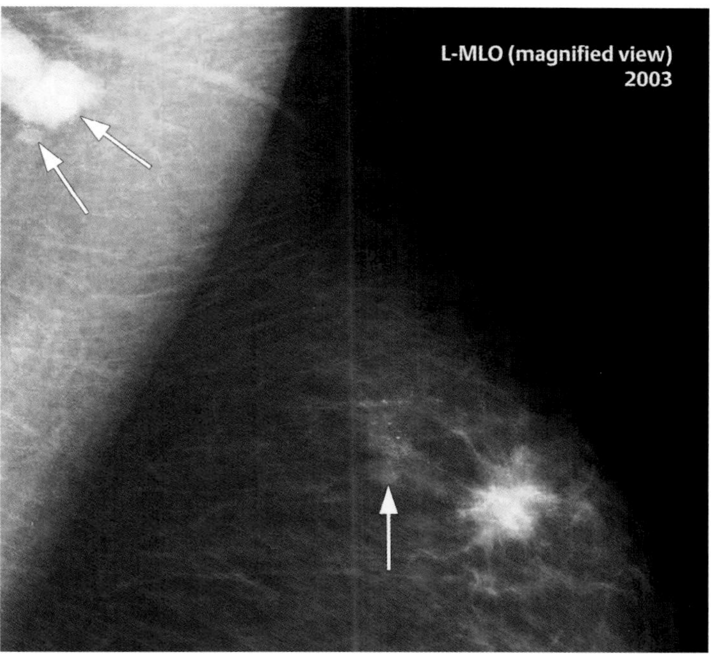


**e** *Oblique mammogram* of the left breast (magnified view of the upper quadrants) shows a 1.2 cm stellate tumor with a deeper satellite lesion (arrow). An enlarged lymph node is visible in the left axilla (double arrows) (ACR 2, BIRADS 5, **P**GMI). *Histology* confirmed that the node was metastatic.

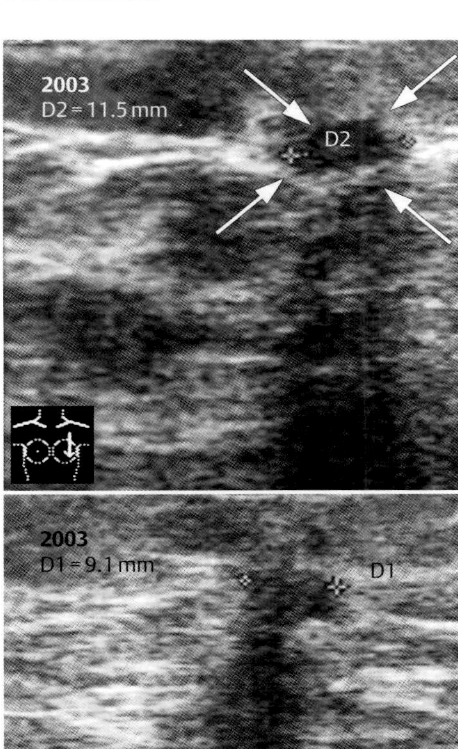


**f** *Sonogram* of the 1 cm × 1.2 cm × 0.9 cm tumor shows typical ill-defined margins, posterior acoustic shadowing, and a fine echogenic halo (arrows). The tumor completely occupies the cyst lumen.

▶ Fig. 5.138 g, h

**Fig. 5.138** *(continued)*

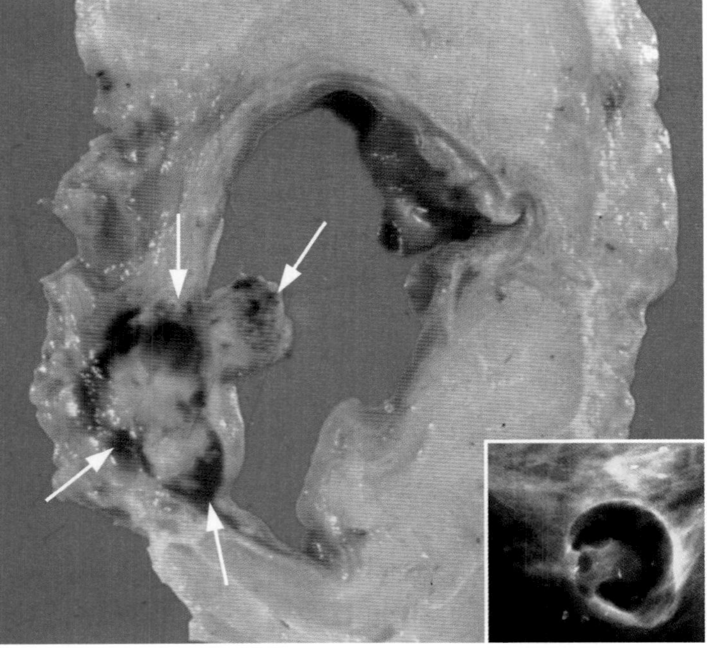

**g** Different patient. *Gross specimen* of *intracystic papillary carcinoma* shows a papilloma-like mass (**B–b/21–23**) extending into the cyst lumen with infiltration and thickening of the cyst walls and foci of peritumoral hemorrhage (arrows). Note the generally irregular margins of the cyst wall (**C–d/20–25**) (image courtesy of Klaus Prechtel, Starnberg). Corresponding pneumocystogram is shown at lower right.

### Answer for Fig. 5.139, Question 1 (p. 275 f)

**Answer (a) is correct. No, the DCIS was not completely removed.** The specimen radiographs show scattered peripheral calcifications in both views (**D/22, h/23, J/22**), indicating that the DCIS was not removed with clear margins. Pathology confirmed this, prompting (also because of the MRI extension) a subcutaneous mastectomy of the right breast in which 150 g of breast parenchyma was removed. An excisional biopsy of the left breast (lateral between the 2-o'clock and 4-o'clock positions) was also performed because MRI showed slight, nonspecific focal gadolinium enhancement (**e**). No residual DCIS was found in either breast—only an area of proliferative fibrocystic change with adenosis, although MRI of the right breast showed gadolinium enhancement extending to the nipple. MRI was unable to distinguish between benign adenosis and DCIS in this case.

**Lesson:** It is not unusual for MRI findings to prompt *overtreatment*, resulting in the unnecessary removal of tissue with innocuous changes. This can cause many patients, such as the relatively young woman in this case, to experience adverse cosmetic and psychological effects.

The **Oxford Overview Analysis** of patients treated with tamoxifen and/or systematic chemotherapy alone over a 15-year period showed a 50% decline in local recurrences and second tumors in the healthy breast. This underscores the importance of avoiding MRI-motivated overtreatment with the removal of presumably malignant tissue, especially in young women who have additionally undergone radiotherapy (Solin 2008; Morrow 2008). Retrospective analysis in the present case shows that the right subcutaneous mastectomy and wide tissue excision from the left breast could have been withheld in favor of a wait-and-see approach.

### Answer for Fig. 5.139, Question 2 (p. 275 f)

**Answer (c) is correct. Mammogram does not show nipple involvement.** The calcifications are located 2–3 cm distant from the nipple. *MRI*, however, shows gadolinium enhancement in and around the area of the calcifications, extending to the nipple. The biopsy was relatively extensive therefore with deformation of the right breast (**f**). Work-up of the mastectomy specimen and the retroareolar biopsy revealed *adenosis* with no residual *DCIS*.

**Lesson:** MRI can detect proliferative tissue by its gadolinium enhancement, but it cannot determine whether the tissue is benign or malignant (high sensitivity, low specificity). DCIS and adenosis both show contrast uptake, with the result that MRI findings may lead to overtreatment. The changes in the lateral portion of the left breast were also consistent with *adenosis*. The surgery caused considerable bilateral disfigurement (**f**). The patient declined silicone implant reconstruction because of her athletic activities. She can live with the status quo. Follow-up mammograms of the residual breast parenchyma showed no new calcifications as of 2009 (8 years after treatment).

**Lesson:** *The local recurrence rate of DCIS after excision with clear margins is only 4.6% (MacDonald et al. 2005). This is less than the recurrence rate of invasive cancer following breast-conserving treatment. Postoperative radiotherapy is still advised, however.*

**Fig. 5.139**

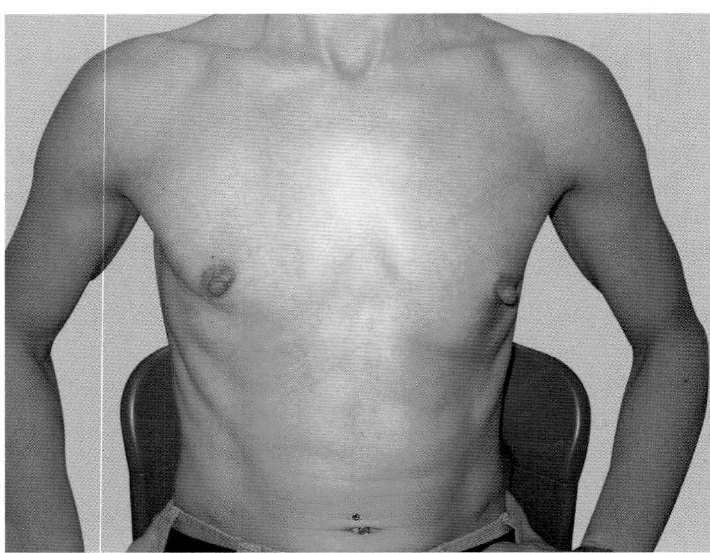

**f** *Clinical appearance* after subcutaneous mastectomy of the right breast and wide excisional biopsy of the left breast, resulting in considerable disfigurement. Six years later the residual glandular tissue in the right breast was still free of recurrence, and no tumorlike changes were detected in the left breast. The patient continues to be active in judo and is satisfied with the condition of her breasts, especially given the demands of her sport.

**Answer for Fig. 5.140, Question 1** (p. 277 f)

**Answer (c) is correct. The nodule is a fibroadenoma, and DCIS has developed at its margins.** The anterior portions of the nodule have smooth margins at mammography consistent with fibroadenoma. The margins become irregular toward the axilla, and the center has an inhomogeneous echo pattern. Some of the cells stem from the fibroadenoma (left image) and some from the *DCIS* (**d**, smaller cluster in the right image). The lesions are not distinguishable by *MRI*, as both *DCIS* and *fibroadenoma* show contrast uptake and the time–density curve is dominated by the fibroadenoma.

The *cytologic* findings exclude *mucinous carcinoma*. The lesion is predominantly round with smooth margins and shows posterior acoustic enhancement. Pure fibroadenoma is a less likely diagnosis based on *ultrasound* and *cytology*.

*Histology: Fibroadenoma* with a 0.2 cm area of DCIS (Van Nuys Index 4, see p. 58, **Fig. 5.140 f**).

**Answer for Fig. 5.140, Question 2** (p. 277 f)

**Answer (a) is correct.** Breast cancer surgery or even DCIS is no reason to avoid pregnancy and breastfeeding. It is good for the breast, the body, and apparently the immune system. Three years after surgery the patient gave birth to her long-desired baby and sent an original birth announcement (**g**). She nursed her baby with both breasts (really the only option), and this did not harm the breast or, obviously, the child. As of 2010, 11 years after therapy and also after a second pregnancy the patient was free of recurrent disease.

**Lesson:** Single-view mammograms are adequate in younger women and can reliably detect or exclude microcalcifications. Ultrasound and MRI are indicated if a malignant process cannot be excluded or the patient is at risk by her family history. In the case shown, MRI was unnecessary to evaluate the nodule, although it did exclude other enhancing foci in the affected breast and the clinically healthy breast.

**Fig. 5.140**

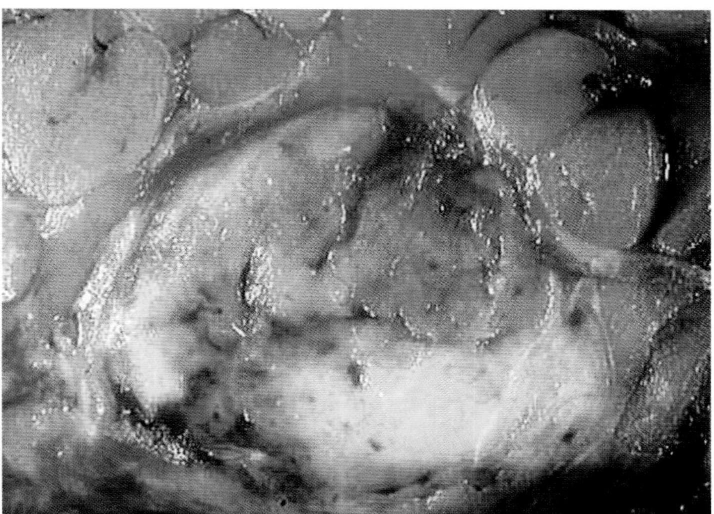

**f** *Macroanatomy* of another fibroadenoma (white areas with smooth margins, see below). There is also associated DCIS (light brown, above) with bleeding into the adjacent parenchyma (image courtesy of Roland Bässler, Fulda).

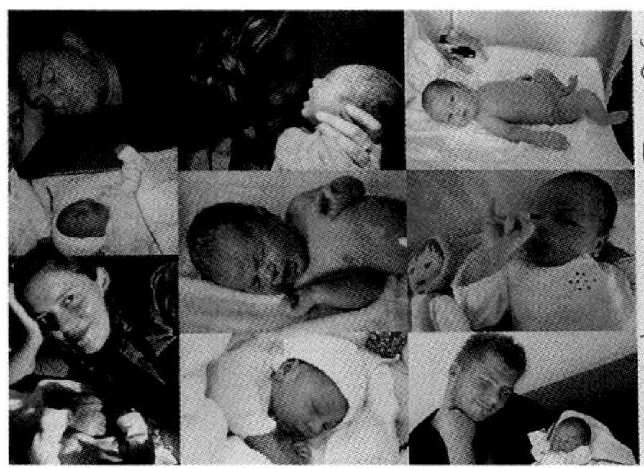


**g** *The birth announcement* from the happy parents proves that breast cancer, including preinvasive disease, is no reason to remain childless. [The note reads "Dear Dr. Barth, here he is, our little son, who makes us so happy. As you recommended, I will make another appointment to see you after our baby has been weaned. If you feel an earlier examination would be better, please let me know. Sincerely, ..."]

**Answer for Fig. 5.141, Question 1** (p. 278 f)

**Answer (c) is correct. Well-differentiated malignant tumor (G1)** that is strongly hormone-receptor-positive. Twenty axillary lymph nodes were free of metastases (no sentinel nodes, as medial tumors drain toward the sternum). The patient underwent breast-conserving therapy that included axillary dissection and postoperative radiation. She declined chemotherapy after consulting with several doctors, as the axillary lymph nodes were clear. Two months after completing radiotherapy she found a lump in the scarred area of her left breast (**e**).

**Answer for Fig. 5.141, Question 2** (p. 278 f)

**Answer (c) is correct. Postoperative oil cyst.** A *local recurrence* would be unusual so soon after the completion of treatment for a G1 tumor. The absence of internal echoes on *sonography*, smooth margins, and posterior acoustic shadowing suggest oily contents. The absence of posterior acoustic enhancement excludes a *seroma*. An *oil cyst* is the most likely diagnosis after such a brief period (confirmed by *FNA*).

**Answer for Fig. 5.141, Question 3** (p. 278 f)

**Answer (c) is correct. Lipoma.** The cytologic features and subcutaneous location of the nodule are typical of lipoma.

**Answer for Fig. 5.141, Question 4** (p. 278 f)

**Answer (b) is correct. No,** because the tumor is located in the lower inner quadrant of the left breast, it most likely drains to the retrosternal nodes and would also metastasize in that direction. Thus, the normal-appearing axilla on that side does not have any real therapeutic implications.

The indication for chemotherapy depends not just on lymph node status but also on tumor characteristics (grade, protease status, immunohistochemical findings, etc.). Thus, the location of the tumor has less bearing on therapeutic decisions than its immunohistochemistry. Protease levels were normal, HER-2/neu status was negative, and hormone receptors of the G1 tumor were greatly increased. It was correct, then, to withhold chemotherapy and treat only with adjuvant antiestrogen therapy (7 years after therapy disease free).

### Answer for Fig. 5.142 (p. 280 f)

**Answer (a) is correct. Sclerosing adenosis.** A marked discrepancy exists between the cytologic features of a hypocellular process with uniform nuclei and compact chromatin (typical of adenosis) and the intense gadolinium enhancement seen at MRI. The latter study was done in the premenstrual phase of the cycle and yielded a false-positive result, as the sclerosing adenosis was more vascular than the rest of the parenchyma due to the cycle phase. It is unclear why a lymph node in the left axilla showed gadolinium enhancement. Nothing was palpable in that area except for a nonspecific firmness in the upper portion of the left breast. The sonogram was suspicious and would have been consistent with well-differentiated lobular carcinoma as well as adenosis. The proliferating TDLUs are located below the ends of the mammary lobes and respect their boundaries.

*Cystosarcoma phylloides* would also be possible on the basis of *ultrasound* and *MRI* findings. The *cytologic* findings do not support this diagnosis, however, as these nodules are very cellular and usually contain atypias.

**Lesson:** MRM and FNA performed during the premenstrual phase of the cycle (or in pregnancy) in young women not taking oral contraceptives will often yield a false-positive diagnosis.

### Answer for Fig. 5.143, Question 1 (p. 281 f)

**Answer (b) is correct. Invasive ductal carcinoma.**

**Fig. 5.143**

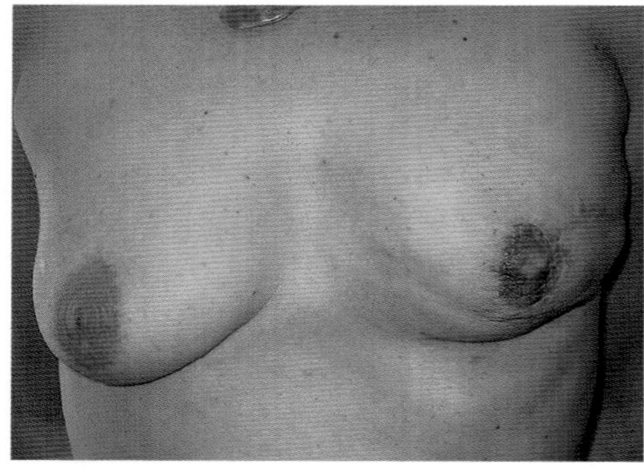

**e** *Clinical inspection* 2 years after mastectomy and reconstruction of the left breast shows good cosmetic results. Augustinus Harjanto Tulusan of Bayreuth (Germany) reconstructed the breast with advancements flaps from the back muscles.

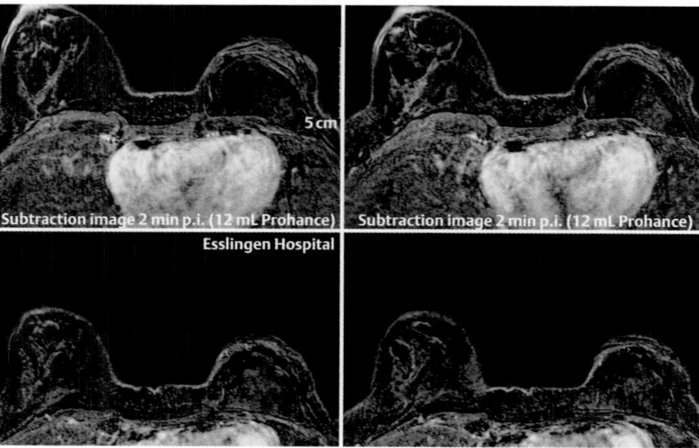


**f** MRM 8 years later. A latissimus dorsi flap together with a Silicon-Pat was used for postmastectomy reconstruction of the left breast. There is no evidence of local recurrence. Atypical gadolinium enhancement is no longer visible in the right breast. All current findings are normal.

### Answer for Fig. 5.143, Question 2 (p. 281 f)

**Answer (a) would be correct** because of the multiple enhancing foci on MRI.

### Answer for Fig. 5.143, Question 3 (p. 281 f)

**Answer (b) is correct. Breast-conserving treatment is not an option.** *MRI* shows multiple additional foci. *Histologic* evaluation of the breast parenchyma also indicates multifocal tumor spread wite EIC and DCIS with one affected lymph node, prompting mastectomy and aesthetic breast reconstruction 6 months later (see **e**). No tumor progression and no second tumor in the right breast were found 8 years after therapy (**f**).

### Answer for Fig. 5.144, Question 1 (p. 283 f)

**Answer (a) is correct. Galactocele,** which is harmless and occurs for a relatively short time during lactation. The nodule resolves spontaneously when aspirated, although it may reform as long as the patient is still lactating. Galactoceles have a predilection for the periphery of the breast, where they form small, padlike subcutaneous masses that are tender to pressure.

The constant hormone levels during lactation inhibit cyst formation and do not support the diagnosis of a benign cyst. The absence of internal echoes and significant posterior acoustic enhancement at ultrasound would not be consistent with *medullary carcinoma.*

### Answer for Fig. 5.144 Question 2 (p. 283 f)

**Answer (b) is correct. Images show a harmless layer of inspissated or "caseated" milk.** This is typical of galactoceles and has nothing to do with intracystic proliferation.

**Lesson:** If the galactocele is not aspirated, the milk will continue to thicken and mimic a solid nodule ("cheese cyst") that may be mistaken at *ultrasound* for carcinoma (**f**).

**Fig. 5.144**

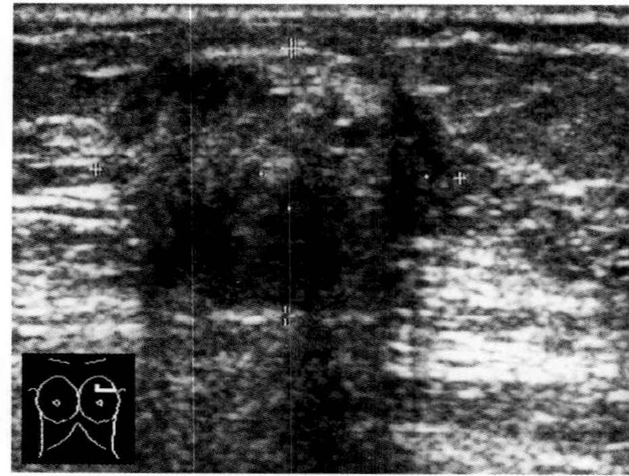

**f** *Sonogram* from a different patient shows a 2 cm mobile nodule that developed in the upper portion of the left breast after the cessation of breastfeeding. CNB identified the nodule as a *cheese cyst*. The cyst resolved spontaneously over the next few months.

### Answer for Fig. 5.145, Question 1 (p. 285 f)

**Answer (d) is correct. This will save costs and reduce the radiation dose by half.** With an atypical clinical presentation, a malignant process should always be excluded *mammographically*, even during pregnancy, because *microcalcifications* are not detectable by ultrasound. A single view of the affected breast (oblique view) is sufficient, however. The oblique projection also directs the x-ray beam upward, protecting the lesser pelvis and the fetus from exposure even to scattered x-rays.

### Answer for Fig. 5.145, Question 2 (p. 285 f)

**Answer (a) is correct. The redness is caused by lactating lobular hyperplasia with associated interstitial inflammation (lactation nodule).**

**Note:** Lactation nodules (circumscribed or diffuse) are relatively rare and produce only mild complaints but may cause conspicuous skin changes. The hyperplasia resolved spontaneously in this case.

### Answer for Fig. 5.146 (p. 286 f)

**Answer (b) is correct.**

**Lactating adenoma** with no evidence of malignancy. Lactating adenomas are easily mistaken for malignancies at *cytology* due to their apparent pleomorphic cells and their prominent nucleoli reflecting increased exocrine activity. The absence of cell clusters and the myriad foam cells in this case do not support a diagnosis of malignancy. The cytologic abnormalities prompted surgical removal of the nodule, but no malignancy was found.

Regression of the lesion from July to September documented *mammographically* and *sonographically*, is not consistent with *medullary carcinoma* or *intracystic ductal papilloma.* Aside from the cytologic findings, all evidence suggests that the lesion is probably not malignant. The lobulated margins would have been consistent with *papilloma*, but the well-defined border visible in **d** and **e** does not support a diagnosis of *medullary carcinoma*.

**Lesson:** Cytologic examinations are very problematic during pregnancy and lactation due to the marked proliferative changes that are present. False-positive findings are almost inevitable. Abnormalities should be investigated by CNB or VB, especially if a diffuse process is suspected (e.g., *inflammatory carcinoma*). The pathologist receiving the biopsy samples should be told if the patient is pregnant or breastfeeding so that he can better interpret the proliferative changes.

### Answer for Fig. 5.147 (p. 288)

**Answer (c) is correct. The postoperative and postpartum swelling can be explained both by postoperative changes and by local recurrence.** *MRI* is more suggestive of a malignant process in the right breast. *PET* scans (**f**) were ordered to narrow the differential diagnosis and detect or exclude distant metastases. The scans reveal a large recurrent tumor in the right breast and two satellite lesions near the axilla (not visible in **f** but visible in **g**). Distant metastases are not found.

**Lesson:** PET scans are useful for detecting or excluding a local recurrence in dense breasts while simultaneously screening for nodal and distant metastases (see **Fig. 5.184**). These findings have major therapeutic implications for the patient.

**Fig. 5.147**

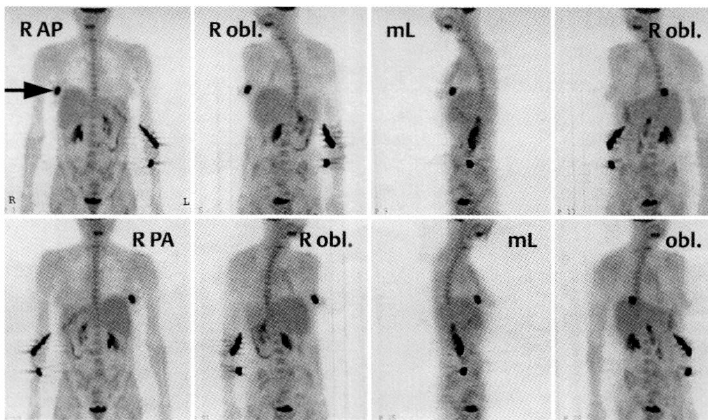


**f** *Whole-body PET* (rotating view) demonstrates a 3 cm hypermetabolic mass in the right breast (arrow). There is no evidence of metastases elsewhere in the body.

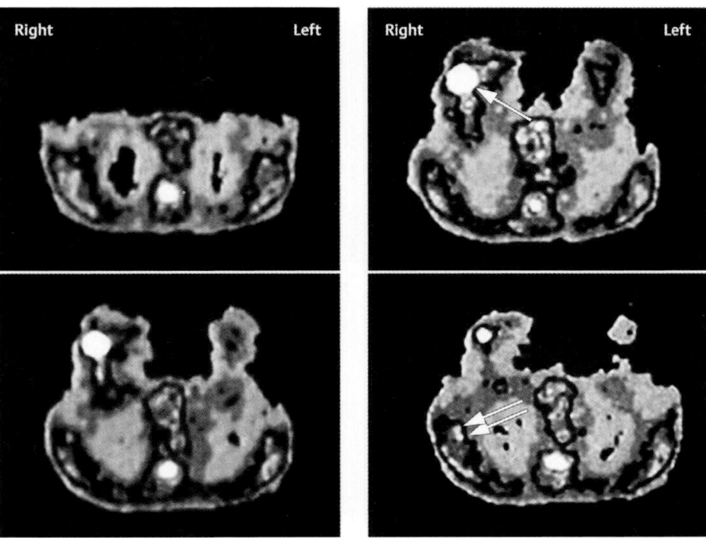


**g** *Transverse PET* scans show an approximately 3 cm mass in the right breast (arrow) and two small metastases in the right axilla (double arrow).

## Answer for Fig. 5.148 (p. 289 f)

**Answer (c) is correct.**

**Inflammatory carcinoma during pregnancy and lactation.** The fact that orange-peel dimpling of the left breast developed 3 months after the cessation of lactation does not support a diagnosis of galactostasis or postpartum mastitis. This fact should have alerted the attending gynecologist, who suspected puerperal mastitis and prescribed a prolactin inhibitor, which did reduce the swelling somewhat. *FNA* of the sonographic change (**e**) yielded large numbers of tumor epithelial cells, and *CNB* showed *moderately differentiated ductal carcinoma with lymphatic invasion.* All level 1–3 lymph nodes showed metastatic involvement. A lymph node metastasis was also found in the *left cervical triangle.* The tumor was receptor-positive.

A partial mastectomy was performed, and the lateral portion of the breast was reconstructed and augmented with a subcutaneous Nova Gold implant (**g**). Tissue was also removed intraoperatively for the production of a *live vaccine.* The patient received chemotherapy and antihormonal therapy; radiotherapy was withheld.

Later a prosthetic infection developed on the left side, accompanied by a cutaneous fistula. The implant was removed (**h**), the infection was eradicated, and an advancement flap reconstruction was performed (**i**). A reduction mammoplasty was performed on the right breast several months later with a relatively good cosmetic outcome (**j**). *Systemic spread occurred as of 2008 (ten years later), valuable time in which to bring up her child* (**k**).

**Lesson:** A detailed history including the time of onset of initial clinical symptoms is important for narrowing the differential diagnosis, especially in postpartum patients.

## Answer for Fig. 5.149, Question 1 (p. 291 f)

**Answer (b) is correct. Yes.** Genetic predisposition is also an important factor in males. Men from families with a history of breast cancer—often first-born males—are at increased risk for developing breast cancer, although this risk is 100 times lower for males than females. In women as well, breast cancer appears to have a predilection for first-borns. This may be because higher estrogen levels are developed during the first pregnancy than in subsequent pregnancies. Thus, intrauterine hyperestrogenism may be considered a risk factor for breast cancer in first-born males and females (Titus-Ernstoff et al. 2002). Both sexes transmit their genetic defects to male and female descendents. Patients with *Klinefelter syndrome* are 50 times more likely to develop breast cancer than men and women without the syndrome.

**Lesson:** The diagnosis of a malignancy is rarely entertained in males, with the result that male breast cancer is often diagnosed at a relatively late stage. Even males with a positive family history of breast cancer should practice self-examination. A genetic predisposition to breast cancer is inherited and transmitted to the same degree in both sexes.

A breast nodule should always raise the possibility of breast cancer, even in males, although a breast nodule in males 15–30 years of age is most likely due to gynecomastia or nodular thickening of the rudimentary gland (80% of male newborns under intrauterine estrogen-stimulus from the mother).

**Fig. 5.148**

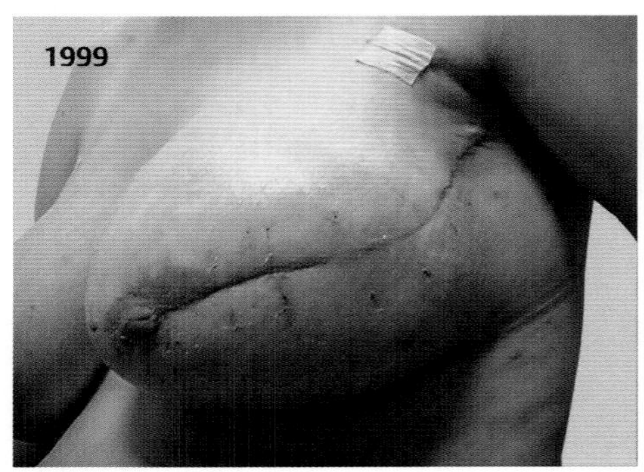


**g** *Clinical inspection:* Postoperative *appearance* of the left breast in 1999 following reconstruction with a subcutaneous implant.

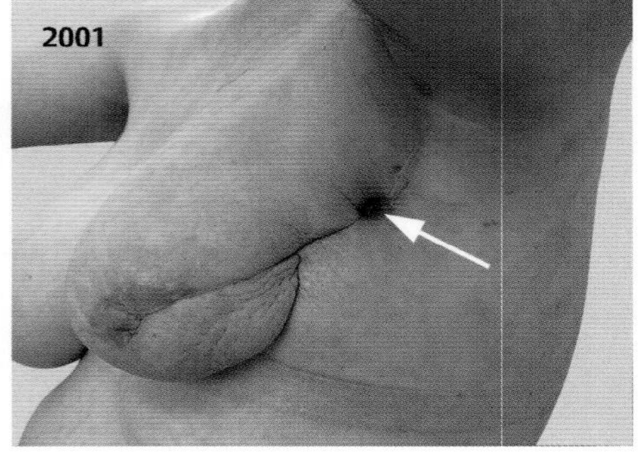


**h** *Appearance* in 2001 with a prosthetic infection and chronic fistula. The infected implant was removed.

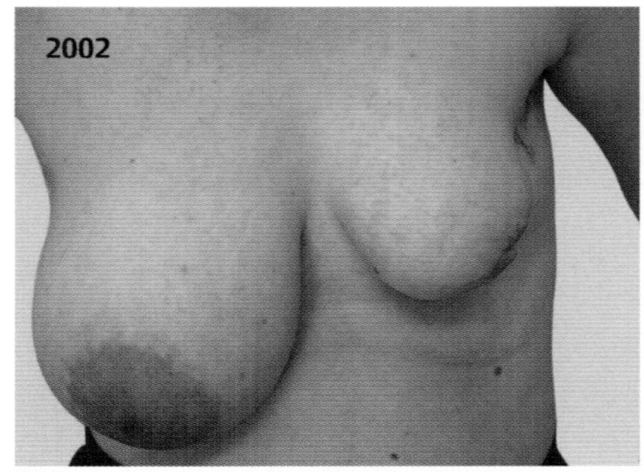


**i** *Appearance* of both breasts in 2002 following partial left mastectomy and fistulous tract removal.

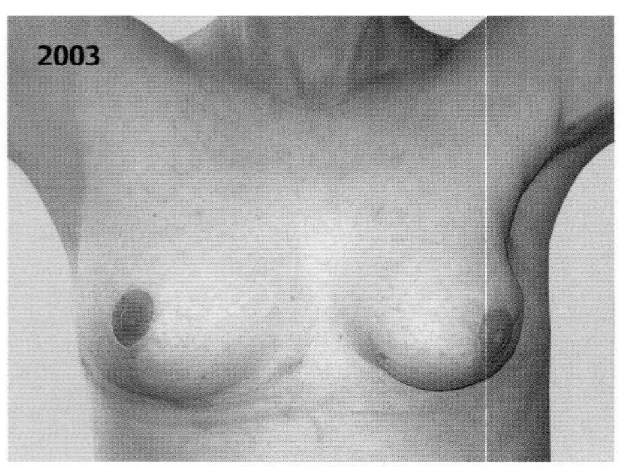


**j** *Appearance* of both breasts in 2003 following reduction mammoplasty of the right breast and reconstruction of the left nipple using portions of the right nipple.

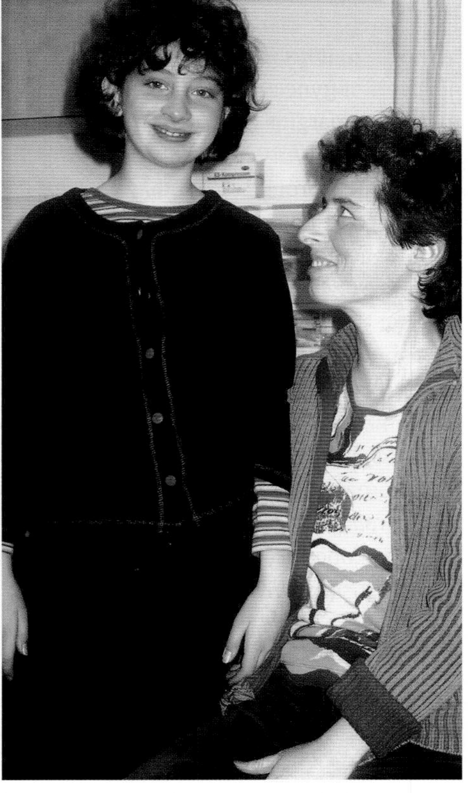

**k** *Extra years of life.* Mother and daughter 10 years after the mother developed an inflammatory neoplasm while pregnant with her daughter. The mother was able to raise her child for over a decade before initial skeletal metastases developed.

Fig. 5.149

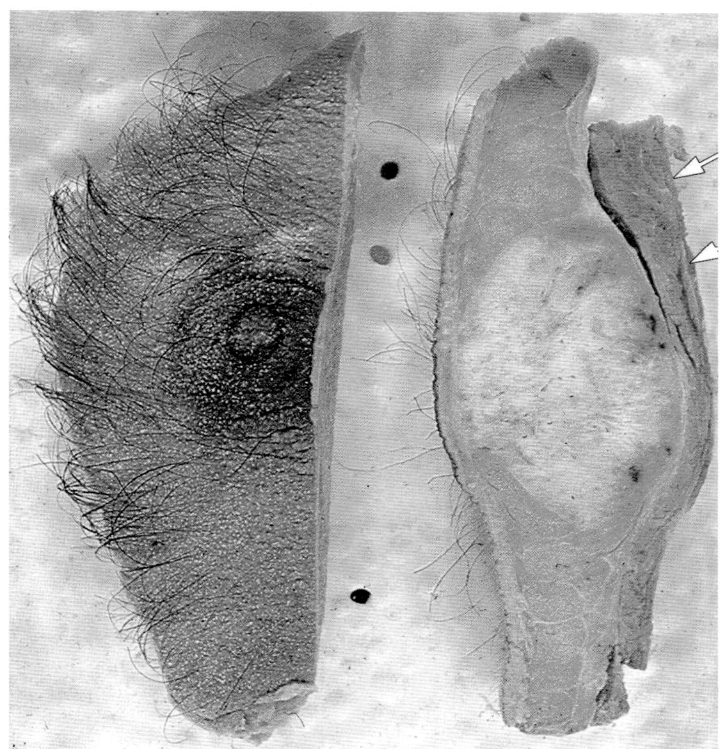

**g** *Anatomic specimen* of *gynecomastia* (different patient from **d–f**) shows a lobulated grayish-white tumor with smooth or scalloped margins. Blood vessels and fat deposits (yellowish) are visible within the tumor, and fatty tissue is also visible around the nodule (yellow). Pectoral muscle is visible at far right (arrows).

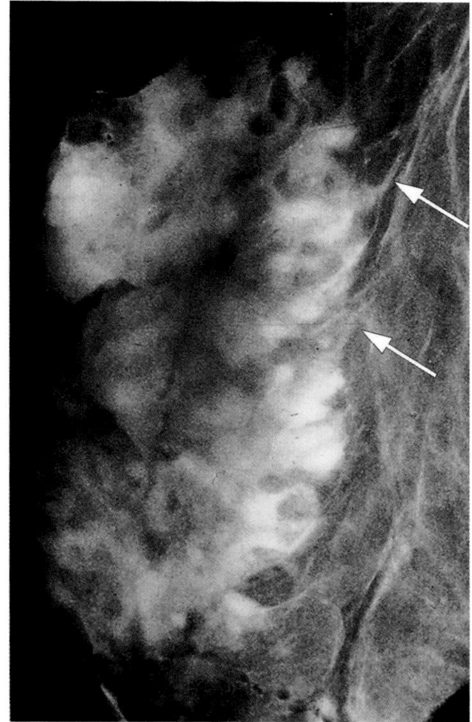

**h** *Specimen radiograph* of *gynecomastia* (same patient as in **g**) shows inhomogeneous opacities with scalloped margins throughout. Individual fibrous septa (part of the suspensory apparatus connecting the breast to the pectoral muscle) are visible at right (arrows).

### Answer for Fig. 5.149, Question 2 (p. 291 f)

**Answer (b) is correct. Gynecomastia.** The nodule displays the classic features of gynecomastia. It has smooth anterior margins, while its posterior margins appear slightly ill-defined due to overlying glandular parenchyma (**g, h**). *Histology* shows obvious demarcation between the fibrous *inter*lobular stroma and periductal *intra*lobular stroma (blue) (**i, j**).

The acute stage of gynecomastia is usually painful, whereas the chronic stage is not. It would be unusual to see carcinoma in a patient of this age. The nodule displays the classic mammographic, sonographic, and cytologic features of gynecomastia. Carcinoma has the same malignancy criteria in males as in females (stellate or lobulated mass, microcalcifications, usually retroareolar, etc.). Papilloma also displays the same features as in females. Bloody nipple discharge may occur in both sexes (see **Fig. 5. 151a**, p. 296). *Ultrasound* and *cytology* after *FNA* do not support a diagnosis of *ductal papilloma*. The concavity and smooth borders of the cellular aggregate are also consistent with a benign process.

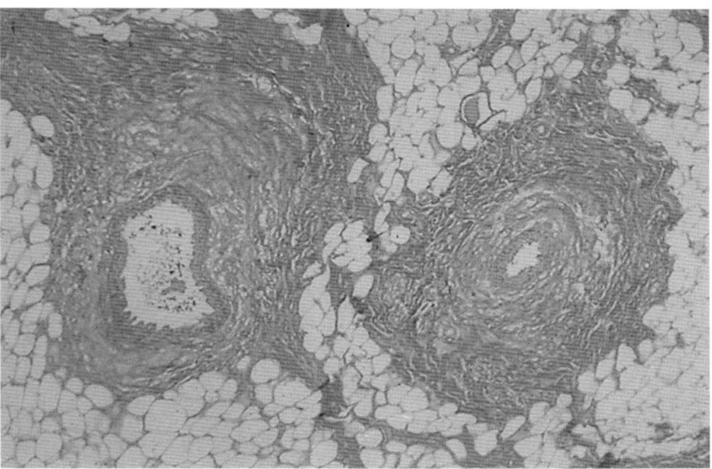

**i** Different patient from **d–h**. *Histologic section* (20×) in the acute stage shows mucopolysaccharide-rich loose intralobular stroma (blue) around the ducts. This architecture may produce a reverse echo pattern with a hyperechoic central duct (see **Fig. 4.5**, p. 27).

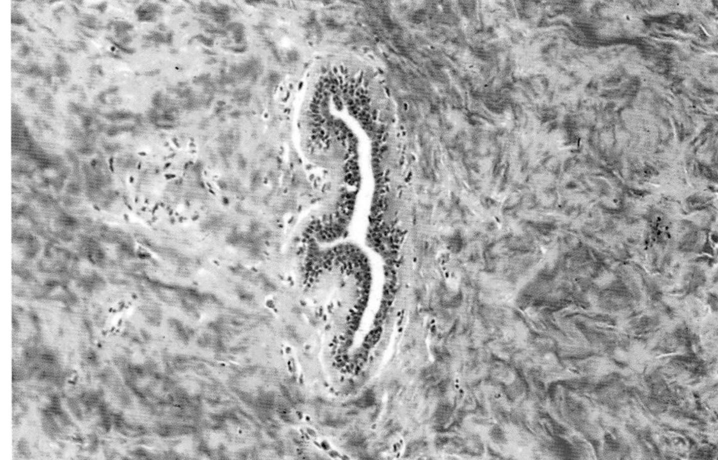

**j** *Histologic section* (120×) (different region from **c**) shows fibrosis (*inter*lobular stroma, red) with no demarcation of periductal *intra*lobular stroma (blue). A duct appears at the center of the section.

**Answer for Fig. 5.150** (p. 293 f)

**Answer (b) is correct. Scarring after subcutaneous mastectomy.** Histological examination of the reexcision specimen from the right breast in 2001 showed retroareolar tissue with *fibrocystic change, focal scarring, and focal fat necrosis with no evidence of malignancy.* The soft-tissue specimen contained fibrotic scarring with some peripheral nerve encasement. It is unclear how scarring developed in areas of fat necrosis even though the previous examination (March, 2000) showed no such change.

This finding is sufficient to account for the increasing retroareolar pain and firmness. It is impossible to remove all the breast parenchyma while leaving the nipple intact. Residual retroareolar parenchyma may continue to proliferate as long as the precipitating cause of gynecomastia (presumably the diuretic in this case) remains. The changes in the left breast are also due to postoperative scarring and fat necrosis; they are not the result of a local recurrence.

The mammograms do not exclude breast cancer. Based on the course, however, it is unlikely that a malignancy would develop after subcutaneous mastectomy. If doubt exists, it would be appropriate to obtain another retroareolar biopsy. This could be accomplished by vacuum biopsy. Gynecomastia is a good indication for vacuum biopsy (but be careful of the nipple!).

**Lesson:** Diuretics (also EADH) may provoke gynecomastia. Fat necrosis and scars after subcutaneous mastectomy may display the same mammographic and clinical features as gynecomastia or breast cancer (nipple retraction, pain from nerve ingrowth, granulation-tissue nodule). Scars are homogeneously dense, contrasting with the branched dendritic pattern of gynecomastia. Vacuum biopsy is an ideal method for the "bloodless" removal of rudimentary glandular tissue in gynecomastia and for the benign–malignant discrimination of postoperative changes. In the case shown, the retroareolar fibrosis would be described as *pseudogynecomastia*. The most common type of *physiologic (true) gynecomastia* in adolescents resolves spontaneously without treatment within 3 years in up to 90% of cases. The gynecomastia that develops in response to antiandrogenic therapy for prostate cancer can be prevented by radiotherapy or tamoxifen (Wimpissinger and Esterbauer 2008).

**Answer for Fig. 5.152** (p. 296 f)

**Answer (c) is correct. Advanced breast carcinoma with carcinomatous lymphangitis and typical orange-peel skin.** The skin pores are especially prominent in the periareolar region (**a**). The lobulated tumor shape suggests a very cellular malignancy (see **Fig. 4.34 c**, p. 64). The *mammogram* shows increased reticular markings extending into the subcutaneous tissue (lymphatic obstruction). The breast therefore is firm to palpation. The axillary lymph nodes are swollen and involved by tumor. Harmless pseudogynecomastia due to hyperplasia of fatty tissue is present on the left side. The sagged position of the areola and the apparent skin retraction in the inframammary fold (**q–r/18** in panel **d**) result from normal loss of skin tone in this 82-year-old man.

**Lesson:** In a "flabby" breast with skin folds, the mammographic technologist should be skilled enough to position the breast so that the skin folds are not visible. Perfect mammographic positioning technique avoids errors of interpretation. Projecting the nipple or areola into the breast can mimic an intramammary mass. Even when a carcinoma is known to be present in one breast, the opposite breast should be imaged just as carefully

**Fig. 5.152**

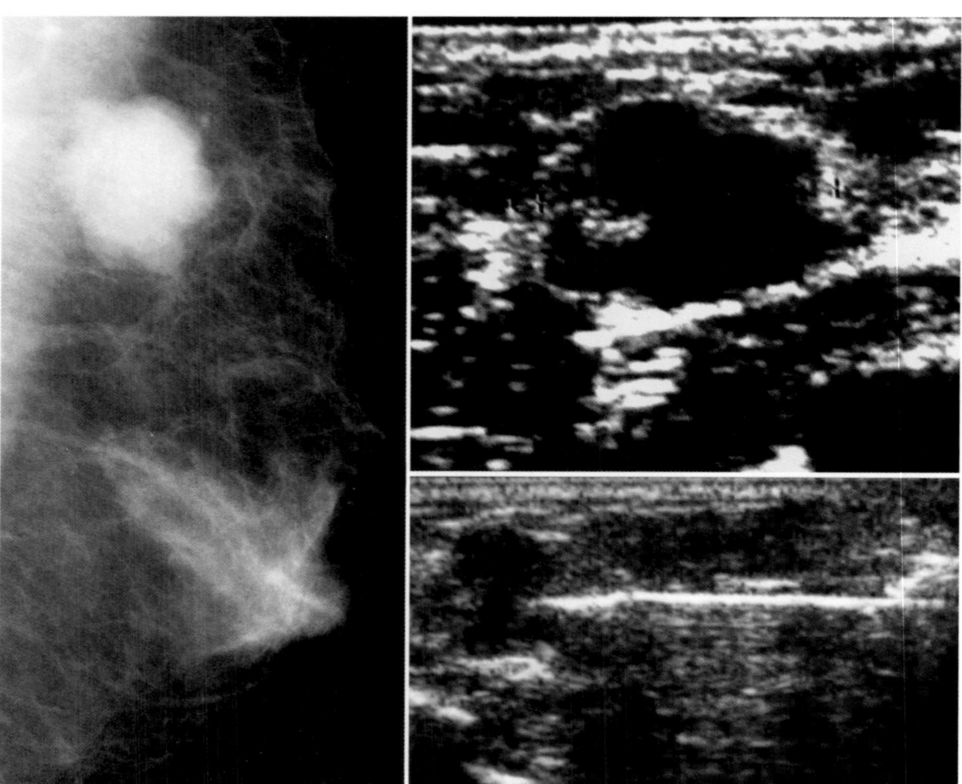

**Male breast cancer does not always develop from gynecomastia as a retroareolar lesion, as the following example shows** (images courtesy of Heinrich Uedelhoven, Haan).

**f** *Oblique mammogram* of the left breast shows gynecomastia with a retroareolar density (**a–c/3–6**). A 1.5 cm homogeneously dense tumor nodule with scalloped margins is visible in the upper prepectoral region of the breast (**a–b/9–11**) (*histology:* adenocarcinoma). The sonographic equivalent is shown on the right side above, image at lower right shows the lesion at **D–d/4** prior to CNB.

### Answer for Fig. 5.153 (p. 298)

**Answer (c) is correct. Shadows from the nipple and areola.** The oblique view *mammography* (not shown) is well positioned and shows mild gynecomastia with no tumorlike densities. Gynecomastia shows some degree of gadolinium enhancement on *MRI* (**d–E/ 9 + 12**).

### Answer for Fig. 5.154 (p. 301)

**Answer (a) is correct. The localization wire should be placed anterior to the calcifications** so that the surgeon first encounters the wire and is then able to resect a generous amount of tissue behind it. If the wire is behind the calcifications or even passing through the lesion, the dissecting surgeon will probably destroy the structures he is trying to remove in a complete, intact state with a healthy tissue margin.

The localization wire in **b** is approximately 2 cm from the microcalcifications, which is too far from the region of interest. It is also *behind* the area to be examined.

### Answer for Fig. 5.156, Question 1 (p. 303)

**Answer (a) is correct. Wire 1.** The adenosis is located at the 11 o'clock position (1), far from the other two calcification clusters. It shows uniform, rounded calcifications in dense glandular tissue (**c**).

The calcifications at 2 and 3 are consistent with foci of *DCIS*. The focus at wire 2 was clinically palpable as a nodule. Because the breast was small, a relatively large amount of tissue had to be removed, causing skin retraction in the inframammary fold (**e**). Seven years later, however, the breast shows a good cosmetic outcome owing to the ingrowth of subcutaneous fat into the surgical bed (**f**, p. 398). The breast received postoperative radiation, and Tamoxifen therapy was recommended.

> ***Lesson:** DCIS accounts for 20–25 % of all breast malignancies. The risk of developing invasive cancer is increased 10- to 12-fold, and there is an approximately 30 % chance of developing invasive cancer during the next 20 years. Every third woman with DCIS undergoes mastectomy—a percentage that is much too high when compared with the risk of invasive disease. Radiotherapy can reduce this risk by 60 %, and adding tamoxifen will reduce it an additional 25 % (SEER database; Baxter et al. 2005). These adjuvant therapies are particularly effective in women under 50 years of age.*

### Answer for Fig. 5.156, question 2 (p. 303)

**Answer (b) is correct. Polychemotherapy is unnecessary for DCIS,** but adjuvant hormonal therapy is indicated (estrogen- and progesterone-receptor-positive tumor). Postoperative radiotherapy to the breast is also indicated for *every* DCIS.

In practical terms, these recommendations are enacted mainly for DCIS lesions larger than 2 cm and for high-grade types of DCIS (Van Nuys Index 7–9, see p. 58). Since this case involved a high-grade (G3) DCIS larger than 2 cm, radiotherapy and antiestrogen therapy were definitely indicated.

### Answer for Fig. 5.156, question 3 (p. 303)

**Answer (b) is correct. Every 6 months.** It depends on the guidelines of the specific country: **USA** (The American College of Radiology, ACR): 6 months after BCT, thereafter annually (for at least 10 years). **Austria** and **Switzerland**: annually for both breasts. The follow-up intervals are the same as for invasive carcinoma. In the case of DCIS, it is better to schedule the follow-ups (for at least 10 years) at even shorter intervals (see p. 35).

**Lesson:** Following DCIS or ADH, bilateral mammograms should be taken every 6 months (for the healthy breast every year) for 3 years and then at 1-year intervals thereafter. Local recurrences are most commonly evidenced by microcalcifications.

> *The local recurrence rate of DCIS after BCT and radiation treatment is 7 % at 5 years, and 12 % at 8 years. After 10 years the recurrence rate is 14.8 % with radiation, and 26.0 % after lumpectomy without radiation (Baxter et al. 2000).*

**Fig. 5.156**

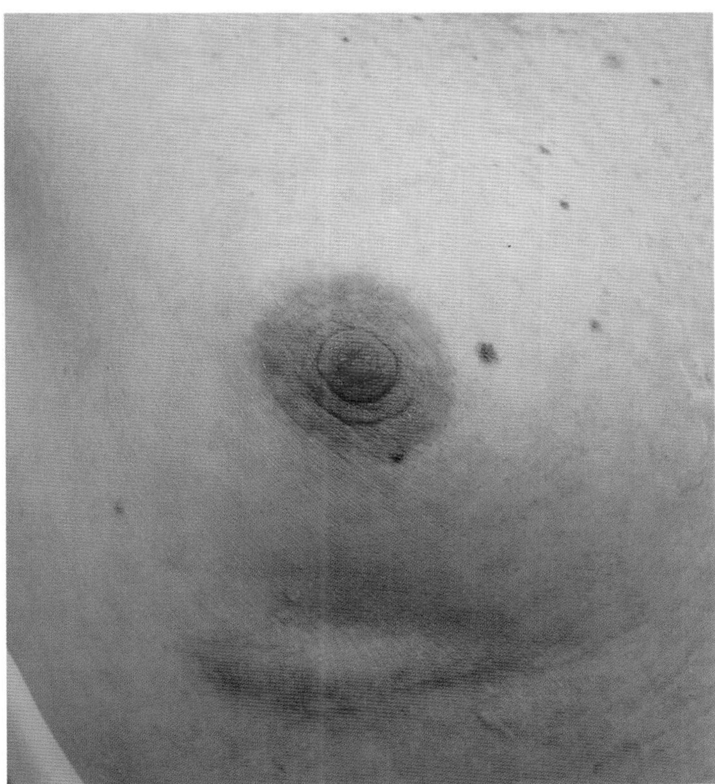

**e** *Clinical inspection* of the right breast 2 years after surgery and radiotherapy.

▶ **Fig. 5.156f**

**Fig. 5.156** *(continued)*

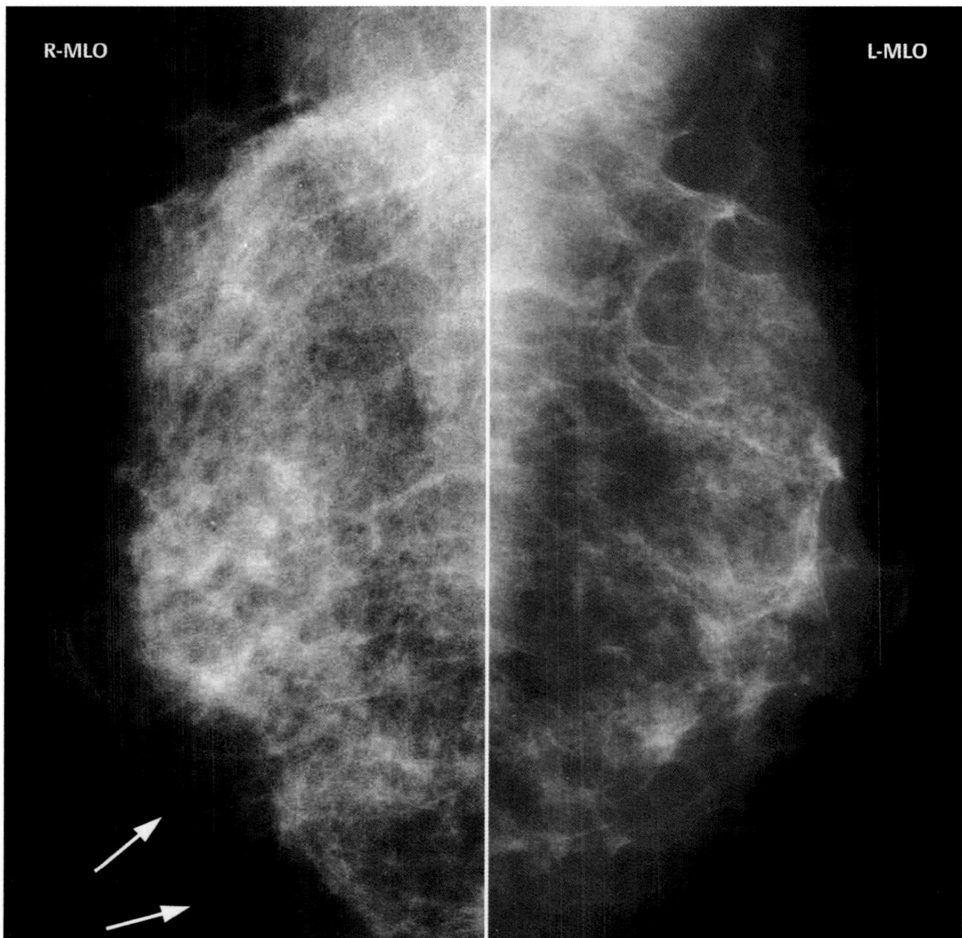


**f** *Bilateral oblique mammograms* 18 months after surgery and radiotherapy show diffuse radiation fibrosis with densities visible in the right breast relative to the left breast (right ACR 3, left ACR 2). Copious subcutaneous fat is present in the lower portion of the operative area (arrows).

### Answer for Fig. 5.157 (p. 304 f)

**Answer (a) is correct. Ultrasound.** The lesion is best visualized with ultrasound, which is also the fastest and cheapest modality for lesion localization. The localization film (**f**) shows the localization wire at the same site where the tumor is visible in **a** and **b** (**F/10, F/22**). This also corresponds to the sonogram.

**Lesson:** The lesion in the left breast is clearly visualized with ultrasound. It is unclear why the lesion was not localized under ultrasound guidance in 1997. At that time the lesion appeared suspicious only on MRI. Because stereotactic and MRI-guided aspiration were not available, contrast bolus CT was performed and provided clear tumor visualization and localization (**e**). If a stereotactic or simple needle guide had been available at that time, the lesion could also have been localized in *one* mammographic plane if it had not been visible in the other view. (When the mammogram was digitized for publication in this book, the tumor was defined more clearly than in the original analog film!).

### Answer for Fig. 5.167, Question 1 (p. 312)

**Answer (a) is correct.** The sentinel lymph node scan gives no more than indirect evidence of a malignant process, being used in both suspected *and* histologically confirmed cases of malignancy. Lymph nodes visualized on the scintigram are *localized* rather than *diagnosed.* Metastases cannot be confirmed or excluded.

**Lesson:** The sentinel lymph node procedure is costly and complex, and hospitals cannot afford it for benign processes. It is essential, therefore, to establish the benign or malignant nature of a lesion prior to surgery.

### Answer for Fig. 5.167, Question 2 (p. 312)

**Answer (a) is correct. Level I.** Because only one prepectoral lymph node group is visualized in the axillary recess and other nodes show uptake toward the clavicle, it is not appropriate to proceed with a level II or level III axillary lymphadenectomy. Indeed, it is questionable whether any axillary dissection should be performed. It would be better to locate and remove the clavicular lymph nodes, although that is difficult in practice. These nodes should definitely be included in the radiotherapy field.

**Lesson:** When a SLN cannot be visualized in the axilla, there is no reason to proceed with an axillary dissection.

### Answer for Fig. 5.168 (p. 312 f)

**Answer (c) is correct. Only radiation without axillary dissection.** The clavicular and retrosternal lymph nodes are inoperable because they are mostly retrosternal or retropectoral. At radiotherapy, then, these nodes should be included in the field for the breast or treated with a separate sternal field (a *PET* scan was negative for lymph node

**Fig. 5.168**

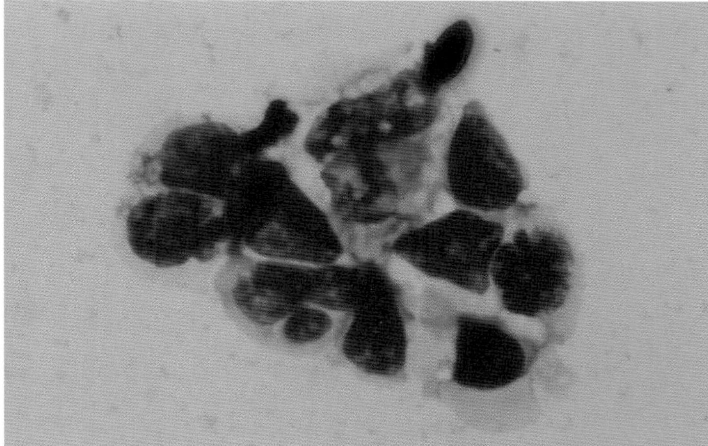

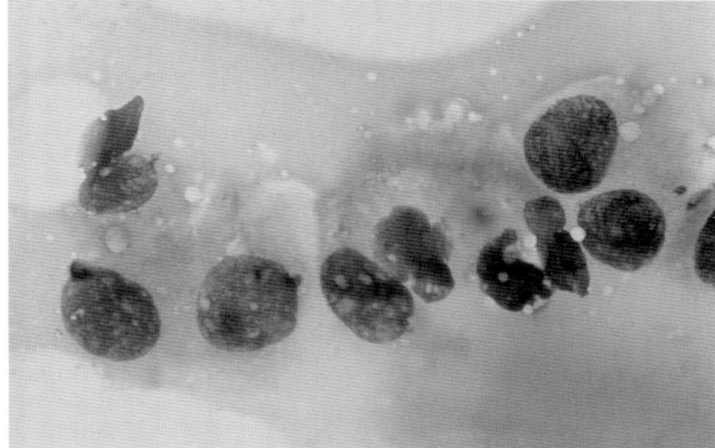

**e** *FNA cytology. Above:* a cluster of pleomorphic ductal carcinoma cells on one side with a finely vacuolated cytoplasm and nuclear degeneration. *Below:* dense cluster of poorly differentiated ductal carcinoma cells showing minimal degenerative change, 3 years after radiotherapy. The cell degeneration indicates that the tumor has no metastatic potential.

metastases). It is essential to avoid overlapping the two radiotherapy fields (see **Fig. 5.181a, b**, p. 330).

Axillary dissection is not appropriate with a sentinel lymph node pattern of this kind. It would constitute overtreatment and would risk lymphedema of the arm.

Three years after the completion of treatment, the patient noticed a small infra-areolar nodule that was visible on *mammograms* (**d**). *FNA* cytology was strongly suspicious for tumor cells (Pap V, **e**), but subsequent *CNB* revealed *radiogenic dysplasia* with no evidence of malignant process.

#### Answer for Fig. 5.169, Question 1 (p. 314 f)

**Answer (b) is correct. About 50%.** A small portion of the calcifications was removed in the first operation but was not described by the pathologist (*histology*: benign adenosis).

#### Answer for Fig. 5.169, Question 2 (p. 314 f)

**Answer (b) is correct. No.** The lesion is not located in the scarred area. Ultrasound localizes it to the 6-o'clock position in the areolar region. When the ultrasound findings were known, the lesion was palpable as a lentil-sized nodule. Despite its palpability, it was localized with ultrasound guidance and removed with clear margins.

#### Answer for Fig. 5.169, Question 3 (p. 314 f)

**Answer (c) is correct. None.** With a *well-differentiated tubular carcinoma* 7 mm in diameter, it is unnecessary to proceed with lymphadenectomy. This tumor does not metastasize, so there is no need to perform preoperative staging or look for metastases later (Kühn 2008).

The sentinel lymph node located in the anterior axilla could be removed. The sternal lymph node is posterior to the sternum and is accessible only through a sternotomy.

In the case shown, definitive histology was established only after the entire tumor was removed. Hence the recommended guidelines could not be followed, and the axillary sentinel lymph node was removed. It proved to be negative.

**Problem 1:** Preoperative localization and specimen radiography. If these are not done according to guidelines, reexcisions will be inevitable. In the case shown, the nature of the calcifications was determined in a second sitting by *digital stereotactic CNB*, and this time the calcifications were described by the pathologist. The diagnosis of "adenosis with calcifications" was upheld, but the left breast was left with a preventable scar.

**Problem 2:** *Ultrasound-guided localization* was not performed in the right breast (3). This step is often omitted with palpable lesions, as some surgeons prefer to rely on their palpable impression. Unfortunately, this method is not always successful. Failure to remove tumors may lead to second and third operations with cosmetically objectionable scarring. The scar at the 3-o'clock position in the right breast was unnecessary. Another biopsy compounded the breast disfigurement (**f**).

**Fig. 5.169**

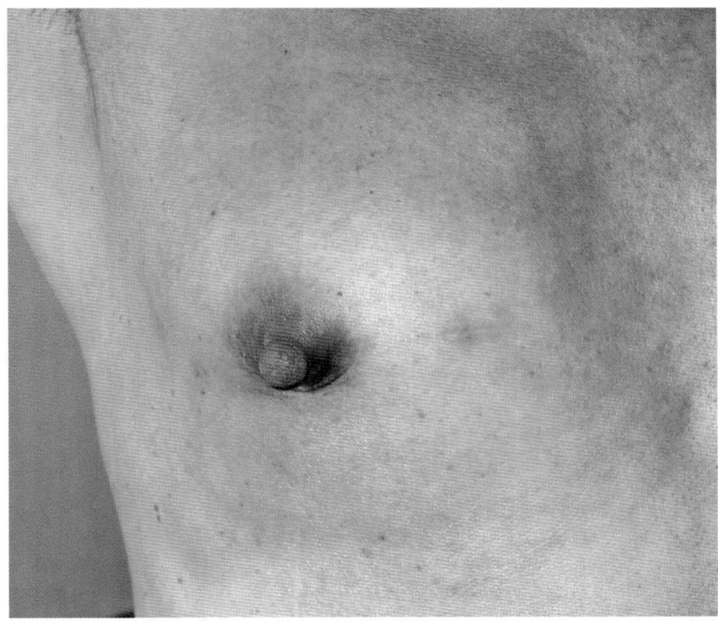

**f** *Clinical appearance* of the right breast after two operations. The breast is small and moderately disfigured.

### Answer for Fig. 5.170 (p. 316 f)

**Answer (c) is correct. Postoperative oil cysts.** It appears that relatively large tissue defects were created, as the density in the operated portions of the breast decreased from ACR 3 to ACR 2.

This presentation would be unusual for *carcinomatous lymphangitis* and *mastitis* because the patient was experiencing no complaints.

*Oil cysts* were confirmed by ultrasound-guided *FNA*. The oil cysts may form coarse calcifications over a period of years (see **Fig. 5.131**, p. 264).

**Lesson:** Operations on the breast complicate the differential diagnosis. This is distressful for patients and may prompt interventional procedures and costly follow-ups. The calcifications in the left breast 2000 could have been investigated by digital stereotactic CNB instead of unnecessary breast surgery.

### Answer for Fig. 5.171 (p. 317 f)

**Answer (a) is correct. Fat necrosis with oil cysts.** Remarkably, this did not occur in the immediate postoperative period but two years later, causing the patient considerable anxiety. The complaints on the left side resolved over the next year, while necrosis and oil cysts were surgically removed from the right breast.

The changes are unrelated to a malignant process. It is unusual to find hematomas two years postoperatively. Similarly, there is nothing to support a diagnosis of epidermal cysts, which are not painful and are usually intradermal or subdermal.

**Lesson:** Postoperative fat necrosis may quickly develop small focal calcifications (especially during adjuvant chemotherapy), mimicking the mammographic appearance of DCIS (see **Fig. 5.174**, p. 321).

### Answer for Fig. 5.172 (p. 319)

**Answer (c) is correct. Both are possible.** The patient declined reexcision. A subsequent PET examination showed no suspicious findings in the operated breast or elsewhere in the body. Because the tumor had been widely excised with clear margins (except posteriorly), the changes could be due to young granulation tissue showing gadolinium enhancement on MRI. The breast subsequently received postoperative radiation and was still free of disease in 2008 (9 years after completion of radiotherapy)

**Lesson:** In the MRI analysis of postoperative changes, it is important to know where the tumor was removed with positive margins or minimal clear margins. This makes it easier to determine whether the changes are malignant or benign. It has been stated in the literature that MRI of the breast is unrewarding for up to 12 months after the completion of radiotherapy, but this is not true. Postoperative analysis would be aided by having preoperative MR images available for comparison, but unfortunately MRM is not always performed before breast-conserving surgery because of the cost.

### Answer for Fig. 5.173 (p. 320)

**Answer (b) is correct. Lymphedema after breast-conserving treatment.** The edema resolved completely with 4 years of lymph drainage therapy (**f, g**). Ultrasound findings also returned to normal (**h**). The treated left breast is still radiodense on mammograms because of diffuse fibrosis (**i**, p. 401). Overall, however, breast density has declined relative to the previous examination in 1999.

**Fig. 5.173**

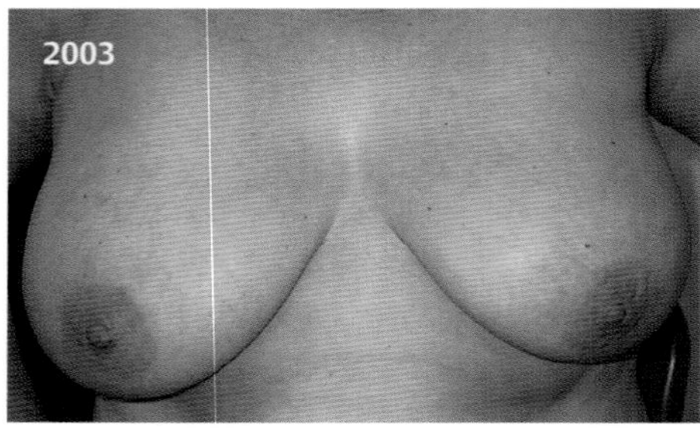


**f** *Clinical appearance.* The left breast appears completely normal on visual inspection.

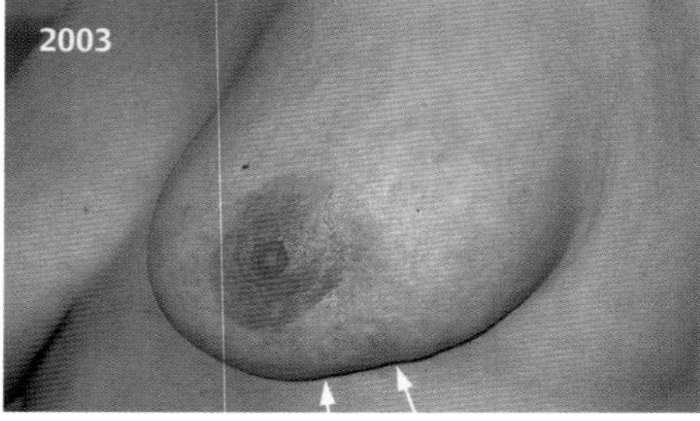


**g** *Clinical appearance* of the left breast shows complete regression of orange-peel dimpling. Post-treatment changes appear as slight contour irregularities in the lower portion of the breast (arrows).

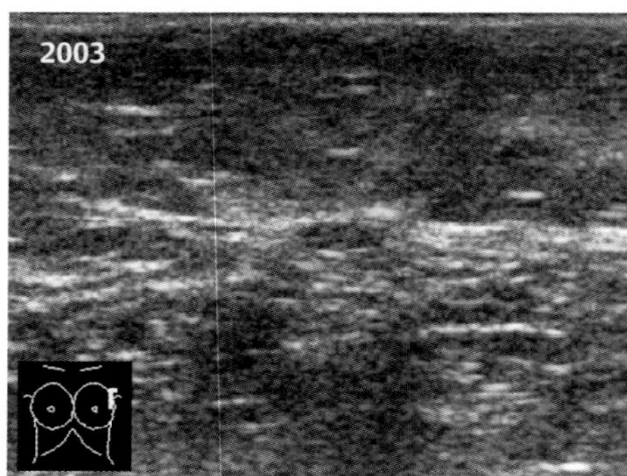


**h** *Sonogram* of the left breast shows normal breast parenchyma with no lobular proliferation. The lymphatic pathways are no longer visible. The skin appears as a thin fine line (compare with **c**, p. 320).

Several findings are inconsistent with *carcinomatous lymphangitis:* the normal *MR* images, the relatively gradual swelling of the left breast, and the normal appearance of subcutaneous structures on *mammograms.* (With inflammatory carcinoma, the Cooper ligaments become enlarged and cause increased reticular markings that are especially prominent in the subcutaneous plane.)

The clinical features are not consistent with *nonpuerperal mastitis,* as the patient did not present with local warmth or pain in the left breast.

**Note:** Lymphedema may develop for up to 3 years after therapy. The reason for this is a gradually progressive fibrosis of the axilla and axillary lymphatics in response to radiotherapy. The enlarged lymphatics are detectable by ultrasound. *Manual lymph drainage* is helpful and should involve not just the breast but also the shoulder girdle and axilla. Sixty percent of patients with lymphedema of the breast also develop swelling of the ipsilateral arm (> 2 cm increase in arm circumference).

**Fig. 5.173** *(continued)*

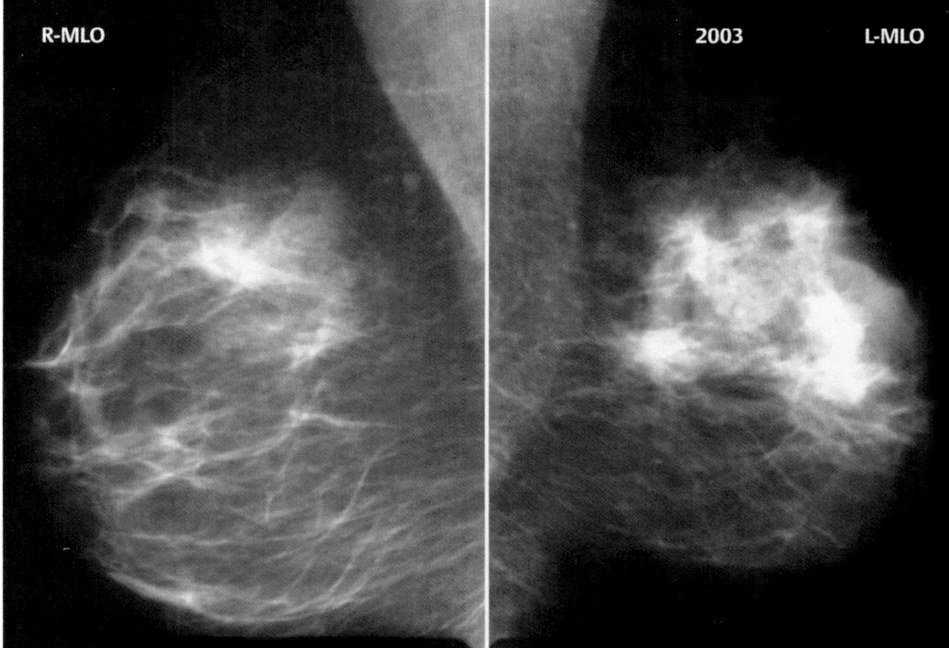


**i** *Bilateral oblique mammograms* in 2003 show greater radiodensity of the left breast with nonspecific scarlike densities (**O–p/22–25**), cc view: compare with prior mammogram in 1999, panel **b**, p. 320. The right breast appears normal (ACR 3 left, ACR 2 right, BIRADS 2 left.

## Answer for Fig. 5.174 (p. 321f)

**Answer (c) is correct. Cannot be determined.** Because previous mammograms are unavailable, we cannot track the development of the calcifications over time. Their morphology and extent would be consistent with DCIS as well as fat necrosis. Digital stereotactic CNB indicates a *focal nonspecific inflammation with chronic scar formation*. It also shows pronounced zones of organizing *fat necrosis* with oil cysts. These findings exclude a malignant process, and treatment is unnecessary.

**Lesson:** Atypical calcifications found after reduction mammoplasty or the operative treatment of benign changes are more likely to result from fat necrosis than from DCIS. Postoperative fat necrosis is more likely to occur after removal of DCIS or carcinoma than malignant calcifications. These published data are not helpful in routine practical situations, however. All atypical calcifications require immediate histologic evaluation. Follow-up is not appropriate for patients with BIRADS 4 lesions.

## Answer for Fig. 5.175 (p. 323)

**Answer (a) is correct. Contrast medium injected into the seroma cavity drains via the ductal system.** Treatment of the skin necrosis and subsequent radiotherapy apparently ruptured the seroma, causing it to drain into the duct system. It is noteworthy that manual compression of the former tumor bed provoked galactorrhea that ceased after the injection of 40% glucose into the seroma cavity.

**Lesson:** Seromas should always be evacuated before radiotherapy is begun. Radiation fibrosis exerts pressure on the seroma that may cause lymphedema of the breast and may occasionally perforate into the duct system, causing recurrent nipple discharge.

**Fig. 5.175** Filling of a seroma may occur via the duct system (**d**) in cases where the seroma has ruptured into the ducts with atypical galactorrhea.

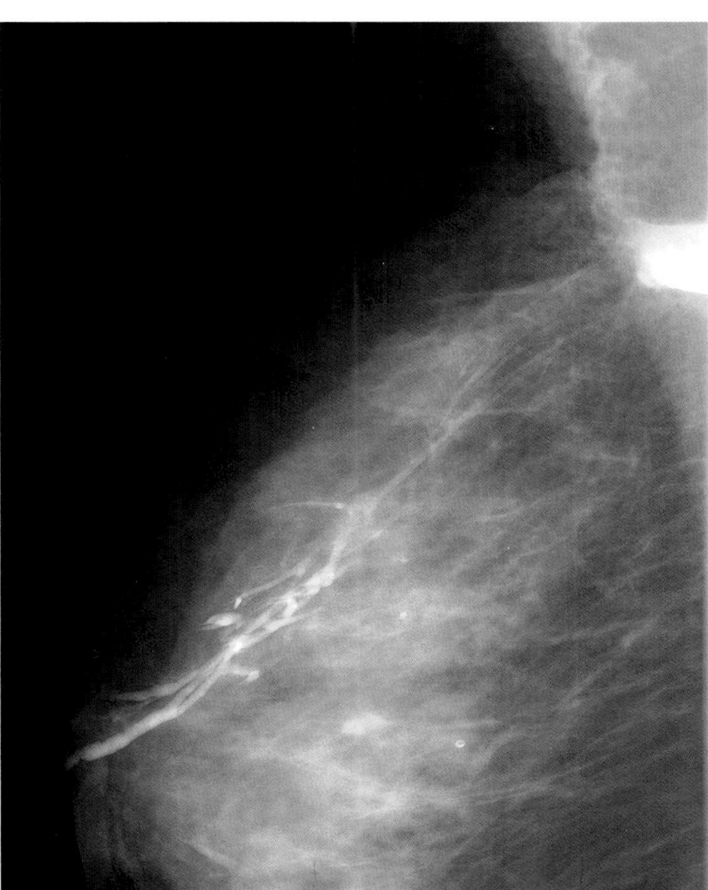

**d** *Ductography* of the right breast of a different patient shows the opacified duct system. Contrast medium has filled a seroma in the axillary recess (image courtesy of Heinrich Uedelhoven, Haan, Germany).

## Answer for Fig. 5.176 (p. 324)

**Answer (b) is correct. The sentinel lymph node procedure after tumor excision.** This did not conform to guidelines because sentinel lymph node imaging was probably done via collaterals that did not reflect the lymphatic drainage of the tumor.

The initial operation, in which a presumably benign tumor was removed without preoperative mammograms and other tests (besides ultrasound), did not conform to guidelines.

Only one axillary lymph node was involved.

**Lesson:** Women should be educated by the media to avoid having breast surgery in hospitals that are not certified and where the physicians on staff do not follow recommended guidelines. The prognosis, especially in younger women, depends critically on receiving optimum primary treatment consistent with established guidelines. SLNE is permissible after a small excision but not after an extensive excision as in the case shown.

*SLNB* is not indicated in patients with suspected lymph node metastasis. (Suspicious lymph nodes at ultrasound should first be investigated by ultrasound-guided FNA or CNB!) SLNB is permissible in patients with multicentric lesions but is not recommended after neoadjuvant (primary) chemotherapy in patients with nodal involvement (Kreienberg 2008).

## Answer for Fig. 5.177 (p. 325)

**Answer (a) is correct. Radiodermatitis** developed 20 days after the completion of radiotherapy. The breast shows exceptionally intense skin redness with absence of epitheliolysis. The redness cleared in 2 months.

This clinical presentation is unusual for *inflammatory breast cancer.* There is no breast swelling or typical orange-peel dimpling of the skin. *MRM* shows focal intramammary gadolinium enhancement and increased subcutaneous reticular markings. *Kaposi sarcoma* does not appear 20 days after radiation therapy and has a different appearance (**c** and **Fig. 5.180**, p. 329; see *inflammatory carcinoma,* p. 64).

**Lesson:** Radiotherapy after the breast-conserving treatment of invasive cancer will reduce local recurrence rates by 25% to approximately 5% in patients with R0 resections. Overall survival is not affected, however. Thus, the value of postoperative radiation should be critically examined in older patients due to its declining benefit with aging. Younger women with BCR and DCIS receive the greatest benefit—especially patients with high-grade (high-risk) disease and resection margins less than 1 cm. Radiodermatitis is an acceptable side-effect for most women (pain, itching, blistering, etc.).

**Fig. 5.177**

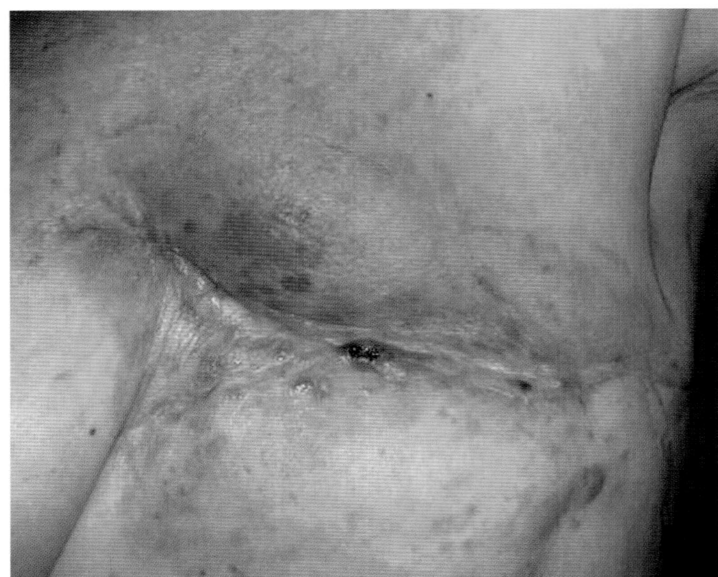

**c** *Clinical appearance* of *Kaposi sarcoma* in a 70-year-old woman who underwent breast-conserving treatment 20 years earlier (pT1c pN1b (2/12) M0 G3, estrogen-receptor-positive, progesterone-receptor-negative; *treatment:* radiotherapy and tamoxifen). Mastectomy was done for a suspected recurrence in May of 2003. *Histology: angiosarcoma (Kaposi sarcoma)* (**d**). Slightly raised reddish-purple nodular skin lesions (**a–c/11–14**) are visible in the scarred area 13 years after mastectomy. This is another aspect of radiodermatitis as seen in panel **a**, p. 325, and *inflammatory local recurrence* as seen in panel **e**.

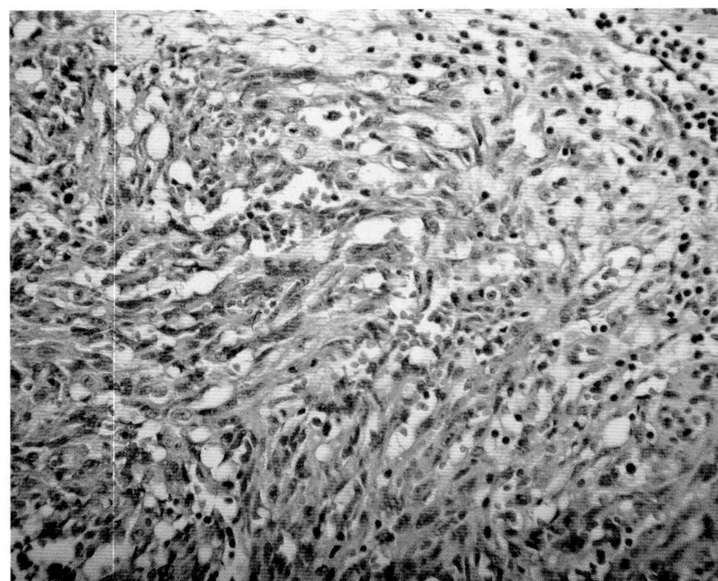

**d** *Histology* of hemangiosarcoma shows a close-packed arrangement of blood-filled capillaries within a stroma that has undergone sarcomatous change (image courtesy of Roland Bässler, Fulda).

**Fig. 5.177** *(continued)*

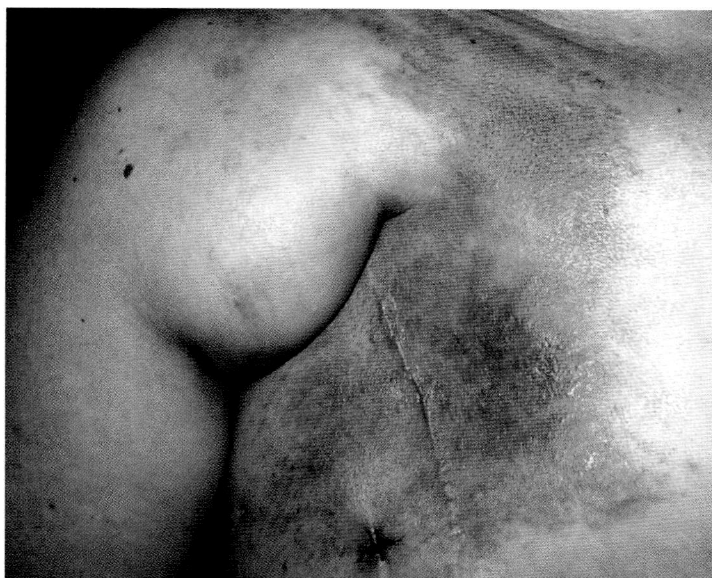

**e** Different patient from **a–c**. *Clinical appearance* of an inflammatory local recurrence 10 years after mastectomy with axillary dissection for locally advanced carcinoma. The patient presented now with swelling of the arm, massive lymph node involvement, and intense flame-shaped redness of the chest wall extending to the clavicle.

## Answer for Fig. 5.178 (p. 325 f)

**Answer (c) is correct. Primary chemotherapy** is the treatment of choice for *inflammatory breast carcinoma* as well as locally advanced neoplasms. *Primary hormonal therapy* may also be tried in older women. In the present case the tumor disappeared within 3 months in response to primary chemotherapy. Subsequent histologic examination of the tumor bed showed only necrotic tumor tissue. *Axillary dissection* was done before chemotherapy in this case to establish the diagnosis and stage the disease **N++** (this is no longer standard practice; current guidelines prescribe *a core biopsy* to determine histology, immunohistochemistry, and proteases).

Ten years later, *mammograms* show radiodense breasts with no signs of recurrent tumor growth (**g**, upper right). *MRI* shows no evidence of malignancy in either breast (**h**). Recurrent lymphedema in the treated breast improves with manual lymph drainage, later on with a special umbrella, very successfully **(l)**. The left nipple shows depigmentation after five years (**i–k**), which is mainly a result of radiotherapy and years of lymphatic obstruction.

**Lesson:** Locally advanced breast cancers are treated by primary chemotherapy. Reduction of tumor size may occur in responders (complete remission may also occur, as in the present case). Micrometastases are simultaneously destroyed by this systemic therapy. Primary operative treatment is obsolete. Good results with advanced tumors such as these are a result of complementary treatment modalities as well as the declining aggressiveness of breast cancer that has been documented in recent decades.

**Fig. 5.178**

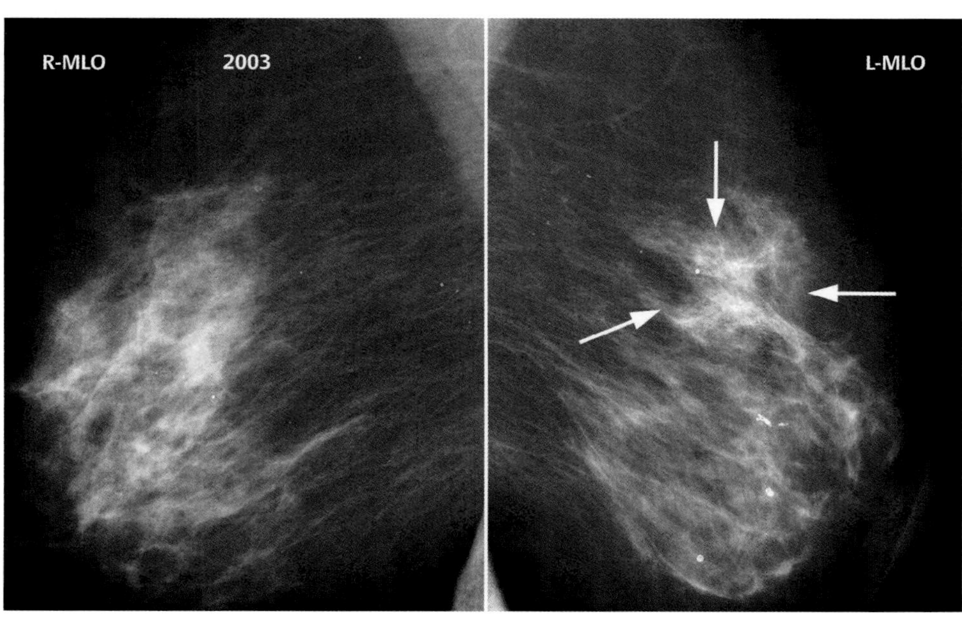


**g** *Bilateral oblique mammograms* show moderately radiodense breasts with coarse calcifications and scarring at the former tumor site (arrows). The areola is still thickened.

▶ Fig. 5.178 h–l

**Fig. 5.178** *(continued)*

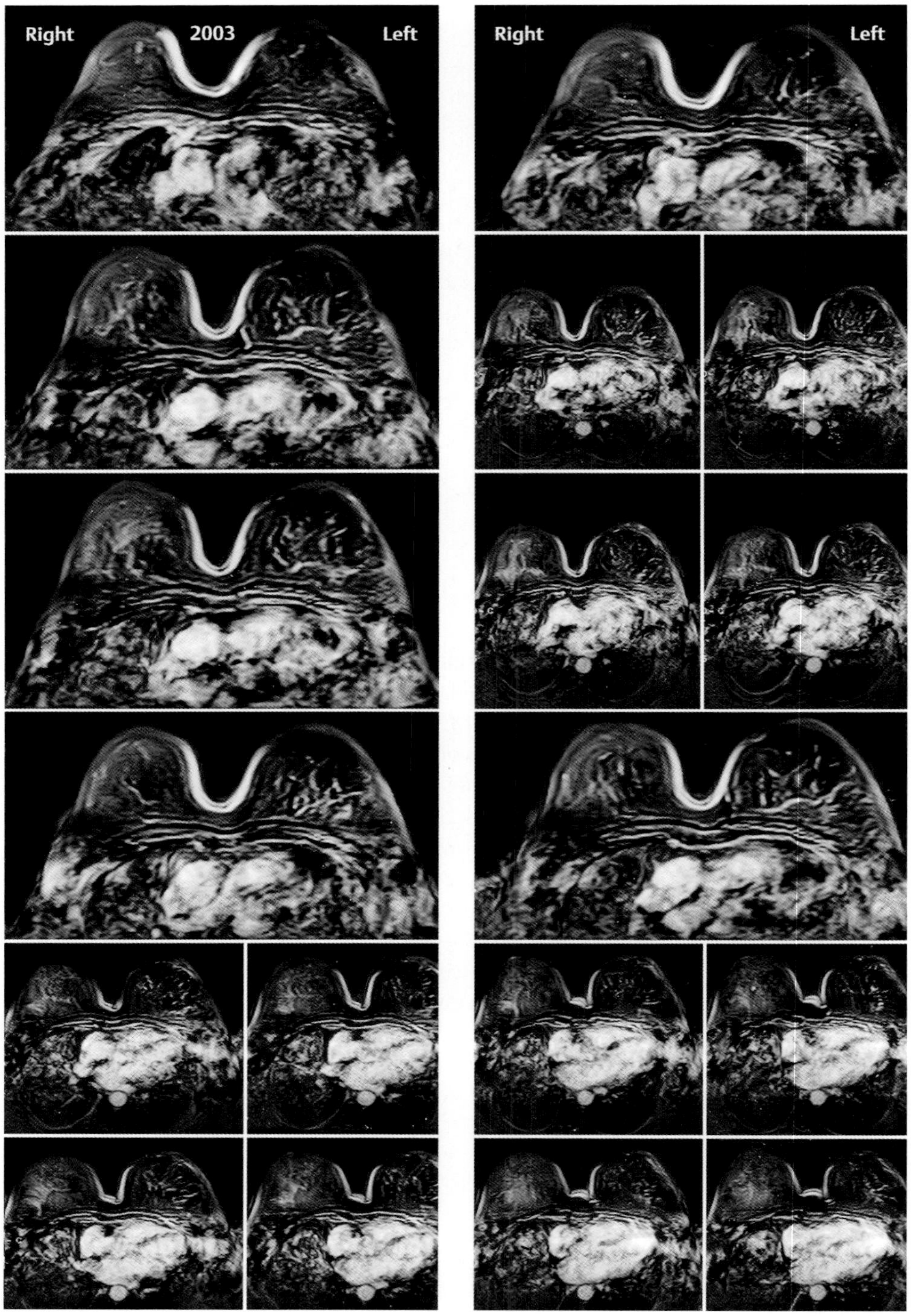

**h** *MRI* in 2003 shows no abnormalities in either breast.

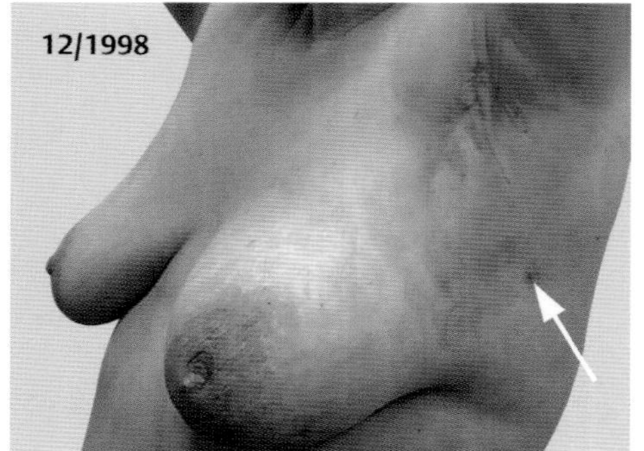


**i** *Clinical appearance* of the left breast in December, 1998. Lymphedema is still present and is now accompanied by slight nipple retraction. A relatively fresh scar is visible in the left axilla. The skin below the scar is reddened following drainage treatment for a seroma (arrow).

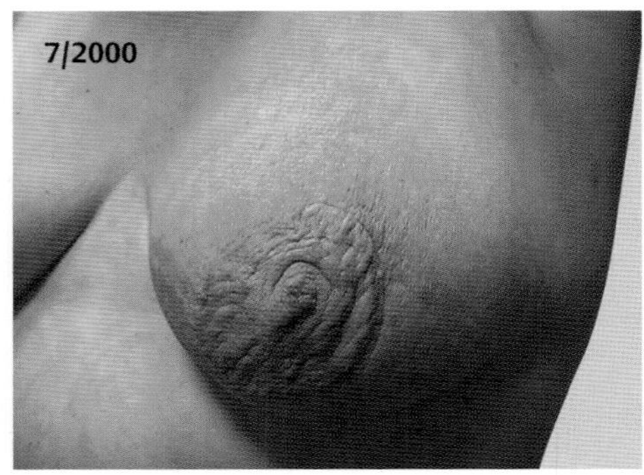


**j** *Clinical appearance* of the left breast in July, 2000. There is still mild lymphedema with slight swelling of the areola and a healthy-looking scar.

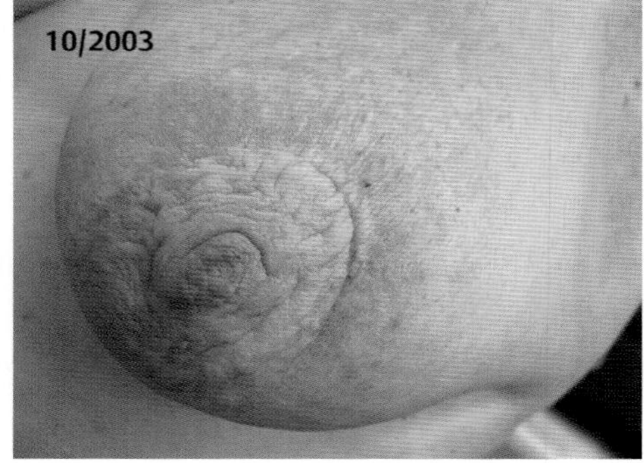


**k** *Clinical appearance* by October, 2003, lymphedema has resolved and the breast appears normal. Depigmentation of the areola is a late sequela of radiation and chemotherapy.

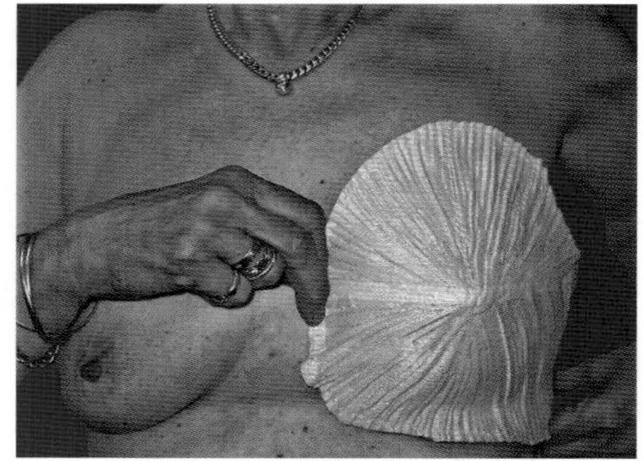

**l** *Clinical appearance:* lymphedema has been treated with a lymph drainage shield that the patient obtained from the Földi Clinic in the Black Forest (Germany). Wearing the device in the brassière provides constant-pressure massage of the lymphatic channels, yielding a very good outcome in this case.

**Answer for Fig. 5.179, Question 1** (p. 327 f)

**Answer (a) is correct. Inflammatory breast cancer.** This case exhibits the classic features with regional lymph node metastases. Cancer was detected in lymph node aspirate but was not confirmed histologically. The patient was discharged home with the presumptive diagnosis of a *systemic inflammatory process (possibly tuberculosis).*

*Nonpuerperal mastitis* may cause lymph node enlargement in the axilla but not in the supraclavicular fossae. A generalized primary *lymphadenopathy (e.g., non-Hodgkin lymphoma)* could cause breast swelling due to obstructed lymphatic drainage in advanced cases.

**Answer for Fig. 5.179, Question 2** (p. 327 f)

**Answer (b) is correct. No.** It is very difficult to confirm or exclude carcinomatous lymphangitis by a simple skin biopsy. Redness and swelling of the skin stem from intramammary edema; this does not mean that tumor cells are necessarily present in the skin.

In the present case the patient was discharged home on the basis of a negative skin biopsy. Several months later she began having dizzy spells and headaches caused by *cerebral metastasis*. Biopsy of the left breast revealed inflammatory carcinoma. The patient died a short time later.

**Lesson:** A simple skin biopsy cannot confirm inflammatory carcinoma. *VB* could have retrieved enough breast parenchyma to establish the correct diagnosis. *PET* was recommended initially but was withheld due to cost. Presumably this study would have detected the breast tumor and the nodal and cerebral metastases at an earlier stage, but without significant therapeutic implications.

**Answer for Fig. 5.180** (p. 329)

**Answer (a) is correct. Angiosarcoma (Kaposi sarcoma) following radiotherapy.** This type of atypical vascular breast lesion is rare following breast-conserving surgery and postoperative radiation, and only a few cases have been reported in the literature (Fineberg and Rosen 1994; Sener et al. 2001). Angiosarcoma also occurs after mastectomy (see **Fig. 5.177c**, p. 402). The retrospective case reports in the literature describe four cases in which atypical vascular skin lesions developed in the irradiated area from 3 to 11 years after radiotherapy. *Local resection* was performed in all four women. One patient had a recurrence of axillary lesions 17 months after the excision. The cases described in the literature were followed for periods of 1–10 years (Dr. Jörg Thomas Hartmann, Center for Soft-Tissue Sarcomas, Tübingen, Germany).

*Shingles* of the breast does not occur as an isolated skin lesion without pain. *Trophic skin changes* would be localized to the lower quadrants, which were treated over a 2-year period.

The patient in this case underwent a right *mastectomy* for Kaposi sarcoma. The angiosarcoma measured 15 cm × 10 cm in size and was removed with a 5 cm safety margin. The surgical defect was covered with a split-thickness skin graft from the right thigh. *Radiotherapy* was withheld.

The angiomatous process in Kaposi sarcoma occurs exclusively in the irradiated skin of the patient. *MRI* and *CT* showed no intramammary abnormalities, and mammograms were also normal. Angiosarcoma shows intense vascularity on *MRI* with associated gadolinium enhancement in the skin (see **c**).

**Lesson:** Kaposi sarcoma is a hemangiosarcoma that was first described by the Viennese physician Moritz Kaposi in 1872. It develops in immunocompromised patients (e.g., HIV or previous organ transplantation). As well as in the breast (approximately 12 years after radiotherapy or in chronic lymphedema-associated angiosarcoma in Stewart–Treves syndrome), Kaposi sarcoma may develop in the skin and mucous membranes of the oral cavity, nose, ear, and lung. Radiotherapy is always indicated, as the lesions are highly radiosensitive (Vogt et al. 2007).

**Answer for Fig. 5.181, Question 1** (p. 330 f)

**Answer (c) is correct. Radiation-induced telangiectasia with fibrosis** from tangential *cobalt-60 irradiation* with an additional sternal field (to saturate the retrosternal nodes). The rectangular boundaries of the field can be seen (**e–F/23–26**). The left side of the radiation field shows little telangiectasia, while the right side that overlapped with the other field shows extensive areas of telangiectasia. **It is unclear why the additional sternal field was applied.** The tumor was located laterally, making it unlikely that it would metastasize to sternal lymph nodes. Overtreatment of this kind does not occur when the patient is irradiated with fast electrons from a linear accelerator. The *mammogram* shows slight spiculated fibrosis in the overtreated area (**I–O/17–23** in **d**), which should not be mistaken for malignancy.

**Lesson:** Sternal field irradiation is used for tumors located in the inner quadrants and for positive retrosternal sentinel nodes. It is also used in cases where more than four axillary lymph nodes are involved. The retrosternal nodes are involved in up to 65% of patients with positive axillary nodes and up to 14% with clear axillary nodes (Singh 2004).

It is reasonable to expect that sternal field radiation would reduce the incidence of distant metastasis and thus prolong survival, but this has not proved to be the case. Indeed, the cure rates with this therapy appear to be lower than without treatment (Fowble et al. 2001; Singh 2004), regardless of the complications (overdose as in the present case, cardiac exposure, sternal marrow irritation, etc.).

**Answer for Fig. 5.181, Question 2** (p. 330 f)

**Answer (b) is correct. No.** Due to the high radiographic density of the scarred area, this relatively young patient should undergo MRI every 1½ years between mammographic and ultrasound examinations to allow for detection and treatment of new proliferative changes. The two local recurrences had been detected by palpation. MRI was withheld because of cost.

**Lesson:** In most cases MRI should be scheduled at regular intervals in the follow-up of scarred, radiodense breasts. Ultrasound generally cannot distinguish between scars and local recurrence.

Fig. 5.182

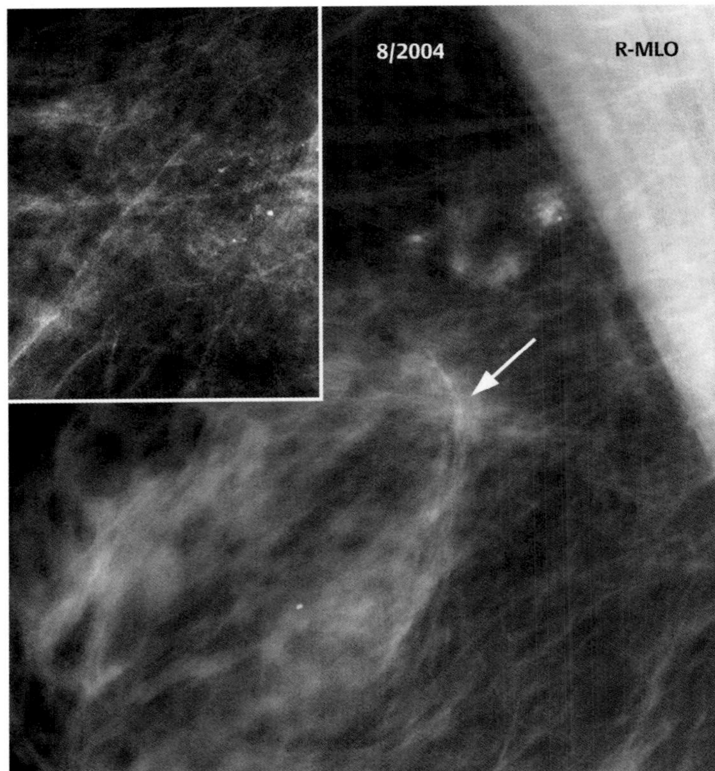


**f** *Oblique mammogram* of the right breast (magnified view) in August, 2004. The scar (arrow) is significantly smaller than in 2002. A cluster of pleomorphic microcalcifications is visible cranial to the scar (inset at upper left). The cluster is not located at the tumor site but is well lateral to it (*histology: atypical ductal hyperplasia* [ADH], excised with clear margins).

### Answer for Fig. 5.182 (p. 331f)

**Answer (a) is correct. Scar after tumorectomy,** commonly mistaken for a local recurrence. *Ultrasound* cannot differentiate these changes, and *MRI* findings were normal. Digital stereotactic or ultrasound-guided *CNB* of the suspicious area could be performed in doubtful cases, but that was not necessary in this case.

**Further course to early 2009** No local recurrence. Microcalcifications (**f**) were not found at the tumor site but in the outer upper quadrant. *Histology* revealed *ADH*, which was removed with clear margins.

**Further course to 2010:** 1.5 cm invasive ductal carcinoma in the right breast near the ADH-localization.

**Lesson:** Many unnecessary reexcisions are done because stellate scars after breast-conserving surgery are mistaken for a local recurrence. Excisional biopsy, vacuum biopsy, or CNB is necessary only if the scar shows gadolinium enhancement on MRI. Otherwise, follow-up examinations (mammography and ultrasound) should be scheduled every 6 months for 3 years and every 12 months thereafter.

Fig. 5.183

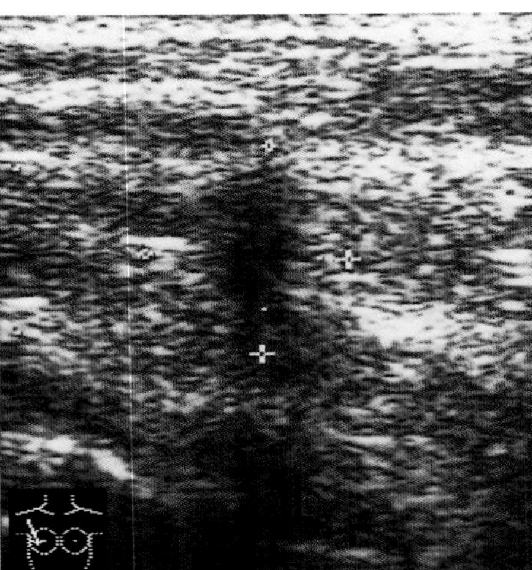

**c** *Sonogram* of the right breast shows an 11 mm × 12 mm hypoechoic area with irregular margins and posterior acoustic shadowing (S-BIRADS 5).

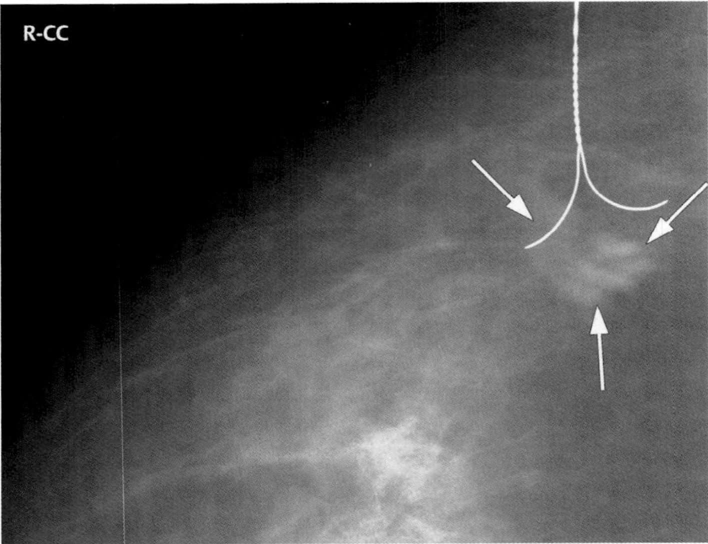


**d** *Craniocaudal mammogram* of the right breast shows the localization wire positioned just lateral to the tumor (arrows).

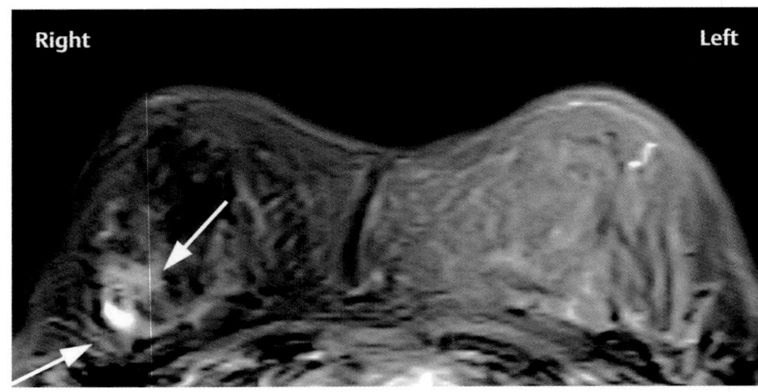


**e** *MRI (subtraction)*of the tumor shows irregular margins and intense gadolinium enhancement (arrows) of the tumor location in the right breast. No abnormalities are visible elsewhere in the breast. The left breast shows no evidence of local recurrence.

### Answer for Fig. 5.183 (p. 334)

**Answer (b) is correct. Inspection and mammography show the tumor.** The tumor is visible on the mammograms (craniocaudal **e/15**, oblique **j/10**). It is manifested clinically by slight skin retraction at the boundary of the outer quadrant (**B/23**). The tumor can be identified *sonographically* (**c**) and by *MRI* (**e**). The localization film demonstrates the localizing wire just lateral to the tumor (**d**).

**Lesson:** *Inspection and palpation* are very important follow-up methods in both the operated breast and the clinically healthy breast. They will even detect changes that are not tumor-related but may cause atypical mammographic findings.

## Answer for Fig. 5.184 (p. 335)

**Patient A has a subcutaneous lipoma** located in the infraclavicular region on the left side. It produces a subcutaneous skin bulge that is freely movable (**N–O/23–25**).

**Patient B has infraclavicular subcutaneous lymph node metastasis on the right side**. This is rare. Usually the enlarged nodes are retropectoral. In contrast to patient A, we see only slight elevation of the skin and pectoralis minor muscle (**Q–q/24–25**) (level III, see panel **j**) with an associated palpable mass. *Ultrasound* shows a large lymph node metastasis (**e**), and *FNA cytology* reveals tumor cells. *PET* shows additional supraclavicular metastases on the left side as well as paravertebral metastases at the level of the dome of the diaphragm (**e**).

**Patient C has a metastasizing breast carcinoma with lymph node metastases located in the supraclavicular region on the left side** in the axilla and at the junction of the left subclavian and internal jugular veins (the tumor was detected by *CT* scan; **f**).

**Patient D has a lymph node metastasis in the supraclavicular region on the right** not from uterine cancer but from the carcinoma in the right breast.

> ***Lesson:*** *Axillary lymph nodes are distributed along the axillary vein and are arranged in three levels:*
> - *Level I (lower axilla): lymph nodes lateral to the lateral border of the pectoralis minor muscle.*
> - *Level II (midaxilla): lymph nodes between the medial and lateral borders of pectoralis minor and interpectoral (Rotter) lymph nodes.*
> - *Level III (apical region): apical lymph nodes and lymph nodes at the medial border of pectoralis minor (excluding the sub-, infra- and supraclavicular nodes) (see panel **j**, diagram of lymph nodes with pectoralis minor).*

**Fig. 5.184**

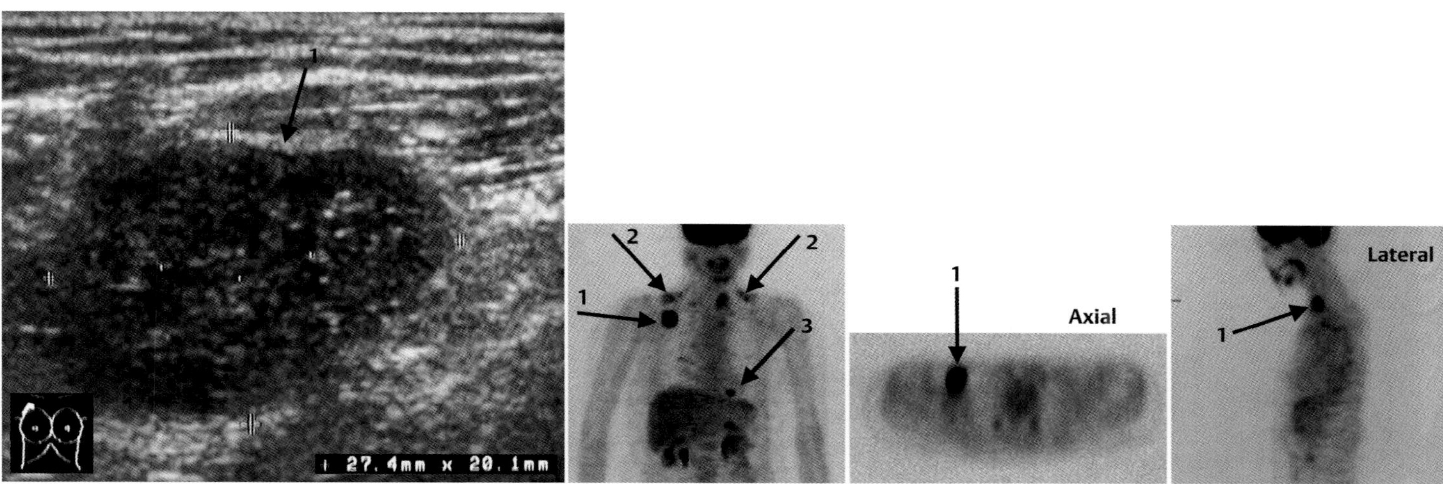


**e Patient B**. Ultrasound shows a large infraclavicular nodal metastasis on the right side (**1**). PET scans show bilateral infra- (**1**) and supraclavicular (**2**) metastases and a paravertebral metastasis in the left costophrenic angle (**3**).

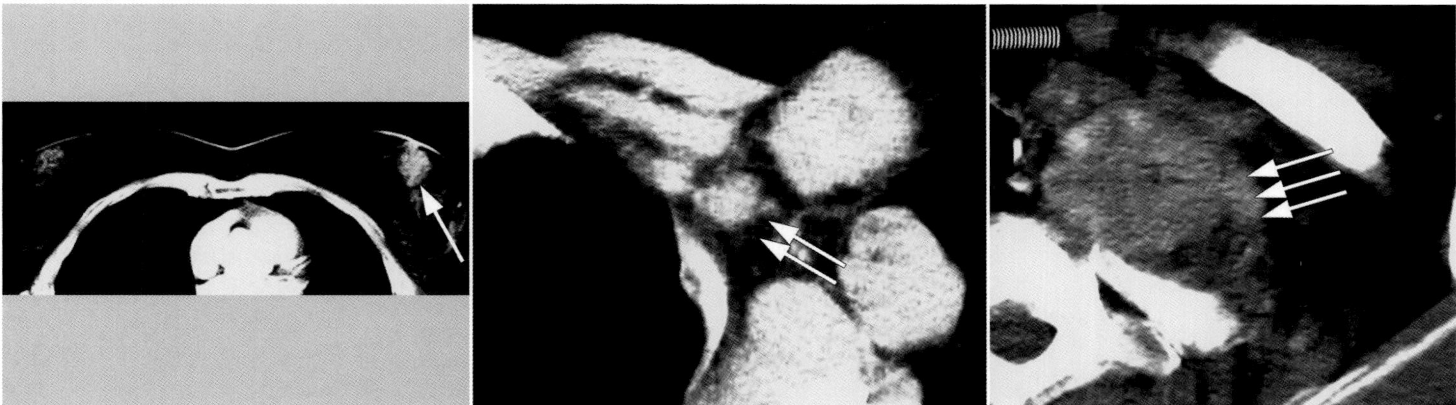

**f Patient C**. CT demonstrates a tumor in the left breast (left image, arrow), axillary lymph node metastases on the left side (middle image, arrows), and large retroclavicular nodal metastases (right image, arrows).

▶ Fig. 5.184 g–j

**Fig. 5.184** *(continued)*

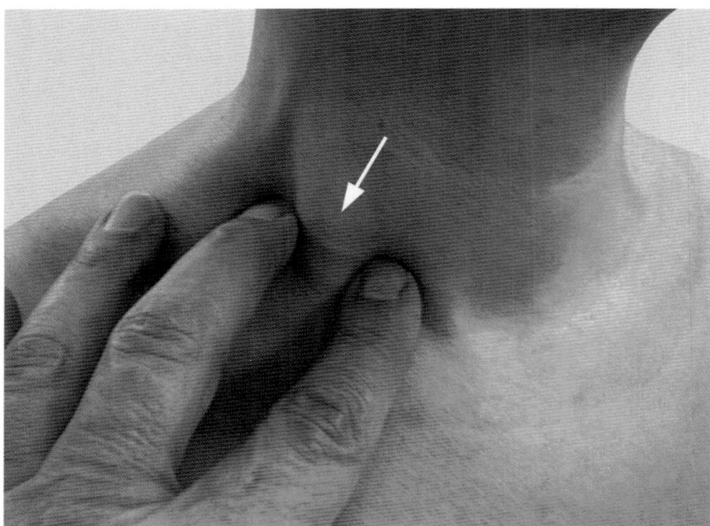

**g Patient D.** Physical examination reveals a palpable nodule at the junction of the right subclavian and internal jugular veins (arrow). Ultrasound (**h**) shows an enlarged lymph node above the subclavicular vein. Cytology (**i**) shows dissociated tumor cells with definite nuclear pleomorphism.

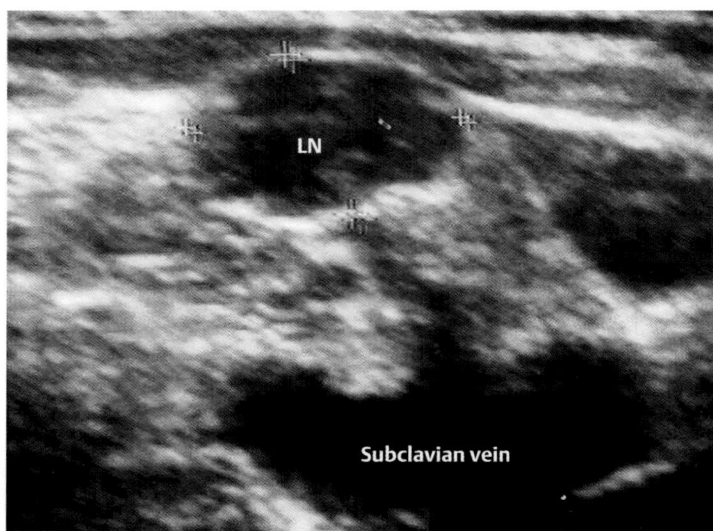


**h** *Sonogram* shows a 1 cm lymph node (LN) at the junction of the right subclavian and internal jugular veins.

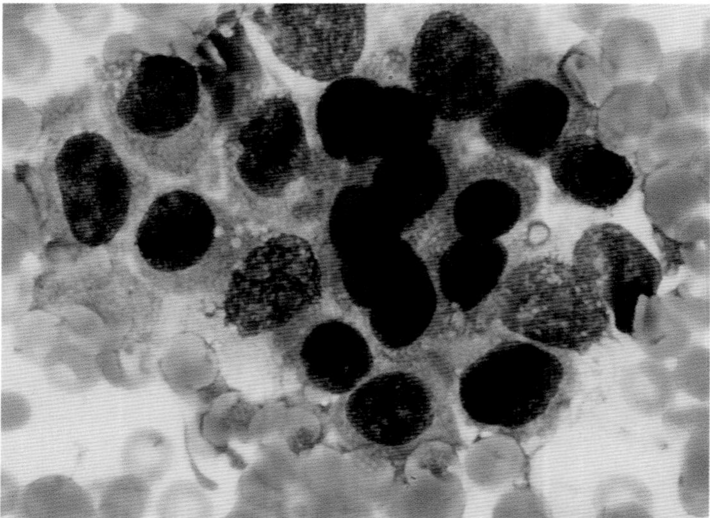

**i** *FNA cytology* shows a loose cluster of ductal carcinoma cells with enlarged nuclei. The nuclear chromatin shows variable density and some premitotic disintegration. Several enlarged nucleoli are visible. The cytologic findings are definitive for malignancy.

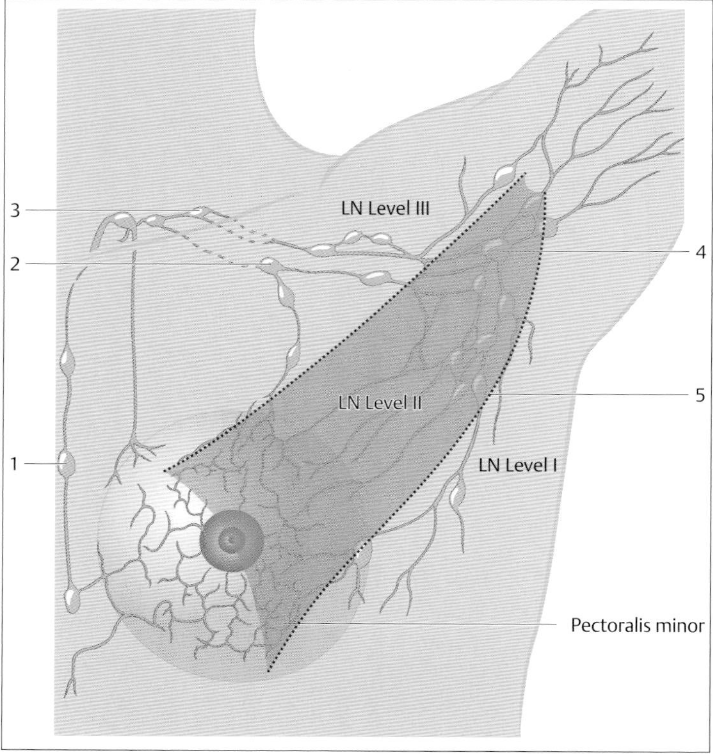


**j** Diagrammatic representation of the regional lymph nodes of the breast in correlation to the minor pectoral muscle.

1 Parasternal lymph nodes
2 Infraclavicular lymph nodes
3 Supraclavicular lymph nodes
4 Axillary lymph nodes
5 Pectoral lymph nodes (Rotter)

Lymph nodes (LN) level I = LN *lateral* to pectoralis minor
Lymph nodes (LN) level II = LN *posterior* to pectoralis minor
Lymph nodes (LN) level III = LN *medial* to pectoralis minor

### Answer for Fig. 5.185 (p. 336)

**Answer (c) is correct. Immediate CNB or vacuum biopsy.** The FNA of scars is unrewarding (showing only regressive changes with debris). *CNB* or *VB* is more reliable and should be done primarily in all patients with suspicious MRI findings. Follow-up is never appropriate when a tumor is suspected, and every suspected tumor should be investigated immediately.

**Further course:** After removal of the *recurrence*, the patient developed another recurrence that necessitated mastectomy. She also had a hepatic metastasis, which was treated by chemotherapy and was later resected. The further course is unknown.

**Lesson:** Local recurrence (LR) has prognostic significance. The relative risk of dying from breast cancer is increased 9-fold in women with LR compared with that in women without LR (Kemperman et al 1995) because 10% of women with LR already have distant metastases. Risk factors for LR are an extensive intraductal component (EIC, see p. 75), a low grade of tumor differentiation, expression of the Ki-67 proliferative index, the absence of progesterone receptors, HER2/neu overexpression, R1 resections, and adolescence (Birrenbach 2003).

### Answer for Fig. 5.186 (p. 339)

**Answer (b) is correct. The cancer was missed in numerous biopsies.** One year later infiltration of the pectoral muscle and shrinking of the breast can be seen (**g, h**).

### Answer for Fig. 5.187, Question 1 (p. 341)

**Answer (b) is correct. No.** There is no plausible connection between the palpable mass with the cytologic features of atypical papilloma and the histologic diagnosis of a lipoma.

### Answer for Fig. 5.187, Question 2 (p. 341)

**Answer (a) is correct.** The chest-wall lesion is a skeletal metastasis, which was resected and removed with a healthy tissue margin. Histology revealed *papillary carcinoma* arising from the primary breast cancer.

### Answer for Fig. 5.188 (p. 342 ff)

**Answer (b) is correct. Cerebral metastases are shielded from the effects of the chemotherapeutic agent and trastuzumab (Herceptin) by the blood–CSF barrier.**

Primary chemotherapy and treatment with trastuzumab led to complete tumor regression within the breast, and the patient was feeling well. Later she developed a dental granuloma in the left maxilla. Before excising it, the oral surgeon ordered a cranial MRI because of the patient's history. That study incidentally revealed multiple cerebral metastases (**m**) at typical peripheral vascular sites and in the left hypothalamus. The cerebral metastases had been completely asymptomatic.

**Fig. 5.186**

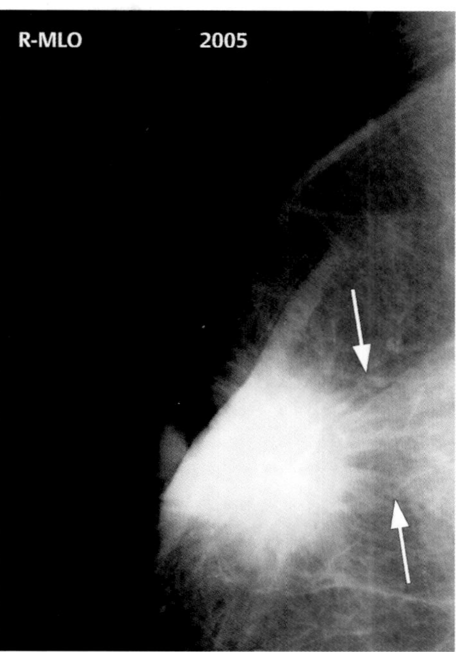


**g** *Oblique mammogram* of the right breast in December, 2005 shows further progression of the spiculated retroareolar density. The lesion now shows fixation and ingrowth into the pectoral muscle.

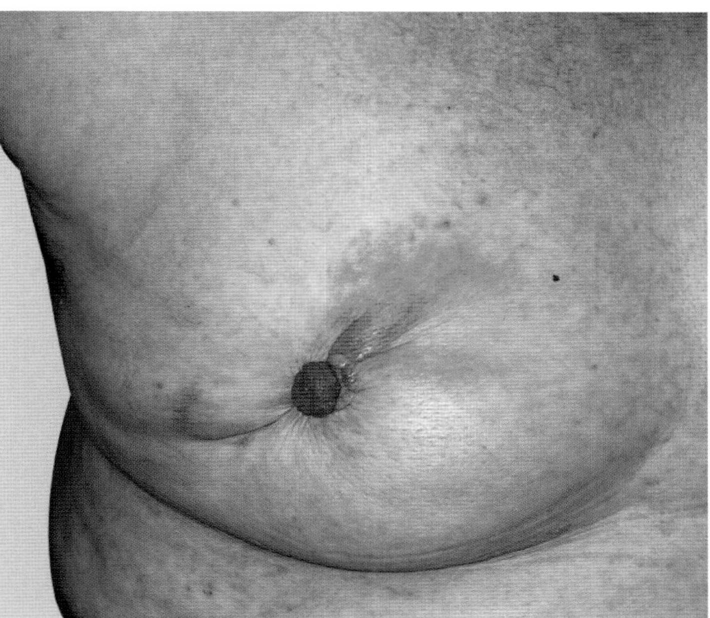

**h** *Clinical appearance* of the right breast in January, 2005. The breast shows significant shrinkage due to repeated biopsies and additional tumor involvement. The latest *CNB* left a large, bloody retroareolar seroma. The collection was removed by percutaneous aspiration and showed no cytologic abnormalities. *Histology:* invasive ductal carcinoma with lymph node involvement.

Any peripheral visceral and skeletal metastases that are present should regress with chemotherapy. However, most chemotherapeutic agents as well as trastuzumab cannot cross the physiologic blood–CSF barrier in the brain and so cannot act there. Cerebral metastases develop in up to 48% of patients treated with trastuzumab (Siekiera 2006). Because these patients died quickly before the trastuzumab era, they usually did not suffer the effects of their cerebral metastases. In the present case, the changing pattern of metastases during trastuzumab therapy should be viewed as a consequence of the longer course of the disease and longer patient survival. We do not fully understand why and to what degree the

Fig. 5.188

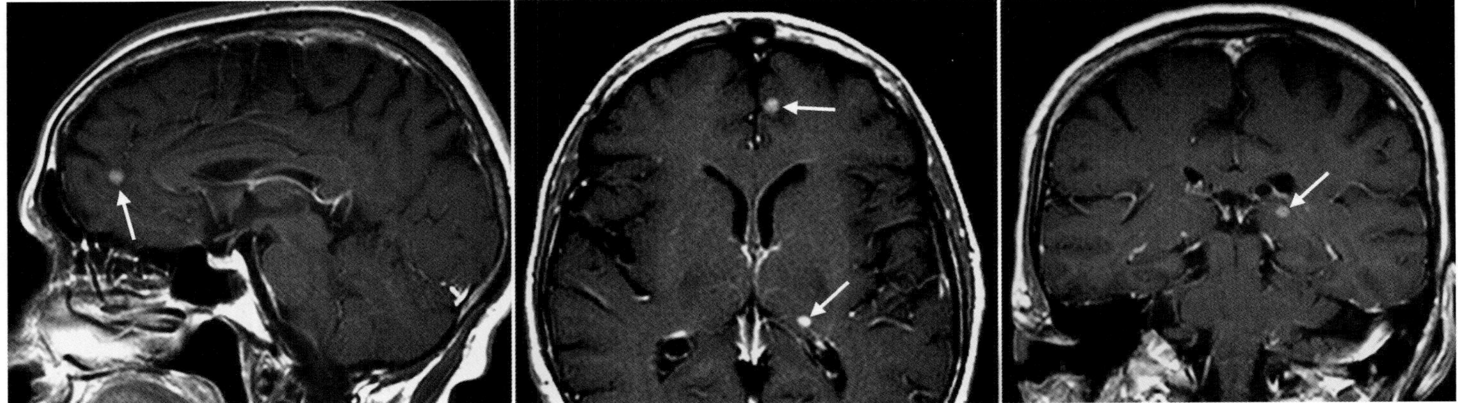

**m** *MRI of the brain* shows multiple round lesions in the cerebral cortex and left basal ganglia with no perifocal edema (arrows). **These metastases disappeared completely six months after radiotherapy.**

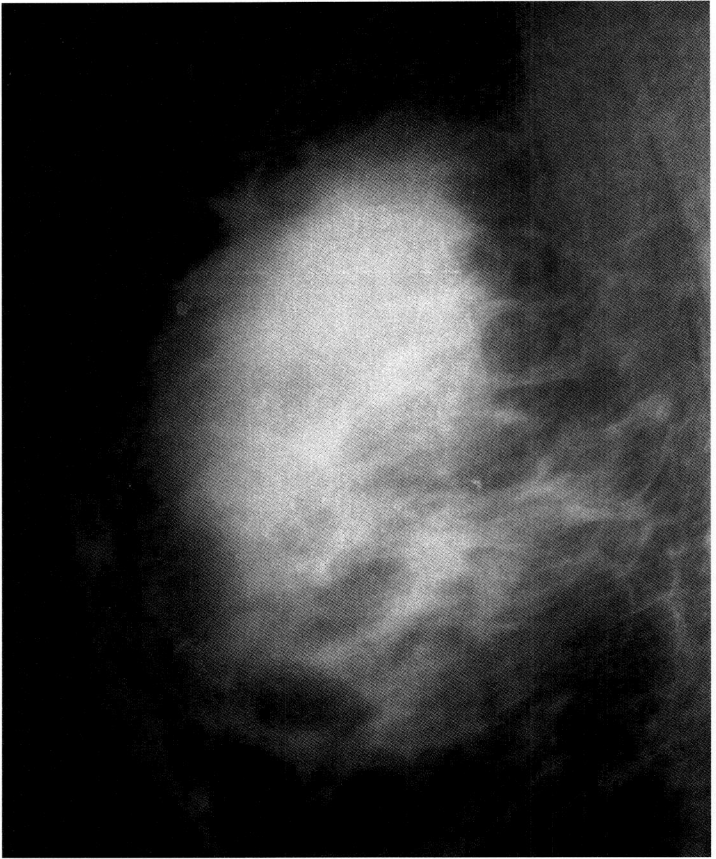

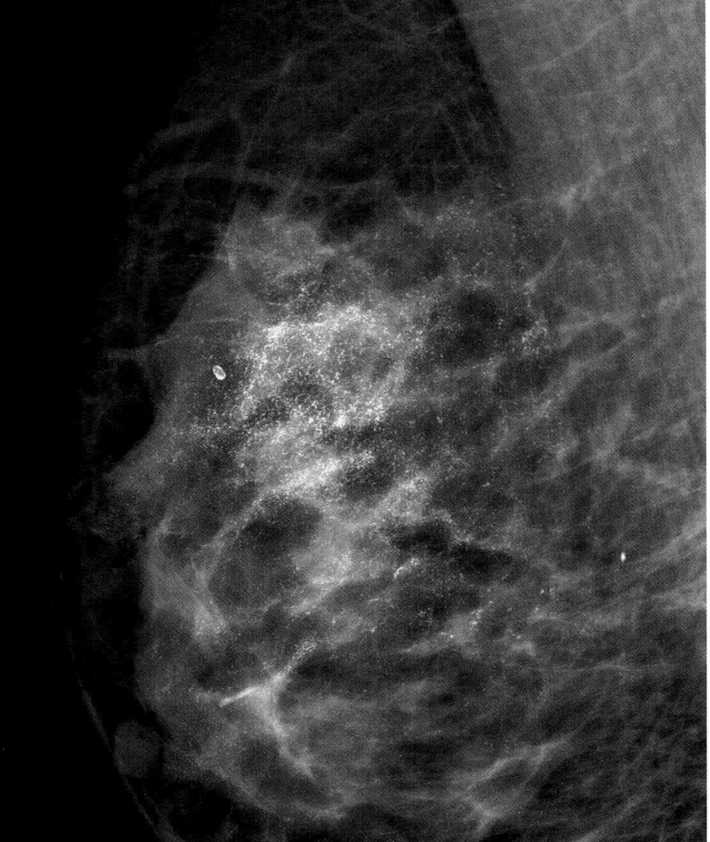

**n, o Another patient with a local progressive tumor** in the right breast from Heinrich Uedelhoeven, (Haan/Germany). After neoadjuvant chemotherapy the density of the breast diminished, though, in contrast to the first patient, not completely. Numerous microcalcifications became visible after therapy. *Histology: extensive comedocarcinoma with regressive changes.* The patient underwent mastectomy with radiation to the chest wall.

*Oblique mammograms* of the right breast (**n**) before and (**o**) 4 months after primary chemotherapy reveal extensive pathologic microcalcifications with a decline in radiographic density. The tumor masses in this case regressed with chemotherapy, exposing the extensive calcifications. **Note** that the calcifications were not new but were invisible due the breast density from the tumor masses and were slower to regress than the tumor cells.

blood–brain barrier inhibits the penetration of cytostatic agents into the cerebral parenchyma, although particle size appears to be an important factor (Kiewe et al. 2008).

This very complex history concludes the case presentations in this atlas. It documents in impressive fashion how evolving treatment strategies can directly and indirectly influence the diagnostic protocol and diagnostic thinking of the physician. *Panta rei* ("everything is in flux") is a concept that applies to all aspects of breast diagnosis.

Treatment in the present case led to a *complete remission* of intramammary disease. The mammograms from a different patient show an example of *incomplete (pathologic) remission* (n, o). Even the cerebral metastases have completely regressed after radiotherapy but recurred 3 years later in 2010.

# 6 Summary

The modern diagnosis and treatment of breast cancer are conducted most effectively in closely linked, certified chains of care in which independent gynecologists, radiologists, pathologists, and hospital-based physicians have assigned roles and are fully responsible for their contribution. These cooperative relationships should be defined in contractual form and should give patients assurance that they are being managed in accordance with guidelines, from their initial screening to follow-up care. The practical implementation of guidelines worldwide is the responsibility of everyone involved in early breast cancer detection. This is not to say that many centers have not already adopted practices that conform to the new guidelines.

The population-wide mammographic screening of all women 50–69 years of age has been practiced for 20–30 years in progressive countries such as the Netherlands, Sweden, Finland, the United Kingdom, and the United States. These programs have had both their advocates and their critics over the years. The U.S. Preventive Services Task Force (USPSTF) issued the following recommendations for breast cancer screening in 2009:

- Biennial screening mammography is recommended for women aged 50 to 74 years.
- The decision to start biennial screening mammography before 50 years of age should be an individual one and take patient context into account, including the patient's values regarding specific benefits and harms.
- Current evidence is insufficient to assess the additional benefits and harms of screening mammography in women 75 years or older.
- The USPSTF recommends against teaching breast self-examination (BSE).
- Current evidence is insufficient to assess the additional benefits and harms of clinical breast examination (CBE) beyond screening mammography in women 40 years or older.
- Current evidence is insufficient to assess the additional benefits and harms of either digital mammography or magnetic resonance imaging (MRI) instead of film mammography as screening modalities for breast cancer.

These recommendations are not entirely consistent with the statements made in this book, particularly with regard to the value of MRI and digital mammography. The USPSTF does not address the benefits of ultrasound in the early detection of breast cancer, as the value of this modality is, unfortunately, not evidence-based. Digital mammography has revolutionized the conduct of screening examinations, while MRI has yielded additional benefits, especially in young women—at least in the investigation of nodular breast lesions and in the examination of younger women at risk. The claim that there is no benefit in screening women 40–49 years of age not only contradicts our own experience (35% of our patients with premalignant and malignant breast lesions are under age 50, with a rising trend!) but also conflicts with ACR recommendations.

A recent article in the *Journal of the American College of Radiology* (Lee et al. 2010) reflects the current change in thinking on the value of other imaging modalities in breast screening:

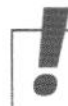

**Screening for breast cancer with mammography has been shown to decrease mortality from breast cancer, and mammography is the mainstay of screening for clinically occult disease. Mammography, however, has well-recognized limitations, and recently other imaging modalities including ultrasound and magnetic resonance imaging have been used as adjunctive screening tools, mainly for women who may be at increased risk for the development of breast cancer. The Society of Breast Imaging and the Breast Imaging Commission of the ACR are issuing these recommendations to provide guidance to patients and clinicians on the use of imaging to screen for breast cancer. Wherever possible, the recommendations are based on available evidence. Where evidence is lacking, the recommendations are based on consensus opinions of the fellows and executive committee of the Society of Breast Imaging and the members of the Breast Imaging Commission of the ACR.**

Presumably these recommendations will provide a basis for more effective screening in the future. The illustrative cases presented in this atlas reflect the limitations of mammography while underscoring the adjunctive capabilities of ultrasound and MRI. If mammographic screening alone can reduce mortality by 30% based on a 30% rate of interval cancers, how effective would it be to screen with new modalities that have only about a 5% rate of false-negative results? We must wait and see. The ACR guidelines already include recommendations on the use of ultrasound in breast examinations, and they will likely prompt a change of strategy in breast screening.

According to the ACR Practice Guideline for the Performance of Breast Ultrasound, appropriate indications for breast ultrasound include, but are not limited to, the following applications:

1. Evaluation and characterization of palpable masses and other breast-related signs and/or symptoms
2. Evaluation of suspected or apparent abnormalities detected on other imaging studies, such as mammography or magnetic resonance imaging (MRI)
3. Initial imaging evaluation of palpable masses in women under 30 years of age and in lactating and pregnant women
4. Evaluation of problems associated with breast implants
5. Evaluation of breasts with microcalcifications and/or architectural distortion suspicious for malignancy or highly suggestive of malignancy in a setting of dense fibroglandular tissue, for detection of an underlying mass that may be obscured on the mammogram
6. Guidance of breast biopsy and other interventional procedures
7. Treatment planning for radiation therapy

Evaluation of the axilla for occult lymph node metastasis in patients with newly diagnosed breast cancer is an area of research. Research is also being done on the efficacy of ultrasound as a screening study for occult masses in dense fibroglandular breasts of high risk women or women with newly diagnosed or suspected breast cancer.

Indeed, screening by mammography alone should be considered obsolete by modern standards. It dates from a time when mammograms were the only tool available for the early detection of breast cancer. Mammography is still the only method that can detect early calcifying stages of breast cancer and preinvasive disease (approximately 25% of cases), but all other noncalcifying tumors (approximately 75%) can be detected equally well by high-resolution ultrasound, and ultrasound is superior to mammography in breasts with a radiographic density of ACR 3 or higher (approximately 60% of our own patients, see p. 372 ff).

The evolution of pure mammographic screening to a combination of single-view digital mammograms (including tomosynthesis) plus ultrasound plus physical examination of the breast would be a better approach as it reduces the radiation dose by half, allowing younger women to be screened. It requires only one breast compression per side and provides greater diagnostic accuracy. In special cases tomosynthesis may become a good alternative to the craniocaudal mammogram in cases where the oblique view appears to show an abnormality. The x-ray dose would be no more than twice the dose received from single-view digital mammograms (Andersson et al. 2008). A combination of high-quality single-view mammography (usually oblique), physical examination, and high-resolution ultrasound could actually reduce breast cancer morality by an additional 25%, and not just in Germany. The author feels that it would not be necessary for physicians alone to perform inspection, palpation, and ultrasound scans in *screening* situations. It has been shown that technologists can be effectively trained in these techniques, and a new generation of automated ultrasound scanners (AFBUS, Siemens) can make this concept a reality. Problem cases should be referred to specialists. Single-view mammography does not mean that a second view cannot be obtained in cases where abnormalities are found.

From a financial standpoint, physicians' fee scales should be adjusted to allow for the extra time required for multimodal screening. Single-view mammography plus ultrasound (including inspection and palpation) should be compensated at a higher rate than two-view mammography. In *curative* applications, ultrasound as an adjunct to single-view mammograms should be performed personally by the same radiologist or gynecologist who interprets the mammograms.

Mammographic systems have undergone a renaissance in recent years worldwide. Since the 1990s older machines in offices and hospitals have been replaced by more advanced systems, with fully digital technology as the modern standard. Unfortunately, this is not yet the case with ultrasound systems. Too many old scanners are still in service, and very few operate at frequencies in the 11–18 MHz range. Even the 7.5 MHz transducers of older machines do not have the resolution needed to detect cancers 4–5 mm in diameter in breasts with a density of ACR 3 or higher, let alone permit a detailed analysis of the breast parenchyma with its physiologic changes and cyclic variations. This is one area in which equipment updates and quality assurance should be pursued with the same vigor as in mammography.

**Fine-needle aspiration (FNA)** is the least costly interventional procedure, but unfortunately it is becoming less widely practiced because too little has been done on its behalf. Anyone who can master this procedure and interpret cytologic smears will become the "king" of their office or department, as this will enable them to tell the patient at once whether a lesion is innocent or suspicious and whether FNA should be followed by **core-needle biopsy** (CNB). Anyone who has not mastered FNA should not perform it (unless learning it again) and should concentrate instead on the more easily acquired techniques of CNB and vacuum biopsy (VB). These minimally invasive procedures supply a confident tissue diagnosis and also allow for additional immunohistochemical tests in malignant lesions. FNA should never be used to confirm a questionable invasive lobular carcinoma, as it is likely to yield a false-negative result. It is valuable for investigating breast lesions during pregnancy.

**Magnetic resonance imaging (MRI)** should be used more frequently as an adjunct than in the past, especially in young women at risk and in patients with confirmed cancer. Currently this is not being done due to budgetary constraints. In patients selected for breast-conserving surgery, MRI is useful for evaluating the residual parenchyma and the healthy breast, especially when radiographic density is in the range of ACR 3–4.

False-positive findings are a common problem in MRI, especially during the second half of the menstrual cycle in women under 40 years of age, and findings at that time should not be overinterpreted. Most true pathology requiring a change in treatment regimen will be found in close proximity to the primary lesion. Magnetic resonance mammography (MRM) is a valuable adjunct to mammography and ultrasound, especially after aesthetic breast reconstructions, after breast implantation, and in breasts with extensive scarring. Any knee joint that has sustained minor trauma may be referred for MRI, but when it comes to breast cancer, with its far-reaching consequences, payors are much more reluctant to provide coverage. It is time for statutory health insurance to cover MRI in every woman with histologically confirmed breast cancer!

**Positron emission tomography (PET)** is another modality that has been underutilized. On the one hand, this is understandable from a cost perspective; but on the other, it is difficult to understand when we consider that primary PET scanning could eliminate the need for other services such as radiography, ultrasound, and endoscopy. This particularly applies to axillary malignancies with no detectable primary tumor (CUP syndrome) and to locally advanced and "missed" breast cancers. PET is also useful for detecting metastatic lesions in the axilla or other organs (lung, liver) as a prelude to the surgical removal of metastases. Critics of the method argue that PET is inappropriate for follow-up because, like the less costly *tumor-marker* assays, it may advance the treatment of metastases without demonstrable benefit for the patient. They feel that conventional tests are generally adequate for symptomatic metastases and that the surgical removal of hepatic and pulmonary metastases does not play a role because treatment would be provided in any case. Critics state that PET is a very costly staging procedure that is not indicated except in patients with advanced disease. Some of these special situations are illustrated in case reports like that in **Fig. 5.147** (pages 288 and 393).

**The genetic tumor profile,** or the genetic code of a tumor, could soon play an important role in the diagnosis and treatment of breast cancer. The capabilities of genetic chip technology were mentioned in an earlier chapter (see Predisposing Genetic Factors, p. 13 ff). This technology will not only affect the screening strategy in special risk groups but will also have therapeutic implications.

As an example, it is hoped that a new prognostic model called the *gene expression test* will meet these expections. By determining the activities of certain genes in a tumor sample from a particular patient, it should be possible to calculate the likelihood that the cancer will recur in that patient. Currently it is believed that many women with breast cancer are "overtreated." Many patients are placed on postoperative chemotherapy based on standard prognostic factors such as tumor size, hormone receptor status, age, or staging in order to kill any remaining tumor cells in the body. But some of these patients are free of residual tumor cells and would not develop a recurrence even if chemotherapy were withheld.

It is hoped that the *gene expression test* can identify this subset of patients. An initial test with the brand name MammaPrint® was approved in early 2007 for clinical use in the U.S. It remains to be seen what impact this technology will have on the utilization of chemotherapy and on cancer screening. One thing is certain, however—the need for an accurate and comprehensive diagnostic approach using both the new and conventional methods described in this book.

The diagnosis and treatment of breast diseases are undergoing a radical change. The incidence of breast cancer is on the rise, but not in every country. In the U.S., for example, the breast cancer incidence has been falling since the 1990s, but the mortality rate has remained constant (approximately 40000 deaths annually in the U.S., compared with 410000 worldwide). This means that we are seeing benefits from the optimization of therapeutic procedures and from screening programs in which many DCIS lesions have been identified and removed. Modifying the screening modalities as recommended above could provide a further reduction in mortality rates, resulting in a major benefit for women.

The only proven safeguard against the **development of breast cancer** appears to be early pregnancy (15–17 years of age), which forces maturation of the lobular breast tissue. But most women today have their first pregnancy at 30–38 years of age and this may be one reason for the rising incidence of breast cancer in young women. It is believed but not proven that oral contraceptive use (combined with heavy smoking) may delay full maturation of the breast lobules, making them more susceptible to the mutagenic effects of nicotine or other potenzially harmful agents (see Chapter 2, Aspects of Tumor Biology, p. 7 ff).

Neither oral contraceptive use after 33 years of age nor estrogen-only hormonal therapy in menopause can definitely be linked to the incidence of breast cancer. Nevertheless, the contraceptive pill should not be taken by carriers of the *BRCA1* mutation because it delays maturation of the follicles–unless the patient became pregnant at an early age.

The link between **hormone replacement therapy (HRT)** and breast cancer risk has been exaggerated. No woman should take hormones if she does not need them. But every woman who suffers from menopausal complaints (hot flushes, depression, insomnia, osteoporosis, etc.) should seriously consider HRT to improve her quality of life. The Million Women Study in the United Kingdom appears to have some significant flaws. From what we know about tumor doubling times, it is not possible for breast cancer to develop in 1.5–2 years as a result of hormonal therapy or any other regimen. At most, hormone therapy could stimulate the growth of receptor-positive neoplasms and allow them to be detected more quickly (it is unclear whether this accelerated growth is associated with earlier metastasis). Because the study is based on the results of a national screening program, we should take seriously the incidence of interval cancers: 30% in the first year, 40% in the second year, and 50% in the third year. Already the study has shown that women who do not use HRT have a higher breast cancer risk than women who take estrogen-only HRT. Thus, transdermal estrogen (gel or patch) and a progestin IUD might be an ideal combination for hormone therapy. Everything now is in a state of flux *(panta rei)*. Perhaps higher-resolution ultrasound probes could be used to identify women whose glandular breast tissue is stimulated by HRT. This is one reason why we have given so much attention in this book to the ability of ultrasound to detect changes in the terminal duct-lobular unit (TDLU; see p. 31).

The current debate about hormone replacement therapy is very disconcerting to many women and their doctors. We must reassure them, advocate early detection, and clarify equivocal findings as quickly as possible. Breast cancer is no longer a death sentence. For reasons still unknown, breast tumors have become less aggressive over the years. Today the breast can be preserved in 80% of new cases detected at an early stage, and the 10-year survival rate exceeds 80%. These numbers are certain to rise in the coming decades as a result of integrated and certified care centers that offer optimized and individualized therapy, disease management programs, and modern optimized screening programs.

At present, digital high-resolution **ultrasound** still has great untapped potenzial and is underrepresented in screening programs. In the U.S., this procedure is usually carried out by technologists without the direct involvement of physicians. But mammography and breast ultrasound need to become a hands-on experience for doctors. A good compromise may be to combine automated full-field breast ultrasound (AFBUS) with other digital modalities such as full-field digital mammography and even digital clinical photographs of localizable breast changes.

High-resolution digital ultrasound is better than mammography for distinguishing cysts from solid tumors and is more accurate for benign-malignant discrimination. Ultrasound can significantly reduce the recall rates in screened populations, despite the 5% false-positive rates that occur with ultrasound screening alone (Buchberger 2005).

Let us look to a future with less mammography and more ultrasound and MRI—especially in younger women and in patients with histologically confirmed breast cancer and its precursors. The capabilities and limitations of each method have been explored in this atlas. Let us satisfy the fans of "mammograms only" by practicing breast tomosynthesis **plus ultrasound**. This combination could have a tremendous impact on disease-free survival.

And now a final word on **guidelines**. There are no legal statutes per se, only recommendations for physicians and their staff to ensure that patients and their families will receive optimum care services that meet the highest international standards. Recommended guidelines cannot be followed in all cases because there are special situations that require a modified or individualized approach. At the same time, this occasional departure from guidelines will broaden our medical experience. Working strictly from guidelines will not advance medical science.

Not every statement that I have made in this book is validated by studies. Consequently, some of the information in this atlas is not evidence-based and is not reflected in guidelines. But everything that I have written in this atlas is derived from almost four decades of personal experience in the use of *complementary breast screening tools*, which had their origin in pathology and continued with the advent of mammographic screening in Germany during the 1970s (Professors Hoeffken, Frischbier, and Hüppe were my scientific companions on this journey). Charles Gros was the "godfather" of mammography in Europe at that time. My "bible" was the monograph *Comparative Anatomy, Pathology and Roentgenology of the Breast* by Ingleby and Gershon-Cohen. This was the first book that compared the anatomy and radiology of breast tissue in a vivid and comprehensive way.

For decades I viewed mammography as *the* method of choice for the early detection of breast cancer (tests such as *luminescence radiography* and *thermography* caused initial euphoria but were ultimately disappointing) until the mid-1990s, when an MRI unit was installed at our institution. By the end of that decade, *ultrasonography* was increasingly gaining the upper hand. Today, in the course of our routine work, we detect more small tumors by ultrasound than by mammography. I learned *fine-needle aspiration* (FNA) during my pathology training in 1972 under Joseph Zajicek at the Karolinska Institute in Stockholm and am still a defender of this simple, low-cost method even though I still perform a great many CNBs and VBs. A good way to advance this oldest, most time-tested interventional procedure and make it more competitive with the dominant market of high-cost VB technology is *contact cytology* (CC) used in conjunction with the CNB of solid breast nodules. When CC is employed, the patient does not have to wait anxiously for days or even weeks for a *histologic* diagnosis but can quickly learn whether the *cytologic* findings suggest a benign or malignant cause. Definitive histology will then confirm this finding and allow for further immunohistochemical tumor analysis.

The journey is the destination, and given the current dominance of mammography, this atlas also could be titled *Back to the Roots*—the roots of a rapid, comprehensive, economical, and accurate diagnosis of breast diseases. No *single* method can provide an early diagnosis (or rapid exclusion) of breast cancer. A *combination* of methods are needed, and one purpose of this atlas was to make that point clear.

Mammography will continue to play an important role in the early detection and diagnosis of breast abnormalities, but it will have to share that role with ultrasound and MRI. Modern screening requires a new way of thinking—a shift away from the complicated and time-consuming handling of conventional mammography and toward the capabilities of *digital* technology. We have explored these issues in this book and have illustrated their potenzial. *Less mammography (using fully digital technology and including tumosynthesis in selected cases) plus the greater utilization of ultrasound/MRI* should reduce the high incidence of interval cancers in screening from the current 30% to approximately 5%. Combined with therapeutic advances, this strategy would significantly increase the life expectancy of women (and men!) with breast cancer. Studies have confirmed that even women under 50 years of age will benefit from screening. Limiting factors in this age group are the added costs of screening younger women plus the higher radiosensitivity of the breast parenchyma, although single-plane mammography combined with high-resolution ultrasound should solve this problem. Breast cancer is no longer the domain of older women. While the worldwide incidence of breast cancer is on the decline, the disease has shown an alarming and unexplained increase in women 30 to 50 years of age. A separate chapter was devoted to this age group and included screening during pregnancy. Considering the possibility of breast cancer in pregnant women with atypical changes and educating younger women in general about the importance of screening examinations is not only a task for gynecologists but also an important social-policy objective in which self-help groups can play a supportive role. Screening points the way to this goal, although it is still practiced with methods from the previous century. Let us optimize it!

As in all areas of medicine, *guidelines* are essential for the optimization of early breast cancer detection and treatment on a broad scale. They are not *laws* that must be rigorously obeyed but are recommendations for the proper management of breast cancer. Guidelines are derived from the results of large-scale studies, and this further underscores their importance in modern medical discoveries. But there are situations in which a patient is better served when her doctor goes beyond guidelines, i.e., when the doctor's own experience promises to yield a better treatment outcome than guideline-based recommendations.

Wendie Berg of Johns Hopkins University, whom I greatly admire for her work in breast ultrasound (as an adjunct to mammography), declined to write a foreword for this book because a great many of my statements have not been validated by studies. I am not angry at her for this, and ultimately she is correct from her own perspective. But in pursuing my own practice, I cannot ignore the wealth of experience that I have gained in over four decades of breast examinations. I must be accountable to my patients, and I (unfortunately) no longer have the time to wait for studies that will analyze and validate my results. Mammography itself was introduced without an evidence base and has become an indispensable tool; yet ultrasound, which is at least as important in screening, cannot gain a foothold because it is not evidence-based. But how shall it become so? There is still a lack of studies to document its value in conjunction with single-plane mammograms. Who will have the courage to finally validate ultrasound in a study?

Leading experts from the American College of Radiology and other scientific societies in the U.S. have spoken to me from the heart in their statement on practice guidelines. I feel that their words provide a fitting conclusion to this atlas:

*These guidelines are an educational tool designed to assist practitioners in providing appropriate radiologic care for patients. They are not inflexible rules or requirements of practice and are not intended, nor should they be used, to establish a legal standard of care. For these reasons and those set forth below, the American College of Radiology cautions against the use of these guidelines in litigation in which the clinical decisions of a practitioner are called into question.*

*The ultimate judgment regarding the propriety of any specific procedure or course of action must be made by the physician or medical physicist in light of all the circumstances presented. Thus, an approach that differs from the guidelines, standing alone, does not necessarily imply that the approach was below the standard of care. To the contrary, a conscientious practitioner may responsibly adopt a course of action different from that set forth in the guidelines when, in the reasonable judgment of the practitioner, such course of action is indicated by the condition of the patient, limitations on available resources, or advances in knowledge or technology subsequent to publication of the guidelines. However, a practitioner who employs an approach substantially different from these guidelines is advised to document in the patient record information sufficient to explain the approach taken.*

*The practice of medicine involves not only the science, but also the art of dealing with the prevention, diagnosis, alleviation, and treatment of disease. The variety and complexity of human conditions make it impossible to always reach the most appropriate diagnosis or to predict with certainty a particular response to treatment. Therefore, it should be recognized that adherence to these guidelines will not assure an accurate diagnosis or a successful outcome. All that should be expected is that the practitioner will follow a reasonable course of action based on current knowledge, available resources, and the needs of the patient to deliver effective and safe medical care. The sole purpose of these guidelines is to assist practitioners in achieving this objective.*

American College of Radiology
American College of Surgeons
College of American Pathologists
Society of Surgical Oncology
Adopted by Board of Chancellors, American College of Radiology
And endorsed by Board of Regents, American College of Surgeons
Society of Surgical Oncology
College of American Pathologists

# Bibliography

Albert U-S, Schulz K-D, Alt D, et al. [A guideline for guidelines—methodological report and use of the guideline women's information.] Zentralbl Gynakol 2003; 125: 484–493

Allgayer B, Lukas P, Loos W, Kersting-Sommerhoff B. [The MRT of the breast with 2D-spin-echo and gradient-echo sequences in diagnostically problematic cases.] RoFo 1993; 158: 423–427

American College of Radiology. ACR Practice Guideline for the Performance of a Breast Ultrasound Examination, 1994 (revised 1998, 2002; amended 2006, revised 2007). Available at http://www.acr.org/secondarymainmenucategories/quality_safety/guidelines/breast/us_breast.aspx. Accessed August 25, 2010

American College of Radiology. BI-RADS® Breast Imaging and Reporting Data System (BI-RADS®) of the American College of Radiology (ACR) 2003. Trans. U. Fischer and G. Pfarl. 4th ed. Stuttgart: Thieme; 2006

Andersson I, Ikeda DM, Zackrisson S, et al. Breast tomosynthesis and digital mammography: a comparison of breast cancer visibility and BIRADS classification in a population of cancers with subtle mammographic findings. Eur Radiol 2008; 18(12): 2817–2825

Arslan A, Ciftçi E, Yildiz F, Cetin A, Demirci A. Multifocal bone tuberculosis presenting as a breast mass: CT and MRI findings. Eur Radiol 1999; 9(6): 1117–1119

Arthur JE, Ellis IO, Flowers C, Roebuck E, Elston CW, Blamey RW. The relationship of "high risk" mammographic patterns to histological risk factors for development of cancer in the human breast. Br J Radiol 1990; 63(755): 845–849

Avril N, Dose J, Ziegler S, Jänicke F, Schwaiger M. Diagnostic evaluation of breast tumors and locoregional lymph node metastases using positron emission tomography. Mamma II. Radiologe 1997; 37(9): 741–748

Baines CJ. Reihenuntersuchungen zur Brustkrebsfrüherkennung: Wie sinnvoll erscheinen sie zu Beginn des 21. Jahrhunderts? Vortrag Internationaler Kongress "Strahlenschutz nach der Jahrhundertwende". Bremen, 9 June 2000

Band PR, Le ND, Fang R, Deschamps M. Carcinogenic and endocrine disrupting effects of cigarette smoke and risk of breast cancer. Lancet 2002; 360(9339): 1044–1049

Barth V. Die Feinstruktur der Brustdrüse im Röntgenbild. Stuttgart: Thieme; 1979a

Barth V. Brustdrüse. In: Frommhold W, ed. Röntgen wie? Wann? Vol. V. Stuttgart: Thieme; 1979b

Barth V. Mammographie—Intensivkurs und Atlas für Fortgeschrittene. Stuttgart: Enke; 1994

Barth V. Radiologische Diagnostik gut- und bösartiger Prozesse in der Brust. In: Klinische Radiologie. Diagnostik mit bildgebenden Verfahren. Heidelberg: Springer Verlag; 1989: 293–384

Barth V, Barth A. Brustkrebs: Schnell verstehen—richtig behandeln. Antworten auf ihre wichtigsten Fragen. Stuttgart: Trias Verlag; 2003

Barth V, Koubenec H-J. BrustkrebsInfo. www.brustkrebs.de. Accessed 5 May, 2005

Barth V, Prechtel K. Pathologie und Radiologie (Röntgendiagnostik und Thermographie) der Brustdrüse. Handbuch der medizinischen Radiologie. Vol. XIX. Part 2: Mammatumoren. Berlin, Heidelberg: Springer Verlag; 1982

Barth V, Prechtel K. Atlas of Breast Disease. Philadelphia: C. Decker; 1991

Barth V, Franz ED, Schöll A. Microcalcifications in mammary glands. Naturwissenschaften 1977; 64: 278–279

Bässler R. Pathologie der Brustdrüse. In: Doerr W, Seifert G, Uehlinger E, eds. Spezielle pathologische Anatomie. Vol. 11. Berlin, Heidelberg, New York: Springer; 1978: 531–553

Baum F, Fischer U, Füzesi L, Obenauer S, Vosshenrich R, Grabbe E. [The radial scar in contrast media-enhanced MR mammography]. RoFo 2000; 172: 817–823

Baxter NN, Virgin BA, Durham SB, Tuttle TM. Radiation after lumpectomy for DCIS to reduce the risk of invasive breast cancer: a population based study. ASCO Annual Meeting Proceedings. 2005. J Clin Oncol 2005; 23(16S): 516

Becker N. [Screening from an epidemiologic perspective.] Radiologe 2008; 48(1): 10–16

Becker N, Junkermann H. Nutzen und Risiko des Mammographie-Screenings. Betrachtung aus epidemiologischer Sicht. Dtsch Arztebl 2008; 105(8): 131–136

Beckmann MW, Niedersacher D, Goecke TO, Bodden-Heinrich R, Schnürch H-G, Bender HG. Hochrisikofamilien mit Mamma- und Ovarialkarzinomen. Möglichkeiten der Beratung, genetische Analyse und Früherkennung. Dtsch Arztebl 1997; 94: B-139–B-145

Beral V, Million Women Study Collaborators. Breast cancer and hormone-replacement therapy in the Million Women Study. Lancet 2003; 362(9382): 419–427

Berg JW, Robbins GF. A late look at the safety of aspiration biopsy. Cancer 1962; 15: 826–827

Berg WA, Blume JD, Cormack JB, et al; ACRIN 6666 Investigators. Combined screening with ultrasound and mammography vs. mammography alone in women at elevated risk of breast cancer. JAMA 2008; 299(18): 2151–2163

Berlin L. The missed breast cancer redux: time for educating the public about the limitations of mammography? AJR Am J Roentgenol 2001; 176(5): 1131–1134

Bernhaus A, Hartmann B, Kubista E, Rudas M. Verschleppte vitale Tumorzellen nach stereotaktischer Mammabiopsie beim DCIS. Fördert Granulationsgewebe die lokale Metastasierung? Senologie 2005; 4: 209

Beyer S. Sport und Brustkrebs. Traumatisierung der weiblichen Brust und deren Bedeutung für die Entstehung von Brustkrebs. Eine epidemiologisch retrospektive Fall-Kontroll-Gruppe. Inaugural dissertation. Tübingen: Eberhard-Karl-Universität; 2004

BfArM [Federal Institute for Drugs and Medical Devices.] Brustimplantate. Eine Informationsbroschüre für Frauen 2. Bonn: Bundesinstitut für Arzneimittel und Medizinprodukte; 2004

Bick U. [Typical and unusual findings in MR mammography.] RoFo 2000; 172: 415–428

Bick U, Diekmann F, Fallenberg EM, Fallenberg EM. [Workflow in digital screening mammography.] Radiologe 2008; 48(4): 335–344

Birkhäuser M, Brändle W, Keller PJ, Kiesel L, Kuhl H, Neulen J. Empfehlungen zur Substitution mit Estrogenen und Gestagenen im Klimakterium und in der Menopause. 33. Arbeitstreffen des "Züricher Gesprächskreises", Oktober 2004

Birrenbach S. Die diagnostische Aussagekraft bildgebender Verfahren in den ersten zwolf Monaten nach brusterhaltender Therapie des Mammakarzinoms. Inaugural dissertation. Tübingen: Eberhard-Karl-Universität; 2003

Bjurstam NG. Radiography of the female breast and axilla. With special reference to diagnosis of mammary carcinoma. Acta Radiol Suppl 1978; 357: 1–31

Blend R, Rideout DF, Kaizer L, Shannon P, Tudor-Roberts B, Boyd NF. Parenchymal patterns of the breast defined by real time ultrasound. Eur J Cancer Prev 1995; 4(4): 293–298

Bloom HJ, Richardson WW. Histological grading and prognosis in breast cancer; a study of 1409 cases of which 359 have been followed for 15 years. Br J Cancer 1957; 11(3): 359–377

Böcker W, Decker T, Rühnke M, Schneider W. [Ductal hyperplasia and ductal carcinoma in situ. Definition—classification—differential diagnosis.] Pathologe 1997; 18(1): 3–18

Bonk U, Gohla G, Sauer U, et al. Zweitbeurteilung: Große Übereinstimmung. Dtsch Ärzteblatt online, www.aerzteblatt.de/aufsaetze/0501; Accessed 4 February, 2005

Brekelmans CT, Wester P, Faber JAJ, Peeters PH, Collette HJ. Age specific sensitivity and sojourn time in a breast cancer screening program (DOM) in the Netherlands: a comparison of different methods. Epidemiol Community Health 1996; 50: 68–71

Brenner RJ, Weitzel JN, Hansen N, Boasberg P. Screening-detected breast cancer in a man with BRCA2 mutation: case report. Radiology 2004; 230(2): 553–555

Brown J, Smith RC, Lee CH. Incidental enhancing lesions found on MR imaging of the breast. AJR Am J Roentgenol 2001; 176(5): 1249–1254

Brücker S, Krainich U, Bamberg M, et al. Brustzentren—Rationale, funktionelles Konzept, Definition und Zertifizierung. Gynakologe 2003; 36: 862–877

Buchberger W. Vortrag: Genetische Beratung. Aktuelle Wertung der Sonographie in der Mammadiagnostik. Österreichische Gesellschaft für Senologie, Maritimer Workshop. Belek; 2005

Buchbinder SS, Leichter IS, Lederman RB, et al. Computer-aided classification of BI-RADS category 3 breast lesions. Radiology 2004; 230(3): 820–823

Burell HC, Sibbering DM, Wilson ARM, et al. Screening intervalbreast cancers: Mammography features and prognostic factors. Radiology 1996; 199: 811–817

Buttenberg D, Werner K. Die Mammographie. Stuttgart: Schattauer; 1962

Butz N. Mammographie-Screening, wenn Wissenschaftler Politik machen. Dtsch Arztebl 2003; 100: A76–A78

Buyer P. Sinn und Unsinn kernspintomographischer Untersuchungen der weiblichen Brustorgane. Dissertation. Tübingen: Eberhard-Karls-Universität; 2002

Byrne C. Studying mammographic density: implications for understanding breast cancer. J Natl Cancer Inst 1997; 89: 531–533

Carter CL, Allen C, Henson DE. Relation of tumor size, lymph node status, and survival in 24, 740 breast cancer cases. Cancer 1989; 63(1): 181–187

Castano-Almendral AH, Glätzner H, Siedentopf HG. [Comparative mammographic and histological findings.] Arch Gynakol 1971; 211: 43

Chen SC, Cheung YC, Lo YF, et al. Sonographic differentiation of invasive and intraductal carcinomas of the breast. Br J Radiol 2003; 76: 600–604

Clade H. Gesundheitsreform: Integration light. Dtsch Arztebl 2004; 101(17): A-1121/B-929/C-905

Clarke CA, Glaser SL, Uratsu CS, Selby JV, Kushi LH, Herrinton LJ. Recent declines in hormone therapy utilization and breast cancer incidence: clinical and population-based evidence. J Clin Oncol 2006; 24(33): e49–e50

Clever K, Hauser R, Hettenbach A. Diskussionsbeitrag der Landesärztekammer Baden-Württemberg (www.aerztekammer-bw.de) zum Mammographie-Screening. Homepage der Ärztekammer Baden-Württemberg vom 1.7.2003

Consensus Conference Committee. Consensus Conference on the classification of ductal carcinoma in situ. The Consensus Conference Committee. Cancer 1997; 80(9): 1798–1802

Daidone MG, Coradini D, Martelli G, Veneroni S. Primary breast cancer in elderly women: biological profile and how it relates to clinical outcome. Crit Rev Oncol Hematol 2003 Mar; 45(3): 313–325

Daland EP. Brustkrebsstudie über Radikalamputation und Frauen ohne Amputation: keine Operation ist auch gut. J Cancer Res 1927; 11: 60

Decker T, Ruhnke M, Schneider W. [Standardized pathologic examination of breast excision specimen. Relevance within an interdisciplinary practice protocol for quality management of breast saving therapy.] Pathologe 1997; 18: 53–59

Decker T, Böcker W. 12 zytologische Begutachtung. In: Fischer U, Baum F. Diagnostische Interventionen der Mamma. Stuttgart: Thieme; 2008: 179

Delorme S. [Breast cancer. Sonography and magnetic resonance mammography.] Radiologe 2004; 44(6): 621–637, quiz 638–639

Destouet JM, Monsees BS, Oser RF, Nemecek JR, Young VL, Pilgram TK. Screening mammography in 350 women with breast implants: prevalence and findings of implant complications. AJR Am J Roentgenol 1992; 159(5): 973–978; discussion 979–981

Destounis SV, DiNitto P, Logan-Young W, Bonaccio E, Zuley ML, Willison KM. Can computer-aided detection with double reading of screening mammograms help decrease the false-negative rate? Initial experience. Radiology 2004; 232(2): 578–584

De Wilde RL, Fehm T, Tchartchin G, et al. Fortschritt in der Therapie des Mammakarzinoms: Optimierte Therapieplanung mit Hilfe von Genprofilen? Senologie 2008; 5: 125–128

Diekmann F, Diekmann S, Beljavskaja M, et al. [Preoperative MRT of the breast in invasive lobular carcinoma in comparison with invasive ductal carcinoma.] RoFo 2004; 176: 544–549

Diekmann S, Diekmann F. [Mammography screening in Germany.] Radiologe 2008; 48(1): 17–25

Dörk T, Bremer M, Karstens JH, Sohn C. Brustkrebs und Strahlensensibilität: eine gemeinsame erbliche Vergangenheit? Eine Übersicht. Geburtshilfe Frauenheilkd 2002; 62: 1162–1169

Duchesne N, Parker SH, Klaus AJ, Mooney ML. Breast biopsy: multicenter study of radiofrequency introducer with US-guided handheld system—initial experience. Radiology 2004; 232(1): 205–210

Duda VF, Schultz-Wendtland R. Mammadiagnostik komplementärer Einsatz aller Verfahren. Berlin: Springer Verlag; 2004

Duijm EM, Fraschbood J. Impact of additional double reading by radiographers on breast cancer-screening; Eur Congress Roentgenol (2007) B-383, Abstract. Zitiert bei Diekmann (2008)

Eiermann W, Kaufmann M, v. Minckwitz G. GABG, German Adjuvant Breast Cancer Study: Pressekonferenz IBIS II—erste Erfahrungen. Frankfurt, 23 November 2004

Egan RL. Roles of mammography in the early detection of breast cancer. Cancer 1969; 24: 1197

Elmore JG, Carney PA, Abraham LA, et al. Obesity increases risk of false-positive mammograms. Arch Intern Med 2004 May 24; 164 (10): 1140–1147

Elmore JG, Armstrong K, Lehman CD, Fletcher SW. Screening for breast cancer. JAMA 2005; 293: 1245–1256

Elston CW, Ellis IO. Pathological prognostic factors in breast cancer. I. The value of histological grade in breast cancer: experience from a large study with long-term follow-up. Histopathology 1991; 19 (5): 403–410

Emons G. Sinkende Mammakarzinominzidenz als Folge reduzierter Verabreichung der peri- und postmeonpausalen HT? Vortrag 28. Jahrestagung der Deutschen Gesellschaft für Senologie: Stuttgart; 2008

Engel J, Hölzel D, Kerr J, Schubert-Fritschle G. Epidemiologie. Empfehlungen zur Diagnostik, Therapie und Nachsorge von Mammakarzinom des Tumorzentrums München. München, Wien, New York: Zuckschwerdt; 2003: 1–11

Eusoma – European Society of Mastology. Breast Unit Guidelines 2000. European Journal of Cancer 2000; 36: 2288–2293

Evans WP III, Starr AL, Bennos ES. Comparison of the relative incidence of impalpable invasive breast carcinoma and ductal carcinoma in situ in cancers detected in patients older and younger than 50 years of age. Radiology 1997; 204(2): 489–491

Everson RB, Li FP, Fraumeni JF Jr, et al. Familial male breast cancer. Lancet 1976; 1(7949): 9–12

Ewen K, Blendl C. Mammographiegeräte-Prüfung. Nationale und internationale Vorschriften. Radiologe 2004; 44: M9–M10

Faverly DR, Bürgers L, Bült P, Holland R. Three dimensional imaging of mammary ductal carcinoma in situ: clinical implications. Semin Diagn Pathol 1994; 11(3): 193–198

Feig SA. Age-related accuracy of screening mammography: how should it be measured? Radiology 2000; 214(3): 633–640

Ferlay J, Autier P, Boniol M, Heanue M, Colombet M, Boyle P. Estimates of the cancer incidence and mortality in Europe in 2006. Ann Oncol 2007; 18(3): 581–592

Fineberg S, Rosen PP. Cutaneous angiosarcoma and atypical vascular lesions of the skin and breast after radiation therapy for breast carcinoma. Am J Clin Pathol 1994; 102(6): 757–763

Fischer U. Deutschland sichert die Qualität in der Mammographie. Radiologe 2004; 4: M58–M60

Fischer U, von Heyden D, Vosshenrich R, Vieweg I, Grabbe E. [Signal characteristics of malignant and benign lesions in dynamic 2D-MRT of the breast.] RoFo 1993; 158: 287–292

Fischer U, Baum F. Mammography Casebook—100 Studies in Breast Imaging. Stuttgart, New York: Thieme; 2006

Fischer U, Baum F. Diagnostische Interventionen der Mamma. Stuttgart: Thieme; 2008

Fischmann A, Pietsch-Breitfeld B, Müller-Schimpfle M, et al. [Radiologic-histopathologic correlation of microcalcifications from 11 g vacuum biopsy: analysis of 3196 core biopsies.] RoFo 2004; 176: 538–543

Fisher BH, Slack N, Bross JDJ. Cancer of the breast: Size of neoplasma and prognosis. Cancer 1969; 24: 1071–1080

Fornage BD, Sneige N, Ross MI, et al. Small (< or = 2-cm) breast cancer treated with US-guided radiofrequency ablation: feasibility study. Radiology 2004; 231(1): 215–224

Foster MC, Helvie MA, Gregory NE, Rebner M, Nees AV, Paramagul C. Lobular carcinoma in situ or atypical lobular hyperplasia at coreneedle biopsy: is excisional biopsy necessary? Radiology 2004; 231(3): 813–819

von Fournier D, Weber E, Hoeffken W, Bauer M, Kubli F, Barth V. Growth rate of 147 mammary carcinomas. Cancer 1980; 45(8): 2198–2207

Fowble BL, Hanlon A, Freedman G, Nicolaou N, Anderson P. Second cancers after conservative surgery and radiation for stages I–II breast cancer: identifying a subset of women at increased risk. Int J Radiat Oncol Biol Phys 2001; 51(3): 679–690

Frankenberg D, Kühn H, Frankenberg-Schwager M. Physikalische und genetische Aspekte: Risiken der Mammographie bei familiär Brustkrebs disponierten Frauen. GYNE 1996; 17: 451–453

Frei KA, Kinkel K, Bonel HM, Lu Y, Esserman LJ, Hylton NM. MR imaging of the breast in patients with positive margins after lumpectomy: influence of the time interval between lumpectomy and MR imaging. AJR Am J Roentgenol 2000; 175(6): 1577–1584

Freund M, Schneider W, Heinlein P, Teichmann A. Telemammographieprojekt – Vorteile regionaler Netzwerke: Qualitätsgerechte Früherkennung, Behandlung und Nachsorge des Mammakarzinoms erfordern integrierte technische Konzepte. Dtsch Arztebl 2004; 101: A247–A250

Fritzsche FR, Dietel M, Kristiansen G. [Flat epithelial neoplasia and other columnar cell lesions of the breast.] Pathologe 2006; 27: 381–386

Frohwein V, Böttcher HW. Frühdiagnostik des Mammakarzinoms. Gynäkol. Praxis. 1998; 22: 685–702

Galea MH, Blamey RW, Elston CE, Ellis IO. The Nottingham Prognostic Index in primary breast cancer. Breast Cancer Res Treat 1992; 22(3): 207–219

Gallager HS, Martin JE. The study of mammary carcinoma by mammography and whole organ sectioning. Early observations. Cancer 1969; 23(4): 855–873

Gatzemeier W, Liersch T, Stylianou A, Buttler A, Becker H, Fischer U. [Preoperative MR mammography in breast carcinoma. Effect on operative treatment from the surgical viewpoint.] Chirurg 1999; 70: 1460–1468

Georgian-Smith D, Lawton TJ. Calcifications of lobular carcinoma in situ of the breast: radiologic-pathologic correlation. AJR Am J Roentgenol 2001; 176(5): 1255–1259

Gerber B. Persönlicher Lebensstil und Brustkrebsrisiko. Journal für Menopause 2003; 10(3): 7–14

Giebel G-B, Nutz V, Jaeger K. Akute Mammanekrose nach Quadranten-Resektion und kombinierter radiologisch/zytologischer Nachbehandlung. In: Neubauer H, ed. Wiederherstellungschirurgie des Alters. Berlin, Heidelberg, New York: Springer; 1986

Giersiepen K, Haartje U, Hentschel S, Katalinic A, Kieschke J. Tumorstadienverteilung in der Zielgruppe für das Mammographie-Screening. Dtsch Arztebl 2004; 101: A2117

Gilles R, Zafrani B, Guinebretière JM, et al. Ductal carcinoma in situ: MR imaging-histopathologic correlation. Radiology 1995; 196(2): 415–419

Gillis CR, Hole DJ. Survival outcome of care by specialist surgeons in breast cancer: a study of 3768 Patients in the West of Scotland. BMJ 1996; 312(7024): 145–148

Glück S. Psychologische Aspekte der Tumornachsorge.Vortrag Maritimer Workshop der Österreichischen Gesellschaft für Senologie. Belek; 2005

Goldhirsch A, Wood WC, Gelber RD, Coates AS, Thürlimann B, Senn HJ. Meeting highlights: updated international expert consensus on the primary therapy of early breast cancer. J Clin Oncol 2003; 21(17): 3357–3365

Golub RM, Bennett CL, Stinson T, Venta L, Morrow M. Cost minimization study of image-guided core biopsy versus surgical excisional biopsy for women with abnormal mammograms. J Clin Oncol 2004; 22(12): 2430–2437

Görse R, Jukasz-Böss I, Ortmann O, Pohl F, Kölbl O, Wenz F. Teilbrust-Bestrahlung nach brusterhaltender Operation des Mammakarzinoms. Frauenheilk up2date 2007; 4: 294–298

Gorczyca DP, Brenner RJ. The Augmented Breast. Radiologic and Clinical Perspectives. Stuttgart: Thieme; 1997

Gordon PD, et al: Proceedings of the Consensus Conference of Sentinel Lymph Node Biopsy in Carcinoma of the Breast. April 19–22 2001, Philadelphia (published 2002 ACS, Dor 10.1002/cncr 10539)

Gordon PB, Goldenberg SL. Malignant breast masses detected only by ultrasound. A retrospective review. Cancer 1995; 76(4): 626–630

Gram IT, Bremnes Y, Ursin G, Maskarinec G, et al: Percentage density, Wolfe's and Tabar's mammographic patterns: agreement and association with risk factors for breast cancer. Eur J Radiol 1997; 24: 131–136

Gros R. Silikon-Implantate. Nutzen, Komplikationen und Alternativen. Stuttgart: Trias; 1996

Gruber R, Bernt R, Hellbig T. Cost effectiviness of percutaneous core needle breast biopsy (CNBB) versus open surgical biopsy (OSB) of nonpalpable breast lesions: metaanalysis and cost evaluation for German-speaking countries. RoFo 2008; 180: 134–142

Hackethal J. Auf Messers Schneide. Kunst und Fehler der Chirurgen. Berlin: Rowohlt Taschenbuch 1977

Haen M, Bokemeyer C, et al. Mammkarzinom. Empfehlung zur Diagnose, Therapie und Nachsorge. Interdisziplinäres Tumorzentrum Tübingen. Tübingen: ITZ, 2003: 22

Hahn M, Walz-Mattmüller R, Hoffmann J, Krainick-Strobel U, Staebler A, Wallwiener D. Stanzbioptisch induzierte AV-Fistel in der Brust. Geburtshilfe Frauenheilkd 2008; 68: 747–748

Hahn SA, Greenhalf B, Ellis I, et al. BRCA2 germline mutations in familial pancreatic carcinoma. J Natl Cancer Inst 2003; 95(3): 214–221

Hall PF. Gynecomastia. Monographs of the Federal Council of the British Medical Association of Australia, New South Wales, Australian Medical Publishing Co; 1959(2): 23–26

Hall-Craggs MA. Interventional MRI of the breast: minimally invasive therapy. Eur Radiol 2000; 10(1): 59–62

Hamperl H. [On the problem of the pathologic anatomical principles of mammography.] Geburtshilfe Frauenheilkd 1968; 28: 901–917

Hankinson SE, Willett WC, Michaud DS, et al. Plasma prolactin levels and subsequent risk of breast cancer in postmenopausal women. J Natl Cancer Inst 1999; 91(7): 629–634

Harbeck N, Kates RE, Look MP, et al. Enhanced benefit from adjuvant chemotherapy in breast cancer patients classified high-risk according to urokinase-type plasminogen activator (uPA) and plasminogen activator inhibitor type 1 (n = 3424). Cancer Res 2002; 62 (16): 4617–4622

Harder von Y, Ratzel R. Das angeblich übersehene Mammakarzinom. Frauenarzt 1999; 10: 1284–1287

Harris JR, Lippman ME, Morrow M, Osborne CK. Disease of the Breast. Philadelphia: Lippincott, Williams and Wilkins; 2004

Harvey JA, Bovbjerg VE. Quantitative assessment of mammographic breast density: relationship with breast cancer risk. Radiology 2004; 230(1): 29–41

Harvey JA, Fechner RE, Moore MM. Apparent ipsilateral decrease in breast size at mammography: a sign of infiltrating lobular carcinoma. Radiology 2000; 214(3): 883–889

Hassler O. Microradiographic investigations of calcifications of the female breast. Cancer 1969; 23(5): 1103–1109

Hata T, Takahashi H, Watanabe K, et al. Magnetic resonance imaging for preoperative evaluation of breast cancer: a comparative study with mammography and ultrasonography. J Am Coll Surg 2004; 198(2): 190–197

Hauth EA, Umutlu L, Quinsten A, Kümmel S, Kimmig R, Forsting M. MRT-gesteuerte Vakuumbiopsie der Brust mit dem ATEC-Brustbiopsie- und Exzisionssystem. Senologie 2008; 5: 156–161

Heidemann E, Rössle S. Qualitätssicherung in der Mammakarzinom-Nachsorge. ÄBW 2004; 4: 156–158

Heidenreich P, Vogt H, Bachter D, et al. Das Konzept des Wächterlymphknotens: Stand und klinische Bedeutung. Dtsch Arztebl 2001; 98(9): A543

Heinlein P, Drexl J, Gössler A, Janssen S, Schneider W. An integrated approach to computer-assisted diagnosis in digital mammography. Int Congr Ser 2001; 1230: 573–579

Helvie MA, Hadjiiski L, Makariou E, et al. Sensitivity of noncommercial computer-aided detection system for mammographic breast cancer detection: pilot clinical trial. Radiology 2004; 231(1): 208–214

Hesch RD, Thommen A, Beckmann WW. Das Mammakarzinom. Workshop der European Society for Clinical Investigations. Molekularpathologie – Molekulargenetik – Präventionsstrategien. Gynakologe 1997; 30: 969–976

Heywang-Köbrunner SH, Schaumlöffel U. Viehweg, Höfer H, Buchmann J, Lampe D. Minimal invasive stereotactic vacuum core breast biopsy. Eur Radiol 1998; 8: 377–385

Heywang SH, Hilbertz T, Beck R, Bauer WM, Eiermann W, Permanetter W. Gd-DTPA enhanced MR imaging of the breast in patients with postoperative scarring and silicon implants. J Comput Assist Tomogr 1990; 14(3): 348–356

Heywang-Köbrunner SH, Huynh AT, Viehweg P, Hanke W, Requardt H, Paprosch I. Prototype breast coil for MR-guided needle localization. J Comput Assist Tomogr 1994; 18(6): 876–881

Heywang-Köbrunner SH, Heinig A, Pickuth D, Alberich T, Spielmann RP. Interventional MRI of the breast: lesion localisation and biopsy. Eur Radiol 2000; 10(1): 36–45

Heywang-Köbrunner SH. Bildgebende Mammadiagnostik: Untersuchungstechnik, Befundmuster, Differenzialdiagnose und Intervention. 2nd ed. Stuttgart: Thieme; 2003

Hille H, Rückner R, Vetter M, Hackeloer BJ. Früherkennung des Mammakarzinoms—was ist gesichert? Frauenarzt 2004a; 45: 642–648

Hille H, Vetter M, Hackelöer BJ. [Re-evaluating the role of breast ultrasound in current diagnostics of malignant breast lesions.] Ultraschall Med 2004b; 25: 411–417

Höffken W, Lanyi M. Röntgenuntersuchung der Brust. Stuttgart: Thieme; 1973

Holland R, Hendriks JH, Vebeek AL, Mravunac M, Schuurmans Stekhoven JH. Extent, distribution, and mammographic/histological correlations of breast ductal carcinoma in situ. Lancet 1990; 335 (8688): 519–522

Hollenhorst M, Hansen C, Hüttebräuker N, et al. Ultrasonographic breast imaging using full angle spatial compounding (FASC): In-vivo Evaluations. 28. Jahrestagung. Deutsche Gesellschaft für Senologie; 2008 [Abstract, p. 194]

Hollerweger A, Macheiner P, Neureiter D, Dietze O. [Uncommon cystic appearance of lymph nodes in malignant lymphoma.] Ultraschall Med 2008; 29(3): 308–310

Horner MJ, Ries LAG, Krapcho M, et al (eds). SEER Cancer Statistics Review, 1975–2006, National Cancer Institute, Bethesda, MD. http://seer.cancer.gov/csr/1975_2006/, based on November 2008 SEER data submission, posted to the SEER web site, 2009

Huang W, Fisher PR, Dulaimy K, Tudorica LA, O'Hea B, Button TM. Detection of breast malignancy: diagnostic MR protocol for improved specificity. Radiology 2004; 232(2): 585–591

Hunt KA, Sickles EA. Effect of obesity on screening mammography: outcomes analysis of 88, 346 consecutive examinations. AJR Am J Roentgenol 2000; 174(5): 1251–1255

Ikeda DM, Andersson I, Wattsgård C, Janzon L, Linell F. Interval carcinomas in the Malmö Mammographic Screening Trial: radiographic appearance and prognostic considerations. AJR Am J Roentgenol 1992; 159(2): 287–294

Ikeda DM, Birdwell RL, O'Shaughnessy KF, Sickles EA, Brenner RJ. Computer-aided detection output on 172 subtle findings on normal mammograms previously obtained in women with breast cancer detected at follow-up screening mammography. Radiology 2004; 230(3): 811–819

Ingleby H, Gershon-Coken J. Comparative Anatomy, Pathology and Roentgenology of the Breast. Philadelphia: University of Pennsylvania Press; 1960

Jakes RW, Duffy SW, Ng FC, et al. Mammographic parenchymal patterns and self-reported soy intake in Singapore Chinese women. Cancer Epidemiol Biomarkers Prev 2002; 11(7): 608–613

Jatoi I, Chen BE, Anderson WS, Rosenberg PS. Breast cancer mortality trends in the United States according to estrogen receptor status and age at diagnosis. J Clin Oncol 2007; May 1; 25(13): 1683–1690

Jöns K. Europäische Erfahrungen und Empfehlungen – Qualitätssicherung in interdisziplinären Brustzentren. Forum 4/2003; 18: 33–35

Julien JP, Bijker N, Fentiman IS, et al; EORTC Breast Cancer Cooperative Group and EORTC Radiotherapy Group. Radiotherapy in breast-conserving treatment for ductal carcinoma in situ: first results of the EORTC randomised phase III trial 10853. Lancet 2000; 355(9203): 528–533

Jung H. [Assessment of usefulness and risk of mammography screening with exclusive attention to radiation risk.] Radiologe 2001; 41: 385–395

Jung H. Aktuelle Diskussion: Haben BRCA-Patientinnen ein erhöhtes Mammographie-Risiko? GYNE 1997; 18: 14–15

Kaiser WA. [MR mammography.] Radiologe 1993; 33(5): 292–299

Kallergi M, Heine JJ, Berman CG, Hersh MR, Romilly AP, Clark RA. Improved interpretation of digitized mammography with wavelet processing: a localization response operating characteristic study. AJR Am J Roentgenol 2004; 182(3): 697–703

Kapur A, Carson PL, Eberhard J, et al. Automated ultrasound scanning on a dual modality breast imaging system. J Ultrasound Med 2007; 26: 645–655

Kaspar S. Die an Brustkrebs erkrankte Frau im Medizinbetrieb. 12 Ziele zur Verbesserung der Situation von Betroffenen. Bonn: Deutsche Krebshilfe e.V. (German Cancer Aid); July 2003

Katalinic A, Bartel C, Raspe H, Schreer I. Beyond mammography screening: quality assurance in breast cancer diagnosis (The QuaMaDi Project). Br J Cancer 2007; 96(1): 157–161

Kaufmann M, Minckwitz G, Eiermann W, Hilfrich J, Jonat W, Kreienberg R. Therapie primärer Mammakarzinome. Kongressbericht: Ergebnis der Konferenz in St. Gallen 2003. Dtsch Arztebl 2004; 101: B163–B169

Kemperman H, Borger J, Hart A, Peterse J, Bartelink H, van Dongen J. Prognostic factors for survival after breast conserving therapy for stage I and II breast cancer. The role of local recurrence. Eur J Cancer 1995; 31: 690–698

Kennedy RJ, Kollias J, Gill PG, Bochner M, Coventry BJ, Farshid G. Removal of two sentinel nodes accurately stages the axilla in breast cancer. Br J Surg 2003; 90(11): 1349–1353

Kerlikowske K, Grady D, Barclay J, Sickles EA, Ernster V. Effect of age, breast density, and family history on the sensitivity of first screening mammography. JAMA 1996; 276(1): 33–38

Kerlikowske K, Miglioretti DL, Ballard-Barbash R, et al. Prognostic characteristics of breast cancer among postmenopausal hormone users in a screened population. J Clin Oncol 2003; 21: 4314–4321

Kettritz U, Rotter K, Schreer I, et al. Stereotactic vacuum-assisted breast biopsy in 2874 patients: a multicenter study. Cancer 2004; 100(2): 245–251

Key TJ, Verkasalo PK. Endogenous hormones and the aetiology of breast cancer. [Commentary] Breast Cancer Res 1999; 1(1): 18–21

Key TJ, Sharp GB, Appleby PN, et al. Soya foods and breast cancer risk: a prospective study in Hiroshima and Nagasaki, Japan. Br J Cancer 1999; 81(7): 1248–1256

Kiechle M, Böttcher B, Ditsch N, et al. Hereditäres Mammakarzinom. Manual Mammakarzinome 2003. Munich: Tumorzentrum München und W. Zuckschwerdt Verlag; 2003: 72–81

Kiewe P, Knorfel A, Weller M. Überwindung der Blut-Hirnschranke. Neue Substanzen zur medikamentösen Hirnmetastasentherapie. Onkologe 2008; 14(3): 260–266

Kleeberg UR. Insulin und insulinartige Wachstumsfaktoren (IGF) in der Onkogenese des Mammakarzinoms: von translationaler Forschung zur Prävention. Vortrag 28. Jahrestagung der Deutschen Gesellschaft für Senologie. Stuttgart; 2008

Koch K. Erstmals Trendwende der Krebsmortalität in USA. Dtsch Arztebl 1996; 93(48): B-2690

Kolb TM, Lichy J, Newhouse JH. Comparison of the performance of screening, mammography, physical examination and breast US and evaluation of factors that influence them: An analysis of 27,825 patient evaluations. Radiology 2002; 225: 165–175

Kopans DB, Moore RH, McCarthy KA, et al. Positive predictive value of breast biopsy performed as a result of mammography: there is no abrupt change at age 50 years. Radiology 1996; 200(2): 357–360

Kopans DB, Feig SA. False positive rate of screening mammography. N Engl J Med 1998; 339(8): 562–564

Koubenec HJ. Mammographie-Screening: Überschätzen wir den Nutzen? Berliner Ärzte 2000; 8(37): 11–16

Kreienberg R, Kopp I, Albrecht K, et al. Interdiziplinäre S3-Leitlinie für die Diagnostik, Therapie und Nachsorge des Mammakarzinoms. München, Wien, New York: Deutsche Krebsgesellschaft, Zuckschwerdt Verlag GmbH; 2008: 24 ff

Kreuzer G, Boqoui E. Zytologie der weiblichen Brustdrüse. Stuttgart: Thieme; 1981

Krokowski E. Betrachtung zur Dynamik des Geschwulstwachstums. In: Gottron HA, ed. Krebsforschung und Krebsbekämpfung. Vol. V. Munich: Urban und Schwarzenberg 1964

Kubba AA. Breast cancer and the pill. J R Soc Med 2003; 96(6): 280–283

Kuehn T, Bembenek A, Decker T, et al; Consensus Committee of the German Society of Senology. A concept for the clinical implementation of sentinel lymph node biopsy in patients with breast carcinoma with special regard to quality assurance. Cancer 2005; 103 (3): 451–461

Kühn T, Kreienberg R. Mammakarzinom. Plastisch-rekonstruktive Techniken in der operativen Therapie. Gynakologe 2005; 38: 1095–1107

Kühn T, Nestle-Krämling C, Roterberg K, Bender HG, Kreienberg R. Optimierung der brusterhaltenden Therapie. Möglichkeiten der Defektdeckung. Gynakologe 2005; 38: 201–208

Kühn T. Sentinel-Lymphknotenmarkierung und -Entfernung. In: Fischer U, Baum F, eds. Diagnostische Interventionen der Mamma. Stuttgart: Thieme; 2008: 171

Kuhl CK. [Familial breast cancer: what the radiologist needs to know.] RoFo 2006; 178: 680–687

Kuhl CK. Familiäre Brustkrebserkrankung: Klinische Grundlagen und Früherkennung. Fortschritt R Röntgenstrahlen 2006; 178: 680–687

Kuhl CK. The “Coming of Age” of Nonmammographic Screening for Breast Cancer. JAMA 2008; 299: 2203–2205

Kuhl CK, Seibert C, Sommer T, Kref B, Gieseke J, Schild HH. [Focal and diffuse lesions in dynamic MR-mammography of healthy probands.] RoFo 1995; 163: 219–224

Kuhl CK, Schmützler RK, Leutner CC, et al. Breast MR imaging screening in 192 women proved or suspected to be carriers of a breast cancer susceptibility gene: preliminary results. Radiology 2000; 215(1): 267–279

Kuhl CK, Schrading S, Bieling HB, et al. MRI for Diagnosis of Pure Ductal Carcinoma in situ. A Prospective Observational study. Lancet 2007; 370(9586): 485–492

Kuhl CK, Braun M. [Magnetic resonance imaging in preoperative staging for breast cancer: pros and contras.] Radiologe 2008; 48: 358–366

Kvistad KA, Rydland J, Vainio J, et al. Breast lesions: evaluation with dynamic contrast-enhanced T1-weighted MR imaging and with T2*-weighted first-pass perfusion MR imaging. Radiology 2000; 216(2): 545–553

Lamarque JL, Rodière MJ, Fontaine A, et al. Approche anatomo-histologique de la radio-anatomie mammaire. J Radiol Electrol Med Nucl 1976; 10(57): 753–766

Langen H-J, Kugel H, Grewe S, et al. [MRI-controlled preoperative wire marking of uncertain breast lesions.] RoFo 2000; 172: 764–769

Langenbeck U. Umwelt und Erbe in der Entstehung des Brustkrebses. Ein Exkurs in Tumorbiologie und molekularer Medizin. Dtsch Arztebl 1995; 92: 1789–1790

Lanyi M. Brustkrankheiten im Mammogramm. Diagnostik und pathomorphologische Bildanalyse. Berlin: Springer; 2003

Lanyi M. Diagnostik und Differenzialdiagnose der Mammaverkalkungen. Berlin: Springer; 1986

Lanyi M, Stiens R, Stiletto M. [The intraductal components and microinvasive foci in ductal breast carcinoma on the mammogram.] RoFo 1994; 161: 195–200

Lattes R. Lobular neoplasia (lobular carcinoma in situ) of the breast – a histological entity of controversial clinical significance. Pathol Res Pract 1980; 166(4): 415–429

Leborgne RA. The Breast in Roentgendiagnostic. London: Constable; 1953

Leconte I, Feger C, Galant C, et al. Mammography and subsequent whole-breast sonography of nonpalpable breast cancers: the importance of radiologic breast density. AJR Am J Roentgenol 2003; 180(6): 1675–1679

Lee CH, Dershaw DD, Kopans D, et al. Breast Cancer Screening With Imaging: Recommendations From the Society of Breast Imaging and the ACR on the Use of Mammography, Breast MRI, Breast Ultrasound, and Other Technologies for the Detection of Clinically Occult Breast Cancer. JACR 2010; 7(1): 18–27

Lee NA, Rusinek H, Weinreb J, et al. Fatty and fibroglandular tissue volumes in the breasts of women 20–83 years old: comparison of X-ray mammography and computer-assisted MR imaging. AJR Am J Roentgenol 1997; 168(2): 501–506

Lee JE, Chung KW, Han W, et al. Effect of estrogen, tamoxifen and epidermal growth factor on the transcriptional regulation of vascular endothelial growth factor in breast cancer cells. Anticancer Res 2004; 24(6): 3961–3964

Leinung S, Horn L-C, Backe J. [Male breast cancer: history, epidemiology, genetic and histopathology.] Zentralbl Chir 2007; 132: 379–385

Lell M, Wenkel E, Aichinger U, Schulz-Wendtland R, Bautz W. [3D ultrasound in core breast biopsy.] Ultraschall Med 2003; 24: 126–130

Levi F, Te V–C, Randimbison L, Vecchia CL. Trends of in situ carcinoma of the breast in Vaud, Switzererland. European Journal of Cancer 1997; 33(6): 903–906

Levi F, Bosetti C, Lucchini F, Negri E, Vecchia CL. Monitoring decrease in breast cancer mortality in Europe. European Journal of Cancer Prevention 2005; 14(6): 497–502

Liberman L, Van Zee KJ, Dershaw DD, Morris EA, Abramson AF, Samli B. Mammographic features of local recurrence in women who have undergone breast-conserving therapy for ductal carcinoma in situ. AJR Am J Roentgenol 1997; 168(2): 489–493

Liberman L, Sama MP. Cost-effectiveness of stereotactic 11-gauge directional vacuum-assisted breast biopsy. AJR Am J Roentgenol 2000; 175(1): 53–58

Liberman L, Morris EA, Dershaer DD, Thornton CM, van Zee KJ, Tan LK. Fast MRI-guided vacuum-assisted-breast biopsy: initial experience. AJR Am J Roentgenol 2003; 181(5): 1283–1293

Liberman L, Gougoutas CA, Zakowski MF, et al. Calcifications highly suggestive of malignancy: comparison of breast biopsy methods. AJR Am J Roentgenol 2001; 177(1): 165–172

Lindholm K. Clinical cytology as cytology in the clinical setting. Acta Cytol 1999; 43(3): 333

Ludwig S, Hauss JPC, Hohlfeld S, Hildebrand G, Horn LC, Leinung S. [The male breast carcinoma: a center experience.] Zentralbl Chir 2007; 132: 386–390

MacDonald HR, Silverstein MJ, Mabry H, et al. Local control in ductal carcinoma in situ treated by excision alone: incremental benefit of larger margins. Am J Surg 2005; 190(4): 521–525

Margolin FR, Kaufman L, Denny SR, Jacobs RP, Schrumpf JD. Metallic marker placement after stereotactic core biopsy of breast calcifications: comparison of two clips and deployment techniques. AJR Am J Roentgenol 2003; 181(6): 1685–1690

Marklund M, Torp-Pedersen S, Bentzon N, Thomsen C, Roslind A, Nolsøe CP. Contrast kinetics of the malignant breast tumour—border versus centre enhancement on dynamic midfield MRI. Eur J Radiol 2008; 65(2): 279–285

Mathews AW. When a mammogram isn't enough. For higher-risk women, the addition of MRI or sonogram may improve detection; a problem with false positives. Wall Street Journal 24.06.2008

Matsubayashi R, Matsuo Y, Edakuni G, Satoh T, Tokunaga O, Kudo S. Breast masses with peripheral rim enhancement on dynamic contrast-enhanced MR images: correlation of MR findings with histologic features and expression of growth factors. Radiology 2000; 217(3): 841–848

McDivitt RW, Stewart FW, Berg JW. Tumors of the Breast. Atlas of Tumor Pathology. Fac. 2, Ser. 2. Washington, DC: Armed Forces Institute of Pathology; 1968: 65

McDivitt RW, Stevens JA, Lee NC, Wingo PA, Rubin GL, Gersell D; The Cancer and Steroid Hormone Study Group. Histologic types of benign breast disease and the risk for breast cancer. Cancer 1992; 69(6): 1408–1414

Meades RT, Svensson WE, Nijran KS, et al. Do radiologists receive a significant radiation dose localising breast lesions ultrasonically following radio-isotope lymphnode imaging? European Radiology Feb 2009 (19, Suppl 1): 533–586

Moon WK, Im J-G, Koh YH, Noh DY, Park IA. US of mammographically detected clustered microcalcifications. Radiology 2000; 217(3): 849–854

Morakkabati N, Leutner CC, Schmiedel A, Schild HH, Kühl CK. Breast MR imaging during or soon after radiation therapy. Radiology 2003; 229(3): 893–901

Morrow M. Magnetic resonance imaging in the breast cancer patient: curb your enthusiasm. J Clin Oncol 2008; 26(3): 352–353

Mueck AO. Hormonersatztherapie (HRT) oder Alternativen: Neuorientierung nach WHI? Geburtshilfe Frauenheilkd 2005; 65: 323–324

Mueck AO, Wallwiener D. Brustkrebsrate und HRT. Differierende Daten aus USA und Europa. Frauenarzt 2007; 48(9): 812–817

Mueck AO, Wallwiener D. Fördert oder verhindert Rauchen Brustkrebs? Deutsche Gesellschaft für Senologie, Newsletter 012004 vom 24.2.2004, 29–30

Mühlhauser I, Höldke B. Mammographie-Screening-Darstellung der wissenschaftlichen Evidenz-Grundlage zur Kommunikation mit der Frau. Arznei-Telegramm 1999; 10: 101–108

Müller RD, Barkhausen J, Sauerwein W, Langer R. Assessment of local recurrence after breast-conserving therapy with MRI. J Comput Assist Tomogr 1998; 22(3): 408–412

Müller-Schimpfle M, Fischmann A, Siegmann K. Digitale Mammographie—Pro und Contra. Med Review 2003; 1: 12–13

Mussurakis S, Gibbs P, Horsman A. Primary breast abnormalities: selective pixel sampling on dynamic gadolinium-enhanced MR images. Radiology 1998; 206(2): 465–473

Narod SA, Dubé MP, Klijn J, et al. Oral contraceptives and the risk of breast cancer in BRCA1 and BRCA2 mutation carriers. J Natl Cancer Inst 2002; 94(23): 1773–1779

Neben K, Hübner G, Folprecht G, Jäger D, Krämer A. Metastasen ohne Primärtumor. Übersichtsarbeit. Dtsch Arztebl 2008; 105 (43): 733–740

Neigmond P. Study: Ultrasound Boosts Breast Cancer Detection; NPR Research News 17. May 2008. http://www.npr.org

OECD. Todesursache Brustkrebs 1995–1999. OECD Gesundheitsdaten; 2002

Ohlinger R, Klaus RG, Oellig F, et al. Diagnostische Wertigkeit von Palpation, Mammographie und Mammasonographie in der präoperativen Diagnostik des Mammakarzinoms. Geburtshilfe Frauenheilkd 2003; 63: 1264–1255

Ohtake T, Abe R, Kimijima I, et al. Intraductal extension of primary invasive breast carcinoma treated by breast-conservative surgery. Computer graphic three-dimensional reconstruction of the mammary duct-lobular systems. Cancer 1995; 76(1): 32–45

Orel SG, Weinstein SP, Schnall MD, et al. Breast MR imaging in patients with axillary node metastases and unknown primary malignancy. Radiology 1999; 212(2): 543–549

Orell SR, Sterrett GF, Walters MN, Whitaker D. Punktionszytologie—Handbuch und Atlas. Stuttgart, New York: Thieme; 1999

Ozzello L. Epithelial-stromal junction of normal and dysplastic mammary glands. Cancer 1970; 25(3): 586–600

Page DL, Dupont WD, Rogers LW, Jensen RA, Schuyler PA. Continued local recurrence of carcinoma 15–25 years after a diagnosis of low grade ductal carcinoma in situ of the breast treated only by biopsy. Cancer 1995; 76(7): 1197–1200

Page DL, Rogers LW. Combined histologic and cytologic criteria for the diagnosis of mammary atypical ductal hyperplasia. Hum Pathol 1992; 23(10): 1095–1097

Page DL, Jensen RA, Simpson JF. Routinely available indicators of prognosis in breast cancer. Breast Cancer Res Treat 1998; 51(3): 195–208

Palesty JA, Foster JM, Hurd TC, Watroba N, Rezaishiraz H, Edge SB. Axillary recurrence in women with a negative sentinel lymph node and no axillary dissection in breast cancer. J Surg Oncol 2006; 93(2): 129–132

Park WW, Lees JC. The absolute curability of cancer of the breast surgery. Gynecol Obstet (Paris) 1951; 93: 129–152

Peer PG, Holland R, Hendriks JH, Mravunac M, Verbeek AL. Age-specific effectiveness of the Nijmegen population-based breast cancer-screening program: assessment of early indicators of screening effectiveness. J Natl Cancer Inst 1994; 86(6): 436–441

Perry N, Broeders M, de Wolf C, Törnberg S, Holland R, von Karsa L, eds. European guidelines for quality assurance in breast cancer screening and diagnosis. 4th ed. Luxembourg: Office for Official Publications of the European Community; 2006

Peters F. Multicentre study of gestrinone in cyclical breast pain. Lancet 1992; 339(8787): 205–208

Pfarl G, Helbich TH. [Breast Imaging Reporting and Data System (BI-RADS)—German version] Rofo 2002; 174(7): 921–926

Pope THL, Fechner RW, Whilhem MC, Wanebo HJ, de Paredes ES. Lobular carcinoma in situ of the breast. Mammographic features. Radiology 1988; 168: 63–66

Poplack SP, Wells WA. Ductal carcinoma in situ of the breast: mammographic-pathologic correlation. AJR Am J Roentgenol 1998; 170 (6): 1543–1549

Poplack SP, Tosteson AN, Grove MR, Wells WA, Carney PA. Mammography in 53,803 women from the New Hampshire mammography network. Radiology 2000; 217(3): 832–840

Powers RW, O'Brien PH, Kreutner A Jr. Lobular carcinoma in situ. J Surg Oncol 1980; 13(3): 269–273

Prechtel K. Mastopathie und altersabhängige Brustdrüsenveränderungen. Fortschr Med 1971; 89: 1312–1315

Prechtel K. [Cytologic diagnosis of breast cancer]. Med Welt 1976; 27: 1028

Prechtel K, Rutzki G. [Microscopic morphological changes of the mammary gland during the biphasic ovarian cycle]. Geburtsh Frauenheilk 1973; 33: 370

Rafnsson V, Sulem P, Tulinius H, Hrafnkelsson J. Breast cancer risk in airline cabin attendants: a nested case–control study in Iceland. Occup Environ Med 2003; 60(11): 807–809

Rahn J. Das Mastion: I. Normale Anatomie, Physiologie und Biomorphose. Zbl Allg Path Path Anat 1972; 115: 326–329

Ramaswamy S, Perou CM. DNA microarrays in breast cancer: the promise of personalised medicine. Lancet 2003; 361(9369): 1576–1577

Rauthe G, de Waal JC, Eiermann W, et al. Behandlung klimakterischer Beschwerden und des post-menopausalen Hormonmangels. In: Manual Mammakarzinome. 9th ed. Tumorzentrum München. München, Wien, New York: Zuckschwerdt 2003: 169–173

Ravdin PM, Cronin KA, Howlader N, et al. The decrease in breast cancer incidence in 2003 in the United States. N Engl J Med 2007; 356: 1670–1674

Reeves GK, Beral V, Green J, Gathani T, Bull D; Million Women Study Collaborators. Hormonal therapy for menopause and breast-cancer risk by histological type: a cohort study and meta-analysis. Lancet Oncol 2006; 7(11): 910–918

Reske SN, Bares N, Bill U, et al. 2. Konsensus-Konferenz PET bei onkologischen Fragestellungen am 12.9.97 in Ulm. Nucl Med (Stuttg) 1997; 36: 45–46

Richards GE. Mammary cancer, the place of surgery and of radiotherapy in its management; a study of some of the factors which determine success or failure in treatment. Br J Radiol 1948; 21 (243): 109–127

Richter K, Hamm B, Heywang-Köbrunner SH, et al. [Automated mammary sonography and mammography: the differentiation of benign and malignant breast lesions.] Rofo 1998; 169(3): 245–252

Rieber A, Merkle E, Zeitler H, et al. Value of MR mammography in the detection and exclusion of recurrent breast carcinoma. J Comput Assist Tomogr 1997; 21(5): 780–784

Robra BP, Dierks ML, Swart E, Frischbier HJ, Hoeffken W. Breast Cancer Screening in Two Regions: The German Mammography Study. In: Pas L, ed. General Practice and Cancer Prevention in Europe. The Involvement of General Practitioners in Cancer Screening Programs. Gent: Mys & Breesch; 1993: 111–112

Rosen EL, Blackwell KL, Baker JA, et al. Accuracy of MRI in the detection of residual breast cancer after neoadjuvant chemotherapy. AJR Am J Roentgenol 2003; 181(5): 1275–1282

Rosen PP. The pathological classification of human mammary carcinoma: past, present and future. Ann Clin Lab Sci 1979; 9(2): 144–156

Rosen PP, Braun DW Jr, Lyngholm B, Urban JA, Kinne DW. Lobular carcinoma in situ of the breast: preliminary results of treatment by ipsilateral mastectomy and contralateral breast biopsy. Cancer 1981; 47(4): 813–819

Rosen PP, Obermann HA. Intraductal carcinoma. In: Rosai J, Sobin LH, et al., eds. Atlas of Tumor Pathology: Tumors of the Mammary Gland. Fasc. 7. Ser. 3. Washington DC: Armed Forces Institute of Pathology; 1993: 143–155

Rosen Y, Papasozomenos SC, Gardner B. Fibromatosis of the breast. Cancer 1978; 41(4): 1409–1413

Roubidoux MA, Bailey JE, Wray LA, Helvie MA. Invasive cancers detected after breast cancer screening yielded a negative result: relationship of mammographic density to tumor prognostic factors. Radiology 2004; 230(1): 42–48

Rossouw JE, Anderson GL, Prentice RL, et al Writing Group for the Women's Health Initiative Investigators. Risks and benefits of estrogen plus progestin in healthy postmenopausal women: principal results from the Women's Health Initiative randomized controlled trial. JAMA 2002; 288(3): 321–333

Runnebaum IB, Wang-Gohrke S, Vesprini D, et al. Progesterone receptor variant increases ovarian cancer risk in BRCA1 and BRCA2 mutation carriers who were never exposed to oral contraceptives. Pharmacogenetics 2001; 11(7): 635–638

Sainsbury JRC, Anderson TJ, Morgan DAL. ABC of breast diseases: breast cancer. BMJ 2000; 321(7263): 745–750

Salomon A. Beiträge zur Pathologie und Klinik der Mammakarzinome. Arch Klin Chir 1913: 103; 573

Saslow D, Boetes C, Burke W, et al American Cancer Society Breast Cancer Advisory Group. American Cancer Society guidelines for breast screening with MRI as an adjunct to mammography. CA Cancer J Clin 2007; 57(2): 75–89

Schätzl M, Schöfer H, Küchler M, Wilhelm M. [Radiation exposure and image sharpness of mammographic units in Bavaria with respect to the European guidelines.] RoFo 2004; 176: 1089–1093

Schering AG. Corporate Communication 13353 Berlin ind. Heft 5, Band 6. München: Interdisziplinäre Onkologie-Fortbildung, 2003: 294–295

Schlag PM. Spezielle Chirurgie, Sentinel Lymphknoten Biopsie. Landsberg/Lech: ecomed Verlagsgesellschaft, 2001: 353

Schleicher UM. [Detection of breast carcinoma: a statistical-epidemiological study of the current situation.] RoFo 1995; 163: 469–473

Schmutzler RK, Beckmann MW, Kiechle M. Prävention – Familiäres Mamma- und Ovarialkarzinom. Dtsch Arztebl 2002; 99: B1146–B1151

Schöndorf H. Die Aspirationszytologie der Brustdrüse. Stuttgart: Schattauer-Verlag; 1977

Schorn C, Fischer U, Döler W, Funke M, Grabbe E. Compression device to reduce motion artifacts at contrast-enhanced MR imaging in the breast. Radiology 1998; 206(1): 279–282

Schreer I, Engel J. Mammographie. In: Schultz K-D, Albert U-S, eds. Stufe-3-Leitlinie Brustkrebs-Früherkennung in Deutschland. Munich, Vienna, New York: Zuckschwerdt-Verlag, 2004: 56

Schuller-Petrovic S. Hautveränderungen im Bereich der Mamma. In: Barth V, ed. Mammographie, Intensivkurs und Atlas für Fortgeschrittene. Stuttgart: Enke; 1994: 358–361

Schulz-Wendtland R. Digitale Mammographie—pro. Hohe Anforderungen an die Bildqualität. Med Review 2003; 1: 9–11

Schulz-Wendtland R, Herrmann K-P, Lell M, et al. Phantomstudie zur Detektion stimulierter Läsionen an fünf verschiedenen digitalen und einem konventionellen Mammographie-System. RoFo 2004; 176: 1127–1132

Schulz K-D, Duda V, Schreer I, Heywang-Köbrunner SH. Möglichkeiten der Brustkrebs-Früherkennung. Gynakologe 1997; 30: 631–636

Schulz K-D, Albert U-S. Stufe-3-Leitlinie Brustkrebs-Früherkennung in Deutschland. Munich: Zuckschwerdt Verlag; 2003

Schwartz GF, Solin LJ, Olivotto IA, Ernster VL, Pressman PI. The Consensus Conference on the treatment of in situ ductal carcinoma of the breast, April 22–25, 1999. Hum Pathol 2000; 31(2): 131–139

Schwartz GF, Giulliano AE, Veronesi U. The Consensus Conference Committee. Proceedings of the Consensus Conference on the role of sentinel lymph node biopsy in carcinoma of the breast, April 19–22, 2001, Philadelphia, Pennsylvania. American Cancer Society 2002; DOI 10.1002/cncr.10539, S2542–2551

Schwartz LM, Woloshin S, Sox HC, Fischhoff B, Welch HG. US women's attitudes to false positive mammography results and detection of ductal carcinoma in situ: cross sectional survey. BMJ 2000; 320(7250): 1635–1640

Schwarz E, Hagen D, Elsäßer M. [The complete disintegration of microcalcification in a ductal invasive breast carcinoma.] RöFo 1999; 170: 514–515

Sehouli J, Lehmacher W, Mirz R, et al. Wie empfinden Patientinnen mit metastasierendem Mammakarzinom ihre Therapie? Forum DKG 2004; 1: 25–28

Seifert J. Das Mammogramm und seine Deutung. Darmstadt: Steinkopf; 1975

Sener SF, Milos S, Feldman JL, et al. The spectrum of vascular lesions in the mammary skin, including angiosarcoma, after breast conservation treatment for breast cancer. J Am Coll Surg 2001; 193 (1): 22–28

Senn HJ, Glaus A, Bolliger B. Chemoprävention des Mammakarzinoms – Stand 2001. Schweiz Med Forum 2001; 14: 359–363

Shalom S, Buchbinder MD, Leichter IS, et al. Computer-aided classification of BI-RADS category 3 breast lesions. Radiology 2004; 230: 820–823

Shetty MK, Shah YP, Sharman RS. Prospective evaluation of the value of combined mammographic and sonographic assessment in patients with palpable abnormalities of the breast. J Ultrasound Med 2003; 22(3): 263–268, quiz 269–270

Sickles EA. Management of probably benign breast lesions. Radiol Clin North Am 1995; 33(6): 1123–1130

Sickles EA. Wolfe Mammographic Parenchymal Patterns and Breast Cancer Risk. AJR 2007; 188: 301–303

Sickles EA, Wolverton DE, Dee KE. Performance parameters for screening and diagnostic mammography: specialist and general radiologists. Radiology 2002; 224(3): 861–869

Siekiera W. Charakteristika von Patientinnen mit Hirnmetastasen beim HER2/neu überexprimierenden, metastasierenden Mammakarzinom. Dissertation. München: Ludwig-Maximilian-Universität; 2006

Sigmund-Schultze N, Zylka-Mehnhorn V, Leinmüller R, Meyer R. Hormontherapie und Brustkrebs. Ein Blick auf die aktuelle Datenlage. Deutsches Ärzteblatt 2008; 105(6): B234–B238

Singer CF. Wechselbeschwerden nach Brustkrebs (Liviell). Vortrag 9. Maritimer Workshop der Österreichischen Gesellschaft für Senologie. Belek: 29.4.–6.5.2005

Singh IM. Langzeitbeobachtung von 1002 adjuvant bestrahlten Mamma-Karzinom-Patientinnen in Hinsicht auf Prognosefaktoren, Bedeutung von Lokalrezidiven und Folgen der Sternalfeldbestrahlung. Inaugural Dissertation. Munich: Technische Universität München; 2004

Sinn HP, Helmcken B, Aulmann S. Konzept und Problematik der lobulären Neoplasie. Pathologe 2006; 27(5): 373–380

Sjönell G, Ståhle L. Mammography screening does not significantly reduce breast cancer mortality in Swedish daily practice. Lakartidningen 1999; 96: 904–913

Skaane P, Young K, Skjennald A. Population-based mammography screening: comparison of screen-film and full-field digital mammography with soft-copy reading—Oslo I study. Radiology 2003; 229(3): 877–884

Smidt ML, Janssen CM, Kuster DM, Bruggink ED, Strobbe LJ. Axillary recurrence after a negative sentinel node biopsy for breast cancer: incidence and clinical significance. Ann Surg Oncol 2005; 12: 29–33

Smith-Bindman R, Chu PW, Miglioretti DL, et al. Comparison of screening mammography in the United States and the United kingdom. JAMA 2003; 290(16): 2129–2137

Smith A. Fundamentals of digital mammography: physics, technology and practical considerations. Radiol Manage 2003; 25(5): 18–24, 26–31, quiz 32–34

Sobin L, Wittekind C. UICC. TNM Classification of Malignant Tumors. 6th ed. New York: Wiley; 2002: 131–141

Soderstrom CE, Harms SE, Copit DS, et al. Three-dimensional RODEO breast MR imaging of lesions containing ductal carcinoma in situ. Radiology 1996; 201(2): 427–432

Soffietti R, Cornu P, Delattre JY, et al. EFNS Guidelines on diagnosis and treatment of brain metastases: report of an EFNS Task Force. Eur J Neurol 2006; 13(7): 674–681

Solin LJ, Orel SG, Hwang WT, Harris EE, Schnall MD. Relationship of breast magnetic resonance imaging to outcome after breast-conservation treatment with radiation for women with early-stage invasive breast carcinoma or ductal carcinoma in situ. J Clin Oncol 2008; 26(3): 386–391

Stang A. Rückgang der postmenopausalen Hormonverordnungen und der Brustkrebsinzidenz. Dtsch Ärztebl 2008; 105(16): 303–309

Steinberg W, Irmscher AK. Hanrath Chr, Böcher E. Feinnadelpunktion von Mammaläsionen—Der Stellenwert der Mamma-Zytologie hat weltweit deutlich zugenommen (Mamma-Zytologie I). GYNE 2000; 3: 45–49

Stemmler HJ, Stieber P, Bauernfeind I, et al. Die Betroffenen wollen mehr Nachsorge – vor allem apparativ. Frauenarzt 2006; 47(10): 916–918

Stomper PC, Geradts J, Edge SB, Levine EG. Mammographic predictors of the presence and size of invasive carcinomas associated with malignant microcalcification lesions without a mass. AJR Am J Roentgenol 2003; 181(6): 1679–1684

Suga K, Yuan Y, Okada M, et al. Breast sentinel lymph node mapping at CT lymphography with iopamidol: preliminary experience. Radiology 2004; 230(2): 543–552

Svane G. Ductal Carcinoma In Situ (DCIS): Incidence, Prognosis, and Diagnostic Aspects of Mammography, Galactography, and Needle Biopsies. In: Ueno E, Shiina T, Kubota M, Sawai K, eds. Research and Development in Breast Ultrasound. Tokyo: Springer; 2004

Symmans WF, Peintinger F, Hatzis C, et al. Measurement of residual breast cancer burden to predict survival after neoadjuvant chemotherapy. J Clin Oncol 2007; 25(28): 4414–4422

Tabar L, Dean PB. Teaching Atlas of Mammography. Stuttgart–New York: Thieme; 2010

Tabar L, Vitak B, et al. Update of the Swedish Two-County Trial of breast cancer screening: histologic grade-specific and age-specific results. Swiss Surg 1999; 5: 199–204

Teboul M, Halliwell M. Atlas of Ultrasound and Ductal Echography of the Breast. Oxford: Blackwell; 1995

Teh W, Wilson ARM. The role of ultrasound in breast cancer screening. A consensus statement by the European Group for Breast Cancer Screening. Eur J Cancer 1998; 34(4): 449–450

Thurfjell E, Lindgren A. Paraffin tissue block radiography of nonpalpable lesions with calcifications detected at mammography: 5-year consecutive series of surgically excised cases. Eur Radiol 1997; 7(7): 1006–1009

Titus-Ernstoff L, Egan KM, Newcomb PA, et al. Early life factors in relation to breast cancer risk in postmenopausal women. Cancer Epidemiol Biomarkers Prev 2002; 11(2): 207–210

Töndury G. Angewandte und topographische Anatomie. 5th ed. Stuttgart, New York: Thieme; 1981

Tonita JM, Hillis JP, Lim CH. Medical radiologic technologist review: effects on a population-based breast cancer screening program. Radiology 1999; 211(2): 529–533

Torosian MH, ed. Breast Cancer: A Guide to Detection and Multidisciplinary Therapy. Totowa, NJ: Humana Press; 2002

Tuschen G, Fries H., v. d. Bergh M. Onkologisches Dokumentationssystem als Basis elektronischer Patientenakten. Qualitätssicherung und Benchmarking von Brustzentren. Onkologie Heute 2004; 3: 8–9

Untch M, Beckmann M, Emons G, et al. SABCS-Libertate Study. Notes from the San Antonio Breast Cancer Meeting Dec 2008. www.Ago-online.org

Urban JA. Excision of the major duct system of the breast. Cancer 1963; 16: 516

Vachon CM, Kushi LH, Cerhan JR, Kuni CC, Sellers TA. Association of diet and mammographic breast density in the Minnesota breast cancer family cohort. Cancer Epidemiol Biomarkers Prev 2000; 9 (2): 151–160

Veronesi U, Marubini E, DelVecchio M, et al. Local recurrences and distant metastases after conservative breast cancer treatments: partly independent events. J Natl Cancer Inst 1995; 87: 19–27

Vignal P, Meslet MR, Roméo JM, Feuilhade F. Sonographic morphology of infiltrating breast carcinoma, relationship with the shape of the hyaluronan extracellular matrix. J Ultrasound Med 2002; 21: 532–538

Völker HU, Langen HJ, Cramer A, et al. Tumorbildende lymphozytische Mastitis (sogenannte diabetische Mastopathie) – eine ungewöhnliche Differenzialdiagnose zum Mammakarzinom bei einer nichtdiabetischen Patientin. Fortschr Röntgenstr. 2008; 180: 150–152

Vogt TH, Brockmeyer N, Kutzner H, Schöfer H. Angiosarkom und Kaposi Sarkom. AWMF online. Kurzleitlinie der Deutschen Dermatologischen Gesellschaft (DDG) und der Deutschen Krebsgesellschaft. AWMF-Leitlinien-Register Nr. 032/025 12/2007. http://www.uni-duesseldorf.de/awmf/awmfengl.htm

Wagner T. Penetranz für Brust- und Eierstockkrebs in österreichischen BRCA1-Mutationsträgerinnen. Vortrag Maritimer Workshop der Österreichischen Gesellschaft für Senologie. Belek: 29.4.–6.5.2005

Wang Y, Abreau M, Hoda S. Mammary duct carcinoma in situ in males: pathological findings and clinical considerations. Mod Pathol 1997; 10: 27A

Warner E, Plewes DB, Shumak RS. Comparison of breast magnetic resonance imaging, mammography, and ultrasound for surveillance of women at high risk for hereditary breast cancer. J Clin Oncol 2001; 19: 3524–3531

Warren R, Lakhani SR. Can the stroma provide the clue to the cellular basis for mammographic density? Breast Cancer Res 2003; 5 (5): 225–227

Weining C. Die Ein-Ebenen-Mammographie in Kombination mit der Mamma-Sonographie versus Zwei-Ebenen-Mammographie zur Untersuchung der weiblichen Brust. Neues Konzept für die Früherkennung von Brustkrebs. Dissertation. Universität Tübingen; 2004

Weining-Klemm O. Vergleich verschiedener Biopsiearten, Feinnadelaspiration (FNA), Feinnadelbiopsie (FNB) und Vakuumbiopsie (VB); Möglichkeiten, Grenzen und Kosten. Dissertation. Universität Tübingen; 2004

Wellings SR, Jentoft VL. Organ cultures of normal, dysplastic, hyperplastic, and neoplastic human mammary tissues. J Natl Cancer Inst 1972; 49(2): 329–338

Wenkel E, Heckmann M, Heinrich M, et al. Automated breast ultrasound: lesion detection and BI-RADS classification—a pilot study. RoFo 2008; 180: 804–808

WHI-Updated Analysis: No Increased Risk of Breast Cancer with Estrogen-Alone. NIH News http://www.nhlbi.nih.gov/new/press/06-04-11a.htm; April 2006

Wilson JMG, Junger G. Principles and Practice of Screening for Disease. Geneva: WHO; 1968

Wilson JMG. Imaging of malignant disease of the breast. Second Utrecht Workshop on Breast Screening in the Framework of "Europe Against Cancer", 1991

Wimpissinger F, Esterbauer B. Leitlinie Gynäkomastie. J Urol Urogynäkol 2008; 15(6): 12–14

Wolf AB, Brem RF. Decreased Mammography Utilization in the United States: Why and How Can We Reverse the Trend? AJR 2009; 192: 400–402

Wolfe JN. Breast patterns as an index of risk for developing breast cancer. AJR Am J Roentgenol 1976; 126(6): 1130–1137

Woodman CB, Threlfall AG, Boggis CR, Prior P. Is the three year breast screening interval too long? Occurrence of interval cancers in NHS breast screening programme's north western region. BMJ 1995; 310(6974): 224–226

Yang WT, Tse GMK. Sonographic, mammographic, and histopathologic correlation of symptomatic ductal carcinoma in situ. AJR Am J Roentgenol 2004; 182(1): 101–110

Yang WT, Whitman GJ, Johnson MM, et al. Needle localization for excisional biopsy of breast lesions: comparison of effect of use of full-field digital versus screen-film mammographic guidance on procedure time. Radiology 2004; 231(1): 277–281

Yi-Hong Chou, Ch–m Tiu, Chen J, Chang R-F. Automated full-field breast ultrasonography: the past and the present. J Med Ultrasound 2007; 15(1): 31–44

Yo LSF, Daniels-Gooszen AW, Duijm LEM, et al. Radioactive seed localization of nonpalpable breast lesions. ECR Wien 2009, Paper B-299

Zajicek J. Monographs in Clinical Cytology Aspiration Biopsy, Cytology, Part I. Basel: Karger; 1974

Zapf S, Halbsguth A, Brunier A, et al. Möglichkeiten der MRT in der Diagnostik nichtpalpabler Mammatumoren. Roefo 1991; 154(1): 106–110

Zeeb H, Razum O, Blettner M, Stegmaier C. Transition in cancer patterns among Turks residing in Germany. Eur J Cancer 2002; 38(5): 705–711

Zonderland HM, Coerkamp EG, Hermans JO, van de Vijver MJ, van Voorthuisen AE. Diagnosis of breast cancer: contribution of US as an adjunct to mammography. Radiology 1999; 213(2): 413–422

Zweifelt E, Payer E. Die Klinik der bösartigen Geschwulste. 3 Vols. Leipzig: Hirzel; 1924/1927

# Index

Page numbers in *italics* refer to figures.

## N

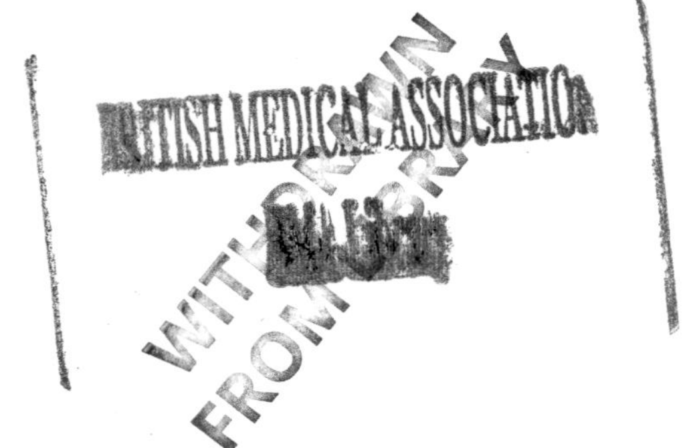
BRITISH MEDICAL ASSOCIATION
WITHDRAWN
FROM LIBRARY